Dedication

This book is dedicated to all faculty, especially clerkship and residency directors, who not only teach medical students and residents but also continue to learn with them. The editors of this book admire those physicians who practice what they teach.

———

CONTRIBUTORS

Joel J. Alpert, MD
Professor and Chairman of Pediatrics Emeritus
Boston University School of Medicine
Professor of Public Health (Health Law) Emeritus
Boston University of Public Health
Pediatrician and Director of Pediatrics Emeritus
Boston Medical Center
Boston, Massachusetts
The Profession of Pediatrics

Robert S. Baltimore, MD
Professor of Pediatrics and Epidemiology
Department of Pediatrics
Yale University School of Medicine
Associate Hospital Epidemiologist and Attending
    Physician
Department of Pediatrics
Yale–New Haven Children's Hospital
New Haven, Connecticut
Infectious Diseases

Warren P. Bishop, MD
Associate Professor, Department of Pediatrics
Roy J. and Lucille A. Carver College of Medicine
University of Iowa
Director, Division of Gastroenterology
Department of Pediatrics
Children's Hospital of Iowa
Iowa City, Iowa
The Digestive System

Kim Blake, MD, MBBS, MRCP, FRCPC
Associate Professor, Department of Pediatrics
Director of Pediatric Undergraduate Program
Division of Medical Education
Dalhousie University
IWK Health Centre
Halifax, Nova Scotia
Adolescent Medicine

Nathan J. Blum, MD
Associate Professor, Department of Pediatrics
University of Pennsylvania School of Medicine
Director, Section of Behavioral Pediatrics
Division of Child Development, Rehabilitation, and
    Metabolic Disease
Children's Hospital of Philadelphia
Philadelphia, Pennsylvania
Psychosocial Issues

Cindy W. Christian, MD
Associate Professor, Department of Pediatrics
University of Pennsylvania School of Medicine
Chair, Child Abuse and Neglect Prevention
Children's Hospital of Philadelphia
Philadelphia, Pennsylvania
Psychosocial Issues

Victoria Davis, MD, FRCSC
Assistant Professor, Department of Obstetrics and
    Gynecology
University of Toronto
Attending Physician, Division of Paediatric and
    Adolescent Gynaecology
Hospital for Sick Children
Toronto, Ontario, Canada
Adolescent Medicine

Jason S. Debley, MD, MPH
Assistant Professor, Department of Pediatrics
University of Washington School of Medicine
Attending Physician, Division of Pulmonary Medicine
Children's Hospital and Regional Medical Center
Seattle, Washington
The Respiratory System

Ramsay Fuleihan, MD
Associate Research Scientist
Department of Pediatrics, Section of Immunology and
    Child Health Research Center
Yale University School of Medicine
New Haven, Connecticut
Immunology

v

Sheila Gahagan, MD, MPH
Clinical Professor, Department of Pediatrics and
    Communicable Diseases
Assistant Research Scientist
Center for Human Growth and Development
University of Michigan
Ann Arbor, Michigan
Behavioral Disorders

Clarence W. Gowen, Jr., MD
Associate Professor, Department of Pediatrics
Director, Pediatric Residency Program
Director, Pediatric Clerkship
Eastern Virginia Medical School
Director of Medical Education
Children's Hospital of the King's Daughters
    Norfolk, Virginia
Fetal and Neonatal Medicine

Larry A. Greenbaum, MD, PhD
Associate Professor, Department of Pediatrics
Medical College of Wisconsin
Attending Physician, Department of Pediatrics
Children's Hospital of Wisconsin
Milwaukee, Wisconsin
Fluids and Electrolytes

Hilary M. Haftel, MD, MHPE
Clinical Associate Professor of Pediatrics, Internal Medicine,
    and Medical Education
University of Michigan Medical School
Attending Physician, University of Michigan Health System
Ann Arbor, Michigan
Rheumatic Diseases of Childhood

Hal B. Jenson, MD
Chair, Department of Pediatrics
Director, Center for Pediatric Research
Professor, Departments of Pediatrics, Microbiology, and
    Molecular Cell Biology
Eastern Virginia Medical School
Senior Vice President for Academic Affairs
Children's Hospital of the King's Daughters
Norfolk, Virginia
Infectious Diseases

Nicholas Jospe, MD
Associate Professor
University of Rochester School of Medicine and Dentistry
Attending Physician, Golisano Children's Hospital at
    Strong Memorial Hospital
Rochester, New York
Endocrinology

Robert M. Kliegman, MD
Professor and Chair, Department of Pediatrics
Medical College of Wisconsin
Pediatrician-in-Chief
Pamela and Leslie Muma Chair in Pediatrics
Children's Hospital of Wisconsin
Milwaukee, Wisconsin
Nephrology and Neurology

Nancy F. Krebs, MD
Professor, Department of Pediatrics
University of Colorado School of Medicine
Medical Director, Department of Nutrition
The Children's Hospital
Denver, Colorado
Pediatric Nutrition and Nutritional Disorders

Mary V. Lasley, MD
Clinical Associate Professor, Department of Pediatrics
University of Washington School of Medicine
Attending Physician
Children's Hospital & Regional Medical Center
Private Practice
Northwest Asthma & Allergy Center
Seattle, Washington
Allergy

Robert M. Lembo, MD
Associate Professor of Clinical Pediatrics
New York University School of Medicine
Attending Physician
Department of Pediatrics
Bellevue Hospital Center
New York, New York
Dermatology

David A. Levine, MD
Chief, Division of Predoctoral Education in Pediatrics
Department of Pediatrics
Morehouse School of Medicine
Atlanta, Georgia
Growth and Development

Paul A. Levy, MD
Assistant Professor of Pediatrics and Pathology,
    Department of Pediatrics
Albert Einstein College of Medicine
Director, Center for Metabolic Disorders
Children's Hospital at Montefiore
Bronx, New York
Human Genetics and Dysmorphology

Donald W. Lewis, MD
Professor of Pediatrics and Neurology
Department of Pediatrics
Eastern Virginia Medical School
Pediatric Neurologist
Children's Hospital of the King's Daughters
Norfolk, Virginia
Neurology

Karen J. Marcdante, MD
Professor and Vice Chair of Education
Department of Pediatrics
Medical College of Wisconsin
Medical Director, Transport Services
Children's Hospital of Wisconsin
Milwaukee, Wisconsin
Nephrology and Neurology
The Acutely Ill or Injured Child

Robert W. Marion, MD
Professor, Departments of Pediatrics,
    Obstetrics/Gynecology, Women's Health
Albert Einstein College of Medicine
Chief, Section of Genetics
Director, Center for Congenital Disorders
Children's Hospital at Montefiore
Bronx, New York
Human Genetics and Dysmorphology

Susan G. Marshall, MD
Associate Professor, Department of Pediatrics
University of Washington School of Medicine
Attending Physician, Division of Pulmonary Medicine
Children's Hospital and Regional Medical Center
Seattle, Washington
The Respiratory System

Thomas W. McLean, MD
Assistant Professor of Pediatrics
Wake Forest University School of Medicine
Winston-Salem, North Carolina
Oncology

Laura E. Primak, RD, CSP, CNSD
Professional Research Assistant and Dietitian
University of Colorado School of Medicine
Denver, Colorado
Pediatric Nutrition and Nutritional Disorders

Russell Scheffer, MD
Division Director, Department of Psychiatry and Behavioral
    Medicine
Medical College of Wisconsin
Medical Director, Child and Adolescent Psychiatry
Children's Hospital of Wisconsin
Milwaukee, Wisconsin
Psychiatric Disorders

Daniel S. Schneider, MD
Assistant Professor, Department of Pediatrics
Eastern Virginia Medical School
Pediatric Cardiologist
Director, Echocardiography Laboratory
Co-Director, Vascular Laboratory
Children's Hospital of the King's Daughters
Norfolk, Virginia
The Cardiovascular System

J. Paul Scott, MD
Professor of Pediatrics
Section of Hematology/Oncology/Transplantation
Medical College of Wisconsin
Medical Director
Wisconsin Sickle Cell Center
Children's Hospital of Wisconsin
Researcher
Blood Center of Wisconsin
Blood Research Institute
Milwaukee, Wisconsin
Hematology

Margretta Seashore, MD
Professor, Department of Genetics and Pediatrics
Yale University School of Medicine
Attending Physician, Department of Pediatrics
Yale–New Haven Hospital
New Haven, Connecticut
Metabolic Disorders

Benjamin S. Siegel, MD
Professor of Pediatrics and Psychiatry, Department of
    Pediatrics
Boston University School of Medicine
Senior Pediatrician, Department of Pediatrics
Boston Medical Center
Boston, Massachusetts
The Profession of Pediatrics

George Thompson, MD
Professor
Departments of Orthopaedic Surgery and Pediatrics
Case Western Reserve University
Director
Department of Pediatric Orthopaedics
Rainbow Babies' and Children's Hospital
Cleveland, Ohio
Orthopedics

Marcia M. Wofford, MD
Associate Professor of Pediatrics
Wake Forest University School of Medicine
Winston-Salem, North Carolina
Oncology

Medical knowledge has grown tremendously in the past decade due to exciting discoveries that have improved our understanding of pathophysiology and led to advances in the diagnosis, treatment, and prevention of diseases in children. As educators and authors, our goal is to deliver these new advances as well as classic pediatrics in a readable and concise text for medical students and residents.

This new edition has been totally revised: topics are reorganized into 203 chapters to offer greater specificity, and new chapters cover topics not addressed in previous editions. These outstanding contributions are written by clerkship directors with expertise in pediatrics and pediatric subspecialties. Faculty with extensive experience teaching medical students and residents and developing curricula at their own medical schools or as part of national organizations present the essentials of pediatric medical and surgical diseases. As in previous editions of this very successful and well-used textbook, we focus our attention on the learner and what is expected of him or her during a pediatric clerkship or residency.

We emphasize the common and classic pediatric disorders in a time-honored, logical format to help the student and resident acquire knowledge and apply that knowledge to their patients. The student and resident will gain the knowledge and skills necessary to succeed during their clerkship or residency training both in caring for patients and in preparing for clerkship or inservice examinations.

We hope this revised edition will continue to serve the thousands of students and residents who rotate through pediatrics as well as those who will become new providers of pediatric care in the years to come.

ROBERT M. KLIEGMAN, MD

KAREN J. MARCDANTE, MD

HAL B. JENSON, MD

RICHARD E. BEHRMAN, MD

ACKNOWLEDGMENTS

The editors could never have published this edition without the assistance and attention to detail of Bill Schmitt and Jacquie Mahon. In addition we are grateful to Carolyn Redman for her outstanding editing, suggestions, organization, and initiative in making this book a reality.

CONTENTS

THE PROFESSION OF PEDIATRICS

Benjamin S. Siegel and Joel J. Alpert

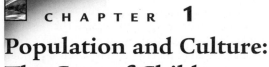

CHAPTER **1**

Population and Culture: The Care of Children in Society

Many medical, developmental, and psychosocial issues challenge pediatricians and their patients in the U.S., which is a nation of cultural and ethnic diversity. We need to appreciate the prevalence of medical conditions and the social and environmental influences associated with such conditions, including health disparities and cultural issues, in providing pediatric care. We depend on the science of pediatrics to expand our ability to practice evidence-based medicine. New technologies and treatments help to improve morbidity, mortality, and the quality of life for children and their families, but also increase the costs of medical care. The challenge for pediatricians is to deliver care that is socially equitable and available for all children.

A BRIEF HISTORY OF PEDIATRICS

In England in 1769, Dr. George Armstrong established a dispensary for the poor children of London in the impoverished Red Lion Square district. Dr. Armstrong, a role model for today's socially conscious pediatricians, authored one of the first pediatric textbooks, *Essay on Diseases Most Fatal to Infants.*

During colonial times, there were a few physicians who were interested in children. Benjamin Rush (a signer of the Declaration of Independence) presented lectures specific to diseases of children. The first formal medical student courses about children's health were at Yale College (1813-1852). The first children's

hospital in the English-speaking world was the Hospital for Sick Children on Great Ormond St. (GOS), London (1852). Charles Dickens lived within a few blocks of the hospital and raised money for GOS with readings from *A Christmas Carol.* The first children's hospital in the U.S. was founded by Dr. Francis W. Lewis, who visited GOS and then established the Children's Hospital of Philadelphia (1855). Dr. Abraham Jacobi was the founder of American pediatrics. He established the first children's clinic in the U.S. (1860), in New York City. The next two children's hospitals were Boston Children's Hospital (1869) and the Children's Hospital National Medical Center, Washington, D.C. (1870). Dr. Jacobi was a founding member of the Section of Pediatrics of the American Medical Association (AMA) and was the first president of the American Pediatric Society (1888). In 1897, Dr. L. Emmet Holt authored his classic American textbook *The Diseases of Infancy and Childhood.*

As the particular problems of children were identified, the federal government responded by accepting responsibility for the care of vulnerable children. In 1909, President Theodore Roosevelt convened the first of many White House conferences on the Care of Dependant Children. In 1912, the federal government established the U.S. Children's Bureau. In 1921, Congress passed the Sheppard-Towner Act, which authorized federal spending to provide direct care for children. The AMA condemned the act as socialized medicine. When the Pediatric Section of the AMA House of Delegates endorsed the renewal of the Sheppard-Towner Act in 1929, the AMA House of Delegates rebuked the Pediatric Section and reversed the Section position, adopting a policy that prohibited any Section from taking any action without endorsement from the AMA House of Delegates. Key members of the Pediatric Section responded by recognizing the need for an independent professional organization and established the American Academy of Pediatrics (AAP) in 1930. The founders of the AAP declared that the core mission would be "to attain optimal physical, mental and social health and well being for all infants, children, adolescents and young adults." Through its many programs and projects, the AAP would seek to address " the needs of children, their families, and their communities . . . through advocacy, education, research, and service." The AAP remains the only national professional health organization whose goal is to serve and advocate for children and not just to serve the needs of its membership.

The Society for Pediatric Research was established for young basic science investigators in 1931. The Ambulatory Pediatric Association was founded in 1960 by a group of hospital outpatient directors interested in developing ambulatory care and health services research.

CURRENT CHALLENGES

Current challenges in the care of children are access to health care; health disparities; children's social, cognitive, and emotional lives; congenital and genetic disorders; and environmental factors that affect optimal outcome of child health. Scientific advances in genetics are particularly relevant to pediatrics. With newer genetic technologies, pediatricians are able to diagnose diseases at the molecular level. Microarray genetic technology can identify the cluster of candidate genes associated with a variety of diseases; this technology is now used for the prognosis of diseases (e.g., cancer). Prenatal diagnosis of a variety of genetic diseases is now possible. Mandatory and recommended newborn screening for genetic and metabolic diseases has improved the accuracy of early diagnosis of these conditions, which, although rare, are often treatable. Giving folic acid to women of childbearing age reduces the risk of neural tube defects. The blood triple or quadruple screen during pregnancy and intrauterine ultrasound as a screening tool to detect fetal malformations and deformations provide information for diagnosis, prognosis, and clinical decision making. Functional magnetic resonance imaging allows a greater understanding of psychiatric and neurologic problems, such as dyslexia and attention-deficit/hyperactivity disorder.

The incidence of many serious bacterial and viral infections has been significantly reduced or eliminated by immunizations. Smallpox has been eliminated worldwide, and polio should be eliminated shortly. The overwhelming success of immunization programs in preventing many of the serious diseases seen in children in the last century has been associated with concerns about minor immunization side effects and rare complications. Pediatricians must continue to seek the safest vaccines possible, but they should oppose vigorously any attempts to limit the use of proven successful immunizations when the risk of complications is remote compared with the serious risk of clinical disease. The inappropriate claim of a causal association of autistic spectrum disorders and the measles vaccine has been disproved, and there have been numerous outbreaks of measles in unimmunized children.

There is increasing concern about environmental toxins in the food chain affecting children's growth and development and the ever-present problem of air pollution adversely affecting children's pulmonary function. Children are subject to physical, emotional, and sexual abuse; they also are victims of and bear witness to violence. Many immigrant families have seen death, destruction, terrorism, and war, all of which affect children's emotional development. Since the September 11, 2001, destruction of the World Trade Center, fear of terrorism has increased the level of anxiety for many families and children.

Pediatricians need to practice as part of an expanded healthcare team. Nurse practitioners provide well-child care and, in collaboration with pediatricians, care for common illnesses. Many pediatricians practice collaboratively with psychiatrists, psychologists, nurses, lawyers, and social workers. School health and school-based health clinics have improved access and outcomes for many common childhood and adolescent conditions.

Childhood antecedents of adult health conditions, such as alcoholism, depression, obesity, hypertension, and hyperlipidemias, are increasingly being recognized. There is an increase in the diagnosis of obesity and type 2 diabetes and a possible increase in the incidence of autistic spectrum disorders, although the latter may be secondary to improved diagnosis. Because of improved neonatal care, a greater percentage of preterm, low birth weight, or very low birth weight newborns are surviving, increasing the number of children with chronic medical conditions and developmental delays. Death from congenital malformations and malignant neoplasms is less common than previously, but these conditions remain the second and third most important causes of death after injuries in the 1- to 4-year-old population.

HEALTH STATUS OF AMERICAN CHILDREN

- In 2002, there were slightly more than **4 million births**. About 33.8% of these were to unmarried women. This percentage increased from 2001-2002 in non-Hispanic whites by 22.9%, in Hispanics by 43.4% and decreased in African Americans by 68%.
- Of the current 72.2 million children (2002), 9.7 million children (13%) have no **health insurance**

coverage for a full year. At any time, 24%, approximately 17 to 18 million children, go without health insurance. Insurance coverage under Medicaid, the State Child Health Insurance Plan (SCHIP), and private employer-based insurance varies by populations: 17% of white, 22% of African American, and 41% of Hispanic children had no health insurance at some time during a year. There is also variation by income: 10% of children with family incomes of 400% or greater above the poverty level had no health insurance, in contrast to 31% of all children with family incomes of 100% to 199% of poverty.

- Access to **primary care** is a major goal for children. In 2000, 87% of all children were reported to have a primary care clinician, with most of this care provided by pediatricians. Ninety-one percent of whites and 75% of Hispanics reported a primary care provider; 93% of high-income families and 81% of poor families identified a primary care provider. The AAP advocates that all children have a medical home where their pediatrician and medical team provide needed preventive and curative services.

- **Prenatal care** in the first trimester has increased by 11% since 1990, with 83.4% of all women receiving prenatal care. Whites (88.7%), Hispanics (76.8%), and African Americans (60.6%) begin prenatal care in the first trimester. Smoking has declined considerably, with only 12% of pregnant women reporting smoking in 2002. Cesarean sections have increased to 26.1% of all births. The incidence of preterm births has been increasing since the 1980s, with an increased rate in whites and a decreased rate in blacks. There has been an increase in low birth weight infants (<2500 g [7.7% of all births]) and a steady rate of very low birth weight infants (<1500 g [1.5% of all births]) since the 1990s.

- The national **birthrate for adolescents** has been steadily dropping since 1990, with more teenagers delaying their first sexual experience or using birth control (or both). There also was a 39% decrease in abortion in adolescents from 1990 to 1999. In 1999, however, there were approximately 487,000 live births to adolescents 19 years old and younger and 556,000 abortions.

- There has been an overall decline in **infant mortality** by 46% since 1980, with equal declines in the rates for white and the nonwhite populations (see Section XI). The disparity between the ethnic groups has not changed. In 2001, the rates per 1000 live births were white, non-Hispanic, 5.7; Hispanic, 5.7; and African American, 14. In 2000, the U.S. ranked 25th in the infant mortality rate, below the Czech Republic, Cuba, Portugal, and Greece. Marked variations in infant mortality also exist by state. New Hampshire and Minnesota had the lowest infant mortality rates in the U.S., whereas West Virginia,

TABLE 1–1.   Causes of Death by Age in the United States, 2001

Age Group (yr)	Causes of Death in Order of Frequency
1-4	Injuries Congenital malformations, deformations, and chromosomal abnormalities Malignant neoplasms Homicide Heart disease
5-9	Injuries Malignant neoplasms Congenital malformations, deformations, and chromosomal abnormalities Homicide Heart disease
10-14	Injuries Malignant neoplasms Suicide Congenital malformations, deformations, and chromosomal abnormalities Homicide
15-19	Injuries Homicide Suicide Malignant neoplasms Heart disease

Data from U.S. Centers for Disease Control and Prevention/NCHS, National Vital Statistics Report, Vol. 52, No. 9, Nov. 7, 2003: Deaths: Leading Causes for 2001.

Louisiana, and Mississippi had the highest, comparable to developing countries.

- The overall **causes of death** in all children (1-19 years old) in the U.S. in 2001, in order of frequency, were injuries, assaults (homicide), malignant neoplasms, suicide, and congenital malformations (Table 1-1). For 2001, there were 25,757 deaths in children age 1 to 19 years. Of that total, 15,726 (61%) deaths of children were violence related secondary to injuries (11,196), homicide (2640), and suicide (1890). Many deaths are associated with alcohol abuse. Two thirds of child passengers (≤14 years old) die in automobile crashes in association with a drunk driver.

- From 2000 to 2001, there were decreases in the rate of injuries in all ages, a decrease in malignant neoplasms, and a decrease in deaths from congenital malformations in the age group 5 to 14 years. There was an increase in the death rate from heart diseases and congenital malformations in the age group 1 to

4 years. Although there was a decrease in the rate of suicide for children (10 to 19 years), there was an increase in deaths caused by assaults and homicide in the age groups 1 to 4 years (35%) and 15 to 19 years (4.4%).

HEALTH DISPARITIES IN HEALTH CARE FOR CHILDREN

Health disparities are defined as the differences that remain after taking into account patients' needs and preferences and the availability of health care. Social conditions, social inequity, discrimination, social stress, language barriers, and poverty are antecedents to and associated causes of health disparities. The disparities in infant mortality relate to poor access to prenatal care during pregnancy and the lack of access and appropriate heath services for women throughout their life span, such as preventive services, family planning, and appropriate nutrition and health care.

- Infant mortality increases as the mother's level of education decreases.
- Poorer children are less likely to be immunized at age 4 years and are less likely to receive dental care.
- Rates of hospital admission for treatable disease are higher for people who live in low-income areas.
- Children of ethnic minorities and children from poor families are less likely to have physician office or hospital outpatient visits and are more likely to have hospital emergency department visits.
- Access to care for children is easier for non-Hispanic whites and for children of higher income families than for minority and low-income families.

Other heath issues that represent challenges for pediatricians include the following:

- Although there was a decline in **cigarette smoking** in high school students from 36% in 1997 to 29% in 2001, more than a quarter of high school students still smoke.
- Among high school students, 38% of girls and 24% of boys do not engage in recommended amounts of moderate or vigorous physical activity.
- The prevalence of **overweight** children among those 6 to 11 years old doubled from 7% to 15% (1976-1980 to 1999-2000), and the prevalence of overweight adolescents among those 12 to 19 years old tripled from 5% to 16% during the same time. Obesity and its associated morbidities are a serious public health concern. It is estimated that 65% of U.S. adults are overweight or obese; this is associated with 300,000 deaths a year and at least $117 billion in healthcare costs.
- In 2000, it was estimated that $64.7 billion was spent treating **injuries** in the U.S., with injury-attributable

medical expenses of $117.2 billion. For children up to 19 years old, the expenses for medical treatment were $24.4 billion, and attributed medical expenses were $29.1 billion. A significant percentage of injuries in adolescents are associated with alcohol abuse.
- In 1999-2000, the **Head Start** program served only 60% of eligible children. There were almost 13 million children in federal Title I reading programs, and greater than 6 million children qualified for disabilities under the Individuals with Disabilities Education Act. The school dropout rate for children was 14.5%.
- In 1999-2000, greater than 800,000 children were **abused**, approximately 500,000 children were in foster care, and 2.3 million were in the care of grandparents; 18.8% of children were living in poverty. In the same years, 1.7 million juveniles were arrested, 112,479 young people were in correctional institutions for juveniles, and 18.8% of these (21,130) were in adult prison facilities.

CHANGING MORBIDITY

Changing morbidity stresses the relationship between environmental, social, emotional, and developmental issues and child health status and outcome. This approach is based on significant interactions of **biopsychosocial** influences on health and illness and stresses that poverty and access to health care should be a major concern of pediatricians. These health issues include the following:

- School problems, learning disabilities, and attention problems
- Child and adolescent mood and anxiety disorders
- Adolescent suicide and homicide
- Firearms in the home
- School violence
- HIV
- The effects of media violence, obesity, and sexual activity
- Substance use and abuse by adolescents, especially the abuse of alcohol

Currently, 20% to 25% of children are estimated to have some mental health problem; 5% to 6% of these problems are severe. Pediatricians are estimated to identify only 50% of mental health problems. Data based on screening in pediatric office settings suggest an overall prevalence of psychosocial dysfunction of preschool and school-age children to be 10% and 13%, respectively. Children from poor families are twice as likely to have psychosocial problems as children from higher income families.

Other important influences on children's health include poverty, homelessness, single-parent families, parental divorce, domestic violence, both parents working, and adequate childcare. Related pediatric challenges include improving the quality of health care, social justice, equality in healthcare access, and improving the public health system. For adolescents, there are special concerns about sexuality, sexual orientation, substance use and abuse, violence, depression, and suicide (see Section XII).

CULTURE

Culture is an active, dynamic, and complex process of the way people interact and behave in the world. Culture encompasses the concepts, beliefs, values (including nurturing of children), and standards of behavior, language, and dress attributable to people that give order to their experiences in the world, give sense and purpose to their interactions with others, and provide meaning for their lives. Culture requires an attempt to understand, from the patient and family perspective, questions such as: What is the nature of health? How does one keep healthy? What is the nature of illness? How does the illness work? Where does it come from (illness attribution, etiology)? What is the approach to treatment? and What is the expected outcome? An appropriate inquiry that addresses this realm includes open-ended questions such as: "What *worries* (concerns) you the most about your child's illness?" or "What do you *think* has caused your child's illness?" These questions facilitate the patient's or family's discussion of their thoughts and feelings about the illness and its causes. Cultural understanding also includes concepts and beliefs about how one interacts with health professionals and what one expects from health professionals. The spiritual and religious aspect of health and health care also can be viewed from this perspective. These differences in perspectives, values, or beliefs may affect the health of the child in an adverse way and may result in differences between the pediatrician and the patient and family. Significant conflicts may arise because religious or cultural practices may lead to the possibility of child abuse and neglect. In this circumstance, the pediatrician is required by law to report the suspected child abuse and neglect to the appropriate social service authorities (see Chapter 22).

Complementary and alternative medicine (CAM) practices constitute a part of the broad cultural perspective. It is estimated that 20% to 30% of all children use some CAM; 50% to 75% of adolescents use CAM. Of children with chronic illness, 30% to 70% use CAM therapies, especially for asthma and cystic fibrosis, whereas only 30% to 60% of children and families tell their physicians about their use of CAM. Therapeutic modalities for CAM include biochemical, lifestyle, biomechanical, bioenergetic, and homeopathy. Some modalities may be effective, whereas others may be ineffective or even dangerous.

By 2020, almost half of U.S. children will be of Latino, African American, Asian, or Native American ethnicity. In many states, this shift already has occurred. Currently, there are immigrants and refugees from Southeast Asia, eastern Europe, the Middle East, Asia, Africa, Central America, South America, and other parts of the world, with a variety of languages and health beliefs. Rapidly changing demographic shifts in populations make it likely that the pediatrician will encounter many different cultural identities. Understanding patient and family health beliefs and practices enables pediatricians to practice better health care.

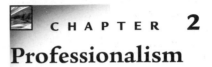

CHAPTER 2
Professionalism

CONCEPT OF PROFESSIONALISM

Society provides a profession with economic, political, and social rewards. Professions have specialized knowledge, and when it is difficult to measure the quality of its work, a profession has the potential to maintain a monopoly on power and control, remaining relatively autonomous. The profession's autonomy can be limited by societal needs. A profession exists as long as it fulfills its responsibilities for the social good. In the past, simply being a physician was considered by many to be a sufficient measure of high-quality health care.

Today the medical professional's activities are subject to explicit public rules of accountability. Governmental and other authorities, whose function is to foster social and distributive justice and the public good, grant limited autonomy to the professional organizations and their membership. City and municipal government departments of public health establish and implement heath standards and regulations. At the state level, boards of registration in medicine, with powers to investigate physician impairment, establish the criteria for obtaining and revoking medical licenses. The federal government has an increasing role in funding direct medical care and regulating the standards of services, which include national programs such as Medicare and Medicaid and the Food and Drug Administration. The Department of Health and Human Services regulates physician behavior in conducting research with the goal of protecting human subjects. The Health Care Quality Act of 1986 authorized the federal government to establish The National Practitioner Data Bank, which began in 1990. This data bank contains information about physicians (and other healthcare clinicians) who have been disciplined by a state licensing board, a professional society (local or national), a hospital, or a health plan. Practitioners who have been named in medical malpractice judgments or settlements also are included. Hospitals are required to review information in this data bank every 2 years as part of clinician recredentialing. There are accrediting agencies for medical schools (Liaison Committee on Medical Education) and postgraduate training (Accreditation Council for Graduate Medical Education [ACGME]). The ACGME includes establishing committees that review residency subspecialty training programs. At the individual physician level, the various specialty boards determine the criteria for competency for practice, including various examinations for board certification. Specialty certification is time limited, and physicians who wish to retain their certification are re-examined periodically. State boards of registration also adjudicate the question of the competence of the physician on an individual basis.

Historically, the most privileged professions have depended for their legitimacy on serving the public interest. The profession should be the guardian of social values emanating from that profession and negotiated with the public. A profession should not become more concerned about its own business, economics, and political interests than the interests of the people it serves. The public trust of physicians is based on the physician's commitment to **altruism**. The ACGME has established competency standards for its accreditation of residency programs. Among numerous required competencies is that of professionalism, which embodies altruism. Many medical schools include variations on the traditional Hippocratic oath as part of the commencement ceremonies as a recognition of a physician's responsibility to put the interest of others ahead of self-interest.

The core of professionalism is embedded in the daily healing work of the physician and encompassed in the patient-physician relationship. The goal in this relationship is to act in the best interest of the patient using all of the technologic, scientific, and humanistic experiences available. Professionalism includes an appreciation for the cultural and religious/spiritual health beliefs of the patient, incorporating the ethical and moral values of the profession and the moral values of the patient. Professionalism includes the family and the community as an important element of the healing perspective. The community perspective includes advocacy for the individual patient and advocacy for the community.

CHALLENGES OF PROFESSIONALISM

The inappropriate actions of a few practicing physicians, physician investigators, and physicians in positions of power in the corporate world, have created a

societal demand to punish those involved and have led to the erosion of respect for the medical profession. These negative physician behaviors include the following:

Abuse of power
Sexual harassment and inappropriate sexual behavior
Conflict of interest and inappropriate financial gain
Professional arrogance and greed
Physician impairment from drugs and alcohol
Fraud in research and practice—misrepresentation
Loss of conscientiousness in fulfilling responsibilities

The AAP, the American Board of Pediatrics, the American Board of Internal Medicine, the Liaison Committee on Medical Education, the Medical Student Objectives Project of the Association of American Medical Colleges, and the ACGME in their Outcomes Project have called for increasing attention to professionalism in the practice of medicine and in the education of physicians.

PROFESSIONALISM FOR PEDIATRICIANS

The American Board of Pediatrics adopted professional standards in 2000, as follows:

1. **Honesty/integrity** is the consistent regard for the highest standards of behavior and the refusal to violate one's personal and professional codes. Honesty and integrity imply being fair, being truthful, keeping one's word, meeting commitments, and being forthright in interactions with patients and peers and in all professional work, whether through documentation, personal communication, presentations, research, or other interactions. Maintaining integrity requires awareness of situations that may result in conflict of interest or that may result in personal gain at the expense of the best interest of the patient.

2. **Reliability/responsibility** means being responsible for and accountable to others. First, there must be accountability to one's patients, not only to children but also to their families. Second, there must be accountability to society to ensure that the public's needs are addressed. Third, the pediatrician must be accountable to the profession to ensure that the ethical precepts of practice are upheld. Inherent in this responsibility is reliability in completing assigned duties or fulfilling commitments. There also must be a willingness to accept responsibility for errors.

3. **Respect for others** is the essence of humanism, and humanism is central to professionalism. This respect extends to all spheres of contact, including, but not limited to, patients, families, other physicians, and professional colleagues, including nurses,

residents, fellows, and medical students. The pediatrician must treat all persons with respect and regard for their individual worth and dignity. The pediatrician must be fair and nondiscriminatory and be aware of emotional, personal, family, and cultural influences on a patient's well-being, rights, and choices of medical care. It is also a professional obligation to respect appropriate patient confidentiality.

4. **Compassion/empathy** is a crucial component of the practice of pediatrics. The pediatrician must listen attentively and respond humanely to the concerns of patients and family members. Appropriate empathy for and relief of pain, discomfort, and anxiety should be part of the daily practice of pediatric medicine.

5. **Self-improvement** is the pursuit of and commitment to providing the highest quality of health care through lifelong learning and education. The pediatrician must seek to learn from errors and aspire to excellence through self-evaluation and acceptance of the critiques of others.

6. **Self-awareness/knowledge of limits** includes recognition of the need for guidance and supervision when faced with new or complex responsibilities. The pediatrician also must be insightful regarding the impact of his or her behavior on others and cognizant of appropriate professional boundaries.

7. **Communication/collaboration** is crucial to providing the best care for patients. Pediatricians must work cooperatively and communicate effectively with patients and their families and with all healthcare providers involved in the care of their patients.

8. **Altruism/advocacy** refers to unselfish regard for and devotion to the welfare of others. It is a key element of professionalism. Self-interest or the interests of other parties should not interfere with the care of one's patients and their families.

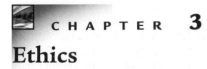

CHAPTER 3

Ethics

ETHICS IN HEALTH CARE

The ethics of health care are embedded in the process whereby patients, family members, and clinicians engage in medical decision making by balancing personal, family, cultural/religious/spiritual, and professional values. These values lead to choices about medical care. In contrast to the scientific method of determining what is factual, which is based on empirical evidence and scientific studies and in which

scientific truth is essentially probabilistic, ethical decision making relies on values to determine what kinds of decisions are best or appropriate for individual patients, family members, and clinicians. In the process of ethical decision making, the clinical question is: What are the values that the parties use to make decisions, weighing the burdens and benefits resulting from each decision, for themselves and others? Sometimes ethical decision making in medical care is a matter of choosing the least harmful option for a patient among many adverse alternatives. In the day-to-day practice of medicine, although all clinical encounters may have an ethical component, major ethical challenges are infrequent.

When a clinician asks the question, "What *can* I do?" the answer is in the scientific realm or based on clinical experience. When the question is, "What *should* I do?" the clinician begins the ethical decision-making process. The legal system influences this process by refining the question to include "What *may* I do?" or "What *must* I do?" The legal system defines the minimal standards of behavior required of physicians and the rest of society through the legislative, regulatory, and judicial systems. The role of the law is to provide for social order and adjudicate disputes. Courts and the legal system may not address ethical concerns, however. An example is a teenager who seeks birth control information and a prescription from her pediatrician and would like to keep this information confidential. The laws are clear and support the principle of **confidentiality** for teenagers who are competent to decide about such issues. Some pediatricians may believe that this request should not be honored, that teenagers should not be having a sexual relationship, or that the parents need to be informed first. This issue becomes more difficult when the pediatrician has had a long-standing relationship with the family, and parents expect to be fully informed about the health of their daughter.

Ethical problems derive from value differences among patients, families, and clinicians about choices and options in the provision of health care. Resolving these value differences involves several important ethical principles. **Autonomy**, which is based on the principle of **respect for persons**, means that competent adult patients can make choices about health care that they perceive to be in their best interests, after being appropriately informed about their particular health condition and the risks and benefits of alternatives of diagnostic tests and treatments. **Paternalism** challenges the principle of autonomy and involves the clinician deciding what is best for the patient and how much information is provided. Paternalism, under certain circumstances, may be more appropriate than autonomy. These circumstances are usually emergency situations, when a patient has a serious life-threatening medical condition or a significant psychiatric disorder, threatening themselves or others. Weighing the values of autonomy and paternalism can challenge the clinician. Other important ethical principles are those of **beneficence** (doing good), **nonmaleficence** (doing no harm or as little harm as possible), and **justice** (the values involved in the equality of the distribution of goods and services and benefits and burdens to the individual, family, or society). In end-of-life decision making, the quality of life and how much suffering is too much (when is life not worth living and who decides) become important considerations for the provision of palliative and hospice care (see Chapter 4). These principles apply to competent patients, who have the capacity for decision making and engaging in the process of informed consent.

ETHICAL PRINCIPLES RELATED TO INFANTS, CHILDREN, AND ADOLESCENTS

Children vary from being totally dependent on parents or guardians to meet their healthcare needs to being more independent. Infants and young children do not have the capacity for making medical decisions for themselves. Paternalism by parents and pediatricians in these circumstances is appropriate. Adolescents (≥18 years old), if competent, have the legal right to make medical decisions for themselves. Children 8 to 9 years old can understand how the body works and the meaning of certain procedures, and by age 14 to 15, young adolescents may be considered autonomous through the process of being designated a mature or emancipated minor or by having certain medical conditions (see later). It is ethical for pediatricians to involve children in the decision-making process with information appropriate to their capacity to understand. The process of obtaining the **assent** of a child is consistent with this goal.

The principle of shared decision making is appropriate, but this process may be limited because of issues of confidentiality in the provision of medical care. Some parents are concerned about the side effects of immunizations for their children, and a few may refuse to have their children immunized. This situation raises a conflict between the need to protect and support the health of the individual and the public with the rights of the individual and involves ethical issues of distributive justice in regard to the costs and distribution of the vaccinations and responsibility for side effects.

LEGAL ISSUES

All competent patients of an age defined legally by each state (usually ≥18 years old) are considered autonomous with regard to their health decisions. To be competent, patients must:

1. Understand the nature of the medical interventions and procedures, understand the risks and benefits of these interventions, and be able to communicate their decision.
2. Reason, deliberate, and weigh the risks and benefits using their understanding about the implications of the decision on their own welfare.
3. Apply a set of personal values to the decision-making process and show an awareness of the possible conflicts or differences in values as applied to the decisions to be made.

These requirements need to be placed within the context of medical care and applied to each case with its specific and possibly unique characteristics. Most young children are not able to meet the noted requirements for competency and need others, usually the parent, to make decisions for them. Legally, parents are given great discretion in making decisions for their children. This discretion is legally limited when there is child abuse and neglect, which triggers a further legal process involving the courts in determining what is in the best interests of the child.

Because laws vary by state, it is important to become familiar with the state laws. State, not federal, law determines when an adolescent can consent to medical care. State laws also determine parental access to confidential adolescent medical information. The Health Insurance Portability and Accountability Act of 1996 (HIPAA), which became effective in 2003, requires a minimal standard of confidentiality protection. The law confers less confidentiality protection to minors than to adults. It is the pediatrician's responsibility to inform minors of their confidentiality rights and help them exercise these rights under the HIPAA regulations.

Under special circumstances, nonautonomous adolescents are granted the legal right to consent under state law when they are considered mature or emancipated minors or because of certain public health considerations, as follows:

1. **Mature minors.** Some states have legally recognized that many adolescents age 14 and older can meet the cognitive criteria and emotional maturity for competence and may decide independently. In these circumstances parents legally do not play a role in decision making. The Supreme Court has decided that pregnant mature minors have the constitutional right to make decisions about abortion without parental consent. Although many state legislatures require parental notification, pregnant adolescents wishing to have an abortion do not have to seek parental consent. The state must provide a judicial procedure to facilitate this decision making for adolescents.

2. **Emancipated minors.** Emancipated minors are children who are legally emancipated from parental control and may seek medical treatment without parental consent. The definition varies from state to state, but generally includes children who have graduated from high school, are members of the armed forces, are married, are pregnant, are runaways, are parents, live apart from their parents and are financially independent, or are declared emancipated by a court.

3. **Interests of the state (public health).** State legislatures have concluded that minors with certain medical conditions, such as sexually transmitted infections and other contagious diseases, pregnancy (including prevention with the use of birth control), certain mental illnesses, and drug and alcohol abuse, may seek treatment for these conditions autonomously without parental consent. States have an interest in limiting the spread of disease that may endanger the public health and in eliminating barriers to access for the treatment of certain conditions.

ETHICAL ISSUES IN PRACTICE

Most often, the parent or guardian is the decision maker for young children. From an ethical perspective, clinicians should engage children and adolescents, based on their developmental capacity, in discussions about medical plans so that they have a good understanding of the nature of the treatments and alternatives, the side effects, and expected outcomes. There should be an assessment of the patient's understanding of the clinical situation, how the patient is responding, and the factors that may influence the patient's decisions. Pediatricians should always listen to and appreciate patients' requests for confidentiality and their hopes and wishes. The ultimate goal is to help nourish children's capacity to become as autonomous as is appropriate to their developmental stage.

Confidentiality

Confidentiality is crucial to the provision of medical care and is an important part of the basis for a trusting patient/family physician relationship. Confidentiality means that information about a patient should not be shared without consent. If confidentiality is broken, patients may experience great harm and may not seek needed medical care. They may not provide a truthful medical history if they believe that others will know about their medical condition. Patient/physician confidentiality is an important value of the medical profession. See Section XII for discussion of confidentiality in the care of adolescents.

Ethical Issues in Genetic Testing and Screening in Children

The goal of **screening** is to identify diseases when there is no clinically identifiable risk factor for disease. Screening should take place only when there is a treatment available or when a diagnosis would benefit the child. **Testing** usually is performed when there is some clinically identifiable risk factor. Genetic testing and screening present special problems because test results have important implications for the individual who is tested and other family members. Some genetic screening (sickle cell anemia or cystic fibrosis) may reveal a carrier state, which may lead to choices about reproduction or create financial, psychosocial, and interpersonal problems (e.g., guilt, shame, social stigma, and discrimination in insurance and jobs). Because carrier screening is important for reproductive choices, screening in childhood does not seem appropriate, unless an adolescent is pregnant or planning a pregnancy. Patients and, when appropriate, families should be in a position to choose what testing is appropriate based on their wishes and ethical beliefs and to choose whom to inform when testing occurs. Confidentiality, beneficence, and the best interests of the child are the ethical principles involved in such decision making. Collaboration with, or referral to, a clinical geneticist is appropriate in helping the family with the complex issues of genetic counseling when a genetic disorder is detected or likely to be detected (see Section IX).

Newborn screening should not be used as a surrogate for parental testing. Examples of diseases that can be diagnosed by genetic screening, even though the manifestations of the disease process do not appear until later in life, are polycystic kidney disease; Huntington disease; certain cancers, such as breast cancer in some ethnic populations; and hemochromatosis. Parents may pressure the pediatrician to order genetic tests when the child is still young, for the parents' purposes. Testing for these disorders should be delayed until the child has the capacity for informed consent or assent and is competent to make decisions, unless there is a direct benefit to the child at the time of testing. Newborn screening to detect carrier status is not ethically appropriate.

Religious Issues and Ethics

Religious knowledge is based on revealed truth, faith, and belief. When religious tenets interfere with the health and well-being of the child, the pediatrician is required to act in the best interests of the child. Freedom of religion does not justify children being harmed. When an infant or child whose parents have a religious prohibition against a blood transfusion needs a transfusion to save his or her life, the courts always have intervened to allow a transfusion. In contrast, parents with strong religious beliefs under some state laws may refuse immunizations for their children. However, state governments can mandate immunizations for all children during disease outbreaks or epidemics. By requiring immunization of all, including individuals who object on religious grounds, the state government is using the principle of distributive justice, which states that all members of society must share in the burdens and the benefits to have a just society.

Children as Human Subjects in Research

The goal of research is to develop new and generalized knowledge. Parents may give informed permission for children to participate in research under certain conditions. Children cannot give consent but may assent or dissent to research protocols. Special federal regulations have been developed to protect child and adolescent participants in human investigation. These regulations provide additional safeguards beyond the safeguards provided for adult participants in research, while still providing the opportunity for children to benefit from the scientific advances of research.

Many parents with seriously ill children hope that the research protocol will have direct benefit for their particular child. The greatest challenge for researchers is to be clear with parents that research is not treatment. This fact should be addressed as sensitively and compassionately as possible.

CHAPTER 4
Palliative Care and End-of-Life Issues

Palliative medical care means alleviating the symptoms of disease without curing the disease; it includes mitigating suffering by alleviating pain and other symptoms. The ultimate goal of medicine is to prevent or cure disease and save or preserve life. Palliation requires caring for the patient when cure is not probable or possible. The palliative care of children includes the comprehensive assessment and management of the medical, psychosocial, cultural, and spiritual concerns before and during the end-of-life process.

The ability to diagnose and to treat many previously untreated diseases has raised the expectations of patients and families for effective cures and the prevention of disease and disability. As a culture, we have denied or suppressed the reality of death; many physicians have difficulty accepting the death of their patients. For parents, the death of a child is one of the most painful and distressing life events, and the related grieving usually lasts longer than all other types of grief and may never be resolved.

Faced with the impending death of a child, the family and the clinician should use palliative care, whether in the home, hospital, or a hospice program. The goal of palliative care is to apply the best available medical care and to maintain, improve, and support the quality of life of children, at their most effective level of functioning, until the time of death. Medical care in this situation is a continuum from curative medicine to palliative care (comfort care); to helping the child, parents, other children, extended family, and community members as the child proceeds through the dying process; to bereavement counseling; and finally to long-term follow-up of the family. Curative care and palliative care can coexist; aggressive pain medication may be provided, while curative treatment is continued in the hopes of a remission or improved health status.

The pediatrician should support the child and the family when death becomes inevitable and provide bereavement counseling and follow-up of families. Most pediatricians care for a very small number of children who die each year and face an unexpected professional challenge when a child dies. The ethical, legal, psychosocial, cultural, and spiritual issues add to the complexity of decision making under these circumstances. Parents usually turn to their pediatricians to discuss issues such as disclosure of information to the child or other family members, changes from curative to palliative care, how to talk with the child who is dying, and the involvement of the child and the family in decision making about treatment options, including withholding and withdrawing treatment. The pediatrician needs to collaborate with other clinicians in an interdisciplinary team to address these complex issues.

Children who are terminally ill or who have a life-threatening illness have (Table 4–1):

1. Conditions for which treatment may be curative, but also may fail; only 75% of all childhood cancers are curable.
2. Conditions that are usually anticipated to be terminal, but excellent treatment may enhance the quality of life for a prolonged period (e.g., HIV/AIDS or severe cystic fibrosis).
3. Progressive diseases for which there is no curative or stabilizing treatment but only palliative care; the course of illness may extend over months or years (e.g., Werdnig-Hoffmann disease).
4. Conditions that create significant neurologic disability (severe developmental delay and severe cerebral palsy) and are associated with an increased risk of death.

TABLE 4–1.   Conditions Appropriate for Pediatric Palliative Care*

Conditions for Which Curative Treatment Is Possible but May Fail

Advanced or progressive cancer or cancer with a poor prognosis
Complex and severe congenital or acquired heart disease

Conditions Requiring Intensive Long-term Treatment Aimed at Maintaining the Quality of Life

Human immunodeficiency virus infection
Cystic fibrosis
Severe gastrointestinal disorders or malformations, such as gastroschisis
Severe epidermolysis bullosa
Severe immunodeficiencies
Renal failure in cases in which dialysis, transplantation, or both are not available or indicated
Chronic or severe respiratory failure
Muscular dystrophy

Progressive Conditions in Which Treatment is Exclusively Palliative after Diagnosis

Progressive metabolic disorders
Certain chromosomal abnormalities, such as trisomy 13 or trisomy 18
Severe forms of osteogenesis imperfecta

Conditions Involving Severe, Nonprogressive Disability, Causing Extreme Vulnerability to Health Complications

Severe cerebral palsy with recurrent infection or difficult-to-control symptoms
Extreme prematurity
Severe neurologic sequelae of infectious disease
Hypoxic or anoxic brain injury
Holoprosencephaly or other severe brain malformations

*Premature death is likely or expected with many of these conditions.
From Himelstein BP, Hilden JM, Morstad Boldt A, Weissman D: Pediatric palliative care. N Engl J Med 350:1752-1762, 2004.

Hospice care is a treatment program for the end of life. It consists of a range of palliative care services, usually provided by an interdisciplinary team, including members of the clergy and specialists in the bereavement and the end-of-life process. Palliative care treatments include symptom relief (e.g., pain, dyspnea, nausea), management of emotional concerns (e.g., depression, anxiety), and addressing end-of-life issues in the context of the patient and family's values, culture, religious or spiritual beliefs, and ethical beliefs. Many insurance companies do not provide coverage for these services; Medicaid uses the adult Medicare model, requiring a prognosis of death within 6 months for children to receive hospice services. Comprehensive, high-quality hospice care, within a specialized inpatient facility, is expensive and can cost $1400 per day.

PRINCIPLES OF PALLIATIVE AND END-OF-LIFE CARE

1. *Respect for the dignity of patients and families.* The clinician should respect and listen to patient and family goals, preferences, and choices. School-age children can articulate a basic understanding of how the body works and have preferences about how they wish to be treated. Adolescents are cognitively more advanced and by the age of 14 can engage in decision making (see Section XII). The pediatrician should assist the patient and the family in understanding the diagnosis, treatment options, and prognosis. The pediatrician should clarify priorities, promote informed choices, allow for the free flow of information, and listen to and discuss the social-emotional concerns. Consideration should be given to the child's cognitive developmental stage and the parent and child's wishes. **Advanced care** (advance directives), as part of hospice care planning, should be instituted with the child and parents participating in discussions about what they would like as treatment options as the end of life nears. When there are differences of opinion between the family and the pediatrician, an attempt to negotiate and clarify issues and concerns should be made so as to prevent the development of an adversarial situation. **Hospital ethics committees** and consultation services are important resources for the pediatrician and family members.

2. *Access to comprehensive and compassionate palliative care.* The clinician should address the physical symptoms, comfort, and functional capacity, with special attention to pain and other symptoms associated with the dying process, and respond empathically to the psychological distress and human suffering. Treatment approaches such as general education, family counseling about grief, peer support, and art and music therapy for the patient, family, and extended family members may be indicated. Respite care should be available at any time during the illness to allow the family caretakers to rest and renew themselves.

3. *Use of interdisciplinary resources.* Because of the complexity of care, no one clinician can provide all the needed services. The team members may include primary and subspecialty physicians, nurses in the hospital/hospice facility or for home visits, the pain management team (palliative care team), psychologists, social workers, clergy, schoolteachers, friends of the family, and peers of the child. The child and

family should be in a position to decide who should know what during all phases of the illness process.

4. *Acknowledging and providing support for caregivers.* The death of a child is difficult to accept and understand. The primary caregivers of the child, family, and friends need opportunities to address their own emotional concerns. Siblings of the child who is dying react emotionally and cognitively based on their developmental level. Opportunities to have team meetings to address the thoughts and feelings of team members are crucial. Soon after the death of the child, the care team should review the experience with the parents and family and share their reactions and feelings. Institutional support may include time to attend funerals, counseling for the staff, opportunities for families to return to the hospital, and scheduled ceremonies to commemorate the death of the child.

5. *Commitment to quality improvement of palliative care through research and education.* Hospitals should develop support systems and staff to monitor the quality of care continually, assess the need for appropriate resources, and evaluate the responses of the patient and family members to the treatment program. Children dying of cancer in the last months of life have substantial suffering, and attempts to control their symptoms are often unsuccessful. Sometimes there are differences between physicians and family members in the timing of the realization that death is imminent. Physicians may realize this earlier than parents or vice versa. When there is recognition by both the family and physician that the end is near, it is easier to move from curative to palliative and hospice care. Consensus results in better palliative care from the medical and psychosocial perspective.

COGNITIVE ISSUES IN CHILDREN AND ADOLESCENTS: UNDERSTANDING OF DEATH AND DYING

The pediatrician should communicate with children about what is happening to them and should use developmental understanding of children's concepts of health and illness to help frame the discussion with children and help parents understand the developmental level of their child. Using a cognitive developmental perspective based on Piaget's work, children's concepts of death and disease can be categorized as sensorimotor, preoperational, concrete operations, and formal operations. Up to 2 years of age (sensorimotor), death is seen as separation, and there is probably no concept of death per se. The associated behaviors usually include protesting and difficulty of attachment to other adults. The degree of difficulty depends on the availability of other nurturing people who have been primary caretakers of the child and with whom the child has had a good previous attachment.

From 2 to 6 years of age (preoperational), sometimes called the **magic years**, death is seen as reversible and only temporary. Because of a developing sense of guilt, death may be viewed as punishment. If the child's younger sibling suddenly died of sudden infant death syndrome, the child may have previously wished the infant to have died or to have gone back where he or she came from. The reality of the sibling's death may be seen psychologically as being caused by the child's wishful thinking. A child of this age may ask questions such as "When is the dead person coming home?" or "How will the dead person drink while in the ground?"

Ages 6 to 11 (school age) are considered the concrete operational stage of cognitive development. Death may be gradually, but not completely, understood as permanent and final. Children have limited capacity to know how the body works. The heart stopped or the lungs did not work are understood as causal to death. Sometimes there is the fear that death is infectious, and if a loved one has died, perhaps other loved ones also will die. Because of the child's uncertainty about the reality of death, it is hard for this age group to understand the loss fully.

The developmental stage of adolescents (≥12 years old) is considered formal operations. Death is a reality and is seen as universal and irreversible. Adolescents handle death issues at the abstract or philosophical level and can be realistic. Adolescents can discuss withholding of treatments. Their wishes, hopes, and fears should be attended to and respected.

ETHICAL ISSUES IN END-OF-LIFE DECISION MAKING

The care of a terminally ill and dying child is a challenging experience for the pediatrician. The ethical principles involved are autonomy, beneficence (doing good), nonmaleficence (not initiating and eliminating or mitigating harm, pain, and suffering), truth telling, confidentiality, and the physician's duty. Technology can prolong life, but the goal of medicine is not only to prolong life. There comes a time when life is no longer worth living, usually when the burdens of treatment or of the medical condition outweigh the benefits as defined by the patient and family. The questions for all family members, including the adolescent, are: What should be done? Who decides?

It is extremely difficult for parents to know when the burdens of continued medical care are no longer appropriate for their child. Pediatricians, patients, and family members may differ on when this time has come, depending on their beliefs and values of what constitutes quality of life, when life ceases to be worth living, and their religious/spiritual, cultural, and philosophical beliefs. This process is highly emotional, and family members vary in the degree to which they can understand and integrate the reality of the impending loss of a loved one. The most important ethical principle is that of what is in the **best interest** of the child as determined through the process of shared decision making, informed permission/consent from the parents, and assent from the child. It is the physician's duty to interpret the medical conditions, including the degree of pain and suffering, to assess the quality of life during the progression of the disease process, and to relieve pain and suffering aggressively.

For the physician, patient, and family, the issues are: What are the goals of continued medical treatment? What are the burdens and benefits of the medical intervention plan? There is no ethical or legal difference between withholding treatment and withdrawing treatment, although many parents and physicians see the latter as more challenging. Physicians must be clear to themselves and to family members that palliative care is not giving up, but another appropriate medical care treatment option. Family members and the patient should agree about what are appropriate **do not resuscitate (DNR)** orders. Clear documentation and understanding of the DNR is essential. When DNR orders are written, there should be clear delineation of the limits of therapy. Obtaining blood cultures or using antibiotics may be limited, but IV fluid for comfort care, pain medication, and sedation may be continued. Nasal oxygen may be continued, but CPR may not be used. Forgoing some measures does not preclude other measures being implemented, based on the needs and wishes of the patient and family. When there are serious differences among parents, children, and physicians on these matters, the physician may consult with the **hospital ethics committee** or as a last resort turn to the legal system by filing a report about potential abuse or neglect.

CULTURAL, RELIGIOUS, AND SPIRITUAL CONCERNS ABOUT PALLIATIVE CARE AND END-OF-LIFE DECISIONS

Parents may engage in religious or complementary and alternative therapies to improve the healing process. Understanding their religious/spiritual or cultural beliefs and values about death and dying can help the pediatrician work with the family to integrate these beliefs, values, and practices into the palliative care plan. Decisions, rituals, and withholding of palliative or lifesaving procedures that could harm the child or are not in the best interests of the child should be addressed. Religious/spiritual or cultural practices may include prayer, anointing, laying on of hands, an exorcism ceremony to undo a curse, amulets, and other religious objects placed on the child or at the bedside. Sometimes clinicians are asked to pray with the patient or family. Cultures vary regarding the roles family members have and the site of treatment for dying people and the preparation of the body. Some ethnic groups expect the clinical team to speak with the oldest family member or only to the head of the family outside the patient's presence. Some families involve the entire extended family in decision making. For some families, dying at home can bring the family bad luck, whereas others believe that the patient's spirit will get lost if the death occurs in the hospital. In some traditions, the healthcare team cleans and prepares the body, whereas in others family members prefer to complete this ritual. Families differ in the idea of organ donation and the acceptance of the autopsy.

SUDDEN DEATH

The sudden death of a child, resulting from injury, homicide, suicide, or the sudden infant death syndrome, does not allow the family or the physician time to prepare for death. Many of these situations occur in emergency departments. These issues should be part of every emergency department educational program. Special attention should be given to the thoughts and feelings of the professional staff, to addressing how families were sensitively cared for, and to the reaction of the professional staff to the sudden death of a pediatric patient. Families who have not had time to prepare for the tragedy of an unexpected death require considerable support. The circumstances of the death must be fully explored. The need to investigate the possibility of child abuse or neglect subjects the family to intense scrutiny and may create guilt and anger directed at the medical team.

SUGGESTED READING

Accreditation Council of Graduate Medical Education: Outcome Project. http://www.acgme.org/outcome/.

Agency for Healthcare Research and Quality: Disparities Report. http://www.ahcpr.gov/qual/nhdr02/nhdrprelim.htm.

Agency for Healthcare Research and Quality: Quality Report. http://www.ahcpr.gov/qual/nhqr03/nhqrsum03.htm.

American Academy of Pediatrics, Committee on Bioethics: Guidelines on foregoing life-sustaining medical treatment. Pediatrics 93:532-536, 1994.

American Academy of Pediatrics, Committee on Bioethics: Informed consent, parental permission, and assent in pediatric practice. Pediatrics 95:314-317, 1995.

American Academy of Pediatrics, Committee on Bioethics: Religious objections to medical care. Pediatrics 99:279-281, 1997.

American Academy of Pediatrics, Committee on Bioethics and Committee on Hospital Care: Palliative care for children. Pediatrics 106:351-357, 2000.

American Academy of Pediatrics, Committee on Bioethics: Ethical issues with genetic testing. Pediatrics 107:1451-1455, 2001.

American Academy of Pediatrics, Committee on Psychosocial Aspects of Child and Family Health: The pediatrician and childhood bereavement. Pediatrics 105:445-447, 2000.

American Academy of Pediatrics, Committee on Psychosocial Aspects of Child and Family Health: The new morbidity revisited: A renewed commitment to the psychosocial aspects of pediatric care. Pediatrics 108:1227-1230, 2001.

American Board of Internal Medicine, American College of Physicians, American Society of Internal Medicine, and the European Federation of Internal Medicine: Medical professionalism in the new millennium: A physician charter. Ann Intern Med 136:243-246, 2002. http://www.abim.org/.

American Board of Pediatrics: Professionalism. http://www.abp.org.

Arias E, MacDorman MF, Strobino DM, et al: Annual summary of vital statistics—2002. Pediatrics 112:1215-1230, 2003.

Barnes LL, Plotnikoff GA, Fox K, et al: Spirituality, religion, and pediatrics: Intersecting worlds of healing. Pediatrics 106(Suppl):899-908, 2000.

Behrman RE, Kliegman RM, Jenson HB (eds): Part I. The Field of Pediatrics. In Nelson Textbook of Pediatrics, 17th ed. Philadelphia, WB Saunders, 2003, pp 1-22.

Bursch B, Zeltzer LK: Pediatric pain management. In Behrman RE, Kliegman RM, Jenson HB (eds): Nelson Textbook of Pediatrics, 17th ed. Philadelphia, WB Saunders, 2003, pp 358-366.

Himelstein BP, Hilden JM, Morstand Boldt A, Weissman D: Pediatric palliative care. N Engl J Med 350:1752-1762, 2004.

Institute of Medicine: When Children Die: Improving Palliative and End-of-Life Care for Children and Their Families. Washington, DC, The National Academy Press, 2003. http://www.iom.edu.

Kleinman A, Eisenberg L, Good B: Culture illness and care: Clinical lessons from anthropologic and cross cultural research. Ann Intern Med 88:251-258, 1978.

Last Acts: Precepts of palliative care of children/adolescents and their families. Last Acts is a campaign to improve end-of-life care by a coalition of professional and consumer organizations. http://www.lastacts.org.

Liaison Committee on Medical Education. http://www.lcme.org/.

Medical School Objectives project of the Association of American Medical Colleges. http://www.aamc.org/meded/msop/start.htm.

National Center for Grieving Children and Families. A site for children and families. http://www.GrievingChild.org.

Sahler OJZ, Frager G, Levetown M, et al: Medical education about end-of life care in the pediatric setting: Principles, challenges and opportunities. Pediatrics 105:575-584, 2000.

Swick HM: Toward a normative definition of medical professionalism. Acad Med 75:612-616, 2002.

Task Force on the Future of Pediatric Education 2000: The future of pediatric education II: Organizing pediatric education to meet the needs of infants, children, adolescents, and young adults in the 21st century. A collaborative project of the pediatric community. Pediatrics 105(Suppl):161-212, 2000.

Wise P: The anatomy of a disparity in infant mortality. Ann Rev Public Health 24:341-362, 2003.

Wolfe J, Grier H, Klar N: Symptoms and suffering at the end-of-life in children with cancer. N Engl J Med 342:326-333, 2000.

Wolfe J, Klar N, Grier H, et al: Understanding of prognosis among parents of children who died of cancer: Impact on treatment goals and integration with palliative care. JAMA 284:2469-2475, 2000.

GROWTH AND DEVELOPMENT

David A. Levine

INTRODUCTION: THE HEALTH MAINTENANCE VISIT

Health maintenance is the centerpiece of pediatric care and a most rewarding aspect of caring for children. The frequent office visits in the first 2 years of life are more than "physicals"; although a somatic history and physical examination are important parts of each visit, many other issues are discussed, including nutrition, development, safety, and behavior.

Knowledge of normal growth and development is essential to medical care. Disorders of growth and development are often associated with chronic or severe illness or may be the only symptom of parental neglect or abuse. Although normal growth and development does not eliminate a serious or chronic illness, in general, it supports a judgment that a child is healthy except for acute, often benign, illnesses that do not affect growth and development.

Although the processes of growth and development are intertwined, it is convenient to refer to **growth** as the increase in the size of the body and **development** as an increase in function of processes related to body and mind. All who care for children must be familiar with normal patterns of growth and development so that they can recognize and manage abnormal variations.

Within the broad limits that characterize normal growth and development, every individual's path through the life cycle is unique, with a range of complex, interrelated changes occurring from the molecular to the behavioral level. The genetic makeup and the physical, emotional, and social environment of the individual determine how a child grows and develops through childhood. One goal of pediatrics is to help each child achieve his or her individual potential for growth and development. Periodically monitoring each child for the normal progression of growth

and development and screening for abnormalities are important means of accomplishing this goal. The AAP recommends routine office visits in the first week of life (depending on nursery discharge); at 2 weeks; at 2, 4, 6, 9, 12, 15, and 18 months; at 2 years and annually up to age 6; and every 2 years between age 6 and adolescence. During adolescence, a complete health maintenance visit is recommended every 2 years and an annual risk-reduction visit every year (see Figure 9–1).

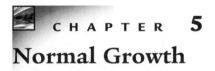

CHAPTER **5**

Normal Growth

Deviations in growth patterns may be nonspecific but may be important indicators of serious and chronic medical disorders. An accurate measurement of height, weight, and head circumference should be obtained at every health supervision visit. Table 5–1 summarizes several convenient benchmarks to evaluate normal growth. It is imperative, however, that growth be measured and compared with statistical norms in a standard fashion on growth charts. When plotting growth, serial measurements are much more useful than single measurements because they can help detect deviations from a particular child's growth pattern even if the value remains within statistically defined normal limits (i.e., between the 3rd and 97th percentiles). Because statistical analysis has defined this normal range, clinically there are some children within the normal range who have growth problems and some children outside the normal range who have normal growth. Following the trend helps to define whether growth is within acceptable limits or warrants further evaluation.

Growth is assessed by plotting accurate measurements on growth charts (Figs. 5–1 to 5–8) and comparing each set of measurements with previous measurements. Measurements are plotted routinely at health maintenance visits or at other visits if there is a concern over the child's growth pattern. The CDC Growth Charts published in 2000 are based on nationally representative data. For ages 0 to 36 months, charts include weight-for-age, length-for-age (measured recumbent), head circumference–by-age, and weight-for-length. For ages 2 to 20, charts include weight-for-age, height-for-age (measured standing), and **body mass index** (BMI)-for age. The BMI is defined as body weight in kilograms divided by height in meters squared. BMI also may be calculated by weight in pounds divided by height in inches, squared, and multiplied by a correction factor of 703. The BMI is an index for classifying adiposity and is recommended as a screening tool for children and adolescents to determine whether an individual is overweight (BMI above the 95th percentile for age) or at risk for being overweight (BMI between the 85th and 95th percentile for age).

Because growth charts are based on a population sample, they make it seem that children grow in a smooth, continuous fashion. Measuring individual

TABLE 5–1. Rules of Thumb for Growth

Weight

1. Weight loss in first few days: 5%-10% of birth weight
2. Return to birth weight: 7-10 days of age
   Double birth weight: 4-5 mo
   Triple birth weight: 1 yr
   Quadruple birth weight: 2 yr
3. Average weights: 3.5 kg at birth
   10 kg at 1 yr
   20 kg at 5 yr
   30 kg at 10 yr
4. Daily weight gain: 20-30 g for first 3-4 mo
   15-20 g for rest of the first yr
5. Average annual weight gain: 5 lb between 2 yr and puberty (spurts and plateaus may occur)

Height

1. Average length: 20 inches at birth, 30 inches at 1 yr
2. At age 3 yr, the average child is 3 ft tall
3. At age 4 yr, the average child is 40 in tall (double birth length)
4. Average annual height increase: 2-3 inches between age 4 yr and puberty

Head Circumference (HC)

1. Average HC: 35 cm at birth (13.5 inches)
2. HC increases: 1 cm/mo for first yr (2 cm/mo for first 3 mo, then slower); 10 cm for rest of life

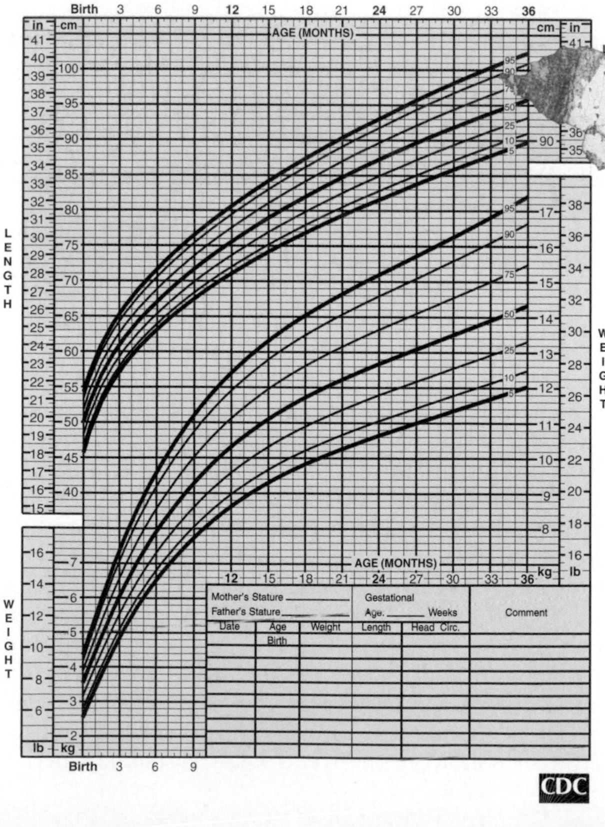

Figure 5–1

length-by-age and weight-by-age percentiles for boys, age birth to 36 months. Developed by the National Center for Health Statistics in collaboration with the National Center for Chronic Disease Prevention and Health Promotion. (From Centers for Disease Control and Prevention, Atlanta, Ga, 2000. Available online at http://www.cdc.gov/growthcharts.)

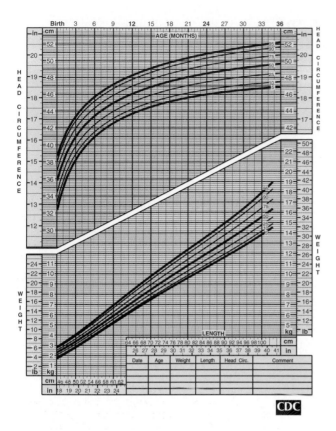

Figure 5-2

Head circumference and weight-by-length percentiles for boys, age birth to 36 months. Developed by the National Center for Health Statistics in collaboration with the National Center for Chronic Disease Prevention and Health Promotion. (From Centers for Disease Control and Prevention, Atlanta, Ga, 2000. Available online at http://www.cdc.gov/growthcharts.)

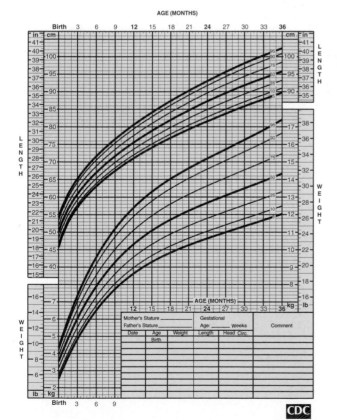

Figure 5-3

Length-by-age and weight-by-age percentiles for girls, age birth to 36 months. Developed by the National Center for Health Statistics in collaboration with the National Center for Chronic Disease Prevention and Health Promotion. (From Centers for Disease Control and Prevention, Atlanta, Ga, 2000. Available online at http://www.cdc.gov/growthcharts.)

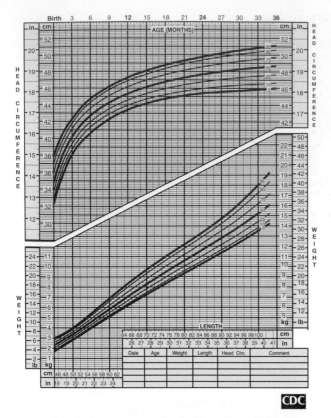

Figure 5–4

Head circumference and weight-by-length percentiles for girls, age birth to 36 months. Developed by the National Center for Health Statistics in collaboration with the National Center for Chronic Disease Prevention and Health Promotion. (From Centers for Disease Control and Prevention, Atlanta, Ga, 2000. Available online at http://www.cdc.gov/growthcharts.)

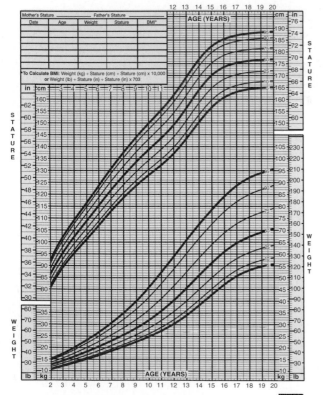

Figure 5–5

Stature-for-age and weight-for-age percentiles for boys, age 2 to 20 years. Developed by the National Center for Health Statistics in collaboration with the National Center for Chronic Disease Prevention and Health Promotion. (From Centers for Disease Control and Prevention, Atlanta, Ga, 2000. Available online at http://www.cdc.gov/growthcharts.)

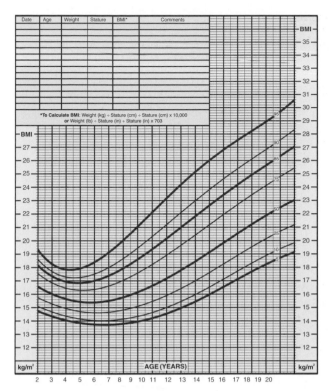

Figure 5–6

Body mass index–for-age percentiles for boys, age 2 to 20 years. Developed by the National Center for Chronic Disease Prevention and Health Promotion. (From Centers for Disease Control and Prevention, Atlanta, Ga, 2000. Available online at http://www.cdc.gov/growthcharts.)

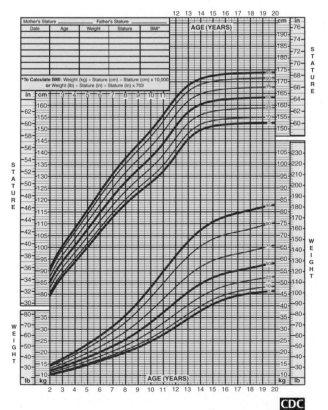

Figure 5–7

Stature-for-age and weight-for-age percentiles for girls, age 2 to 20 years. Developed by the National Center for Health Statistics in collaboration with the National Center for Chronic Disease Prevention and Health Promotion. (From Centers for Disease Control and Prevention, Atlanta, Ga, 2000. Available online at http://www.cdc.gov/growthcharts.)

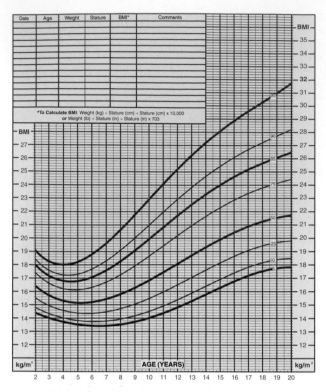

CDC

Figure 5–8

Body mass index–for-age percentiles for girls, age 2 to 20 years. Developed by the National Center for Health Statistics in collaboration with the National Center for Chronic Disease Prevention and Health Promotion. (From Centers for Disease Control and Prevention, Atlanta, Ga, 2000. Available online at http://www.cdc.gov/growthcharts.)

children shows, however, that normal growth patterns have spurts and plateaus, so some shifting on percentile graphs can be expected. Nonetheless, large shifts in percentiles warrant attention, as do large discrepancies among height, weight, and head circumference percentiles. Pediatricians follow longitudinal growth carefully by plotting measurements on standardized growth charts. When caloric intake is inadequate, the weight percentile falls first, then the height, and last the head circumference (Fig. 5-9). Caloric intake may be poor because the parents are not feeding the child enough or because the child is not receiving adequate attention and stimulation ("nonorganic" failure to thrive [see Chapter 21]).

Caloric intake also may be inadequate because of increased caloric needs. Children with chronic illness, such as congestive heart failure from a ventricular septal defect or cystic fibrosis (with malabsorption with or without repeated respiratory infections), may require a significantly higher caloric intake for growth. An increasing weight percentile in the face of a falling height percentile suggests hypothyroidism (Fig. 5-10). Head circumference may be disproportionately large when there is familial megalocephaly (knowing the size of the parents' heads is essential), hydrocephalus, or merely "catch-up" growth in a neurologically normal premature infant. A child is considered microcephalic if head circumference is at less than the 3rd percentile, even if length and weight measurements also are proportionately low. Serial measurements of head circumference are crucial during infancy, a period of rapid brain development, and should be plotted regularly until the child is 3 years old. Any suspicion of abnormal growth warrants at least close follow-up or further evaluation or both.

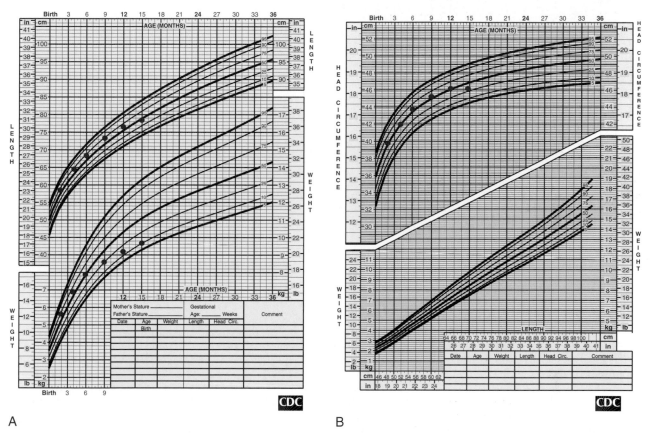

A

B

Figure 5-9

Failure to thrive due to insufficient caloric intake. A, Length-by-age and weight-by-age percentiles for boys, age birth to 36 months. **B,** Head circumference and weight-by-length percentiles for boys, age birth to 36 months. When caloric intake is inadequate, the weight percentile falls first, then the height, and finally the head circumference. Caloric intake may be poor because the child is not taking in enough (so-called nonorganic failure to thrive) or because of increased caloric needs, such as in children with congestive heart failure from a cardiac defect or cystic fibrosis (with malabsorption or tachypnea or both).

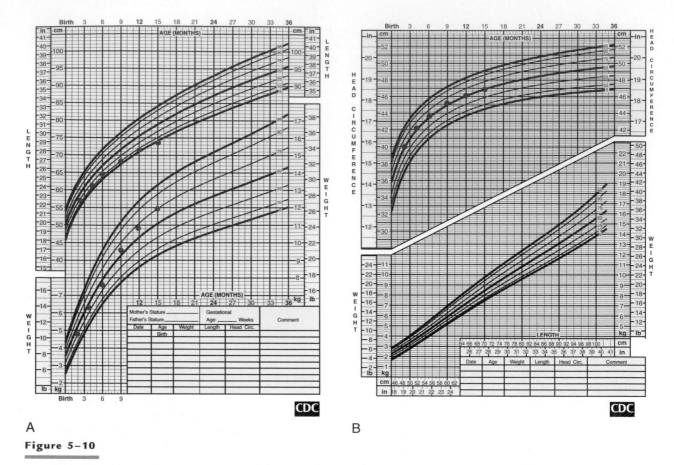

A

B

Figure 5–10

Growth pattern with hypothyroidism. A, Length-by-age and weight-by-age percentiles for boys, age birth to 36 months. **B,** Head circumference and weight-by-length percentiles for boys, age birth to 36 months. This different pattern (contrast with pattern in Figure 5–9) shows an increasing weight percentile in the face of a falling height percentile, which suggests hypothyroidism. There are other patterns that clinicians interpret to give diagnostic clues as to the etiology of the growth problem.

CHAPTER 6
Disorders of Growth

The most common reasons for deviant measurements are technical (i.e., faulty equipment and human errors in measurement or plotting, including errors related to trying to measure a squirming or screaming child). The first step in investigating a deviant measurement should be to repeat it. Separate growth charts are available for very low birth weight infants (weight <1500 g) and for children with Turner syndrome, Down syndrome, achondroplasia, and other dysmorphology syndromes.

Variability in body proportions also occurs from fetal to adult life. This variability is important for newborns because their heads are significantly larger in proportion to the rest of their body, and they can lose a significant amount of body heat through their heads. Wearing hats prevents heat loss. This head circumference difference gradually disappears as the child gets older. There also is considerable variation in body form among normal children, often following familial patterns. Children may still be normal, even if their weight is at the 50th percentile, length is at the 25th percentile (as long as the weight-for-length is in the normal range), and head circumference is at the 90th percentile. Differences in body proportions depend on variations in the growth rates of parts of the body or

TABLE 6–1. **Specific Growth Patterns Requiring Further Evaluation**		
Pattern	**Representative Diagnoses to Consider**	**Further Evaluation**
Weight, length, head circumference all <5th percentile	Familial short stature Constitutional short stature Intrauterine insult Genetic abnormality	Mid-parental heights Evaluation of pubertal development Examination of prenatal records Chromosome analysis
Discrepant percentiles (e.g., weight 5th, length 5th, head circumference 50th, or other discrepancies)	Normal variant (familial or constitutional) Endocrine growth failure Caloric insufficiency	Mid-parental heights Evaluation of pubertal development Thyroid hormone Growth factors, provocative GH testing
Declining percentiles	"Catch-down" growth	Complete history and physical examination Dietary and social history Failure to thrive evaluation

GH, growth hormone.

organ systems. Certain growth disturbances result in characteristic changes in the proportional sizes of the trunk, extremities, and head. Patterns requiring further assessment are summarized in Table 6–1.

Evaluating a child over time often elucidates the growth pattern as normal or abnormal much better than a single point. This evaluation of the growth pattern should be coupled with a careful history and physical examination. Parental heights are an important aspect of the history to evaluate growth problems because they may determine whether to observe rather than evaluate immediately other diagnostic possibilities and proceed with a further evaluation.

For a girl, mid-parental height is calculated as follows:

$$\frac{\left[\begin{array}{c}\text{Paternal height (inches)}\\ + \text{ maternal height (inches)} - 2.5\end{array}\right]}{2}$$

For a boy, mid-parental height is calculated as follows:

$$\frac{\left[\begin{array}{c}\text{Paternal height (inches)}\\ + \text{ maternal height (inches)} + 2.5\end{array}\right]}{2}$$

As in other "rules of thumb," mid-parental height should be considered only a gross approximation. Actual growth depends on too many variables to make an accurate prediction for every child. The growth pattern of a child with small weight, length, and head circumference (or with a larger head) is commonly associated with **familial short stature** (see Chapter 173). These children are genetically normal, but are smaller than most children. A child who is preadolescent or adolescent by age and starts puberty later than others may have the normal variant called **constitutional short stature** (see Chapter 173). These "late

bloomers" must be examined closely for abnormalities of pubertal development, although most are normal. Girls are considered normal if there is any development of secondary sexual characteristics (e.g., breast budding) on or before the 14th birthday and menarche by age 16. Girls who do not start menstruation until age 16 usually are smaller than their peers at ages 12 and 13. Similar patterns are observed in boys who start puberty later (see Chapter 174).

In many children, growth moves to lower percentiles during their first year of life. These children, whose mothers usually have had excellent prenatal care and provide appropriate nurturing, often start out in high growth percentiles. Between 6 and 18 months, they assume a lower percentile, until they match their genetic "programming," then begin to grow along new, lower percentiles. They usually do not decrease more than two major percentiles. They have normal developmental, behavioral, and physical examination. These children with "catch-down growth" should be followed closely, but no further evaluation is warranted.

Children recovering from neonatal illnesses often exhibit "catch-up growth." Infants who were born small for gestational age or premature ingest more breast milk or formula and, unless there are complications that require extra calories, usually catch up in the first half of the first year. It is important to counsel the family that the infant may require large amounts of milk until he or she catches up. Families should be taught to feed these infants on demand and as much as they want unless they are vomiting (not just spitting up [see the Chapter 128]). Some of these infants may benefit from a higher caloric content formula if they are formula-fed. Many of the risk factors that may have led to the infant being born small or early are the same psychosocial risks that may contribute to nonorganic failure to thrive (see Chapter 21).

The distinctive patterns of proportionate growth rates for several body systems correlate closely with function. Growth of the nervous system is most rapid in the first 2 years, correlating with increasing physical, emotional, behavioral, and cognitive development. Osseous maturation (bone age) is determined from radiographs on the basis of the number and size of calcified epiphyseal centers; the size, shape, density, and sharpness of outline of the ends of bones; and the distance separating the epiphyseal center from the zone of provisional calcification. Functional correlations also exist with changes in osseous maturation. Bone age corresponds more closely to sexual maturity, which depends on the maturation of the endocrine system, than to chronologic age. The heart, relatively large at birth, increases in size in parallel with the general growth spurt of puberty. Pulse rate, respiratory rate, and blood pressure vary with age and growth, as do many metabolic processes (with consequent nutritional requirements) (see Chapters 21, 27, and 28).

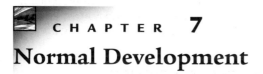

CHAPTER 7
Normal Development

PHYSICAL ASSESSMENT

Parallel to the changes in the developing brain and mind are changes in the physical development of the body. Various crucial bodily changes occur at different ages.

NEWBORN PERIOD

Primitive neonatal reflexes are unique in the newborn period, a consequence of the continued development of the CNS after birth. Any asymmetry, increase, or decrease in tone elicited by passive movement may indicate a significant CNS abnormality and requires further evaluation. Similarly a delay in the expected disappearance of the reflexes may warrant an evaluation of the CNS. The most important reflexes to assess during the newborn period are as follows:

The **Moro reflex** is elicited by allowing the infant's head gently to move back suddenly (from a few inches off the crib mattress). This results in abduction and upward movement of the arms followed by adduction and flexion. The Moro reflex disappears by 4 to 6 months.

The **rooting reflex** is elicited by touching the corner of the infant's mouth, resulting in the lowering of the lower lip on the same side with tongue movement toward the stimulus. The face may turn to the stimulus. The rooting reflex disappears at 4 to 6 months.

The **sucking reflex** occurs with almost any object placed in the newborn's mouth. The infant responds with vigorous sucking. The sucking reflex is replaced later by voluntary sucking only.

The **grasp reflex** occurs when placing an object, such as a finger, onto the infant's palm (palmar grasp) or sole (plantar grasp). The infant responds by flexing fingers or curling the toes. The palmar grasp usually disappears by 3 to 4 months and the plantar grasp by 6 to 8 months.

The **asymmetric tonic neck reflex** is elicited by placing the infant supine and turning the head to the side. This placement results in ipsilateral extension of the arm and the leg into a "fencing" position. The contralateral side flexes as well. This reflex disappears by 2 to 3 months of age.

See Sections XI, XIX, and XXVI for additional information on the newborn period.

LATER INFANCY

With the development of gross motor skills, the infant is first able to control his or her posture, then proximal musculature, and lastly distal musculature. As the infant progresses through these developmental stages, the parents may notice orthopedic deformities (see Chapters 200 and 201). In the newborn period, the infant also may have deformities that are related to intrauterine positioning. Physical examination should reveal whether the deformity is fixed or able to be moved passively into the proper position. When the infant positions a joint in an abnormal fashion, but the examiner is able to move the extremity passively into the proper position, this deformity has a high likelihood of resolving with the progression of gross motor development. Fixed deformities warrant immediate pediatric orthopedic consultation (see Section XXVI).

Continuous evaluation of vision and ocular movements also is important to prevent the serious outcome of strabismus. The cover test and light reflex should be examined at every health maintenance visit (see Chapter 179).

LATE SCHOOL-AGE/EARLY ADOLESCENT CHILD

Older school-age children, who begin to participate in competitive sports, should have a comprehensive sports physical examination, including an evaluation of the cardiovascular system. The AAP sports preparticipation form is excellent for documenting cardiovascular and other risks. Before the examination, the patient (and preferably the parent as well) should be interviewed to assess cardiovascular risk. Any history of heart disease or a murmur must be referred and evaluated by a pediatric cardiologist. Similarly a child with a history of dyspnea or chest pain on exertion, irregular heart rate (skipped beats, palpitations), syncope, or seizure should be referred to a pediatric cardiologist for further evaluation. A family history of a primary (immediate family) or secondary (immediate family's immediate family) atherosclerotic disease (myocardial infarction or cerebrovascular disease) before age 50 years or sudden unexplained death at any age also requires additional assessment.

Patients interested in contact sports should be assessed for special vulnerabilities. A history of renal disease, such as having a single kidney, is a contraindication for contact sports. Similarly, vision should be assessed as a crucial part of a comprehensive history and physical examination before participation in sports.

ADOLESCENT

Other than during the first year of life, there is no time of greater bodily change than during adolescence. Adolescents need a comprehensive health assessment to ensure that they progress through puberty without major problems (see Chapters 67 and 68). The provider who shows sensitivity to adolescent issues, including appearance, often has better communication with the adolescent and establishes a therapeutic alliance.

Other issues in physical development include scoliosis, obesity, and trauma (see Chapters 29 and 202). Most scoliosis is mild and requires only observation to see if it progresses. Obesity may first become manifest during adolescence and is an issue for many adolescents. Orthopedic problems may arise from trauma to developing joints and bones (see Chapter 197).

Sexual maturity is another important adolescent issue. All adolescents should be assessed to determine the sexual maturity rating (see Chapter 67). Monitoring the progression through sexual maturity rating stages provides an ongoing evaluation of puberty. It is approximately 2 years from the start of breast budding (beginning of puberty in girls) to menarche. Girls should be assessed as to their menstrual cycles, especially for dysmenorrhea or menometrorrhagia. Boys should be assessed for gynecomastia.

DEVELOPMENTAL MILESTONES

The use of developmental milestones to assess development focuses on discrete behaviors that the clinician can observe or accept as present by parental report. This approach is based on comparing the patient's behavior with that of many normal children whose behaviors evolve in a uniform sequence within specific age ranges (see Chapter 8). A behavior is the response of the neuromuscular system to a specific situation. The development of the neuromuscular system, similar to that of other organ systems, is determined first by genetic endowment and then molded by environmental influences.

Norms for discrete behaviors provide a convenient way to monitor development, but are an incomplete picture. Although a sequence of specific, easily measured behaviors can adequately represent some areas of development (**gross motor**, **fine motor**, and **language**), other areas, particularly social and emotional development, are not adequately assessed. Easily measured developmental milestones are well established only through age 6 years. Other types of assessment (intelligence tests, achievement tests, school performance, personality profiles, and neurodevelopmental assessments) that expand the developmental milestone approach beyond the age of 6 years are available for older children; these tests generally require time and expertise in administration and interpretation that are not available in the primary care setting. Pediatricians need to supplement their screening of developmental milestones with less precise but important surveillance of psychosocial issues that are pertinent at each age.

PSYCHOSOCIAL ASSESSMENT
Bonding and Attachment in Infancy

The terms bonding and attachment describe the affectional relationships between parents and infants. **Bonding** occurs shortly after birth and reflects the feelings of the parents toward the newborn (unidirectional); **attachment** involves reciprocal feelings between parent and infant and develops gradually over the first year. Effective bonding in the postpartum period may enhance the development of attachment. The importance of bonding has led to increased postpartum parent-infant contact, such as rooming in with the parents in the postpartum unit.

Attachment of infants outside of the newborn period is crucial for optimal development. Infants who received "extra" attention, such as parents responding immediately to any crying or fussiness, showed much less crying and fussiness at the end of the first year. **Stranger anxiety** develops between ages 9 and 18 months, when infants normally become insecure about separation from the primary caregiver. The infant is beginning to understand simple, immediate, cause-and-effect relationships and can anticipate separations (when the parents get a coat), but still has an inadequate appreciation of time and delayed gratification. The infant's new motor skills and attraction to novelty may lead to headlong plunges into new adventures that result in fright or pain followed by frantic efforts to find and cling to the primary caregiver. The result is dramatic swings from stubborn independence to clinging dependence that can be frustrating and confusing to parents. With a secure attachment, this period of ambivalence may be shorter and less tumultuous.

Developing Autonomy in Early Childhood

Toddlers build on attachment and begin developing autonomy that allows separation from parents. In times of stress, toddlers often cling to their parents, but in their usual activities they may be actively separated (frequently saying "No!" to their parents). Ages 2 to 3 years are a time of major accomplishments in fine motor skills, social skills, cognitive skills, and language skills. The dependency of infancy yields to developing independence, and the "I can do it myself" age. Limit setting is essential to balance the child's emerging independence.

School Readiness

When a toddler has achieved autonomy and independence, school readiness should be assessed. Awareness of available resources in the community aids with determination of school readiness and in the appropriate school fit. Readiness for preschool depends on the development of autonomy and the ability of the parent and the child to separate for hours at a time. Preschool experiences help 3- to 4-year-old children develop socialization skills; improve language; increase skill building in areas such as colors, numbers, and letters; and increase problem solving (puzzles).

Readiness for school (kindergarten) requires emotional maturity, peer group and individual social skills, cognitive abilities, and fine and gross motor skills (Table 7–1). Other issues include chronologic age and gender. Although not a perfect association, children do better in kindergarten if their fifth birthday is at least 4 to 6 months before the beginning of school. In addition, girls usually are ready earlier than boys. Knowledge of the prior developmental status also helps. If the child is in less than the average developmental range, he or she should not be forced into early school. Holding a child back for reasons of developmental delay, in the false hope that the child will catch up, also can lead to difficulties, however. The child should enroll on schedule, and educational planning should be initiated to address any deficiencies. Pushing a child into an environment for which he or she is not prepared can contribute to school refusal, poor school achievement, and behavioral problems.

Physicians should be able to identify children at risk for school difficulties, such as developmental delays or physical disabilities. These children may require specialized school services. Federal law mandates these

TABLE 7–1.   Evaluating School Readiness
Physician Observations (Behaviors Observed in the Office)

Ease of separation of the child from the parent
Speech development and articulation
Understanding of and ability to follow complex directions
Specific preacademic skills
    Knowledge of colors
    Counts to 10
    Knows age, first and last name, address, and phone number
    Ability to copy shapes
Motor skills
    Stand on one foot, skip, and catch a bounced ball
    Dress and undress without assistance

Parent Observations (Questions Answered by History)
Does the child play well with other children? Does the child separate well, such as a child playing in the backyard alone with occasional monitoring by the parent? Does the child show interest in books, letters, and numbers? Can the child sustain attention to quiet activities? How frequent are toilet-training "accidents" ?

services for children who qualify; services may include speech-language therapy, occupational therapy, or physical therapy (see Chapter 10).

Adolescence

Although the Society for Adolescent Medicine defines adolescence as ages 10 to 25 years, adolescence is characterized better by developmental stages (*early, middle,* and *late* adolescence) that all teens must negotiate to develop into healthy, functional adults. Different behavioral and developmental issues characterize each stage. The age at which each issue becomes manifest and the importance of these issues vary widely among individuals, as do the rates of cognitive, psychosexual, psychosocial, and physical development.

During **early adolescence**, attention is focused on the present and on the peer group. Concerns are primarily related to the body's physical changes and normality. Exploratory, undifferentiated sexual behavior resulting in physical contact with same-sex peers is normal during early adolescence, although heterosexual interests also can develop. Strivings for independence are ambivalent. These young adolescents are difficult to interview because they often respond with short, clipped conversation and may have little insight.

Middle adolescence can be a difficult time for adolescents and the adults who have contact with them. Cognitive processes are more sophisticated. Through abstract thinking, middle adolescents can experiment with ideas, consider things as they might be, develop insight, and reflect on their own feelings and the feelings of others. As they mature cognitively and psychosocially, these adolescents focus on issues of identity not limited solely to the physical aspects of their body. These teenagers explore their parents' and the culture's values, and they may do this by expressing the contrary side of the dominant value. Many middle adolescents explore these values only in their minds; others do so by challenging their parents' authority. Many engage in high-risk behaviors, including unprotected sexual intercourse, substance abuse, or dangerous driving. The strivings of middle adolescents for independence, testing of limits, and need for autonomy are often distressing to their families, teachers, or other authority figures. These adolescents are at higher risk for morbidity and mortality from accidents, homicide, or suicide.

Late adolescence usually is marked by formal operational thinking, including thoughts about the future (educationally, vocationally, and sexually). Late adolescents are usually more committed to their sexual partners than are middle adolescents. Unresolved separation anxiety from previous developmental stages may emerge at this time as the young person begins to move physically away from the family of origin to college or vocational school, a job, or military service.

MODIFYING PSYCHOSOCIAL BEHAVIORS

Child behavior is determined by heredity (genetics) and by the environment. Behavioral theory postulates that behavior is primarily a product of external environmental determinants and that manipulation of the environmental antecedents and consequences of behavior can be used to modify maladaptive behavior and to increase desirable behavior (operant conditioning). The four major methods of operant conditioning are positive reinforcement, negative reinforcement, extinction, and punishment. Many common behavioral problems of children can be ameliorated by these methods.

Positive reinforcement increases the frequency of a behavior by following the behavior with a favorable event. Praising a child for his or her excellent school performance and rewarding an adolescent with a later curfew hour are examples. **Negative reinforcement** increases the frequency of a behavior by following the behavior with the removal, cessation, or avoidance of an unpleasant event (a child avoids a remedial after-school study period by doing school work accurately and on time). Conversely, sometimes, this reinforcement may occur unintentionally, increasing the frequency of an undesirable behavior. A toddler may purposely try to stick a pencil in a light socket to obtain attention, be it positive or negative. **Extinction** occurs when there is a decrease in the frequency of a previously reinforced behavior because the reinforcement is withheld. Extinction is the principle behind the common advice to ignore such behavior as crying at bedtime or temper tantrums, which parents may unwittingly reinforce through attention and comforting. **Punishment** decreases the frequency of a behavior through unpleasant consequences. Many families overvalue punishment. Positive reinforcement has been proved to be more effective than punishment. Punishment is more effective when combined with positive reinforcement. A toddler who draws on the wall with a crayon may be punished, but he or she learns much quicker when positive reinforcement is given for proper use of the crayon, on paper, not the wall. Interrupting and modifying behaviors are discussed in detail in Section III.

TEMPERAMENT

Significant individual differences exist within the normal development of temperament (behavioral style). Temperament must be appreciated because if an expected pattern of behavior is too narrowly defined, normal behavior may be inappropriately labeled as abnormal or pathologic. There are three common constellations of temperamental characteristics:

1. The "**easy child**" (about 40% of children) is characterized by regularity of biologic functions (consistent, predictable times for eating, sleeping, and elimination), a positive approach to new stimuli, high adaptability to change, mild or moderate intensity in responses, and a positive mood.
2. The "**difficult child**" (about 10%) is characterized by irregularity of biologic functions, negative withdrawal from new stimuli, poor adaptability, intense responses, and a negative mood.
3. The "**slow to warm up child**" (about 15%) is characterized by a low activity level, withdrawal from new stimuli, slow adaptability, mild intensity in responses, and a somewhat negative mood.

The remaining children have more mixed temperaments. The individual temperament of a child has important implications for parenting and for the advice a pediatrician may give in anticipatory guidance or behavioral problem counseling.

Although temperament may be to some degree "hard wired" (nature) in each child, the environment (nurture) in which the child grows has a strong effect on the child's adjustment. Social and cultural factors can have marked effects on the child through differences in parenting style, educational approaches, and behavioral expectations.

CHAPTER 8

Disorders of Development

DEVELOPMENTAL SURVEILLANCE AND SCREENING

Developmental and behavioral problems are more common than any category of problems in pediatrics except acute infections and trauma. Approximately 15% to 18% of children in the U.S. have developmental or behavioral disabilities. As many as 25% of children have serious psychosocial problems. Parents often neglect to mention these problems because they think the physician is uninterested or cannot help. It is necessary to monitor development and screen for the presence of such problems at every health supervision visit, particularly in the preschool years, when the pediatrician may be the only professional to evaluate the child (Table 8–1).

After the child's sixth birthday and until adolescence, developmental surveillance is largely done by inquiring about school performance (academic achievement and behavior). Inquiring about concerns raised by teachers or other adults who care for the child (after-school program counselor, coach, religious leader) is prudent. Surveillance by milestones and history may seriously underestimate the number of children with developmental or behavioral problems. Although formal developmental testing of children is beyond the scope of the primary care pediatrician, the healthcare provider should be the coordinator of testing and evaluation done by other specialists (e.g., psychology, education).

Although developmental surveillance based on milestones is an informal, continuous process that may or may not involve the use of formal measures, **developmental screening** involves the use of standardized screening tests. Developmental screening is a brief evaluation comparing the developmental skills of a particular child with skills of a population of children to identify children with suspected delays who require further diagnostic assessment. Although screening tests are often used after a clinician notices a developmental problem on surveillance, the AAP recommends the use of standardized screening tools at each health maintenance visit. A failed developmental screening test indicates the need for further evaluation. Developmental evaluations for children with suspected developmental delays and intervention services for children with diagnosed disabilities are available in the U.S. free to families through a combination of state and federal funds.

Screening tests can be categorized as general screening tests that cover all behavioral domains or as targeted screens that focus on one area of development. Some may be administered in the office by professionals, and others may be completed at home (or in a waiting room) by parents. Because of the variability of child development, standards for abnormality in developmental/behavioral screening tests are set lower than what is usually accepted for other types of medical screening. Even with this limitation, good developmental/behavioral screening instruments have sensitivity of 70% to 80% to detect suspected problems and specificity of 70% to 80% to detect normal development. Although 30% of children screened may be "over-referred," this group also includes children whose skills are below average and who may benefit from definitive testing that may help address relative developmental deficits. The 20% to 30% of children who have disabilities that are not detected by the single administration of a screening instrument are likely to be identified on repeat screening at subsequent health maintenance visits.

The **Denver Developmental Screening Test II** is commonly used by general pediatricians (Figs. 8–1 and 8–2). The Denver II assesses the development of children from birth to 6 years in four domains: (1) **personal-social**, (2) **fine motor–adaptive**, (3) **language**, and (4) **gross motor**. Items on the Denver II are carefully selected for their reliability and consistency of norms across subgroups and cultures. The Denver II is a useful screening instrument, but it cannot assess adequately the complexities of socioemotional development. Children with "suspect" or "untestable" scores must be followed carefully.

The pediatrician asks questions (items labeled with an "R" may be asked of parents to document the task "by report") or directly observes behaviors. On the scoring sheet, a line is drawn at the child's chronologic age. All tasks that are entirely to the left of the line that the child has not accomplished are considered delayed (at least 90% of the population accomplished the task). If the test instructions are not followed accurately or if items are omitted, the validity of the test becomes much poorer. To assist physicians in using the Denver II, the scoring sheet also features a table to document confounding behaviors, such as interest, fearfulness, or apparent short attention span. Repeat screening at subsequent health maintenance visits often detects abnormalities that a single screen was unable to detect.

Other developmental screening tools include parent-completed Ages and Stages Questionnaires, Child Development Inventories, and Parents' Evaluations of Developmental Status. Parent-reported screens have good validity compared with office-based screening measures. They may have the added benefit of promoting parental involvement with the child's development. These measures have validity that simple developmental surveillance does not because these

TABLE 8–1. Developmental Milestones

Age	Gross Motor	Fine Motor–Adaptive	Personal-Social	Language	Other Cognitive
2 wk	Moves head side to side		Regards face	Alerts to bell	
2 mo	Lifts shoulder while prone	Tracks past midline	Smiles responsively	Cooing	
				Searches for sound with eyes	
4 mo	Lifts up on hands	Reaches for object	Looks at hand	Laughs and squeals	
	Rolls front to back	Raking grasp	Begins to work toward toy		
	If pulled to sit from supine, no head lag				
6 mo	Sits alone	Transfers object hand to hand	Feeds self	Babbles	
			Holds bottle		
9 mo	Pulls to stand	Starting to pincer grasp	Waves bye-bye	Says Dada and Mama, but nonspecific	
	Gets into sitting position	Bangs 2 blocks together	Plays pat-a-cake	2-syllable sounds	
12 mo	Walks	Puts block in cup	Drinks from a cup	Says Mama and Dada, specific	
	Stoops and stands		Imitates others	Says 1-2 other words	
15 mo	Walks backward	Scribbles	Uses spoon and fork	Says 3-6 words	
		Stacks 2 blocks	Helps in housework	Follows commands	
18 mo	Runs	Stacks four blocks	Removes garment	Says at least 6 words	
	Kicks a ball		"Feeds" doll		
2 yr	Walks up and down stairs	Stacks 6 blocks	Washes and dries hands	Puts 2 words together	Understands concept of "today"
	Throws overhand	Copies line	Brushes teeth	Points to pictures	
			Puts on clothes	Knows body parts	
3 yr	Walks steps alternating feet	Stacks 8 blocks	Uses spoon well, spilling little	Names pictures	Understands concepts of "tomorrow" and "yesterday"
	Broad jump	Wiggles thumb	Puts on t-shirt	Speech understandable to stranger 75%	
				Says 3-word sentences	
4 yr	Balances well on each foot	Copies O, maybe +	Brushes teeth without help	Names colors	
	Hops on one foot	Draws person with 3 parts	Dresses without help	Understands adjectives	
5 yr	Skips	Copies □		Counts	
	Heal-to-toe walks			Understands opposites	
6 yr	Balances on each foot 6 sec	Copies △		Defines words	Begins to understand "right" and "left"
		Draws person with 6 parts			

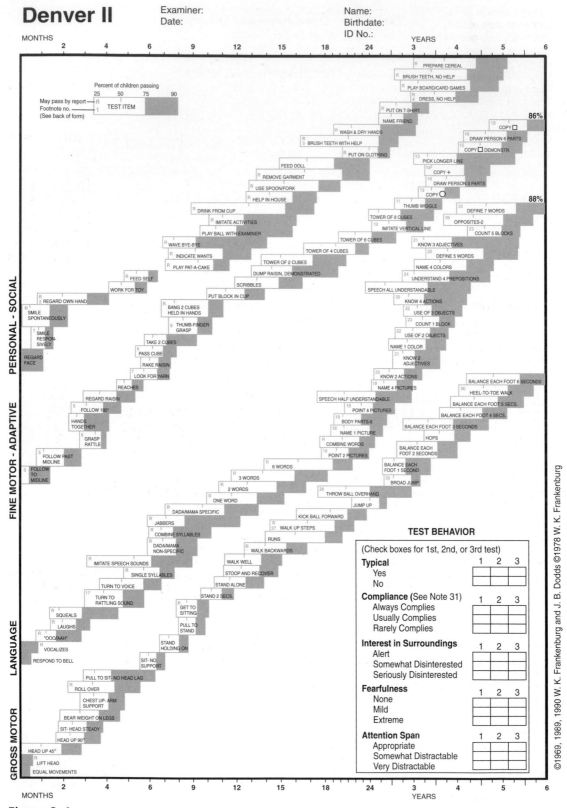

Figure 8–1

Scoring form for Denver II. (From Frankenburg WK: Denver II Developmental Screening Test, 2nd ed. Denver, Denver Developmental Materials, 1990.)

1. Try to get child to smile by smiling, talking or waving. Do not touch him/her.
2. Child must stare at hand several seconds.
3. Parent may help guide toothbrush and put toothpaste on brush.
4. Child does not have to be able to tie shoes or button/zip in the back.
5. Move yarn slowly in an arc from one side to the other, about 8" above child's face.
6. Pass if child grasps rattle when it is touched to the backs or tips of fingers.
7. Pass if child tries to see where yarn went. Yarn should be dropped quickly from sight from tester's hand without arm movement.
8. Child must transfer cube from hand to hand without help of body, mouth, or table.
9. Pass if child picks up raisin with any part of thumb and finger.
10. Line can vary only 30 degrees or less from tester's line. ✓
11. Make a fist with thumb pointing upward and wiggle only the thumb. Pass if child imitates and does not move any fingers other than the thumb.

               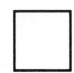

12. Pass any enclosed form. Fail continuous round motions.
13. Which line is longer? (Not bigger.) Turn paper upside down and repeat. (pass 3 of 3 or 5 of 6)
14. Pass any lines crossing near midpoint.
15. Have child copy first. If failed, demonstrate.

When giving items 12, 14, and 15, do not name the forms. Do not demonstrate 12 and 14.

16. When scoring, each pair (2 arms, 2 legs, etc.) counts as one part.
17. Place one cube in cup and shake gently near child's ear, but out of sight. Repeat for other ear.
18. Point to picture and have child name it. (No credit is given for sounds only.)
    If less than 4 pictures are named correctly, have child point to picture as each is named by tester.

     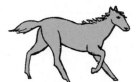   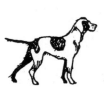   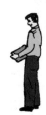

19. Using doll, tell child: Show me the nose, eyes, ears, mouth, hands, feet, tummy, hair. Pass 6 of 8.
20. Using pictures, ask child: Which one flies?... says meow?... talks?... barks?... gallops? Pass 2 of 5, 4 of 5.
21. Ask child: What do you do when you are cold?... tired?... hungry? Pass 2 of 3, 3 of 3.
22. Ask child: What do you do with a cup? What is a chair used for? What is a pencil used for?
    Action words must be included in answers.
23. Pass if child correctly places <u>and</u> says how many blocks are on paper. (1, 5).
24. Tell child: Put block **on** table; **under** table; **in front of** me, **behind** me. Pass 4 of 4.
    (Do not help child by pointing, moving head or eyes.)
25. Ask child: What is a ball?... lake?... desk?... house?... banana?... curtain?... fence?... ceiling? Pass if defined in terms of use, shape, what it is made of, or general category (such as banana is fruit, not just yellow). Pass 5 of 8, 7 of 8.
26. Ask child: If a horse is big, a mouse is __? If fire is hot, ice is __? If the sun shines during the day, the moon shines during the __? Pass 2 of 3.
27. Child may use wall or rail only, not person. May not crawl.
28. Child must throw ball overhand 3 feet to within arm's reach of tester.
29. Child must perform standing broad jump over width of test sheet (8 1/2 inches).
30. Tell child to walk forward, ⚬⚬⚬➝ heel within 1 inch of toe. Tester may demonstrate.
    Child must walk 4 consecutive steps.
31. In the second year, half of normal children are non-compliant.

OBSERVATIONS:

Figure 8–2

Instructions for the Denver II. Numbers are coded to scoring form (see Fig. 8–1). "Abnormal" is defined as two or more delays (failure of an item passed by 90% at that age) in two or more categories or two or more delays in one category with one other category having one delay and an age line that does not intersect one item that is passed. (From Frankenburg WK: Denver II Developmental Screening Test, 2nd ed. Denver, Denver Developmental Materials, 1990.)

TABLE 8–2.　Rules of Thumb for Speech Screening

Age (yr)	Speech Production	Articulation (Amount of Speech Understood by a Stranger)	Following Commands
1	1-3 words		One-step commands
2	2- to 3-word phrases	$1/2$	Two-step commands
3	Routine use of sentences	$3/4$	
4	Routine use of sentence sequences; conversational give-and-take	Almost all	
5	Complex sentences; extensive use of modifiers, pronouns, and prepositions	Almost all	

questions are standardized. In addition to these full screens, there may be a concern about only one area of development. This area may be identified by parents or an abnormal screen on the Denver II or other standardized screening tool.

Language screening is important because it correlates best with cognitive development in the early years. Table 8–2 provides some rules of thumb for language development that focus on speech production (expressive language). Although expressive language (speech) is the most obvious language element, the most dramatic changes in language development in the first years involve recognition and understanding (receptive language). Also, much language up to age 2 years is visually mediated (pointing). One useful tool is the Early Language Milestone Scale, which screens visual and auditory receptive and expressive skills.

Whenever there is a language delay, a **hearing deficit** must be considered. The implementation of universal newborn hearing screening detects many, if not most, of these children in the newborn period, and appropriate early intervention services may be provided. Conditions that present a high risk for an associated hearing deficit are listed in Table 8–3. Dysfluency ("stuttering") is common in 3- and 4-year-olds. Unless the dysfluency is severe, is accompanied by tics or unusual posturing, or occurs after the age of 4, parents should be counseled that it is normal and transient and to accept it calmly and patiently. Comments such as "relax," "slow down," or "think before you speak" may be counterproductive for a child who already may be too anxious about a behavior over which he or she has little control.

OTHER ISSUES IN ASSESSING DEVELOPMENT AND BEHAVIOR

The environment in which the child grows and develops is a crucial component of the causes, manifestations, and management of developmental and behavioral problems. Ignorance of the context may result in ineffective or inappropriate management (or both). Table 8–4 lists some contextual factors that should be considered in the etiology of a child's behavioral or developmental problem.

Building rapport with the parents and the child is a prerequisite for obtaining the often-sensitive information that is essential for understanding a behavioral or developmental issue. Rapport usually can be established quickly if the parents sense that the clinician respects them and is genuinely interested in listening to their concerns. The clinician develops rapport with the child by engaging the child in developmentally appropriate conversation or play, providing toys while interviewing the parents, and being sensitive to the fears the child may have. Too often the child is ignored until it is time for the physical examination. Similar to their parents, children feel more comfortable if they are greeted by name and involved in pleasant interactions before they are asked sensitive questions or threatened with examinations. Young children can be engaged in conversation on the parent's lap, which provides

TABLE 8–3.　Conditions Considered High Risk for Associated Hearing Deficit

Congenital hearing loss in first cousin or closer relative
Bilirubin level of ≥20 mg/dL
Congenital rubella or other nonbacterial intrauterine infection
Defects in the ear, nose, or throat
Birth weight of ≤1500 g
Multiple apneic episodes
Exchange transfusion
Meningitis
5-min Apgar score of ≤5
Persistent fetal circulation (primary pulmonary hypertension)
Treatment with ototoxic drugs (e.g., aminoglycosides and loop diuretics)

TABLE 8–4. Context of Behavioral Problems

Child Factors

Health (past and current)
Developmental status
Temperament (e.g., difficult, slow to warm up)
Coping mechanisms

Parental Factors

Misinterpretations of stage-related behaviors
Mismatch of parental expectations and characteristics of
   child
Parental characteristics (e.g., depression, lack of interest,
   rejection, overprotectiveness)
Coping mechanisms

Environmental Factors

Stress (e.g., marital discord, unemployment, personal loss)
Support (e.g., emotional, material, informational, child
   care)

Parent-Child Interactions

The common pathway through which the listed factors
   interact to influence the development of a behavior
   problem
The key to resolving the behavior problem

security and places the child at the eye level of the examiner.

With adolescents, emphasis should be placed on building a physician-patient relationship that is distinct from the relationship with the parents. The parents should not be excluded; however, the adolescent should have the opportunity to express concerns to and ask questions of the physician in confidence. Two intertwined issues must be taken into consideration—consent and confidentiality. Although laws vary from state to state, in general, adolescents who are able to give informed consent (mature minors) may consent to visits and care related to high-risk behaviors (i.e., substance abuse; sexual health, including prevention, detection, and treatment of sexually transmitted infections; and pregnancy). Pediatricians should become familiar with the governing law in the state where they practice (see http://www.guttmacher.com/statecenter/index.html.) Most physicians who regularly work with adolescents believe that confidentiality is crucial to providing adolescents with optimal care (especially for obtaining a history of risk behaviors). States vary in the law governing confidentiality rights for adolescents, although most states support the physician who wishes the visit to be confidential. When assessing development and behavior, confidentiality can be achieved by meeting with the adolescent alone for at least part of each visit. Parents must be informed, however, when the clinician has significant concerns about the health and safety of the child. Often the clinician can convince the adolescent to inform the parents directly about a problem or can reach an agreement with the adolescent about how the parents will be informed by the physician.

SERIAL VISITS AND INTERVIEWING

Because the time to assess development in an initial health supervision visit is often short and the assessment usually is only part of what needs to be accomplished during an office visit, it may be best to explore developmental and behavioral problems during subsequent visits when more comprehensive information and observations can be obtained. Specific interviewing practices enhance the collection of behavioral information. Responses to open-ended questions often provide clues to underlying, unstated problems and identify the appropriate direction for further, more directed questions. The interviewer may restrict the scope of the discussion unintentionally by prematurely using directed questions. Histories about developmental and behavioral problems are often vague and confusing; to reconcile apparent contradictions, the interviewer frequently must request clarification (to ascertain the meaning of a word to the patient), more detail, or mere repetition. By summarizing an understanding of the information at frequent intervals and by recapitulating at the close of the visit, the interviewer and patient and family can ensure that they understand each other.

To build trust and to encourage family members to talk about difficult issues, the physician should communicate respect and empathy for the patient. Empathy is apparent when the physician recognizes the emotions that underlie the patient's responses and communicates this understanding verbally and nonverbally.

If the clinician's impression of the child differs markedly from the parent's description, there may be a crucial parental concern or issue that has not yet been expressed. The parent may fail to express a concern for several reasons: because it may be difficult to talk about (e.g., marital problems), because it is unconscious, or because the parent overlooks its relevance to the child's behavior. Alternatively the physician's observations may be atypical, even with multiple visits. The observations of teachers, relatives, and other regular caregivers may be crucial in sorting out this possibility. The parent also may have a distorted image of the child, rooted in parental psychopathology. A sensitive, supportive, and noncritical approach to the parent is crucial to appropriate intervention.

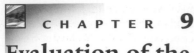

CHAPTER 9
Evaluation of the Well Child

Health maintenance or supervision visits should consist of a comprehensive assessment of the child's health and of the parent's/guardian's role in providing an environment for optimal growth, development, and health. Elements of the visit include evaluation and management of parental concerns, growth, development, and nutrition; anticipatory guidance (including safety information and counseling); physical examination; screening tests; and immunizations (Table 9–1). Figure 9–1 indicates the ages that specific prevention measures should be undertaken (by testing, such as vision and hearing; by physician history and physical examination; or by laboratory screening, such as the neonatal metabolic screening test or lead screening).

TABLE 9–1.　Topics for Health Supervision Visits

Focus on the Child

Concerns (parent's or child's)
Past problem follow-up
Immunization and screening test update
Routine care (e.g., eating, sleeping, elimination, and health habits)
Developmental progress
Behavioral style and problems

Focus on the Child's Environment

Family
Caregiving schedule for caregiver who lives at home
Parent-child and sibling-child interactions
Extended family role
Family stresses (e.g., work, move, finances, illness, death, marital and other interpersonal relationships)
Family supports (relatives, friends, groups)

Community
Caregivers outside the family
Peer interaction
School and work
Recreational activities

Physical Environment
Appropriate stimulation
Safety

SCREENING TESTS

Children usually are quite healthy, especially after 1 year of age, and only the following screening tests are recommended: newborn metabolic screening with hemoglobin electrophoresis, hearing and vision evaluation, anemia and lead screening, urinalysis, and tuberculosis testing. Children born to families with dyslipidemias or early heart disease also may be screened for lipid disorders. Sexually experienced adolescents should be screened for sexually transmissible infections. When an infant or child begins care after the newborn period, the pediatric provider should perform any missing screening tests and immunizations.

Newborn Screening

Metabolic Screening

Every state in the U.S. mandates newborn metabolic screening. Phenylketonuria (PKU) is the prototypic illness to be screened for and prevented. PKU is an unusual metabolic illness with a low prevalence. If PKU is detected early, however, a modified diet (a highly specialized phenylalanine-free formula) can be provided, and the disease-related developmental and growth problems can be prevented. Each state determines its own priorities and procedures, but the following diseases are usually included in metabolic screening: PKU, galactosemia, congenital hypothyroidism, and maple sugar urine disease (see Section X).

Hemoglobin Electrophoresis

Children with hemoglobinopathies are at higher risk of infection and complications from anemia. Early detection may prevent or ameliorate these complications. Children with sickle cell disease are begun on oral penicillin prophylaxis to prevent sepsis, the major cause of mortality in these children (see Chapter 150).

Hearing Evaluation

Hearing disorders are poorly detected by a physician's developmental surveillance. Because speech and language are central to a child's cognitive development, screening is done before discharge from the newborn nursery. Children who have an abnormal test should be referred for definitive testing before the consequences of abnormal hearing become apparent. An infant's hearing is tested by placing headphones over the infant's ears and electrodes on the head. Standard sounds are played, and the transmission of the impulse to the brain is documented. If this screening test is abnormal, a further evaluation is indicated using evoked response technology of sound transmission, similar to an EEG.

Hearing and Vision Screening of Older Children

Infants and Toddlers

Inferences about hearing are drawn from asking parents about responses to sound and speech and by examining speech and language development closely. Inferences about vision may be made by examining gross motor milestones (children with vision problems may have a delay) and by physical examination of the eye. Parents should be queried as to any concerns about vision until the child is 3 years old and about hearing until the child is 4 years old. If there are concerns, definitive testing should be arranged. Hearing can be screened by audio evoked responses as mentioned for infants. For toddlers and older children who cannot cooperate with formal audiologic testing with headphones, behavioral audiology may be used. Sounds of a specific frequency or intensity are provided in a standard environment within a soundproof room, and responses are assessed by a trained audiologist. Vision may be assessed by referral to a pediatric ophthalmologist and by visual evoked responses (VER).

Children 3 Years Old and Older

At various ages, hearing and vision should be screened objectively using standard techniques. In Figure 9-1, any age marked O requires objective screening; S denotes that a subjective assessment is adequate at that age. Asking the family and child about any concerns or consequences of poor hearing or vision accomplishes this subjective evaluation. At age 3 years, children are screened for vision for the first time if they are developmentally able to be tested. Many children at this age do not have the language or interpersonal skills to perform a vision screen; these children should be re-examined at a 3- to 6-month interval to ensure that vision is normal. Because most of these children do not identify letters yet, using a Snellen Eye Chart with standard shapes is recommended. When a child is able to identify letters, the more accurate letter-based chart should be used. Audiologic testing of sounds with headphones and children identifying sounds heard should be begun on the fourth birthday (although Head Start requires that pediatricians attempt hearing screening at age 3 years). Any suspected audiologic problem should be evaluated by a careful history and physical examination, and the children should be referred for comprehensive testing. Children who have a documented vision problem, failed screening, or parental concern should be referred to a pediatric ophthalmologist.

Anemia Screening

After the newborn period, when hemoglobin electrophoresis is used to detect inherited abnormalities, children are screened for anemia at ages when there is a higher incidence of iron deficiency anemia. Anemic infants do not perform as well on standard developmental testing. Infants are screened at birth if there is a documented risk, such as low birth weight or prematurity. Healthy term infants usually are screened at 9 months old because this is when a high incidence of iron deficiency is noted. Children are assessed at other visits for risks or concerns related to anemia (denoted by an asterisk in Fig. 9-1). Routine testing resumes during adolescence, once for boys and yearly for menstruating girls. Any abnormalities detected should be evaluated for etiology. When iron deficiency is strongly suspected, a therapeutic trial of iron may be used (see Chapter 150).

Urinalysis

It is uncommon to detect significant problems by urinalysis. Dipstick or biochemical screening is recommended, with microscopy if hemoglobin (RBCs) or leukocyte esterase (WBCs) is positive (see Chapter 161).

Lead Screening

Lead intoxication may cause developmental and behavioral abnormalities that are not reversible even if the hematologic and other metabolic complications are treated. Although the CDC recommends environmental investigation at blood lead levels of 10 mg/dL, levels of 5 to 10 mg/dL may cause learning problems. Areas of high risk for lead intoxication include older residences with cracked or peeling lead-based paint, industrial exposures, use of foreign remedies (diarrhea remedies in Mexico), or use of pottery with lead paint glaze. Each state usually mandates screening by measuring the blood lead level at 9 to 12 months or 2 years or both. Because of the significant association of lead intoxication with poverty and the numerous children living in poverty, the CDC recommends blood lead screening at both ages. In addition, all children should be screened for risk of lead intoxication between 6 months and 6 years by asking standardized screening questions (Table 9-2). Any positive or suspect response is an indication for obtaining a blood lead level. Because capillary blood sampling produces false-positive results, a venous blood sample should be obtained. County health departments and private companies provide lead inspection and detection services to determine the source of the lead. Standard decontamination techniques should be used to remove the lead, while avoiding aerosolizing the toxic metal that a child might breathe or creating dust that a child might ingest. (Also see Chapters 149 and 150.)

Recommendations for Preventive Pediatric Health Care
Committee on Practice and Ambulatory Medicine

Each child and family is unique; therefore, these **Recommendations for Preventive Pediatric Health Care** are designed for the care of children who are receiving competent parenting, have no manifestations of any important health problems, and are growing and developing in satisfactory fashion. **Additional visits may become necessary if** circumstances suggest variations from normal.

These guidelines represent a consensus by the Committee on Practice and Ambulatory Medicine in consultation with national committees and sections of the American Academy of Pediatrics. The Committee emphasizes the great importance of **continuity of care** on comprehensive health supervision and the need to avoid **fragmentation of care.**

Continued

INFANCY / EARLY CHILDHOOD

AGE[5]	PRENATAL[1]	NEWBORN[2]	2-4d[3]	By 1mo	2mo	4mo	6mo	9mo	12mo	15mo	18mo	24mo	3y	4y
HISTORY Initial/Interval	•	•	•	•	•	•	•	•	•	•	•	•	•	•
MEASUREMENTS Height and Weight		•	•	•	•	•	•	•	•	•	•	•	•	•
Head Circumference		•	•	•	•	•	•	•	•	•	•	•	•	
Blood Pressure													•	•
SENSORY SCREENING Vision		S	S	S	S	S	S	S	S	S	S	S	O[8]	O
Hearing		O[7]	S	S	S	S	S	S	S	S	S	S	S	O
DEVELOPMENTAL/ BEHAVIORAL ASSESSMENT[8]		•	•	•	•	•	•	•	•	•	•	•	•	•
PHYSICAL EXAMINATION[9]		•	•	•	•	•	•	•	•	•	•	•	•	•
PROCEDURES-GENERAL[10] Hereditary/Metabolic Screening[11]		←→	←→	←→										
Immunization[12]		•	•	•	•	•	•	• ↑	↑	•	•	•	•	•
Hematocrit or Hemoglobin[13]						•		• ★	↑ ★	★	★	★ ★	★ ★	★ ★
Urinalysis														
PROCEDURES-PATIENTS AT RISK Lead Screening[16]						•	•	•	•			★	★	★
Tuberculin Test[17]														
Cholesterol Screening[18]														
STD Screening[19]														
Pelvic Exam[20]														
ANTICIPATORY GUIDANCE[21] Injury Prevention[22]		•	•	•	•	•	•	•	•	•	•	•	•	•
Violence Prevention[23]		•	•		•	•	•	•	•	•	•	•	•	•
Sleep Positioning Counseling[24]		•	•											
Nutrition Counseling[25]		•	•											
DENTAL REFERRAL[26]									↓				•	

MIDDLE CHILDHOOD / ADOLESCENCE

AGE[5]	5y	6y	8y	10y	11y	12y	13y	14y	15y	16y	17y	18y	19y	20y	21y
HISTORY Initial/Interval	•	•	•	•	•	•	•	•	•	•	•	•	•	•	•
MEASUREMENTS Height and Weight	•	•	•	•	•	•	•	•	•	•	•	•	•	•	•
Head Circumference															
Blood Pressure	•	•	•	•	•	•	•	•	•	•	•	•	•	•	•
SENSORY SCREENING Vision	O	O	O	O	S	O	S	S	O	S	S	O	S	S	S
Hearing	O	O	O	O	S	O	S	S	O	S	S	O	S	S	S
DEVELOPMENTAL/ BEHAVIORAL ASSESSMENT[8]	•	•	•	•	•	•	•	•	•	•	•	•	•	•	•
PHYSICAL EXAMINATION[9]	•	•	•	•	•	•	•	•	•	•	•	•	•	•	•
PROCEDURES-GENERAL[10] Hereditary/Metabolic Screening[11]	• ★	•	•	•	•	•	• [14]	•	•	•	•	•	•	•	• ↑
Immunization[12]															↑
Hematocrit or Hemoglobin[13]						• [15]									
Urinalysis															

Figure 9-1

For legend see following page

PROCEDURES—PATIENT AT RISK

Lead Screening[16]			★	★	★	★	★	★	★	★	★	★	★
Tuberculin Test[17]			★	★	★	★	★	★	★	★	★	★	★
Cholesterol Screening[18]										★	★	★	★
STD Screening[19]										★	★	★	★
Pelvic Exam[20]										← →			

ANTICIPATORY GUIDANCE[21]

Injury Prevention[22]	•	•	•	•	•	•	•	•	•	•	•	•	•
Violence Prevention[23]	•	•	•	•	•	•	•	•	•	•	•	•	•
Sleep Positioning Counseling[24]	•	•	•	•									
Nutrition Counseling[25]	•	•	•	•	•	•	•	•	•	•	•	•	•
DENTAL REFERRAL[26]													

1. A prenatal visit is recommended for parents who are at high risk, for first-time parents, and for those who request a conference. The prenatal visit should include anticipatory guidance, pertinent medical history, and a discussion of benefits of breastfeeding and planned method of feeding per AAP statement "The Prenatal Visit" (1996).
2. Every infant should have a newborn evaluation after birth. Breastfeeding should be encouraged and instruction and support offered. Every breastfeeding infant should have an evaluation 48-72 hours after discharge from the hospital to include weight, formal breastfeeding evaluation, encouragement, and instruction as recommended in the AAP statement "Breastfeeding and the Use of Human Milk" (1997).
3. For newborns discharged in less than 48 hours after delivery per AAP statement "Hospital Stay for Healthy Newborns" (1995).
4. Developmental, psychosocial, and chronic disease issues for children and adolescents may require frequent counseling and treatment visits separate from preventive care visits.
5. If a child comes under care for the first time at any point on the schedule, or if any items are not accomplished at the suggested age, the schedule should be brought up to date at the earliest possible time.
6. If the patient is uncooperative, rescreen within 6 months.
7. All newborns should be screened per the AAP Task Force on Newborn and Infant Hearing Loss: Detection and Intervention" (1999).
8. By history and appropriate physical examination; if suspicious, by specific objective developmental testing. Parenting skills should be fostered at every visit.
9. At each visit, a complete physical examination is essential, with infant totally unclothed, older child undressed and suitably draped.
10. These may be modified, depending upon entry point into schedule and individual need.
11. Metabolic screening (e.g., thyroid, hemoglobinopathies, PKU, galactosemia) should be done according to state law.
12. Schedule(s) per the Committee on Infectious Diseases, published annually in the January edition of Pediatrics. Every visit should be an opportunity to update and complete a child's immunizations.
13. See AAP Pediatric Nutrition Handbook (1998) for a discussion of universal and selective screening options. Consider earlier screening for high-risk infants (e.g., premature infants and low birth weight infants). See also "Recommendations to Prevent and Control Iron Deficiency in the United States". MMWR. 1998;47 (RR-3):1-29.
14. All menstruating adolescents should be screened annually.
15. Conduct dipstick urinalysis for leukocytes annually for sexually active male and female adolescents.
16. For children at risk for lead exposure consult the AAP statement "Screening for Elevated Blood Levels" (1998). Additionally, screening should be done in accordance with state law where applicable.
17. TB testing per recommendations of the Committee on Infectious Diseases, published in the current edition of Red Book: Report of the Committee on Infectious Diseases. Testing should be done upon recognition of high-risk factors.
18. Cholesterol screening for high-risk patients per AAP statement "Cholesterol in Childhood" (1998). If family history cannot be ascertained and other risk factors are present, screening should be at the discretion of the physician.
19. All sexually active patients should be screened for sexually transmitted diseases (STDs).
20. All sexually active females should have a pelvic examination. A pelvic examination and routine pap smear should be offered as part of preventive health maintenance between the ages of 18 and 21 years.
21. Age-appropriate discussion and counseling should be an integral part of each visit for care per the AAP Guidelines for Health Supervision III (1998).
22. From birth to age 12, refer to the AAP injury prevention program (TIPP) as described in A Guide to Safety Counseling in Office Practice (1994).
23. Violence prevention and management for all patients per AAP statement "The Role of the Pediatrician in Youth Violence Prevention in Clinical Practice and at the Community Level" (1999).
24. Parents and caregivers should be advised to place healthy infants on their backs when putting them to sleep. Side positioning is a reasonable alternative but carries a slightly higher risk of SIDS. Consult the AAP statement "Changing Concepts of Sudden Infant Death Syndrome: Implications for Infant Sleeping Environment and Sleep Position" (2000).
25. Age-appropriate nutrition counseling should be an integral part of each visit per the AAP Handbook of Nutrition (1998).
26. Earlier initial dental examinations may be appropriate for some children. Subsequent examinations as prescribed by dentist.

Key: • = to be performed ★ = to be performed for patients at risk
S = subjective, by history O = objective, by a standard testing method
←——→ = the range during which a service may be provided, with the dot indicating the preferred age.

NB: Special chemical, immunologic, and endocrine testing is usually carried out upon specific indications. Testing other than newborn (e.g., inborn errors of metabolism, sickle disease, etc) is discretionary with the physician.

The recommendations in this statement do not indicate an exclusive course of treatment or standard of medical care. Variations, taking into account individual circumstances, may be appropriate. Copyright© 2000 by the American Academy of Pediatrics. No part of this statement may be reproduced in any form or by any means without prior written permission from the American Academy of Pediatrics except for one copy for personal use.

Figure 9-1

Recommendations for preventive pediatric health care. (From the Committee on Practice and Ambulatory Medicine, American Academy of Pediatrics. Pediatrics 105:645, 2000.)

TABLE 9–2. Lead Poisoning Risk Assessment Questions to Be Asked Between 6 Months and 6 Years

Does the child spend any time in a building built before 1960 that has cracked or peeling paint (e.g., home, school, barn)?

Is there a brother, sister, housemate, playmate, or community member being followed or treated (or even rumored to be) for lead poisoning?

Does the child live with an adult whose job or hobby involves exposure to lead (e.g., lead smelting and automotive radiator repair)?

Does the child live near an active lead smelter, battery recycling plant, or other industry likely to release lead?

Does the family use home remedies or pottery from another country?

Tuberculosis Testing

The prevalence of tuberculosis is increasing largely as a result of the adult HIV epidemic; children often present with serious and multisystem disease (miliary tuberculosis). All children should be assessed for tuberculosis at health maintenance visits after 1 year of age. The high-risk groups as defined by the CDC are listed in Table 9–3. The standardized PPD intradermal test is used. Because parents may misinterpret the test, a healthcare provider (nurse or physician) should evaluate the test 48 to 72 hours after injection. The size of induration (hardness to the skin), not the color of any mark, denotes a positive test. For most patients, 10 mm of induration is a positive test. For HIV-positive patients, recent tuberculosis contacts, patients with evidence of old healed tuberculosis on chest film, or immunosuppressed patients, 5 mm is a positive test (see Chapter 124).

TABLE 9–3. Groups High Risk for Tuberculosis

Close contact with persons known or suspected to have TB (Do you or your child know anyone with TB, with a positive TB test, or suspected to have TB?)

Foreign-born persons from areas with high TB rates (Asia, Africa, Latin America, Eastern Europe, Russia)

Healthcare workers

High-risk racial or ethnic minorities or other populations at higher risk (Asian, Pacific Islander, Hispanic, African American, Native American, groups living in poverty [e.g., Medicaid recipients], migrant farm workers, homeless persons, substance abusers)

Infants, children, and adolescents exposed to adults in high-risk categories

TABLE 9–4. Selective Cholesterol Screening Recommendations

1. Screen children and adolescents whose parents or grandparents, at ≤55 years old, were found to have coronary atherosclerosis; this includes individuals who have undergone balloon angioplasty or coronary artery bypass surgery
2. Screen children and adolescents whose parents or grandparents, at ≤55 years old, had a myocardial infarction, angina, peripheral vascular disease, cerebrovascular disease, or sudden cardiac death
3. Screen the children of a parent with an elevated blood cholesterol level (≥240 mg/dL)
4. For children and adolescents whose parental history is unobtainable or for children and adolescents with risk factors such as smoking, obesity, or diabetes, physicians at least should consider measuring cholesterol levels

Cholesterol

Children and adolescents who have a family history of premature cardiovascular disease or have at least one parent with a high blood cholesterol level are at increased risk of having high blood cholesterol levels as adults and increased risk of coronary heart disease. The AAP recommends selective screening in the context of regular health care for at-risk populations (Table 9–4).

Children who are being assessed because of a parent with an elevated cholesterol test or because of unavailable information or other risk factors should have a random total cholesterol level. If the random level is greater than 200 mg/dL, a fasting (12-hour) lipoprotein analysis should be done. If the total cholesterol is borderline (170 to 199 mg/dL), the test should be repeated and the two total cholesterol values averaged. If the average is borderline or higher, the children should have a fasting lipoprotein analysis. Children with a family history of atherosclerotic disease should have a fasting lipoprotein analysis.

Sexually Transmissible Infection Testing

Annual office visits are recommended for adolescents, at least after age 12. A full adolescent psychosocial history should be obtained in confidential fashion, with the parent excused from the examination room and confidentiality discussed. Part of this evaluation is a comprehensive sexual history. Often adolescents must be questioned creatively to elicit information on sexual activity. Not all adolescents identify oral sex as sex, and some adolescents misinterpret the term *sexually active* to mean that one has many sexual partners or is very vigorous during intercourse. The questions "Are you having sex?" and "Have you ever had sex?" should be asked. Any child or adolescent who has had any form of sexual intercourse should have at least an annual evaluation (if not more often if there is a history of high-risk sex) for sexually transmitted diseases by physical examination (genital warts, genital herpes, and pediculosis) and laboratory testing (chlamydia, gonorrhea, syphilis, and HIV). Adolescent girls should be assessed for human papillomavirus and precancerous lesions by Papanicolaou smear 3 years after beginning vaginal intercourse or at age 21 years.

IMMUNIZATIONS

Another important aspect of the health maintenance visit is the provision of age-appropriate vaccinations. Immunization records should be checked at each office visit, regardless of the reason, and appropriate vaccinations should be administered (see Chapter 94).

DENTAL CARE

Many families in the U.S., particularly poor families and ethnic minorities, underuse dental health care. Pediatricians may identify gross abnormalities, such as large caries, gingival inflammation, or significant malocclusion. All children should have a dental examination by a dentist at least annually and a dental cleaning by a dentist or hygienist every 6 months. Dental healthcare visits should include instruction as to preventive care practiced at home (brushing and flossing). Other prophylaxis methods shown to be effective at preventing caries are fluoride topical treatments and acrylic sealants on the molars provided by dentists. Pediatric dentists recommend beginning visits at age 1 year to educate families and to screen for milk bottle caries. General or family dentists generally recommend starting care at age 3 years (see Chapter 127).

NUTRITIONAL ASSESSMENT

Plotting a child's growth on the standard charts is a vital component of the nutritional assessment. A general assessment of behavior and development also may be relevant to detecting children at risk for nutritional problems. A dietary history should be obtained because the content of the diet may suggest a risk of nutritional deficiency (see Chapters 27 and 28).

ANTICIPATORY GUIDANCE

Anticipatory guidance is information conveyed to parents verbally or by written materials (or even directing parents to certain websites on the Internet) that is meant to assist them in facilitating optimal growth and development for their children. Figure 9–1 calls for discussions in four arenas: injury prevention, violence prevention, sleep position counseling (until 6 months old), and nutrition counseling. Table 9–5 summarizes representative issues that might be discussed within the four areas and a fifth area, fostering optimal development and behavior. In addition to the age-relevant topics, it is important to review briefly safety topics previously discussed at other visits for reinforcement. Age-appropriate discussions should occur at each visit.

Safety Issues

Two topics warrant special attention: car safety and sleep position for infants. The most common cause of death for infants 1 month to 1 year old is motor vehicle crashes. Car safety is paramount. No newborn should be discharged from a nursery unless the parents have a functioning and properly installed car seat. Many automobile dealerships offer services to parents to ensure that safety seats are installed properly in their specific model. Most states now have traffic laws that mandate safety seats until age 4 years or 40 lb. Repeat offenses may lead to suspension of driving privileges. The following are age-appropriate recommendations for car safety.

- Infants younger than 1 year old and weighing less than 20 lb—use a rear-facing infant seat
- Children older than 1 year and 20 to 40 lb—use a front-facing infant seat
- Children 4 to 8 years and 40 to 80 lb—use a booster seat (for as long as the child fits comfortably)
- If the shoulder belt lies across the child's neck or the lap belt is across the abdomen, the child is not ready for seat belts.
- Children age 12 and younger should always be in the back seat, seat belt buckled 100% of the time; front seat air bags are dangerous for younger and smaller children.

The **"Back to Sleep" initiative** has reduced the incidence of sudden infant death syndrome (SIDS). Before the initiative, infants routinely were placed prone to sleep. Since 1992 when the AAP recommended this program, the annual SIDS rate has decreased by more than 50%. Another initiative is aimed at daycare providers because 20% of SIDS deaths occur in daycare settings.

Fostering Optimal Development

See Figure 9–1 and Table 9–5 for presentation of age-appropriate activities that the pediatrician may advocate for families.

TABLE 9–5.   Anticipatory Guidance Topics Suggested by Age

Ages	Injury Prevention	Violence Prevention	Sleep Position	Nutritional Counseling	Fostering Optimal Development
Birth	Crib safety	Assess bonding and attachment	Back to sleep	Exclusive breastfeeding encouraged	Discuss parenting skills
	Hot water heaters <120°F	Identify family strife, lack of support, pathology	Crib safety	Formula as a second-best option	Refer for parenting education
	Car safety seats	Educate parents on nurturing			
	Smoke detectors				
2 wk	Falls	Reassess	Back to sleep	Assess breastfeeding and offer encouragement, problem solving	Recognize and manage postpartum blues
		Discuss sibling rivalry			Childcare options
		Assess if guns in the home			
2 mo	Burns/hot liquids	Reassess	Back to sleep		Parent getting enough rest and managing returning to work
		Firearm safety			
4 mo	Infant walkers	Reassess	Back to sleep	Introduction of solid foods	Discuss central to peripheral motor development
	Choking/ suffocation				Praise good behavior
6 mo	Changing car seats	Reassess		Assess status	Consistent limit-setting versus "spoiling" an infant
	Burns/hot surfaces				Praise good behavior
9 mo	Water safety	Assess parents' ideas on discipline and "spoiling"		Assess anemia, discuss iron-rich foods	Assisting infants to sleep through the night if not accomplished
	Home safety review Ingestions/ poisoning				Praise good behavior
12 mo	Firearm hazards	Discuss timeout versus corporal punishment		Introduction of whole cow's milk (and constipation with change discussed)	Avoiding walkers
	Auto-pedestrian safety	Avoiding media violence			Safe exploration
		Review firearm safety			Proper shoes
					Praise good behavior
15 mo	Review and reassess topics	Encourage nonviolent punishments (timeout or natural consequences)		Discuss decline in eating with slower growth	Fostering independence
				Assess food choices and variety	Reinforce good behavior
					Ignore annoying but not unsafe behaviors
18 mo	Review and reassess topics	Limit punishment to high yield (not spilled milk!)		Discuss food choices, portions, "finicky" feeders	Preparation for toilet training
		Parents consistent in discipline			Reinforce good behavior

TABLE 9–5.   Anticipatory Guidance Topics Suggested by Age—cont'd

Ages	Injury Prevention	Violence Prevention	Sleep Position	Nutritional Counseling	Fostering Optimal Development
2 yr	Falls—play equipment	Assess and discuss any aggressive behaviors in the child		Assess body proportions and consider low-fat milk Assess family cholesterol and atherosclerosis risk	Toilet training and resistance
3 yr	Review and reassess topics	Review, especially avoiding media violence		Discuss optimal eating and the food pyramid Healthy snacks	Read to child Socializing with other children Head Start if possible
4 yr	Booster seat versus seat belts			Healthy snacks	Read to child Head Start or Pre-K options
5 yr	Bicycle safety	Developing consistent, clearly defined family rules and consequences		Assess for anemia	Reinforcing school topics
	Water/pool safety	Avoiding media violence		Discuss iron-rich foods	Read to child Library card Chores begun at home
6 yr	Fire safety	Reinforce consistent discipline Encourage nonviolent strategies Assess domestic violence Avoiding media violence		Assess content, offer specific suggestions	Reinforcing school topics After-school programs Responsibility given for chores (and enforced)
7-10 yr	Sports safety	Reinforcement		Assess content, offer specific suggestions	Reviewing homework and reinforcing school topics
	Firearm hazard	Assess domestic violence Assess discipline techniques Avoiding media violence Walking away from fights (either victim or spectator)			After-school programs Introduce smoking and substance abuse prevention (concrete)
11-13 yr	Review and reassess	Discuss strategies to avoid interpersonal conflicts Avoiding media violence Avoiding fights and walking away Discuss conflict resolution techniques		Junk food versus healthy eating	Reviewing homework and reinforcing school topics Smoking and substance abuse prevention (begin abstraction) Discuss and encourage abstinence; possibly discuss condoms and contraceptive options Avoiding violence Offer availability

Continued

TABLE 9–5.   Anticipatory Guidance Topics Suggested by Age—cont'd

Ages	Injury Prevention	Violence Prevention	Sleep Position	Nutritional Counseling	Fostering Optimal Development
14-16 yr	Motor vehicle safety	Establish new family rules related to curfews, school, and household responsibilities		Junk food versus healthy eating	Review school work
	Avoiding riding with substance abuser				Begin career discussions and college preparation (PSAT)
					Review substance abuse, sexuality, and violence regularly
					Discuss condoms, contraception options, including emergency contraception
					Discuss sexually transmitted diseases, HIV
					Providing no-questions-asked ride home from at-risk situations
17-21 yr	Review and reassess	Establish new rules related to driving, dating, substance abuse		Heart healthy diet for life	Continuation of above topics
					Off to college or employment
					New roles within the family

Discipline means to teach, not merely to punish. The ultimate goal is the child's self-control. Overbearing punishment to control a child's behavior interferes with the learning process and focuses on external control at the expense of the development of self-control. Parents who set too few reasonable limits may be frustrated by children who cannot control their own behavior. Discipline should teach a child exactly what is expected by supporting positive behaviors and responding appropriately to negative behaviors with proper limits. It is more important to reinforce good behavior than to punish bad behavior.

Commonly used and seemingly effective techniques to control undesirable behaviors in children include scolding, physical punishment, and threats. These techniques have potential adverse effects, however, on children's sense of security and self-esteem. The effectiveness of scolding diminishes the more it is used. Scolding should not be allowed to expand from an expression of displeasure about a specific event to derogatory statements about the child. Scolding also

may escalate to the level of psychological abuse. It is important to educate parents that they have a "good child who does bad things from time to time," so they do not think and tell the child that he or she is "bad."

Corporal punishment is one method of punishment. Frequent mild physical punishment may become less effective over time and tempt the parent to escalate the physical punishment, increasing the risk of child abuse. Corporal punishment teaches a child that in certain situations it is proper to strike another person. Commonly, in households that employ spanking, older children who have been raised with this technique are seen responding to younger sibling behavioral problems by hitting their siblings.

Threats by parents to leave or to give up the child are perhaps the most psychologically damaging ways to control a child's behavior. Children of any age may remain fearful and anxious about loss of the parent long after the threat is made. Many children are able to see through "empty" threats, however. A family vacation that has been planned for months (and would cost significant resources if cancelled) is unlikely to be cancelled regardless of the child's behavior. Threatening a mild loss of privileges (no video games for 1 week or "grounding" a teenager) may be appropriate, but the consequence must be enforced if there is a violation.

Parenting involves a dynamic balance between *setting limits* on the one hand and allowing and encouraging freedom of expression and exploration on the other. Children whose behavior is out of control improve when clear limits on their behavior are set and enforced. Children find comfort and security in clear limits. Parents must agree, however, on where the limit will be set and how it will be enforced. The limit and the consequence of breaking the limit must be clearly presented to the child. Enforcement of the limit should be consistent and firm. Too many limits are hard to learn and may thwart the normal development of autonomy. The limit must be reasonable in terms of the child's age, temperament, and developmental level. To be effective, both parents must enforce limits. Otherwise, children may effectively "split" the parents and seek to test the limits with the more indulgent parent. In all situations, to be effective, punishment must be brief and linked directly to a behavior. More effective behavioral change occurs when punishment also is linked to praise of the intended behavior. Two effective punishment techniques are discussed next, "extinction" and "timeout."

Extinction is a systematic way to eliminate a frequent, annoying, and relatively harmless behavior by ignoring it. First, parents should note the frequency of the behavior to appreciate realistically the magnitude of the problem and to evaluate progress. It also is important to help parents determine what reinforces the child's behavior and what needs to be consistently eliminated. An appropriate behavior is identified to give the child a positive alternative that the parents can reinforce. Parents should be warned that the annoying behavior usually increases in frequency and intensity (and may last for weeks) before it decreases when the parent ignores it (removes the reinforcement). A child who has an attention-seeking temper tantrum should be ignored or placed in a secure environment (e.g., a playpen). This action may anger the child more, however, and the behavior may get louder and angrier (the child is again seeking more attention; a parent responding to this reinforces the behavior, even if responding by scolding). Eventually, as the child realizes on a conscious or unconscious level that there is no audience for the tantrum, the tantrums decrease in intensity and frequency. In each specific instance, when the child has begun to play with a favorite toy in a quiet and appropriate fashion, he or she should be praised, and extra attention should be given. This is an effective technique for early toddlers, before their capacity to understand and adhere to a timeout.

The *timeout* consists of a short period of isolation *immediately* after a problem behavior is observed. Timeout interrupts the behavior and immediately links it to an unpleasant consequence. At the outset, this method requires considerable effort by the parents because the child does not wish to be isolated. A parent may need to hold the child physically in timeout. In this situation, the parent should become part of the furniture and should not respond to the child until the timeout period is over. When established, a simple isolation technique, such as making a child stand in the corner or sending a child to his or her room, may be effective. If such a technique is not helpful, a more systematic procedure may be needed. One effective protocol for the timeout procedure involves interrupting the child's play when the behavior occurs and having the child sit in a dull, isolated place for a brief period, measured by a portable kitchen timer (kitchen timers are valuable because the clicking noises document that time is passing and the bell alarm at the end signals the end of the punishment; this obviates responding to the inevitable question, "is time up yet?") Timeout is simply punishment. It is not a time for a young child to "think" about the behavior (because these children do not possess the capacity for abstract thinking) or a time to de-escalate the behavior. The amount of timeout should be appropriate to the child's short attention span. One minute per year of a child's age is recommended. This inescapable and unpleasant consequence of the undesired behavior motivates the child to learn to avoid the behavior. If used matter-of-factly and with a minimum of expressed anger by the parent, a timeout procedure is a potent teaching tool with less chance for adverse side effects than other commonly used discipline techniques. Parents often report that they have tried limit setting, extinction, and timeout, but that the child responds angrily when parents impose their wills. The child's foreseeable frustration can be minimized if the parents are prepared to *redirect* the child to more acceptable activities and then follow-up with attention and other rewards.

CHAPTER **10**

Evaluation of the Child with Special Needs

Children with disabilities (cerebral palsy [CP]), severe chronic illnesses (diabetes or AIDS), congenital defects (cleft lip and palate), and health-related educational and behavioral problems (attention-deficit/hyperactivity disorder or a learning disability) are **children with**

special healthcare needs. Many of these children share a broad group of experiences and encounter similar problems, such as school difficulties and family stress. The term *children with special healthcare needs* defines these children noncategorically, without regard to specific diagnoses, in terms of increased service needs. Approximately 18% of children in the U.S. younger than age 18 have a physical, developmental, behavioral, or emotional condition requiring services of a type or amount beyond that required by children generally. If the definition of chronic illness is restricted to a condition that lasts or is expected to last more than 3 months and limits age-appropriate social functioning, such as school performance or recreational activities, about 6% of children are affected in the U.S.

The goal in managing a child with special healthcare needs is to maximize the child's potential for productive adult functioning by treating the primary diagnosis and by helping the patient and family deal with the stresses and secondary impairments incurred because of the disease or disability. Whenever a chronic disease is diagnosed, family members typically grieve similar to that seen at the time of death; they show anger, denial, negotiation (in an attempt to forestall the inevitable), and depression. Because the child with special healthcare needs is a constant reminder of the object of this grief, however, it may take family members a long time to accept the condition. An understanding and supportive physician can facilitate the process of acceptance by sharing the known and the unknown and by allaying guilty feelings and fear. To minimize denial, it is helpful to confirm the family's observations about the child. Also, in discussions when a new diagnosis of a special healthcare need has been presented, the family may not be able to absorb any additional information at that moment, so written material and the option for further discussion at a later date should be offered. Parents often recount that they did not remember anything after the pediatrician shared the devastating news.

The primary pediatrician should provide a **medical home** to maintain close oversight of treatments and subspecialty services, provide preventive care, and facilitate interactions with school and community agencies. The pediatrician also must recognize that the family is the one constant in a child's life, whereas service systems and support personnel within those systems fluctuate. A major goal of "family-centered care" is for the family and child to feel in control of the situation. Although the medical management team usually directs treatment in the acute healthcare setting, the locus of control should shift to the family as the child moves into a more routine, home-based life. Treatment plans should be organized to allow the greatest degree of normalization of the child's life. As the child matures, self-management programs that provide health education, self-efficacy skills, and techniques such as symptom monitoring help promote good long-term health habits. These programs should be introduced at age 6 or 7 years, or when a child is at a developmental level to take on chores and benefit from being given responsibility. Self-management minimizes "learned helplessness" and the "vulnerable child syndrome," both of which occur commonly in families with chronically ill or disabled children.

MULTIFACETED TEAM ASSESSMENT OF COMPLEX PROBLEMS

When developmental screening and surveillance suggest the presence of significant developmental lags, the pediatrician should take responsibility for coordinating the further assessment of the child by the team of professionals that is indicated and provide continuity in the care of the child and family. The physician should become aware of the facilities and programs for assessment and treatment in the local area. If the child is at high risk because of prematurity or another identified illness that might have long-term developmental impact, a structured follow-up program to monitor the child's progress already may exist. Under federal law, children are entitled to developmental assessments regardless of income if there is a suspected developmental delay or a risk factor for delay (e.g., prematurity, failure to thrive, and parental mental retardation [MR]). Up to age 3 years, special programs are developed by states to implement this policy. Developmental interventions are arranged in conjunction with third-party payers (insurance companies, Medicaid, state children's health insurance program), with the local program funding the cost only when there is no insurance coverage. After age 3 years, development programs usually are administered by school districts. Federal laws also mandate that special education programs be provided for all children with developmental disabilities from birth through 21 years of age.

Children with special needs may be enrolled in pre-K programs with a therapeutic core, including visits to the program by therapists to work on challenges in the context of the pre-K schedule. Children who are of traditional school age (kindergarten through secondary school) should be evaluated by the school district and provided an **individualized educational plan (IEP)** to address any deficiencies. An IEP may feature individual tutoring time (so-called resource time), placement in a special education program, placement in classes with children with severe behavioral problems, or other strategies to address deficiencies. As part of the comprehensive evaluation of developmental/behavioral issues, all children should receive a thorough medical assessment. Depending on the issue, a variety of other specialists may assist in the assessment and intervention for children with special needs, including sub-specialist pediatricians (e.g., neurology, orthopedics, psychiatry, developmental/behavioral), therapists (e.g., occupational, physical, oral-motor), and others (e.g., psychologists, early childhood development specialists).

Medical Assessment

The physician's main goals in team assessment are to identify the cause of the developmental dysfunction, if possible (often a specific cause is not found), and identify and interpret other medical conditions that have a developmental impact. The comprehensive history (Table 10-1) and physical examination (Table 10-2) include a careful graphing of growth parameters and an accurate description of dysmorphic features. Many of the diagnoses are rare or unusual diseases or syndromes, beyond the level of someone beginning in pediatrics. Many of these diseases and syndromes are discussed further in Sections IX and XXIV.

Motor Assessment

The comprehensive neurologic examination is an excellent basis for evaluating motor function, but it should be supplemented by an adaptive functional evaluation (see Chapter 179). Watching the child at play aids in the assessment. Specialists in early childhood development and therapists (especially occupational and physical therapists who have experience with children) can provide excellent input into the evaluation of age-appropriate adaptive function.

Psychological Assessment

Psychological assessment includes the testing of cognitive ability (Table 10-3) and the evaluation of personality and emotional well-being. The IQ and mental age scores, taken in isolation, are only partially descriptive of a person's functional abilities, which are a combination of cognitive, adaptive, and social skills. Tests of achievement are subject to variability based on culture, educational exposures, and experience and must be standardized for social factors. Projective and nonprojective tests are useful in understanding the child's emotional status. Although a child should not be labeled as having a problem solely on the basis of a standardized test, such tests do provide important and reasonably objective data for evaluating a child's growth within a particular educational program.

Educational Assessment

The educational assessment involves the evaluation of areas of specific strengths and weaknesses in reading, spelling, written expression, and mathematical skills.

Schools routinely screen children with group tests to aid in problem identification and program evaluation. For the child with special needs, this screening ultimately should lead to individualized testing and the development of an IEP that would enable the child to progress comfortably in school. Diagnostic teaching, in which the child's response to various teaching techniques is assessed, also may be helpful.

Social Environment Assessment

Assessment of the environment in which the child is living, working, playing, and growing is important in understanding the child's development. A home visit by a social worker, community health nurse, or home-based intervention specialist can provide valuable information about the child's social milieu. If there is a suspicion of inadequate parenting and, especially, if there is a suspicion of neglect or abuse (including emotional abuse), the child and family must be referred to the local child protection agency. Information about reporting hotlines and local child protection agencies usually is found inside the front cover of local telephone directories (see Chapter 22).

MANAGEMENT OF DEVELOPMENTAL PROBLEMS

Intervention in the Primary Care Setting

The clinician must decide whether a problem requires referral for further diagnostic workup and management or whether management in the primary care setting is appropriate. Counseling roles required in caring for these children are listed in Table 10-4. When a child is young, much of the counseling interaction takes place between the parents and the clinician; as the child matures, direct counseling shifts increasingly toward the child.

The assessment process may be therapeutic in itself. By assuming the role of a nonjudgmental, supportive listener, the clinician creates a climate of trust in which the family feels free to express difficult or painful thoughts and feelings. Expressing emotions may allow the parent or caregiver to move on to the work of understanding and resolving the problem.

Interview techniques also may facilitate clarification of the problem for the family and for the clinician. The family's ideas about the causes of the problem and descriptions of attempts to deal with it can provide a basis for developing strategies for problem management that are much more likely to be implemented successfully because they emanate in part from the family. The clinician shows respect by endorsing the parent's ideas when appropriate; this can increase self-esteem and sense of competency.

TABLE 10–1.   Information to Be Sought During the History Taking of a Child with Suspected Developmental Disabilities

Item	Possible Significance
Parental Concerns	Parents are quite accurate in identifying development problems in their children
Current Levels of Developmental Functioning	Should be used to monitor child's progress
Temperament	May interact with disability or may be confused with developmental delay
Prenatal History	
Alcohol ingestion	Fetal alcohol syndrome; an index of care-taking risk
Exposure to medication, illegal drug, or toxin	Development toxin (e.g., phenytoin); may be an index of care-taking risk
Radiation exposure	Damage to CNS
Nutrition	Inadequate fetal nutrition
Prenatal care	Index of social situation
Injuries, hyperthermia	Damage to CNS
Smoking	Possible CNS damage
HIV exposure	Congenital HIV infection
Maternal PKU	Maternal PKU effect
Maternal illness	Toxoplasmosis, rubella, cytomegalovirus, herpesvirus infections
Perinatal History	
Gestational age, birth weight	Biologic risk from prematurity and small for gestational age
Labor and delivery	Hypoxia or index of abnormal prenatal development
Apgar scores	Hypoxia, cardiovascular impairment
Specific perinatal adverse events	Increased risk for CNS damage
Neonatal History	
Illness—seizures, respiratory distress, hyperbilirubinemia, metabolic disorder	Increased risk for CNS damage
Malformations	May represent syndrome associated with developmental delay
Family History	
Consanguinity	Autosomal recessive condition more likely
Mental functioning	Increased hereditary and environmental risks
Illnesses (e.g., metabolic disease)	Hereditary illness associated with developmental delay
Family member died young or unexpectedly	May suggest inborn error of metabolism or storage disease
Family member requires special education	Hereditary causes of developmental delay
Social History	
Resources available (e.g., financial, social support)	Necessary to maximize child's potential
Educational level of parents	Family may need help to provide stimulation
Mental health problems	May exacerbate child's conditions
High-risk behaviors (e.g., illicit drugs, sex)	Increased risk for HIV infection; index of care-taking risk
Other stressors (e.g., marital discord)	May exacerbate child's conditions or compromise care
Other History	
Gender of child	Important for X-linked conditions
Developmental milestones	Index of developmental delay; regression may indicate progressive condition
Head injury	Even moderate trauma may be associated with developmental delay or learning disabilities

TABLE 10–1. Information to Be Sought During the History Taking of a Child with Suspected Developmental Disabilities—cont'd

Item	Possible Significance
Serious infections (e.g., meningitis)	May be associated with developmental delay
Toxic exposure (e.g., lead)	May be associated with developmental delay
Physical growth	May indicate malnutrition; obesity, short stature associated with some conditions
Recurrent otitis media	Associated with hearing loss and abnormal speech development
Visual and auditory functioning	Sensitive index of impairments in vision and hearing
Nutrition	Malnutrition during infancy may lead to delayed development
Chronic conditions such as renal disease	May be associated with delayed development or anemia

From Liptak G: Mental retardation and developmental disability. In Kliegman RM, editor: Practical Strategies in Pediatric Diagnosis and Therapy. Philadelphia, WB Saunders, 1996.

TABLE 10–2. Information to Be Sought During the Physical Examination of a Child with Suspected Developmental Disabilities

Item	Possible Significance
General Appearance	May indicate significant delay in development or obvious syndrome
Stature	
Short stature	Williams syndrome, malnutrition, Turner syndrome; many children with severe retardation have short stature
Obesity	Prader-Willi syndrome
Large stature	Sotos syndrome
Head	
Macrocephaly	Alexander syndrome, Sotos syndrome, gangliosidosis, hydrocephalus, mucopolysaccharidosis, subdural effusion
Microcephaly	Virtually any condition that can retard brain growth (e.g., malnutrition, Angelman syndrome, de Lange syndrome, fetal alcohol effects)
Face	
Coarse, triangular, round, or flat face; hypotelorism or hypertelorism, slanted or short palpebral fissure; unusual nose, maxilla, and mandible	Specific measurements may provide clues to inherited, metabolic, or other diseases such as fetal alcohol syndrome, cri du chat syndrome (5p– syndrome), or Williams syndrome
Eyes	
Prominent	Crouzon syndrome, Seckel syndrome, fragile X syndrome
Cataract	Galactosemia, Lowe syndrome, prenatal rubella, hypothyroidism
Cherry-red spot in macula	Gangliosidosis (GM_1), metachromatic leukodystrophy, mucolipidosis, Tay-Sachs disease, Niemann-Pick disease, Farber lipogranulomatosis, sialidosis III
Chorioretinitis	Congenital infection with cytomegalovirus, toxoplasmosis, or rubella
Corneal cloudiness	Mucopolysaccharidosis I and II, Lowe syndrome, congenital syphilis

Continued

TABLE 10–2.   Information to Be Sought During the Physical Examination of a Child with Suspected Developmental Disabilities—cont'd

Item	Possible Significance
Ears	
Pinnae, low set or malformed	Trisomies such as 18, Rubinstein-Taybi syndrome, Down syndrome, CHARGE association, cerebro-oculofacial-skeletal syndrome, fetal phenytoin effects
Hearing	Loss of acuity in mucopolysaccharidosis; hyperacusis in many encephalopathies
Heart	
Structural anomaly or hypertrophy	CHARGE association, CATCH-22, velocardiofacial syndrome, glycogenosis II, fetal alcohol effects, mucopolysaccharidosis I; chromosomal anomalies such as Down syndrome; maternal PKU; chronic cyanosis may impair cognitive development
Liver	
Hepatomegaly	Fructose intolerance, galactosemia, glycogenosis types I-IV, mucopolysaccharidosis I and II, Niemann-Pick disease, Tay-Sachs disease, Zellweger syndrome, Gaucher disease, ceroid lipofuscinosis, gangliosidosis
Genitalia	
Macro-orchidism	Fragile X syndrome
Hypogenitalism	Prader-Willi syndrome, Klinefelter syndrome, CHARGE association
Extremities	
Hands, feet, dermatoglyphics, and creases	May indicate specific entity such as Rubinstein-Taybi syndrome or be associated with chromosomal anomaly
Joint contractures	Sign of muscle imbalance around joints—e.g., with meningomyelocele, cerebral palsy, arthrogryposis, muscular dystrophy; also occurs with cartilaginous problems such as mucopolysaccharidosis
Skin	
Café au lait spots	Neurofibromatosis, tuberous sclerosis, Bloom syndrome
Eczema	Phenylketonuria, histiocytosis
Hemangiomas and telangiectasia	Sturge-Weber syndrome, Bloom syndrome, ataxia-telangiectasia
Hypopigmented macules, streaks, adenoma sebaceum	Tuberous sclerosis, hypomelanosis of Ito
Hair	
Hirsutism	de Lange syndrome, mucopolysaccharidosis, fetal phenytoin effects, cerebro-oculofacial-skeletal syndrome, trisomy 18
Neurologic	
Asymmetry of strength and tone	Focal lesion, cerebral palsy
Hypotonia	Prader-Willi syndrome, Down syndrome, Angelman syndrome, gangliosidosis, early cerebral palsy
Hypertonia	Neurodegenerative conditions involving white matter, cerebral palsy, trisomy 18
Ataxia	Ataxia-telangiectasia, metachromatic leukodystrophy, Angelman syndrome

CHARGE, coloboma, heart defects, atresia choanae, retarded growth, genital anomalies, ear anomalies (deafness); CATCH-22, cardiac defects, abnormal face, thymic hypoplasia, cleft palate, hypocalcemia, defects on chromosome 22.

From Liptak G: Mental retardation and developmental disability. In Kliegman RM (ed): Practical Strategies in Pediatric Diagnosis and Therapy. Philadelphia, WB Saunders, 1996.

TABLE 10–3. Tests of Cognition

Test	Age Range	Special Features
Infant Scales		
Bayley Scales of Infant Development (2nd ed)	2-42 mo	Mental, psychomotor scales, behavior record; weak intelligence predictor
Cattell Infant Intelligence Scale	Birth-30 mo	Used to extend Stanford-Binet downward
Gesell Developmental Schedules	Birth-3 yr	Used by many pediatricians
Ordinal Scales of Infant Psychological Development	Birth-24 mo	Six subscales; based on Piaget's stages; weak in predicting later intelligence
Preschool Scales		
Stanford-Binet Intelligence Scale (4th ed)	2 yr-adult	Four area scores, with subtests and composite IQ score
McCarthy Scales of Children's Abilities	$2^{1}/_{2}$-8 yr	6-18 subtests; good at defining learning disabilities; strengths/weaknesses approach
Wechsler Primary and Preschool Test of Intelligence–Revised (WPPSI-R)	3-6$^{1}/_{2}$ yr	11 subtests; verbal, performance IQs; long administration time; good at defining learning disabilities
Merrill-Palmer Scale of Mental Tests	2-4$^{1}/_{2}$ yr	General test for young children
Differential Abilities Scale	$2^{1}/_{2}$ yr-adult	Special nonverbal composite; short administration time
School-Age Scales		
Stanford-Binet Intelligence Scale (4th ed)	2 yr-adult	See above
Wechsler Intelligence Scale for Children (3rd ed) (WISC III)	6-16 yr	See comments on WPPSI-R
Leiter International Performance Scale	2 yr-adult	No verbal abilities needed
Wechsler Adult Intelligence Scale–Revised (WAIS-R)	16 yr-adult	See comments on WPPSI-R
Differential Abilities Scale	$2^{1}/_{2}$ yr-adult	See above
Adaptive Behavior Scales		
Vineland Adaptive Behavior Scale	Birth-adult	Interview/questionnaire; typical persons and blind, deaf, and retarded
American Association on Mental Retardation (AAMR) Adaptive Behavioral Scale	3 yr-adult	Useful in retardation, other disabilities

Educating parents about normal and aberrant development and behavior may prevent problems through early detection and anticipatory guidance. Such education also communicates the physician's interest in hearing parental concerns. Early detection is important because intervention can be started before the problem becomes entrenched, and associated problems develop (e.g., depression over poor school performance leading to further school failure).

Many parents expect and need specific, detailed advice from the clinician. Specific suggestions for changes in the family environment often are useful, such as arranging for respite and increased emotional support for the primary caregiver, who usually is discouraged and exhausted by the time the clinician hears about the problem. The clinician also may suggest other community services to relieve pressure and to improve the coping ability of the family (e.g., nursery school, tutors, recreational programs, and parent support and education groups).

The severity of developmental and behavioral problems ranges from variations of normal, to problematic responses to stressful situations, to frank disorders. The clinician must try to establish the severity and scope of the patient's symptoms so that appropriate intervention can be planned.

TABLE 10–4. Primary Care Counseling Roles

Allow ventilation
Facilitate clarification
Support patient problem solving
Provide specific reassurance
Provide education
Provide specific parenting advice
Suggest environmental interventions
Provide follow-up
Facilitate appropriate referrals
Coordinate care and interpret reports after referrals

Most developmental and behavioral problems seem simple when initially presented, and often a small amount of education and reassurance and a few simple suggestions are sufficient. Follow-up is crucial, however, because complex problems often present as simple problems. Clinicians must be ready to accept failure of their suggestions without attributing the failure to inadequacy in the parents' application of the recommendations. Indications for referral to developmental disability or mental health specialists vary according to the expertise of the primary care clinician, but children should not be followed for long periods in the hope that they will "outgrow" the problem. After referral, the clinician is needed to help coordinate and interpret the evaluations and recommendations.

Counseling Principles

Behavioral change is difficult in any situation. For the child, behavioral change must be learned, not simply imposed. It is easiest to learn when the lesson is simple, clear, and consistent and presented in an atmosphere free of fear or intimidation. Parents often try to impose behavioral change in an emotionally charged atmosphere, most often at the time of a behavioral "violation." Clinicians often try to "teach" parents with hastily presented advice when the parents are distracted by other concerns or not engaged in the suggested behavioral change.

Apart from management strategies directed specifically at the problem behavior, regular times for positive parent-child interaction should be instituted. Frequent, brief, affectionate physical contact over the day provides opportunities for positive reinforcement of desirable child behaviors and for building a sense of competence in the child and the parent. The clinician must be careful of using developmental or behavioral labels, even though they may be helpful in diagnosis and management. These labels can become self-fulfilling prophecies as the people in the child's environment treat the child as a disorder or disability, which becomes part of the child's self-concept.

Most parents feel guilty when their children have a developmental/behavioral problem. This guilt may be caused by the assumption or fear that the problem was caused by inadequate parenting or guilt about previous angry responses to the child's behavior (excessive physical punishment or derogatory comments). The clinician should not unwittingly contribute to parental guilt with insensitive comments that may be construed as criticism by the parents. If possible and appropriate, the clinician should find ways to alleviate guilt, which may be a serious impediment to problem solving. The clinician can diffuse this guilt by honestly pointing out how often other parents have similar problems and by empathizing with the difficulties of coping with the problem. Often parents benefit from a problem-specific or general parenting support group.

Interdisciplinary Team Intervention

In many cases, a team of professionals is required to provide the breadth and quality of services needed to serve appropriately the child who has developmental problems. This is commonly the case in follow-up programs for infants leaving intensive care nurseries. The physician may play a key role in guiding the child and family to available services. When the child reaches school age, the public school system takes increasing responsibility for developmental and educational services, and the physician's role becomes primarily one of consultation on medically related issues. The primary care physician should monitor the progress of the child and continually reassess that the requisite therapy is being accomplished. If the family reports that the publicly supported early intervention project is not accomplishing the objectives for the child, the physician may advocate for better services or refer to the private sector for additional services (depending on family health coverage and resources).

Educational intervention for a young child begins as home-based infant stimulation, often with an early childhood educator; nurse; or occupational, speech, or physical therapist providing direct stimulation for the child and training the family to provide the stimulation. As the child matures, a center-based nursery program may be indicated. For the school-age child, special services may range from extra attention given by the classroom teacher to a self-contained special education classroom. Home-based tutoring or residential programs typically are reserved for only the most behaviorally or cognitively impaired children in this age range.

Psychological intervention may take several forms. Therapy may be parent or family directed or may become, with an older child, primarily child directed. Examples of therapeutic approaches are guidance therapies, such as directive advice giving, counseling the family and child in their own solutions to problems, psychotherapy, behavioral management techniques, psychopharmacologic methods, and cognitive therapy.

Motor intervention may be performed by a physical or occupational therapist or by another professional under the therapist's direction. All therapies suggested should be evidence based and reviewed by the pediatrician. Two commonly employed methods serve as examples. *Neurodevelopmental therapy* (NDT), the most commonly used method, is based on the concept that nervous system development is hierarchical and subject to some plasticity. The focus of NDT is on gait training and motor development, including daily living skills and perceptual abilities, such as eye-hand coordination,

Problem	Ask About or Check
Motor	Range of motion examination; scoliosis check; assessment of mobility; interaction with orthopedist, physiatrist, and PT/OT as needed
Diet	Dietary history, feeding observation, growth parameter measurement and charting, supplementation as indicated by observations
Sensory impairments	Functional vision and hearing screening; interaction as needed with ophthalmologist, audiologist
Dermatology	Examination of *all* skin areas for decubitus ulcers or infection
Dentistry	Examination of teeth and gums; confirmation of access to dental care
Behavioral problems	Aggression, self-injury, pica; sleep problems; psychotropic drug levels and side effects
Advocacy	Educational program, family supports, financial supports
Seizures	Major motor, absence, other suspicious symptoms; monitoring of anticonvulsant levels and side effects
Infectious diseases	Ear infections, diarrhea, respiratory symptoms, aspiration pneumonia, immunizations (especially hepatitis B and influenza)
GI problems	Constipation, gastroesophageal reflux, GI bleeding (stool for occult blood)
Sexuality	Sexuality education, hygiene, contraception (when appropriate), genetic counseling
Other syndrome-specific problems	Ongoing evaluation of other "physical" problems as indicated by known MR/DD etiology

TABLE 10–5. Recurring Medical Issues in Children with Developmental Disabilities

GI, gastrointestinal; MR/DD, mental retardation/developmental disability; PT/OT, physical therapist/occupational therapist.

spatial relationships, and motor sequencing, that help guide motor activity. *Sensory integration therapy* also is used sometimes by occupational therapists to structure sensory experience from the tactile, proprioceptive, and vestibular systems to allow for adaptive motor responses.

Speech-language intervention by a speech therapist (oral-motor therapist) is usually part of the overall educational program and is based on the tested language strengths and weaknesses of the child. Children needing this type of intervention may show difficulties in reading and other academic areas and develop social and behavioral problems because of their difficulties in being understood and in understanding others. **Hearing intervention**, performed by an audiologist (or an otolaryngologist), includes monitoring hearing acuity, providing amplification when necessary via hearing aids, and assessing the aftereffects of ear infections by objective tests of middle ear function (tympanometry and acoustic impedance testing).

Social and environmental intervention generally takes the form of nursing or social work involvement with the family. Frequently the task of coordinating the services of other disciplines falls to these specialists. These case managers may be in the private sector or part of the child protection agency. The child protection agency may assess the environment and provide targeted interventions (transportation to appointments or case management) rather than placing a child outside of the parents' home.

Medical intervention for a child with a developmental disability involves providing primary care and specific treatment of conditions associated with disability. Although curative treatment often is not possible because of the irreversible nature of many disabling conditions, functional impairment can be minimized through thoughtful medical management. Certain general medical problems are found more frequently in mentally retarded and developmentally disabled people (Table 10–5). Many of these children have more than developmental issues, especially if the delay is part of a known syndrome of malformations (Down syndrome or VATER association). These latter children may have a limited life expectancy. Supporting the family through palliative care, hospice, and bereavement is another important role of the primary care pediatrician.

SELECTED CLINICAL PROBLEMS IN THE SPECIAL NEEDS CHILD
Mental Retardation

MR is defined as significantly subnormal intellectual functioning for a child's developmental stage, existing concurrently with deficits in adaptive behaviors (self-care, home living, communication, and social interactions). MR is defined statistically as cognitive performance that is 2 SD below the mean (roughly below the 3rd percentile) of the general population as measured on standardized intelligence testing; this

TABLE 10–6. Levels of Mental Retardation

Level of Retardation	Stanford-Binet IQ Score	WISC-III IQ Score	Educational Label
Mild	67-52	70-55	"Educable (EMR)"
Moderate	51-36	54-40	"Trainable (TMR)"
Severe	35-20	39-25	
Profound	<20	<24	Severe-profound

WISC-III, Wechsler Intelligence Scale for children (3rd ed.).

implies that 8.5 million persons in the U.S. can be characterized as having MR; clinical estimates range from 2.2 to 10 million (the higher number includes persons with so-called borderline intelligence and poor social adaptation).

Levels of MR from IQ scores derived from two typical tests are shown in Table 10–6. Caution must be exercised in interpretation, however, because these categories do not reflect the actual functional level of the tested individual. In school, a child with mild MR, because of poor social (adaptive) abilities, may be better served in a class for children defined as "trainable," whereas another child who tests in the moderate range of retardation but who has especially good language abilities may be more stimulated in a class for children defined as "educable." Persons who perform in the severe or profound ranges of MR also are capable of responding to some educational interventions. A greater emphasis should be placed on descriptions of functional deficits, especially in the adaptive skill areas (activities of daily living), rather than on IQ scores.

The etiology of the CNS insult resulting in MR may involve genetic disorders, teratogenic influences, perinatal insults, acquired childhood disease, and environmental and social factors (Table 10–7). The potential mechanisms and causes are listed in declining frequency. Mild MR correlates with socioeconomic status, although profound MR does not. Although a single organic cause may be found, each individual's performance should be considered a function of the interaction of environmental influences with the individual's organic substrate. It is common for a child with MR to have behavioral difficulties resulting from the MR itself and from the family's reaction to the child and his or her condition. More severe forms of MR can be traced to biologic factors, and the earlier the cognitive slowing is recognized, the more severe the deviation from normal is likely to be. The pattern of an individual's development can aid in making a diagno-

sis, but at any given point in time, it may be difficult to predict future performance.

The first step in the diagnosis and management of a child with MR is to obtain evaluations from several disciplines to identify functional strengths and weaknesses for purposes of medical and habilitative therapies. When the developmental lags have been identified, the history and physical examination may suggest the point in development at which a CNS insult may have occurred and minimize the need for laboratory tests. Frequently used laboratory tests include chromosomal analysis and MRI of the brain. Almost one third of individuals with MR do not have readily identifiable reasons for their disability. In many cases, enough factors can be ruled out, however, to allay the guilt and anxiety of families about their responsibility in causing the disability.

Vision Impairment

Significant visual impairment is a problem in many children. *Partial vision* (defined as visual acuity between 20/70 and 20/200) occurs in 1 in 500 school-age children in the U.S., with about 35,000 children having visual acuity between 20/200 and total blindness. *Legal blindness* is defined as distant visual acuity of 20/200 in the better eye or a visual field that subtends an angle not greater than 20 degrees. Although this definition allows for considerable residual vision, such impairment can be a major barrier to optimal educational development.

The most common cause of *severe visual impairment* in children is retinopathy of prematurity (see Chapter 61). Congenital cataracts resulting from a variety of causes occur in 1 of 250 newborns and can lead to significant amblyopia. Cataracts also are associated with other ocular abnormalities and developmental disabilities. *Amblyopia* is defined as a pathologic alteration of the visual system characterized by a reduction in visual acuity in one or both eyes with no clinically apparent organic abnormality that can completely account for the visual loss. Amblyopia is due to a distortion of the normal clearly formed retinal image (from congenital cataracts or severe refractive errors), abnormal binocular interaction between the eyes with one eye competitively inhibiting the other (strabismus), or a combination of both mechanisms. Optic atrophy, retinal degeneration (retinitis pigmentosa), retinoblastoma, and congenital glaucoma are other, less common causes of significant visual impairment.

Children with *mild to moderate visual impairment* usually are discovered to have an uncorrected refractive error. The most common presentation is myopia or nearsightedness. Other causes are hyperopia (farsightedness) and astigmatism (alteration in the shape of the cornea leading to visual distortion). In children younger than 6 years old, high refractive errors in one or both eyes also may cause amblyopia, which aggravates the vision impairment.

TABLE 10–7. Differential Diagnosis of Mental Retardation*

Early Alterations of Embryonic Development

Sporadic events affecting embryogenesis, usually a stable developmental challenge
   Chromosomal changes (e.g., trisomy 21)
   Prenatal influences (e.g., substance abuse, teratogenic medications, intrauterine TORCH infections)

Unknown Causes

No definite issue is identified, or multiple elements present, none of which is diagnostic (may be multifactorial)

Environmental and Social Problems

Dynamic influences, commonly associated with other challenges
   Deprivation (neglect)
   Parental mental illness
   Environmental intoxications (e.g., significant lead intoxication)[†]

Pregnancy Problems and Perinatal Morbidity

Impingement on normal intrauterine development or delivery; neurologic abnormalities frequent, challenges are stable or
   occasionally worsening
   Fetal malnutrition and placental insufficiency
   Perinatal complications (e.g., prematurity, birth asphyxia, birth trauma)

Hereditary Disorders

Preconceptual origin, variable expression in the individual infant, multiple somatic effects, frequently a progressive or
   degenerative course
   Inborn errors of metabolism (e.g., Tay-Sachs disease, Hunter disease, PKU)
   Single-gene abnormalities (e.g., neurofibromatosis or tuberous sclerosis)
   Other chromosomal aberrations (e.g., fragile X syndrome, deletion mutations such as Prader-Willi syndrome)
   Polygenic familial syndromes (pervasive developmental disorders)

Acquired Childhood Illness

Acute modification of developmental status, variable potential for functional recovery
   Infections (all can ultimately lead to brain damage, but most significant are encephalitis and meningitis)
   Cranial trauma (accidental and child abuse)
   Accidents (e.g., near-drowning, electrocution)
   Environmental intoxications (prototype is lead poisoning)

*Some health problems fit in several categories (e.g., lead intoxication may be involved in several areas).
[†]This also may be considered as an acquired childhood disease.
TORCH, toxoplasmosis, other (congenital syphilis and viruses), rubella, cytomegalovirus, and herpes simplex virus

The diagnosis of severe visual impairment commonly is made when an infant is 4 to 8 months old. Clinical suspicion is based on parental concerns aroused by unusual behavior, such as lack of smiling in response to appropriate stimuli, the presence of nystagmus, wandering eye movements, or motor delays in beginning to reach for objects. On physical examination, fixation and visual tracking behavior can be seen in most infants by 6 weeks of age. This behavior can be assessed by moving a brightly colored object (or the examiner's face) across the visual field of a quiet but alert infant at a distance of 1 ft. The eyes also should be examined for red reflexes and pupillary reactions to light, although optical alignment (binocular vision with both eyes consistently focusing on the same spot) should not be expected until the infant is beyond the newborn period. Persistent nystagmus is abnormal at any age. If ocular abnormalities are identified, referral to a pediatric ophthalmologist is indicated.

During the newborn period, vision may be assessed by physical examination and by VER. VER evaluates the conduction of electrical impulses from the optic nerve to the occipital cortex of the brain. The eye is stimulated by a bright flash of light (flash VER), and the resulting electrical response is recorded from electrodes strategically placed on the scalp, similar to an EEG. Instead of a flash, the stimulus used also may consist of an alternating checkerboard of black-and-white squares, which the patient observes. This is known as a pattern VER.

There are many developmental implications of visual impairment. Perception of body image is abnormal, and imitative behavior, such as smiling, is delayed. Delays in mobility may occur in children who are visually impaired from birth, although their postural milestones (ability to sit) usually are achieved appropriately. Social bonding with the parents also is affected.

Visually impaired children can be helped in various ways. Classroom settings may be augmented with resource-room assistance to present material in a nonvisual format; some schools consult with an experienced teacher of the blind. Fine motor activity development, listening skills, and Braille reading and writing are intrinsic to successful educational intervention with the child who has severe visual impairment.

Hearing Impairment

The clinical significance of hearing loss varies with its type (conductive versus sensorineural), its frequency (recurrent otitis media), and its severity as measured in number of decibels heard. The most common cause of mild to moderate hearing loss in children is a conduction abnormality caused by acquired middle ear disease. This abnormality may have a significant effect on the development of speech and other aspects of language development, particularly if there is chronic fluctuating middle ear fluid. When hearing impairment is more severe, sensorineural hearing loss is more common. Causes of sensorineural deafness include congenital infections (e.g., rubella or cytomegalovirus), meningitis, birth asphyxia, kernicterus, ototoxic drugs (especially aminoglycoside antibiotics), and tumors and their treatments. Genetic deafness may be either dominant or recessive in inheritance; this is the main cause of hearing impairment in schools for the deaf. In Down syndrome, there is a predisposition to conductive loss caused by middle ear infection and sensorineural loss caused by cochlear disease. Any hearing loss may have a significant effect on the child's developing communication skills. These skills then affect all areas of the child's cognitive and skills development (Table 10–8).

It is sometimes quite difficult to determine accurately the presence of hearing in infants and young children. Using developmental surveillance to inquire about an infant's response to parental sounds or even observing the infant's response to sounds in the office is unreliable for identifying hearing-impaired children. An improvement in detecting hearing impairment has resulted from the implementation of universal screening of newborns. Two tests that are used to screen a newborn's hearing are as follows:

- **Auditory brainstem response.** This test measures how the brain responds to sound. Clicks or tones are played through soft earphones into the infant's ears. Three electrodes placed on the infant's head measure the brain's response.
- **Otoacoustic emissions.** This test measures sound waves produced in the inner ear. A tiny probe is placed just inside the infant's ear canal. It measures the response (echo) when clicks or tones are played into the infant's ears.

Both of these tests are quick (5 to 10 minutes), painless, and may be done while the infant is sleeping or lying still. The tests are sensitive, but not as specific as more definitive tests. Infants who fail these tests are referred for more comprehensive testing. Many of these infants have normal hearing on definitive testing. Infants who do not are immediately referred for etiologic diagnosis and early intervention programs. Most states now have early hearing detection and intervention programs.

For children not screened at birth or children with suspected acquired hearing loss, later testing may allow early appropriate intervention. Hearing can be screened by means of an office audiogram, but other techniques are needed (auditory evoked brainstem potential) for young, neurologically immature or impaired, behaviorally difficult, or severely cognitively impaired children. The typical audiologic assessment includes pure-tone audiometry over a variety of sound frequencies (pitches), especially over the range of frequencies in which most speech occurs. Tympanometry is used in the assessment of middle ear function and the evaluation of tympanic membrane compliance for pathology in the middle ear, such as fluid, ossicular dysfunction, and eustachian tube dysfunction (see Chapter 9).

The treatment of conductive hearing loss (largely due to otitis media and middle ear effusions) is discussed in Chapter 105. Treatment of sensorineural hearing impairment may be medical or surgical. The audiologist may believe that amplification is indicated, in which case hearing aids can be tuned preferentially to amplify the frequency ranges in which the patient has decreased acuity. Educational intervention typically includes speech-language therapy and teaching American Sign Language. Even with amplification, many hearing-impaired children show deficits in processing information presented through the auditory pathway, requiring special educational services for helping to read and for other academic skills. Cochlear implants may benefit some children. A cochlear implant is a surgically implantable device that provides hearing sensation to individuals with severe to profound hearing loss who do not benefit from hearing aids. The implants are designed to substitute for the function of the middle ear, cochlear mechanical motion, and sensory cells, transforming sound energy into electrical energy that initiates impulses in the auditory nerve. The indications for cochlear implants

TABLE 10–8. Neurodevelopmental-Behavioral Complications of Hearing Loss

Severity of Hearing Loss	Possible Etiologic Origins	Complications			Types of Therapy
		Speech-Language	*Educational*	*Behavioral*	
Slight 15-25 dB (ASA)	Serous otitis media Perforation of tympanic membrane Sensorineural loss Tympanosclerosis	Difficulty with distant or faint speech	Possible auditory learning dysfunction May reveal a slight verbal deficit	Usually none	May require favorable class setting, speech therapy, or auditory training Possible value in hearing aid
Mild 25-40 dB (ASA)	Serous otitis media Perforation of tympanic membrane Sensorineural loss Tympanosclerosis	Difficulty with conversational speech over 3-5 ft May have limited vocabulary and speech disorders	May miss 50% of class discussions Auditory learning dysfunction	Psychological problems May act inappropriately if directions are not heard well Acting out behavior Poor self-concept	Special education resource help Hearing aid Favorable class setting Lip reading instruction Speech therapy
Moderate 40-65 dB (ASA)	Chronic otitis media Middle ear anomaly Sensorineural loss	Conversation must be loud to be understood Defective speech Deficient language use and comprehension	Learning disability Difficulty with group learning or discussion Auditory processing dysfunction Limited vocabulary	Emotional and social problems Behavioral reactions of childhood Acting out Poor self-concept	Special education resource or special class Special help in speech-language development Hearing aid and lip reading Speech therapy
Severe 65-95 dB (ASA)	Sensorineural loss Middle ear disease	Loud voices may be heard 2 ft from ear Defective speech and language No spontaneous speech development if loss present before 1 yr	Marked educational retardation Marked learning disability Limited vocabulary	Emotional and social problems that are associated with handicap Poor self-concept	Full-time special education for deaf children Hearing aid, lip reading, speech therapy Auditory training Counseling Cochlear implant
Profound ≥95 dB (ASA)	Sensorineural or mixed loss	Relies on vision rather than hearing Defective speech and language Speech and language will not develop spontaneously if loss present before 1 yr	Marked learning disability because of lack of understanding of speech	Congenital and prelingually deaf may show severe emotional problems	As above Oral and manual communication Counseling

ASA, Acoustical Society of America.
From Gottleib MI: Otitis media. In Levine MD, Carey WB, Crocker AC, et al (eds): Developmental-Behavioral Pediatrics. Philadelphia, WB Saunders, 1983.

TABLE 10–9. Indications for Cochlear Implants in Children

Age 12 mo to 17 yr
Profound bilateral sensorineural hearing loss
Limited benefit from hearing aids
Failure to progress in auditory skill development
No radiologic or medical contraindications

are presented in Table 10–9. Implanting children as young as possible gives them the most advantageous auditory environment for speech-language learning. Cochlear implants also may result in serious complications, however, such as pneumococcal meningitis.

Speech-Language Impairment

Parents often bring the concern of speech delay to the physician's attention when they compare their young child with others of the same age (Table 10–10). The most common causes of the speech delay are MR, hearing impairment, social deprivation, autism, and oral-motor abnormalities. If a problem is suspected based on screening with tests such as the Denver II or other standard screening test (Early Language Milestone Scale), a referral to a specialized hearing and speech center is indicated. While awaiting the results of testing or initiation of speech-language therapy, parents should be advised to speak slowly and clearly to the child (and avoid "baby talk"). Parents and older siblings should read to the speech-delayed child frequently.

Speech disorders include **articulation**, **fluency**, and **resonance disorders**. Articulation disorders include difficulties producing sounds in syllables or saying words incorrectly to the point that other people cannot understand what is being said. Fluency disorders include problems such as **stuttering**, the condition in which the flow of speech is interrupted by abnormal stoppages, repetitions ("st-st-stuttering") or prolonging sounds and syllables ("ssssstuttering"). Resonance or voice disorders include problems with the pitch, volume, or quality of a child's voice that distract listeners from what is being said.

Language disorders can be either receptive or expressive. Receptive disorders refer to difficulties understanding or processing language. Expressive disorders include difficulty putting words together, limited vocabulary, or inability to use language in a socially appropriate way.

Speech-language pathologists (speech therapists) are professionals educated in the study of human communication, its development, and its disorders. By assess-

TABLE 10–10. Clues to When a Child with a Communication Disorder Needs Help

0-11 Months

Before 6 months, the child does not startle, blink, or change immediate activity in response to sudden, loud sounds
Before 6 months, the child does not attend to the human voice and is not soothed by his or her mother's voice
By 6 months, the child does not babble strings of consonant and vowel syllables or imitate gurgling or cooing sounds
By 10 months, the child does not respond to his or her name
At 10 months, the child's sound-making is limited to shrieks, grunts, or sustained vowel production

12-23 Months

At 12 months, the child's babbling or speech is limited to vowel sounds
By 15 months, the child does not respond to "no," "bye-bye," or "bottle"
By 15 months, the child does not imitate sounds or words
By 18 months, the child is not consistently using at least six words with appropriate meaning
By 21 months, the child does not respond correctly to "Give me . . . ," "Sit down," or "Come here" when spoken without gestural cues
By 23 months, two-word phrases have not emerged that are spoken as single units ("Whatszit," "Thank you," "Allgone")

24-36 Months

By 24 months, at least 50% of the child's speech is not understood by familiar listeners
By 24 months, the child does not point to body parts without gestural cues
By 24 months, the child is not combining words into phrases ("Go bye-bye," "Go car," "Want cookie")
By 30 months, the child does not show understanding of on, in, under, front, and back
By 30 months, the child is not using short sentences ("Daddy went bye-bye.")
By 30 months, the child has not begun to ask questions, using where, what, why
By 36 months, the child's speech is not understood by unfamiliar listeners

All Ages

At any age, the child is consistently dysfluent with repetitions, hesitations; blocks or struggles to say words. Struggle may be accompanied by grimaces, eye blinks, or hand gestures

Adapted from Weiss CE, Lillywhite HE: Communication Disorders: A Handbook for Prevention and Early Detection. St Louis, Mosby, 1976.

ing the speech, language, cognitive-communication, and swallowing skills of children, speech-language pathologists can determine what types of communication problems exist and the best way to treat these challenges. Speech-language pathologists skilled at working with infants and young children also are vital in training parents and infants in other oral-motor skills, such as teaching the parent of an infant born with cleft lip and palate how to feed the infant appropriately.

Speech-language therapy involves having a speech-language specialist work with a child on a one-on-one basis, in a small group, or directly in a classroom to overcome a specific disorder. Speech-language therapy uses a variety of therapeutic strategies, including language intervention activities and articulation therapy. Language intervention activities involve having a speech-language specialist interact with a child by playing and talking to him or her. The therapist may use pictures, books, objects, or ongoing events to stimulate language development. The therapist also may model correct pronunciation and use repetition exercises to build speech and language skills. Articulation therapy involves having the therapist model correct sounds and syllables for a child, often during play activities. The level of play is age appropriate and related to the child's specific needs. This therapy involves physically showing a child how to make certain sounds, such as the "r" sound. A speech-language therapist may show how a child should move his or her tongue to produce specific sounds.

Children enrolled in therapy early in their development (<3 years old) tend to have better outcomes than children who begin therapy later. This does not mean that older children cannot make progress in therapy; they may progress at a slower rate because they often have learned patterns that need to be modified or changed. Parental involvement is crucial to the success of a child's progress in speech-language therapy.

Cerebral Palsy

CP refers to a group of nonprogressive, but often changing, motor impairment syndromes secondary to anomalies or lesions of the brain usually arising in the early stages of development. A total of 2 to 2.5 of every 1000 live-born children in developed countries have CP; incidence is higher in premature and twin births. Although perinatal asphyxia and kernicterus are causes, occult infection or inflammation is increasingly implicated. Risk factors associated with CP are summarized in Table 10–11. Nearly 50% of children with CP have no identifiable risk factors.

Most children with CP, except in its mildest forms, are diagnosed in the first 18 months when they fail to attain motor milestones or when they show abnormal-

TABLE 10–11. Risk Factors for Cerebral Palsy
Before Pregnancy
Maternal thyroid disorder
History of fetal wastage
Family history of mental retardation
Pregnancy and Birth
Low socioeconomic status
Maternal seizures/seizure disorder
Treatment with thyroid hormone, estrogen, or progesterone
Pregnancy complications
Polyhydramnios
Eclampsia
Third trimester bleeding (including threatened abortion and placenta previa)
Multiple births
Fetal growth retardation
Abnormal fetal presentation
Congenital malformation
Postnatal Period
Newborn hypoxic-ischemic or bilirubin (kernicterus) encephalopathy

ities such as asymmetric gross motor function, increased muscle tone, or floppiness. CP can be characterized further by the affected parts of the body (Table 10-12) and descriptions of the predominant type of motor disorder (Table 10-13). A severity scale ranging from level I, with limitations in only advanced motor skills, but normal walking, to level V, where self-mobility is severely limited even with the use of supporting technology, helps characterize the degree of involvement. Comorbidities in these children often include epilepsy, learning difficulties, behavioral challenges, and sensory impairments.

Treatment depends on the pattern of dysfunction that is present. Physical and occupational therapy can

TABLE 10–12. Descriptions of Cerebral Palsy by Site of Involvement
Hemiparesis (hemiplegia)—predominantly unilateral impairment of the arm and leg on the same (e.g., right or left) side
Diplegia—motor impairment primarily of the legs (often with some limited involvement of the arms; some authors challenge this specific type as not being different from quadriplegia)
Quadriplegia—all four limbs (whole body) are functionally compromised

TABLE 10–13. Classification of Cerebral Palsy by Type of Motor Disorder

Spastic cerebral palsy—the most common form of CP, occurring in 70%-80%. It results from injury to the upper motor neurons of the pyramidal tract. It may occasionally be bilateral. It is characterized by at least two of the following:
 Abnormal movement pattern
 Increased tone
 Pathologic reflexes (e.g., Babinski response, hyperreflexia)
Dyskinetic cerebral palsy—occurs in 10%-15% of cases of CP. It is dominated by abnormal patterns of movement and involuntary, uncontrolled, recurring movements
Ataxic cerebral palsy—accounts for <5% of CP cases. This form of CP results from cerebellar injury and features abnormal posture or movement and loss of orderly muscle coordination or both
Dystonic cerebral palsy—also uncommon. It is characterized by reduced activity and stiff movement (hypokinesia) and hypotonia
Choreoathetotic cerebral palsy—rare now that excessive hyperbilirubinemia is aggressively prevented and treated. This form is dominated by increased and stormy movements (hyperkinesia) and hypotonia
Mixed cerebral palsy (10%-15% of all cases)—term used when more than one type of motor pattern is present and when one pattern does not clearly dominate another. It typically is associated with more complications, including sensory deficits, seizures, and cognitive-perceptual impairments.

facilitate optimal positioning and movement patterns, increasing function of the affected parts. Spasticity management also may include oral medications, botulinum toxin injections, and implantation of intrathecal baclofen pumps. Management of seizures, spasticity, orthopedic impairments, and sensory impairments all may help improve educational attainment. CP cannot be cured, but a host of interventions can improve functional abilities, participation in society, and quality of life. These interventions must involve the whole family and must be in the context of family needs, values, and abilities.

SUGGESTED READING

Anderson L, Shinn C, Fulilove M, et al: The effectiveness of early childhood development programs: A systematic review. Am J Prev Med 24:32-46, 2003.

Behrman RE, Kliegman RM, Jenson HB (eds): Nelson Textbook of Pediatrics, 17th ed. Philadelphia, WB Saunders, 2004, pp 23-66.

Committee on Children with Disabilities: Developmental surveillance and screening of infants and young children. Pediatrics 108:192-196, 2001.

Committee on Injury and Poison Prevention: Office-based counseling for injury prevention (RE9427). Pediatrics 94:566-567, 1994.

Committee on Psychosocial Aspects of Child and Family Health 1995-1996: Guidelines for Health Supervision III. Elk Grove Village, Ill, American Academy of Pediatrics, 1997.

Culbertson J, Newman J, Willis D: Childhood and adolescent psychologic development. Pediatr Clin North Am 50:1-20, 2003.

Glascoe F: Early detection of developmental and behavioral problems. Pediatr Rev 21:272, 2000.

Green M, Palfrey J, Clark E, Anastasi J (eds): Bright Futures: Guidelines for Health Supervision of Infants, Children, and Adolescents, 2nd ed. Arlington, Va, National Center for Education in Maternal and Child Health, 2001.

Kliegman RM, Greenbaum LA, Lye PS (eds): Practical Strategies in Pediatric Diagnosis and Therapy, 2nd ed. Philadelphia, WB Saunders, 2004.

Kuczmarski R, Ogden C, Grummer-Strawn L, et al: CDC growth charts: United States. Advance Data 314:1-8, 2000.

Regalado M, Halfon N: Primary care services promoting optimal child development from birth to age 3 years. Arch Pediatr Adolesc Med 155:1311-1322, 2001.

Rosenbaum P: Cerebral palsy: What parents and doctors want to know. BMJ 326:970-974, 2003.

BEHAVIORAL DISORDERS

Sheila Gahagan

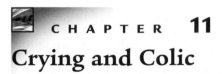

CHAPTER 11

Crying and Colic

All infants cry. Crying can be a sign of pain, distress, hunger, or tiredness, and it is often difficult to interpret the meaning of an infant's cry. Humans interpret their infants' cries according to the context of the crying. The cry of a newborn at the time of delivery heralds the health and vigor of the infant. The screams of the same infant at 6 weeks of age after feeding, changing, and soothing may be interpreted as a sign of illness, difficult temperament, or poor parenting. Crying is a manifestation of infant arousal influenced by the environment and interpreted through the lens of the family, social, and cultural context.

NORMAL DEVELOPMENT

Understanding average normal crying behavior and individual variation includes attention to the characteristics of timing, duration, frequency, intensity, and modifiability of the cry (Fig. 11–1). Most infants cry little during the first 2 weeks of life. Between 2 and 6 weeks, total daily crying duration increases from an average of 2 hours per day to 3 hours per day. By 12 weeks of age, the average daily duration of crying is 1 hour.

Cry duration differs by culture and infant care practices; the duration of crying is 50% lower in the !Kung San hunter gatherers, who continuously carry their infants and feed them four times per hour, compared with infants in the U.S. Premature infants cry little before 40 weeks' gestational age and tend to cry more than term infants around 6 weeks' corrected age. Crying behavior in former premature infants also may be influenced by ongoing medical conditions, such as bronchopulmonary dysplasia, visual impairments, and feeding disorders. At 6 weeks of age, the mean frequency of combined crying and fussing is 9.5 to 10.5 episodes in 24 hours (assessed by parental diary and voice-activated radiotelemetric tape recordings).

Frequency of crying has less individual variability and less variability between cultural groups than duration of crying. Diurnal variation in crying is the norm, with crying concentrated in the late afternoon and evening. The **intensity** of infant cries varies, with descriptions ranging from fussing to crying to screaming. An infant who cries more intensely (pitch and loudness) is more likely to elicit concern or even alarm from the parents and caregivers than an infant who frets more quietly. The mean pitch for the cries of healthy term newborns ranges from 425 to 600 Hz. Pain cries have a higher frequency than hunger cries (510 Hz compared with 450 Hz). Pain cries of newborns are remarkably loud: 80 dB at a distance of 30.5 cm from the infant's mouth. This is 20 dB louder than adult speech. Hunger cries, when not attended to for a protracted period, become acoustically similar to pain cries. Most infant crying is of a lesser intensity, consistent with fussing. The duration of crying is modifiable by caregiving strategies.

COLIC

Colic often is diagnosed using Wessel's "rule of threes"—crying for more than 3 hours per day for more than 3 days per week for more than 3 weeks. The limitations of this definition include the lack of definition of crying (does this include fussing?) and the necessity to wait 3 weeks to make a diagnosis in an infant who has excessive crying. The crying of colic is often described as paroxysmal and may be characterized by facial grimacing, drawing up of the legs, and passing flatus.

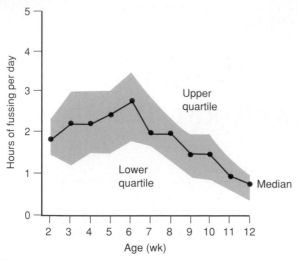

Figure 11–1

Distribution of total crying time among 80 infants studied from 2 to 12 weeks old. Data derived from daily crying diaries recorded by mothers. (From Brazelton TB: Crying in infancy. Pediatrics 29:582, 1962.)

Etiology

Less than 5% of infants evaluated for excessive crying have an organic etiology. Because the etiology of colic is unknown, this syndrome may be the extreme of the normal phenomenon of infant crying. Nonetheless, evaluation of infants with excessive crying is warranted.

Epidemiology

Cumulative incidence rates of colic vary from 5% to 19% in different studies. Girls and boys are affected equally. Studies vary by how colic is defined and by data collection methodology, such as maintaining a cry diary or actual recording of infant vocalizations. Concern about infant crying also varies by culture; this may influence what is recorded as crying or fussing.

Clinical Manifestations

The clinician who evaluates a crying infant must differentiate rare organic disease from colic, which has no identifiable etiology. The family should be asked first to describe the crying, including duration, frequency, intensity, and modifiability. Does the infant have associated symptoms, such as pulling up of the legs, facial grimacing, vomiting, or back arching? When did the crying first begin? Has the crying changed? Does anything relieve the crying? Does anything exacerbate the crying? Is there a diurnal pattern to the crying? A review of systems is essential because crying in an

infant is a systemic symptom that can herald disease in any organ system. Past medical history also is important because infants with perinatal problems are at increased risk for neurologic causes of crying. Attention to the feeding history is crucial because some causes of crying are related to feeding problems, including hunger, air swallowing (worsened by crying), gastroesophageal reflux, and food intolerance. Questions concerning the family's ability to handle the stress of the infant's crying and their knowledge of infant soothing strategies assist the clinician in assessing risk for mental health comorbidities and developing an intervention plan suitable for the family.

The **physical examination** is an essential component of the evaluation of an infant with colic. The diagnosis of colic is made only when the physical examination reveals no organic cause for the infant's excessive crying. The examination begins with vital signs, weight, length, and head circumference, looking for effects of systemic illness on growth, such as occur with infection or malnutrition. A thorough inspection of the infant is important to identify possible sources of pain, including skin lesions, **corneal abrasions**, **hair tourniquets**, **skeletal infections**, or signs of child abuse such as **fractures** (see Chapters 22 and 197). Infants with common conditions such as otitis media, urinary tract infections, mouth sores, and insect bites may present with crying. A neurologic examination may reveal previously undiagnosed neurologic conditions, such as perinatal brain injuries, as the cause of irritability and crying. Observation of the infant during a crying episode is invaluable to assess the infant's potential for calming and the parent's skill in soothing the infant.

Laboratory and imaging studies are reserved for infants in whom there are history or physical examination findings suggesting an organic cause for excessive crying. An algorithm for the medical evaluation of an infant with excessive crying inconsistent with colic is presented in Figure 11–2.

Differential Diagnosis

Excessive crying of infancy is multifactorial in origin. The differential diagnosis for colic is broad and includes any condition that can cause pain or discomfort in the infant and conditions associated with "nonpainful" distress, such as fatigue or sensory overload (Table 11–1).

Cow's milk protein intolerance, maternal drug effects (including fluoxetine hydrochloride via breastfeeding), and anomalous left coronary artery all have been reported as causes of persistent crying. In addition, situations associated with poor infant regulation, including fatigue, hunger, parental anxiety, and chaotic environmental conditions, may increase the

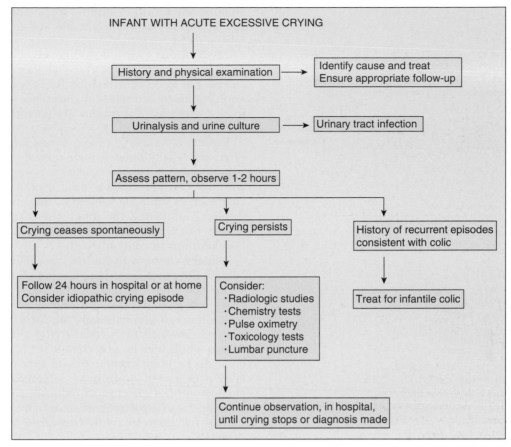

INFANT WITH ACUTE EXCESSIVE CRYING

History and physical examination → Identify cause and treat
Ensure appropriate follow-up

Urinalysis and urine culture → Urinary tract infection

Assess pattern, observe 1-2 hours

Crying ceases spontaneously

Crying persists

History of recurrent episodes consistent with colic

Follow 24 hours in hospital or at home
Consider idiopathic crying episode

Consider:
· Radiologic studies
· Chemistry tests
· Pulse oximetry
· Toxicology tests
· Lumbar puncture

Treat for infantile colic

Continue observation, in hospital, until crying stops or diagnosis made

Figure 11–2

Algorithm for medical evaluation of infants with acute excessive crying. (From Barr RG, et al: Crying complaints in the emergency department. In Crying as a Sign, a Symptom, and a Signal. London, MacKeith Press, 2000.)

risk for excessive crying. In most cases, the cause of crying in infants is unexplained. If the condition began before 3 weeks' corrected age, the crying has a diurnal pattern consistent with colic (afternoon and evening clustering), the infant is otherwise developing and thriving, and no organic cause is found, a diagnosis of colic is indicated.

Treatment

The management of colic begins with education and demystification. When the family and the physician are reassured that the infant is healthy, and no infection, trauma, or underlying disease is present, education about the normal pattern of infant crying is appropriate. Learning about the temporal pattern of colic can be reassuring; the mean crying duration begins to decrease at 6 weeks of age and decreases by half by 12 weeks of age. Parents should not be told that colic resolves by 3 months of age, however, when at that point the mean duration of crying is 1 hour per day. Approximately 15% of infants with colic continue to have excessive crying after 3 months of age.

Helping families develop caregiving schedules that accommodate the infant's fussy period is useful. For most families, it is important to have someone available who can attend to the infant during the afternoon and evening fussy periods. Techniques for soothing infants include soothing vocalizations or singing, swaddling, slow rhythmic rocking, walking, white noise, and gentle vibration (e.g., a ride in a car). Products are available that simulate the effects of a car ride in the infant's crib. Giving caretakers permission to allow the infant to rest when soothing strategies are not working may alleviate overstimulation in some infants; this also relieves families of guilt and allows them a wider range of responses to infant crying. **Avoidance** of dangerous soothing techniques, such as

TABLE 11–1.   Diagnoses in 56 Infants Presenting to the Denver Children's Hospital Emergency Department with an Episode of Unexplained, Excessive Crying

Diagnosis	No. with Diagnosis
Idiopathic	10
Infectious	
Otitis media*	10
Viral illness with anorexia, dehydration*	2
Urinary tract infection*	1
Mild prodrome of gastroenteritis	1
Herpangina*	1
Herpes stomatitis*	1
Trauma	
Corneal abrasion*	3
Foreign body in eye*	1
Foreign body in oropharynx*	1
Tibial fracture (from child abuse)*	1
Clavicular fracture (accidental)*	1
Brown recluse spider bite*	1
Hair tourniquet syndrome (hair wrapped tightly around digit)	1
Gastrointestinal	
Constipation	3
Intussusception*	1
Gastroesophageal reflux*	1
CNS	
Subdural hematoma (bleeding around the brain from child abuse)*	1
Encephalitis*	1
Pseudotumor cerebri*	1
Drug reaction/overdose	
DTP reaction†	1
Inadvertent pseudoephedrine (cold medication) overdose	1
Behavioral	
Night terrors	1
Overstimulation	1
Cardiovascular	
Supraventricular tachycardia*	2
Metabolic	
Glutaric aciduria type 1*	1
Total	56

*Indicates conditions considered serious.
†From diphtheria/tetanus/pertussis (DTP) vaccine.
From Barr RG, et al: Crying complaints in the emergency department. In Crying as a Sign, a Symptom, and a Symbol. London, MacKeith Press, 2000; with permission.

shaking the infant or placing the infant on a vibrating clothes dryer (which has resulted in injury from falls), should be stressed.

Medications, including phenobarbital, diphenhydramine, alcohol, simethicone, dicyclomine, and lactase, are of no benefit in reducing colic. Sedatives, antihistamines, antireflux medications, alcohol, and motion sickness medications are potentially harmful and should be avoided.

Parents, especially from Mexico and Eastern Europe, often use chamomile, fennel, vervain, licorice, and balm-mint teas. These teas have not been studied scientifically as remedies for colic. Families should be counseled to limit the volume of tea given because it displaces milk from the infant's diet and may limit caloric intake. Teas may be lead contaminated or botulinum toxin contaminated.

Dietary changes should be considered in certain specific circumstances. There is rationale for change to a non–cow's milk formula if the infant has signs of cow's milk protein colitis. If the infant is breastfeeding, the mother can eliminate dairy products from her diet. Another rare cause of excessive crying is fructose intolerance, which may be suspected if the onset of crying coincides with the introduction of fruit juice or black current or fennel tea. In most circumstances, dietary changes are not effective in reducing colic, but they may appear to help because their use coincides with the natural reduction in crying between 6 and 12 weeks of age.

Prognosis

Infants with colic have not been shown to have adverse long-term outcomes in health or temperament after the neonatal period. Similarly, infantile colic does not have untoward long-term effects on maternal mental health. When the colic subsides, the maternal distress resolves. Infantile colic can lead to early discontinuation of breastfeeding and premature introduction of infant solids. Family distress is a common complication of excessive infant crying. Cases of child abuse have been associated with inconsolable infant crying, including death due to child abuse. In these latter cases, other risk factors interact with the infant's crying to result in death of the infant.

Prevention

Much can be done to prevent colic, beginning with education of all prospective parents about the normal pattern of infant crying. Prospective parents often imagine that they will not "let their infant cry," not realizing that some of the infant's behavior and state regulation are beyond their control. Instead, new parents can plan realistically how they will manage the hours late in the day when they may be tired and hungry themselves with an infant who may be crying inconsolably. Increased contact and carrying of the infant in the weeks before the onset of colic may decrease the duration of crying episodes. Similarly, other soothing strategies may be more effective if the infant has experienced them before the onset of the excessive crying. Infants who have been tightly swaddled for sleep and rest during the first weeks of life often calm to swaddling during a crying episode; this is not true for infants who have not experienced swaddling before a crying episode. Parents also can be coached to learn to read their infant's cues and ask themselves if the infant is hungry, uncomfortable, bored, or overstimulated. Parents also should be counseled that there are times when the infant's cry is not interpretable, and caregivers can only do their best.

CHAPTER 12
Temper Tantrums

A temper tantrum is defined as out of control behavior, including screaming, stomping, hitting, head banging, falling down, and other violent displays of frustration. In the extreme, tantrums can include breath holding, vomiting, conjunctival hemorrhages, and serious aggression, including biting. Such behavior is seen most often when the young child experiences frustration, anger, or simple inability to cope with a situation. Temper tantrums can be considered normal behavior in 1- to 3-year-old children, when the temper tantrum period is of short duration and the tantrums are not manipulative in nature. Some reserve the term *temper tantrum* for pathologic behavior.

ETIOLOGY

Temper tantrums are believed to be a normal human developmental stage. Child temperament may be a determinant of tantrum behavior.

EPIDEMIOLOGY

This behavior is common in children age 18 months to 4 years. In U.S. studies, 50% to 80% of 2- to 3-year-old children have had regular tantrums, and 20% are reported to have daily tantrums. The behavior appears to peak late in the third year of life. Approximately 20% of 4-year-olds are still having regular temper tantrums, and explosive temper occurs in approximately 5% of school-age children. Tantrums occur equally in boys and girls during the preschool period.

CLINICAL MANIFESTATIONS

Temper tantrums are the most commonly reported behavioral problem in 2- and 3-year-old children. The typical frequency of tantrums is approximately one per week with a great deal of variability (Fig. 12–1). The duration of each tantrum is 2 to 5 minutes, and duration increases with age (Fig. 12–2). Helping the family to identify the typical antecedents of the child's tantrums is essential to evaluation and intervention. A child who has tantrums only when he or she misses a routine nap can be treated differently than a child who has frequent tantrums related to minor difficulties or disappointments.

The **evaluation** of a child who is having temper tantrums requires a complete history, including perinatal and developmental information. Describing behavioral patterns can aid in the identification of a genetic disorder. Careful attention to the child's daily routines may reveal problems associated with hunger, fatigue, inadequate physical activity, or overstimulation. A social history is important because family stress can exacerbate or prolong what begins as a normal developmental phase. When this normal behavior is frequent or occurs beyond age 3, the possibility of family stress or conditions that reinforce the tantrum behavior should be considered. Some children may be exposed to violence in the home and may be exhibiting learned behavior. The coexistence of other behavioral problems, such as sleep problems, learning problems, and social problems, suggests the possibility of a more serious mental health disorder.

The physical examination focuses on discovering underlying illness that could decrease the child's ability to self-regulate. Thorough examination of the skin to

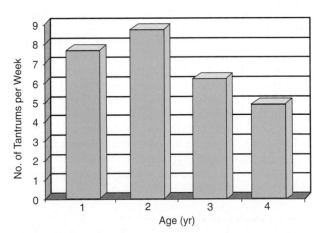

Figure 12–1

Mean tantrum frequency per week. Children 1 to 4 years old who have tantrums typically have four to nine tantrums per week.

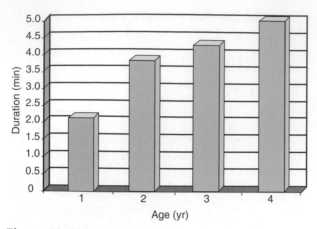

Figure 12–2

Mean duration of tantrums. The typical duration of a tantrum increases with the age of the child.

identify child abuse is recommended (see Chapter 22). The neurologic examination identifies underlying brain disorders. Dysmorphic features may reveal a genetic syndrome. Behavioral observations reveal a child's ability to follow instructions, play with age-appropriate toys, and interact with parents and clinician.

Laboratory studies screening for iron deficiency anemia and lead exposure are important. Other laboratory and imaging studies are performed only when the history and physical examination suggest a possible underlying etiology.

DIFFERENTIAL DIAGNOSIS

Most children who have temper tantrums have no underlying medical problem. In rare instances, seizures may mimic a tantrum. Hearing loss and language delay are associated with temper tantrums. Children with brain injury and other brain disorders are at increased risk for prolonged temper tantrum behavior (in terms of actual tantrum duration and continued manifestation after the normal tantrum age). These children include former premature infants and children with autism, traumatic brain injury, cognitive impairment, and Prader-Willi and Smith-Magenis syndromes. Children with rare conditions, such as congenital adrenal hyperplasia and precocious puberty, also may present with severe and persistent tantrums.

TREATMENT

Intervention begins with parental education about temper tantrums, stressing that tantrums are a normal developmental phase (Table 12–1). Parents may have

unwarranted fears about their own parenting skills or their child's mental health. The clinician can allay their fears and move them toward more effective parenting. Preventing temper tantrums is a realistic goal. Parents can understand that their role is to help the child move toward self-regulation of frustration and anger. Young toddlers do not have highly developed frontal lobe control. Parents and other caregivers can provide some external control of the child's behavior by preventing hunger, fatigue, loneliness, or hyperstimulation. The environment can be structured to limit toddler frustration and age-inappropriate demands on the child. When the inevitable event occurs, the parent can take a moment to look at the big picture and ask what can be done to move the child quickly back into a state of control without reinforcing an unreasonable 2-year-old's demand. It is important to review the child's daily routine to understand whether the child's behavior is communicating an essential unmet need. Children who behave well all day at daycare and exhibit temper tantrums at home in the evening may be signaling that they need parental attention at that moment. It is possible that the child is tired from the day and simply needs to go to bed earlier. Identification of underlying stress is the cornerstone of treatment because many stressors can be eliminated. If the child is required to put away toys before a snack and always has a tantrum, the parent could consider switching the order of the activities. It is possible that the child is hungry at that moment and cannot handle the delay in nourishment. Parents may consider some changes in the home environment so that they do not have to say "No" to the child as frequently. A child who is intent on playing with the parent's CD player may have fewer tantrums if the CD player is out of sight in a locked cabinet.

In some cases, parents inadvertently reinforce tantrum behavior by complying with the child's

---

TABLE 12–1. Intervention for Temper Tantrums

Explain age-appropriate norms for tantrum behavior
Review child's daily routine—adequate sleep, food, nurturing?
Review antecedents to tantrums—pattern?
Clarify parental expectations and restrictions
Remedy unmet needs
Eliminate unnecessary antecedents
Consistent age-appropriate expectations
Reinforce desired behavior with parental attention
Behavioral therapy designed to decrease tantrum behavior (usually not necessary)

demands. A 2-year-old who has learned that her mother will give her soda pop when she screams may repeat this behavior to get what she wants. The child's behavior can be seen as manipulative, but it may be learned behavior from a prior successful experience. Parental ambivalence about acceptable toddler behavior also may lead to inconsistent expectations and restrictions. Helping parents to clarify what their child is allowed to do and what behavior is off limits can avert the temptation to give in when the child screams loudly or publicly.

Distraction from the frustrating object or event is an effective means of short-circuiting impending tantrums. Physically removing the child from an environment that is associated with the child's difficulty is sometimes helpful. Children who have difficulty with noisy or visually stimulating environments can be protected from that type of overstimulation until they are more mature.

Further behavioral interventions are recommended only after strategies to help the child gain control by meeting basic needs, altering the environment, and anticipating meltdowns are in place. Behavioral strategies employed by mental health professionals include behavior modification with positive and negative reinforcement, extinction, and pharmacotherapy.

During the first week of any behavioral intervention, a child may increase tantrum behavior. Parents must be warned that it will probably get worse before it gets better. At the same time that parents are working to extinguish or decrease the tantrums, it is important that they provide positive reinforcement for good behavior. It also is advisable to spend time with the child when his or her behavior is desirable, reinforcing behavior that the parents enjoy.

COMPLICATIONS

The complications of tantrums include minor bruises and lacerations. There are no case reports of self-inflicted subdural hemorrhage or other serious injuries from a temper tantrum. Child abuse can be a complication of temper tantrums.

PREVENTION

Providing parents with knowledge about the temper tantrum stage and strategies for assisting the child with emotional regulation is recommended at a healthcare maintenance visit between 12 and 18 months. Regular routines for sleeping, eating, and physical activity in a childproofed home (or daycare center) provided by well-rested and psychologically healthy parents (or caregivers) usually result in a quick transition through this challenging period.

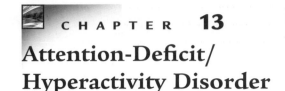

CHAPTER 13
Attention-Deficit/Hyperactivity Disorder

Attention-deficit/hyperactivity disorder (ADHD) is a neurobehavioral disorder defined by symptoms of inattention, hyperactivity, and impulsivity. Current clinical guidelines emphasize the use of the *Diagnostic and Statistical Manual of Mental Health Disorders, Fourth Edition,* criteria to diagnose ADHD (Table 13–1). These criteria require that the child have symptoms in at least two environments and functional impairment in addition to the symptoms of the disorder for diagnosis.

ETIOLOGY

ADHD is a complex of symptoms with diverse etiology. There is evidence that ADHD runs in some families, but no evidence of any single gene that determines ADHD type. ADHD can be seen in children who have other forms of brain developmental disorder, including fetal alcohol syndrome and Down syndrome, and in children who have had varying levels of brain injury, including perinatal brain damage. Most commonly, there is no identified cause for ADHD. It is likely that the symptoms of ADHD represent a final common pathway for diverse causes, including genetic, organic, and environmental etiologies (perhaps in combination).

EPIDEMIOLOGY

The estimated prevalence of ADHD in U.S. school-age community populations is 8% to 10%, with boys having a two to three times higher prevalence than girls. Girls are more likely to be diagnosed with inattentive-type ADHD. Symptoms of ADHD persist into adolescence in 60% to 80% of patients. Many continue to have symptoms into adulthood.

CLINICAL MANIFESTATIONS

The diagnosis of ADHD is made by **history**. The clinician should elicit the history by interview using open-ended questions focused on specific behaviors or by using ADHD-specific rating scales. ADHD rating scales are sensitive and specific for diagnosing ADHD. The Conners Questionnaires and the Vanderbilt forms are two commonly used parent and teacher questionnaires. Other types of child behavior rating scales, such

TABLE 13–1. Diagnostic Criteria for Attention-Deficit/Hyperactivity Disorder

A. Either 1 or 2
  1. Six (or more) of the following symptoms of **inattention** have persisted for at least 6 mo to a degree that is maladaptive and inconsistent with developmental level
  Inattention
     a. Often fails to give close attention to details or makes careless mistakes in schoolwork, work, or other activities
     b. Often has difficulty sustaining attention in tasks or play activities
     c. Often does not seem to listen when spoken to directly
     d. Often does not follow through on instructions and fails to finish schoolwork, chores, or duties in the workplace (not due to oppositional behavior or failure to understand instructions)
     e. Often has difficulty organizing tasks and activities
     f. Often avoids, dislikes, or is reluctant to engage in tasks that require sustained mental effort (e.g., schoolwork or homework)
     g. Often loses things necessary for tasks or activities (e.g., toys, school assignments, pencils, books, or tools)
     h. Is often easily distracted by extraneous stimuli
     i. Is often forgetful in daily activities
  2. Six (or more) of the following symptoms of **hyperactivity-impulsivity** have persisted for at least 6 mo to a degree that is maladaptive and inconsistent with developmental level
  Hyperactivity
     a. Often fidgets with hands or feet or squirms in seat
     b. Often leaves seat in classroom or in other situations in which remaining seated is expected
     c. Often runs about or climbs excessively in situations in which it is inappropriate (in adolescents or adults, may be limited to subjective feelings of restlessness)
     d. Often has difficulty playing or engaging in leisure activities quietly
     e. Is often "on the go" or often acts as if "driven by a motor"
     f. Often talks excessively
  Impulsivity
     g. Often blurts out answers before questions have been completed
     h. Often has difficulty awaiting turn
     i. Often interrupts or intrudes on others (e.g., butts into conversations or games)
B. Some hyperactive-impulsive or inattentive symptoms that caused impairment were present <7 yr of age
C. Some impairment from the symptoms is present in two or more settings (e.g., at school [or work] and at home)
D. There must be clear evidence of clinically significant impairment in social, academic, or occupational functioning
E. The symptoms do not occur exclusively during the course of a pervasive developmental disorder, schizophrenia, or other psychotic disorder and are not better accounted for by another mental disorder (e.g., mood disorder, anxiety disorder, dissociative disorder, or personality disorder)

Code based on type:
314.01 Attention-Deficit/Hyperactivity Disorder, Combined Type: if both criteria A1 and A2 are met for the past 6 mo
314.00 Attention-Deficit/Hyperactivity Disorder, Predominantly Inattentive Type: if criterion A1 is met but criterion A2 is not met for the past 6 mo
314.01 Attention-Deficit/Hyperactivity Disorder, Predominantly Hyperactive, Impulsive Type: if criterion A2 is met but criterion A1 is not met for the past 6 mo
314.9 Attention-Deficit/Hyperactivity Disorder Not Otherwise Specified

From the American Psychiatric Association: Diagnostic and Statistical Manual of Mental Disorders, 4th ed (DSM-IV). Arlington, Va, American Psychiatric Association, 1994.

as the Auchenbach Child Behavior Checklist, are not specific for the diagnosis of ADHD.

The **physical examination** is essential to rule out possible underlying medical or developmental problems. The examination should include the observation of the child and the parents and their relationship. It is a mistake to interpret absence of hyperactivity in the office as a sign that the child does not have ADHD. It is common for children with ADHD to focus without hyperactivity in an environment that has low stimulation and little distraction.

Laboratory and imaging studies are not routinely recommended. The clinician may consider thyroid function studies, blood lead levels, genetic karyotyping, and brain imaging studies if any of these studies are indicated by past medical history, environmental history, or physical examination. These studies do not confirm ADHD, but are useful in excluding other conditions.

DIFFERENTIAL DIAGNOSIS

The differential diagnosis includes hyperactivity and distractibility secondary to hyperthyroidism or lead intoxication. Chaotic living situations also can lead to symptoms of hyperactivity, distractibility, and inattention. Children who have symptoms of ADHD in only one setting may be having problems secondary to cognitive level, level of emotional maturity, or feelings of well-being in that particular setting.

Comorbid conditions commonly occur with ADHD, including speech-language delay and learning disabilities (see Chapter 8). Psychiatric conditions, such as conduct disorder, depression, and anxiety disorder, also are more common in children with ADHD than in the general population (see Section IV).

TREATMENT

Management begins with recognizing ADHD as a chronic condition and educating affected children and their parents about the symptoms of ADHD and mechanisms to control the adverse effects of the condition on learning, school functioning, social relationships, and family life. Children with ADHD benefit from **behavioral approaches** to accommodate their condition. It is helpful to providing structure, routine, and appropriate behavioral goals. Some children benefit from social skills counseling or mental health treatment to assist behavior change or to preserve self-esteem.

Stimulant medication is effective for managing the symptoms of inattention, hyperactivity, and distractibility in most children with ADHD. Stimulant medications do not treat the comorbid conditions and do not improve intelligence. Short-acting, intermediate-acting, and long-acting methylphenidate and long-acting dextroamphetamine are widely used stimulant medications. Nonstimulant medications, including tricyclic antidepressants and bupropion, may be helpful for children who have not responded to stimulant medications, but should be prescribed by health professionals with significant experience using these medications. Clonidine also can be helpful for children with ADHD, especially for children with sleep disorders. Dosing for ADHD medications is listed in Table 13-2. Common side effects of stimulant medication include appetite suppression and sleep disturbance.

TABLE 13–2. Medications Used in the Treatment of Attention-Deficit/Hyperactivity Disorder

Generic Class (Brand Name)	Daily Dosage Schedule	Duration	Prescribing Schedule
Stimulants (First-Line Treatment)			
Methylphenidate			
Short-acting (Ritalin, Metadate, Methylin)	bid-tid	3-5 hr	5-20 mg bid-tid
Intermediate-acting (Ritalin-SR, Metadate ER, Methylin ER)	qd-bid	3-8 hr	20-40 mg qd or 40 mg in the morning and 20 mg in the early afternoon
Extended release (Concerta, Metadate CD, Ritalin LA*)	qd	8-12 hr	18-72 mg qd
Amphetamine			
Short-acting (Dexedrine, Dextrostat)	bid-tid	4-6 hr	5-15 mg bid or 5-10 mg tid
Intermediate-acting (Adderall, Dexedrine Spansule)	qd-bid	6-8 hr	5-30 mg qd or 5-15 mg bid
Extended Release (Adderall XR*)	qd		10-30 mg qd
Antidepressants (Second-Line Treatment)			
Tricyclics			
Imipramine, desipramine	bid-tid		2-5 mg/kg/day†
Bupropion			
Wellbutrin	qd-tid		50-100 mg tid
Wellbutrin SR	bid		100-150 mg bid

†Prescribing and monitoring information in Physicians' Desk Reference; currently FDA approved.
From American Academy of Pediatrics: Clinical Practice Guideline: Treatment of the school-aged child with attention-deficit/hyperactivity disorder. Pediatrics 108:1033-1044, 2001.

These side effects usually can be managed by careful adjustment of dosage and timing of the medication.

Many parents worry that their child may develop illicit drug use and even addiction because of taking stimulant medication. Children with ADHD may be at increased risk for drug use during adolescence because of their impulsivity. Nonetheless, there is a decreased risk of drug abuse in children with ADHD who are well managed medically.

COMPLICATIONS

ADHD may be associated with academic under-achievement, difficulties in interpersonal relationships, and poor self-esteem.

PREVENTION

Little is known about prevention of ADHD. Child-rearing practices that include promoting calm environments and opportunities for increasing length of focus on age-appropriate activities may be helpful. Limiting time spent watching television and playing rapid-response video games also may be prudent because these activities reinforce short attention span. Prevention of secondary disabilities can be achieved by education of medical professionals and educators about the signs and symptoms of ADHD and the most appropriate interventions (behavioral and pharmaceutical).

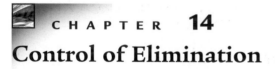

CHAPTER 14
Control of Elimination

NORMAL DEVELOPMENT OF ELIMINATION

Development of control of urination and defecation involves physical and cognitive maturation and is strongly influenced by cultural norms and practices. Toilet training practices differ in various cultural and economic groups in the U.S. There is even greater diversity of toilet training practices and age of acquisition of toilet mastery throughout the world and historically. In the first half of the 20th century, toilet mastery by 18 months of age was the norm in the U.S. Concern about harsh toilet training and possible later psychological distress led to professional endorsement of later toilet training. In 1962, Brazelton introduced the *child-centered approach,* which respects the child's autonomy and pride in mastery. The invention of disposable diapers also facilitated later toilet training. Changes in

family life, including maternal work and the use of daycare centers, also have influenced this trend because most childcare centers do not teach toilet mastery, leaving this task to families. Families in which both parents work often choose to wait until the child is older because the duration of the training period is shorter. Toilet training usually begins after the second birthday and is achieved at about age 3 years in middle-class white U.S. populations. Toilet training between 12 and 18 months continues to be accepted in lower income families.

Prerequisites for achieving elimination in the toilet include the child's ability to recognize the sensation of urination and defecation, get to the toilet, maintain adequate attention span to sit for the necessary time, take pride in achievement or parental pleasure, understand the sequence of tasks required, and avoid oppositional behavior. The entire process of toilet training can take 6 months and need not be hurried. Successful parent-child interaction around the goal of toilet mastery can set the stage for future active parental teaching and training (e.g., manners, kindness, rules and laws, and limit setting). Toilet training is often most successful when the child wears a minimum of loose-fitting clothing without snaps, buttons, or zippers. Some parents favor a "no pants" approach in their own home or backyard. Keeping the child clean and dry is important so that the child is accustomed to and happiest in this condition. Modern highly absorbent diapers may remove much of the discomfort that motivates the child toward achievement of toilet mastery. Getting the child out of diapers for the training experience may be helpful. Praise for accomplishment of any step of the process bolsters the child's feeling of accomplishment. The child may be praised for getting to the toilet, even if the urination happens on the floor in front of the toilet. Other opportunities for praise include recognition of impending urination or defecation, removal of clothing, using toilet paper, or hand washing. Parents must understand that there will be accidents. Homes that can accommodate an occasional accident are ideal. If the home is entirely carpeted, outdoor toilet training in the summertime may provide a less stressful option. Regressions or occasional accidents are normal, and the child's self-esteem should be preserved on these occasions.

ENURESIS

Enuresis is urinary incontinence in a child who is considered adequately mature to have achieved continence. Enuresis is classified as diurnal (daytime) or nocturnal (nighttime). Daytime dryness is expected in the U.S. by age 4 years. Nighttime dryness is expected by age 6 years. Another useful classification of enuresis is **primary** (incontinence in a child who has never achieved dryness) and **secondary** (incontinence in a child who has been dry for at least 6 months).

Etiology

Enuresis is a symptom with multiple possible etiologic factors, including developmental difference, organic illness, or psychological distress. Primary enuresis often is associated with a family history of delayed acquisition of bladder control. A genetic etiology has been hypothesized, and familial groups with autosomal dominant phenotypic patterns for nocturnal enuresis have been identified. Although most children with enuresis do not have a psychiatric disorder, stressful life events can trigger loss of bladder control. Sleep physiology may play a role in the etiology of nocturnal enuresis with a high arousal threshold commonly noted. In a subgroup of enuretic children, nocturnal polyuria relates to a lack of a nocturnal vasopressin peak. Another possible etiology is malfunction of the detrusor muscle such that it has a tendency for involuntary contractions even when the bladder contains small amounts of urine. Reduced bladder capacity can be associated with enuresis and is commonly seen in children who have chronic constipation with a large dilated distal colon, which impinges on the bladder.

Epidemiology

Enuresis is the most common urologic condition in children. Nocturnal enuresis has a reported prevalence of 7% in 8-year-olds and 1% in 15-year-olds. The spontaneous remission rate is reported to be 15% per year. The odds ratio of nocturnal enuresis in boys compared with girls is 1.4:1. The prevalence of daytime enuresis is lower than nocturnal enuresis but has a female predominance. Estimates of prevalence are 2% in boys and 3% in girls at age 7 years. Of children with enuresis, 22% wet only during the day, 17% wet during the day and at night, and 61% wet at night only. Large family size and father absence were independently associated with enuresis.

Clinical Manifestations

The **history** begins with elucidating the pattern of voiding: How often does wetting occur? Does it occur during the day, night, or both? Are there any associated conditions with wetting episodes (e.g., bad dreams, consumption of caffeinated beverages, or exhausting days)? Has the child had a period of dryness in the past? Was a change in wetting pattern preceded by a stressful event, such as a family move, birth of a sibling, or death of a family member? A review of systems should include a developmental history and detailed information about the neurologic, urinary, and gastrointestinal systems (including patterns of defecation). A history of sleep patterns also is important, including snoring, parasomnias, and timing of nighttime urination, if known. A family history often reveals that one or both parents had enuresis as children. Although enuresis is rarely associated with child abuse, physical and sexual abuse history should be included as part of the psychosocial history. Many families have tried numerous interventions before seeking a physician's help. Identifying these interventions and how they were carried out assists the physician's understanding of the child's condition and its role within the family.

The **physical examination** begins with observation of the child and the parent for clues about child developmental and parent-child interaction patterns. Special attention is paid to the abdominal, neurologic, and genital examination. A rectal examination is recommended if the child has chronic constipation. Observation of voiding is recommended if a history of voiding problems, such as hesitancy or dribbling, is elicited. The lumbosacral spine should be examined for signs of spinal dysraphism or a tethered cord.

For most children with enuresis, the only laboratory test recommended is a clean catch urinalysis to look for chronic urinary tract infection (UTI), renal disease, and diabetes mellitus. Further testing, such as urine culture, is based on the urinalysis. Children with complicated enuresis, including children with previous UTI, severe voiding dysfunction, positive urine culture, or a neurologic finding, are evaluated with a renal sonogram and a voiding cystourethrogram. If vesicoureteral reflux, hydronephrosis, or posterior urethral valves are found, the child is referred to an urologist for further evaluation and treatment.

Differential Diagnosis

Most children with enuresis have no identified cause of their condition. In most cases, enuresis resolves by adolescence without treatment. Children with primary nocturnal enuresis are most likely to have a family history and are least likely to have an identified etiology. Children with secondary diurnal and nocturnal enuresis are more likely to have an organic etiology, such as UTI, diabetes mellitus, or diabetes insipidus, to explain their symptoms. Children with primary diurnal and nocturnal enuresis may have a neurodevelopmental condition or a problem with bladder function. Children with secondary nocturnal enuresis may have a psychosocial stressor as a predisposing condition for enuresis.

Treatment

Treatment of underlying organic causes of enuresis, including UTIs, diabetes mellitus, sleep disorders, and urologic abnormalities, is essential. Elimination of underlying chronic constipation is often curative. For a child whose enuresis is not associated with an identifiable disorder, all therapies must be considered in terms of cost in time, money, disruption to the family, the treatment's known success rate, and the child's likelihood to recover spontaneously from the condition without treatment. Treatment options include **conditioning therapy**, **pharmacotherapy**, and **hypnotherapy**. The clinician also should assist the family in making a plan to help the child cope with this problem until it is resolved. Many children have to live with enuresis for months to years before a cure is achieved, and a few children have symptoms into adulthood. A plan for handling wet garments and linens in a non-humiliating and hygienic manner preserves the child's self-esteem. Considering aesthetics to ensure that the child's bedroom and clothing do not smell badly is helpful to families. Simple recommendations include the use of plastic mattress covers, protective pads over the sheets, and a covered laundry pail for bed linens and pajamas. The child should take as much responsibility as he or she is able, depending on age, development, and family culture.

The most widely used **conditioning therapy** for nocturnal enuresis is the **enuresis alarm**. Enuresis alarms have an initial success rate of 70% with a relapse rate of 10%. The use of an alarm requires commitment from the parent and the child. The alarm has a probe that is placed in the underpants or pajamas in front of the urethra. The alarm sounds when the first drop of urine contacts the probe. The alarm is worn on the wrist or clipped onto a layer of clothing. The child is instructed to get up and finish voiding in the bathroom when the alarm sounds. After 3 to 5 months, 70% of children are sleeping through the night without nighttime wetting. **Conditioned awakening** to a full bladder is an equally successful outcome. Although these devices are inexpensive, they are often unavailable to low-income families because most insurance companies do not cover the cost of purchase.

Children with daytime enuresis and small bladder capacity often are treated with **bladder stretching exercises**, in which the child is asked to practice holding urination for longer and longer periods. A reward system often is used in conjunction with this practice. Anticholinergic drugs, such as oxybutynin (5 mg two to three times a day for children 5 years and older) often are used for 2 to 3 months during "bladder stretching." There are no controlled trials of this intervention.

Pharmacotherapy for nighttime enuresis includes tricyclic antidepressants and desmopressin acetate. **Imipramine** reduces the frequency of nighttime wetting. The initial dose for children 6 years and older is 25 mg 1 hour before bedtime. The dose may be increased to 50 mg after 1 week. The maximum dose for children younger than 12 years is 50 mg; it is 75 mg for those 12 years and older. The initial success rate is 50%. Imipramine is effective only during treatment, with a relapse rate of 90% on discontinuation of the medication. The most important contraindication is risk for overdose (associated with fatal cardiac arrhythmia). **Desmopressin** is also used to treat enuresis and has proved to be safe. It is available in an oral form, which is more acceptable than the nasal spray formulation. The oral medication is started at 0.2 mg per dose (one dose at bedtime) and on subsequent nights is increased to 0.4 mg and then to 0.6 mg if needed. Desmopressin decreases the number of wet nights per week by 1.34. This treatment must be considered symptomatic, not curative, and has a relapse rate of 90% when the medication is discontinued.

Hypnotherapy has a reported 44% success rate without relapse; an additional 31% showed significant improvement in the number of dry nights. Hypnotherapy for enuresis should be offered by health or mental health professionals who are qualified to evaluate and treat enuresis by other modalities and who have training in pediatric hypnotherapy.

Complications

There are no medical complications to enuresis that is not caused by other organic underlying conditions or treatments. The psychological consequences can be severe, however. Families can minimize the impact on the child's self-esteem by avoiding punitive approaches and ensuring that the child is competent to handle issues of their own comfort, hygiene, and aesthetics.

Prevention

Although there are no studies on prevention of enuresis, prevention and early identification of chronic constipation can eliminate one common cause of enuresis. Early diagnosis and treatment of sleep disorders can eliminate another cause of nocturnal enuresis. Appropriate anticipatory guidance concerning toilet training to educate parents that 15% of 5-year-olds and 7% of 8-year-olds regularly wet the bed helps to alleviate considerable anxiety about children who do not achieve nighttime dryness early in childhood.

FUNCTIONAL CONSTIPATION AND SOILING

Constipation is decreased frequency of bowel movements usually associated with a hard stool consistency. The occurrence of pain at defecation frequently accompanies constipation. Although underlying gastrointestinal, endocrinologic, or neurologic disorders can cause constipation, *functional constipation* implies that there is no identifiable causative organic condition. *Encopresis* is the regular, voluntary or involuntary passage of feces into a place other than the toilet after 4 years of age. Encopresis without constipation is uncommon and may be a symptom of oppositional defiant disorder or other psychiatric illness. *Soiling* is the involuntary passage of stool and often is associated with fecal impaction. The normal frequency of bowel movements declines between birth and 4 years of age, beginning with greater than four stools per day to approximately one per day.

Etiology

The etiology of functional constipation and soiling includes a low-fiber diet, slow gastrointestinal transit time for neurologic or genetic reasons, and withholding of bowel movements because of pain, discomfort, or psychological distress. Approximately 95% of children referred to a subspecialist for encopresis have no other underlying pathologic condition.

Epidemiology

In U.S. studies, 16% to 37% of children experience constipation between ages 5 and 12. Constipation with overflow soiling occurs in 1% to 2% of preschool children and 4% of school-age children. The incidence of constipation and soiling is equal in preschool girls and boys, whereas there is a male predominance during school age.

Clinical Manifestations

The presenting complaint for constipation with soiling is typically a complaint of uncontrolled defecation in the underwear. Parents often report that the child has diarrhea because of soiling of liquid stool. Soiling may be frequent or continuous. On further questioning, the clinician learns that the child is passing large-caliber bowel movements that occasionally may block the toilet. Children younger than age 3 years often present with painful defecation, impaction, and withholding. The history should include a complete review of systems for gastrointestinal, endocrine, and neurologic disorders and a developmental and psychosocial history.

Stool impaction can be felt on abdominal examination in about 50% of patients at presentation. Firm packed stool in the rectum is highly predictive of fecal impaction. A rectal examination allows assessment of sphincter tone and size of the rectal vault. Evaluation of anal placement and existence of anal fissures also is

helpful in considering etiology and severity. A neurologic examination, including lower extremity reflexes, anal wink, and cremasteric reflexes, may reveal underlying spinal cord abnormalities.

Abdominal x-ray is not required. It can be helpful, however, to show to the family the degree of colonic distention and fecal impaction. In obese children or children who cannot cooperate with a physical examination, a flat plate provides the evidence needed to make the diagnosis. In general, further studies, such as barium enema and rectal biopsy, are indicated only if an organic cause for the constipation is indicated by history or physical examination. Similarly, although endocrinologic conditions such as hypothyroidism can cause chronic constipation, laboratory studies are not indicated without history or physical examination suggesting such a disorder.

Differential Diagnosis

The differential diagnosis for functional constipation and soiling includes organic causes of constipation (e.g., neurogenic, anatomic, endocrinologic, gastrointestinal, and pharmacologic). A child with chronic constipation and soiling who had delayed passage of meconium and has an empty rectum and a tight sphincter may have Hirschsprung disease (see Chapter 129). Spinal cord abnormalities, such as a spinal cord tumor or a tethered cord, may present with chronic constipation. Physical examination findings of altered lower extremity reflexes, absent anal wink, or a sacral hairy tuft or pilonidal dimple may be a clue to these anomalies. Hypothyroidism can present with chronic constipation and typically is accompanied by poor linear growth and bradycardia. Anal stenosis may lead to chronic constipation. The use of opiates, phenothiazine, antidepressants, and anticholinergics also may lead to chronic constipation. Developmental problems, including mental retardation and autism, may be associated with chronic constipation.

Treatment

Treatment begins with education and demystification for the child and family about chronic constipation and soiling, emphasizing the chronic nature of this condition and the good prognosis with optimal management. Explaining the physiologic basis of constipation and soiling to the child and the family alleviates blame and enlists cooperation. Education may improve adherence to the long-term treatment plan (Table 14-1). One half to two thirds of children with functional constipation recover completely, meaning that they no longer require medication support. The younger the child is when diagnosis and treatment

TABLE 14–1. Education About Chronic Constipation and Soiling

Constipation affects 16%-37% of children, and 1%-4% of children have functional constipation and soiling

Functional constipation with or without soiling begins early in life for most children owing to a combination of common factors:

Uncomfortable/painful stool passage

Withholding of stool to avoid discomfort

Diets higher in constipating foods and lower in fiber and fluid intake*

Use of medications that are constipating

Developmental features—increasing autonomy and perhaps toilet avoidance

Perhaps family genetic factors—slower colonic transit

When chronic impaction of stool has occurred, physiologic changes at the rectum reduce a child's ability to control his/her bowel movements

Rectal vault is dilated resulting in reduced sensation to standard fecal volume

Rehabilitation of rectal musculature and strength requires several months. Until then, the dilated rectal musculature may be less able to expel stool effectively

Some children have paradoxical anal sphincter contraction when the urge to defecate is felt; this can lead to incomplete emptying of stool at defecation attempt

Many children do not recognize their soiling accidents owing to olfactory accommodation

Although children frequently present with low self-esteem or other behavioral concerns, these symptoms are improved for most with education and management for the constipation and soiling

Effective management of functional constipation requires a substantial commitment of the child and family, usually for 6-24 mo

Degree of child and family adherence is likely a predictor of the child's success

*The common features of the transition to the toddler diet (decreased fluid intake, continued high dairy intake, and "finicky" eating patterns) make this a high-risk time during development for constipation problems.

begin, the higher the success rate. Treatment involves a combination of behavioral training and laxative therapy. Successful treatment requires 6 to 24 months. The next step is adequate colonic clean out or disimpaction. Clean-out methods include enemas alone or combinations of enema, suppository, and oral laxatives. High-dose oral mineral oil is a slower approach to clean out. Choice of disimpaction method depends on the age of the child, family choice, and the clinician's experience with a particular method. Methods, side effects, and costs are summarized in Table 14–2. The child and family should be included in the process of choosing the clean-out method. Because enemas may be invasive and oral medication may be unpleasant, allowing points of choice and control for the child and praising all signs of cooperation are important.

Behavioral training is essential to the treatment of chronic constipation and soiling. The child and family are asked to monitor and document stool output. Routine toilet sitting is instituted for 5 to 10 minutes three to four times per day. The child is asked to demonstrate proper toilet sitting position with the upper body flexed forward slightly and feet on the floor or foot support. The child should be praised for all components of cooperation with this program, and punishment and embarrassment should be avoided. As symptoms resolve, toilet sitting is decreased to twice daily and finally to once a day.

When disimpaction is achieved, the child begins the maintenance phase of treatment. This phase promotes regular stool production and prevents reimpaction. It involves attention to diet, medications to promote stool regularity, and behavioral training. Increasing dietary fiber and fluid are recommended. The recommended daily dose of fiber in grams is calculated as 5 plus the child's age in years (e.g., a 10-year-old should take 15 g of fiber per day). For children with chronic constipation, the recommended grams are 10 plus the child's age in years. Families need to learn to read food labels and to plan for their child's daily intake of fiber. At least 2 oz of nondairy fluid intake per gram of fiber intake is recommended. Sorbitol-based juices, including prune, pear, and apple juice, increase the water content of bowel movements. Lubricants or osmotic laxatives are used to promote regular soft bowel movements. The use of medication during the maintenance phase is more effective than behavioral therapy alone. Maintenance medications, including side effects and costs, are listed in Table 14–3. Polyethylene glycol powder is well tolerated because the taste and texture are palatable. Some children may require the use of a lubricant in addition to an osmotic laxative, and children with severe constipation may require a stimulant laxative. Treatment failure occurs in approximately one in five children secondary to problems with adherence or poor recognition of inadequate treatment resulting in reimpaction.

Complications

Chronic constipation and soiling interfere with social functioning and self-esteem. Discomfort and fear of accidents may distract children from their schoolwork and other important tasks. Children also may develop unusual eating habits in response to chronic constipation and their beliefs about this condition. Case reports of child abuse related to soiling have been published.

TABLE 14–2. Clean-Out Disimpaction

Medication	Side Effects/Comments	Cost*
Infants		
Glycerin suppositories	No side effects	25/$3
Enema—6 mL/kg up to 4.5 oz (135 mL)	If enemas are considered, administer first in physician's office	25.5 oz/$3
Children		
Rapid Cleanout		
Enema—6 mL/kg up to 4.5 oz (135 mL) every 12-24 hr × 1-3	Invasive. Risk of mechanical trauma Large impaction: mineral oil enema followed 1-3 hr later by normal saline or phosphate enema Small impaction: normal saline or phosphate enema	25.5 oz/$3
Mineral oil	Lubricates hard impaction. May not see return after administration	16 oz/$5
Normal saline	Abdominal cramping; may not be as effective as hypertonic phosphate	
Hypertonic phosphate	Abdominal cramping; risk or hyperphosphatemia, hypokalemia, and hypocalcemia especially with Hirschsprung or renal insufficiency or if retained. Some experts do not recommend phosphate enema for children <4 yr, others for children <2 yr	1.5 oz/$4
Milk of molasses: 1:1 milk:molasses	For difficult to clear impaction	
Combination: enema, suppository, oral laxative		
Day 1: Enema q12-24 h	See enemas above	25.5 oz/$3
Day 2: Biscodyl suppository (10 mg) q12-24 h	Abdominal cramping, diarrhea, hypokalemia	12/$3
Day 3: Biscodyl tablet (5 mg) q12-24 h	Abdominal cramping, diarrhea, hypokalemia	25/$3
Repeat 3-day cycle if needed × 1-2		
Oral/nasogastric tube: Polyethylene glycol electrolyte solution (GoLYTELY or NuLytely)—25 mL/kg/hr up to 1000 mL/hr × 4 hr/day	Nausea, cramping, vomiting, bloating, aspiration. Large volume. Usually requires nasogastric tube and hospitalization to administer	GoLYTELY4L/ $17 NuLytely4L/ $21
Slower Cleanout		
Oral high-dose mineral oil—15-30 mL per year of age per day up to 8 oz × 3-4 days	Aspiration—lipoid pneumonia. Give chilled	16 oz/$5
X-Prep (senna): 15 mL q12 h × 3	Abdominal cramping. May not see output until dose 2 or 3	2.5 oz/$15
Magnesium citrate: 1 oz/yr of age to maximum of 10 oz per day for 2-3 days	Hypermagnesemia	10 oz/$2
Maintenance medications—also may be used for cleanout		255 g/$20

*Approximate retail cost—may vary from store to store. The cost of brand name products is calculated as AWP − 10% based on pricing obtained from the 4/1/03 Amerisource Bergen product catalog. The cost of generic products is calculated as MAC plus $3.00 based on the 1/27/03 BCBSM MAC list.

TABLE 14–3. Maintenance Medications

Medication	Side Effects/Comments	Cost*
Infants		
Oral Medications/Other		
Juices containing sorbitol	Pear, prune, apple	
Lactulose or sorbitol: 1-3 mL/kg/day ÷ doses bid	See below	Lactulose 480 mL/$13 Sorbitol 70% 480 mL/$10
Corn syrup (light or dark): 1-3 mL/kg/day ÷ doses bid	Not considered risk for *Clostridium botulinum* spores	
Per Rectum		
Glycerin suppository	No side effects	25/$3
Children		
Oral Medications		
Lubricant	Softens stool and eases passage	
Mineral oil: 1-3 mL/kg day as one dose or ÷ bid	Aspiration—lipoid pneumonia Chill or give with juice. Adherence problems. Leakage: dose too high or impaction	16 oz/$5
Osmotic	Retains water in stool aiding bulk and softness	
Lactulose: 10 g/15 mL, 1-3 cc/kg/day ÷ doses bid	Synthetic disaccharide: abdominal cramping, flatus	480 mL/$13
Magnesium hydroxide (milk of magnesia): 400 mg/5 mL, 1-3 mL/kg/day ÷ bid 800 mg/5 mL, 0.5 mL/kg ÷ bid	Risk of hypermagnesemia, hypophosphatemia, secondary hypocalcemia with overdose or renal insufficiency	12 oz/$4
Miralax (polyethylene glycol powder): 17 g/240 cc water or juice stock, 1.0 g/kg/day ÷ doses bid (approximately 15 cc/kg/day)	Titrate dose at 3-day intervals to achieve mushy stool consistency May make stock solutions to administer over 1-2 days. Excellent adherence	255 g/$22
Sorbitol: 1-3 mL/kg/day ÷ doses bid	Less costly than lactulose	480 mL/$10
Stimulants†	Improves effectiveness of colonic and rectal muscle contractions	
Senna: syrup—8.8 g sennoside/5 mL 2-6 yr: 2.5-7.5 cc/day ÷ doses bid 6-12 yr: 5-15 cc/day ÷ doses bid (Tablets and granules available)	Idiosyneratic hepatitis, melanosis coli, hypertrophic osteoarthropathy, analgesic nephropathy. Abdominal cramping. Melanosis coli improves after medication stopped	2.5 oz/$9 tab: 20/$8 grn: 2 oz/$10
Bisacodyl: 5-mg tablets, 1-3 tablets/dose 1-2 × daily	Abdominal cramping, diarrhea, hypokalemia	25/$3
Per Rectum		
Glycerin suppository	No side effects	25/$3
Bisacodyl: 10-mg suppositories, 0.5-1 suppository, 1-2 × daily	Abdominal cramping, diarrhea, hypokalemia	12/$3

Note: Single agent may suffice to achieve daily, comfortable stools.

*Approximate retail cost—may vary from store to store. The cost of brand name products is calculated as AWP − 10% based on pricing obtained from the 4/1/03 Amerisource Bergen product catalog. The cost of generic products is calculated as MAC plus $3.00 based upon the 1/27/03 BCBSM MAC list.

†Stimulants should be reserved for short-term use.

Prevention

The primary care physician should pay attention to fiber intake in all children and encourage families to help their children to institute regular toileting habits at an early age as preventive measures. Earlier diagnosis of chronic constipation can prevent much secondary disability and shorten the length of treatment required.

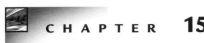

CHAPTER 15

Normal Sleep and Pediatric Sleep Disorders

Sleep is a complex physiologic and behavioral process in which the person achieves a reversible state of disengagement from the environment and partial unresponsiveness. Sleep physiology rapidly changes from fetal life through infancy and childhood. Polysomnographic recordings show two broad categories of sleep: random eye movement sleep (REM) and nonrandom eye movement sleep (NREM). NREM sleep is divided into four stages—from stage 1, which has relatively low voltage with mixed frequency activity, to stage 4, which has greater than 50% high-amplitude waves with slow frequency activity. In the fetus and neonate, sleep is categorized into active sleep and quiet sleep. Active sleep becomes REM sleep in the child and adult. There is significant motor activity during active sleep. Periodic breathing and rapid eye movements accompany active sleep. Quiet sleep matures into NREM sleep.

Full-term infants sleep two thirds of the day. The longest sleep period at 6 weeks of age is variable, with 2 standard deviations ranging between 3 and 11 hours. It is typical of neonates to start their sleep cycle in active sleep, whereas older children and adults begin sleep in NREM sleep. Sleep cycles typically last 60 minutes in newborns compared with 90 minutes in children and adults. Slow-wave sleep (stages 3 and 4) is not seen before 3 to 6 months of age. Between 6 and 12 months, active sleep shifts toward the last third of the night and continues this pattern into adulthood.

One-year-olds sleep on average 15 hours a day. Most U.S. children sleep 2 to 3 hours during the day and the remainder at night. By 12 years of age, the average child sleeps 9 hours a day. During adolescence, sleep physiology changes with decreased stages 3 and 4 NREM sleep and decreased REM sleep. Adolescents continue to need on average 9 hours of sleep per day. Cultural influences strongly determine whether children sleep independently (the norm in the U.S.) or with parents, other siblings, or grandparents (the norm in other cultures).

ETIOLOGY

Numerous sleep disorders exist (Table 15–1). Many are sleep-onset association disorders (infancy), parasomnias, or circadian rhythm disorders (adolescence); other disorders are associated with difficulty falling asleep. Sudden infant death syndrome (SIDS), obstructive sleep apnea (OSA), and sleep disorders associated with mental and physical illness are included in the discussion of the differential diagnosis.

EPIDEMIOLOGY

Childhood sleep disorder is a common complaint in the pediatrician's office. Almost half of mothers of infants complain to the pediatrician about their infants' sleep rhythms. OSA is reported in 2% of children. Adolescent insomnia is much more common. Night talking is the most common parasomnia experienced by almost all people at one time in their life. Sleepwalking occurs in approximately 15% of children at least once between the ages of 5 and 12 years. Night terrors also are common.

CLINICAL MANIFESTATIONS

The assessment of sleep complaints begins with a detailed **history** of sleep habits, including bedtime and bedtime rituals, times of achieving sleep, and waking. A detailed description of the sleep environment, including the type of bed, who shares it, and the ambient light, noise, and temperature can lead to a dynamic understanding of the challenges to and resources for achieving normal sleep. Parental work patterns may be important because some children resist sleep until a parent is at home, and infants have been known to reverse their day-night cycle to breast-feed during the night when the mother is at home. Dietary practices, including timing of meals, undernutrition and overnutrition, and caffeine intake, influence sleep patterns. Documentation of snoring and breathing pauses during sleep can lead to a diagnosis related to OSA. New-onset sleep disorders may be associated with a psychological trauma. When the history does not reveal the cause of the sleep disorder, a sleep diary can be helpful.

A complete **physical examination** is important to rule out medical causes of sleep disturbance, such as conditions that cause pain, neurologic conditions that could be associated with seizure disorder, and other CNS disorders. Children with genetic syndromes associated with developmental delay may have sleep disorder. Similarly, children with attention-deficit/

TABLE 15–1.   Childhood Sleep Disruption Disorders

Type	Cause	Symptoms	Treatment
Organic			
Colic	Unknown	Crying, irritability	Rocking, pacifier, nursing Support until resolution
Medications	Stimulants Bronchodilators Anticonvulsants	Failure to fall asleep; restless sleep	Adjust dosage/timing; change medication
Illness	Any chronically irritating disorder (e.g., otitis, dermatitis, asthma, or esophageal reflux)	Painful crying out	Treat disease symptomatically
CNS disorders	Variable; rule out seizures	Decreased sleep	Evaluate environment Sedatives as last resort
Parasomnias			
Sleepwalking, sleep terrors Confusional arousals	Stage 4 (deep) sleep instability	Awakening 1-3 hr after falling asleep Intense crying, walking, disorientation, talking	Reassurance; protective environment
Enuresis	? Stage 4 instability Metabolic disease (e.g., diabetes) Urinary tract infection Urinary anatomic anomaly	Bed-wetting	Rule out medical conditions Fluid limitation Prebed voiding Behavioral approaches (bell and pad) Emotional support Medication (e.g., imipramine, DDAVP) Reassurance
Sleep-wake Schedule Disorders			
Irregular sleep-wake pattern	No defined schedule	Variable waking and sleeping	Regularize schedule
Regular but inappropriate sleep-wake schedule	Napping at wrong times Prematurely eliminated nap	Morning sleepiness Night wakenings	Rework schedule
Delayed sleep phase	Late sleep onset with resetting of circadian rhythm	Late sleep onset Morning sleepiness Not sleepy at bedtime	Enforce wake-up time Gradually move bedtime earlier or keep awake overnight to create drowsy state
Environmental and Psychosocial Factors			
Inappropriate sleep-onset associations	No defined bedtime routine Child falls asleep in conditions different from those of the rest of the night	Night wakings requiring intervention	Regularize routine Minimize nocturnal parental response
Excessive nocturnal fluid	Child gets food/drink with each awakening	Night waking or wanting drink	Gradually decrease nocturnal fluid
Inconsistent limit setting	Parental anxiety	Delayed bedtime Excessive expression of "needs" by child	Modify parental behavior to improve limit setting Gradually increase limits
Anxieties; fears	Separation anxieties	Night waking Refusal to sleep	Reassurance when appropriate Counseling in severe cases
Social disruptions	Family stressors	Night waking Refusal to sleep	Family counseling Regularize routines

hyperactivity disorder and fetal alcohol syndrome are at higher risk for sleep disorder than children without these conditions. Careful attention to the upper airway and pulmonary examination may reveal enlarged tonsils or adenoids or other signs of obstruction.

A **polysomnogram** is used to detect obstructive and central apnea, excessive limb movements, and seizure disorder. Children can be admitted for an overnight polysomnogram, and 24-hour ambulatory recordings are available. Children who have a history consistent with a behavioral sleep disorder, such as sleep-onset association disorder and difficulty falling asleep, do not need a polysomnogram, unless they do not improve with intervention.

DIFFERENTIAL DIAGNOSIS

Infancy

The incidence of **SIDS** has decreased by 60% as a result of placing infants on their backs to sleep and reducing overbundling and cigarette smoke exposure (see Chapter 134). Although SIDS is probably a final common pathway for a variety of different etiologies, decreased arousal to hypoxia or hypercapnia may be a mechanism in some cases.

Sleep-onset association disorders are common in the U.S. where a high degree of independence is expected for infant sleep. Infants experience arousal during each sleep cycle as they go back into light sleep (stage 1). Infants who wake under conditions different from those they experienced as they fell asleep are likely to become more aroused. An infant who falls asleep in the parent's arms in front of the television with the light on may awaken 1 hour later in his or her crib in a silent, darkened room. This infant can be expected to cry. Infants can become conditioned to expect certain conditions to achieve sleep. This mechanism underlies many of the interventions for frequent night waking.

Childhood

Difficulty falling asleep includes bedtime resistance, delayed sleep onset, sleep anxiety, and fears. Bedtime resistance is most common in preschool children. Psychologically, bedtime is experienced as separation from parents, with morning being a reunion experience. Children with insecure attachment may be more prone to distress at bedtime. Bedtime resistance does not rule out other sleep pathology and is more common in children with sleep-disordered breathing.

OSA in childhood is not always obvious or easy to diagnose. OSA is commonly caused by tonsillar or adenoidal hypertrophy. Some authors prefer the term *sleep-disordered breathing* because obstruction is often partial.

These children typically present with a history of snoring, and some may have excessive daytime sleepiness. Obese children are at increased risk for OSA. In toddlers, OSA often is associated with poor growth, which improves when the obstruction is relieved by tonsillectomy or adenoidectomy. Many children with OSA experience cognitive difficulties and school problems. Hyperactivity also is more common in these children than in age-matched controls.

Parasomnias include night terrors, sleepwalking, and sleep talk and involve movement from stage 3 or 4 sleep into REM. Night terrors are common, occur in preschool children, and are likely to resolve with time and developmental maturation. Night terrors are differentiated from nightmares, which occur later in the night and result from arousal from REM or dreaming sleep. Children typically remember their nightmares, but have no recollection of night terrors. Parents often report distress at their child's night terrors because the child may scream and not recognize them during the episode.

Adolescence

Circadian rhythm disorder in adolescence is caused by irregularities in sleep hygiene and leads to delayed sleep phase syndrome. Many adolescents stay up late and sleep 7 hours or less a night during the week with attempts to recoup lost sleep on the weekend. This schedule disrupts the biologic clock. Teens then develop bedtime insomnia and difficulty maintaining sleep during the night with inability to arouse in the morning. Sleep deprivation leads to cognitive problems and problems of emotional regulation.

Primary sleep disorders must be differentiated from sleep disorders associated with psychiatric and medical disorders. Psychoses, anxiety disorders, and substance abuse can present with disordered sleep. The clinician also should consider sleep-related epilepsy, sleep-related headaches, and degenerative and developmental disorders. Asthma and gastroesophageal reflux also can disrupt sleep.

TREATMENT

The management of sleep-onset association disorder, difficulty falling asleep, and circadian rhythm disorder is challenging. Evaluation for medical and psychiatric causes is important before beginning a behavioral treatment plan. Family dynamics may be important in perpetuating a child's sleep problem. A couple who prefer not to be intimate may subconsciously reinforce night waking and parental bed sharing with their child. Treatment involves the behavioral management principles of (1) education and demystification, (2) setting objectives and a timetable, (3) positive reinforcement and rewards, and (4) negative reinforcement and withdrawal of attention or privileges.

Infants who have become habituated to parental soothing for achieving sleep are put in bed slightly awake after they have had a diaper change, food, and comfort. Parents understand that the infant will cry in protest, and over the course of several weeks, they gradually lengthen the amount of crying that they tolerate. During this period, they also allow increased duration of crying during the night rather than immediate attention. It is important that the infant is developmentally able to go without feeding and drinking. Children younger than 4 months old need nighttime feeding. Safety and comfort also are essential. It is difficult to follow this type of behavioral intervention if the infant is sleeping in the parental bedroom.

Difficulty falling asleep and bedtime resistance are treated by meticulous attention to sleep hygiene of the youngster. Removing televisions and VCRs from the bedroom is advised because children who fall asleep with the television require the television for soothing during the night. Watching television at bedtime also may delay sleep onset. Children who are experiencing separation anxiety can benefit from behavioral therapy aimed at reinforcing feelings of safety and parental presence. Objects of attachment, such as a favorite blanket or stuffed animal, are helpful. Children with minor brain injury secondary to fetal alcohol syndrome or complications of prematurity may be more resistant to behavioral treatment. Similarly, children with attention-deficit/hyperactivity disorder may have significant problems settling for sleep at bedtime. Paradoxically, some children with attention-deficit/hyperactivity disorder have improved sleep after beginning stimulant therapy.

Rarely, children with difficulty falling asleep are treated pharmacologically. Melatonin (dose 2.5 to 10 mg) has soporific properties useful in treating delayed sleep phase syndrome. Developmentally normal and developmentally delayed children have been treated successfully with melatonin for difficulty falling asleep. Melatonin is available without prescription in stores that sell dietary supplements. The α-agonist clonidine acts preferentially on presynaptic α_2 neurons to inhibit noradrenergic activity. Somnolence is a side effect of clonidine, which can be put to use in cases of refractory sleep difficulties. Clonidine usually is started in a dose of 0.05 mg at bedtime and increased to 0.1 mg at bedtime if needed. There are data on treating children age 4 years with clonidine; this is an "off-label" use in children. Weaning off clonidine is recommended at the end of treatment.

Night terrors are best managed by minimal intervention. The child can be laid down and quietly comforted. Conversation with the child is not possible at the time of the night terror. Children who have frequent or prolonged night terrors have been treated successfully with soporific medications and with clinical hypnosis. Children with atypical night terrors may need a sleep study to evaluate possible coexisting sleep disorders.

Circadian rhythm disorder in adolescents can be treated by meticulous attention to sleep hygiene and gradual resetting of the biologic clock. Advancing the bedtime forward is one treatment. This therapy requires the adolescent to stay awake for 1 night followed by going to bed at the desired time the next day. He or she then is required to go to bed at the same time (including weekend nights) for the duration of treatment and maintenance. The adolescent also is required to arise at a consistent time on the weekends, not more than several hours after their weekday wake-up time. Another method of resetting the biologic clock involves gradually shifting the bedtime and waking times earlier over the course of several weeks. Both therapies are supplemented by attention to regular mealtimes, avoidance of caffeine, exclusion of the television from the bedroom, and use of soporific medications if needed. Families require a great deal of support and counseling during this intervention.

COMPLICATIONS

The most obvious and serious complication associated with childhood sleep disorders is impairment of cognitive ability and emotional regulation. This impairment puts children at risk for school failure, family difficulties, and social problems. It is likely that sleep-deprived children are at increased risk for acute illness and psychiatric disorders.

PREVENTION

The principles of prevention for pediatric behavioral sleep disorders are outlined in Table 15–2. Sleep-onset association disorder in infancy usually can be pre-

---

TABLE 15–2. Prevention of Pediatric Behavioral Sleep Disorders

Consistent ambient noise, light, temperature in bedroom
Adequate food, liquid, socialization, and physical activity during the day
Caffeine avoidance
Regular bedtime
Regular wake-up time
Consistent bedtime routine (15-30 min) to cue sleep
No television in bedroom
Child feels safe and protected
Child allowed to develop self-soothing strategies
Parents are comfortable setting limits/boundaries

vented by parental understanding of infant sleep physiology, developmentally appropriate expectations, and planning the infant sleep environment to coincide with family needs. Infants can adapt to sleeping with a parent or sleeping independently in a crib. Cosleeping is often chosen by breastfeeding mothers for ease of feeding the infant throughout the night. The mother is advised to consider how long she will want the infant to continue sleeping in her bed because the transition to independent sleeping may be difficult for the infant, especially at certain developmental periods, such as the period of separation anxiety, which peaks between 10 and 18 months and fades by 2 years of age. Cosleeping is not advised in case of alcohol or drug use by the parent. Soft bedding, pillows, and blankets, which may cover the infant, also can increase the risk of SIDS in an infant sleeping in the parent's bed. The infant quickly habituates to the sleeping environment and becomes dependent on that environment to cue sleep. It is important for parents to understand that it is normal for their infant to wake frequently for the first 6 weeks before settling into a routine of waking every 3 to 4 hours for feeding. Infants typically do not sleep through the night before 6 months of age, and many do not sleep through the night before age 18 months. Rocking an infant to sleep is pleasurable for the infant and the parent. Families who prefer not to get up in the night to rock their infant back to sleep are advised to put the infant into the bed slightly awake to promote the development of some self-soothing. Infant night waking is particularly difficult for families in which both parents are working. Sleep-deprived parents may not function optimally at home or at work.

Difficulty falling asleep in toddlers and preschool children can be largely prevented by a structured daily routine, including good sleep hygiene at a bedtime that takes into account the child's needs for sleep and for time with the parents. Including physical activity in the daily routine is advised so that the child is physically and mentally tired at bedtime. Children crave time and attention from their parents. For families in which both parents work, this time occurs in the evening along with dinner, parental socialization, and bedtime routines. Designating special parent-child time can alleviate the child's need to delay bedtime. Bedtime routines should last no more than 30 minutes and include a set combination of activities that might include bath, teeth brushing, story, and cuddle. A consistent bedtime ensures that the child's circadian rhythm matches the parental expectation. Parents should understand that this is an activity that may test their ability to set limits firmly. These recommendations may not be necessary for families whose culture and environment allow children to stay up late with the family and sleep later in the morning.

Young children may begin to sleep in their parent's bed during times of illness or stress in the family. Proactively considering the desirability of bed sharing allows parents to be in control rather than ceding this control to the young child.

Requiring a consistent bedtime during the week can prevent circadian rhythm disorders in adolescence; this may require limiting extracurricular activities, television, and video games. Similarly, setting a weekend wake-up time can prevent significant shifting of the biologic clock. Setting limits with adolescents is challenging. Beginning to lay the groundwork for these expectations earlier in the adolescent years is often helpful (e.g., "When you are in high school your weeknight bedtime will be 11:00 PM, and you will be allowed to sleep in until 11:00 AM on weekends."). Some professionals believe that adolescents would be less likely to have sleep disorders if high schools started at 9:00 AM instead of 7:30 AM. This is not the norm in the U.S., however, because many adolescents are employed, and many participate in athletic and other extracurricular activities after school.

SUGGESTED READING

American Academy of Pediatrics: Clinical Practice Guideline: Diagnosis and evaluation of the child with attention-deficit/hyperactivity disorder. Pediatrics 105:1158-1170, 2000.

Barr RG: Colic and crying syndromes in infants. Pediatrics 102(5 Suppl E):1282-1286, 1998.

Behrman RE, Kliegman RM, Jenson HB (eds): Nelson Textbook of Pediatrics, 17th ed. Philadelphia, WB Saunders, 2004.

Blass EM, Camp CA: Changing determinants of crying termination in 6- to 12-week-old human infants. Dev Psychobiol 42:312-316, 2003.

Brazelton TB: Toddlers and Parents: A Declaration of Independence. New York, Delacorte Press/Seymour Lawrence, 1989.

Halbower AC, Marcus CL: Sleep disorders in children. Curr Opin Pulm Med 9:471-476, 2003.

Issenman RM, Filmer RB, Gorski PA: A review of bowel and bladder control development in children: How gastrointestinal and urologic conditions relate to problems in toilet training. Pediatrics 103(6 Pt 2):1346-1352, 1999.

Mikkelsen EJ: Enuresis and encopresis: Ten years of progress. J Am Acad Child Adolesc Psychiatry 40:1146-1158, 2001.

Potegal M, Davidson RJ: Temper tantrums in young children: 1. Behavioral composition. J Dev Behav Pediatr 24:140-147, 2003.

PSYCHIATRIC DISORDERS

Russell Scheffer

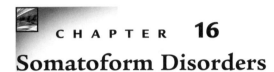

CHAPTER **16**

Somatoform Disorders

The somatoform disorders are a group of conditions that involve a complaint of physical symptoms (pain or loss of function) that suggest a medical condition, but are not fully explained by a medical condition, a pharmacologic effect, or another psychiatric condition (Table 16–1). The symptoms are usually recurrent involving multiple, clinically significant complaints. In evaluating somatoform complaints, the evidence for medical disorders should be sought while evaluating evidence for psychological disorders. The use of physical complaints as signals of distress is common and may not indicate a serious psychiatric illness.

Treatment approaches for somatoform problems are complex. The patient must believe that the physician, in finding no evidence of disease, will not judge the symptoms to be feigned or imaginary ("all in your head"). The physician must have the patient's trust and confidence for treatment to be effective. Even if the physician and the patient agree that psychological factors are playing some role, there still may be an organic pathologic cause underlying the symptoms. When a diagnosis of a somatoform disorder is made, efforts to decrease morbidity by avoiding unnecessary medical procedures are important. One physician should serve as the team leader in treatment; this helps coordinate the findings and concerns from multiple consultants.

Somatization disorder involves multiple unexplained physical complaints, including pain and gastrointestinal, sexual, and pseudoneurologic symptoms (Table 16–2). These physical symptoms are not caused by known physiologic or pathologic mechanisms and may be related to the patient's need to maintain the sick role. The patient is convinced that the symptoms are unrelated to psychological factors. The criteria to diagnose this disorder are listed in Table 16–3.

The onset of the condition is common during adolescence, onset generally occurs before age 30, and the condition typically lasts for years. Prevalence estimates range from 0.2% to 2% in women and less than 0.2% in men. The course of the illness is chronic and waxes and wanes. The symptoms tend to persist or to change character despite ongoing treatment. There is an increased risk of the disorder in first-degree relatives, especially female relatives (10% to 20%). Other conditions that occur at higher rates in patients with somatization disorder and their family members are substance abuse and dependence, antisocial personality disorder, histrionic and borderline personality disorders, major depression, and anxiety symptoms. Medical conditions that should be ruled out include systemic lupus erythematosus, Lyme disease, multiple sclerosis, hemochromatosis, hyperparathyroidism, and other conditions that have multiple systemic symptoms. Somatization disorder is not a factitious disorder or malingering. These syndromes commonly coexist, however.

Patients with somatization disorder often undergo multiple medical procedures and tests without significant findings. It is common for patients to come under the care of many providers, often at the same time. When a diagnosis is made, limiting morbidity from medical procedures is a major goal. The prognosis is typically guarded, and poor outcomes are common.

Undifferentiated somatoform disorder includes one or more unexplained physical complaints lasting for at least 6 months. The number of physical complaints is less than that required for a diagnosis of somatization disorder (Table 16–4). These symptoms are not explained by medical conditions or drugs. Patients may recognize an association between their symptoms and stress. The course of undifferentiated somatoform

TABLE 16–1. Features of Somatoform Disorders of Children and Adolescents

Psychophysiologic Disorder

Presenting complaint is a physical symptom
Physical symptom caused by a known physiologic mechanism
Physical symptom is stress induced
Patient may recognize association between symptom and stress
Symptom responds to medication, biofeedback, and stress reduction

Conversion Reaction

Presenting complaint is physical (loss of function, pain, or both)
Physical symptom not caused by a known physiologic mechanism
Physical symptom related to unconscious idea, fantasy, or conflict
Patient does not recognize association between symptom and the unconscious
Symptom responds slowly to resolution of unconscious factors

Somatization Disorder

Presenting complaint is >13 physical symptoms in girls, >11 in boys
Physical symptoms not caused by a known physiologic or pathologic mechanism
Physical symptoms related to need to maintain the sick role
Patient convinced that symptoms unrelated to psychological factors
Symptoms tend either to persist or to change character despite treatment

Hypochondriasis

Presenting complaint is a physical sign or symptom
Physical sign or symptom is normal
Patient interprets physical symptom to indicate disease
Conviction regarding illness may be related to depression or anxiety
Symptom does not respond to reassurance; medication directed at underlying psychological problems often helps

Malingering

Presenting complaint is a physical symptom
Physical symptom is under voluntary control
Physical symptom is used to gain reward (e.g., money, avoidance of military service)
Patient consciously recognizes symptom as factitious
Symptom may not lessen when reward is attained (need to retain reward)

Factitious Disorder (e.g., Munchausen Syndrome)

Presenting complaint is symptom complex mimicking known syndrome
Symptom complex is under voluntary control
Symptom complex is used to attain medical treatment (including surgery)
Patient consciously recognizes symptom complex as factitious, but is often psychologically disturbed so that unconscious factors also are operating
Symptom complex often results in multiple diagnoses and multiple operations

disorder varies. If the condition does not progress to somatization disorder, it may have a good outcome if medical procedures do not lead to complications.

This syndrome most commonly occurs in young women of low socioeconomic status. It can occur in both sexes, however, and in all races and socioeconomic classes. Treatments include medication, biofeedback, and stress reduction.

Conversion disorder includes motor and sensory symptoms that suggest neurologic or other medical illness (Table 16–5). The symptoms are referred to as *pseudoneurologic* because they mimic neurologic symptoms. Conversion symptoms typically are not consistent with neuroanatomic and physiologic knowledge. Also, they are often inconstant; for instance, a patient moves a "paralyzed" extremity when he or she thinks no one is watching. *Falling out syndrome* (falling down with consciousness alteration) is common in several cultures throughout the world. *Stocking glove (nonanatomic) anesthesia* is another common finding. Onset of symptoms in childhood and adolescence is common. In prepubertal children, gait abnormalities

TABLE 16–2. Somatoform Symptoms
Pain Symptoms (Site or Function)
Head Back Joints Chest Rectum Abdomen Extremities Menstruation Urination Sexual intercourse
Gastrointestinal Symptoms
Nausea Bloating Food intolerance Vomiting Diarrhea
Sexual Symptoms
Sexual indifference Erectile dysfunction Vomiting throughout pregnancy Irregular menses Ejaculatory dysfunction Excessive menstrual bleeding
Pseudoneurologic Symptoms
Difficulty swallowing Loss of touch or pain sensation Hallucinations Aphonia Seizures Double vision Blindness Deafness Urinary retention Loss of consciousness Dissociative symptoms (e.g., amnesia) Impaired coordination or balance Paralysis or localized weakness

sclerosis, dystonias, and dyskinesias (abnormal movements) are conditions commonly mistaken for conversion disorder. The cause of conversion symptoms may be related to an unconscious idea, fantasy, or conflict. The patient does not recognize an association between the symptoms and the unconscious conflict. A common example is a fearful soldier losing use of his or her weapon-firing arm or hand.

Conversion disorders are uncommon, ranging from 11 to 500 per 100,000 in the general population. The prevalence increases in psychiatric (1% to 3%) and surgical (1% to 14%) patients. Conversion symptoms are more common in first-degree relatives than the general population. A family history of unexplainable medical problems in the family may serve as a clue to the diag-

TABLE 16–3. Criteria for Diagnosis of Somatization Disorder

Each of the following criteria must have been met, with individual symptoms occurring at any time during the course of disturbance
  1. *Four pain symptoms:* a history of pain related to at least four different sites or functions (e.g., head, abdomen, back, joints, extremities, chest, rectum, during menstruation, during sexual intercourse, or during urination)
  2. *Two gastrointestinal symptoms:* a history of at least two gastrointestinal symptoms other than pain (e.g., nausea, bloating, vomiting other than during pregnancy, diarrhea, or intolerance of several different foods)
  3. *One sexual symptom:* a history of at least one sexual or reproductive symptom other than pain (e.g., sexual indifference, erectile or ejaculatory dysfunction, irregular menses, excessive menstrual bleeding, vomiting throughout pregnancy)
  4. *One pseudoneurologic symptom:* a history of at least one symptom or deficit suggesting a neurologic condition not limited to pain (conversion symptoms such as impaired coordination or balance, paralysis or localized weakness, difficulty swallowing or lump in throat, aphonia, urinary retention, hallucinations, loss of touch or pain sensation, double vision, blindness, deafness, seizures; dissociative symptoms such as amnesia; or loss of consciousness other than fainting)
Either (1) or (2)
  1. After appropriate investigation, each of the symptoms from above criteria cannot be fully explained by a known general medical condition or the direct effects of a substance (e.g., a drug of abuse, a medication)
  2. When there is a related general medical condition, the physical complaints or resulting social or occupational impairment are in excess of what would be expected from the history, physical examination, or laboratory findings

and pseudoseizures are the most common expressions of the condition.

The **diagnosis** should be made only after thorough and repeated physical examinations. Previously, 25% of patients diagnosed with conversion disorder were found to have a medical cause for their symptoms. Now, this "misdiagnosis" of conversion disorders is less common. This change is probably due to increased awareness of the diagnosis and improved medical diagnostics. When the diagnosis is suspected or made, medical procedures should be limited to decrease associated morbidity. Myasthenia gravis, multiple

---

TABLE 16–4. Criteria for Diagnosis of Undifferentiated Somatoform Disorder

A. One or more physical complaints (e.g., fatigue, loss of appetite, gastrointestinal or urinary complaints)
B. Either (1) or (2)
  1. After appropriate investigation, the symptoms cannot be fully explained by a known general medical condition or the direct effects of a pharmacologic substance (e.g., a drug of abuse, a medication)
  2. When there is a related general medical condition, the physical complaints or resulting social occupational impairment is in excess of what would be expected from the history, physical examination, or laboratory findings
C. The symptoms cause clinically significant distress or impairment in social, occupational, or other important areas of functioning
D. The duration of disturbance is at least 6 mo
E. The disturbance is not better accounted for by another mental disorder (e.g., another somatoform disorder, sexual dysfunction, mood disorder, anxiety disorder, sleep disorder, or psychotic disorder)
F. The symptom is not intentionally produced or feigned (as in factitious disorder or malingering)

---

onset, severity, and maintenance of this symptom (Table 16–6). Chronic, recurrent pain syndromes in childhood most commonly involve abdominal pain, headache, limb pain, or chest pain. It is unusual for children to exhibit more than one such pain syndrome at the same time, although they often may have had chronic, recurrent pain in a different location of the body in the past. An organic etiology is found in only about 10% of children. The diagnosis of psychogenic pain should be based, however, not only on the absence of adequate physical findings to explain the pain, but also on evidence specific to the etiologic role of psychological factors. Most chronic, recurrent pain syndromes have no clear organic or emotional origin.

Diagnosis is based on a careful history and physical examination, including a comprehensive psychosocial assessment. In addition to the location, quality, and chronology of the pain, attention must be focused on the circumstances in which the pain is felt. Signs and symptoms indicating increased likelihood of an organic etiology include constant pain, pain that awakens the child from sleep, well-localized pain, and physical findings such as fever, weight loss, jaundice,

nosis. People in rural areas and people with lower socioeconomic status are more commonly affected.

The course of the condition is often benign. Twenty percent to 25% of patients experience a recurrence. Good prognostic characteristics include acute onset, above-average intelligence, presence of an identifiable stressor, short time to diagnosis and psychiatric treatment, and symptoms of paralysis, aphonia, and blindness. Poor prognostic characteristics include tremor and pseudoseizures. Pseudoseizures also are common in patients who have epilepsy.

Treatment is best accomplished by reassuring patients that the symptoms usually go away. Prevention of unnecessary medical interventions can decrease morbidity. Direct confrontation usually is not helpful. Allowing the patient to "save face" and letting the symptom resolve on its own is helpful. Multiple medical treatments and diagnostic interventions can lead to solidifying the symptoms and delaying recovery. Hypnotherapy and amobarbital sodium (Amytal Sodium) interviews may uncover conflicts and assist the patient's recovery. In some cases, exploring these conflicts has proved helpful. In cases in which a clear conflict exists, symptoms often respond slowly to resolution of the conflict. In other cases, a conflict is never identified.

Pain disorder features pain as the predominant complaint. Psychological factors are important in the

---

TABLE 16–5. Criteria for Diagnosis of Conversion Disorder

A. One or more symptoms or deficits affecting voluntary motor or sensory function that suggest a neurologic or other general medical condition
B. Psychological factors are judged to be associated with the symptom or deficit because the initiation or exacerbation of the symptom or deficit is preceded by conflicts or other stressors
C. The symptom or deficit is not intentionally produced or feigned (factitious disorder or malingering)
D. After appropriate investigation, the symptom or deficit cannot be fully explained by a general medical condition, by the direct effects of a substance, or as a culturally sanctioned behavior or experience
E. The symptom or deficit causes clinically significant distress or impairment in social, occupational, or other important areas of functioning or warrants medical evaluation
F. The symptom or deficit is not limited to pain or sexual dysfunction, does not occur exclusively during the course of somatization disorder, and is not better accounted for by another mental disorder

Specify type of symptom or deficit
  With motor symptom or deficit
  With sensory symptom or deficit
  With seizures or convulsions
  With mixed presentation

TABLE 16–6. Criteria for Diagnosis of Pain Disorder

A. Pain in ≥1 anatomic sites is the predominant focus of the clinical presentation and is of sufficient severity to warrant clinical attention
B. The pain causes clinically significant distress or impairment in social, occupational, or other important areas of functioning
C. Psychological factors are judged to have an important role in the onset, severity, exacerbation, or maintenance of the pain
D. The symptom or deficit is not intentionally produced or feigned (as in factitious disorder or malingering)
E. The pain is not better accounted for by a mood, anxiety, or psychotic disorder and does not meet criteria for dyspareunia

Code as follows
Pain disorder associated with psychological factors: psychological factors are judged to have a major role in the onset, severity, exacerbation, or maintenance of the pain. (If a general medical condition is present, it does not have a major role in the onset, severity, exacerbation, or maintenance of the pain.) This type of pain disorder is not diagnosed if criteria also are met for somatization disorder

Specify if
Acute: duration <6 mo
Chronic: duration ≥6 mo
Pain disorder associated with psychological factors and a general medical condition: psychological factors and a general medical condition are judged to have important roles in the onset, severity, exacerbation, or maintenance of the pain

Specify if
Acute: duration <6 mo
Chronic: duration of ≥6 mo

Note: The following is not considered to be a mental disorder and is included here to facilitate differential diagnosis
Pain disorder associated with a general medical condition: a general medical condition has a major role in the onset, severity, exacerbation, or maintenance of the pain. (If psychological factors are present, they are not judged to have a major role in the onset, severity, exacerbation, or maintenance of the pain.) The diagnostic code for the pain is selected based on the associated general medical condition if one has been established or on the anatomic location of the pain if the underlying general medical condition is not yet clearly established (e.g., low back, joint, bone, abdominal, breast, renal, ear, eye, throat, tooth, and urinary)

changes in stools (color, consistency, or frequency), and urinary tract symptoms.

Psychological conditions that preceded the onset of the recurrent pain syndrome must be distinguished from conditions that followed the pain onset because by the time the child exhibits a chronic problem, evidence of psychological stress usually is found. The nurturing responses of the family may provide secondary gain that prolongs the pain complaints. Alternatively, frustration with failure to find a specific cause may lead to accusations of malingering and to increased stress on the child, which may exacerbate the problem. Diagnostic studies should be undertaken in response to specific findings that suggest an organic etiology.

Counseling with reassurance of the benign nature of the pain is the primary treatment. Symptom diaries, including the events that immediately precede and follow the pain episode, are helpful in the initial assessment and the ongoing management of the problem. Minimizing secondary psychological consequences of recurrent pain syndromes is important.

Hypochondriasis is the preoccupation with the fear of having a serious disease based on misinterpretation of bodily symptoms and functions (Table 16–7). The presenting complaint is a physical sign or symptom, which is normal but is interpreted by the patient to indicate disease. A headache resulting in a marked concern about a brain tumor is a common

TABLE 16–7. Criteria for Diagnosis of Hypochondriasis

A. Preoccupation with fears of having, or the idea that one had, a serious disease based on the person's misinterpretation of bodily symptoms
B. The preoccupation persists despite appropriate medical evaluation and reassurance
C. The belief in criterion A is not of delusional intensity (as in delusional disorder, somatic type) and is not restricted to a circumscribed concern about appearance (as in body dysmorphic disorder)
D. The preoccupation causes clinically significant distress or impairment in social, occupational, or other important areas of functioning
E. The duration of the disturbance is at least 6 mo
F. The preoccupation is not better accounted for by generalized anxiety disorder, obsessive-compulsive disorder, panic disorder, major depressive episode, separation anxiety, or another somatoform disorder

Specify if
With poor insight: if, for most of the time during the current episode, the person does not recognize that the concern about having a serious illness is excessive or unreasonable

example of hypochondriasis. An underlying depression or anxiety disorder may be related to the symptoms. These symptoms typically do not respond to reassurance. Psychotropic medications directed at underlying psychiatric problems can be helpful. Limiting medical procedures can help to decrease morbidity.

Somatoform disorder not otherwise specified is used to describe somatoform symptoms that do not meet criteria for a specific somatoform disorder but still cause significant distress or dysfunction.

Psychological factors affecting physical condition is a diagnosis in which a physical illness is exacerbated by psychological or behavioral factors. These factors can worsen the underlying illness or affect its treatment. This diagnosis is commonly made in patients with chronic medical conditions. An example is a child with insulin-dependent diabetes mellitus whose stressors and maladaptive behaviors interfere with his or her ability to monitor blood glucose levels.

Chronic fatigue syndrome may occur in adolescents and is frequently a postviral phenomenon. In other cases, its etiology is undetermined. It is often associated with depression. The condition can be incapacitating and include numerous physical complaints of fatigue. Chronic fatigue syndrome usually is considered when vague symptoms exist, and no significant findings are present on examination or laboratory studies. Treatment is nonspecific, unless a psychological or general medical cause is uncovered.

Malingering is a condition in which patients present with a complaint of a physical symptom that is under voluntary control and is used to gain reward (money or avoidance of school, jail, or military service). In many cases, the motivation is not readily apparent, but the patient consciously recognizes the symptom as factitious. Symptoms may not lessen when the reward is attained because of a need to retain the reward. Malingering is difficult to prove unless the patient is directly observed or confesses. It is a serious matter that may have legal consequences.

Factitious disorder is a condition in which physical or psychological symptoms are produced intentionally to assume the sick role (Table 16–8). This diagnosis is made either by direct observation or by eliminating other possible causes. The presenting complaint is often a symptom complex that mimics a known syndrome. The presentation can include subjective complaints (abdominal pain), falsified objective signs (blood in urine), or self-inflicted injury. In addition, it is common to have exaggeration of symptoms of existing conditions (pseudoseizures and epilepsy). This condition often leads to unnecessary medical tests, procedures, and treatments (including surgeries). The patient consciously recognizes that the symptom complex is factitious, but is often psychologically disturbed. The evaluation of factitious disorder must

---

TABLE 16–8. Criteria for Diagnosis of Factitious Disorder

A. Intentional production or feigning of physical or psychological signs or symptoms
B. The motivation for the behavior is to assume the sick role
C. External incentives for the behavior (e.g., economic gain, avoiding legal responsibility, or improving physical well-being, as in malingering) are absent

Code based on type

With predominantly psychological signs and symptoms: if psychological signs and symptoms predominate in the clinical presentation

With predominantly physical signs and symptoms: if physical signs and symptoms predominate in the clinical presentation

With combined psychological and physical signs and symptoms: if psychological and physical signs and symptoms are present, but neither predominates in the clinical presentation

---

include a thorough medical evaluation or a psychiatric evaluation if the symptoms are psychiatric. Somatoform disorders and malingering are other disorders to be considered. The patient may not know the motivation for the feigning of symptoms; this differs from malingering, in which symptoms are feigned for secondary gain.

Factitious disorder occurs more commonly in females. *Approximate answers* reported during a mental status examination are most commonly found in factitious disorders. This term is applied when patients give close answers (e.g., $20 - 3 = 18$). The use of psychoactive substances also can complicate the physical findings. The most common comorbid condition is substance abuse. The prevalence of the disorder is unknown. In large general hospitals, approximately 1% of patients who receive psychiatric consultation are diagnosed with factitious disorder.

Munchausen syndrome by proxy is a form of factitious disorder by proxy, where a parent mimics symptoms in his or her child. It is a type of child abuse (see Chapter 22). The symptoms are often inconsistent with the healthy appearance of the child. The motivation of the perpetrator is believed to be a psychological need to assume a sick role through the child. Usually external incentives for the behavior are absent. The child may not be aware of the parent's actions. This phenomenon is more common in parents with some healthcare background. The most common presenting symptoms include vomiting, diarrhea, respiratory arrest, asthma, seizures, uncoordination, loss of consciousness, fever, bleeding, failure to thrive, rash, and hypoglycemia. Simulation of psychiatric disorders occurs, but is less frequent than those already mentioned. Preschoolers and neonates are the most common victims. Older children and teenagers may be assisting the parent. Boys are more commonly abused in this way. When confronted with the facts of the case, the parent may become distraught or angry and may initiate legal action. Video surveillance of the patient's room may detect episodes. Charges frequently are pressed. This situation should be reported to child protective services. Treatment involves protecting the child from further abuse. Unnecessary medical tests and treatments can cause significant morbidity.

CHAPTER 17

Anxiety and Phobias

ANXIETY DISORDERS

Anxiety disorders tend to be chronic, recurring conditions that wax and wane in intensity over time. They are among the most common psychiatric illnesses and affect more than 10% of the population.

Panic disorder is the presence of recurrent, unexpected panic attacks. At least 1 month of persistent worrying about having another panic attack is required to make the diagnosis (Table 17–1). Panic disorder is eight times more common in family members of affected individuals than the general population. Onset during childhood and adolescence increases the likelihood that a first-degree family member will be affected. Twin studies suggest a genetic component to the illness. More than half of all affected individuals do not have an affected family member (spontaneous cases). Children with *separation anxiety disorder* seem to be at risk for subsequent development of panic disorder.

Panic disorder is described in all racial groups. Lifetime prevalence rates range from 1% to 3.5% of the general population. In psychiatric samples, the rate approaches 10% of patients. In some medical settings, the rates are higher still. Common clinical settings for presentation include otolaryngology (vestibular), pulmonary, neurology, and cardiology.

A **panic attack** is a sudden onset of intense fear associated with a feeling of impending doom. These attacks are time-limited and accompanied by physical symptoms of anxiety. They occur in the absence of real danger. Characteristic symptoms include shortness of breath, palpitations, chest pain, a choking or smothering sensation, and a fear of losing control or going

TABLE 17–1. Criteria for Diagnosis of Panic Disorder

A. Both (1) and (2)
 1. Recurrent unexpected panic attacks
 2. At least one of the attacks has been followed by ≥1 month of ≥1 of the following:
  a. Persistent concern about having additional attacks
  b. Worry about the implications of the attack or its consequences (e.g., losing control, having a heart attack, "going crazy")
  c. A significant change in behavior related to the attacks
B. The presence or absence of agoraphobia
C. The panic attacks are not due to the direct physiologic effects of a drug of abuse or a medication or a general medical condition (e.g., hyperthyroidism)
D. The panic attacks are not better accounted for by another mental disorder, such as social phobia (e.g., occurring on exposure to feared social situations), specific phobia (e.g., on exposure to a specific phobic situation), obsessive-compulsive disorder (e.g., on exposure to dirt in someone with an obsession about contamination), post-traumatic stress disorder (e.g., in response to stimuli associated with a severe stressor), or separation anxiety disorder (e.g., in response to being away from home or close relatives)

"crazy" (Table 17–2). It is common for patients to present to the emergency department secondary to fear of having a heart attack, thinking that they are about to die. Panic attacks can occur in a variety of conditions involving numerous organ systems, including

TABLE 17–2. Criteria for Diagnosis of a Panic Attack
A discrete period of intense fear or discomfort, in which ≥4 of the following symptoms developed abruptly and reached a peak within 10 min Palpitations, pounding heart, or accelerated heart rate Sweating Trembling or shaking Sensations of shortness of breath or smoldering Feeling of choking Chest pain or discomfort Nausea or abdominal distress Feeling dizzy, unsteady, lightheaded, or faint Derealization (feelings of unreality) or depersonalization (being detached from oneself) Fear of losing control or going crazy Paresthesias (numbness or tingling sensations) Chills or hot flashes

cardiovascular, respiratory, vestibular, and gastrointestinal. These symptoms may occur when an individual is frightened but not having a panic attack.

Panic attacks are classified as unexpected, bound to situations (occur immediately on exposure), and predisposed to situations (attacks occur while at school, but not every time). Triggers can be external (life-threatening situation) or internal (worries about a situation). Situational attacks are common and occur in many patients with other anxiety disorders. Panic attacks must occur unexpectedly to diagnose a panic disorder. Panic disorder may occur with or without *agoraphobia*. Agoraphobia is present in approximately half of the patients with panic disorder.

Panic disorder most often begins in the adolescent or early adult years. Onset before puberty is significantly less common. The course of illness tends to be chronic with waxing and waning of symptom severity over time.

There are no diagnostic laboratory or neuroimaging studies for panic disorder or any other anxiety disorder. Patients experiencing a panic attack may present with respiratory alkalosis (decreased carbon dioxide). Infusions of sodium lactate and breathing into a paper bag have been used as provocative tests in laboratory settings. Mitral valve prolapse, seen on echocardiogram, also can mimic symptoms of panic attacks. The major illnesses to be differentiated from panic disorder are the other anxiety disorders. It is necessary to exclude anxiety disorders secondary to general medical conditions and substance-induced anxiety disorders.

Anxiety disorder due to a general medical condition is characterized by impairing symptoms of anxiety that are judged to be the direct consequence of another medical illness. Medical illnesses that can mimic panic disorder and other anxiety disorders include cardiovascular disease (dysrhythmias, mitral valve prolapse), hyperthyroidism, asthma, irritable bowel syndrome, chronic obstructive pulmonary disease, and pheochromocytoma. **Substance-induced anxiety disorder** is characterized by impairing symptoms of anxiety that are judged to be the direct consequence of a drug (caffeine or other stimulants).

The selective serotonin reuptake inhibitors (SSRIs) are commonly used to treat panic disorder and other anxiety disorders. In the initial phases of treatment, anxiety symptoms may be exacerbated by SSRIs. Benzodiazepines are used more frequently in adults with anxiety disorders. In children and adolescents, it is much more common for patients to become disinhibited on benzodiazepines. Patients with anxiety disorders are often less tolerant of medication side effects and need extra support in maintaining their treatment regimens.

Cognitive and behavioral therapy can be beneficial in a variety of anxiety disorders. The individual components of cognitive therapy and behavioral therapy can be used alone in some patients. Reassurance that the patient does not have a life-threatening illness and cognitive reframing of the symptoms can be important. Other psychosocial treatments include stress management, supportive therapies, and biofeedback.

A variety of psychiatric illnesses occur concurrently with panic disorder, including major depression, obsessive-compulsive disorder (OCD), and other anxiety disorders. Patients with anxiety disorders abuse substances at rates higher than the general population. Panic disorder can have a significant morbidity. Patients frequently use more healthcare resources, have significant functional impairment, and often have a reduced quality of life.

Panic disorder tends to be chronic, but usually is responsive to treatment. Anxiety disorders typically wax and wane over time. There are no proven primary prevention techniques. Emphasis is placed on decreasing morbidity and mortality through proper treatment.

Agoraphobia literally means fear of the marketplace. In common usage, the term is applied to a pathologic condition describing fear of conditions where escape is difficult or would draw unwanted attention to the person (Table 17–3). Agoraphobia can occur on its own or in relationship to panic disorder; 95% of

---

TABLE 17–3. Criteria for Diagnosis of Agoraphobia

Anxiety about being in places or situations from which escape might be difficult (or embarrassing) or in which help may not be available in the event of having an unexpected or situationally predisposed panic attack or panic-like symptoms

Agoraphobic fears typically involve characteristic clusters of situations that include being outside the home alone; being in a crowd or standing in line; being on a bridge; and traveling in a bus, train, plane, or automobile

Note: Consider the diagnosis of specific phobia if the avoidance is limited to one or only a few specific situations or social phobia if the avoidance is limited to social situations in general

The anxiety or phobic avoidance is not better accounted for by another mental disorder, such as social phobia (e.g., avoidance limited to social situations because of fear of embarrassment), specific phobia (e.g., avoidance limited to a single situation, such as elevators), obsessive-compulsive disorder (e.g., avoidance of dirt in someone with an obsession about contamination), post-traumatic stress disorder (e.g., avoidance of stimuli associated with a severe stressor), or separation anxiety disorder (e.g., avoidance of leaving home or relatives)

patients with agoraphobia also have panic disorder. The condition is far more common in females than males. Agoraphobia is often persistent and can leave people homebound.

Generalized anxiety disorder (GAD) includes **overanxious disorder of childhood.** GAD is characterized by 6 or more months of persistent and excessive anxiety and worry (Table 17–4). The etiology of GAD is unknown. Biologic relatives have an increased risk for developing GAD. Family studies also have shown an increased risk for major depression in biologic relatives. The lifetime prevalence rate for GAD is 5%. It is a common diagnosis in patients referred to a psychiatrist.

TABLE 17–4.   Criteria for Diagnosis of Generalized Anxiety Disorder

A. Excessive anxiety and worry (apprehensive expectation), occurring more days than not for at least 6 mo, about numerous events or activities (e.g., work or school performance)
B. The person finds it difficult to control the worry
C. The anxiety and worry are associated with ≥3 of the following 6 symptoms (with at least some symptoms present for more days than not for the past 6 mo).
   Note: Only one symptom is required in children
   1. Restlessness or feeling keyed up or on edge
   2. Being easily fatigued
   3. Difficulty concentrating or mind going blank
   4. Irritability
   5. Muscle tension
   6. Sleep disturbance (difficulty falling or staying asleep or restless, unsatisfying sleep)
D. The focus of the anxiety and worry is not confined to features of a disorder (e.g., the anxiety or worry is not about having a panic attack, as in panic disorder; being embarrassed in public, as in social phobia; being contaminated, as in obsessive-compulsive disorder; being away from home or close relatives, as in separation anxiety disorder; gaining weight, as in anorexia nervosa; having multiple physical complaints, as in somatization disorder; or having a serious illness, as in hypochondriasis), and the anxiety and worry do not occur exclusively during post-traumatic stress disorder
E. The anxiety, worry, or physical symptoms cause clinically significant distress or impairment in social, occupational, or other important areas of functioning
F. The disturbance is not due to the direct physiologic effects of a drug (e.g., a drug of abuse or a medication) or a general medical condition (e.g., hyperthyroidism) and does not occur exclusively during a mood disorder, a psychotic disorder, or a pervasive developmental disorder

---

The anxiety must be accompanied by at least three of the following symptoms to diagnose GAD: restlessness, easy fatigability, difficulty concentrating, irritability, muscle tension, and disturbed sleep. The fear or anxiety must be out of proportion to what is realistic for the situation. Physical signs of anxiety are often present, including shakiness, trembling, and myalgias. Gastrointestinal symptoms (nausea, vomiting, diarrhea) and autonomic symptoms (tachycardia, shortness of breath) commonly coexist. In children and adolescents, the symptoms often are related to school performance or sports. Children with GAD may be perfectionists and overly concerned about the approval of others. GAD, similar to other anxiety disorders, tends to be chronic. Many patients with GAD describe having been anxious all their lives. The onset of the illness is usually in childhood or adolescence. There are no laboratory or imaging studies that are diagnostic for GAD.

The **differential diagnosis** for GAD is broad and includes normal anxiety that does not interfere with daily living, other anxiety disorders (OCD, separation anxiety disorder, social phobia), anorexia nervosa (worries about gaining weight), and somatoform disorders (worries about health). Substance-induced anxiety disorder also must be considered (caffeine intoxication, and sedative-hypnotic withdrawal). Essential tremor can start in adolescence and is often accompanied by social fears. Self-medication with alcohol is common. Common causes of anxiety due to a general medical condition include hyperthyroidism, irritable bowel syndrome, pheochromocytoma, and essential tremor. The anxiety symptoms must persist beyond when the patient is depressed or psychotic.

Treatment for GAD is two-pronged—medications and psychotherapy. SSRIs have been used frequently to treat GAD. Benzodiazepines have been used in adults but generally are avoided in children and adolescents because of frequent behavioral disinhibition. Cognitive, behavioral, and supportive psychotherapy all are commonly used techniques for GAD.

GAD tends to be a chronic illness with symptom intensity waxing and waning over time. There is no known primary prevention. Prevention goals focus on decreasing the morbidity associated with GAD.

Post-traumatic stress disorder (PTSD) is characterized by re-experiencing an extremely traumatic event. The re-experiencing is accompanied by avoidance of stimuli that remind the person of the trauma and by autonomic hyperarousal. A diagnosis of PTSD requires that the person has been exposed to a trauma in which actual or threatened death or serious injury was possible. Witnessing or learning about such an event also can be the cause of the trauma. Stressors of human design, including rape and torture, are particularly traumatic (Table 17–5). The genetic or

TABLE 17–5.   Criteria for Diagnosis of Post-Traumatic Stress Disorder

A. The person has been exposed to a traumatic event in which both of the following were present:
 1. The person experienced, witnessed, or was confronted with an event or events that involved actual or threatened death or serious injury or a threat to the physical integrity of self or others
 2. The person's response involved intense fear, helplessness, or horror. **Note:** In children, this may be expressed instead by disorganized or agitated behavior
B. The traumatic event is persistently re-experienced in ≥1 of the following ways:
 1. Recurrent and intrusive distressing recollections of the event, including images, thoughts, or perceptions. **Note:** In young children, repetitive play may occur in which themes or aspects of the trauma are expressed
 2. Recurrent distressing dreams of the event. **Note:** In children, there may be frightening dreams without recognizable content
 3. Acting or feeling as if the traumatic event were recurring (includes a sense of reliving the experience, illusions, hallucinations, and dissociative flashback episodes, including flashbacks that occur on awakening or when intoxicated). **Note:** In young children, trauma-specific reenactment may occur
 4. Intense psychological distress at exposure to internal or external cues that symbolize or resemble an aspect of the traumatic event
 5. Physiologic reactivity on exposure to internal or external cues that symbolize or resemble an aspect of the traumatic event
C. Persistent avoidance of stimuli associated with the trauma and numbing of general responsiveness (not present before the trauma), as indicated by ≥3 of the following:
 1. Efforts to avoid thoughts, feelings, or conversations associated with the trauma
 2. Efforts to avoid activities, places, or people that arouse recollections of the trauma
 3. Inability to recall an important aspect of the trauma
 4. Markedly diminished interest or participation in significant activities
 5. Feeling of detachment or estrangement from others
 6. Restricted range of affect (e.g., unable to have loving feelings)
 7. Sense of a foreshortened future (e.g., does not expect to have a career, marriage, children, or a normal life span)
D. Persistent symptoms of increased arousal (not present before the trauma), as indicated by ≥2 of the following:
 1. Difficulty falling or staying asleep
 2. Irritability or outbursts of anger
 3. Difficulty concentrating
 4. Hypervigilance
 5. Exaggerated startle response
E. Duration of the disturbance (symptoms in criteria B, C, and D) is >1 mo
F. The disturbance causes clinically significant distress or impairment in social, occupational, or other important areas of functioning

Specify if
 Acute: if duration of symptoms is <3 mo
 Chronic: if duration of symptoms is ≥3 mo

Specify if
 With delayed onset: if onset of symptoms is at least 6 mo after the stressor

psychosocial factors that may predispose a person who is traumatized to develop PTSD are unknown. The lifetime prevalence estimates of PTSD vary, but 8% is most commonly cited. There are increased risks of developing PTSD in family members of patients with PTSD; this is likely due to inherited genetic vulnerability for developing the disorder.

The clinical manifestations of PTSD fall into four general categories. The *first criterion* is that the person had to have experienced a trauma. *Trauma* is defined as an event in which actual or threatened death or serious injury is personally experienced or witnessed or learning about such a violent event. Severity, duration, and proximity of the event are the most likely predictors of developing PTSD.

The *second criterion* is that the trauma must be re-experienced by the person. This re-experiencing can be manifest as recurrent and intrusive recollections of the event or recurrent distressing dreams. In children, the dreams may be nonspecific to the trauma (e.g., monsters). In addition, children's play may be repetitive revolving around the circumstances of the trauma.

Dissociative states, in which the person relives the traumatic event, are referred to as *flashbacks*. These can last a few seconds to many hours.

The *third criterion* is that the person attempts to avoid situations that remind him or her of the original trauma. The *fourth criterion* is that the person must experience physical signs of anxiety or increased arousal, including difficulty falling or staying asleep, hypervigilance, exaggerated startle response, irritability, angry outbursts, and difficulty concentrating.

PTSD can occur from one dramatic incident (e.g., a motor vehicle accident). PTSD in children is often the result of repeated trauma. These repeatedly traumatized children may be more difficult to treat.

Most of the symptoms of PTSD are adaptive until they reach the point that they interfere with the person's functioning. Remembering a trauma, avoiding situations similar to the trauma, and increased vigilance are adaptive until they lead to dysfunction in daily life. The course of the illness usually begins within 3 months of the trauma. Delay in symptom expression can occur, with symptoms arising many months later. Typically an acute stress disorder is present immediately after the trauma.

No laboratory or imaging studies diagnose PTSD. Autonomic arousal (e.g., increased heart rate, dilated pupils) may be evident on physical examination. The **differential diagnosis** includes other anxiety disorders, adjustment disorders, acute stress disorder, OCD (because of the intrusive thoughts in OCD), psychotic disorders, substance-induced disorders, and psychotic disorders secondary to general medical conditions. If financial compensation is at issue, malingering should be ruled out, although this is relatively rare in children.

The **treatment** for PTSD includes antidepressants, mood stabilizers, and antipsychotics. Psychosocial treatments, including cognitive and behavioral therapies, supportive therapy, and group therapy, have been used. Group therapy is the most controversial because it is in conflict with the diagnostic criterion of avoidance. Many patients do not participate in group therapy because it is a reminder of the traumatic event.

Major depression is commonly associated with PTSD. In adults, loss of employment and personal relationships often occurs. In children, the inability to form secure relationships and decreased school performance are common. The prognosis for PTSD varies. Some patients have excellent recovery, and others have significant functional decline. There is no proven prevention for PTSD. Early intervention to decrease morbidity is important.

Acute stress disorder is characterized by the same signs and symptoms as PTSD, but occurring immediately after a traumatic event. These symptoms do not always progress to PTSD. If impaired function persists after 1 month, the diagnosis of PTSD is made.

Anxiety disorder not otherwise specified is a common condition in clinical practice. This diagnosis is used when there are impairing anxiety or phobic symptoms that do not meet full criteria for another anxiety disorder.

School phobia and **separation anxiety disorder** are often intertwined. Children and adolescents who avoid or refuse to go to school may have histories of separation anxiety and multiple vague somatic complaints, such as headaches, abdominal pain, and fatigue. They often have been seen by numerous specialists and undergo elaborate medical evaluations. Their absence from school often is mistakenly seen as a consequence of their symptoms.

The expression of the somatic symptoms is a means of avoiding school and gaining the attention of a parent. These patients may have either a valid or an irrational concern about a parent and refuse to leave home. They also may have had an unpleasant experience in school. These patients rarely have a true phobia related to schoolwork. When challenged with the prospect of returning to school, these children often become extremely anxious and incapacitated with escalating symptoms. School phobia that first becomes manifest during adolescence may be an expression of a severe underlying psychopathologic condition. If there is no medical contraindication for the adolescent to return to school, and if he or she refuses to return, psychiatric consultation may be indicated.

The most effective **treatment** for school refusal is for the child to go to school (exposure). It does not become easier for the child to attend school after extended absences. It is common for parents, usually coerced by the child, to ask for retrospective "excuses" for already missed school days. The best way to avoid this problem is for parents to send the child to school.

SPECIFIC PHOBIAS

Specific phobias are marked persistent fears of things or situations, which often lead to avoidance behaviors (Table 17-6). Exposure to the feared object or situation leads to anxiety. The closer the person is to the fear-provoking stimulus, the greater the anxiety. The response to the fear can range from full panic attacks to more limited symptoms of anxiety. Although adults and adolescents usually can recognize that their fears are out of proportion to the circumstances, children may not. The anticipation of fear or actual fear must interfere with their daily living to make the diagnosis. Many patients have had actual fearful experiences with the object or situation (traumatic event).

Approximately 10% of people are affected with a diagnosable phobia. The ratio of females to males is

TABLE 17–6.   Criteria for Diagnosis of Specific Phobia

A. Marked and persistent fear that is excessive or unreasonable, cued by the presence or anticipation of a specific object or situation (e.g., flying, heights, animals, receiving an injection, seeing blood)
B. Exposure to the phobic stimulus almost invariably provokes an immediate anxiety response, which may take the form of a situationally bound or situationally predisposed panic attack. **Note:** In children, the anxiety may be expressed by crying, tantrums, freezing, or clinging
C. The person recognizes that the fear is excessive or unreasonable. **Note:** In children, this feature may be absent
D. The phobic situation is avoided or else is endured with intense anxiety or distress
E. The avoidance, anxious anticipation, or distress in the feared situation interferes significantly with the person's normal routine, occupational (or academic) functioning, or social activities or relationships, or there is marked distress about having the phobia
F. In children <18 yr, the duration is at least 6 mo
G. The anxiety, panic attacks, or phobic avoidance associated with the specific object or situation are not better accounted for by another mental disorder, such as obsessive-compulsive disorder (e.g., fear of dirt in someone with an obsession about contamination), post-traumatic stress disorder (e.g., avoidance of stimuli associated with a severe stressor), separation anxiety disorder (e.g., avoidance of school), social phobia (e.g., avoidance of social situations because of fear of embarrassment), panic disorder with agoraphobia, or agoraphobia without history of panic disorder

Specify type:
  Animal type is fear elicited by animals or insects
  Natural environment type (e.g., heights, storms, water)
  Blood/injection/injury type is fear related to seeing blood, injuries, injections, or having an invasive medical procedure
  Situational type is fear caused by specific situations (e.g., airplanes, elevators, enclosed places)
  Other type (e.g., fear of choking, vomiting, or contracting an illness; in children, fear of loud sounds or costumed characters)

2:1 for specific phobias. There is an increased risk for specific phobias in first-degree relatives of patients with specific phobias.

The associated anxiety is almost always felt immediately when confronted with the feared object or situation. The severity of the anxious response generally is related to the proximity of the situation or object and the ability to escape easily. The greater the proximity or the harder it is to escape, the higher the person's phobic anxiety. Fears of objects and situations are common. Often the severity of impairment does not interfere with the person's daily functioning. If function is not impaired, a disorder should not be diagnosed. Many people do not like spiders and are afraid of them, yet few are impaired in daily functioning because of this. The focus of the fear may be anticipated harm from the object or situation (fear of being bitten by dogs). Children may express their anxiety as crying, tantrums, freezing, or clinging. The onset of phobias commonly is during childhood.

No laboratory or imaging studies can diagnose a specific phobia. Specific phobias share many symptoms with other anxiety disorders. A feared object or situation usually can be identified. Concurrent illnesses often include major depression and *substance-related disorders*. More than half of all patients with a specific phobia meet diagnostic criteria for another psychiatric disorder.

Social phobia is a common (3% to 13% prevalence) type of phobia characterized by a marked and persistent fear of social or performance situations in which embarrassment might occur (Table 17–7). The focus of the person's fears are interpersonal and performance situations. In other ways, social phobia is similar to specific phobias.

Cognitive and behavioral techniques are frequently successful in **treating** phobias. Rapid exposure (flooding) or systematic desensitization (slowly getting closer to the feared object) are common techniques. Medications, including SSRIs or benzodiazepines, are used in more extreme or urgent cases. The psychotherapeutic techniques are more likely to have persistent effects after they are discontinued.

Left untreated or poorly treated, phobias can become immobilizing and result in significant morbidity. People with specific phobias often significantly restrict their lives. A vasovagal fainting response is common in *blood/injection/injury-type* phobias. In addition, blood/injection/injury-type phobias may lead patients to avoid needed medical care.

If a phobia persists into adulthood, there is only a 20% chance of remission. There are no well-studied primary prevention techniques. Preventing a cycle of exposure and escape (which reinforces the phobic response) can decrease the likelihood of prolonged impairment.

TABLE 17–7. Criteria for Diagnosis of Social Phobia

A. A marked and persistent fear of ≥1 social or performance situations in which the person is exposed to unfamiliar people or to possible scrutiny by others. The individual fears that he or she will act in a way (or show anxiety symptoms) that will be humiliating or embarrassing. **Note:** In children, there must be evidence of the capacity for age-appropriate social relationships with familiar people, and the anxiety must occur in peer settings, not just in interactions with adults

B. Exposure to the feared social situation almost invariably provokes anxiety, which may take the form of a situationally bound or situationally predisposed panic attack. **Note:** In children, the anxiety may be expressed by crying, tantrums, freezing, or shrinking from social situations or unfamiliar people

C. The person recognizes that the fear is excessive or unreasonable. **Note:** In children, this feature may be absent

D. The feared social or performance situations are avoided or else are endured with intense anxiety or distress

E. The avoidance, anxious anticipation, or distress in the feared social or performance situation interferes significantly with the person's normal routine, occupational (academic) functioning, or social activities or relationships, or there is marked distress about having the phobia

F. In children <18 yr, the duration is at least 6 mo

G. The fear or avoidance is not due to the direct physiologic effects of a drug of abuse, a medication, or a general medical condition and is not better accounted for by another mental disorder (e.g., panic disorder with or without agoraphobia, separation anxiety disorder, body dysmorphic disorder, pervasive developmental disorder, or schizoid personality disorder)

H. If a general medical condition or another mental disorder is present, the fear in criterion A is unrelated to it (e.g., the fear is not of stuttering, trembling in Parkinson's disease, or exhibiting abnormal eating behavior in anorexia nervosa or bulimia nervosa)

Specify if
  Generalized: if the fears include most social situations (e.g., initiating or maintaining conversations, participating in small groups, dating, speaking to authority figures, attending parties). **Note:** Also consider the additional diagnosis of avoidant personality disorder

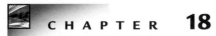

CHAPTER 18

Depression and Bipolar Disorders

DEPRESSION

Major depression is a diagnosis that requires a minimum of 2 weeks of depressive symptoms. A depressed mood or loss of interest or pleasure in nearly all activities is required. Four additional symptoms also must be present (Table 18–1).

The cause of depression is unknown. Neurochemical studies consistently have shown a decreased turnover of CNS serotonin. There is a genetic component as shown by twin and adoption studies. People with affected family members are at increased risk to develop depression. Sporadic (nonfamilial) cases are common, however. Depression affects all races and socioeconomic groups. In addition, psychosocial stressors are commonly involved in the precipitation of a depressive episode, and environmental stressors play a role. Early parental loss is one of the stressors that correlates most specifically with subsequent major depression. The World Health Organization estimates that depression will be the number one cause of morbidity throughout the world in the 21st century. Depression is a relatively common condition, occurring in 2% of children and 8% of adolescents.

Major depression is a condition whose prominent symptom is depressed mood. In children, irritable mood can serve as a proxy for depressed mood. Besides depressed (or irritable) mood or loss of interest or pleasure, the patient must have four additional symptoms. Other symptoms of depression are early morning awakening, middle and terminal insomnia or hypersomnia, changes in appetite, loss of sexual interest, psychomotor retardation or fatigue, inability to concentrate, and feelings of excessive guilt, worthlessness, and hopelessness. Typically, patients with depression have disturbed sleep with middle and terminal insomnia and decreased appetite with weight loss or failure to gain appropriate weight. In atypical depression, patients sleep and eat excessively. In this condition, a craving for carbohydrates is common. **Seasonal affective disorder** is a condition in which depressive

TABLE 18–1. Criteria for Diagnosis of Major Depressive Episode

A. Five or more of the following symptoms have been present during the same 2-wk period and represent a change from previous functioning; at least one of the symptoms is either (1) depressed mood or (2) loss of interest or pleasure. **Note:** Do not include symptoms that are clearly due to a general medical condition or mood-incongruent delusions or hallucinations
  1. Depressed mood most of the day, nearly every day, as indicated by either subjective report (e.g., feels sad or empty) or observation made by others (e.g., appears tearful). **Note:** In children and adolescents, mood can be irritable
  2. Markedly diminished interest or pleasure in all, or almost all, activities most of the day, nearly every day (as indicated by either subjective account or observation made by others)
  3. Significant weight loss when not dieting or weight gain (e.g., a change of >5% of body weight in 1 mo) or decrease or increase in appetite nearly every day. **Note:** In children, consider failure to make expected weight gains
  4. Insomnia or hypersomnia nearly every day
  5. Psychomotor agitation or retardation nearly every day (observable by others, not merely subjective feelings of restlessness or being slowed down)
  6. Fatigue or loss of energy nearly every day
  7. Feelings of worthlessness or excessive or inappropriate guilt (which may be delusional) nearly every day (not merely self-reproach or guilt about being sick)
  8. Diminished ability to think or concentrate or indecisiveness nearly every day (either by subjective account or as observed by others)
  9. Recurrent thoughts of death (not just fear of dying), recurrent suicidal ideation without a specific plan, or a suicide attempt or a specific plan for committing suicide
B. The symptoms do not meet criteria for a mixed manic episode
C. The symptoms cause clinically significant distress or impairment in social, occupational, or other important areas of functioning
D. The symptoms are not due to the direct physiologic effects of a drug of abuse, a medication, or a general medical condition (e.g., hypothyroidism)
E. The symptoms are not better accounted for by bereavement (i.e., after the loss of a loved one), and the symptoms persist >2 mo or are characterized by marked functional impairment, morbid preoccupation with worthlessness, suicidal ideation, psychotic symptoms, or psychomotor retardation

symptoms occur in the late fall and early winter when the hours of daylight are shortening. It is most common in northern latitudes.

The signs and symptoms of major depression can be remembered using the mnemonic *SIGECAPS*:

S—Sleep disturbance (usually decreased, can be increased)
I—Interests (decreased, for usual activities)
G—Guilt (excessive or inappropriate)
E—Energy (decreased)
C—Concentration problems
A—Appetite change (usually decreased, can be increased)
P—Pleasure (decreased)
S—Suicidal thoughts or actions

Depressed children and adolescents may not be able to identify their affective state. Depression can be indicated by "boredom," restlessness, difficulty in concentrating, decreasing school performance, preoccupation with somatic complaints (fatigue or vague or localized pains), running away, fights with peers, and other "acting-out" behaviors. Older adolescents may be better able to reflect on their feelings of depression and sadness. The characteristic sleep architecture abnormalities in adolescents and adults include decreased REM latency and middle and terminal insomnia. It is uncertain if these patterns occur in children.

Suicidal thoughts and behavior are common in depressed patients. Discussion of suicidal thoughts is important when counseling depressed patients. There is no evidence that discussing suicide leads to increased suicidal thoughts. There has been a large increase in the number of patients prescribed antidepressants since the 1990s. Some decrease in suicides has occurred over the same time. An increased risk of suicidal thoughts and behavior in children and youth receiving antidepressants has been reported, however.

No laboratory or imaging studies can diagnose major depression. Screening for hypothyroidism should be performed if indicated by clinical symptoms. *Dysthymia* and other *affective disorders* are the primary psychiatric disorders in the differential diagnosis for major depression. *Adjustment disorders* are common and respond to psychosocial interventions, including brief hospitalizations and supportive therapy. In addition, *mood disorder due to a general medical condition* (e.g., hypothyroidism) and *substance-induced mood disorders* (e.g., alcohol abuse and dependence, sedative-hypnotics) should be considered.

The **treatment** of depression in children and adolescents has developed amidst controversy. The results of large-scale studies of SSRIs for Food and Drug Administration (FDA) pediatric exclusivity have been disappointing. Of the eight SSRIs currently available in the U.S., only fluoxetine was found to be safe and efficacious. Six other SSRIs were found to be no better than placebo. One reason for the inability to differentiate their effects from placebo is the large placebo response rates. Paroxetine and venlafaxine were found to increase the risk for developing suicidal thoughts. This increase was on the order of 2% for the medication-treated groups. As a result of these findings, the FDA is cautioning clinicians to monitor patients for suicidal thoughts and behaviors.

Clinicians are not able to determine in advance which medication might work in which individual patient. All of the SSRIs are effective in some individuals. An antidepressant should be given an adequate trial before switching or discontinuing. An adequate trial would be 6 weeks at "therapeutic" doses. Serious side effects are the major reason to stop a medication before an adequate trial has been completed.

Medication selection should be based on several criteria. The first is efficacy. On the basis of efficacy and safety, fluoxetine is FDA approved for children and adolescents. A second criterion is effectiveness. This information could include knowledge of prior response to specific medications by the patient or family members. Also, minor differences in side-effect profiles and drug-drug interactions affect choice in patients taking multiple medications. Common side effects of SSRIs include gastrointestinal distress, sexual dysfunction (adolescents), activation, akathisia, and occasionally precipitation of mania.

The duration of treatment with antidepressants also is controversial. In adults, depression typically is treated for 6 to 9 months after remission of depressive symptoms. Some studies found that longer durations of treatment (≥2 years) lead to decreased numbers of relapses. For a first episode of depression in children and adolescents, it also is recommended to continue therapy for 6 to 9 months after full remission of symptoms. Patients with recurrent or chronic depression may need to take antidepressants for extended periods (years or lifetime).

Psychotherapy is another potential treatment for depression. Cognitive-behavioral therapy, interpersonal therapy, and dialectic behavioral therapy all show promise in the treatment of children and adolescents. In referring patients for therapy, identifying what approach the therapist uses can be helpful. The combination of psychotherapy and antidepressants has been studied to a small extent in pediatrics and holds promise for the treatment of depression.

If a patient does not respond to adequate trials of two or more antidepressants, a child psychiatrist should be consulted. The psychiatrist's evaluation should focus on diagnostic clarity and psychosocial issues that might be preventing full response. An initial evaluation by a child psychiatrist to confirm diagnosis also may be helpful. In many cases, starting an SSRI and subsequently referring to a child psychiatrist can decrease the time it takes for the child to receive adequate treatment.

Objective measures of the severity of depression and its response to intervention are required. A variety of clinician-administered (Hamilton Depression Rating Scale, Child Depression Rating Scale) and patient self-administered scales (Child Depression Inventory, Beck Depression Inventory) can be used to assess the patient's response to treatment. Using a formal scale or a clinician-rated Liekert scale (1 to 10) to assess and monitor the severity of depression is recommended.

Suicide is a **complication** of major depression. Fifteen percent to 20% of patients commit suicide. The risk for suicide may increase as a patient recovers from depression. Before full symptom resolution, the patient has increased energy and motivation, and this may lead to more suicide attempts. Major depression may be a chronic recurrent illness. There are no known primary prevention interventions. Treatment is targeted toward decreasing morbidity and suicide.

Dysthymia is a chronic form of depressed mood that has not reached full threshold symptoms for major depression. In children and adolescents, symptoms must be present more days than not for 1 year. In adults, the time criterion is 2 years. **Depressive disorder not otherwise specified** is a diagnosis used when patients have functionally impairing depressive symptoms that do not meet criteria for another condition.

MANIA AND DEPRESSION

Bipolar disorder, previously called *manic-depressive disorder*, often has its onset during childhood or adolescence. Mania consists of distinct periods of elevated, expansive, or irritable moods associated with hyperactivity and distractibility that may alternate rapidly with periods of severe depression lasting several days or weeks.

The family history of children with bipolar disorder is often positive for mental illness (major depression, bipolar disorder, schizophrenia, or attention-deficit/hyperactivity disorder [ADHD]). Having a first-degree relative with bipolar disorder leads to a 10-fold increase in the patient's chance of developing it as well. No gene has been identified as the cause of bipolar disorder; however, family and adoption studies indicate a significant genetic contribution. Sleep deprivation and substance abuse may precipitate the onset of the illness. Antidepressants have been shown to trigger mania.

Bipolar disorder may occur in 3.7% of the general population. It is estimated that 1% of children and adolescents meet diagnostic criteria for bipolar disorder. To **diagnose** bipolar disorder, the *Diagnostic and Statistical Manual of Mental Disorders, Fourth Edition,* requires

TABLE 18–2. Mania Symptoms

A. A distinct period of abnormally and persistently elevated, expansive, or irritable mood, lasting at least 1 wk (or any duration if hospitalization is necessary)
B. During the period of mood disturbance, ≥3 of the following symptoms have persisted (4 if the mood is only irritable) and have been present to a significant degree
   1. Inflated self-esteem or grandiosity
   2. Decreased need for sleep (e.g., feels rested after only 3 hr of sleep)
   3. More talkative than usual or pressure to keep talking
   4. Flight of ideas or subjective experience that thoughts are racing
   5. Distractibility (i.e., attention too easily drawn to unimportant or irrelevant external stimuli)
   6. Increased goal-directed activity (socially, at work or school, or sexually) or psychomotor agitation
   7. Excessive involvement in pleasurable activities that have a high potential for painful consequences (e.g., engaging in unrestrained buying sprees, sexual indiscretions, or foolish business investments)
C. The symptoms do not meet criteria for a mixed episode
D. The mood disturbance is sufficiently severe to cause marked impairment in occupational functioning or in usual social activities or relationships with others or to necessitate hospitalization to prevent harm to self or others, or there are psychotic features
E. The symptoms are not due to the direct physiologic effects of a substance (e.g., a drug of abuse, a medication, or other treatment) or a general medical condition (e.g., hyperthyroidism). **Note:** Manic-like episodes that are clearly caused by somatic antidepressant treatment (e.g., medication, electroconvulsive therapy, light therapy) should not count toward a diagnosis of bipolar I disorder

elevated or expansive mood and three additional symptoms or irritable mood and four additional manic symptoms (Table 18-2). The term *euphoria* describes elevated and expansive mood. Children and adolescents with euphoric mood are bubbly, giggly, "over-the-top" happy, to a degree that it is socially unacceptable and irritating to others.

A decreased need for sleep is a hallmark of *mania*. Although decreased sleep is not absolutely required to make the diagnosis, there are no other diagnoses where a child has a greatly decreased amount of total sleep (compared with age-appropriate norms) and is not tired.

Grandiosity in children is often expressed as being better than everyone else. Children behave as if they are superior even in situations in which it is obvious that this is not true. Behaving as if the laws of nature do not apply to them (attempting to get out of moving motor vehicles) and telling adults (other than their parents) what to do or how to do their jobs are common types of grandiosity in children.

Irritability can substitute for elated mood as a cardinal symptom of mania. Irritability is common in people of all ages. This irritability is so severe that often parents are unable to console the patient. This causes family members to "walk on eggshells" for fear of aggravating the child. Another common feature of bipolar disorder is *racing thoughts*. Racing thoughts are when thoughts are generated too quickly for a patient to keep up with them. Periods of extreme *rage* also are common in children with bipolar disorder. These rages or tantrums are not diagnostic criteria, however. Many children with bipolar disorder do not exhibit this symptom.

Mixed mania is a term used to describe the co-occurrence of manic and depressive symptoms in the same week. **Dysphoric mania** is another term used to describe periods of mania that are accompanied by "bad feelings." Continuous symptoms, as opposed to discrete episodes, also are common in children with bipolar disorder. *Hypomania* is used to describe a period of more than 4 but less than 7 days of manic symptoms. It also is used to describe less intense mania.

Suicidal thoughts and behaviors are common in affective disorders. Fifteen percent to 20% of patients with bipolar disorder ultimately commit suicide; 50% of adolescents with bipolar disorder make a suicide attempt or gesture. Significant impairment at home, school, and with peers is common.

Bipolar II disorder includes at least one full major depressive episode and at least one period of hypomania. This is in contrast to **bipolar I disorder**, in which impairing symptoms of mania have to be present for at least 7 days. **Bipolar disorder NOS** is used to describe prominent symptoms of bipolar disorder that do not meet full diagnostic criteria. It also is used when historical information is unclear or contradictory. **Cyclothymic disorder** is characterized by 2 years or more (1 year in children) of numerous periods of hypomania and depression that do not meet full criteria for either a manic or a major depressive episode.

Patients with bipolar disorder often have concurrent conditions that warrant treatment. **ADHD** occurs in approximately 70% of children with bipolar disorder. ADHD is primarily a disorder of inattention, hyperactivity, and impulsivity that by definition must occur before age 7 years (see Chapter 13). It is not a mood disorder. Typically, patients with untreated ADHD are demoralized and not grandiose. Symptoms of grandiosity, decreased need for sleep, and euphoria can be used to help differentiate between mania and

ADHD. Medications used to treat mania do not treat the inattentive symptoms of ADHD.

Anxiety disorders also commonly co-occur with bipolar disorder. They are often quite impairing and generally do not respond to antimanic agents. *Substance abuse problems* can precipitate and perpetuate mania and depression.

No laboratory or imaging studies can diagnose bipolar disorder. Periodic monitoring of blood levels for select medications (lithium and divalproex sodium) can help ensure the safety of the treatment and ensure that the patient is receiving therapeutic amounts of the medication. The **differential diagnosis** for bipolar disorder includes ADHD, major depression, conduct disorder, schizophrenia, mood disorder due to a general medical condition, and substance-induced mood disorder.

Many patients with bipolar disorder are aggressive. They often damage property and impulsively commit other crimes. They may meet criteria for conduct disorder. Prominent symptoms of mania assist in differentiating between conduct disorder and bipolar disorder.

The term *mood stabilizer* is used to refer to a medication that treats mania. This term implies effectiveness against depression as well. The FDA has approved lithium, divalproex sodium, olanzapine, risperidone, quetiapine, ziprasidone, and aripiprazole for adults with bipolar disorder. Studies of most of these agents are under way in adolescents. Lithium is the oldest proven treatment for mania. It has been used effectively in children and adolescents clinically for years. Common side effects of lithium include hypothyroidism, polyuria, and acne. The FDA has approved lamotrigine in adults to maintain remission for depressive and manic symptoms. A medication-related rash, which can progress to Stevens-Johnson syndrome, limits its use in patients younger than age 16.

Combination treatments commonly are required to stabilize mania and to treat comorbid conditions. ADHD is a common concurrent illness. There is concern about precipitating mania when stimulants or antidepressants are used to treat ADHD (see Chapter 13). New evidence suggests that if the manic symptoms are stabilized first, a stimulant often can be added safely and effectively.

Anxiety symptoms also are common in patients with bipolar disorder. SSRIs can destabilize patients and precipitate mania. Depression is the other pole of bipolar illness. Controversy currently surrounds the use of antidepressants in pediatric bipolar disorder (see discussion of major depression). These agents often destabilize patients, even when added to effective antimanic agents.

Cognitive and behavioral therapies are aimed at improving adherence to medication treatments and ameliorating anxiety and depressive symptoms. These therapies may be the treatment of choice for concurrent anxiety and depressive symptoms.

Untreated or poorly treated bipolar disorder can lead to many problems. Suicide, school and occupational failures, social difficulties, and arrest are common in patients who do not obtain or adhere to good treatment regimens. Developmental delays are common in young children with bipolar disorder because they are not cognitively "available" to learn.

The prognosis for bipolar disorder is guarded. Persons with bipolar disorder tend to have a chronic course of illness. The response to treatment can be robust. There are no known primary prevention interventions. Emphasis is on decreasing morbidity by decreasing the amount of time the patient stays ill.

CHAPTER 19
Obsessive-Compulsive Disorder

Obsessive-compulsive disorder (OCD) is characterized by obsessions (thoughts that cause marked anxiety) or compulsions (actions aimed at counteracting anxiety) or both. The person generally recognizes that the obsessions or compulsions are unreasonable (Table 19–1). Children may not be able to recognize this and often do not complain about the symptoms.

Family studies reflect a genetic component in OCD, with monozygotic twins affected more commonly than dizygotic twins. OCD may be related to group A streptococcal infection (see Chapter 103). When this is the case, the onset is often before puberty and frequently is associated with neurologic abnormalities. The adult disorder is equally distributed between men and women. With childhood onset, OCD is more common in boys. It occurs in 1% to 2% of the general population.

Obsessions are persistent ideas, thoughts, impulses, or images that are experienced as intrusive and cause marked anxiety and distress. The most common obsessions are fears of contamination, repeated doubts, need for orderliness, aggressive or horrific impulses, and sexual imagery. *Compulsions* are repetitive behaviors that serve to decrease anxiety and distress. The most common compulsions are hand washing, ordering, checking, requesting or demanding reassurance, praying, counting, and repeating words silently.

The disorder most commonly starts in adolescence or the early 20s. The onset is usually gradual; however, abrupt onset does occur. Similar to other anxiety disorders, the course of illness waxes and wanes over time.

TABLE 19–1. Criteria for Diagnosis of Obsessive-Compulsive Disorder

A. Either obsessions or compulsions
    Obsessions are defined by (1), (2), (3), and (4)
    1. Recurrent and persistent thoughts, impulses, or images that are experienced, at some time during the disturbance, as intrusive and inappropriate and that causes marked anxiety or distress
    2. The thoughts, impulses, or images are not simply excessive worries about real life problems
    3. The person attempts to ignore or suppress such thoughts, impulses, or images or to neutralize them with some other thought or action
    4. The person recognizes that the obsessional thoughts, impulses, or images are a product of his or her own mind (not imposed from without as in thought insertion)
    Compulsions are defined by (1) and (2)
    1. Repetitive behaviors (e.g., hand washing, ordering, checking) or mental acts (e.g., praying, counting, repeating words silently) that the person feels driven to perform in response to an obsession or according to rules that must be applied rigidly
    2. The behaviors or mental acts are aimed at preventing or reducing distress or preventing some dreaded event or situation; however, these behaviors or mental acts either are not connected in a realistic way with what they are designed to neutralize or prevent or are clearly excessive
B. At some point during the course of the disorder, the person has recognized that the obsessions or compulsions are excessive or unreasonable. **Note:** This does not apply to children
C. The obsessions or compulsions cause marked distress; are time-consuming (taking >1 hr a day); or significantly interfere with the person's normal routine, occupational (or academic) functioning, or usual social activities or relationships
D. If another Axis I disorder is present, the content of the obsessions or compulsions is not restricted to it (e.g., preoccupation with food in the presence of an eating disorder, hair pulling in the presence of trichotillomania, concern with appearance in the presence of body dysmorphic disorder, preoccupation with drugs in the presence of a substance use disorder, preoccupation with having a serious illness in the presence of hypochondriasis, preoccupation with sexual urges or fantasies in the presence of a paraphilia, or guilty ruminations in the presence of major depressive disorder)
E. The disturbance is not due to the direct physiologic effects of a drug of abuse, a medication, or a general medical condition

Specify if
With poor insight: if, for most of the time during the current episode, the person does not recognize that the obsessions and compulsions are excessive or unreasonable

About 15% of patients deteriorate significantly over time. No laboratory or imaging studies confirm or disprove the diagnosis. Physical examination may reveal evidence of excessive hand washing (rough, cracked skin).

The **differential diagnosis** for OCD includes psychotic disorders, other anxiety disorders, and **obsessive-compulsive personality disorder**. Obsessive-compulsive personality disorder is a character structure involving preoccupation with orderliness, perfectionism, and control. No obsessions or compulsions are present. OCD is present in approximately 50% of patients with Tourette disorder. **Tic disorders** also can be thought of as anxiety-relieving compulsive behaviors. In this case, the motor movements indicate a tic. **Body dysmorphic disorder**, a delusional fixation on appearance, can be confused with OCD. *Trichotillomania* or hair pulling to relieve anxiety or tension also can be confused with OCD. Schizophrenia can co-occur with OCD. The intrusive thoughts of OCD can be confused with hallucinations.

SSRIs, sometimes at high doses, have shown positive results in large clinical trials. Antipsychotics may be needed in severe or treatment refractory cases. Cognitive and behavioral therapy has shown clinical efficacy; neuroimaging studies show similar brain changes in patients successfully treated with medications and cognitive and behavioral therapy. Intravenous penicillin and other techniques aimed at the streptococcal related cases are being investigated. Psychosurgical interventions, including ablation of the cingulate gyrus, have been used in extreme cases.

Major depression, other anxiety disorders, eating disorders, and obsessive-compulsive personality disorder commonly co-occur with OCD. Learning disorders and disruptive behavior disorders are also common.

The prognosis for OCD is guarded. It is generally possible to obtain significant symptomatic response with treatment. There are no proven primary prevention interventions. Secondary and tertiary prevention is aimed at decreasing morbidity associated with the illness.

CHAPTER **20**

Pervasive Developmental Disorders and Psychoses

Autism and other pervasive developmental disorders typically have their onset in infancy and preschool years. The hallmarks of these disorders include impaired social interaction, impaired communication, and stereotypic behaviors, interests, and activities. Mental retardation is common in patients with pervasive developmental disorders.

AUTISTIC DISORDER

Autistic disorder is characterized by marked impairment in social interaction and communication and a restricted range of activities and interests (Table 20–1). Impaired reciprocal social interactions are the hallmark of the illness. Patients with autism often are not able to understand nonverbal communication (eye contact) and do not interact with people as significantly different from objects. Communication difficulties can arise from lack of spoken or nonverbal language or may present as stereotyped and repetitive language. Their repetitive language can be mistaken as a sign of OCD or as perseveration that is associated with psychosis.

The **etiology** of autistic disorder is unknown. There is an increased risk of autistic disorder in siblings compared with the general population (0.05% to 0.5%). Siblings of an individual with autistic disorder also are at greater risk for other developmental problems.

There have been concerns about an increasing frequency of autism. **Epidemiologic** surveys suggest that the rate has remained relatively constant at 5 per 10,000 children. It is likely that more children with mental retardation have been diagnosed with autistic disorder or pervasive developmental disorders. Males are affected four to five times more frequently than females. When females are affected, they usually exhibit severe mental retardation.

Clinical manifestations of the disorder should be present by 3 years of age. Approximately 20% of parents report relatively normal development until age 1 or 2, followed by a steady or sudden decline. If the delays occur later than age 3, a different developmental disorder should be considered (Rett syndrome or childhood disintegrative disorder).

As an infant, the autistic child is often noticeably "uncuddly," with delayed or absent smiling. Later the young child may spend hours in solitary play and be withdrawn in the presence of other children or adults and indifferent to attempts at communication. Intense, absorbing interests, ritualistic behavior, and compulsive routines are characteristic, and disruption of these may invoke tantrum or rage reactions. Eye contact is abnormal or absent. Head banging, teeth grinding, rocking, diminished responsiveness to pain and external stimuli, and self-mutilation may be noted. Speech often is delayed; when present, it is frequently dominated by echolalia, pronoun reversal, nonsense rhyming, and other unusual language forms.

The severity and character of the symptoms are likely to change over time. Although the expression of

---

TABLE 20–1. Criteria for Diagnosis of Autistic Disorder

A. Six or more items from (1), (2), and (3), with at least 2 from (1) and 1 each from (2) and (3)
   1. Qualitative impairment in social interaction, as manifested by at least 2 of the following:
      a. Marked impairment in the use of multiple nonverbal behaviors, such as eye-to-eye gaze, facial expression, body postures, and gestures to regulate social interaction
      b. Failure to develop peer relationships appropriate to developmental level
      c. A lack of spontaneous seeking to share enjoyment, interests, or achievements with other people (e.g., by a lack of showing, bringing, or pointing out objects of interest)
      d. Lack of social or emotional reciprocity
   2. Qualitative impairments in communication as manifested by at least 1 of the following:
      a. Delay in, or total lack of, the development of spoken language (not accompanied by an attempt to compensate through alternative modes of communication, such as gesture or mime)
      b. In individuals with adequate speech, marked impairment in the ability to initiate or sustain a conversation with others
      c. Stereotyped and repetitive use of language or idiosyncratic language
      d. Lack of varied, spontaneous make-believe play or social imitative play appropriate to developmental level
   3. Restricted repetitive and stereotyped patterns of behavior, interests, and activities, as manifested by at least 1 of the following:
      a. Encompassing preoccupation with ≥1 stereotyped and restricted patterns of interest that is abnormal either in intensity or focus
      b. Apparently inflexible adherence to specific, nonfunctional routines or rituals
      c. Stereotyped and repetitive motor mannerisms (e.g., hand or finger flapping or twisting or complex whole body movements)
      d. Persistent preoccupation with parts of objects
B. Delays or abnormal functioning in at least 1 of the following areas, with onset before age 3 yr
   1. Social interaction
   2. Language as used in social communication
   3. Symbolic or imaginative play
C. The disturbance is not better accounted for by Rett syndrome or childhood disintegrative disorder

---

symptoms may fluctuate, children with autistic disorder remain continuously impaired. Adolescence may bring an improvement or worsening of impairment. Language skills and IQ are the best predictors of long-term function. The better the person can communicate, the more likely he or she will be able to live independently or in less structured group living situations. Some children with autism spectrum disorders show remarkable isolated abilities (*savant* or *splinter skills*). Mental retardation ranging from mild to profound is present in most cases. Seizure disorders are common, occurring in 25% of patients, and often start in early adolescence.

There are no definitive laboratory studies for autistic disorder. Hearing should be tested to determine if there is a deficit that may account for the language problems. Chromosomal abnormalities, genetic polymorphisms, congenital infections, and structural brain abnormalities all should be evaluated as possible etiologic causes of these symptoms. There is no specific MRI pattern to identify autism. Speech pathology consultation can be helpful in evaluating the communication difficulties. Nonspecific electroencephalographic abnormalities are common even without seizures.

The **differential diagnosis** includes CNS developmental abnormalities, fragile X syndrome, and tuberous sclerosis. Expressive and mixed receptive and expressive language disorders also should be considered. The main diagnoses that can be confused with autistic disorder are the other pervasive developmental disorders. **Asperger disorder** can be distinguished from autistic disorder by a preservation of language development. **Childhood disintegrative disorder** has a distinctive pattern of severe developmental regression. This regression occurs after milestones are achieved relatively normally in the first 2 years of life. A rapid deterioration in multiple functional areas is the hallmark of the disorder. **Rett syndrome** has been diagnosed only in girls; autistic disorder is more common in boys. Rett syndrome is one of the only psychiatric disorders in which a specific genetic abnormality has been identified. There is a characteristic pattern of developmental regression that occurs after relatively normal development in the first few months of life. Head circumference growth dramatically decelerates, and a characteristic hand-wringing stereotyped movement exists. Motor coordination problems also are prominent. **Pervasive developmental disorder not otherwise specified** is a diagnosis made when significant impairment exists in developmental trajectory, but the patient does not meet full criteria for one of the aforementioned disorders.

When autistic disorder is suspected, referral to a specialist is required for further evaluation and treatment. There is no specific medical or psychotherapeutic treatment for autism. Treatments are directed toward target symptoms or syndromes. Aggression, inattention, self-stimulatory behavior, and hyperactivity are the most common targets of medication management. Psychostimulants can be used with caution for symptoms of attention-deficit/hyperactivity disorder (ADHD).

The newer antipsychotics (risperidone, olanzapine, quetiapine, ziprasidone, and aripiprazole) and α_2-agonists (clonidine and guanfacine) can be used for aggression. Severe self-stimulatory behavior occasionally responds to naltrexone. Families with severely ill children often need counseling and supportive services. Many parents are desperate for assistance and may spend significant amounts of money on unproven treatments.

The prognosis for autism is guarded. The condition is chronic, with few patients "growing out of it." At present, there are no known methods of primary prevention. Treatment and educational interventions are aimed at decreasing morbidity and maximizing function.

SCHIZOPHRENIA

Schizophrenia generally presents in adolescence or early adulthood. The onset of schizophrenia in adolescents resembles that in adults. Onset of schizophrenia before puberty is rare. The same diagnostic criteria are applied, but must be interpreted in terms of the developmental stage of the child. Schizophrenia prevalence rates are 0.5% to 1.5% of the adult population; this is regardless of ethnic or other cultural factors. The etiology of schizophrenia is unknown. Numerous studies have shown genetic predisposition and linkages for the disorder. In addition, family studies consistently have shown higher risk for monozygotic twins compared with dizygotic twins and siblings. First-degree relatives of patients with schizophrenia are at a 10-fold higher risk to be affected than the general population. Although genetics plays a strong role, many patients diagnosed with schizophrenia have sporadic or nonfamilial histories.

Psychosis is the hallmark of schizophrenia and consists of hallucinations and delusions. Hallucinations are auditory or visual misperceptions that occur without external stimuli. This is in contrast to illusions, which are misperceptions of sensory stimuli. Delusions are fixed false beliefs. Delusions can be classified as bizarre or nonbizarre. The determination of whether a delusion is bizarre or not is based on cultural norms. If the false belief is within cultural boundaries, it is nonbizarre. The determination of bizarreness generally is made if the belief is implausible, not understandable, or outside cultural norms. An example of a bizarre delusion would be a child who fears aliens have taken over his or her actions. Healthcare providers frequently see adolescents in the early stages of psychosis because of behavioral or somatic symptoms. It is important to take cultural norms into account when assessing whether a phenomenon is abnormal or not; for example, in some cultures it is not abnormal to converse with dead relatives.

To meet criteria for diagnosing schizophrenia, clinical symptoms should be present for at least 6 months. It is possible to meet other diagnostic criteria for schizophrenia but not the time criteria. This happens in two different circumstances. The first is that not enough time has elapsed. The second is when symptoms resolve before 6 months. If symptoms are present less than 1 month, the condition is called **brief psychotic disorder**. If symptoms are present more than 1 month but less than 6 months, a diagnosis of **schizophreniform disorder** is made. Psychotic symptoms that do not meet full diagnostic criteria for schizophrenia but are clinically significant are diagnosed as **psychotic disorder not otherwise specified**.

Schizophrenia is characterized by hallucinations, delusions, disorganization, loosening of associations, inappropriate affect, ambivalent emotional state, and gradual but marked withdrawal from family, school, and peers (Table 20–2). Perceptual disturbances are frequent. These symptoms must cause marked social and functional impairment, and some signs must be present for at least 6 months to make a diagnosis of schizophrenia.

The symptoms of schizophrenia typically fall into four broad categories. *Positive symptoms* are symptoms that a patient with schizophrenia has that are added to usual function. These typically include hallucinations and delusions. *Negative symptoms* are functions that are normally present but are frequently absent in patients with schizophrenia. These include a lack of motivation and social interactions and flat affect. *Disorganization of thoughts and behavior* is another category of symptoms that cause significant impairment. *Cognitive impairment* also is common. These cognitive impairments are perhaps the most disabling features of schizophrenia, and until more recently, the treatment of these symptoms received little attention.

The course of illness for schizophrenia varies. Rarely a patient may respond well initially and have no

---

TABLE 20–2.   Criteria for Diagnosis of Schizophrenia

A. *Characteristic symptoms:* ≥2 of the following, each present for a significant portion of time during a 1-mo period (or less if successfully treated)
   1. Delusions
   2. Hallucinations
   3. Disorganized speech (e.g., frequent derailment or incoherence)
   4. Grossly disorganized or catatonic behavior
   5. Negative symptoms (i.e., affective flattening, alogia, or avolition)
   Note: Only 1 criterion A symptom is required if delusions are bizarre or hallucinations consist of a voice keeping up a running commentary on the person's behavior or thoughts or two or more voices conversing with each other
B. *Social/occupational dysfunction:* For a significant portion of the time since the onset of the disturbance, ≥1 major areas of functioning, such as work, interpersonal relations, or self-care, are markedly below the level achieved before the onset (or when the onset is in childhood or adolescence, failure to achieve expected level of interpersonal, academic, or occupational achievement)
C. *Duration:* Continuous signs of the disturbance persist for at least 6 mo. This 6-mo period must include at least 1 mo of symptoms (or less if successfully treated) that meet criterion A (i.e., active-phase symptoms) and may include periods of prodromal or residual symptoms. During these prodromal or residual periods, the signs of disturbance may be manifested by only negative symptoms or ≥2 symptoms listed in criterion A present in an attenuated form (e.g., odd beliefs, unusual perceptual experiences)
D. *Schizoaffective and mood disorder exclusion:* Schizoaffective disorder and mood disorder with psychotic features have been ruled out because either (1) no major depressive, manic, or mixed episodes have occurred concurrently with the active-phase symptoms or (2) if mood episodes have occurred during active-phase symptoms, their total duration has been brief relative to the duration of the active and residual periods
E. *Substance/general medical condition exclusion:* The disturbance is not due to the direct physiologic effects of a drug of abuse, a medication, or a general medical condition
F. *Relationship to a pervasive developmental disorder:* If there is a history of autistic disorder or another pervasive developmental disorder, the additional diagnosis of schizophrenia is made only if prominent delusions or hallucinations also are present for at least 1 mo (or less if successfully treated)

Classification of longitudinal course (can be applied only after at least 1 yr has elapsed since the initial onset of active-phase symptoms)
Episodic with interepisode residual symptoms (episodes are defined by the re-emergence of prominent psychotic symptoms); *also specify if:* **with prominent negative symptoms**
Episodic with no interepisode residual symptoms
Continuous (prominent psychotic symptoms are present throughout the period of observation); *also specify if:* **with prominent negative symptoms**

additional psychotic episodes. Other patients respond but have intermittent episodes throughout their lives. Still others have a chronic deteriorating course.

There are five subtypes of schizophrenia: paranoid, disorganized, catatonic, undifferentiated, and residual. *Paranoid type* has prominent hallucinations and delusions with relatively normal cognition. The delusions are often persecutory, but other types also may occur. *Disorganized type* features disorganized speech, disorganized behavior, and flat or inappropriate affect. *Catatonic type* includes prominent psychomotor abnormalities that may include extreme inactivity or excessive motor activity. *Cataplexy* (waxy flexibility) was common in earlier times; this is rare in children and adolescents. In *undifferentiated type,* a patient meets the diagnostic criteria for schizophrenia, but not paranoid, disorganized, or catatonic type. *Residual type* describes a clinical situation in which full diagnostic criteria have been met previously, but currently there are no prominent positive symptoms.

No diagnostic tests or imaging studies are specific for schizophrenia. It is a diagnosis of exclusion to be made when all other causes have been eliminated. The clinician must rule out medical and psychiatric conditions that could mimic these symptoms. Structural brain imaging studies typically reveal large cerebral ventricles and an increased ventricle-to-brain ratio (less cortex, more CSF). Also, numerous neurochemical and neuropsychological abnormalities have been reported in patients with schizophrenia. None of these studies are specific enough to be considered diagnostic. MRI of the brain should be performed for new-onset psychosis to evaluate for intracranial lesions that could mimic schizophrenia. Temporal lobe epilepsy is a condition that mimics symptoms of schizophrenia but is etiologically related to the seizure disorder. Owing to the seizure activity being in deep temporal lobe structures, special EEG lead placement may be necessary to diagnose this condition.

The differential diagnosis for schizophrenia in children or adolescents is long and includes other psychotic disorders, medical conditions with psychosis as a consequence, and variants of normalcy. Isolated psychotic symptoms also may be encountered in children. The long-term prognostic importance of these symptoms is not well delineated. They may be signs of schizophrenia or another psychiatric illness. The first episode of psychosis commonly occurs in adolescence. The following conditions should be considered in the differential diagnosis:

Substance-induced psychotic disorders have psychotic symptoms that are related to drug or alcohol ingestion.

Schizoaffective disorder is diagnosed when a person has clear symptoms of schizophrenia for at least 2 weeks without active symptoms of depression or mania. These affective syndromes occur at other times, even when psychotic symptoms are present.

Delusional disorder consists of at least 1 month of nonbizarre delusions without other symptoms of schizophrenia.

Major depression with psychotic features and **bipolar disorder with psychotic features** are diagnoses made when psychotic symptoms occur only during the course of depression or mania.

Psychotic disorder due to a general medical condition describes psychotic symptoms that are judged to be the direct result of a general medical condition.

Shared psychotic disorder, *folie à deux,* occurs when delusional symptoms from one person influence delusions, with similar content, in another person.

Five new antipsychotic drugs—risperidone, olanzapine, quetiapine, ziprasidone, and aripiprazole—have been approved by the Food and Drug Administration for the treatment of schizophrenia in adults. None of these medications has been approved in children or younger adolescents. These drugs are better tolerated than previously available antipsychotics, but they have specific side effects that limit their use, such as weight gain and accompanying diabetes mellitus, sedation, neuromotor effects, and akathisia. Neuromotor side effects, including dystonia (severe painful muscle contractions), pseudoparkinsonism (signs and symptoms induced by medications that mimic Parkinson disease), and akathisia (an uncomfortable sense of motor restlessness), all were more common with the older (typical) antipsychotics. These side effects also can occur with the newer antipsychotics. It is important to choose an antipsychotic by side-effect profile geared toward a specific patient.

There is strong evidence that suggests the longer a patient is psychotic (or manic, depressed, or anxious), the more difficult the condition is to treat. For schizophrenia, more than 6 months of untreated psychosis dramatically decreases the rate of response to treatment. If there is any question about the possibility of psychosis, or impending psychosis, early psychiatric evaluation is indicated. If untreated or poorly treated, patients can experience a significant decline in social, occupational, and intellectual function. Many patients with schizophrenia commit suicide. Command hallucinations to harm oneself should be treated as a psychiatric emergency.

The prognosis of schizophrenia varies. Most patients have recurrent illness. Some have interepisode residual symptoms, whereas others return to a more normal baseline. Many patients with schizophrenia end up unemployed and homeless. Many others are productive members of society with only occasional serious difficulties.

Little is known about effective primary prevention. Reducing avoidable stressors and education about the illness can help to limit recurrences.

SUGGESTED READING

American Psychiatric Association: Diagnostic and Statistical Manual of Mental Disorders, 4th ed, Text Revision. Washington, D.C., American Psychiatric Association, 2000.

Behrman RE, Kliegman RM, Jenson HB (eds): Nelson Textbook of Pediatrics, 17th ed. Philadelphia, WB Saunders, 2003, pp 67-112.

Eth S: PTSD in Children and Adolescents. In Oldham JM, Riba MB (eds): Review of Psychiatry, Vol. 20. Arlington, Va, American Psychiatric Publishing, 2001, pp 1-216.

Hales RE, Yudofsky SC (eds): The American Psychiatric Publishing Textbook Essentials of Clinical Psychiatry, 2nd ed. Arlington, Va, American Psychiatric Publishing, 2004.

Kliegman RM, Greenbaum LA, Lye PS: Practical Strategies in Pediatric Diagnosis and Therapy, 2nd ed. Philadelphia, WB Saunders, 2004.

Ozonoff S, Rogers SJ, Hendren RL (eds): Autism Spectrum Disorders: A Research Review for Practitioners. Arlington, Va, American Psychiatric Publishing, 2003.

Phillips KA: Somatoform and Factitious Disorders. In Oldham JM, Riba MB (eds): Review of Psychiatry, Vol. 20. Arlington, Va, American Psychiatric Publishing, 2001, pp 1-216.

Schatzberg AF, Nemeroff CB (eds): The American Psychiatric Publishing Textbook of Psychopharmacology, 3rd ed. Arlington, Va, American Psychiatric Publishing, 2004.

Shaffer D, Waslick B: The Many Faces of Depression in Children and Adolescents. In Oldham JM, Riba RB (eds): Review of Psychiatry, Vol. 21. Arlington, Va, American Psychiatric Publishing, 2002, pp 1-206.

Weiner JM, Dulcan MK (eds): The American Psychiatric Publishing Textbook of Child and Adolescent Psychiatry, 3rd ed. Arlington, Va, American Psychiatric Publishing, 2004.

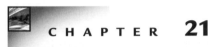

CHAPTER 21

Failure to Thrive

Failure to thrive (FTT) is a term given to malnourished infants and young children who fail to meet expected standards of growth. The term *FTT* is most often used to describe malnutrition that is related to environmental or psychosocial causes, although in most children with inadequate growth, organic and environmental contributors coexist. FTT may be due to various problems that have little in common except for their damaging effect on growth. In evaluating FTT, it is important to assess the potential medical, nutritional, developmental, psychosocial, and environmental contributors to the problem.

FTT is most commonly diagnosed using the Centers for Disease Control and Prevention growth charts (see Chapter 5). FTT is diagnosed by weight that falls or remains below the 3rd percentile for age, that decreases crossing two major percentile lines on the growth chart over time, or that is less than 80% of the median weight for the height of the child. Caveats to these definitions exist. According to growth chart standards, 3% of the population naturally falls below the 3rd percentile. These children, who typically have short stature or constitutional delay of growth, usually are proportional (normal weight for height). Additionally, in the first few years of life, large fluctuations in percentile position can occur in normal children. Changes in weight should be assessed in relation to height (length) and head circumference.

Weight that decreases from a disproportionately high percentile to one that is proportional with the height and head circumference causes no concern, but weight that decreases to a percentile that is disproportionately low is of concern. Allowances must be made for prematurity; weight corrections are needed until 24 months of age, height corrections are needed until 40 months of age, and head circumference corrections are needed until 18 months of age. Although some growth variants can be difficult to distinguish from FTT, growth velocity and height-for-weight determinations can be useful in distinguishing the cause of growth failure. In children with FTT, malnutrition initially results in wasting (deficiency in weight gain). Stunting (deficiency in linear growth) generally occurs after months of malnutrition, and head circumference generally is spared except with chronic, severe malnutrition. FTT that is *symmetric* (weight, height/length, and head circumference are proportional) suggests long-standing malnutrition, chromosomal abnormalities, congenital infection, or teratogenic exposures. FTT is a common problem in pediatrics, affecting 5% to 10% of young children and approximately 3% to 5% of children admitted to teaching hospitals. FTT is more common in children living in poverty and foster care and affects 15% of the latter group.

ETIOLOGY

Diseases of any organ system can cause malnutrition; poor growth can be an important clue to chronic illness. Because the possible causes of growth failure are so diverse and often multifactorial, the management of FTT begins with a careful search for its etiology (Table 21-1). The common causes of FTT vary by age, which should be reflected in the evaluation (Table 21-2). In most cases, a comprehensive history and physical examination are sufficient to suggest or eliminate medical disease as the primary cause for FTT. Relatively few children with FTT have a primary medical etiology for their growth failure. Medical diseases are diagnosed in less than 50% of children hospitalized for growth failure and even less frequently in children managed in the outpatient setting. Growth failure is often a manifestation of more extensive family problems.

TABLE 21–1.   Causes of Failure to Thrive

Environmental (common)
  Emotional deprivation
  Rumination
  Child maltreatment
  Maternal depression
  Poverty
  Poor feeding techniques
  Improper formula preparation
  Improper mealtime environment
  Unusual parental nutritional beliefs
Gastrointestinal
  Cystic fibrosis and other causes of pancreatic
    insufficiency
  Celiac disease
  Other malabsorption syndromes
  Gastrointestinal reflux
Congenital/anatomic
  Chromosomal abnormalities, genetic syndromes
  Congenital heart disease
  Gastrointestinal abnormalities (e.g., pyloric stenosis,
    malrotation)
  Vascular rings
  Upper airway obstruction
  Dental caries
  Congenital immunodeficiency syndromes
Infections
  HIV
  Tuberculosis
  Hepatitis
  Urinary tract infection
  Chronic sinusitis
  Parasitic infection
Metabolic
  Thyroid disease
  Adrenal or pituitary disease
  Aminoaciduria, organic aciduria
  Galactosemia
Neurologic
  Cerebral palsy
  Hypothalamic and other CNS tumors
  Hypotonia syndromes
  Neuromuscular diseases
  Degenerative and storage diseases
Renal
  Chronic renal failure
  Renal tubular acidosis
  Urinary tract infection
Hematologic
  Sickle cell disease
  Iron deficiency anemia

DIAGNOSIS AND CLINICAL MANIFESTATIONS

A medical history should address prenatal and postnatal factors that influence growth, including the history of prenatal care, maternal illnesses during pregnancy, identified fetal growth problems, prematurity, and birth size (weight, length, and head circumference). Indicators of medical diseases, such as vomiting, diarrhea, fever, respiratory symptoms, and fatigue, should be noted. A careful diet history is essential to the evaluation. Lactation problems in breastfed infants and improper formula preparation are frequent causes of growth failure early in infancy; the adequacy of the maternal milk supply or the precise preparation of formula should be evaluated. For older infants and young children, a detailed diet history is helpful, although it may be difficult to obtain. It is essential to evaluate intake of solid foods and liquids. Because of parental dietary beliefs, some children have inappro-

TABLE 21–2.   Common Causes of Malnutrition in Early Life

Neonate

Failed breastfeeding
Improper formula preparation
Congenital syndromes
Prenatal infections
Teratogenic exposures

Early Infancy

Maternal depression
Improper formula preparation
Gastroesophageal reflux
Poverty
Congenital heart disease
Cystic fibrosis
Neurologic abnormalities
Child neglect

Later Infancy

Celiac disease
Food intolerance
Child neglect
Delayed introduction of age-appropriate foods
Juice consumption

After Infancy

Acquired diseases
Highly distractible child
Juice consumption
Autonomy struggles
Inappropriate mealtime environment
Inappropriate diet

priately restricted diets. Other children with FTT drink excessive amounts of fruit juice, leading to malabsorption or anorexia for more nutrient-dense foods. The child's daily schedule, including the timing, frequency, and location of meals, is important to evaluate. Mealtime practices, especially distractions that interfere with completing meals, can influence growth. A complete psychosocial assessment of the child and family is required. Child factors (temperament, development), parental factors (depression, domestic violence, social isolation, mental retardation, substance abuse), and environmental and societal factors (poverty, unemployment, illiteracy, lead toxicity) all may contribute to growth failure. In some cases, the history provided by parents of children with FTT is inaccurate, which complicates the evaluation and management of the problem.

A complete physical examination and developmental screening should assess signs of inflicted injury; oral or dental problems that may interfere with feeding; indicators of pulmonary, cardiac, or gastrointestinal disease; and dysmorphic features that may suggest a genetic or teratogenic cause for growth failure. A complete neurologic examination may reveal spasticity or hypotonia, both of which can have untoward effects on feeding and growth. Some children may have physical findings related to malnutrition, such as dermatitis, hepatomegaly, cheilosis, or edema (see Section VI). Additionally, children with FTT have more otitis media and more respiratory and gastrointestinal infections than age-matched controls; severely malnourished children are at risk for a variety of serious infections.

The history and physical examination findings are used to guide the laboratory evaluation. An extensive laboratory search for medical diseases has no merit. Simple screening tests are recommended to screen for the common illnesses that may cause growth failure and to search for medical problems that result from malnutrition. Recommended laboratory tests include screening for iron deficiency anemia and lead toxicity; urinalysis, urine culture, and serum electrolytes to assess renal infection or dysfunction; and a PPD to screen for tuberculosis. HIV testing may be indicated for selected children. For children with diarrhea, abdominal pain, or malodorous stools, stool sample for culture and ova and parasites may be indicated. Observation during feeding and home visitation, if possible, are of great diagnostic value in assessing feeding problems, food preferences, mealtime distractions, unusual or disruptive parent-child interactions, and the home environment.

TREATMENT

The treatment for children with FTT must address the nutritional requirements of the child and the social issues of the family. Initial treatment should focus on the nutritional and medical management of the child, while engaging the family in the treatment plan. Parents of malnourished children may feel personally responsible and threatened by the diagnosis of FTT. Parents may be so depressed or dysfunctional that they cannot focus on their child's needs; they may not recognize the psychosocial and family contributors to the malnutrition. These issues can have a profound effect on the success of treatment, and in the course of therapy, they need to be addressed.

Children with mild malnutrition whose cause is easily identified can be managed by the primary care physician and family. In more challenging cases, however, a multidisciplinary team approach is warranted. A team approach to therapy, including pediatricians, nutritionists, developmental specialists, nurses, and social workers, has been shown to improve nutritional outcome in children with FTT compared with treatment by primary care physicians alone. Most children with FTT can be treated in the outpatient setting. Children with severe malnutrition, children with underlying diagnoses that require hospitalization for evaluation or treatment, and children whose safety is in jeopardy because of maltreatment require hospitalization. Admitting children to the hospital to induce and document weight gain is not recommended, unless intensive outpatient evaluation and intervention has failed, or the social circumstances of the family are a contraindication for attempting outpatient management.

Nutritional management is the cornerstone of treatment of FTT, regardless of the etiology. Children with FTT may require more than 1.5 times the expected calorie and protein intake for their age for catch-up growth. Children with FTT who are anorexic and picky eaters may not be able to consume this amount in volume and require calorically dense foods. For formula-fed infants, the concentration of formula can be changed from 20 cal/oz to 24 or 27 cal/oz (Table 21–3). For toddlers, dietary changes should include increasing the caloric density of favorite foods by adding butter, oil, sour cream, peanut butter, or other high-calorie foods. High-calorie oral supplements that provide 30 cal/oz are often well tolerated by toddlers. In some cases, specific carbohydrate, fat, or protein additives are used to boost calories. These additives have the advantage of increasing calories without increasing volume requirements and can be used to supplement formulas for infants and older children. In addition, vitamin and mineral supplementation is needed, especially during catch-up growth. In general, the simplest and least costly approach to dietary change is warranted.

Depending on the severity of the malnutrition, initiation of catch-up growth may take 2 weeks. Initial weight gain of more than double normal growth can

TABLE 21-3.   Infant Formula Preparation*

Amount of Powder/Liquid	Amount of Water (oz)	Final Concentration
1 cup powdered formula	29	20 kcal/oz
4 scoops powdered formula	8	20 kcal/oz
13 oz liquid concentrate	13	20 kcal/oz
1 cup powdered formula	24	24 kcal/oz
5 scoops powdered formula	8	24 kcal/oz
13 oz liquid concentrate	9	24 kcal/oz
1 cup powdered formula	21	27 kcal/oz
5.5 scoops powdered formula	8	27 kcal/oz
13 oz liquid concentrate	6	27 kcal/oz

*Final concentrations are reached by adding formula to water. One scoop of powdered formula = one measuring tablespoon. For healthy infants, formulas are prepared to provide 20 kcal/oz.

From Jew R (ed): Department of Pharmacy Services Pharmacy Handbook and Formulary, 2000-2001. Hudson, Ohio, Department of Pharmacy Services, 2000, p 422.

be seen. Weight improvement precedes improvement in stature. For children with chronic, severe malnutrition, many months are needed to reverse all trends in growth. Although many children with FTT eventually reach normal size, they continue to be at risk for developmental, learning, and behavioral problems.

COMPLICATIONS

Malnutrition causes defects in host defenses. Conversely, infection increases the metabolic needs of the patient and often is associated with anorexia. Children with FTT may suffer from a malnutrition-infection cycle, in which recurrent infections exacerbate malnutrition, which leads to greater susceptibility to infection. Children with FTT must be evaluated and treated promptly for infection and followed closely. Treatment regimens should be appropriate for the infection, but made as simple as possible to improve success with compliance.

During starvation, the body slows metabolic processes and growth to minimize the need for nutrients and uses its stores of glycogen, fat, and protein to maintain normal metabolic requirements. During starvation, the body also generally can maintain homeostasis and normal serum concentrations of electrolytes. With the rapid reinstitution of feeding after starvation, fluid and electrolyte homeostasis may be lost, and the body may be unable to maintain normal serum concentrations of vital electrolytes. Changes in serum electrolyte concentrations and the associated complications resulting from these changes are collectively termed **refeeding syndrome**. These changes typically affect phosphorus, potassium, calcium, and magnesium and can result in life-threatening cardiac,

pulmonary, or neurologic problems. Infants and children with marasmus, kwashiorkor, and anorexia nervosa and who have had prolonged fasting are at risk for refeeding syndrome. Refeeding syndrome can be avoided by slow institution of nutrition for children with severe malnutrition, close monitoring of serum electrolytes during the initial days of feeding, and prompt replacement of depleted electrolytes.

Occasionally, children who live in psychological deprivation develop short stature with or without concomitant FTT or delayed puberty, a syndrome called **psychosocial short stature**. The signs and symptoms found in children with psychosocial short stature include polyphagia, polydipsia, hoarding and stealing of food, gorging and vomiting, drinking from toilet bowls, and other notable behaviors. Although these behaviors may not be present, their identification in a child with abnormal growth should raise the possibility of psychosocial short stature. Affected children are often shy and passive and are typically depressed and socially withdrawn. Endocrine dysfunction is often identified in affected children, who may have decreased growth hormone secretion and a muted response to exogenous growth hormone. Removal of the child from the adverse environment typically results in rapid improvement in endocrine function and subsequent rapid somatic and pubertal growth of the child. The prognosis for children with psychosocial short stature depends on the age at diagnosis and the degree of psychological trauma the child has experienced. Early identification and removal from the detrimental environment portends a healthy prognosis. Children who are diagnosed in later childhood or adolescence may not reach their genetic potential for growth and have a poorer psychosocial prognosis.

CHAPTER 22

Child Abuse and Neglect

Few social problems have as profound an impact on the well-being of children as child abuse and neglect. Each year in the U.S., 3 million reports of suspected maltreatment are made to child welfare agencies. Approximately 1 million of these reports can be substantiated after investigation by Child Protective Services (CPS). These reports represent only a small portion of the children who suffer from maltreatment. Parental surveys indicate that several million adults admit to physical violence against their children each year, and many more adults report abusive experiences as children. Federal and state laws define child abuse and neglect, but each state determines the process of investigating abuse, protecting children, and punishing perpetrators for their crimes. Much of the abuse that is recognized by mandated reporters does not get reported to CPS for investigation. Adverse childhood events, such as child abuse and neglect, increase the risk of the individual developing behaviors that predict adult morbidity and early mortality. The ability to recognize child maltreatment and effectively advocate for the protection and safety of a child is a great challenge in pediatric practice that can have a profound influence on the health and future well-being of a child.

Child abuse is parental behavior destructive to the normal physical or emotional development of a child. Because personal definitions of abuse vary according to religious and cultural beliefs, individual experiences, and family upbringing, various physicians have different thresholds for reporting suspected abuse to CPS. In every state, however, physicians are mandated by law to protect children by identifying and reporting all cases of *suspected* child abuse and neglect. It is the responsibility of CPS to investigate reports of suspected abuse to determine whether abuse has occurred and to ensure the ongoing safety of the child. State laws also define as crimes intentional or reckless acts that cause harm to a child. Law enforcement investigates crimes such as sexual abuse and serious physical abuse or neglect for possible prosecution of the perpetrator.

Child abuse and neglect are often considered in broad categories that include physical abuse, sexual abuse, emotional abuse, and neglect. Of these, neglect is the most common, accounting for approximately half of the reports made to child welfare agencies. **Child neglect** is defined by omissions that prevent a child's basic needs from being met. These needs include adequate food, clothing, supervision, housing, health care, education, and nurturance. Child abuse and neglect result from a complex interaction of individual, family, and societal risk factors. Although some risk factors, such as parental substance abuse, maternal depression, and domestic violence in the household, are strong risk factors for maltreatment, these and other risk factors are better considered as broadly defined markers to alert a physician to a potential risk, rather than determinants of specific abuse and neglect. These risk factors, although important for developing public policies and prevention strategies for maltreatment, should not be used to determine whether a specific patient is a victim of child maltreatment.

The ability to identify victims of child abuse varies by the age of the patient and the type of maltreatment sustained. Children who are victims of sexual abuse are often brought for medical care after the child makes a disclosure, and the diagnosis is obvious. Physically abused infants may be brought for medical evaluation of irritability or lethargy, without a disclosure of trauma. If the infant's injuries are not severe or visible, the diagnosis may be missed. Approximately one third of infants with inflicted head trauma initially are misdiagnosed by unsuspecting physicians, only to be identified after sustaining further injury. Although physicians are inherently trusting of parents, a constant awareness of the possibility of abuse is needed.

PHYSICAL ABUSE

The physical abuse of children by parents affects children of all ages, from an infant who sustains inflicted head injury to an adolescent who is beaten by the parent in the name of discipline. It is estimated that 1% to 2% of children are physically abused during their childhood, and approximately 2000 children are fatally injured each year. Although mothers are most frequently reported as the perpetrators of physical abuse, serious injuries, such as head or abdominal trauma, are more likely to be inflicted by fathers or maternal boyfriends. The diagnosis of physical abuse can be made easily if the child is battered, has obvious external injuries, or is capable of providing a history of the abuse. In many cases, the diagnosis is not obvious. The history provided by the parent is often inaccurate because the parent is unwilling to provide the correct history or is a nonoffending parent who is unaware of the abuse. The child may be too young or ill to provide a history of the assault. An older child may be too scared to do so or may have a strong sense of loyalty to the perpetrator.

A **diagnosis** of physical abuse initially is suggested by a history that seems incongruent with the clinical presentation of the child (Table 22–1). Although injury to any organ system can occur from physical abuse, some injuries are more common. Bruises are universal findings in nonabused ambulatory children, but also are among the most common injury identified in abused children. Bruises that raise concern for abuse

TABLE 22–1. Clues to the Diagnosis of Physical Abuse

A child presents for medical care with significant injuries, and a history of trauma is denied, especially if the child is an infant or toddler

The history provided by the caregiver does not explain the injuries identified

The history of the injury changes significantly over time

A history of self-inflicted trauma does not correlate with the child's developmental abilities

There is an unexpected or unexplained delay in seeking medical care

Multiple organ systems are injured, including injuries of various ages

The injuries are pathognomonic for child abuse

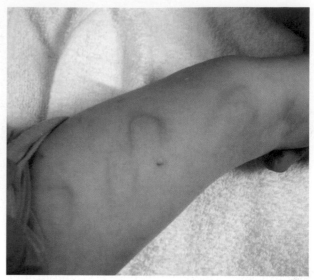

Figure 22–1

Multiple looped cord marks on a 2-year-old abused child who presented to the hospital with multiple untreated burns to the back, arms, and feet.

include those that are patterned, such as a slap mark on the face or looped extension cord marks on the body (Fig. 22–1). Bruises in healthy children generally are distributed over bony prominences; bruises that occur in an unusual distribution, such as isolated to the trunk or neck, should raise concern. Bruises in non-ambulatory infants are unusual, occurring in less than 2% of healthy infants seen for routine medical care. They should always be evaluated. Occasionally a subtle bruise may be the only external clue to abuse and can be associated with more significant internal injury.

Burns are common pediatric injuries and usually represent preventable nonintentional trauma (see Chapter 44). Approximately 10% of children hospitalized with burns are victims of abuse. Inflicted burns can be the result of contact with hot objects, such as irons, radiators, or cigarettes, but more commonly result from scalding injuries (Fig. 22–2). Hot tap water burns in infants and toddlers are sometimes the result of immersion injury, which often occur around toilet training issues. These burns have clear lines of demarcation, uniformity of burn depth, and characteristic pattern.

Inflicted fractures occur more commonly in infants and young children. Although diaphyseal fractures are most common in abuse, they are nonspecific for inflicted injury. Fractures that should raise suspicion for abuse include fractures that are unexplained, fractures that occur in young, nonambulatory children, and fractures that involve multiple bones. Certain fractures have a high specificity for abuse, such as rib, metaphyseal, scapular, vertebral, or other unusual fractures (Fig. 22–3).

Abdominal injury is an uncommon but serious form of physical abuse. Blunt trauma to the abdomen is the primary mechanism of injury, and toddlers are the most common victims. Injuries to solid organs, such as the liver or pancreas, predominate. Hollow viscus injury

occurs more commonly with inflicted trauma than accidental, and injury to solid and hollow organs occurs almost exclusively with abuse. Even in severe cases of trauma, there may be no bruising to the abdominal wall. The lack of external trauma, along with the usual inaccurate history, can cause delay in diagnosis. A careful evaluation often reveals additional injuries. Abdominal

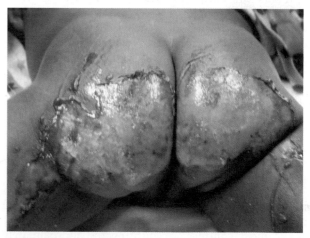

Figure 22–2

A 1-year-old child brought to the hospital with a history that she sat on a hot radiator. Suspicious injuries such as this require a full medical and social investigation, including a skeletal survey to look for occult skeletal injuries and a child welfare evaluation.

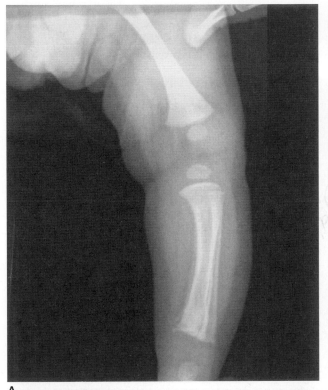

A

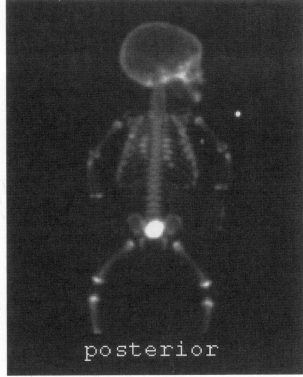

B

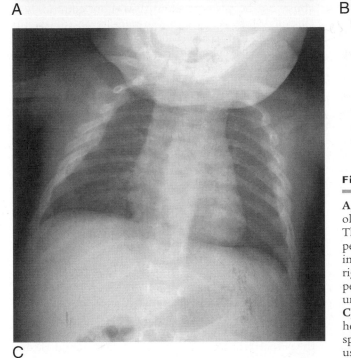

C

Figure 22–3

A, Metaphyseal fracture of the distal tibia in a 3-month-old infant admitted to the hospital with severe head injury. There also is periosteal new bone formation of that tibia, perhaps from a previous injury. **B,** Bone scan of same infant. Initial chest x-ray showed a single fracture of the right posterior fourth rib. A radionuclide bone scan performed 2 days later revealed multiple previously unrecognized fractures of the posterior and lateral ribs. **C,** Follow-up radiographs 2 weeks later showed multiple healing rib fractures. This pattern of fracture is highly specific for child abuse. The mechanism of these injuries is usually violent squeezing of the chest.

trauma is the second leading cause of mortality from physical abuse, although the prognosis is generally good for children who survive the acute assault.

Inflicted head injury is the leading cause of mortality and morbidity from physical abuse. Most victims are young; infants predominate. Shaking, blunt impact trauma, or both cause injuries. The perpetrators are most commonly fathers and boyfriends, and the trauma typically is precipitated by the perpetrator's intolerance to a crying, fussy infant. Victims with head injury present with neurologic symptoms ranging from lethargy and irritability to seizures, apnea, and coma. Unsuspecting physicians misdiagnose approximately one third of infants, and of these, more than 25% are reinjured before diagnosis. Infants most likely to be misdiagnosed include infants with mild injuries, infants who are younger than 6 months old, and white infants who live in two-parent households. A common finding on presentation is subdural hemorrhage, often associated with progressive cerebral edema (Fig. 22–4). Secondary hypoxic injury is a significant contributor to the pathophysiology of the brain injury. Associated findings include retinal hemorrhages (seen in many, but not all, victims) and skeletal trauma, including rib and metaphyseal fractures. At the time of diagnosis,

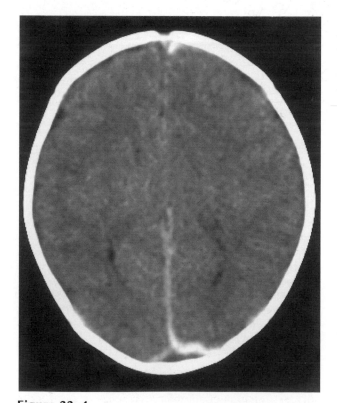

Figure 22–4

Acute subdural hemorrhage in the posterior interhemispheric fissure in an abused infant.

many head-injured infants have evidence of previous injury. Mortality is usually due to uncontrollable increased intracranial pressure, and survivors are at high risk for permanent neurologic sequelae.

The **differential diagnosis** of physical abuse depends on the type of injury the child sustains and is extensive (Table 22–2). For children who present with pathognomonic injuries to multiple organ systems, an exhaustive search for medical diagnoses is unwarranted. Children with unusual medical diseases have been incorrectly diagnosed as victims of abuse, however, emphasizing the need for careful, objective assessments of all children. All infants and young toddlers who present with suspicious injuries should undergo a skeletal survey looking for occult or healing fractures. One third of young infants with multiple fractures, facial injuries, or rib fractures may have occult head trauma, and consideration should be given to obtaining brain imaging for some asymptomatic infants.

SEXUAL ABUSE

Child sexual abuse is defined as the involvement of children in sexual activities that they cannot understand, are developmentally unprepared for, and cannot give consent to and that violate societal taboos. Sexual abuse can be a single event, but more commonly is chronic. Most perpetrators are adults or adolescents who are known to the child and who have real or perceived power over the child. Most sexual abuse involves manipulation and coercion of the child and is typically a physically nonviolent assault. Although stranger assaults occur, they are infrequent. Perpetrators are more often male than female and include parents, relatives, teachers, family friends, members of the clergy, and other individuals who have access to children. All perpetrators strive to keep the child from disclosing the abuse and often do so with coercion or threats.

Each year, more than 150,000 cases of sexual abuse are substantiated by CPS, which is likely to be a significant underestimation of the incidence. Approximately 80% of victims are girls, although the sexual abuse of boys is underrecognized and underreported. Children generally come to attention after they have made a disclosure of their abuse. They may disclose to a non-offending parent, sibling, relative, friend, or teacher. Children seldom disclose their abuse after a single event, and it is common for children to delay their disclosure for many weeks, months, or years, especially if the perpetrator has ongoing access to the child. Sexual abuse also should be considered in children who have behavioral problems, although no behavior is pathognomonic for sexual abuse. Sexually abused children can be withdrawn, aggressive, angry, or depressed, or they may show no behavioral manifestation of their abuse. Hypersexualized behaviors should raise the possibility of abuse, although some children with these behaviors

TABLE 22–2.   Differential Diagnosis of Physical Abuse*

Bruises

Accidental injury (common)
Dermatologic disorders
  Mongolian spots
  Erythema multiforme
  Phytophotodermatitis
Hematologic disorders
  Idiopathic thrombocytopenic purpura
  Leukemia
  Hemophilia
  Vitamin K deficiency
  Disseminated intravascular coagulopathy
Cultural practices
  Cao gio (coining)
  Quat sha (spoon rubbing)
Infection
  Sepsis
  Purpura fulminans (meningococcemia)
Genetic diseases
  Ehlers-Danlos syndrome
  Familial dysautonomia (with congenital indifference
    to pain)
  Vasculitis
  Henoch-Schönlein purpura

Burns

Accidental burns (common)
Infection
  Staphylococcal scalded skin syndrome
  Impetigo

Dermatologic
  Phytophotodermatitis
  Stevens-Johnson syndrome
  Fixed drug eruption
  Epidermolysis bullosa
  Severe diaper dermatitis
Cultural practices
  Cupping
  Moxibustion

Fractures

Accidental injury
Birth trauma
Metabolic bone disease
  Osteogenesis imperfecta
  Copper deficiency
Rickets
Infection
  Congenital syphilis
  Osteomyelitis

Head Trauma

Accidental head injury
Hematologic disorders
  Vitamin K deficiency (hemorrhagic disease of the newborn)
  Hemophilia
Intracranial vascular abnormalities
Infection
Metabolic diseases
  Glutaric aciduria type I

*The differential diagnosis of physical abuse varies by the type of injury and organ system involved.
Data from Christian CW: Child abuse physical. In Schwartz MW (ed): The 5-Minute Pediatric Consult, 3rd ed. Philadelphia, Lippincott Williams & Wilkins, 2003.

are exposed to inappropriate sexual behaviors on television or videos or by witnessing adult sexual activity. Sexual abuse occasionally is recognized by the discovery of an unexplained vaginal, penile, or anal injury or by the discovery of a sexually transmitted disease.

In most cases, the diagnosis of sexual abuse is made by the history obtained from the child. In cases in which the sexual abuse has been reported to CPS or the police (or both), and the child has been interviewed before the medical visit, a complete, forensic interview is not needed. Many communities have systems in place to ensure quality investigative interviews of sexually abused children, and repetitive interviewing of the child should be avoided. If no other professional has spoken to the child about the abuse, or the child makes a spontaneous disclosure to the physician, the child should be interviewed with questions that are open-ended and nonleading. In all cases, the child should be questioned about medical issues related to the abuse, such as the timing of the assault and symptoms, such as bleeding, discharge, or genital pain.

The physical examination should be complete, with careful inspection of the genitals and anus. Most sexually abused children have a normal genital examination at the time of the medical evaluation. Genital injuries are seen more commonly in children who present for medical care within 72 hours of their most recent assault and in children who report genital bleeding, but they are diagnosed in only 5% to 10% of sexually abused children. Many types of sexual abuse (fondling, vulvar coitus, oral-genital contact) do not injure genital tissue, and genital mucosa heals so rapidly and completely that minor injuries have healed by the time of the medical examination. For children who present within 72 hours of the most recent assault, special attention should be given to identifying acute injury to the child and the presence of blood or semen on the child. Injuries to the oral mucosa, breasts, or thighs should not be overlooked. Forensic evidence collection is needed in a few cases and has the greatest yield when collected in the first 24 hours after an acute assault. Highest yields come from the child's clothing or bed

TABLE 22–3. Proper Testing Methods for Sexually Transmitted Diseases in Children and Adolescents

Organism	Infants and Prepubertal Children	Adolescents
Neisseria gonorrhoeae	Culture*	Culture, NAAT[†]
Chlamydia trachomatis	Culture	Culture, NAAT[†]
Trichomonas vaginalis	Vaginal wet mount and culture	Vaginal wet mount and culture
Syphilis, HIV, hepatitis B, C	Serum tests	Serum tests
Herpes simplex virus	Culture	Culture

*Culture from pharynx, anus, vagina, or urethra (boys) positive for gram-negative, oxidase-positive diplococcus, with two of three confirmatory tests positive (e.g., carbohydrate utilization, direct fluorescent antibody testing, enzyme substrate testing).
[†]Nucleic acid amplification test (NAAT) can be substituted, with positive test confirmed by second NAAT test. Non-NAAT, direct fluorescent antibody, and enzyme immunoassay are *not* recommended.

linens, and efforts should be made to secure these items. Few findings are diagnostic of sexual assault, but findings with the most specificity include acute, unexplained lacerations or ecchymoses of the hymen, posterior fourchette or anus, complete transection of the hymen, unexplained anogenital scarring, or pregnancy in an adolescent with no other history of sexual activity.

The **laboratory evaluation** of a sexually abused child is dictated by the child's age, history, and symptoms. Universal screening for sexually transmitted diseases is unnecessary because the risk of infection is low in asymptomatic prepubertal children. The type of assault, the identity and known medical history of the perpetrator, and the epidemiology of sexually transmitted diseases in the community also are considered. Because of the medicolegal implications of the diagnosis, proper methods must be used for testing. In prepubertal children, culture diagnosis is the gold standard; nonculture diagnosis of *Neisseria gonorrhoeae* and *Chlamydia trachomatis* do not meet medical or legal standards at this time (Table 22–3). The diagnosis of most sexually transmitted infections in young children requires an investigation for sexual abuse (Table 22–4) (see Chapter 116).

MANAGEMENT

The management of child abuse includes medical treatment for injuries and infections, careful medical documentation of verbal statements and findings, and ongoing advocacy for the safety and health of the child (Fig. 22–5). Parents always should be informed of the suspicion of abuse and the need to report to CPS. The discussion should focus on the need to ensure the safety and well-being of the child. Accusatory outbursts

TABLE 22–4. AAP Recommendations for the Diagnosis and Reporting of Sexually Transmitted Diseases in Infants and Prepubertal Children

STD Confirmed	Sexual Abuse	Suggested Action
Gonorrhea*	Diagnostic[†]	Report[‡]
Syphilis*	Diagnostic	Report
HIV[§]	Diagnostic	Report
*Chlamydia**	Diagnostic[†]	Report
Trichomonas vaginalis	Highly suspicious	Report
Condylomata acuminata* (anogenital warts)	Suspicious	Report
Herpes (genital location)	Suspicious	Report[¶]
Bacterial vaginosis	Inconclusive	Medical follow-up

*If not perinatally acquired.
[†]Use definitive diagnostic methods, such as culture or DNA probes.
[‡]To agency mandated in community to receive reports of suspected sexual abuse.
[§]If not perinatally or transfusion acquired.
[¶]Unless there is a clear history of autoinoculation. Primary and secondary herpes and are difficult to differentiate by current techniques.
From American Academy of Pediatrics Committee on Child Abuse and Neglect: Guidelines for the evaluation of sexual abuse of children: Subject review. Pediatrics 103:186-191, 1999.

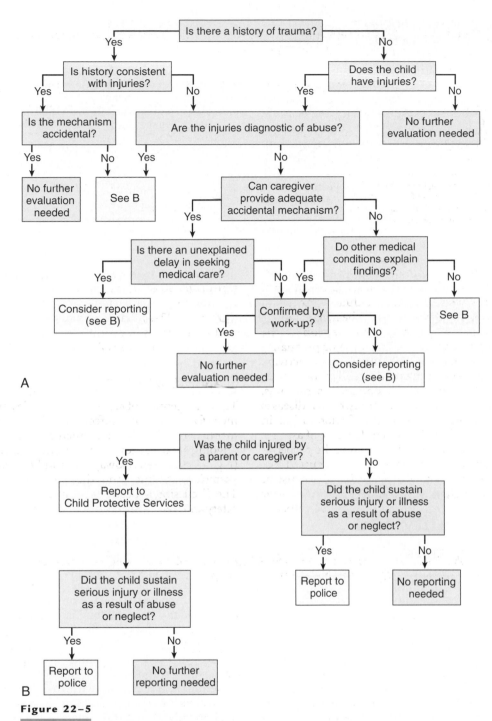

Figure 22–5

A, Approach to initiating the civil and criminal investigation of suspected abuse.
B, Reporting to Child Protective Services (CPS) or law enforcement or both in child
abuse cases. CPS reports are required when a child is injured by a parent, by an adult
acting as a parent, or by a caregiver of the child. The police investigate crimes
against children committed by any person, including parents or other caregivers.
(From Christian CW: Child abuse. In Schwartz MW [ed]: Clinical Handbook of
Pediatrics, 3rd ed. Baltimore, Lippincott Williams & Wilkins, 2003, pp 192-193.)

or apportioning blame is neither professional nor appropriate and does not help the child. Crimes that are committed against children also are investigated by law enforcement, so the police become involved in some, but not all, cases of suspected abuse. Physicians occasionally are called to testify in court hearings regarding civil issues, such as dependency and custody, or criminal issues. Careful review of the medical records and preparation for court are needed to provide an educated, unbiased account of the child's medical condition and diagnoses.

The need to prevent child abuse is obvious, yet it is premature to consider the primary prevention of maltreatment an attainable goal because of the complexity of factors that contribute to the problem and the limited resources available to reduce the contributing risks. Much of what we consider prevention is in reality reactive: High-risk families are identified and monitored, counseling and therapy are provided when available, and the criminal justice system assists in protecting children and attempting to modify behavior. There are a few partially successful primary prevention programs. Visiting home nursing programs that begin during pregnancy and continue through early childhood may reduce the risk of abuse and neglect. Physicians who care for children always need to remain cognizant of the diagnosis, aware of their professional mandates, and willing to advocate on behalf of these vulnerable patients.

CHAPTER 23
Homosexuality and Gender Identity

The development of sexuality occurs throughout a child's life. Sexuality includes gender roles, gender identity, sexual orientation, and sexual behaviors and is influenced by biologic and social factors and individual experience. Pediatricians are likely to be consulted if parents have a concern about their child's sexual development. A pediatrician who provides an open and nonjudgmental environment may be a valuable resource for an adolescent with questions about heterosexual behaviors, homosexuality, or gender identity (Table 23–1).

DEVELOPMENT OF SEXUAL IDENTITY

Sexual behaviors occur throughout childhood. Male infants can have erections in the first few days of life. During the preschool period, masturbation is common

TABLE 23–1.   Terminology
Gender Identity
Perception of oneself as male or female
Gender Role
Behaviors and appearance that signal to others being male or female
Heterosexual
Sexual attraction to members of the opposite sex with weak attraction to members of the same sex
Homosexual
Sexual attraction to members of the same sex with weak attraction to members of the opposite sex

in both sexes. Between 2 and 3 years of age, children identify themselves as a boy or a girl, but the understanding that one is always a male or always a female may not develop until 4 to 5 years of age. Stating that one wants to be a member of the opposite sex and pretending to be a member of the opposite sex are not unusual behaviors in this age group. Preschool children need to begin to learn that genitals and sexual behaviors are private; it is common for preschool children to touch their genitals in public, show their genitals to others, or undress in public. It would be highly unusual for a preschool child to imitate intercourse or other adult sexual behaviors. If this behavior is occurring, the child should be evaluated for exposure to inappropriate sexual material and possible sexual abuse (see Chapter 22).

Most elementary school–age children show a strong and consistent **gender identity**, and their behaviors (**gender roles**) reflect this gender identity. If a child this age is engaging in gender role behaviors typical of the opposite sex, parents may be concerned about teasing and about the possibility of the child having a homosexual sexual orientation. This concern is particularly true if a boy is engaged in effeminate behaviors because this is generally viewed as less socially acceptable than a girl acting as a "tomboy." By this age, dressing as a member of the opposite sex and particularly stating a desire to be the opposite sex are uncommon, but playing with toys "designed" for the opposite sex remains common. In assessing parental concerns about atypical gender role behaviors, pediatricians should consider the type of behavior exhibited and the consistency of these behaviors. Reassurance that the behavior is consistent with typical child development is appropriate when these behaviors are part of a flexible repertoire of male and female gender role behaviors. Reassurance is appropriate if the behaviors occur in response to a stress, such as the birth of an infant of the opposite sex from the child or divorce of the parents. In contrast, if these behaviors occur as a consistent and persistent pattern of nearly exclusive interest in behaviors typical of the gender role opposite that of the child's anatomic sex, referral for evaluation for **gender identity disorder** (GID) would be appropriate.

The biologic, social, and cognitive changes during adolescence place a focus on sexuality. Becoming comfortable with one's sexuality is one of the principal developmental tasks of this period. The development of the adolescent's sexual identity is likely to include questioning and experimentation. Of adolescents, 10% to 25% have at least one homosexual experience, with this behavior being reported more commonly by boys than girls. Although many adolescents have sexual experiences with a same-sex partner, only a few have a homosexual sexual orientation by late adolescence. When adolescents develop a consistent sexual orientation is probably affected by many different factors (societal, family, individual). Some adolescents report that they are certain of their sexual orientation in the early teenage years, whereas for others this does not develop until later. By age 18, only a small proportion of individuals report being uncertain of their sexual orientation.

GENDER IDENTITY DISORDER

GID is characterized by a persistent cross-gender identification and discomfort with one's own sex. In children, these feelings may be manifested by behaviors such as cross-dressing, stating that one wants to be or is the opposite sex, and a strong and almost exclusive preference for cross-sex roles, games, and playmates. The onset of this behavioral pattern often can be traced back to the preschool period, but children are most likely to be referred for evaluation at school age, when it becomes clear that the behaviors do not represent a transient phase, and the behaviors may begin to interfere with social relationships.

In adults, GID may be characterized by a belief that one was born the wrong sex and by a persistent desire to live and be treated as the opposite sex. Adults may request hormones or surgical procedures to alter sexual characteristics to simulate the other sex. Long-term follow-up studies suggest that only about 10% of children with GID become adults with GID. At least in males (who have been studied more than females), about two thirds of boys with GID become homosexual men, whereas about a quarter become heterosexual men. Parents of children with GID often express a desire to know if their child will develop a homosexual orientation in adulthood. Although an honest answer must acknowledge that these children are significantly more likely to have a homosexual orientation than the general population, there is no reliable way to predict the sexual orientation of any one particular child. There is no evidence that parental behavior would alter the developmental pathway toward homosexual or heterosexual behavior (see Chapter 24).

HOMOSEXUALITY

Homosexuality has existed in all societies and among all cultures. Biologic and social factors play a role in determining sexual orientation. Identical twins (even twins raised in separate families) show a higher concordance rate for sexual orientation than would be expected by chance alone, but nowhere near 100%, as would be expected if genetics alone determined sexual orientation. Some studies have found differences in the size of certain brain regions in homosexual individuals, but the findings are inconsistent. Even if such differences are confirmed, further research is required to clarify whether the differences are the cause or the result of homosexuality. The levels of androgens and estrogens have not been found to differ in homosexual and heterosexual adults. Whether prenatal exposure to sex steroids influences sexual orientation is unknown. Even less is known about how social factors may influence sexual orientation. Although it is well documented that parents tend to treat boys and girls differently, if, or how, these interactions affect sexual orientation is unknown.

It is currently estimated that about 1% to 5% of adults identify themselves as homosexual. Given the prevalent negative societal attitudes toward homosexuality, these children are at high risk for having a negative self-esteem, being isolated, being verbally harassed, and often being physically assaulted. Although sexual behaviors, not sexual orientation, determine risk for sexually transmitted diseases, homosexual male adolescents engage in high-risk behaviors despite the threat of infection from HIV. For medical and psychosocial reasons, healthcare providers need to provide an environment in which adolescents feel comfortable discussing their sexual orientation. Table 23–2 lists measures that healthcare providers can take to ensure a safe and supportive environment for homosexual youth.

Acknowledging that one is homosexual and disclosing it to one's parents is often extremely stressful. This is especially true when the adolescent has reason to believe that the parents are not likely to be supportive. Although many parents come to accept their child's homosexuality, some parents, particularly those who view this behavior as immoral, may reject their child. Homosexual youth are at a high risk of homelessness. Adolescents need to be made aware that even parents who eventually come to accept their child's homosexuality initially may be shocked, fearful

TABLE 23–2.   Providing Supportive Healthcare Environments for Homosexual Youth

Ensure confidentiality

Implement policies against homophobic jokes and remarks

Ensure information-gathering forms use gender-neutral language (e.g., *partner* as opposed to *husband/wife*)

Ensure that one uses gender-neutral questions when asking about dating or sexual behaviors

Display posters, brochures, and information that show concern for issues important to homosexual youth and their families

Provide information about support groups and other resources for homosexual youth and their families

Adapted from Perrin EC: Sexual Orientation in Child and Adolescent Health Care. New York, Kluwer Academic/Plenum Publishers, 2002.

about their child's well-being, or upset about the loss of the adulthood they had expected for their child. Parents may need to be reassured that they did not cause their child to have a homosexual orientation. Likewise, they may need to be informed that therapies designed to change sexual orientation not only are unsuccessful, but also they often lead to the child having more feelings of guilt and a lower self-esteem. The healthcare provider should have knowledge of support groups and counselors who can discuss these issues with the adolescent or his or her parents when the information the healthcare provider offers is not sufficient.

The homosexual youth is affected by how homosexuality is addressed in schools, by peers, and by other community groups. Unbiased information about homosexuality is often not available in these settings, and homophobic jokes, teasing, and violence are common. It is not surprising that homosexual youth and adults have higher rates of anxiety and mood disorders than are found in the general population. Increased rates of substance abuse and suicide are reported. Healthcare providers have an important role in detecting these problems.

Although education about safe sexual practices should be part of all adolescent well-child visits, healthcare providers should be aware that certain sexual behaviors of homosexual males increase the risk for certain types of sexually transmitted diseases. Anal intercourse is an efficient route for infection by hepatitis B virus, cytomegalovirus, and HIV. Proctitis caused by gonorrhea, chlamydia, herpes simplex virus, syphilis, or human papillomavirus may occur (see Chapter 116).

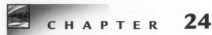

CHAPTER **24**

Family Structure and Function

A family is a dynamic system of interactions among biologically, socially, or legally related individuals. By virtue of these interactions, families have their unique power to promote or interfere with health and development. Every member of the family affects each individual in the family. A problem for one member of a family has an influence on every other member of the family.

When a family functions well, the interactions among members support the physical and emotional needs of all family members, and the family serves as a resource for an individual member who is having difficulty. Alternatively, the problems of an individual member or the interactions among members may prevent the family from meeting the physical or emotional needs of one or more family members or, in the worst-case scenario, may cause physical or emotional harm to a member of the family. These situations are often referred to as **family dysfunction**. Families have crucial roles that must be filled for children.

FAMILY FUNCTIONS

The functions that families carry out in support of their children can be categorized broadly as providing for physical needs, emotional support, education, and socialization (Table 24–1). Within these categories, all families have strengths and weaknesses; there is not one "correct" amount of support for all children. The amount of support that an individual child needs in these categories varies with the child's development, personality, temperament, health status, family stressors, experiences, and other factors.

Although the appropriate amount of support for a child varies, at the extremes too much and too little support can interfere with optimal child health and development. Most cases of child abuse involve the failure of the family to provide a safe environment for the child. Overprotective parents may limit friendships and other growth-promoting experiences or seek excessive health care, as may occur in the vulnerable child syndrome. Child neglect is an extreme form of understimulation, whereas overstimulation and parental perfectionism may create intense pressure on children related to achievement that may contribute to problems such as anxiety disorders.

TABLE 24–1. Important Roles Families Play in Supporting Children

Physical Needs

Safety
Food
Shelter
Health and health care

Emotional Support

Affection
Stimulation
Communication
Guidance/discipline

Education and Socialization

Values
Relationships
Community
Formal schooling

FAMILY STRUCTURE

The traditional family consists of a married mother and father and their biologic children. The diversity in the structure of the family in the U.S. has increased dramatically, however, and less than half of children now live in the traditional nuclear family. Today, children may live with unmarried parents, single parents of either gender, a parent and a stepparent, grandparents, parents living as a same-sex couple, or foster care families. There is little evidence that family structure alone is a significant predictor of child health or development. Regardless of family structure, the presence of a loving adult or adults serving as a parent or parents committed to the fulfilling of a child's physical, emotional, and socialization needs is the best predictor of a child's optimal health and development. Different family structures create different types of family stresses.

Single-Parent Families

Some children live in single-parent families because of divorce or the death of a parent (see Chapter 26). More than 20% of children are born to unmarried mothers, and many of these children live in single-parent families for some, if not all, of their childhood. Although some women elect to have children without getting married, in many situations the single parent is a young mother who had an unplanned pregnancy.

Single parents must work and raise the child and often have fewer financial resources and social supports. The mean income of single mother–headed households is only 40% of that of two-parent families.

More than half of these households live in poverty. Single parents also must rely to a greater extent on other adults for childcare. Although these adults may be sources of support for the single parent, they also may criticize the parent, decreasing confidence in parenting skills. This decreased confidence, in combination with the fatigue associated with working and raising a child, makes consistent discipline harder to maintain, which may exacerbate behavioral problems. These parents are likely to have less time for a social life or other activities, which may increase their isolation. When the increased burdens of being a single parent are associated with exhaustion, isolation, and depression, optimal child development is less likely.

When the parent is a teenage mother, problems of parenting may be exacerbated further (see Section XII). Being a teenage parent is associated with lower educational attainment, lower paying jobs without much opportunity for autonomy or advancement, and lower self-esteem. Teenagers also have less knowledge of normal child development and may be more impatient with their children. They are even less likely than other single mothers to have any support from the child's father. Children of adolescent mothers are at high risk for cognitive delays, behavioral problems, and difficulties in school. Referral to early intervention services or Head Start programs is important in these situations.

When a single parent has good social supports, is able to collaborate well with other care providers, and has sufficient financial resources, he or she is likely to be successful in raising a child. Pediatricians can improve parental confidence through education about child development and behavior and validation of parenting behaviors. Empathetic understanding of the difficulties of being a single parent can have a healing effect or help a parent to discuss difficulties that may suggest the need for a referral to other professionals.

Children Living with Grandparents or Other Family Members

In most cases when a child is living with a grandparent or other family member, it is related to an event that already has caused significant emotional distress for the child and other family members. The new living situation may arise out of legal intervention related to neglect or abuse, may be agreed on by the parents because of parental illness, or may occur because of parental death. Additional factors that may exacerbate the child's stress further in these situations include family conflict about where the child should live, moving to a new neighborhood and school, or having one's primary caretaker change frequently.

The grandparents' or other family members' health and emotional concerns related to the caring for the child are important to consider. Grandparents may not have the energy required to raise a child, may feel isolated from parents of similar-age children, and are likely to have a decreased ability to participate in the typical social activities they enjoyed before taking on the child's care. If the child's change in living arrangements was related to parental substance abuse, violence, or other antisocial behavior or significant emotional illness, there may be concerns about the implications of these behaviors for the child. Common child misbehaviors may be misinterpreted as precursors of problems similar to the parents' problems. In response, the caretaker may be overly critical or use harsh discipline to "prevent" similar problems from developing in the child. These responses may interfere further with the child's ability to develop a secure emotional bond with the family member. Children and grandparents or other family members in these situations may need significant support from social service agencies and other professionals.

Despite the many potential difficulties outlined here, many children adapt well to living with a grandparent or other family member. The child is most likely to adapt well when the family member can give an unambiguous message to the child that he or she loves and will care for the child. It also is helpful if the child has had a good previous relationship with the family member, and the family has sufficient financial and social resources to care for the child. If the biologic parents are going to continue to be involved in the child's life, there should be a plan for how this will occur in a manner that is consistent and clear to the child about each family member's role.

Children Living with Homosexual Parents

Most children with a gay or lesbian parent were conceived in the context of a heterosexual relationship. Some parents were unaware of their homosexuality at the time that they married, whereas others may view themselves as bisexual or marry despite the recognition that they are gay. Some of these parents may continue to live with a heterosexual spouse, but others divorce. When a divorce occurs, a homosexual parent may live as a single parent or in a relationship with a same-sex partner. Gay men and lesbian women also become parents on their own or in the context of an already established relationship with a same-sex partner. Children living with homosexual parents may encompass many possible family structures.

Parents in these families are likely to have concerns about how disclosure of the homosexuality and the associated social stigma will affect the child. In general, earlier disclosure of a parent's homosexuality to children, especially before adolescence, is associated with better acceptance. Most children of homosexual parents experience some social stigma associated with having a gay or lesbian parent; this may occur in the form of teasing by peers, disapproval from adults, and stress or isolation related to keeping the parent's homosexuality a "secret."

Evidence suggests that having a homosexual parent does not cause increased problems in the parent-child relationship or the child's social-emotional development. Gender and gender role behaviors are typical for the child's age. Nonetheless, distress related to teasing or maintaining the parent's secret may be great for some children, especially in early adolescence when issues of peer acceptance, sexual identity, and separation from one's parents are especially strong.

Adoption

Adoption is a legal and social process that provides full family membership to a child not born to the adoptive parents. Approximately 2% of children in the U.S. are adopted. A significant proportion of legal and informal adoptions are by stepparents or relatives of the child. Most adoptions in the U.S. involve U.S. parents adopting U.S. children, but shifting cultural trends and a shortage of healthy U.S. children available for adoption have increased the diversity in the ways in which adoptions occur (e.g., international adoptions, privately arranged adoptions, and the use of a surrogate parent). These types of adoption each raise unique issues for families and healthcare providers. *Open adoptions* in which the biologic parents and birth parents agree to interact are occurring with increased frequency and create new issues for the adoption triad (biologic parent, adoptive parent, and child). Adoptions by single parents create another set of issues.

Pediatricians are in an ideal position to help adoptive parents. In addition to providing standard health supervision, pediatricians can help parents obtain and evaluate medical information, consider the unique medical needs of the adopted child, and provide a source of advice and counseling from the preadoption period through the issues that may arise when the child is an adolescent. The physician's involvement may begin with a *preadoption visit*. The physician may be able to help the family interpret the medical information they have received about the child. The physician also can help identify important pieces of the medical history that may be missing, such as the medical history of the biologic family and the educational and social history of the biologic parents. The preadoption period is the time that families are most likely to be able to obtain this information. When children are adopted from another country, there may be risks of infections, in utero substance exposure, poor nutrition, or inadequate infant care that are specific to individual countries and should be discussed with parents.

When the adopted child is first seen, the pediatrician should consider screening for medical disorders beyond the typical age-appropriate screening tests. If the child has not had the standard newborn screening tests, the pediatrician may need to obtain these tests. Documented immunizations should be reviewed, and, if needed, a plan should be developed to complete the needed immunizations (see Chapter 94). Children may be at high risk for infection based on the biologic mother's social history or the country from which the child was adopted. The pediatrician specifically should consider the need to test for infection with HIV, hepatitis B, cytomegalovirus, tuberculosis, syphilis, and parasites. A complete blood count may be needed to screen for iron deficiency.

A knowledgeable pediatrician also can be a valuable source of support and advice about psychosocial issues. The pediatrician should help the adoptive parents think about how they will raise the child in their family while helping the child to understand the fact that he or she is adopted. Neither denial of nor intense focus on the adoption is healthy. Parents should use the term *adoption* around their children during the toddler years and explain the simplest facts first. Children's questions should be answered honestly and can help inform parents as to what information the child is ready to hear. Parents should expect that children will ask the same or similar questions repeatedly, and that during the preschool period the child's cognitive limitations make it likely the child will not fully understand the meaning of adoption. As children get older, they may have fantasies of being reunited with their biologic parents, and there may be new challenges as the child begins to interact more with individuals outside the family. Families may want advice about difficulties created by school assignments such as creating a genealogical chart or teasing by peers. During the teenage years, the child may have questions about his or her identity and a desire to find his or her biologic parents. Adoptive parents may need reassurance that these desires do not represent rejection of the adoptive family, but the child's desire to understand more about his or her life. In general, adopted adolescents should be supported in efforts to learn about their past, but most experts recommend encouraging children to wait until late adolescence before deciding to search actively for the biologic parents.

Adoptive parents experience the same pleasures and difficulties of parenting that people raising their biologic children experience. Although adopted children have a higher rate of school, learning, and behavioral problems, much of this increase is likely to be related to biologic and social influences before the adoption. The pediatrician can play an important role in helping families distinguish developmental and behavioral variations from problems that may require recommendations for early intervention, counseling, or other services.

Foster Care

Foster care is a means of providing protection for children who require out-of-home placement, most commonly because of homelessness, parental inability to care for the child, parental substance abuse, or child neglect or abuse. The number of children in foster care doubled between 1987 and 2001, and currently more than 0.5 million children live in foster care. For these children, reunification with the biologic family is the goal for approximately 40%, and adoption or placement with relatives is the goal for 25% to 35%. Ten percent of children are in long-term foster care. For the remaining 20%, no long-term goal has been established.

Children in foster care are at extremely high risk for medical, nutritional, developmental, behavioral, and mental health problems. At the time of placement in foster care, most of these children have received incomplete medical care and have had multiple detrimental life experiences. When comprehensive assessments are done at the time of placement, many children are found to have untreated acute medical problems, and 40% to 70% are found to have chronic illnesses. More than half have significant developmental delays, and behavioral disorders are common. Ideally, foster care provides a healing service for these children and families, leading to reunification or adoption. Too often, however, inadequately resourced programs contribute to the ongoing difficulties of the children.

Given the complex needs of children entering foster care, these children need consistent, multidisciplinary, and coordinated care. For children in foster care for more than 1 year, more than 40% experience three or more home placements, and for children in foster care for more than 4 years, this figure is approximately 60%. Poor case coordination in conjunction with these multiple placements leads to frequent changes in schools and medical providers, further fragmenting the health care and education these children receive. In some locations, one third of children received no immunizations while in foster care. Frequent changes in placement exacerbate the problems foster children often have in forming a secure relationship with adult caregivers. Children may manifest this difficulty by resisting foster parents' attempts to develop a close relationship. This detachment from the foster parent may be difficult for the foster parent to endure, which may perpetuate a cycle of placement failures. Although the "protections" of the foster care system end at age 18 years, these adolescents rarely have the skills and maturity that allow them to live independently.

When healthcare providers see a child in foster care, it is crucial that they perform a comprehensive health assessment for acute and chronic medical problems and developmental and behavioral disorders. When children are placed with competent and nurturing foster parents and provided coordinated care from skilled professionals, significant improvements in a child's health status, development, and academic achievement usually occur.

FAMILY DYSFUNCTION
Physical Needs

Failure to meet a child's physical needs for protection or nutrition results in some of the most severe forms of family dysfunction (see Chapters 21 and 22). There are many other ways in which parent behaviors can interfere with a child having a healthy and safe environment, such as prenatal and postnatal substance abuse. Prenatal use of alcohol exposes children to potentially devastating consequences of this teratogen. Children with **fetal alcohol syndrome** have in utero and postnatal growth retardation, microcephaly, mental retardation, and a characteristic dysmorphic facial appearance. Even in the absence of growth retardation and a dysmorphic appearance, some children exposed to alcohol in utero develop problems with coordination, attention, hyperactivity, impulsivity, and other learning or behavioral problems related to the alcohol exposure. In the past, these children have been described as having fetal alcohol effects, but the currently recommended terminology is *alcohol-related neurodevelopmental disorder*.

Other substances also may affect the fetus, but investigation of these effects is complicated by the fact that often more than one substance is used, and nutrition and prenatal care are not optimal. Cigarette smoking during pregnancy is associated with lower birth weight and increased child behavioral problems. Use of cocaine in the perinatal period has been associated with intracranial hemorrhages and abruptio placentae, but persistent cognitive deficits in infants related solely to prenatal cocaine exposure have not been found consistently. Similarly, although exposure to opiates in utero can result in a neonatal withdrawal syndrome, significant cognitive deficits do not seem to be associated with the use of opiates alone. Cocaine-exposed and opiate-exposed infants often have other coexisting high risk factors for cognitive deficits, such as low birth weight.

Parental substance abuse after the child's birth is associated with increased family conflict, decreased organization, increased isolation, and increased family stress related to marital and work problems. Family violence may be more frequent. Despite the fact that these parents often have difficulty providing discipline and structure for their children, they have been found to expect their children to be competent at a variety of tasks at a younger age than non–substance-abusing parents. This situation may set the children up for failure and contribute to increased rates of depression, anxiety, and low self-esteem. The parents' more accepting attitude toward alcohol and drugs seems to increase the chance that their children will use substances during adolescence.

Parents also may expose children directly to the harmful effects of other substances, such as occurs through exposure to *second-hand cigarette smoke*. Exposure to environmental tobacco smoke is consistently associated with increased rates of childhood respiratory illnesses, otitis media, and sudden infant death syndrome. Despite these effects, only a few parents restrict smoking in their homes. There are many other ways in which parents may not physically protect their children. Failing to immunize children, to childproof the home adequately, and to provide adequate supervision are other examples.

Parents' attempts to provide too much protection for their child also can cause problems. One example of this is the **vulnerable child syndrome**. A child who is ill early in life continues to be viewed as vulnerable by the parents despite the fact that the child has fully recovered. Behavioral difficulties may result if parents are overindulgent and fail to set limits. Parental reluctance to leave the child may contribute to the child having separation anxiety. Parents may be particularly attentive to minor variations in bodily functions, leading them to seek excess medical care. If the physician does not recognize this situation, the child may be exposed to unnecessary medical procedures.

Emotional Support, Education, and Socialization

Failure to meet a child's emotional or educational needs can have a severe and enduring negative impact on child development and behavior. Infants need a consistent adult who learns to understand their signals and early in life meets the infant's needs for attention as well as food. As the adult caregiver learns these signals, he or she responds more rapidly and appropriately to the infant's attempts at communication. Through this process, often referred to as **attachment**, the special relationship between parent and child develops. When affectionate and responsive adults are not consistently available, infants often are less willing to explore the environment and may become unusually clingy, angry, or hard to comfort.

Appropriate stimulation also is vital for a child's cognitive development. Children whose parents do not read to them and do not play developmentally appropriate games with them have lower scores on intelligence tests and more school problems. In these situations, early intervention has been shown to be particularly effective in improving skill development and subsequent school performance. At the other extreme, there are increasing concerns that some parents may provide too much stimulation and scheduling of the child's day. There may be such emphasis on achievement that children come to feel that parental love is contingent on achievement. There are concerns that this narrow definition of success may contribute to problems with anxiety and self-esteem for some children.

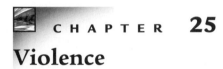

CHAPTER 25

Violence

DOMESTIC VIOLENCE AND CHILDREN

Intimate partner violence between adults affects the lives of millions of children each year. Children experience domestic violence by seeing or hearing the violence or seeing its aftermath. Children who live in households with domestic violence often develop psychological and behavioral problems that interfere with their ability to function normally in school, at home, and with peers. They may be injured during violent outbursts, sometimes while attempting to intervene on behalf of a parent. Many children are victims of abuse themselves. It is estimated that there is at least a 50% concurrence rate between domestic violence and child abuse. Children who grow up in violent households learn that violence is appropriate in intimate relationships. A history of having witnessed domestic violence as a child is a strong predictor for becoming a batterer in adulthood. Children who live with domestic violence have experienced more than sporadic outbursts of violence. They live in households in which one partner, usually the mother, is isolated, belittled, made to feel worthless, and the victim of physical violence. This type of environment is filled with disruptive events that can overtly or subtly affect the child's normal development. Although domestic violence occurs between heterosexual and homosexual partners and can be perpetrated by women, most domestic violence is perpetrated by men against women. When asked, most parents underestimate their children's exposure to domestic violence.

There is no particular behavioral consequence or disturbance that is specific to children who witness domestic violence. Some children are traumatized by fear for their mother's safety and feel helpless to protect her. Others may blame themselves for the violence. Children may have symptoms of **post-traumatic stress disorder**, depression, anxiety, aggression, or hypervigilance. Older children may have conduct disorders, poor school performance, low self-esteem, or other nonspecific behaviors. Infants and young toddlers are at risk for disrupted attachment and routines around eating and sleeping. Preschoolers may show signs of regression, irritable behavior, or temper tantrums. During school-age years, gender differences begin to emerge, although any given child may not follow these patterns. Boys who have witnessed violence tend to be more aggressive or disruptive, whereas girls become more withdrawn and passive. Boys and girls may have loss of confidence or academic problems. Because of family isolation, some children have no opportunity to participate in extracurricular activities at school and do not form friendships outside of the family. Adolescent girls who have lived with domestic violence are at risk for becoming victims of physical violence by their boyfriends; adolescent boys may become victimizers. Although some adolescents learn to assume the parent role, others turn on the victimized parent and identify themselves with the abusive parent.

Because of the high concurrence of domestic violence and child abuse, asking about domestic violence is part of the screening for violence against children. Many women's advocates suggest that intervening on behalf of battered women is an active form of child abuse prevention. Recognizing the importance of domestic violence screening in pediatric practice, the AAP has endorsed universal domestic violence screening in this setting.

Screening for domestic violence in pediatric offices identifies women who have been victims in the past and, less often, women who remain involved in an abusive relationship. Without standardized screening, pediatricians may underestimate the prevalence of domestic violence in their practices. Screening is recommended for all families intermittently, especially in the first few years of the child's life. Physical violence against women is high during pregnancy and in the postpartum period. Parents should not be screened together. Questions about family violence should be direct, nonjudgmental, and done in the context of child safety and anticipatory guidance. Table 25-1 lists approaches to questions for children and adults.

Intervention is needed for women who disclose domestic violence. It is appropriate to show concern and to inform the woman of available community resources. It is important to assess her safety and inquire about whether the children are in physical danger. In some states, physicians are mandated to report domestic violence. Information for women that provides details about community resources and state laws is helpful.

TABLE 25–1. Questions for Adults and Children Related to Family Violence

For the Child

How are things at home, at school?
Who lives with you?
How do you get along with your family members?
What do you like to do with them?
What do you do if something is bothering you?
Do you feel safe at home?
Do people fight at home? What do they fight about?
  How do they fight?

Additional Questions for the Adolescent

Do your friends get into fights often? How about you?
When was your last physical fight?
Have you ever been injured during a fight?
Has anyone you know been injured or killed?
Have you ever been forced to have sex against your will?
Have you ever been threatened with a gun? A knife?
How do you avoid getting in fights?
Do you carry a weapon for self-defense?

For the Parent

Do you have any concerns about your child?
Who helps with your children?
How do you feel about your neighborhood?
Do you feel safe at home?
Is there any fighting or violence at home?
Does anyone at home use drugs?
Have you been frightened by your partner?
Does your partner ever threaten you? Hurt you?

YOUTH VIOLENCE

Youth violence is a leading cause of pediatric mortality in the U.S. Each year, more than 2500 children, primarily adolescents, are victims of homicide; almost 2000 more commit suicide. Youth violence is a problem in urban, suburban, and rural communities and affects children of all races and both genders. Surveys of adolescents show that 30% to 40% of boys and 15% to 30% of girls report having committed a serious violent offense during childhood, including robbery, rape, aggravated assault, or homicide. Most of these crimes are not reported to the police, and the perpetrator is arrested in only a few cases. Although boys commit more crimes than girls, this gap has narrowed. Boys are much more likely to be arrested for their crimes. Self-reported violent events do not differ much between white and minority adolescents; the latter are more likely to be arrested for their crimes.

Most violent youth begin to exhibit their violent behaviors during early adolescence. More mild forms of aggression, such as **bullying**, which can involve verbal and physical aggression, peak during middle school years. Children who bully others are more likely to be involved with other problem behaviors, such as smoking and alcohol use. Although most bullies do not progress into serious violent offenders, violent behavior that continues into high school years indicates the potential for severe violent behavior in adulthood. Another subset of violent youth begins at a very young age. These children tend to be more serious offenders, perpetrate more crimes, and more often continue their violence into adulthood. The peak age of onset for serious violence is 15 to 16 years for boys and a few years earlier for girls. Most adolescent violence ends by young adulthood. Most violent youth are only intermittently violent; frequent acts of violence are committed more commonly by youth who start their violence before the onset of puberty. These violent youth need to be evaluated for cognitive impairments or mental illness.

Serious youth violence is not an isolated problem, but usually coexists with other adolescent risk-taking behaviors, such as drug use, truancy and school dropout, early sexual activity, and gun ownership. Risk factors for youth violence are slightly different for children who begin their violence early in life compared with youth who begin during adolescence. Often, these risk factors exist in clusters, and they tend to be additive. Although understanding risk factors for violence is crucial for developing prevention strategies, the risk factors do not predict whether an individual will become violent. For children who begin their violence early in life, the strongest risk factors are early substance abuse (<12 years old) and perpetration of nonviolent, serious crimes during childhood. Additional risk factors include poverty, male gender, and antisocial behavior. For children who begin their violence during adolescence, individual risk factors are less important, whereas factors related to peer groups are most important. Membership in a gang, associating with antisocial or delinquent friends, being unpopular in school, and having weak ties to conventional peer groups are important risk factors for adolescent-onset violence. Table 25–2 lists individual, family, school, peer group, and community risk factors for early-onset and later onset youth violence. The strength of the listed risk factors is not uniform, and some factors show only a small effect. Table 25–2 also lists protective factors, conditions that seem to buffer the effects of risk factors. Although the research on protective factors is limited, these factors are thought to be an important tool in violence prevention strategies. One important protective factor is the child's level of school connectedness, such as involvement in class and extracurricular activities, and how positively the child regards the school's personnel. Another protective factor is

TABLE 25–2. Risk and Protective Factors for Serious Youth Violence by Age of Onset

Factors	Early Onset (<12 yr)	Later Onset (>12 yr)	Protective Factors
Individual	**Substance use*** **General offenses** Being male Antisocial behavior Aggression[†] Hyperactivity Exposure to TV violence Low IQ Antisocial attitudes Dishonesty[†]	General offenses Aggression[†] Being male Physical violence Antisocial attitudes Crimes against persons Low IQ Substance abuse Risk-taking behaviors	Intolerance toward deviance High IQ Being female Positive social orientation Perceived sanctions for transgressions
Family	Low SES/poverty Antisocial parents Poor parent-child relations Broken home Abusive, neglectful parents	Poor parent-child relations Low parent involvement Antisocial parents Broken home Low SES/poverty Abusive parents	Supportive parents or other adults Parental monitoring Parents' positive evaluation of peers
School	Poor attitude Poor performance	Poor attitude Poor performance Academic failure	Commitment to school Recognition for involvement in school activities
Peer	Weak social ties Antisocial peers	**Weak social ties** **Antisocial delinquent peers** **Gang membership**	Friends who engage in conventional behavior
Community		Neighborhood crime Neighborhood drugs Neighborhood disorganization	

*****Bold** = factors with strongest effect.
[†]Males only.
SES, socioeconomic status.
From National Center for Injury Prevention and Control, Substance Abuse and Mental Health Services Administration: Youth Violence: A Report of the Surgeon General. Rockville, Md, U.S. Department of Health and Human Services, 2001.

the support of nonviolent family members and close friends.

Violence prevention efforts that target risk and protective factors need to be developmentally appropriate. Education about the dangers of substance abuse should begin before the onset of puberty, whereas adolescent programs must consider the importance of peer group identification. Many violence prevention programs fail to show long-term effects. Effective violence prevention programs must address simultaneously individual, family, and environmental (school, peer group, social) risk factors; capitalize on the child's strengths; involve family and other supports; and be implemented over an extended period.

DATING VIOLENCE AND DATE RAPE

Dating violence and date rape are relatively common problems in society. It is estimated that 15% to 40% of adolescents have experienced violence in a dating relationship; adolescent and young adult women experience higher rates of sexual assault than any other age group. An acquaintance or partner of the victim perpetrates most adolescent sexual assaults; stranger assaults are the exception. Risk factors for date rape include initiating dating at a young age, initiating early sexual activity, and having a history of past sexual abuse or victimization. A history of child abuse or sexual abuse by parents or siblings increases the risk for being a perpetrator or a victim of dating violence. Adolescent boys who hold opinions that are accepting of dating violence are at risk for becoming perpetrators. These opinions include believing that it is appropriate to strike a girl if she insulted or embarrassed him or intentionally tried to make him jealous. Date-specific factors put some teens at risk for date rape, including issues such as who initiated the date, the activities of the date, which person drove, and who paid for the date.

Alcohol use is extremely common in episodes of adolescent sexual assault, occurring in approximately

50% of cases. Drugs such as benzodiazepines, cocaine, and marijuana also contribute to the problem in some cases. Flunitrazepam (Rohypnol) and gamma hydroxybutyrate are two commonly implicated drugs that cause sedation and amnesia, especially when used in conjunction with alcohol.

Relatively few victims of date rape report the assault to law enforcement. Reporting rates are even lower when the victim knows the perpetrator rather than when the perpetrator is a stranger. Women who report assaults to the police are more likely to receive timely medical care; it is likely that many sexually assaulted adolescents do not receive medical attention, putting them at risk for physical and mental health consequences. Routine adolescent health care should screen for adolescent dating violence and sexual assault, provide routine sexually transmitted disease evaluation, and be able to identify counseling resources for teens who are victims or perpetrators of dating violence (see Chapter 116).

CHAPTER 26
Divorce, Separation, and Bereavement

The family is the child's principal resource for meeting his or her needs for protection, emotional support, education, and socialization. A variety of different events can result in disruptions that cause the child to be separated from his or her parents. At times, these separations may be relatively brief but unexpected, as may occur with a parent's acute illness or injury. The separation may occur in the context of significant parental discord, as often occurs with a divorce. The death of a parent results in a permanent separation that may be anticipated or unanticipated. All of these disruptions cause significant stress for the child with the potential for long-term adverse consequences. The child's adaptation to these stresses is affected by the reasons for the separation and the child's age, temperament, and available support systems.

DIVORCE

Approximately 40% of first marriages end in divorce. About half of these divorces occur in the first 7 years of marriage, so there are often young children in the family when the parents divorce. At least 25% of children experience the divorce or separation of their parents. Few events in childhood are as dramatic and challenging for the child as divorce.

Divorce is a painful process that is likely to be accompanied by changes in behavioral and emotional adjustment. Children from divorced families require psychological help two to three times more frequently than children with married parents. Long-term studies suggest that few children have sustained emotional or behavioral difficulties after a divorce. When groups of children from divorced families are compared with groups of children from married families on standardized measures of psychological adjustment, the children from divorced families are found to have only a relatively small increase in problems.

Divorce is not a single event, but a process that occurs over time. In most cases, marital conflict begins long before the physical or legal separation, and the divorce brings about permanent changes in the family structure. Multiple potential stresses for the child are associated with divorce, including parental discord before and after the divorce, changes in living arrangements and sometimes location, and changes in the child's relationship with both parents.

The child's relationship with each parent is changed by the divorce. In the short-term, the parent is likely to experience new burdens and feelings of guilt, anger, or disappointment that may disrupt parenting skills and family routines. Parents often are perceived by their children as being unaware of the child's distress around the time of the divorce. Pediatricians can help parents to understand things they can do that will be reassuring to the child. Maintaining contact with both parents, seeing where the noncustodial parent is living, and in particular maintaining familiar routines are comforting to the child in the midst of the turmoil of a separation and divorce. The child should attend school and continue to have opportunities to interact with friends. Given the parents' distress, assistance from the extended family can be helpful, but often these family members do not offer to help for fear of "interfering." It may be helpful for pediatricians to encourage parents to ask for this assistance. Pediatricians should look for maladaptive coping responses. Some parents may respond to their increased burdens and distress by treating their children as friends with whom they share their distress. Alternatively, they may place excessive responsibilities on the child or leave the child unsupervised for longer periods of time. Responses such as these increase the burdens on the child and increase the chance that the child will develop behavioral or emotional problems.

Reaction to Divorce at Different Ages

The child's reaction to the divorce is influenced by the child's age and developmental level. Infants do not react directly to the divorce, but if the divorce results in prolonged or more frequent separations from a primary caretaker, developing a secure relationship with this individual may be more difficult. Infants require special consideration in relation to custody and visitation. Separations from a primary caretaker should be brief. Preschool children are characterized by having magical beliefs about cause and effects and an egocentric view of the world. They may believe that something they did caused the divorce, leading them to be particularly upset. They may engage in unusual behaviors that they believe will bring the parents back together again. At this age, parents need to deliver a clear message that the divorce was related to disagreements between the parents, that nothing the child did caused the divorce, and that nothing the child could do would bring the parents back together again. Preschool children may reason that if the parents left each other they also might leave the child. To counteract this fear of abandonment, children may need to be reassured that although parents separated, they will not abandon the child and that the child's relationship with both parents will endure.

School-age children have a concrete understanding of cause and effect; if something bad happened, they understand that something caused it to happen. They are not likely to understand fully the subtleties of parental conflict, however, or the idea that multiple factors contribute to a conflict. Children at this age may express more anger than younger children and often feel rejected. Many young school-age children worry about what will happen to one or both parents. School performance often deteriorates. Older elementary school–age children may believe that one parent was wronged by the other, further contributing to their anger. This belief in conjunction with their concrete understanding of cause and effect allows children to be easily co-opted by one parent to take sides against the other. Parents need to understand this vulnerability and resist the temptation to support their child in taking sides.

Adolescents may respond to the divorce by engaging in acting-out behaviors, becoming depressed, or experiencing somatic symptoms. Adolescents also are in the process of developing a sense of autonomy, a sense of morality, and the capacity for intimacy. The divorce may lead adolescents to question previously held beliefs. They may be concerned about what the divorce means for their future and whether they too will experience marital failure. Questioning of previous beliefs in conjunction with decreased supervision may set the stage for risk-taking behaviors, such as truancy, sexual behaviors, and alcohol or drug use.

Outcome of Divorce

One of the best predictors of children's adaptation to divorce is whether the physical separation is associated with a decrease in the child's exposure to parental discord. In most cases, divorced parents still must interact with each other around the child's schedule, child custody and support, and other parenting issues. If one parent tends to keep the child up much later than the bedtime at the other parent's house, sleep problems may develop. If one parent does not require the child to do homework when he or she is with the child after school, the other parent may be left to deal with a tired child who still has homework to do. There is the potential for the child to have ongoing exposure to significant discord between the parents. When children feel caught in the middle of ongoing conflicts between their divorced parents, child behavior or emotional problems are much more likely. Regardless of how angry parents are with each other, the pediatrician should counsel the parents that they must shield their child from this animosity. Clear rules about schedules, discipline, and other parenting roles often are helpful in minimizing conflicts. When parents have trouble resolving these issues, mediation may be helpful. Pediatricians also need to be wary of parents' attempts to recruit them into custody battles to substantiate claims of poor parenting, unless the pediatrician has first-hand knowledge that the concerns are valid.

Issues related to visitation and custody can be quite complex. Although the primary physical residence for most children is still with the mother, the court's bias toward preferring mothers in custody decisions has decreased. Most states now allow joint physical or legal custody. In joint physical custody, the child spends an approximately equal amount of time with both parents, and in joint legal custody, parents share authority in decision making. Although joint custody arrangements may promote the involvement of both parents in the child's life, they also can be a vehicle through which parents continue to express their anger at each other. When parents have severe difficulty working together, joint custody is an inappropriate arrangement and has been associated with deterioration in the child's psychological and social adjustment.

Divorce often creates financial difficulties for the mother and child. The mother's family income declines by an average of almost 60% in the year after the divorce. Only about half of mothers who have child support awards receive the full amount they are due, and a quarter receive no money at all. These financial changes may have multiple adverse affects on the child. The family may have to move to a new house or new neighborhood, and the child may have to attend a new school, disrupting peer and family relationships. The child may spend more time in childcare if the mother has to return to work or increase her work hours.

Role of the Pediatrician

Pediatricians may be confronted with issues related to marital discord before the divorce, may be consulted around the time of the divorce, or may be involved in helping the family to manage issues in the years after the divorce. The pediatrician can be an important voice in helping the parents to understand and meet the child's needs. Before the divorce, parents may wonder what they should tell their children. Children should be told of the parents' decision before the physical separation. The separation should be presented as a rational step in managing marital conflict and should prepare the child for the changes that will occur. Parents should be prepared to answer children's questions, and they should expect that the questions will occur repeatedly over the next weeks and months. When parents have told children of the separation, it may be confusing to the child if the parents continue to appear to live together and may raise false hopes that the parents will not divorce.

Pediatricians can make many recommendations to help children and families around the time of the divorce (Table 26–1). After the acute distress of the separation has decreased, however, there is still a need for ongoing support. Many parents report not feeling like their life had stabilized until 2 to 3 years or more after the divorce, and for some the divorce remains a painful issue 10 years later. Children's

understanding of the divorce changes at different developmental stages, and their questions may change as they try to understand their family's history. Although most children ultimately show good adjustment to the divorce, some have significant acting-out behaviors or depression that requires referral to a mental health professional. Some parents need the assistance of a mediator or family therapist to help them stay focused on their child's needs. In the most contentious situations, a guardian *ad litem* may need to be appointed by the court. This individual is usually a lawyer or mental health professional with the power to investigate the child and family's background and relationships to make a recommendation to the court as to what would be in the best interests of the child.

SEPARATIONS FROM PARENTS

Children experience separations from their primary caretaker for a variety of reasons. Brief separations, such as those to attend school, camp, or other activities, are nearly a universal experience. Many children experience longer separations for a variety of reasons, including parental business trips, military service, or hospitalization. Child adjustment to the separation is affected by child factors, such as the age of the child and the child's temperament; factors related to the separation, such as the length of the separation, reason for the separation, and whether the separation was planned or unplanned; and factors related to the caregiving environment during the separation, such as how familiar the child is with the caregiver and whether the child has access to friends and familiar toys and routines.

Children between 6 months and 3 or 4 years old often have the most difficulty adjusting to a separation from their primary caregiver. Older children have cognitive and emotional skills that help them adjust. They may be better able to understand the reason for the separation, communicate their feelings to others, and comprehend the passage of time, allowing them to anticipate the parent's return. For older children, the period immediately before a planned separation may be particularly difficult if the reason for the separation causes significant family tension, as it may in the case of hospitalization or military service.

If parents can anticipate a separation, they should explain the reason for the separation to the child and to the extent possible give them concrete information on when they will be in contact with the child and when they will return home. If the child can remain at home with a familiar and responsive caregiver, this is likely to help adjustment. If the child cannot remain at home, he or she should be encouraged to take with

TABLE 26–1. General Recommendations for Pediatricians to Help Children During Separation, Divorce, or Death of a Close Relative

Acknowledge and provide support for grief the parent/caregiver is experiencing
Help parent/caregiver to consider child's needs
Encourage parent/caregiver to maintain routines familiar to the child
Encourage continued contact between child and his or her friends
If primary residence changes, the child should take transitional objects, familiar toys, and other important objects to the new residence
Minimize frequent changes in caregivers, and for infants keep times away from primary caregiver brief
Have parent/caregiver reassure the child that he or she will continue to be cared for
Have parent/caregiver reassure the child that he or she did not cause the separation, divorce, or death (especially important in preschool children)
Encourage parent/caregiver to create times or rituals that allow the child to discuss questions and feelings if the child wishes

them transitional objects, such as a favorite pillow, blanket, or stuffed animal. Familiar toys and important objects such as a picture of the parent should be taken to the new environment. Maintenance of familiar family routines and relationships with friends should be encouraged.

DEATH OF A PARENT OR FAMILY MEMBER AND BEREAVEMENT

Death of a close family member is a sad and difficult experience. When a child loses a parent, it is a devastating experience. This experience is not rare. By 15 years of age, 4% of children in the U.S. experience the death of a parent. This experience is likely to alter forever the child's view of the world as a secure and safe place. Similar to the other separations, a child's cognitive development and temperament along with the available support systems affect the child's adjustment after the death of a parent. Many of the recommendations in Table 26–1 are helpful. The death of a parent or close family member also brings up some unique issues.

Explaining Death to a Child

Children's understanding of death changes with their cognitive development and experiences (see Chapter 4). Preschool children often do not view death as permanent and may have magical beliefs about what caused death. As children become older, they understand death as permanent and inevitable, but the concept that death represents the cessation of all bodily functions and has a biologic cause may not be fully appreciated until adolescence.

Death should not be hidden from the child. It should be explained in simple and honest terms that are consistent with the family's beliefs. The explanation should help the child to understand that the dead person's body stopped functioning and that the dead person will not return. Preschool children should be reassured that nothing they did caused the individual to die. One should be prepared to answer questions about where the body is and let the child's questions help determine what information the child is prepared to hear. False or misleading information should be avoided. Comparisons of death to sleep may contribute to sleep problems in the child.

There are many possible reactions of children to the death of a parent or close relative. Sadness and a yearning to be with the dead relative are common. Sometimes a child might express a wish to die so that he or she can visit the dead relative, but a plan or desire to commit suicide is uncommon and would need immediate evaluation. A decrease in academic functioning, lack of enjoyment with activities, and changes in appetite and sleep can occur. About half of children have their most severe symptoms about 1 month after the death, but for many the most severe symptoms in reaction to the death do not occur until 6 to 12 months after the death.

Should the Child Attend the Funeral?

Children often find it helpful to attend the funeral. It may help the child to understand that the death occurred and provide an opportunity to say good-bye. Seeing others express their grief and sadness may help the child to express these feelings. Going to the funeral helps prevent the child from having fears or fantasies about what happened at the funeral. If the child is going to attend the funeral, he or she should be informed of what will happen at the funeral. If a preschool-age child expresses a desire not to attend the funeral, he or she should not be encouraged to attend. For older children, it may be appropriate to encourage attendance, but a child who feels strongly about not wanting to go to the funeral should not be required to attend.

SUGGESTED READING

American Academy of Pediatrics Committee on Early Childhood, Adoption, and Dependent Care: Health care of young children in foster care. Pediatrics 109:536-541, 2002.

American Academy of Pediatrics Committee on Child Abuse and Neglect: Shaken baby syndrome: Rotational cranial injuries—technical report. Pediatrics 108:206-210, 2001.

Behrman RE, Kliegman RM, Jenson HB (eds): Social issues. In Nelson Textbook of Pediatrics, 17th ed. Philadelphia, WB Saunders, 2004, pp 113-132.

Christian CW: Assessment and evaluation of the physically abused child. Clin Fam Pract 5:21-46, 2003.

Fein JA, Mollen CJ: Interpersonal violence. Curr Opin Pediatr 11:588-593, 1999.

Felitti VJ, Anda RF, Nordenberg D, et al: Relationship of childhood abuse and household dysfunction to many of the leading causes of death in adults: The adverse childhood experiences (ACE) study. Am J Prev Med 14:245-258, 1998.

Jenista JA: The immigrant, refugee, or internationally adopted child. Pediatr Rev 22:419-429, 2001.

Johnson JL, Leff M: Children of substance abusers: Overview of research findings. Pediatrics 103:1085-1099, 1999.

Keane V, Feigelman S: Failure to thrive and malnutrition. In Kliegman RM, Greenbaum LA, Lye PS (eds): Practical Strategies in Pediatric Diagnosis and Therapy, 2nd ed. Philadelphia, WB Saunders, 2004, pp 233-248.

Perrin EC: Sexual Orientation in Child and Adolescent Health Care. New York, Kluwer Academic/Plenum Publishers, 2002.

Reece RM: Child abuse. In Kliegman RM, Greenbaum LA, Lye PS (eds): Practical Strategies in Pediatric Diagnosis and Therapy, 2nd ed. Philadelphia, WB Saunders, 2004, pp 611-630.

U.S. Department of Health and Human Services: Youth Violence: A Report of the Surgeon General. Rockville, Md, U.S. Department of Health and Human Services, Centers for Disease Control and Prevention, National Center for Injury Prevention and Control; Substance Abuse and Mental Health Services Administration, Center for Mental Health Services; and National Institutes of Health, National Institute of Mental Health, 2001.

Visher JS, Visher EB: Beyond the nuclear family: Resources and implications for pediatricians. Pediatr Clin North Am 42:31-43, 1995.

Wallerstein JS: Separation, divorce, and remarriage. In Levine MD, Carey WB, Crocker AC (eds): Developmental-Behavioral Pediatrics, 3rd ed. Philadelphia, WB Saunders, 1999, pp 149-161.

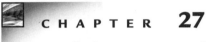

CHAPTER **27**

Diet of the Normal Infant

Infancy, especially the first 6 months, is a period of exceptionally rapid growth and high nutrient requirements relative to body weight (see Chapter 5). For approximately the first 6 months, the infant also is uniquely dependent on a single food source. These factors imply a vulnerability to inadequate nutrition, such that if inadequate total intake or inappropriate choice of food occurs, there is risk of rapid deterioration in growth and nutritional status, with potential for adverse consequences on neurocognitive development.

BREASTFEEDING

Human milk is the ideal and **uniquely superior** food for infants for the first year of life and as the sole source of nutrition for the first 6 months. This recommendation stems from the compelling advantages that breastfeeding offers infants, mothers, and society. Human milk feeding decreases the incidence or severity of diarrhea, respiratory illnesses, otitis media, bacteremia, bacterial meningitis, and necrotizing enterocolitis. Breastfeeding advantages to mothers include decreased risk for postpartum hemorrhage, longer period of amenorrhea, reduced risk of ovarian and premenopausal breast cancers, and possibly a reduced risk of osteoporosis. Advantages to society include **reduced healthcare costs** owing to lower incidence of illness in breastfed infants and reduced employee absenteeism for care attributable to infant illness. Human milk may reduce the incidence of food allergies and eczema. It also contains protective bacterial and viral antibodies (secretory IgA) and nonspecific immune factors, including macrophages and nucleotides, which also help limit infections.

Breastfeeding initiation rates in 2002 were at an all-time high of approximately 70%. The number of infants still breastfeeding by 6 months decreased to 33%, however, and was even lower by 1 year (approximately 15%). Breastfeeding rates are lower among several subpopulations of women, especially low-income, minority, and young mothers. Many mothers face obstacles in maintaining lactation because of lack of support from healthcare professionals and family and the need to return to work. Skilled use of a breast pump, particularly an electric one, may help to maintain lactation in many circumstances. Primary lactation failure is rare; most women can succeed at breastfeeding if given adequate information and support, especially in the early postpartum period. Human milk has several nutritional and non-nutritional advantages over infant formula. The nutrient composition of human milk is summarized and compared with infant formulas in Table 27–1. Outstanding characteristics include the relatively low but highly bioavailable protein content, a generous quantity of essential fatty acids, the presence of long-chain unsaturated fatty acids of the ω-3 series (docosahexaenoic acid is thought to be especially important), a relatively low sodium and solute load, and low but highly bioavailable concentrations of calcium, iron, and zinc, which provide adequate quantities of these nutrients to a normal breastfed infant for approximately 6 months. From a practical point of view, breast milk does not need to be warmed, does not require a clean water supply, and is generally free of microorganisms.

Breastfeeding Initiation

The mother should be comfortable and the infant positioned so that nothing interferes with mouth-to-breast

TABLE 27–1. Composition of Breast Milk and Infant Formulas

	Breast Milk (per dL)	Standard Formula (per dL)	Premature Formula (per dL)	Soy Formula (per dL)	Nutramigen (per dL)	Pregestimil (per dL)
Calories (kcal)	67	67	67-81	67	67	67
Protein (g)	1.1	1.5	2.0-2.4	1.7	1.9	1.9
(% calories)	(6%)	(9%)	(12%)	(10%)	(11%)	(11%)
Whey/casein protein ratio	80/20	60/40, 18/82	60/40	Soy protein, methionine	Casein hydrolysate plus L-cystine, L-tyrosine, and L-tryptophan	Casein hydrolysate plus L-cystine, L-tyrosine, and L-tryptophan
Fat (g)	4.0	3.6	3.4-4.4	3.6	3.3	3.8
(% calories)	(55%)	(50%)	(45%)	(48%)	(45%)	(48%)
MCT (%)	0	0	40-50	0	0	55
Carbohydrate	7.2	6.9-7.2	8.5-8.9	6.8	7.3	6.9
(% calories)	(40%)	(41%)	(42%)	(40%)	(44%)	(41%)
Source	Lactose	Lactose	Lactose, corn syrup	Corn syrup, sucrose	Corn syrup solids, cornstarch	Corn syrup solids, cornstarch, dextrose
Minerals (per L)						
Calcium (mg)	290	420-550	1115-1452	700	635	777
Phosphorus (mg)	140	280-390	561-806	500	420	500
Sodium (mEq)	8.0	6.5-8.3	11-15	13	14	14
Vitamin D	Variable	400	1000-1800	400	400	400
Osmolality (mOsm/L)	253	270	230-270	200-220	290	290
Renal solute load (mOsm/L)	75	100-126	175-213	126-150	175	125
Comments	Reference standard, deficient in vitamin K; may be deficient in Na+, Ca2+, protein, vitamin D for VLBW infants	Risk of milk protein intolerance—gastrointestinal bleeding, anemia, wheezing, eczema	Specifically fortified with additional protein, Ca2+, P, Na+, vitamin D, and MCT oil	Useful for lactose and milk protein intolerance; may lead to soy protein intolerance; rickets develops in VLBW infants	Useful for lactose and milk protein intolerance (allergy)	Useful for malabsorption states, lactose and milk protein intolerance (allergy)

MCT, medium-chain triglyceride; VLBW, very low birth weight.

contact. The breast from which the infant nurses should be supported with the opposite hand, with the thumb and index finger above the nipple to allow the infant easy access to the nipple. The rooting reflex should be explained to the parents to make initiation of breast-feeding easier. The nipple is stroked against the infant's cheek nearest the nipple. The infant turns toward the nipple (rooting reflex) and open the mouth, allowing the introduction of the nipple and areola. The entire nipple and most of the areola should be placed in the infant's mouth. The infant "latches on" by compressing the lips. The mechanics of normal suckling include suction of 4 to 6 cm of the areola, compression of the nipple against the palate, stimulation of milk ejection by initial rapid non-nutritive sucking, and extraction of milk from the lactiferous sinuses by a slower suck-swallow rhythm of approximately one per second. The infant may be removed from the breast by placing a clean finger between the infant's gums and the areola to release suction. The mean feeding frequency during the early weeks postpartum is 8 to 12 times per day.

Exclusive Breastfeeding

Breastfeeding is the recommended method for feeding normal infants during approximately the first 6 months of life. Colostrum, a high-protein, low-fat fluid, is produced in small amounts during the first few postpartum days. It has some nutritional value but primarily has important immunologic and maturational properties. Primiparous women often experience breast **engorgement** as the milk comes in around the third postpartum day; the breasts become hard and are painful, the nipples become nonprotractile, and the mother's temperature may increase slightly. Enhancement of milk flow is the best management. If severe engorgement occurs, areolar rigidity may prevent the infant from grasping the nipple and areola. Attention to proper latch-on and hand expression of milk assist in drainage.

Adequacy of milk intake can be assessed by voiding and stooling patterns of the infant. A well-hydrated infant voids six to eight times a day. Each voiding should soak, not merely moisten, a diaper, and urine should be colorless. By 5 to 7 days, loose yellow stools should be passed at least four times a day. Rate of weight gain provides the most objective indicator of adequate milk intake. Total weight loss after birth should not exceed 7%, and birth weight should be regained by 10 days. An infant may be adequately hydrated while not receiving enough milk to achieve adequate energy and nutrient intake. Telephone follow-up is valuable during the interim between discharge and the first pediatric visit to monitor the progress of lactation. A follow-up visit should be scheduled by 3 to 5 days of age.

The characteristics of the stools of breastfed infants often alarm parents. Stools are unformed, yellow, and seedy in appearance. Parents commonly think their breastfed infant has diarrhea. Stool frequencies vary; during the first 4 to 6 weeks, breastfed infants tend to produce stool more frequently than formula-fed infants. After 6 to 8 weeks, breastfed infants may go several days without passing a stool.

In the newborn period, elevated concentrations of serum bilirubin are present more often in breastfed infants than in formula-fed infants (see Chapter 62). Feeding frequency during the first 3 days of life of breastfed infants is inversely related to the level of bilirubin; frequent feedings stimulate meconium passage and excretion of bilirubin in the stool. Infants who have insufficient milk intake and poor weight gain may have an increase in unconjugated bilirubin secondary to an exaggerated enteropathic circulation of bilirubin. This is known as **breastfeeding jaundice**. Attention should be directed toward improved milk production and intake. The use of water supplements in breastfed infants has no effect on bilirubin levels and is not recommended. In an older breastfed infant, prolonged elevated serum bilirubin may be due to presence of an unknown factor in milk that enhances intestinal absorption of bilirubin. This is termed **breast milk jaundice**, which is a diagnosis of exclusion and should be made only if an infant is otherwise thriving, with normal growth and no evidence of hemolysis, infec-

tion, or metabolic disease (see Chapter 62). Exclusively breastfed infants should be supplemented with vitamin D (200 IU/day starting at 2 months of age), and possibly fluoride after 6 months.

Common Breastfeeding Problems

Breast tenderness, engorgement, and cracked nipples are the most common problems encountered by breastfeeding mothers. Engorgement, one of the most common causes of lactation failure, should receive prompt attention because milk supply can decrease quickly if the breasts are not adequately emptied. Applying warm or cold compresses to the breasts before nursing and hand expression or pumping of some milk can provide relief to the mother and make the areola easier to grasp by the nursling. Nipple tenderness requires attention to proper latch-on and positioning of the infant. Supportive measures include nursing for shorter periods, beginning feedings on the less sore side, air drying the nipples well after nursing, and applying lanolin cream after each nursing session. Severe nipple pain and cracking usually indicate improper latch-on. Temporary pumping, which is well tolerated, may be needed. Meeting with a lactation consultant may help minimize these problems and allow the successful continuation of breastfeeding.

If a lactating woman reports fever, chills, and malaise, **mastitis** should be considered. Treatment includes frequent and complete emptying of the breast and antibiotics. Breastfeeding usually should not be stopped because the mother's mastitis commonly has no adverse effects on the breastfed infant, and abrupt weaning may increase the risk of development of a breast abscess. Untreated mastitis also may progress to a **breast abscess**. If an abscess is diagnosed, treatment includes incision and drainage, antibiotics, and regular emptying of the breast. Nursing from the contralateral breast can be continued with the healthy infant. If maternal comfort allows, nursing also can continue on the affected side.

Maternal infection with HIV is considered a contraindication for breastfeeding in developed countries. When the mother has active tuberculosis, syphilis, or varicella, restarting breastfeeding may be considered after therapy is initiated. If a woman has herpetic lesions on her breast, nursing and contact with the infant on that breast should be avoided. Women with genital herpes can breastfeed. Proper hand-washing procedures should be stressed. Galactosemia in the infant also is a contraindication to breastfeeding.

Maternal Drug Use

Any drug prescribed therapeutically to newborns usually can be consumed via breast milk without ill effect. The factors that determine the effects of maternal drug therapy on the nursing infant include the route of administration, dosage, molecular weight, pH, and protein binding. Few therapeutic drugs are absolutely contraindicated; these include radioactive compounds, antimetabolites, lithium, and certain antithyroid drugs. The mother should be advised against the use of unprescribed drugs, including alcohol, nicotine, caffeine, or "street drugs."

Maternal use of illicit or recreational drugs is a contraindication to breastfeeding. If a woman is unable to discontinue drug use, she should not breastfeed. Expression of milk for a feeding or two after use of a drug is not acceptable. Breastfed infants of mothers taking methadone (but no alcohol or other drugs) as part of a treatment program generally have not experienced ill effects.

FORMULA FEEDING

Cow's Milk–Based Formulas

The alternative to human milk is iron-fortified formula, which permits adequate growth of most infants and is formulated to mimic human milk. No vitamin or mineral supplements (other than possibly fluoride after 6 months) are needed with such formulas. Cow's milk formulas (Table 27–2; see also Table 27–1) are composed of reconstituted, skimmed cow's milk or a mixture of skimmed cow's milk and electrolyte-depleted cow's milk whey or casein proteins. The fat used in infant formulas is a mixture of vegetable oils, commonly including soy, palm, coconut, corn, oleo, or safflower oils. The carbohydrate is generally lactose, although lactose-free cow's milk–based formulas are available. The caloric density of formulas is 20 kcal/oz (0.67 kcal/mL), similar to that of human milk. Formula-fed infants often gain weight more rapidly than breastfed infants, especially after the first 3 to 4 months of life. Formula-fed infants are at higher risk for obesity later in childhood; this may be related to differences in feeding practices for formula-fed infants compared with breastfed infants. Cow's milk–based infant formulas are used as substitutes for breast milk for infants whose mothers choose not to or cannot breastfeed or as supplements for breastfeeding. Human milk fortifiers, which when mixed with breast milk boost the caloric (24 kcal/oz) and nutrient content, also are available for use in special situations, such as for a premature infant, for whom nutrient requirements are relatively high and for whom nutrient content of human milk alone is inadequate for optimal growth.

Soy Formulas

Soy protein–based formulas provide an alternative to cow's milk–based formula when intolerance occurs from immune reactions to cow's milk proteins. A sig-

nificant proportion of infants allergic to cow's milk protein also are allergic to soy protein, however. The soy formulas are nutritionally safe alternatives to cow's milk–based formulas. The soy protein is supplemented with methionine to improve its nutritional qualities. The carbohydrates in soy formulas are glucose oligomers (smaller molecular weight corn starches) and sometimes sucrose. The fat mixture is similar to that used in cow's milk formulas. Caloric density is the same as for cow's milk formulas.

Soy protein formulas do not prevent the development of allergic disorders in later life, and clinical intolerance to soy protein or cow's milk protein occurs with similar frequency. Soy protein formulas can be recommended for use by vegetarian families choosing not to serve animal protein formulas and in the management of galactosemia and primary and secondary lactose intolerance. Soy formulas should not be used indiscriminately to "treat" poorly evaluated patients with colic, formula intolerance, or more serious diseases. Soy protein–based formulas are not recommended for premature infants with birth weights less than 1800 g.

Therapeutic Formulas

The composition of specialized infant and pediatric formulas is modified to meet specific therapeutic requirements (Tables 27–2 and 27–3). Therapeutic formulas are designed to treat digestive and **absorptive insufficiency** or protein hypersensitivity. Semielemental formulas include protein hydrolysate formulas. The major nitrogen source of each of these products is a casein or whey hydrolysate, supplemented with selected amino acids. These formulas contain an abundance of essential fatty acids from vegetable oil. Certain brands also provide substantial amounts (25% to 50% of total fat) of medium chain triglycerides, which are water soluble and are more easily absorbed than long chain fatty acids; this is a useful feature for patients with malabsorption resulting from such conditions as short gut syndrome, intestinal mucosal atrophy or injury, chronic diarrhea, or cholestasis. Elemental formulas also are available that contain synthetic free amino acids and varying quantities and types of fat components. These are especially designed for patients with protein allergy or sensitivity. The carbohydrate content of these specialized formulas varies, but all are lactose free; some contain glucose oligomers and soluble starches.

COMPLEMENTARY FOODS AND WEANING

By approximately 6 months, complementary feeding of semisolid foods is suggested. By this age, an exclusively breastfed infant requires additional sources of several nutrients, including protein, iron, and zinc. If the

TABLE 27–2. Infant Feedings and Formulas

Formula Category	Example Formulas	Features and Typical Uses
Human milk		"Gold standard." Expressed milk can be delivered by gavage or nasogastric tube
Cow's milk–based (with lactose)	Enfamil Similac Carnation Good Start	Standard substitute for breast milk
Cow's milk–based (without lactose)	Lactofree Similac Lactose Free	Useful for transient lactase deficiency or lactose intolerance
Soy protein–based/lactose-free	Prosobee Isomil	Alternative to milk protein–based formulas. Not recommended for premature infants
Premature formula: cow's milk (reduced lactose)	Similac Special Care Enfamil Premature	Indicated for premature and LBW infants. Fat is 50% MCT, higher in many micronutrients
Predigested	Pregestimil (50% fat MCT) Nutramigen (no MCT) Alimentum (50% fat MCT)	Casein hydrolysate, useful for protein allergies and malabsorptive disorders
Elemental	Neocate Elecare	Free amino acids for severe protein allergy or malabsorption
Premature transitional	Enfacare Neosure	Standard at 22 kcal/oz, intermediate in protein and micronutrients to promote growth post discharge
Fat modified	Lipisorb Portagen	High MCT, useful for chylous effusions and for some malabsorptive disorders
Prethickened	Enfamil AR	May be useful for dysphagia, mild GER
Carbohydrate intolerance	3232A Ross Carbohydrate Free	All monosaccharides and disaccharides removed; can titrate dextrose or fructose additives to tolerance

GER, gastroesophageal reflux; LBW, low birth weight; MCT, medium chain triglyceride.

TABLE 27–3. Pediatric Enteral Formulas

Formula Category	Formula Examples	Typical Uses
Standard, milk protein–based	Nutren Junior Pediasure (with/without fiber) Kindercal (with/without fiber)	Nutritionally complete for ages 1-10. Can be used for tube feeds or oral supplements
Food-based	Compleat Pediatric	Made with beef protein, fruits, and vegetables—contains lactose. Fortified with vitamins/minerals
Semielemental	Peptamen Jr.	Indicated for impaired gut function with peptides as protein source, high MCT content with lower total fat percentage than standard pediatric formulas
Elemental	Pediatric Vivonex (24 kcal/oz) Elecare Neocate One Plus	Indicated for impaired gut function or protein allergy, contains free amino acids. Lower fat, with most as MCT

MCT, medium chain triglyceride.

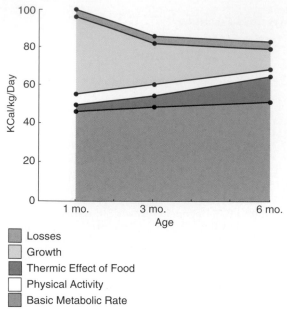

Figure 27–1

Energy requirements of infants. (From Waterlow JC: Basic concepts in the determination of nutritional requirements of normal infants. In Tsang RC, Nichols BL [eds]: Nutrition During Infancy. Philadelphia, Hanley & Belfus, 1988.)

introduction of solid foods is delayed, nutritional deficiencies can develop, and oral sensory issues (texture and oral aversion) may occur. General signs of **readiness** include the ability to hold the head up and sit unassisted, bringing objects to the mouth, showing interest in foods, and the ability to track a spoon and open the mouth. Although the growth rate of the infant is decreasing, energy needs for activity increase (Fig. 27–1). A relatively high-fat and calorically dense diet (human milk or formula) is needed to deliver adequate calories. The choice of complementary foods to meet micronutrient needs is less critical for formula-fed infants because of the nutrient fortification of formula. The exposure to different textures and the process of self-feeding are important developmental experiences for formula-fed infants.

Commercially prepared or homemade foods help meet the nutritional needs of the infant. Because infant foods are usually less energy dense than human milk and formula, they should not be used in young infants to compensate for inadequate intake from breastfeeding or formula. Oropharyngeal coordination is immature before 3 months, making feeding with solid foods difficult. Vitamin-fortified and iron-fortified dry cereals are often used as a source of calories and micronutrients (particularly iron) to supplement the diet of infants whose needs for these nutrients are not met by human milk after about 6 months of age. Cereals commonly are mixed with breast milk, formula, or water

and later with fruits. To help identify possible allergies or food intolerances that may arise when new foods are added to the diet, single-grain cereals (rice, oatmeal, barley) are recommended as starting cereals. New single-ingredient foods generally can be offered approximately every week. Mixed cereal (oat, corn, wheat, and soy) provides greater variety to older infants.

Puréed fruits, vegetables, and meats are available in containers that provide an appropriate serving size for infants. By approximately 6 months, the infant's gastrointestinal tract is mature, and the order of introducing complementary foods is not critical. Introduction of single-ingredient meats (versus combination dinners) as an early complementary food provides an excellent source of bioavailable iron and zinc, both of which are important for the older breastfed infant. Parents who prefer to make homemade infant foods using a food processor or food mill should be encouraged to practice safe food handling techniques and avoid flavor additives such as salt. Juice frequently is given to infants, although it is not a necessary "food" for infants. If given, juice should be started only after 6 months of age, be given in a cup (as opposed to a bottle), and limited to 4 oz daily. An infant should never be put to sleep with a bottle or sippy cup filled with milk, formula, or juice because this can result in **infant bottle tooth decay** (see Chapter 127). Foods with high allergic potential that should be avoided during infancy, especially for infants with a strong family history of food allergy, including fish, peanuts, nuts, dairy products, and eggs. Hot dogs, grapes, and nuts also present a risk of aspiration and airway obstruction. All foods with the potential to obstruct the young infant's airway should be cut into sizes smaller than an infant's main airway. Honey (risk of infant botulism) should not be given before 1 to 2 years of age.

CHAPTER **28**

Diet of the Normal Child and Adolescent

Nutrient needs for children and adolescents are summarized in Table 28–1.

NUTRITION ISSUES FOR TODDLERS AND OLDER CHILDREN

Cow's milk ideally is not introduced until approximately 1 year of age to avoid occult intestinal blood loss. Excessive milk (>24 oz/day) intake should be avoided in toddlers because larger intakes may reduce the intake of

TABLE 28–1. Food and Nutrition Board, Institute of Medicine, National Academy of Sciences Dietary Reference Intakes: Recommended Intakes for Individuals

Life Stage Group	Calcium (mg/day)	Phosphorus (mg/day)	Magnesium (mg/day)	Vitamin D (μg/day)*†	Fluoride (mg/day)	Thiamine (mg/day)	Riboflavin (mg/day)	Niacin (mg/day)‡	Vitamin B6 (mg/day)	Folate (μg/day)§	Vitamin B12 (μg/day)	Pantothenic Acid (mg/day)	Biotin (pg/day)	Choline (mg/day)‖
Infants														
0-6 mo	210	100	30	5	0.01	0.2	0.3	2	0.1	65	0.4	1.7	5	125
7-12 mo	270	275	75	5	0.5	0.3	0.4	4	0.3	80	0.5	1.8	6	150
Children														
1-3 yr	500	460	80	5	0.7	0.5	0.5	6	0.5	150	0.9	2	8	200
4-8 yr	800	500	130	5	1	0.6	0.6	8	0.6	200	1.2	3	12	250
Males														
9-13 yr	1300	1250	240	5	2	0.9	0.9	12	1	300	1.8	4	20	375
14-18 yr	1300	1250	410	5	3	1.2	1.3	16	1.3	400	2.4	5	25	550
19-30 yr	1000	700	400	5	4	1.2	1.3	16	1.3	400	2.4	5	30	550
31-50 yr	1000	700	420	5	4	1.2	1.3	16	1.3	400	2.4	5	30	550
51-70 yr	1200	700	420	10	4	1.2	1.3	16	1.7	400	2.4¶	5	30	550
>70 yr	1200	700	420	15	4	1.2	1.5	16	1.7	400	2.4¶	5	30	550
Females														
9-13 yr	1300	1250	240	5	2	0.9	0.9	12	1	300	1.8	4	20	375
14-18 yr	1300	1250	360	5	3	1	1	14	1.2	400#	2.4	5	25	400
19-30 yr	1000	700	310	5	3	1.1	1.1	14	1.3	400#	2.4	5	30	425
31-50 yr	1000	700	320	5	3	1.1	1.1	14	1.3	400#	2.4	5	30	425
51-70 yr	1200	700	320	10	3	1.1	1.1	14	1.5	400	2.4¶	5	30	425
>70 yr	1200	700	320	15	3	1.1	1.1	14	1.5	400	2.4¶	5	30	425

Continued

TABLE 28-1. Food and Nutrition Board, Institute of Medicine, National Academy of Sciences Dietary Reference Intakes: Recommended Intakes for Individuals—cont'd

Life Stage Group	Calcium (mg/day)	Phosphorus (mg/day)	Magnesium (mg/day)	Vitamin D (µg/day)*†	Fluoride (mg/day)	Thiamine (mg/day)	Riboflavin (mg/day)	Niacin (mg/day)‡	Vitamin B6 (mg/day)	Folate (µg/day)§	Vitamin B12 (µg/day)	Pantothenic Acid (mg/day)	Biotin (pg/day)	Choline (mg/day)∥
Pregnancy														
≤18 yr	1300	1250	400	5	3	1.4	1.4	18	1.9	600**	2.6	6	30	450
19-30 yr	1000	700	350	5	3	1.4	1.4	18	1.9	600**	2.6	6	30	450
31-50 yr	1000	700	360	5	3	1.4	1.4	18	1.9	600**	2.6	6	30	450
Lactation														
≤18 yr	1300	1250	360	5	3	1.4	1.6	17	2	500	2.8	7	35	550
19-30 yr	1000	700	310	5	3	1.4	1.6	17	2	500	2.8	7	35	550
31-50 yr	1000	700	320	5	3	1.4	1.6	17	2	500	2.8	7	35	550

Note: This table presents recommended dietary allowances (RDAs) in **bold type** and adequate intakes (AIs) in ordinary type. RDAs and AIs may be used as goals for individual intake. RDAs are set to meet the needs of almost all (97-98%) individuals in a group. For healthy breastfed infants, the AI is the mean intake. The AI for other life-stage and gender groups is believed to cover needs of all individuals in the group, but lack of data or uncertainty in the data prevents being able to specify with confidence the percentage of individuals covered by this intake.

*As cholecalciferol. 1 pg cholecalciferol = 40 IU vitamin D.

†In the absence of adequate exposure to sunlight.

‡As niacin equivalents (NE). 1 mg of niacin = 60 mg of tryptophan; 0-6 months = preformed niacin (not NE).

§As dietary folate equivalents (DFE). 1 DFE = 1 µg food folate = 0.6 µg of folic acid from fortified food or as a supplement consumed with food = 0.5 mg of a supplement taken on an empty stomach.

∥Although AIs have been set for choline, there are few data to assess whether a dietary supply of choline is needed at all stages of the life cycle, and it may be that the choline requirement can be met by endogenous synthesis at some of these stages.

¶Because 10-30% of older people may malabsorb food-bound B₁₂, it is advisable for those ≥50 years old to meet their RDA mainly by consuming foods fortified with B₁₂ or a supplement containing B₁₂.

#In view of evidence linking folate intake with neural tube defects in the fetus, it is recommended that all women capable of becoming pregnant consume 400 µg from supplements or fortified foods in addition to intake of food folate from a varied diet.

**It is assumed that women will continue consuming 400 µg from supplements or fortified foods until their pregnancy is confirmed and they enter prenatal care, which ordinarily occurs after the end of the periconceptional period—the critical time for formation of the neural tube.

a good variety of nutritionally important solid foods; large intakes also may contribute to excessive caloric intake. Juice intake for toddlers and young children should be limited to 4 to 6 oz/day, and juice intake for children 7 to 18 years old should be limited to 8 to 12 oz/day. By 1 year of age, infants should be eating meals with the family, have a regular schedule of meals and snacks, and be encouraged to self-feed with appropriate finger foods. The Food Guide Pyramid by the U.S. Department of Agriculture can provide parents with a general guideline for the types of foods to be offered on a regular basis. A general rule for the quantity of food to offer is 1 tablespoon of each food provided per meal, with more given if the toddler requests. Power struggles over eating are common between parents and toddlers. The **parent's role** is to decide the what, when, and where of the meals. The **child's role** is to decide if, what, and how much to eat. Breastfeeding of the older infant can continue as long as mutually desired, with care taken to ensure the infant is consuming a variety of other foods and is not depending excessively on breastfeeding for nutritional or comfort needs.

Iron intake may be inadequate in some children between 1 and 3 years old in the U.S. The incidence of iron deficiency anemia has decreased in young children in the U.S., in part as a result of participation of children in the Women, Infants and Children (WIC) program. Significant iron deficiency and iron deficiency anemia exist, however, in some high-risk minority or poor populations of young children.

Among families who participate in federal assistance programs, higher than the expected number of children have weight/height measurements below the 5th percentile. In addition, 10% of 2- to 5-year-old children have weight-for-length or body mass index (BMI) percentiles at or above the 95th percentile for age. The relatively high prevalences of **underweight** and **overweight** emphasize the importance of surveillance of growth velocity in all young children to allow early detection of abnormal rates of weight gain relative to linear growth.

Learning healthy eating behaviors at an early age is an important preventive measure because of the association of diet with several chronic adult diseases, such as obesity, diabetes, and cardiovascular disease. Table 28–2 provides guidelines for a **prudent diet** appropriate for most children older than 2 years. After 2 years, it is recommended that the fat intake gradually be reduced to approximately 30% and not less than 20% of calories.

NUTRITION ISSUES FOR ADOLESCENTS

Adolescence can be a time when poor eating habits develop. Skipped meals (especially breakfast), binge eating with friends or alone, dieting, and consumption

---

TABLE 28–2. Prudent Diet Guidelines for Children Older than 2 Years

General Recommendations

Consume 3 regular meals daily with healthful snacks according to appetite, activity, and growth needs
Include a variety of foods with abundant vegetables and fruits

Key Nutrients

Carbohydrates
Complex carbohydrates should provide ≥55-60% of daily calories; emphasis should be on whole-grain, high-fiber foods
Simple sugars should be limited to <10% daily calories

Fat
<30% of total calories should come from dietary fat
Saturated and polyunsaturated fats should make up <10% total calories each
Monounsaturated fats should provide at least 10% total calories
Encourage lean cuts of meat, fish, low-fat dairy products, vegetable oils
Cholesterol intake should approximate 100 mg/1000 kcal/day (maximum of 300 mg/day)
Severe fat restriction (<15-20% total calories) should be avoided because it may result in growth failure

Sodium
Limit sodium intake by choosing fresh over highly processed foods

Behavioral

Limit grazing behavior, eating while watching television, and regular consumption of high-calorie, low-nutrient foods

---

of nutrient-poor, calorically dense foods are common problems. Excessive consumption of sugar from soda, fruit drinks, and specialty coffee and tea drinks may contribute to excess weight gain and tooth decay and may displace other needed nutrients. Poor calcium intake during adolescence may predispose adults to osteoporotic hip fractures in later life. **Osteoporosis** (osteopenia) caused by poor dietary calcium or vitamin intake or poor absorption of ingested calcium in children and adolescents is becoming more clinically recognized and treated. Inadequate iron intake may result in symptoms of fatigue and iron deficiency anemia. Student athletes may be especially vulnerable to inadequate iron intakes, severely restrictive eating patterns, and use of inappropriate nutritional and vitamin supplements. Adolescents should be counseled on appropriate dietary recommendations (see Chapter 70).

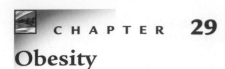

CHAPTER 29

Obesity

EPIDEMIOLOGY AND DEFINITIONS

The prevalence of obesity in children has increased dramatically. Data from 1999-2000 indicate that 15% of American children age 6 to 19 years were considered **overweight** (body mass index [BMI] ≥95th percentile). The prevalence of obesity has increased to approximately 10% in children 4 to 5 years old. The largest increases in the prevalence of obesity were seen in the most overweight classifications and in certain ethnic groups, such as African American and Mexican American children, of whom more than 20% are overweight.

Many obese children become obese adults. The risk of remaining obese increases with age and the degree of obesity. Eleven-year-old children who are overweight are more than twice as likely to remain overweight at age 15 than are 7-year-old overweight children. The risk of becoming obese as a child and remaining obese as an adult also is influenced by family history. If one parent is obese, the odds ratio for the child to be obese in adulthood is 3, but this increases to 10 if both parents are obese.

Obesity runs in families; this could be related to genetic influences or the influence of a common, shared environment. In comparisons of adopted twin pairs, 80% of the variance in weight for height or skinfold thickness may be explained on the basis of genetics. A strong relationship exists between the BMI of adoptees and that of their biologic parents; a weaker relationship exists between the BMI of adoptees and that of their adoptive parents. These relationships support the influence of genetics. The association between obesity and television watching and dietary intake, the different rates of obesity observed in urban versus rural areas, and changes in obesity with seasons also support the important influence of environment.

CLINICAL MANIFESTATIONS

Complications of obesity in children and adolescents can affect virtually every major organ system. The clinician should direct the history and physical examination toward screening for many potential complications noted among obese patients (Table 29–1) in addition to specific diseases associated with obesity (Table 29–2). Medical complications usually are related to the degree of obesity and usually decrease in severity or resolve with weight reduction.

TABLE 29–1.	Complications of Obesity
Complication	**Effects**
Psychosocial	Peer discrimination, teasing, reduced college acceptance, isolation, reduced job promotion*
Growth	Advance bone age, increased height, early menarche
CNS	Pseudotumor cerebri
Respiratory	Sleep apnea, pickwickian syndrome
Cardiovascular	Hypertension, cardiac hypertrophy, ischemic heart disease,* sudden death*
Orthopedic	Slipped capital femoral epiphysis, Blount disease
Metabolic	Insulin resistance, type 2 diabetes mellitus, hypertriglyceridemia, hypercholesterolemia, gout,* hepatic steatosis, polycystic ovary disease, cholelithiasis

*Complications unusual until adulthood.

The **diagnosis** of obesity depends on the measurement of excess body fat. Actual measurement of body composition is not practical in most clinical situations. **BMI** is a convenient screening tool that correlates fairly strongly with body fatness in children and adults. **BMI age-specific and gender-specific percentile curves** (for 2- to 20-year-olds) allow an assessment of BMI percentile (available online at http://www.cdc.gov/growthcharts). Table 29–3 provides BMI interpretation guidelines. For children younger than 2 years old, weight for length greater than 95th percentile may indicate overweight or obesity and warrants further assessment.

ASSESSMENT

Early recognition of at risk for overweight or overweight children is essential because family counseling and treatment interventions are more likely to be successful before obesity becomes severe. Routine evaluation at well-child visits should include the following:

1. Anthropometric data, including weight, height, and calculation of BMI. Data should be plotted on age-appropriate and gender-appropriate growth charts and assessed for weight gain trends and upward crossing of percentiles.
2. Dietary and physical activity history (Table 29–4). Assess patterns and potential areas for change.
3. **Physical examination.** Assess blood pressure, adiposity distribution (central versus generalized),

TABLE 29–2.   Diseases Associated with Childhood Obesity*

Syndrome	Manifestations
Alström syndrome	Hypogonadism, retinal degeneration, deafness, diabetes mellitus
Carpenter syndrome	Polydactyly, syndactyly, cranial synostosis, mental retardation
Cushing syndrome	Adrenal hyperplasia or pituitary tumor
Fröhlich syndrome	Hypothalamic tumor
Hyperinsulinism	Nesidioblastosis, pancreatic adenoma, hypoglycemia, Mauriac syndrome (poor diabetic control)
Laurence-Moon-Bardet-Biedl syndrome	Retinal degeneration, syndactyly, hypogonadism, mental retardation; autosomal recessive
Muscular dystrophy	Late onset of obesity
Myelodysplasia	Spina bifida
Prader-Willi syndrome	Neonatal hypotonia, normal growth immediately after birth, small hands and feet, mental retardation, hypogonadism; some have partial deletion of chromosome 15
Pseudohypoparathyroidism	Variable hypocalcemia, cutaneous calcifications
Turner syndrome	Ovarian dysgenesis, lymphedema, web neck; XO chromosome

*These diseases represent <5% of cases of childhood obesity.

markers of comorbidities (acanthosis nigricans, hirsutism, hepatomegaly, orthopedic abnormalities), and physical stigmata of genetic syndrome (Prader-Willi syndrome).

4. **Laboratory studies.** These are generally reserved for children who are overweight (BMI >95th percentile) or who have evidence of comorbidities or both. Useful laboratory tests may include a fasting lipid profile, fasting insulin and glucose levels, liver function tests, and thyroid function tests (if evidence of plateau in linear growth). Other studies should be guided by findings in the history and physical examination.

TREATMENT

The approach to therapy and aggressiveness of treatment should be based on risk factors, including age, severity of obesity and comorbidities, and family history and support. The primary goal for all children with uncomplicated overweight is to achieve **healthy eating and activity patterns**. For children with a secondary complication, improvement of the complication is an important goal. For children 2 to 7 years old with BMI greater than or equal to 95th percentile and without complications, the goal is **maintenance** of baseline weight, allowing the child to "**grow into**" their height, with a gradual normalization of BMI. For children 2 to 7 years old with BMI greater than or equal

TABLE 29–3.   Body Mass Index (BMI) Interpretation

BMI/Age percentile	Interpretation
<5th	Underweight
5-85th	Normal
85-95th	At risk for overweight
>95th	Overweight or obese

TABLE 29–4.   Key Areas of Assessment for Overweight/Obesity Evaluation

Diet

Meal and snack pattern: structured versus grazing, skipping meals; where and with whom are meals/snacks eaten; eating in front of TV?
Portion sizes: are portions age-appropriate; portions for child same as adult?
Frequency of meals away from home (restaurants, takeout, childcare setting)
Frequency and amounts of caloric beverages (soda, juice, milk, energy drinks, specialty coffee and tea drinks)
Frequency of eating fruits and vegetables

Activity

Hours per day spent in sedentary activity: television, computer games/Internet, video games
Daily or weekly time spent in vigorous (i.e., generating sweating!) activity: organized sports, physical education, free play
Activities of daily living: walking, free unstructured play, chores
Activity levels of parents

to 95th percentile and secondary complications, weight loss is indicated. For children older than 7 years with BMI between 85th and 95th percentile, without complications, weight maintenance is an appropriate goal. Weight loss is recommended if secondary complications are present; an appropriate goal is 1 lb weight loss per month until a BMI less than 85th percentile is achieved. Because children and young adolescents are still growing, excessive acute weight loss should be avoided, as this may contribute to linear growth stunting and nutrient deficiencies.

Childhood and adolescent obesity treatment programs can lead to sustained weight loss and decreases in BMI when treatment focuses on behavioral changes and is family centered. **Concurrent changes in dietary and physical activity patterns** are most likely to provide success. Healthy eating patterns need to be adopted by the whole family, with parents modeling healthy food choices, controlling foods brought into the home, and guiding appropriate portion sizes. Limiting sedentary activity has been found to be more effective than specifically promoting increased physical activity. The AAP recommends no **television** for children younger than 2 years old and a maximum of 2 hours per day of television and video/computer games for older children.

When considering treatment, three options can be considered depending on the severity of the problem, the age of the child, the ability and readiness of the family to make changes, the preferences of the parents and child, and the skills of the healthcare provider:

1. **General guidelines:** Counseling regarding problem areas identified by dietary and physical activity history should be provided (see Table 29–4); emphasis should be on healthy eating and physical activity patterns. This is especially appropriate for preventing further weight gain and for mildly overweight children. Advice that is appropriate for all children includes encouragement to increase active play, reduce television and other screen time, increase intake of fruits and vegetables, and limit intake of soda and juice drinks.
2. **Structured advice:** This approach provides more specific dietary guidance, such as meal and menu planning, and an exercise prescription and behavioral change goals. This may be done in the primary care setting or by referral to a more specialized treatment center.
3. **Group treatment programs:** This type of program generally works best for older children or adolescents, with varying level of parental involvement depending on the age of the child. Several published programs are available. The Weight Information Network is a service available through the National Institutes of Health, which disseminates information on weight control programs (available at http://www.niddk.nih.gosv//NutritionDocs.html).

There is no single course of treatment that is likely to be effective for all patients. The physician would do best to assess the severity of overweight/obesity with attention to comorbidities, the child's treatment needs in the context of the family's preferences and abilities, and access to resources, such as registered dietitians with expertise in pediatric weight management and behavioralists or family therapists. Pharmacotherapy and bariatric surgery are treatment options for adults and are being studied as treatment options for older children and adolescents, but evidence from controlled trials is insufficient to justify specific recommendations.

PREVENTION

Obesity is challenging to treat and can cause significant medical and psychosocial issues for young children and adolescents. Families need to be counseled on age-appropriate and healthy eating patterns beginning in infancy with the promotion of **breastfeeding**. For infants, transition to complementary and table foods and the importance of regularly scheduled meals and snacks versus grazing behavior should be emphasized. Age-appropriate **portion sizes** for meals and snacks should be encouraged. Children should be taught to recognize hunger and satiety cues, guided by reasonable portions and healthy food choices by parents. Children should never be forced to eat when they are not willing, and overemphasis of food as a reward should be avoided. The U.S. Department of Agriculture Food Guide Pyramid provides a good framework for a healthy diet, with an emphasis on whole grains, fruits, and vegetables and with age-appropriate portion sizes. After age 2 years, most children should change from whole or 2% milk to skim milk because other food sources provide adequate fat for growth and development.

The importance of physical activity should be emphasized. For some children, organized sports and school-based activities provide opportunities for vigorous activity and fun, whereas for others a focus on activities of daily living, such as increased walking, using stairs, and more active play may be better received. Time spent in **sedentary behavior**, such as television viewing and video/computer games, should be limited. Television in children's rooms is associated with more television time and with higher rates of overweight, and the risks of this practice should be discussed with parents. Clinicians may need to help families identify alternatives to sedentary activities, especially for families with deterrents to activity, such as unsafe neighborhoods or lack of supervision after school.

CHAPTER 30
Pediatric Undernutrition

Worldwide, protein-energy malnutrition (PEM) is a leading cause of death among children younger than 5 years old. PEM is a spectrum of conditions caused by varying levels of protein and calorie deficiencies. Primary PEM is caused by social or economic factors that result in a lack of food. Secondary PEM occurs in children with various conditions associated with increased caloric requirements (infection, trauma, cancer) (Fig. 30–1), increased caloric loss (malabsorption), reduced caloric intake (anorexia, cancer, oral intake restriction, social factors), or a combination of these three variables. See Table 30–1 for guidelines on the classification of pediatric undernutrition. Protein and calorie malnutrition may be associated with other nutrient deficiencies, which may be evident on the physical examination (Table 30–2).

FAILURE TO THRIVE

The most common diagnosis of pediatric undernutrition in the U.S. is often termed *failure to thrive* and is estimated to have a prevalence of 5% to 10% among young children (see Chapter 21). Psychosocial risk factors may develop as a result of medical problems or may be a primary cause of undernutrition. In the U.S., most factors that contribute to poor growth are likely to be due to behavioral and psychosocial factors. The terms *organic* and *nonorganic* failure to thrive have lost favor in recognition of the frequent interplay between underlying medical conditions that may cause maladaptive behaviors. Similarly, social and behavioral factors that initially may have been associated with feeding problems and poor growth also may be associated with medical problems, including frequent minor acute illnesses. For information on diagnosis and treatment of failure to thrive, see Chapter 21.

MARASMUS

Marasmus is the term used for **severe PEM** and is relatively common on a global basis. Many secondary forms of marasmic PEM are associated with chronic

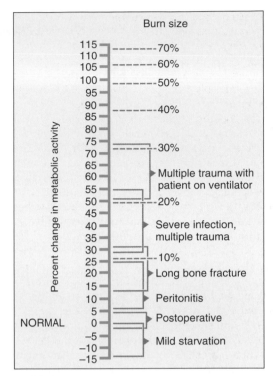

Figure 30–1

Increased energy needs with stress. (Adapted from Wilmore D: The Metabolic Management of the Critically Ill. New York, Plenum Publishing, 1977. Revised in Walker W, Watkins J [eds]: Nutrition in Pediatrics: Basic Science and Clinical Application. Boston, Little, Brown, 1985.)

TABLE 30–1. Classification Guidelines for Pediatric Undernutrition

Nutrition Status	Weight/Age	Height/Age	Weight/Height	% IBW
Wasting	Normal or low	Normal	<5th percentile	<85-90%
Stunting	<5th percentile	<5th percentile	Normal	Normal
Mild malnutrition	Normal or low	Normal	<5th percentile	81-90%
Moderate malnutrition	Normal or low	Normal	<5th percentile	70-80%
Kwashiorkor	Normal or low	Normal or low	Normal (edema)	Normal
Marasmus (severe wasting)	Low	Normal or low	<5th percentile	<70%

IBW, ideal body weight.

TABLE 30–2.   Physical Signs of Nutritional Deficiency Disorders

System	Sign	Deficiency
General appearance	Reduced weight for height	Calories
Skin and hair	Pallor	Anemias (iron, vitamin B_{12}, vitamin E, folate, and copper)
	Edema	Protein, thiamine
	Nasolabial seborrhea	Calories, protein, vitamin B_6, niacin, riboflavin
	Dermatitis	Riboflavin, essential fatty acids, biotin
	Photosensitivity dermatitis	Niacin
	Acrodermatitis	Zinc
	Follicular hyperkeratosis (sandpaper-like)	Vitamin A
	Depigmented skin	Calories, protein
	Purpura	Vitamins C, K
	Scrotal, vulval dermatitis	Riboflavin
	Alopecia	Zinc, biotin, protein
	Depigmented, dull hair, easily pluckable	Protein, calories, copper
Subcutaneous tissue	Decreased	Calories
Eye (vision)	Adaptation to dark	Vitamins A, E, zinc
	Color discrimination	Vitamin A
	Bitot spots, xerophthalmia, keratomalacia	Vitamin A
	Conjunctival pallor	Nutritional anemias
	Fundal capillary microaneurysms	Vitamin C
Face, mouth, and neck	Angular stomatitis	Riboflavin, iron
	Cheilosis	Vitamins B_6, niacin, riboflavin
	Bleeding gums	Vitamins C, K
	Atrophic papillae	Riboflavin, iron, niacin, folate, vitamin B_{12}
	Smooth tongue	Iron
	Red tongue (glossitis)	Vitamins B_6, B_{12}, niacin, riboflavin, folate
	Parotid swelling	Protein
	Caries	Fluoride
	Anosmia	Vitamins A, B_{12}, zinc
	Hypogeusia	Vitamin A, zinc
	Goiter	Iodine
Cardiovascular	Heart failure	Thiamine, selenium, nutritional anemias
Genital	Hypogonadism	Zinc
Skeletal	Costochondral beading	Vitamins D, C
	Subperiosteal hemorrhage	Vitamin C, copper
	Cranial bossing	Vitamin D
	Wide fontanel	Vitamin D
	Epiphyseal enlargement	Vitamin D
	Craniotabes	Vitamin D, calcium
	Tender bones	Vitamin C
	Tender calves	Thiamine, selenium, vitamin C
	Spoon-shaped nails (koilonychia)	Iron
	Transverse nail line	Protein
Neurologic	Sensory, motor neuropathy	Thiamine, vitamins E, B_6, B_{12}
	Ataxia, areflexia	Vitamin E
	Ophthalmoplegia	Vitamin E, thiamine
	Tetany	Vitamin D, Ca^{2+}, Mg^{2+}
	Retardation	Iodine, niacin
	Dementia, delirium	Vitamin E, niacin, thiamine
	Poor position sense, ataxia	Thiamine, vitamin B_{12}

diseases (cystic fibrosis, tuberculosis, cancer, AIDS, celiac disease). The principal **clinical manifestation** in a child with severe malnutrition is **emaciation** with a body weight less than 60% of the median (50th percentile) for age or less than 70% of the ideal weight for height and depleted body fat stores. Although growth stunting may be observed with longer term malnutrition, the ratio of observed-to-expected weight relative to height reveals a reduction in body mass exceeding that caused by any coexisting growth stunting. Loss of muscle mass and subcutaneous fat stores is confirmed by inspection or palpation and quantified by anthropometric measurements. The head may appear large, but generally is proportional to the body length. Edema usually is absent. The skin is dry and thin, and the hair may be thin, sparse, and easily pulled out. Marasmic children may be apathetic and weak. Bradycardia and hypothermia signify severe and life-threatening malnutrition. Atrophy of the filiform papillae of the tongue is common, and monilial stomatitis is frequent. Inappropriate or inadequate weaning practices and chronic diarrhea are common findings in developing countries.

KWASHIORKOR

Kwashiorkor is **hypoalbuminemic, edematous malnutrition** and presents with pitting edema that starts in the lower extremities and ascends with increasing severity. It is classically described as being caused by inadequate protein intake in the presence of fair to good caloric intake. Other factors, such as acute infection, toxins, and possibly specific micronutrient or amino acid imbalances, are likely to contribute to the etiology. The major **clinical manifestation** of kwashiorkor is that the body weight of the child ranges from 60% to 80% of the expected weight for age; weight alone may not accurately reflect the nutritional status because of edema. **Physical examination** reveals a relative maintenance of subcutaneous adipose tissue and a marked atrophy of muscle mass. Edema varies from a minor pitting of the dorsum of the foot to generalized edema with involvement of the eyelids and scrotum. The hair is sparse, is easily plucked, and appears dull brown, red, or yellow-white. Nutritional repletion restores hair color, leaving a band of hair with altered pigmentation followed by a band with normal pigmentation (flag sign). Skin changes are common and range from hyperpigmented hyperkeratosis to an erythematous macular rash (pellagroid) on the trunk and extremities. In the most severe form of kwashiorkor, a superficial desquamation occurs over pressure surfaces ("flaky paint" rash). Angular cheilosis, atrophy of the filiform papillae of the tongue, and monilial stomatitis are common. Enlarged parotid glands and facial edema result in moon facies; apathy and

disinterest in eating are typical of kwashiorkor. Examination of the abdomen may reveal an enlarged, soft liver with an indefinite edge. Lymphatic tissue commonly is atrophic. Chest examination may reveal basilar rales. The abdomen is distended, and bowel sounds tend to be hypoactive.

TREATMENT OF MALNUTRITION

The basal metabolic rate and immediate nutrient needs decrease in cases of malnutrition. When nutrients are provided, the metabolic rate increases, stimulating anabolism and increasing nutrient requirements. The body of the malnourished child may have compensated for micronutrient deficiencies with lower metabolic and growth rates; refeeding may unmask these deficiencies. The gastrointestinal tract may not tolerate a rapid increase in intake. Nutritional rehabilitation should be initiated and advanced slowly to minimize these complications. Intravenous fluid should be avoided if possible to avoid excessive fluid and solute load and resultant congestive heart failure or renal failure. **Overzealous refeeding has been documented to cause life-threatening abnormalities** of these and other nutrients. If edema develops in the child during refeeding, caloric intake should be kept stable until the edema begins to resolve.

When nutritional rehabilitation is initiated, calories can be safely started at 20% above the child's recent intake. If no estimate of the caloric intake is available, 50% to 75% of the normal energy requirement is safe. Following these guidelines should help to avoid the **refeeding syndrome**, which is characterized by fluid retention, hypophosphatemia, hypomagnesemia, and hypokalemia. Careful monitoring of laboratory values and clinical status with severe malnutrition is essential.

When nutritional rehabilitation has begun, caloric intake can be increased 10% to 20% per day, with monitoring for electrolyte imbalances, poor cardiac function, edema, or feeding intolerance. If any of these occurs, further caloric increases are not made until the child's status stabilizes. Caloric intake is increased until appropriate regrowth or catch-up growth is initiated. Catch-up growth refers to gaining weight at greater than 50th percentile for age and may require 150% or more of the recommended calories for an age-matched, well-nourished child. A general "rule of thumb" for infants and children up to 3 years old is to provide 100 to 120 kcal/kg based on ideal weight for height. Protein needs also are increased as anabolism begins and are provided in proportion to the caloric intake. Vitamin and mineral intake in excess of the daily recommended intake is provided to account for the increased requirements; this is frequently accomplished by giving an age-appropriate daily multiple vitamin, with other individual micronutrient supplements as warranted by history, physical examination, or laboratory studies. Iron supplements are not recommended during the acute rehabilitation phase, especially for children with kwashiorkor, for whom ferritin is often high. Additional iron may pose an oxidative stress, and iron supplementation has been associated with higher morbidity and mortality.

In most cases, cow's milk–based formulas are tolerated and provide an appropriate mix of nutrients. Other easily digested foods, appropriate for the age, also may be introduced slowly. If feeding intolerance occurs, lactose-free or semielemental formulas should be considered.

COMPLICATIONS OF MALNUTRITION

Malnourished children are more susceptible to **infection**, especially sepsis, pneumonia, and gastroenteritis. Hypoglycemia is common after periods of severe fasting, but also may be a sign of sepsis. Hypothermia may signify infection or, with bradycardia, may signify a decreased metabolic rate to conserve energy. Bradycardia and poor cardiac output predispose the malnourished child to heart failure, which is exacerbated by acute fluid or solute loads. **Micronutrient deficiencies** also can complicate malnutrition. Vitamin A and zinc deficiencies are common in the developing world and are an important cause of altered immune response and increased morbidity and mortality. Depending on the age at onset and the duration of the malnutrition, malnourished children may have permanent growth stunting (from malnutrition in utero, infancy, or adolescence) and delayed development (from malnutrition in infancy or adolescence). Environmental (social) deprivation may interact with the effects of the malnutrition to impair further development and cognitive function.

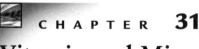

CHAPTER 31
Vitamin and Mineral Deficiencies

Micronutrients comprise 13 vitamins and 17 essential minerals. In industrialized societies, frank clinical deficiencies are unusual in healthy children, but they can and do occur in certain high-risk circumstances. Risk factors include diets that are consistently limited in variety, especially with the exclusion of whole food groups, malabsorption syndromes, and conditions causing high physiologic requirements. Various common etiologies of vitamin and nutrient deficiency

TABLE 31–1.   Etiology of Vitamin and Nutrient Deficiency States

Etiology	Deficiency
Diet	
Vegans (strict)	Protein, vitamins B$_{12}$, D, riboflavin
Breast fed infant	Vitamins K, D
Cow's milk–fed infant	Iron
Bulimia, anorexia nervosa	Electrolytes, other deficiencies
Parenteral alimentation	Essential fatty acids, trace elements
Alcoholism	Calories, vitamin B$_1$, B$_6$, folate
Medical Problems	
Malabsorption syndromes	Vitamins A, D, E, K, zinc, essential fatty acids
Cholestasis	Vitamins E, D, K, A, zinc, essential fatty acids
Medications	
Sulfonamides	Folate
Phenytoin, phenobarbital	Vitamins D, K, folate
Mineral oil	Vitamins A, D, E, K
Antibiotics	Vitamin K
Isoniazid	Vitamin B$_6$
Antacids	Iron, phosphate, calcium
Digitalis	Magnesium, calcium
Penicillamine	Vitamin B$_6$
Specific Mechanisms	
Transcobalamin II or intrinsic factor deficiency	Vitamin B$_{12}$
Other digestive enzyme deficiencies	Carbohydrate, fat, protein
Menkes kinky hair syndrome	Copper
Acrodermatitis enteropathica	Zinc
Reduced exposure to direct sunlight	Vitamin D

states are highlighted in Table 31–1, and characteristics of vitamin deficiencies are outlined in Table 31–2.

WATER-SOLUBLE VITAMINS

Water-soluble vitamins are not "stored" in the body except for vitamin B$_{12}$; intake alters tissue levels. Absorption from the diet is usually high, and the compounds exchange readily between intracellular and extracellular fluids; excretion is via the urine. Water-soluble vitamins typically function as coenzymes in

TABLE 31–2. Characteristics of Vitamin Deficiencies

Vitamin	Purpose	Deficiency	Comments	Source
Water Soluble				
Thiamine (B$_1$)	Coenzyme in ketoacid decarboxylation (e.g., pyruvate → acetyl-CoA transketolase reaction)	*Beri-beri:* polyneuropathy, calf tenderness, heart failure, edema, ophthalmoplegia	Inborn erros of lactate metabolism; boiling milk destroys B$_1$	Liver, meat, milk, cereals, nuts, legumes
Riboflavin (B$_2$)	FAD coenzyme in oxidation-reduction reactions	Anorexia, mucositis, anemia, cheilosis, nasolabial seborrhea	Photosensitizer	Milk, cheese, liver, meat, eggs, whole grains, green leafy vegetables
Niacin (B$_3$)	NAD coenzyme in oxidation-reduction reactions	*Pellagra:* photosensitivity, dermatitis, dementia, diarrhea, death	Tryptophan is a precursor	Meat, fish, live, whole grains, green leafy vegetables
Pyridoxine (B$_6$)	Cofactor in amino acid metabolism	Seizures, hyperacusis, microcytic anemia, nasolabial seborrhea, neuropathy	Dependency state: deficiency secondary to drugs	Meat, liver, whole grains, peanuts, soybeans, meat
Pantothenic acid	CoA in Krebs cycle	None reported		Meat, vegetables
Biotin	Cofactor in carboxylase reactions of amino acids	Alopecia, dermatitis, hypotonia, death	Bowel resection, inborn error of metabolism,* and ingestion of raw eggs	Yeast, meats; made by intestinal flora
B$_{12}$	Coenzyme for 5-methyl-tetrahydrofolate formation; DNA synthesis	Megaloblastic anemia, peripheral neuropathy, posterior lateral spinal column disease, vitiligo	Vegans; fish tapeworm; transcobalamin or intrinsic factor deficiencies	Meat, fish, cheese, eggs
Folate	DNA synthesis	Megaloblastic anemia	Goat milk deficient; drug antagonists; heat inactivates	Liver, greens, vegetables, cereals, cheese
Ascorbic acid (C)	Reducing agent; collagen metabolism	*Scurvy:* irritability, purpura, bleeding gums, periosteal hemorrhage, aching bones	May improve tyrosine metabolism in preterm infants	Citrus fruits, green vegetables; cooking destroys it
Fat Soluble				
A	Epithelial cell integrity; vision	Night blindness, xerophthalmia, Bitot spots, follicular hyperkeratosis	Common with protein-calorie malnutrition; malabsorption	Liver, milk, eggs, green and yellow vegetables, fruits
D	Maintain serum calcium, phosphorus levels	*Rickets:* reduced bone mineralization	Prohormone of 25- and 1,25-vitamin D	Fortified milk, cheese, liver
E	Antioxidant	Hemolysis in preterm infants; areflexia, ataxia, ophthalmoplegia	May benefit patients with G6PD deficiency	Seeds, vegetables, germ oils, green leafy vegetables
K	Post-translation carboxylation of clotting factors II, VII, IX, X and proteins C, S	Prolonged prothrombin time; hemorrhage; elevated PIVKA (protein induced in vitamin K absence)	Malabsorption; breastfed infants	Liver, green vegetables; made by intestinal flora

*Biotinidase deficiency.

CoA, coenzyme A; FAD, flavin adenine dinucleotide; G6PD, glucose-6-phosphate dehydrogenase; NAD, nicotinamide adenine dinucleotide.

energy, protein, amino acid, and nucleic acid metabolism; as cosubstrates in enzymatic reactions; and as structural components.

Ascorbic Acid

The principal forms of vitamin C are ascorbic acid and the oxidized form, dehydroascorbic acid. Ascorbic acid accelerates hydroxylation reactions in many biosynthetic reactions, including hydroxylation of proline in the formation of collagen. The needs of full-term infants for ascorbic acid and dehydroascorbic acid are calculated by estimating the availability in human milk.

A deficiency of ascorbic acid results in the clinical manifestations of **scurvy**. Infantile scurvy is manifested by irritability, bone tenderness with swelling, and pseudoparalysis of the legs. The disease may occur if infants are fed unsupplemented cow's milk in the first year of life or if the diet is devoid of fruits and vegetables. Subperiosteal hemorrhage, bleeding gums and petechiae, hyperkeratosis of hair follicles, and a succession of mental changes characterize the progression of the illness. Anemia secondary to bleeding, decreased iron absorption, or abnormal folate metabolism also is seen in chronic scurvy. **Treatment** of scurvy and several of the following disorders is presented in Table 31–3.

B Vitamins

The B vitamins thiamine, riboflavin, and niacin are routinely added to enriched grain products; deficiencies in normal hosts are rare in the U.S. Levels from human milk reflect maternal intake, and deficiency can develop in breastfed infants of deficient mothers.

Thiamine

Vitamin B_1 functions as a coenzyme in biochemical reactions related to carbohydrate metabolism, to decarboxylation of α-ketoacids and pyruvate, and to transketolase reactions of the pentose pathway. Thiamine also is involved in the decarboxylation of branched-chain amino acids. Thiamine is lost during milk pasteurization and sterilization. **Infantile beriberi** occurs between 1 and 4 months of age in breastfed infants whose mothers have a thiamine deficiency (alcoholism), in infants with protein-calorie malnutrition, in infants receiving unsupplemented hyperalimentation fluid, and in infants receiving boiled milk. Thiamine deficiency occurs in alcoholics and has been reported in adolescents who have undergone bariatric surgery for severe obesity. Acute **"wet beriberi"** with cardiac symptoms and signs predominates in infantile beriberi. Anorexia, apathy, vomiting, restlessness, and pallor progress to dyspnea, cyanosis, and death from congestive heart failure. Infants with beriberi have a characteristic aphonic cry; they appear to be crying, but no sound is uttered. Other signs include peripheral neuropathy and paresthesias.

Riboflavin

Vitamin B_2 is a constituent of two coenzymes, riboflavin 5'-phosphate and flavin-adenine dinucleotide. These

---

TABLE 31–3. Recommended Daily Dose Ranges for Treatment of Vitamin-Related Diseases

Vitamin	Treatment of Vitamin Deficiency	Treatment of Deficiency in Patients with Malabsorption	Treatment of Dependency Syndrome
A (IU)	5,000-10,000	10,000-25,000	—
D (IU)	400-5,000	4,000-20,000	50,000-200,000
Calcifediol (μg)	—	20-100	50-100
Calcitriol (1,25-[OH]$_2$-D) (μg)	—	1-3	1-3
E (IU)	—	100-1,000	—
K (mg)	1*	5-10*	—
Ascorbic acid (C) (mg)	250-500	500	—
Thiamine (mg)	5-25	5-25	25-500
Riboflavin (mg)	5-25	5-25	—
Niacin (mg)	25-50	25-50	50-250
B$_6$ (mg)	5-25	2-25	10-250
Biotin (mg)	0.15-0.3	0.3-1.0	10
Folic acid (mg)	1	1	—†
B$_{12}$ (μg)	—*	—*	1-40

*To be used parenterally as needed.
†To be used only in conjunction with multivitamin mixtures.
From AMA Council on Scientific Affairs: Vitamin preparations as dietary supplements and as therapeutic agents. JAMA 257:1929-1936, 1987.

coenzymes are essential components of glutathione reductase and xanthine oxidase, which are involved in electron transport. A deficiency of riboflavin affects glucose, fatty acid, and amino acid metabolism. Riboflavin and its phosphate are decomposed by exposure to light and by strong alkaline solutions.

Ariboflavinosis is characterized by an angular stomatitis, glossitis, cheilosis, seborrheic dermatitis around the nose and mouth, and eye changes that include reduced tearing, photophobia, corneal vascularization, and the formation of cataracts. Subclinical riboflavin deficiencies have been found in diabetic subjects, children in families with low socioeconomic status, children with chronic cardiac disease, and infants undergoing prolonged phototherapy for hyperbilirubinemia.

Niacin

Niacin consists of the compounds nicotinic acid and nicotinamide (niacinamide). Nicotinamide, the predominant form of the vitamin, functions as a component of the coenzymes nicotinamide adenine dinucleotide (NAD) and nicotinamide adenine dinucleotide phosphate (NADP). Niacin is involved in multiple metabolic processes, including fat synthesis, intracellular respiratory metabolism, and glycolysis.

In determining the needs for niacin, the content of tryptophan in the diet must be considered because tryptophan is converted to niacin. Niacin is stable in foods and can withstand heating and prolonged storage. Approximately 70% of the total niacin equivalents in human milk are derived from tryptophan. **Pellagra**, or niacin deficiency disease, is characterized by weakness, lassitude, dermatitis, photosensitivity, inflammation of mucous membranes, diarrhea, vomiting, dysphagia, and, in severe cases, dementia.

Vitamin B₆

Vitamin B_6 refers to three naturally occurring pyridines: pyridoxine (pyridoxol), pyridoxal, and pyridoxamine. The phosphates of the latter two pyridines are metabolically and functionally related and are converted in the liver to the coenzyme form, pyridoxal phosphate. The metabolic functions of vitamin B_6 include interconversion reactions of amino acids, conversion of tryptophan to niacin and serotonin, metabolic reactions in the brain, carbohydrate metabolism, immune development, and the biosynthesis of heme and prostaglandins. The pyridoxal and pyridoxamine forms of the vitamin are destroyed by heat; heat treatment was responsible for vitamin B_6 deficiency and seizures in infants fed improperly processed formulas. Goat's milk is deficient in vitamin B_6.

Dietary deprivation or malabsorption of vitamin B_6 in children results in hypochromic microcytic anemia, vomiting, diarrhea, failure to thrive, listlessness, hyper-irritability, and seizures. Children receiving isoniazid or penacillamine may require additional vitamin B_6 because the drug binds to the vitamin. Vitamin B_6 is unusual as a water-soluble vitamin in that **very large doses (≥500 mg/day) have been associated with a sensory neuropathy**. Megadoses have been claimed to promote improved neurocognitive development in children with Down syndrome, but data from controlled trials are lacking, and the practice is not currently justified.

Folate

A variety of chemical forms of folate are nutritionally active as long as the parent molecule of pteroylglutamic acid is present. Folate functions in transport of single-carbon fragments in synthesis of nucleic acids and for normal metabolism of certain amino acids and in conversion of homocysteine to methionine. Food sources include green leafy vegetables, oranges, and whole grains; folate fortification of grains is now routine in the U.S.

Folate deficiency, characterized by **hypersegmented neutrophils**, **macrocytic anemia**, and glossitis, may result from a low dietary intake, malabsorption, or vitamin-drug interactions. Deficiency can develop within a few weeks of birth because infants require 10 times as much folate as adults relative to body weight but have scant stores of folate in the newborn period. Folate is particularly heat labile, and heat-sterilizing home-prepared formula can decrease the folate content by half. Evaporated milk and goat's milk are low in folate. Patients with chronic hemolysis (sickle cell anemia, thalassemia) may require extra folate to avoid deficiency because of the relatively high requirement of the vitamin to support erythropoiesis. Other conditions with risk of deficiency include pregnancy, alcoholism, and treatment with anticonvulsants (phenytoin) or antimetabolites (methotrexate). First occurrence and recurrence of **neural tube defects** are reduced significantly by maternal supplementation during embryogenesis. Because closure of the neural tube occurs before usual recognition of pregnancy, all women of reproductive age are recommended to have a folate intake of at least 400 μg/day as prophylaxis.

Vitamin B₁₂

Vitamin B_{12} is one of the most complex of the vitamin molecules, containing an atom of cobalt held in a "corrin ring" (similar to that of iron in hemoglobin). The cobalt ion is at the active center of the ring and serves as the site for attachment of alkyl groups during their transfer. The vitamin functions in single-carbon transfers and is intimately related to folate function and interconversions. Vitamin B_{12} is essential for normal lipid and carbohydrate metabolism in energy production and in protein biosynthesis and nucleic acid synthesis.

In contrast to the other water-soluble vitamins, the absorption of vitamin B_{12} is complex, involving cleavage of the vitamin from dietary protein and binding to a glycoprotein called *intrinsic factor* secreted by the gastric mucosa (parietal cells). The cobalamin–intrinsic factor complex is efficiently absorbed from the distal ileum. As vitamin B_{12} is absorbed into the portal circulation, it is transported bound to a specific protein, transcobalamin II. Its large stores in the liver also are unusual as water-soluble vitamin, and efficient enterohepatic circulation normally protects from deficiency for months to years. Dietary sources of the vitamin are animal products only, and **strict vegetarians should take a vitamin B_{12} supplement**.

Vitamin B_{12} deficiency is rare. Early diagnosis and treatment of this disorder in childhood are important because of the danger of irreversible neurologic damage. Most cases in childhood result from a specific defect in absorption (see Table 31–2). Such defects include **congenital pernicious anemia** (absent intrinsic factor), **juvenile pernicious anemia** (autoimmune), and deficiency of transcobalamin II transport. Gastric or intestinal resection and small bowel bacterial overgrowth also cause vitamin B_{12} deficiency. Exclusively breastfed infants ingest adequate vitamin B_{12} unless the mother is a strict vegetarian without supplementation.

Depression of serum vitamin B_{12} and the appearance of hypersegmented neutrophils and macrocytosis (indistinguishable from folate deficiency) are early clinical manifestations of deficiency. Vitamin B_{12} deficiency also causes **neurologic manifestations**, including depression, peripheral neuropathy, posterior spinal column signs, dementia, and eventual coma. The neurologic signs do not occur in folate deficiency, but administration of folate may mask the hematologic signs of vitamin B_{12} deficiency, while the neurologic manifestations progress. Patients with vitamin B_{12} deficiency also have increased urine levels of methylmalonic acid. Most cases of vitamin B_{12} deficiency in infants and children are not of dietary origin and require treatment throughout life. Maintenance therapy consists of repeated monthly intramuscular injections, although a form of vitamin B_{12} is administered intranasally.

FAT-SOLUBLE VITAMINS

Fat-soluble vitamins generally have stores in the body, and dietary deficiencies generally develop more slowly than for water-soluble vitamins. Absorption of fat-soluble vitamins depends on normal fat intake, digestion, and absorption. The complexity of normal fat absorption and the potential for perturbation in many disease states explains the more common occurrence of deficiencies of these vitamins.

Vitamin A

The basic constituent of the vitamin A group is retinol. Ingested plant carotene or animal tissue retinol esters release retinol after hydrolysis by pancreatic and intestinal enzymes. Chylomicron-transported retinol esters are stored in the liver as retinol palmitate. Retinol is transported from the liver to target tissues by retinol-binding protein. After free retinol is delivered to the target tissues, the kidney excretes the retinol-binding protein. Diseases of the kidney diminish excretion of retinol-binding protein, whereas liver parenchymal disease or malnutrition lowers the synthesis of retinol-binding protein. Specific cellular binding proteins facilitate the uptake of retinol by target tissues. In the eye, retinol is metabolized to form **rhodopsin**; the action of light on rhodopsin is the first step of the visual process. Retinol also influences the growth and differentiation of epithelia. The clinical manifestations of vitamin A deficiency in humans appear as a group of ocular signs termed **xerophthalmia**. The earliest symptom is **night blindness**, which is followed by **xerosis** of the conjunctiva and cornea. Untreated, xerophthalmia can result in ulceration, necrosis, keratomalacia, and a permanent corneal scar. Clinical and subclinical vitamin A deficiencies are associated with **immunodeficiency**; increased risk of infection, especially measles; and increased risk of mortality, especially in developing nations. Xerophthalmia and vitamin A deficiency should be urgently treated.

Treatment is summarized in Table 31–3. Hypervitaminosis A also has serious sequelae, including headaches, pseudotumor cerebri, hepatotoxicity, and **teratogenicity**; death may occur (Table 31–4).

Vitamin E

Eight naturally occurring compounds have vitamin E activity. The most active of these, α-tocopherol, accounts for 90% of the vitamin E present in human tissues and is commercially available as an acetate or succinate. Vitamin E acts as a biologic **antioxidant** by inhibiting the peroxidation of polyunsaturated fatty acids present in cell membranes. It scavenges free radicals generated by the reduction of molecular oxygen and by the action of oxidative enzymes.

Human milk has a lower content of α-tocopherol and a lower ratio of vitamin E to polyunsaturated fatty acids compared with formulas. Nevertheless, term and preterm infants have higher serum α-tocopherol levels when fed human milk. The vitamin E requirement is increased in diets that have high concentrations of

TABLE 31–4. Toxic Effects of Vitamins and Other Nutrients

Nutrient	Effects	Comments
Fat-Soluble Vitamins		
		Toxicity noted at lower multiples of RDA than water-soluble vitamins
A		
Acute	Lethargy, headache, papilledema, bulging fontanel	Megadoses used to prevent cancer,* treat acne
Chronic	Scaly, dry skin; alopecia; sore tongue; hyperostoses; anorexia; increased intracranial pressure (pseudotumor cerebri); teratogenic	Consumption of polar bear liver; toxicity with chronic 20,000-50,000 IU/24 hr
D		
Acute	Hypercalcemia, muscle weakness, anorexia, emesis, headache, polyuria	Hypercalcemia produces arrhythmias, hypertension, renal water wasting
Chronic	Nephrocalcinosis, bone pain, vascular calcification, renal insufficiency; idiopathic infantile hypercalcemia	Toxicity with chronic 3000-4000 IU/24 hr
E	Muscle weakness, diarrhea, antagonism of vitamin K, enhanced anticoagulant drug action	Megadoses used to improve libido and prevent heart disease and cancer*; toxicity with 300-800 IU/24 hr
K	Water-soluble analogues produce neonatal jaundice	Menadione induces neonatal hemolysis
Water-Soluble Vitamins		
C	Uricosuria, oxalate stones, G6PD-deficient hemolysis, rebound scurvy in infants; false-positive test for glycosuria; false-negative test for hematochezia	Prevention of upper respiratory tract infections*
Niacin	Histamine release, ulcers, asthma, flushing, pruritus, gout, hepatotoxic	Used to treat hypercholesterolemia; orthomolecular treatment of schizophrenia; toxicity with 200-1000 mg/24 hr
Pyridoxine (B_6)	Peripheral sensory neuropathy; fetal-neonatal dependency and seizures	Treat depression and premenstrual syndrome; toxicity with 2-6 g/24 hr
Tryptophan	Eosinophilia, myositis, fasciitis, scleroderma	Treat depression* and premenstrual syndrome*; possible toxic metabolite; toxicity with 0.5-4.0 g/24 hr

*No established benefit.
G6PD, glucose-6-phosphate dehydrogenase; RDA, recommended daily allowance.

polyunsaturated fatty acids or iron, both of which facilitate membrane peroxidation and generation of free radicals.

Vitamin E deficiency occurs in children with fat malabsorption secondary to liver disease, untreated celiac disease, cystic fibrosis, and abetalipoproteinemia. In these children, without vitamin E supplementation, a syndrome of progressive **sensory and motor neuropathy** develops; the first sign of deficiency is loss of deep tendon reflexes. Deficient preterm infants at 1 to 2 months old have hemolytic anemia characterized by an elevated reticulocyte count, an increased sensitivity of the erythrocytes to hemolysis in hydrogen peroxide, peripheral edema, and thrombocytosis. All the abnor-malities are corrected after oral, lipid, or water-soluble vitamin E therapy. Toxic conditions caused by excess vitamin E are noted in Table 31–4.

Vitamin D

Cholecalciferol (vitamin D_3) is the mammalian form of vitamin D and is produced by UV irradiation of inactive precursors in the skin. Ergocalciferol (vitamin D_2) is derived from plants. Vitamin D_2 and vitamin D_3 require further metabolism to become active. They are of equivalent potency. Clothing, lack of sunlight exposure, and skin pigmentation decrease the generation of vitamin D in the epidermis and dermis.

Vitamin D (D_2 and D_3) is metabolized in the liver to calcidiol, or 25-hydroxyvitamin D (25-[OH]-D); this metabolite, which has little intrinsic activity, is transported by a plasma-binding globulin to the kidney, where it is converted to the most active metabolite calcitriol, or 1,25-dihydroxyvitamin D (1,25-[OH]$_2$-D). The action of 1,25-(OH)$_2$-D results in a decrease in the concentration of messenger RNA (mRNA) for collagen in bone and an increase in the concentration of mRNA for vitamin D–dependent calcium-binding protein in the intestine (directly mediating increased intestinal calcium transport). The antirachitic action of vitamin D probably is mediated by provision of appropriate concentrations of calcium and phosphate in the extracellular space of bone and by enhanced intestinal absorption of these minerals. Vitamin D also may have a direct anabolic effect on bone. 1,25-(OH)$_2$-D also has direct feedback to the parathyroid gland and inhibits secretion of parathyroid hormone.

Vitamin D deficiency appears as **rickets** in children and as **osteomalacia** in postpubertal adolescents. Inadequate direct sun exposure and vitamin D intake are sufficient causes, but other factors, such as various drugs (phenobarbital, phenytoin) and malabsorption, also may increase the risk of development of vitamin-deficiency rickets. Breastfed infants, especially infants with dark-pigmented skin, also are at risk for vitamin D deficiency.

The pathophysiology of rickets results from defective bone growth, especially marked at the epiphyseal cartilage matrix, which fails to mineralize. The uncalcified osteoid results in a wide, irregular zone of poorly supported tissue, the rachitic metaphysis. This soft rather than hardened zone produces many of the skeletal deformities through compression and lateral bulging or flaring of the ends of bones.

The **clinical manifestations** of rickets are most common during the first 2 years of life and may become evident only after several months of a vitamin D–deficient diet. **Craniotabes** is caused by thinning of the outer table of the skull, which when compressed feels to the touch like a Ping-Pong ball. Enlargement of the costochondral junction (the **rachitic rosary**) and thickening of the wrists and ankles may be palpated. The anterior fontanel is enlarged, and its closure may be delayed. In advanced rickets, scoliosis and exaggerated lordosis may be present. Bowlegs or knock-knees may be evident in older infants, and greenstick fractures may be observed in long bones.

The **diagnosis** of rickets is based on a dietary history of poor vitamin D intake and a history of little exposure to direct UV sunlight. The serum calcium usually is normal but may be low, the serum phosphorus level usually is reduced, and the serum alkaline phosphatase activity is elevated. When serum calcium levels decline to less than 7.5 mg/dL, tetany may occur.

Levels of 24,25-(OH)$_2$-D are undetectable, and serum 1,25-(OH)$_2$-D levels are commonly less than 7 ng/mL, although 1,25-(OH)$_2$-D levels also may be normal. The best measure of vitamin D status is the level of 25-(OH)-D. Characteristic **radiographic** changes of the distal ulna and radius include widening, concave cupping, and frayed, poorly demarcated ends. The increased space between the distal ends of the radius and ulna and the metacarpal bones is the enlarged, nonossified metaphysis.

The **treatment** of vitamin D–deficiency rickets and osteomalacia is presented in Table 31–3. Breastfed infants born of mothers with adequate vitamin D stores usually maintain adequate serum vitamin D levels for at least 2 months, but rickets may develop subsequently if these infants are not exposed to the sun or do not receive supplementary vitamin D. The AAP recommends **vitamin D supplementation of all breastfed infants** in the amount of 200 IU/day, started in the first 2 months of life and given until the infant is taking more than 500 mL/day of formula or vitamin D–fortified milk (for age >1 year). Toxic effects of vitamin D are noted in Table 31–4.

Vitamin K

The plant form of vitamin K is phylloquinone, or vitamin K_1. Another form is menaquinone, or vitamin K_2; this is one of a series of compounds with unsaturated side chains synthesized by the intestinal bacteria. Plasma factors II (prothrombin), VII, IX, and X in the cascade of blood coagulation factors depend on vitamin K for synthesis and for post-translational conversion of their precursor proteins. The post-translational conversion of glutamyl residues to carboxyglutamic acid residues of a prothrombin molecule creates effective calcium-binding sites, making the protein active.

Other vitamin K–dependent proteins include proteins C, S, and Z in plasma and γ-carboxyglutamic acid–containing proteins in several tissues. Bone contains a major vitamin K–dependent protein, osteocalcin, and lesser amounts of other glutamic acid–containing proteins.

Phylloquinone is absorbed from the intestine and transported by chylomicrons. The rarity of dietary vitamin K deficiency in humans with normal intestinal function suggests that the absorption of menaquinones is possible. Vitamin K deficiency has been observed in subjects with impaired fat absorption caused by obstructive jaundice, pancreatic insufficiency, and celiac disease; often these problems are combined with the use of antibiotics that change intestinal flora.

Hemorrhagic disease of the newborn, a disease more common among breastfed infants, occurs in the first few weeks of life. It is rare in infants who receive prophylactic intramuscular vitamin K on the first day of life. Hemorrhagic disease of the newborn usually is marked by generalized ecchymoses, gastrointestinal hemorrhage, or bleeding from a circumcision or umbilical stump; intracranial hemorrhage can occur, but is uncommon. The AAP recommends that **parenteral vitamin K (0.5 to 1 mg) be given to all newborns** shortly after birth.

MINERALS

The major minerals are minerals that require intakes of more than 100 mg/day and contribute at least 0.1% of total body weight. There are seven essential minerals: calcium, phosphorus, magnesium, sodium, potassium, chloride, and sulfur. Ten trace minerals, which comprise less than 0.1% of body weight, have essential physiologic roles. Characteristics of trace mineral deficiencies are listed in Table 31–5.

Calcium

Calcium is the most abundant major mineral. Ninety-nine percent of calcium is in the skeleton; the remaining 1% is in extracellular fluids, intracellular compartments, and cell membranes. The 1% nonskeletal calcium has a role in nerve conduction, muscle contraction, blood clotting, and membrane permeability. There are two distinct bone calcium phosphate pools—a large, crystalline form and a smaller, amorphous phase. Bone calcium constantly turns over, with concurrent bone resorption and formation. Approximately **half of bone mineral accretion occurs during adolescence**. Bone mineral density peaks in early

TABLE 31–5. Characteristics of Mineral Deficiencies

Mineral	Function	Manifestations of Deficiency	Comments	Sources
Iron	Heme-containing macromolecules (e.g., hemoglobin, cytochrome, and myoglobin)	Anemia, spoon nails, reduced muscle and mental performance	History of pica, cow's milk, gastrointestinal bleeding	Meat, eggs, grains
Copper	Redox reactions (e.g., cytochrome oxidase)	Hypochromic anemia, neutropenia, osteoporosis, hypotonia, hypoproteinemia	Inborn error, Menkes kinky hair syndrome	Liver, oysters, meat, nuts, grains, legumes, chocolate
Zinc	Metalloenzymes (e.g., alkaline phosphatase, carbonic anhydrase, DNA polymerase); wound healing	*Acrodermatitis enteropathica:* poor growth, acro-orificial rash, alopecia, delayed sexual development, hypogeusia, infection	Protein-calorie malnutrition; weaning; malabsorption syndromes	Meat, grains, cheese, nuts
Selenium	Antioxidant; glutathione peroxidase	Keshan cardiomyopathy in China	Endemic areas; long-term TPN	Meat, vegetables
Chromium	Insulin cofactor	Poor weight gain, glucose intolerance, neuropathy	Protein-calorie malnutrition, long-term TPN	Yeast, breads
Fluoride	Strengthening of dental enamel	Caries	Supplementation during tooth growth, narrow therapeutic range, fluorosis may cause staining of the teeth	Seafood, water
Iodine	Thyroxine, triiodothyronine production	Simple endemic goiter *Myxedematous cretinism:* congenital hypothyroidism *Neurologic cretinism:* mental retardation, deafness, spasticity, normal thyroxine level at birth	Endemic in New Guinea, the Congo; endemic in Great Lakes area before use of iodized salt	Seafood, iodized salt, most food in nonendemic areas

TPN, total parenteral nutrition.

adulthood and is influenced by prior and concurrent dietary calcium intake, exercise, and hormone status (testosterone, estrogen).

Calcium intake can come from a variety of sources, with dairy products providing the most common and concentrated source. The calcium equivalent of 1 cup of milk (about 300 mg of calcium) is $^3/_4$ cup of plain yogurt, 1.5 oz of cheddar cheese, 2 cups of ice cream, $^4/_5$ cup of almonds, and 2.5 oz of sardines. Other sources of calcium include some leafy green vegetables (broccoli, kale, collards), lime-processed tortillas, calcium-precipitated tofu ("bean curd" from soybeans), and calcium-fortified juices, cereals, and breads.

There is no classic calcium deficiency syndrome because blood and cell levels are closely regulated. The body can mobilize skeletal calcium and increase the absorptive efficiency of dietary calcium. **Osteoporosis** that occurs in childhood is related to protein-calorie malnutrition, vitamin C deficiency, steroid therapy, endocrine disorders, immobilization and disuse, osteogenesis imperfecta, or calcium deficiency (in premature infants). It is believed that the primary method of prevention of **postmenopausal osteoporosis** is to ensure maximum peak bone mass by providing optimal calcium intake during childhood and adolescence. Bone mineral status can be monitored by dual-energy x-ray absorptiometry.

No adverse effects are observed in adults with dietary calcium intakes of 2.5 g/day. There is concern that higher intakes may increase the risk for urinary stone formation, constipation, and decreased renal function and may inhibit intestinal absorption of other minerals (iron, zinc).

Iron

Iron, the most abundant trace mineral, is used in the synthesis of hemoglobin, myoglobin, and enzyme iron. Body iron content is regulated primarily through modulation of iron absorption, which depends on the state of body iron stores, the form and amount of iron in foods, and the mixture of foods in the diet. There are two categories of iron in food. The first is **heme iron**, present in hemoglobin and myoglobin, which is supplied by meat and rarely accounts for more than a quarter of the iron ingested by infants. The absorption of heme iron is relatively efficient and is not influenced by other constituents of the diet. The second category is **nonheme iron**, which represents the preponderance of iron intake consumed by infants and exists in the form of iron salts. The absorption of nonheme iron is influenced by the composition of consumed foods. Enhancers of nonheme iron absorption are ascorbic acid, meat, fish, and poultry. Inhibitors are bran, polyphenols (including the tannates in tea), and phytic acid, a compound found in legumes and whole grains.

The percent intestinal absorption of the small amount of iron in human milk is 50%; 4% is absorbed from iron-fortified cow's milk formula and from iron-fortified infant dry cereals.

In a normal term infant, there is little change in total body iron and little need for exogenous iron before 4 months of age. Iron deficiency is rare among term infants during the first 4 months, unless there has been substantial blood loss (see Chapter 62). After about 4 months of age, iron reserves become marginal, and, unless exogenous sources of iron are provided, the infant becomes progressively at risk for anemia as the iron requirement to support erythropoiesis and growth increases (see Chapter 150). Premature or low birth weight infants have a lower amount of stored iron because significant amounts of iron are transferred from the mother in the third trimester. In addition, their postnatal iron needs are greater because of rapid rates of growth and frequent phlebotomy. Iron needs can be met by supplementation (ferrous sulfate) or by iron-containing complementary foods. Under normal circumstances, iron-fortified formula should be the only alternative to breast milk in infants younger than 1 year old. Premature infants fed human milk may develop iron deficiency anemia earlier unless they receive iron supplements. Formula-fed preterm infants should receive iron-fortified formula.

In older children, iron deficiency may result from inadequate intake with excessive cow's milk intake or from intake of foods with poor iron bioavailability. Iron deficiency also can result from blood loss from such sources as menses or gastric ulceration. Iron deficiency affects many tissues (muscle and CNS) in addition to producing anemia. **Iron deficiency and anemia** have been associated with lethargy and decreased work capacity and **impaired neurocognitive development**, the deficits of which may persist into adolescence.

The **diagnosis** of iron deficiency anemia is established by the presence of a microcytic hypochromic anemia, low serum ferritin levels, low serum iron levels, reduced transferrin saturation, normal to elevated red blood cell width distribution, and enhanced iron-binding capacity. The mean corpuscular volume and red blood cell indices are reduced, and the reticulocyte count is low. Iron deficiency may be present without anemia. Clinical manifestations are noted in Table 31–5.

Treatment of iron deficiency anemia requires changes in the diet to provide adequate iron and the administration of 2 to 6 mg iron/kg/24 hr (as ferrous sulfate). Reticulocytosis is noted within 3 to 7 days of starting treatment. Oral treatment should be continued for 5 months. Rarely, intramuscular or intravenous iron therapy is needed if oral iron cannot be given. Parenteral therapy carries the risk of anaphylaxis and should be administered according to a strict protocol, including a test dose.

Zinc

Zinc is the second most abundant trace mineral and is important in protein metabolism and synthesis, in nucleic acid metabolism, and in stabilization of cell membranes. Zinc functions as a cofactor for more than 200 enzymes and is essential to numerous cellular metabolic functions. Adequate zinc status is especially crucial during periods of growth and for tissue proliferation (immune system, wound healing, skin and gastrointestinal tract integrity); physiologic functions for which zinc is essential include normal growth, sexual maturation, and immune function.

Dietary zinc is absorbed (20% to 40%) in the duodenum and proximal small intestine The best dietary sources of zinc are animal products, including human milk, from which it is readily absorbed. Whole grains and legumes also contain moderate amounts of zinc, but factors such as phytic acid and fiber inhibit absorption from these sources. On a global basis, poor bioavailability secondary to phytic acid is thought to be a more important factor than low intake in the widespread occurrence of zinc deficiency. Excretion of zinc occurs from the gastrointestinal tract. In the presence of ongoing losses, such as in chronic diarrhea, requirements can drastically increase.

Zinc deficiency dwarfism syndrome was first described in a group of children in the Middle East with low levels of zinc in their hair, poor appetite, diminished taste acuity, hypogonadism, and short stature. Zinc supplementation reduces morbidity and mortality from **diarrhea** and **pneumonia** and enhances growth in developing countries. Mild to moderate zinc deficiency is considered to be highly prevalent in developing countries, particularly in populations with high rates of **stunting**. Mild zinc deficiency occurs in older breastfed infants without adequate zinc intake from complementary foods or in young children with poor total or bioavailable zinc intake in the general diet. A high infectious burden also may increase the risk of zinc deficiency in developing countries. Acute acquired severe zinc deficiency occurs in patients receiving total parenteral nutrition without zinc supplementation and in premature infants fed human milk without fortification. **Clinical manifestations** of mild zinc deficiency include **anorexia, growth faltering**, and **immune impairment**. Moderately severe manifestations include delayed sexual maturation, rough skin, and hepatosplenomegaly. The signs of severe deficiency include acral and periorificial erythematous, scaling dermatitis; growth and immune impairment; diarrhea; mood changes; alopecia; night blindness; and photophobia.

Diagnosis of zinc deficiency is challenging. Plasma zinc concentration is most commonly used, but levels are frequently normal in conditions of mild deficiency; levels in moderate to severe deficiency are typically less than 60 µg/dL. Acute infection also can result in depression of circulating zinc levels. The standard for the diagnosis of deficiency is response to a trial of supplementation, with outcomes such as improved linear growth or weight gain, improved appetite, and improved immune function. Because there is no pharmacologic effect of zinc on these functions, a positive response to supplementation is considered evidence of a preexisting deficiency. Clinically an empirical trial of zinc supplementation (1 mg/kg/day) is a safe and reasonable approach in situations in which deficiency is considered possible.

Acrodermatitis enteropathica is an autosomal recessive disorder that begins within 2 to 4 weeks after infants have been weaned from breast milk. It is characterized by an acute perioral and perianal dermatitis, alopecia, and failure to thrive. The disease is caused by severe zinc deficiency from a specific defect of intestinal zinc absorption. Plasma zinc levels are markedly reduced, and serum alkaline phosphatase activity is low. **Treatment** is with high-dose oral zinc supplements. A relatively uncommon condition associated with presentation of severe zinc deficiency is due to a defect in the secretion of zinc from the mammary gland, resulting in abnormally low milk zinc concentrations. Breastfed infants, especially if they were born prematurely, present with classic signs of zinc deficiency: growth failure, diarrhea, and dermatitis. Because there is no defect in the infant's ability to absorb zinc, treatment consists of supplementing the infant with zinc for the duration of breastfeeding, which can be successfully continued. Subsequent infants born to the mother will also need zinc supplementation if breastfed. Zinc is relatively nontoxic. Excess intake produces nausea, emesis, abdominal pain, headache, vertigo, and seizures.

Fluoride

Dental enamel is strengthened when fluoride is substituted for hydroxyl ions in the hydroxyapatite crystalline mineral matrix of the enamel. The resulting fluoroapatite is more resistant to chemical and physical damage. Fluoride is incorporated into the enamel during the mineralization stages of tooth formation and by surface interaction after the tooth has erupted. Fluoride is similarly incorporated into bone mineral and may protect against osteoporosis later in life.

Because of concern about the risk of **fluorosis**, infants should not receive fluoride supplements before 6 months of age. Commercial formulas are made with defluoridated water and contain small amounts of fluoride. An infant older than 6 months who receives only ready-feed formula or is exclusively breastfed may benefit from supplemental fluoride. The fluoride content of human milk is low and is not influenced significantly by maternal intake. Fluoride levels of the water supply to which the child is exposed should be determined before fluoride supplements are prescribed. If the concentration of fluoride in the drinking water is less than 0.3 ppm, a supplement of 0.25 mg/day is recommended for infants and children 6 months to 3 years old. Fluorosis commonly stains the teeth.

SUGGESTED READING

American Academy of Pediatrics Committee on Drugs: The transfer of drugs and other chemicals to human milk. Pediatrics 108:776-789, 2001.

Behrman RE, Kliegman, RM, Jenson HB (eds): Nelson Textbook of Pediatrics, 17th ed. Philadelphia, WB Saunders, 2003.

Dewey KG: Nutrition, growth, and complementary feeding of the breastfed infant. Pediatr Clin North Am 48:87-104, 2001.

Gartner LM, Greer FR: Section on Breastfeeding and Committee on Nutrition, American Academy of Pediatrics: Prevention of rickets and vitamin D deficiency: New guidelines for vitamin D intake. Pediatrics 111:908-910, 2003.

Kavey RE, Daniels SR, Lauer RM, et al: American Heart Association guidelines for primary prevention of atherosclerotic cardiovascular disease beginning in childhood. J Pediatr 142:368-372, 2003.

Kleinman RE (ed): Pediatric Nutrition Handbook, 5th ed. Washington, DC, American Academy of Pediatrics, 2004.

Kramer MS, Guo T, Platt RW, et al: Infant growth and health outcomes associated with 3 compared with 6 mo of exclusive breastfeeding. Am J Clin Nutr 78:291-295, 2003.

Krebs NF, Hambidge KM: Trace elements. In Walker WA, Watkins JB, Duggan C (eds): Nutrition in Pediatrics: Basic Science and Clinical Applications, 3rd ed. Hamilton, Ontario, BC Decker, 2003, pp 86-110.

Penny ME: Protein-energy malnutrition: Pathophysiology, clinical consequences, and treatment. In Walker WA, Watkins JB, Duggan C (eds): Nutrition in Pediatrics: Basic Science and Clinical Applications, 3rd ed. Hamilton, Ontario, BC Decker, 2003, pp 174-194.

FLUIDS AND ELECTROLYTES

Larry A. Greenbaum

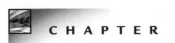

CHAPTER 32

Maintenance Fluid Therapy

BODY COMPOSITION

Water is the most plentiful constituent of the human body. **Total body water** (TBW) as a percentage of body weight varies with age. The fetus has a high TBW, which gradually decreases to about 75% of birth weight for a term infant. Premature infants have a higher TBW content than term infants. During the first year of life, TBW decreases to about 60% of body weight and basically remains at this level until puberty. At puberty, the fat content of females increases more than males, who acquire more muscle mass than females. Because fat has low water content, and muscle has high water content, by the end of puberty TBW in males remains at 60%, but it decreases to 50% of body weight in females. The high fat content in overweight children causes a decrease in TBW as a percentage of body weight. During dehydration, the TBW decreases and is a smaller percentage of body weight.

TBW is divided between two main compartments: **intracellular fluid (ICF)** and **extracellular fluid (ECF)**. In the fetus and newborn, the ECF volume is larger than the ICF volume. The normal postnatal diuresis causes an immediate decrease in the ECF volume. This decrease in ECF volume is followed by continued expansion of the ICF volume owing to cellular growth. By 1 year of age, the ratio of the ICF volume to the ECF volume approaches adult levels. The ECF volume is 20% to 25% of body weight, and the ICF volume is 30% to 40% of body weight (Fig. 32–1). With puberty, the increased muscle mass of males causes them to have a higher ICF volume than

females. There is no significant difference in the percentage of ECF volume between postpubertal females and males.

The ECF is divided further into **plasma water** and **interstitial fluid** (see Fig. 32–1). Plasma water is about 5% of body weight. The blood volume, given a hematocrit of 40%, is usually 8% of body weight, although it is higher in newborns and young infants. In premature newborns, it is around 10% of body weight. The volume of plasma water can be altered by pathologic conditions, including dehydration, anemia, polycythemia, heart failure, abnormal plasma osmolality, and hypoalbuminemia. The interstitial fluid, normally 15% of body weight, can increase dramatically in diseases associated with edema, such as heart failure, protein-losing enteropathy, liver failure, and nephrotic syndrome.

The composition of the solutes in the ICF and ECF is different (Fig. 32–2). Sodium and chloride are the dominant cation and anion in the ECF. Potassium is the most abundant cation in the ICF, and its concentration within the cells is approximately 30 times higher than in the ECF. Proteins, organic anions, and phosphate are the most plentiful anions in the ICF. The dissimilarity between the anions in the ICF and the ECF is determined largely by the presence of intracellular molecules that do not cross the cell membrane, the barrier separating the ECF and the ICF. In contrast, the difference in the distribution of cations—sodium and potassium—is due to the activity of the Na^+,K^+-ATPase pump, which uses cellular energy to actively extrude sodium from cells and move potassium into cells.

REGULATION OF INTRAVASCULAR VOLUME AND OSMOLALITY

Proper cell functioning requires close regulation of plasma osmolality, intravascular volume, and intracellular and extracellular electrolytes; these are controlled

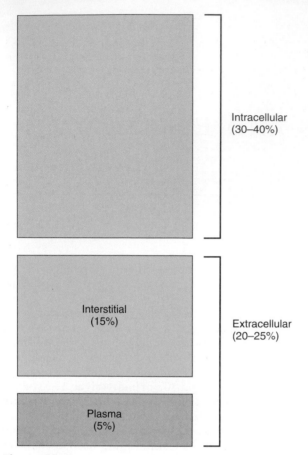

Figure 32–1

Compartments of total body water, expressed as percentage of body weight, in an older child or adult. (From Greenbaum LA: Pathophysiology of body fluids and fluid therapy. In Behrman RE, Kliegman RM, Jenson HB [eds]: Nelson Textbook of Pediatrics, 17th ed. Philadelphia, WB Saunders, 2004, p 191).

by independent systems for water balance, which determines osmolality, and sodium balance, which determines volume status. Maintenance of a normal *osmolality* depends on control of water balance. Although sodium concentration is the dominant determinant of plasma osmolality, the body does not control osmolality by regulating sodium balance. Control of *volume status* depends on regulation of sodium balance. When volume depletion is present, however, this takes precedence over regulation of osmolality, and retention of water contributes to maintenance of intravascular volume.

The plasma osmolality is tightly regulated to maintain it between 285 and 295 mOsm/kg. Modification of water intake and excretion maintains a normal plasma osmolality. In the steady state, water intake and water produced by the body from oxidation balances water losses from the skin, lungs, urine, and gastrointestinal tract. Only water intake and urinary losses can be regulated. A small increase in the plasma osmolality stimulates thirst. Urinary water losses are regulated by the secretion of **antidiuretic hormone** (ADH), which increases in response to an increasing plasma osmolality. ADH, by stimulating renal tubular reabsorption of water, decreases urinary water losses. Control of osmolality is subordinate to maintenance of an adequate intravascular volume. When significant volume depletion is present, ADH secretion and thirst are stimulated, regardless of the plasma osmolality.

An appropriate intravascular volume is crucial for survival; volume depletion and volume overload may cause significant morbidity and mortality. Because sodium is the principal extracellular cation, and sodium is restricted to the ECF, adequate body sodium is necessary for maintenance of intravascular volume.

The kidney determines sodium balance because there is little homeostatic control of sodium intake, although salt craving occasionally occurs, typically in children with chronic renal salt loss. The kidney regulates sodium balance by altering the percentage of filtered sodium that is reabsorbed along the nephron. Given the importance of sodium balance, it is not surprising that many systems are involved in the regulation of renal sodium excretion.

The **renin-angiotensin system** is an important regulator of renal sodium reabsorption and excretion. The juxtaglomerular apparatus produces renin in response to decreased effective intravascular volume. Specific stimuli for renin release are decreased perfusion pressure in the afferent arteriole of the glomerulus, decreased delivery of sodium to the distal nephron, and increased β_1-adrenergic agonists in response to intravascular volume depletion. Renin, a proteolytic enzyme, cleaves angiotensinogen, producing angiotensin I. Angiotensin-converting enzyme converts angiotensin I into angiotensin II. The actions of angiotensin II include direct stimulation of the proximal tubule to increase sodium reabsorption and stimulation of the adrenal gland to increase aldosterone secretion. Through its actions in the distal nephron, aldosterone increases sodium reabsorption.

Volume expansion stimulates the synthesis of **atrial natriuretic peptide**, which is produced by the atria in response to atrial wall distention. Along with increasing glomerular filtration rate, atrial natriuretic peptide inhibits sodium reabsorption, facilitating an increase in urinary sodium excretion.

MAINTENANCE FLUIDS

Maintenance IV fluids are used in children who cannot be fed enterally. Along with maintenance fluids, children may require concurrent **replacement fluids** if

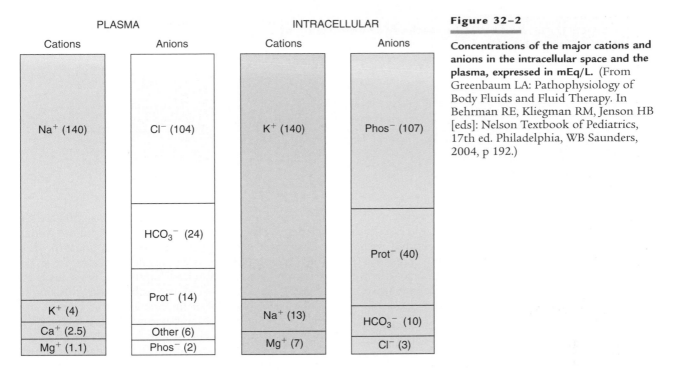

PLASMA   INTRACELLULAR

Cations   Anions   Cations   Anions

Na$^+$ (140)   Cl$^-$ (104)   K$^+$ (140)   Phos$^-$ (107)

                HCO$_3^-$ (24)   Prot$^-$ (40)

                Prot$^-$ (14)

K$^+$ (4)   Na$^+$ (13)   HCO$_3^-$ (10)
Ca$^+$ (2.5)   Other (6)
Mg$^+$ (1.1)   Phos$^-$ (2)   Mg$^+$ (7)   Cl$^-$ (3)

Figure 32–2

Concentrations of the major cations and anions in the intracellular space and the plasma, expressed in mEq/L. (From Greenbaum LA: Pathophysiology of Body Fluids and Fluid Therapy. In Behrman RE, Kliegman RM, Jenson HB [eds]: Nelson Textbook of Pediatrics, 17th ed. Philadelphia, WB Saunders, 2004, p 192.)

they have excessive **ongoing losses**, such as may occur with drainage from a nasogastric tube. In addition, if dehydration is present, the patient also needs to receive deficit replacement (see Chapter 33).

Children can tolerate significant variations in intake because of the many homeostatic mechanisms that can adjust absorption and excretion of water and electrolytes. The calculated water and electrolyte needs that form the basis of maintenance therapy are not absolute requirements. Rather, these calculations provide reasonable guidelines for IV therapy.

Maintenance fluids are composed of a solution of water, glucose, sodium potassium, and chloride. This solution replaces electrolyte losses from the urine and stool and water losses from the urine, stool, skin, and lungs. The glucose in maintenance fluids provides approximately 20% of the normal caloric needs of the patient. This percentage is enough to prevent the development of starvation ketoacidosis and diminishes the protein degradation that would occur if the patient received no calories. Glucose also provides added osmoles, avoiding the administration of hypotonic fluids, which may cause hemolysis.

Maintenance fluids do not provide adequate calories, protein, fat, minerals, or vitamins. Because of inadequate calories, a child on maintenance IV fluids loses 0.5% to 1% of real weight each day. Patients should not remain on maintenance therapy indefinitely; parenteral nutrition (see Chapter 34) should be used for children who cannot be fed enterally for more than a few days. Parenteral nutrition is especially important in a patient with underlying malnutrition.

Daily water losses are measurable (urine and stool) and not measurable (*insensible losses* from the skin and lungs). Failure to replace these losses leads to a thirsty, uncomfortable child and, ultimately, a dehydrated child. Table 32–1 provides a system for calculating **24-hour maintenance water** needs based on the patient's weight. Sodium and potassium are given in maintenance fluids to replace losses from urine and stool. Maintenance requirements are 2 to 3 mEq/kg/day for sodium and 1 to 2 mEq/kg/day for potassium.

Maintenance fluids usually contain 5% dextrose (D5). After calculation of water needs and electrolyte needs, children typically receive either D5 in quarter normal saline (NS) plus 20 mEq/L of potassium chloride or D5 in half NS plus 20 mEq/L of potassium chloride. NS is isotonic to plasma; quarter or half NS is not isotonic. Children weighing less than about 20 to 25 kg do best with the solution containing quarter NS (38.5 mEq/L) because of their high water needs per kilogram. In contrast, larger children and adults may receive the solution with half NS (77 mEq/L). These guidelines assume that there is no disease process present that would require an adjustment in either the volume or the electrolyte composition of maintenance fluids (children with renal insufficiency may be hyperkalemic or unable to excrete potassium and may not tolerate 20 mEq/L of potassium). These solutions work

TABLE 32–1.   Body Weight Method for Calculating Maintenance Fluid Volume and Rate

Body Weight (kg)	Volume Per Day	Hourly Rate
0-10	100 mL/kg	4 mL/kg/hr
11-20	1000 mL + 50 mL/kg for each 1 kg >10 kg	40 mL/hr + 2 mL/kg/hr × (wt − 10)
>20	1500 mL + 20 mL/kg for each 1 kg >20 kg*	60 mL/hr + 1 mL/kg/hr × (wt − 20)[†]

*The maximum total fluid per day is normally 2400 mL.
[†]The maximum fluid rate is normally 100 mL/hr.

well in children who have normal homeostatic mechanisms for adjusting urinary excretion of water, sodium, and potassium. In children with complicated pathophysiologic derangements, it may be necessary to adjust the electrolyte composition and rate of maintenance fluids empirically based on electrolyte measurements and assessment of fluid balance.

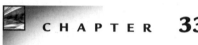

CHAPTER   33

Dehydration and Replacement Therapy

REPLACEMENT THERAPY

The calculation of maintenance water (see Chapter 32) is based on standard assumptions regarding water losses. In some patients, these assumptions are incorrect, however. To identify such situations, it is helpful to understand the source and magnitude of normal water losses. Table 33–1 lists the three sources of normal water loss—the components of maintenance water. **Insensible losses**, composed of evaporative losses from the skin and lungs, represent approximately one third of total maintenance water. Sweating is not insensible and, in contrast to evaporative losses, contains water and electrolytes.

Table 33–2 lists a variety of clinical situations that modify normal maintenance water balance. Evapora-

tive skin water losses can be especially significant in neonates, especially premature infants who are under radiant warmers or who are receiving phototherapy (see Chapter 62). Burns can result in massive losses of water and electrolytes (see Chapter 44). Fever leads to a predictable increase in insensible losses, causing a 10% to 15% increase in maintenance water needs for each 1°C increase in temperature greater than 38°C. Tachypnea or a tracheostomy increases evaporative losses from the lungs. A humidified ventilator or a mist tent causes decreases in insensible losses from the lungs. The gastrointestinal tract is potentially a source of considerable water and electrolyte losses. Because normal gastrointestinal losses of water and electrolytes are quite small, perceivable gastrointestinal losses are considered excessive, and the increase in the water requirement is equal to the volume of fluid losses. Precise measurement of gastrointestinal electrolyte

TABLE 33–1.   Components of Maintenance Water

Urine	60%
Insensible losses (skin and lungs)	35%
Stool	5%

TABLE 33–2.   Adjustments in Maintenance Water

Source	Causes of Increased Water Needs	Causes of Decreased Water Needs
Skin	Radiant warmer	Mist tent
	Phototherapy	Incubator
	Fever	(premature
	Sweat	infants)
	Burns	
Lungs	Tachypnea	Humidified
	Tracheostomy	ventilator
		Mist tent
Gastrointestinal	Diarrhea	
	Emesis	
	Nasogastric	
	suction	
Renal	Polyuria	Oliguria/anuria
Miscellaneous	Surgical drain	Hypothyroidism
	Third space losses	

TABLE 33–3. Adjusting Fluid Therapy for Gastrointestinal Losses	
Average Composition	**Approach to Replacement**
Diarrhea	**Replacement of Ongoing Stool Losses**
Sodium: 55 mEq/L	Solution: 5% dextrose in $\frac{1}{4}$ normal saline + 15 mEq/L bicarbonate + 25 mEq/L potassium chloride
Potassium: 25 mEq/L	Replace stool mL/mL every 1-6 hr
Bicarbonate: 15 mEq/L	
Gastric Fluid	**Replacement of Ongoing Gastric Losses**
Sodium: 60 mEq/L	Solution: 5% dextrose in half normal saline + 10 mEq/L potassium chloride
Potassium: 10 mEq/L	Replace output mL/mL every 1-6 hr
Chloride: 90 mEq/L	

TABLE 33–4. Adjusting Fluid Therapy for Altered Renal Output	
Oliguria/Anuria	**Polyuria**
Place the patient on insensible fluids ($\frac{1}{3}$ maintenance)	Place the patient on insensible fluids ($\frac{1}{3}$ maintenance)
Replace urine output mL/mL with half normal saline	Measure urine electrolytes
	Replace urine output mL/mL with a solution that is based on the measured urine electrolytes

and water losses is possible, permitting the use of an appropriate replacement solution.

It is impossible to predict gastrointestinal losses for the next 24 hours. The child should receive an appropriate maintenance fluid (see Chapter 32) that does not consider the gastrointestinal losses. The losses should be replaced after they occur, using a solution with the same approximate electrolyte concentration as the gastrointestinal fluid. The losses usually are replaced every 1 to 6 hours, depending on the rate of loss, with rapid losses being replaced more frequently. **Replacement solutions** should have approximately the same electrolyte composition as the fluid that is lost. Electrolyte content can be measured directly, or a solution can be selected based on the typical electrolyte composition of diarrhea or gastric losses (Table 33–3).

Urine output is normally the largest cause of water loss. Diseases such as renal failure and the syndrome of inappropriate ADH (SIADH), can lead to a decrease in urine volume. A patient with oliguria or anuria has a decreased need for water and electrolytes; continuation of maintenance fluids produces fluid overload. In contrast, other conditions produce an increase in urine volume. The polyuric phase of acute tubular necrosis, diabetes mellitus, and diabetes insipidus are examples. The patient must receive more than standard maintenance fluids when the urine output is excessive to prevent dehydration.

The approach to decreased or increased urine output is similar (Table 33–4). The patient receives a maintenance fluid that replaces insensible losses. This replacement is accomplished by a rate of fluid administration that is one third of the normal maintenance rate. Placing the **anuric** child on "insensibles" theoretically maintains an even fluid balance, with the caveat that one third of maintenance fluids is only an *estimate* of insensible losses. In the individual patient, this rate may need to be adjusted based on monitoring of the patient's weight and hydration status. An **oliguric** child needs to receive a urine replacement solution.

Most children with **polyuria** (except for children with diabetes mellitus [see Chapter 171]) should be placed on insensible fluids plus urine replacement. When urine output is excessive, it is important to measure the sodium and potassium concentration of the urine to determine the electrolyte composition of the urine replacement solution.

Output from surgical drains and chest tubes, when significant, should be measured and replaced. **Third space losses** manifest with edema and ascites and are due to a shift of fluid from the intravascular space into the interstitial space. Third space losses cannot be quantitated easily. Nonetheless, these losses can be large and lead to intravascular volume depletion, despite weight gain because of edema. Replacement of third space fluid is empirical but should be anticipated in patients who are at risk, such as children who have burns or abdominal surgery. Third space losses and chest tube output are isotonic and usually require replacement with an isotonic fluid, such as normal saline or Ringer's lactate. Adjustments in the amount of replacement fluid for third space losses are based on continuing assessment of the patient's intravascular volume status.

DEHYDRATION

Dehydration, most often due to gastroenteritis, is common in children. The first step in caring for a child with dehydration is to assess the degree of dehydration.

TABLE 33–5. Assessment of Degree of Dehydration

	Mild	Moderate	Severe
Infant	5%	10%	15%
Adolescent	3%	6%	9%
Infants and young children	Thirsty; alert; restless	Thirsty; restless or lethargic but irritable or drowsy	Drowsy; limp, cold, sweaty, cyanotic extremities; may be comatose
Older children	Thirsty; alert; restless	Thirsty; alert (usually)	Usually conscious (but at reduced level), apprehensive; cold, sweaty, cyanotic extremities; wrinkled skin on fingers and toes; muscle cramps
Signs and Symptoms			
Tachycardia	Absent	Present	Present
Palpable pulses	Present	Present (weak)	Decreased
Blood pressure	Normal	Orthostatic hypotension	Hypotension
Cutaneous perfusion	Normal	Normal	Reduced and mottled
Skin turgor	Normal	Slight reduction	Reduced
Fontanel	Normal	Slightly depressed	Sunken
Mucous membrane	Moist	Dry	Very dry
Tears	Present	Present or absent	Absent
Respirations	Normal	Deep, may be rapid	Deep and rapid
Urine output	Normal	Oliguria	Anuria and severe oliguria

Data from World Health Organization.

The degree of dehydration dictates the urgency of the situation and the volume of fluid needed for rehydration. Table 33–5 summarizes the clinical features that are present with varying degrees of dehydration.

An infant with **mild dehydration** (3% to 5% of body weight dehydrated) has few clinical signs or symptoms. The infant may be thirsty; the alert parent may notice a decline in urine output. The history describes the intake and fluid losses. An infant with **moderate dehydration** has clear physical signs and symptoms. Intravascular space depletion is evident by an increased heart rate and reduced urine output. The patient is 10% dehydrated and needs fairly prompt intervention. An infant with **severe dehydration** is gravely ill. The decrease in blood pressure indicates that vital organs may be receiving inadequate perfusion (shock) (see Chapter 40). The infant is approximately 15% dehydrated and should receive immediate and aggressive IV therapy. Mild, moderate, and severe dehydration represent 3%, 6%, and 9% of body weight lost in older children and adults. This difference is because water is a higher percentage of body weight in infants (see Chapter 32). Clinical assessment of dehydration is only an estimate; the patient must be continually re-evaluated during therapy. The degree of dehydration is underestimated in hypernatremic dehydration because the osmotically driven shift of water from the intracellular space to the extracellular space helps to preserve the intravascular volume. The opposite occurs with hyponatremic dehydration.

Laboratory Evaluation

Serum **BUN** and creatinine concentrations are useful in assessing a child with dehydration. Volume depletion without renal insufficiency may cause a disproportionate increase in the BUN, with little or no change in the creatinine concentration. This situation is secondary to increased passive reabsorption of urea in the proximal tubule caused by appropriate renal conservation of sodium and water. This increase in the BUN may be absent or blunted in a child with poor protein intake because urea production depends on protein degradation. Conversely, the BUN may be disproportionately increased in a child with increased urea production, as occurs in a child with a gastrointestinal bleed or a child who is receiving glucocorticoids, which increase catabolism. A significant elevation of the creatinine concentration suggests renal insufficiency.

The **urine specific gravity** is usually elevated (≥1.025) in cases of significant dehydration, but decreases after rehydration. With dehydration, a urinalysis may show hyaline and granular casts, a few white blood cells and red blood cells, and 30 to 100 mg/dL of proteinuria. These findings usually are not associated with significant renal pathology, and

TABLE 33–6. Calculation of Deficit Water and Electrolytes
Water Deficit
Percent dehydration × weight
Sodium Deficit
Water deficit × 80 mEq/L
Potassium Deficit
Water deficit × 30 mEq/L

TABLE 33–7. Fluid Management of Dehydration
Restore intravascular volume
Normal saline: 20 mL/kg over 20 min (repeat until intravascular volume restored)
Calculate 24-hr water needs
Calculate maintenance water
Calculate deficit water
Calculate 24-hr electrolyte needs
Calculate maintenance sodium and potassium
Calculate deficit sodium and potassium
Select an appropriate fluid (based on total water and electrolyte needs)
Administer half the calculated fluid during the first 8 hr, first subtracting any boluses from this amount
Administer the remainder over the next 16 hr
Replace ongoing losses as they occur

they remit with therapy. Hemoconcentration from dehydration causes an increase in the hematocrit and hemoglobin.

Calculation of Deficits

A child with dehydration has lost water; there is usually a concurrent loss of sodium and potassium. Most patients have isotonic dehydration (normal serum sodium). The guidelines in Table 33–6 are used for calculating the deficits in isotonic dehydration secondary to gastroenteritis. The water deficit is the percentage of dehydration multiplied by the patient's weight (for a 10-kg child, 10% of 10 kg = 1 L deficit). The sodium and potassium deficits are derived from the water deficit (see Table 33–6).

Approach to Dehydration

The child with dehydration requires acute intervention to ensure that there is adequate tissue perfusion (see Chapter 40). This resuscitation phase requires rapid restoration of the circulating intravascular volume. This restoration should be done with an isotonic solution, such as normal saline or Ringer's lactate. Blood is an appropriate fluid choice for a child with acute blood loss. The child is given a **fluid bolus**, usually 20 mL/kg of the isotonic solution, over about 20 minutes. A child with mild dehydration does not usually require a fluid bolus. In contrast, a child with severe dehydration may require multiple fluid boluses and may need to receive fluid at a faster rate. The initial resuscitation and rehydration is complete when the child has an adequate intravascular volume. Typically the child has some general clinical improvement, including a lower heart rate, normalization of the blood pressure, improved perfusion, and a more alert affect.

With adequate intravascular volume, it is now appropriate to plan the fluid therapy for the next 24 hours (Table 33–7). The child receives normal maintenance fluids and the remaining fluid deficit. The total

amount of water and electrolytes are added together, then an appropriate fluid is selected. For a patient with isotonic dehydration, D5 half NS with 20 mEq/L of potassium chloride is usually an appropriate fluid. For a child weighing less than 10 to 20 kg with mild dehydration, a reduction of the sodium concentration is usually reasonable (quarter NS) because the sodium deficit is small. Potassium usually is not included in the IV fluids until the patient voids, unless significant hypokalemia is present. Half of the total fluid is given over the first 8 hours; previous boluses are subtracted from this volume. The remainder is given over the next 16 hours. Children with significant ongoing losses need to receive an appropriate replacement solution (see earlier).

Monitoring and Adjusting Therapy

The formulation of a plan for correcting a child's dehydration is only the beginning of management. All calculations in fluid therapy are only approximations. The patient needs to be monitored during treatment with therapy modifications based on the clinical situation (Table 33–8).

Hyponatremic dehydration occurs in children who have diarrhea and consume a hypotonic fluid (water or diluted formula). Volume depletion stimulates secretion of ADH, preventing the water excretion that should correct the hyponatremia. Hyponatremic dehydration produces a more substantial intravascular volume depletion owing to the shift of water from the extracellular space into the intracellular space. In addition, some patients develop symptoms, predominantly neurologic, from the hyponatremia (see Chapter 35). Most patients with hyponatremic dehydration do well

TABLE 33–8. Monitoring Therapy
Vital/signs
Pulse
Blood pressure
Intake and output
Fluid balance
Urine output and specific gravity
Physical examination
Weight
Clinical signs of depletion or overload
Electrolytes

TABLE 33–9. Treatment of Hypernatremic Dehydration
Restore intravascular volume
Normal saline: 20 mL/kg over 20 min (repeat until intravascular volume restored)
Determine time for correction based on initial sodium concentration
[Na] 145-157 mEq/L: 24 hr
[Na] 158-170 mEq/L: 48 hr
[Na] 171-183 mEq/L: 72 hr
[Na] 184-196 mEq/L: 84 hr
Administer fluid at a constant rate over the time for correction
Typical fluids: 5% dextrose in $\frac{1}{4}$ normal saline or 5% dextrose in half normal saline (both with 20 mEq/L potassium chloride unless contraindicated)
Typical rate: 1.25-1.5 times maintenance
Follow serum sodium concentration
Adjust fluid based on clinical status and serum sodium concentration
Signs of volume depletion: administer normal saline (20 mL/kg)
Sodium decreases too rapidly
Increase sodium concentration of IV fluid *or*
Decrease rate of IV fluid
Sodium decreases too slowly
Decrease sodium concentration of IV fluid *or*
Increase rate of IV fluid
Replace excessive ongoing losses as they occur

with the same general approach outlined in Table 33-7. Overly rapid correction of hyponatremia (>12 mEq/L/24 hr) should be avoided because of the remote risk of **central pontine myelinolysis**.

Hypernatremic dehydration is usually a consequence of an inability to take in fluid, owing to a lack of access, a poor thirst mechanism (neurologic impairment), intractable emesis, or anorexia. The movement of water from the intracellular space to the extracellular space during hypernatremic dehydration partially protects the intravascular volume. Children with hypernatremic dehydration often appear less ill than children with a similar degree of isotonic dehydration. Urine output may be preserved longer, and there may be less tachycardia. Children with hypernatremic dehydration are often lethargic and irritable when touched. Hypernatremia may cause fever, hypertonicity, and hyperreflexia. More severe neurologic symptoms may develop if cerebral bleeding or thrombosis occurs.

Too-rapid treatment of hypernatremic dehydration may cause significant morbidity and mortality. **Idiogenic osmoles** are generated within the brain during the development of hypernatremia. These idiogenic osmoles increase the osmolality within the cells of the brain, providing protection against brain cell shrinkage secondary to movement of water out of cells into the hypertonic ECF. These idiogenic osmoles dissipate slowly during correction of hypernatremia. With rapid lowering of the extracellular osmolality during correction of hypernatremia, there may be a new gradient created that causes water movement from the extracellular space into the cells of the brain, producing **cerebral edema**. Symptoms of the resultant cerebral edema can produce seizures, brain herniation, and death.

To minimize the risk of cerebral edema during correction of hypernatremic dehydration, the serum sodium concentration should not decrease more than 12 mEq/L every 24 hours. The deficits in severe hyper-

natremic dehydration may need to be corrected over 2 to 4 days (Table 33-9). The choice and rate of fluid are not nearly as important as vigilant monitoring of the serum sodium concentration and adjustment of the therapy based on the result. Nonetheless, the initial resuscitation-rehydration phase of therapy remains the same as for other types of dehydration.

Oral Rehydration

Mild to moderate dehydration from diarrhea of any cause can be treated effectively using a simple, oral rehydration solution (ORS) containing glucose and electrolytes (see Chapter 112). The ORS relies on the coupled transport of sodium and glucose in the intestine. Oral rehydration therapy is used in many countries and has significantly reduced the morbidity and mortality from acute diarrhea and has lessened diarrhea-associated malnutrition. Oral rehydration is underused in developed countries, but should be attempted for most patients with mild to moderate diarrheal dehydration. Oral rehydration therapy is less expensive than IV therapy and has a lower complication rate. IV therapy still may be required for patients with severe dehydration; patients with uncontrollable vomiting; patients unable to drink because of extreme fatigue, stupor, or coma; or patients with gastric or intestinal distention.

As a guideline for oral rehydration, 50 mL/kg of the ORS should be given within 4 hours to patients with mild dehydration, and 100 mL/kg should be given over 4 hours to patients with moderate dehydration. Supplementary ORS is given to replace ongoing losses from diarrhea or emesis. An additional 10 mL/kg of ORS is given for each stool. Fluid intake should be decreased if the patient appears fully hydrated earlier than expected or develops periorbital edema. Breastfeeding should be allowed after rehydration in infants who are breastfed; in other patients, their usual formula, milk, or feeding should be offered after rehydration.

When rehydration is complete, maintenance therapy should be started, using 100 mL of ORS/kg/24 hr until the diarrhea stops. Breastfeeding or formula-feeding should be maintained and not delayed for more than 24 hours. Patients with more severe diarrhea require continued supervision. The volume of ORS ingested should equal the volume of stool losses. If stool volume cannot be measured, an intake of 10 to 15 mL of ORS/kg/hr is appropriate.

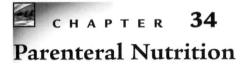

CHAPTER 34
Parenteral Nutrition

Parenteral nutrition (PN) is necessary when enteral feeding is inadequate to meet the nutritional needs of a patient. Enteral nutrition is always preferred because it is more physiologic, less expensive, and associated with fewer complications. In some children, PN supplements enteral nutrition. In other children, PN is the only source of nutrition, although there are fewer complications if some nutrition can be provided enterally.

INDICATIONS

A variety of clinical situations necessitate PN (Table 34–1). Acute PN is frequently given in an ICU; this is due to poor tolerance of enteral feeds, potentially secondary to a transient ileus, or concerns regarding bowel ischemia or the risk of aspiration pneumonia. **Short bowel syndrome** is the most common indication for long-term PN; it may be caused by a congenital gastrointestinal anomaly or acquired after necrotizing enterocolitis (see Chapter 63). Some

TABLE 34–1. Indications for Parenteral Nutrition
Acute
Prematurity
Trauma
Burns
Bowel surgery
Multiorgan system failure
Bone marrow transplantation
Malignancy
Chronic
Short bowel
Intractable diarrhea
Intestinal pseudo-obstruction
Inflammatory bowel disease
Immunodeficiency

patients with a chronic indication for PN eventually may be transitioned to partial or full enteral feedings.

ACCESS FOR PARENTERAL NUTRITION

PN can be given via either a peripheral IV line or a central venous line. Long-term PN should be given via a central venous line. Acute PN may be given peripherally, although a temporary central venous line often is used in patients in an ICU. Most children with cancer or receiving a bone marrow transplant have a central venous line. A **peripherally inserted central catheter** is an excellent source of central access for acute PN because there are fewer complications with a peripherally inserted central catheter than with a standard central venous line.

A peripheral IV has two major limitations. First, a peripheral IV frequently fails, necessitating interruption of PN and potentially painful placement of a new IV. Second, high-osmolality solutions cause **phlebitis** of peripheral veins; this limits the dextrose and amino acid content of peripheral PN. The dextrose content of peripheral PN cannot be greater than 12%, with a lower limit if the amino acid concentration is high. Lipid emulsion has a low osmolality, so it can be administered peripherally via the same IV as the dextrose and amino acid solution. Patients still can receive adequate nutrition via a peripheral IV, but the volume of PN needs to be higher than is necessary when a central venous line is available because of the limitations on dextrose and amino acid concentration. This situation may be problematic in patients who cannot tolerate larger fluid volumes.

COMPOSITION OF PARENTERAL NUTRITION

PN provides calories, amino acids, electrolytes, minerals, essential fatty acids, vitamins, iron, and trace elements. The **calories** in PN are from dextrose and fat. The amino acids in PN are a potential source of calories, but they should be used predominantly for protein synthesis. PN is given as two separate solutions: a dextrose and amino acid solution and a 20% lipid emulsion. The dextrose solution has all of the other components of PN except for fat.

The dextrose concentration of peripheral PN is typically 10% to 12%, whereas central PN has a concentration of about 20%, although it may be increased to 25% to 30% in patients who are fluid restricted. To avoid hyperglycemia, the dextrose delivery is increased gradually when starting total PN. Protein delivery in PN is via amino acids in the dextrose solution. The goal is 0.8 to 2 g protein/kg/24 hr for older children, 1.5 to 3 g/kg/24 hr for full-term and older infants, and 2.5 to 3.5 g/kg/24 hr for preterm infants.

The electrolyte and mineral composition of PN, which includes sodium, potassium, chloride, acetate, calcium, phosphate, and magnesium, is based on the patient's age, the volume of PN, and the nature of the underlying disease process. Vitamins, iron, and trace element delivery depend on age, with some adjustment necessary in certain diseases (decreased in renal failure or increased if stool losses). The 20% lipid emulsion provides essential fatty acids and calories. The lipid emulsion is started at a rate of 0.5 to 1 g/kg/24 hr, gradually increasing the rate so that the patient receives adequate calories; this typically requires 2.5 to 3.5 g/kg/24 hr. The lipid emulsion usually provides 30% to 40% of the required calories; it should not exceed 60%. The serum triglyceride concentration is monitored as the rate of lipid emulsion is increased, with reduction of the lipid emulsion rate if significant hypertriglyceridemia develops.

COMPLICATIONS

There are protean potential complications of PN. Central venous lines are associated with complications during insertion (pneumothorax or bleeding) and long-term issues (thrombosis). **Catheter-related sepsis**, most commonly due to coagulase-negative staphylococci, is common and may necessitate catheter removal. Other potential pathogens are *Staphylococcus aureus,* gram-negative bacilli, and fungi. Electrolyte abnormalities, nutritional deficiencies, hyperglycemia, and complications from excessive protein intake (azotemia or hyperammonemia) can be detected with careful monitoring.

The most concerning complication of long-term PN is **cholestatic liver disease**, which can lead to cirrhosis and liver failure. Ultimately, some patients with short bowel syndrome become candidates for combined small bowel–liver transplantation. Current PN decreases the risk of liver disease by including reduced amounts of hepatotoxic amino acids. The best preventive strategy is early use of the gastrointestinal tract, even if only trophic feeds are tolerated.

CHAPTER **35**

Disorders of Sodium

The kidney regulates sodium balance and is the principal site of sodium excretion. Sodium is unique among electrolytes because **water balance**, not sodium balance, usually determines its concentration. When the sodium concentration increases, the resultant higher plasma osmolality causes increased thirst and increased secretion of ADH, which leads to renal conservation of water. Both of these mechanisms increase the water content of the body, and the sodium concentration returns to normal. During hyponatremia, the fall in plasma osmolality decreases ADH secretion, and consequent renal water excretion leads to an increase in the sodium concentration. Although water balance usually is regulated by osmolality, volume depletion stimulates thirst, ADH secretion, and renal conservation of water. Volume depletion takes precedence over osmolality; volume depletion stimulates ADH secretion, even if a patient has hyponatremia. This principle is crucial for understanding the pathophysiology of many causes of hyponatremia.

The excretion of sodium by the kidney is not regulated by the plasma osmolality. The patient's effective plasma volume determines the amount of sodium in the urine. This volume is mediated by a variety of regulatory systems, including the renin-angiotensin-aldosterone system and intrarenal mechanisms. In hyponatremia or hypernatremia, the underlying pathophysiology determines the urinary sodium concentration, not the serum sodium concentration.

HYPONATREMIA

Etiology

Different mechanisms can cause hyponatremia (Fig. 35-1). **Pseudohyponatremia** is a laboratory artifact that is present when the plasma contains high concentrations of protein or lipid. It does not occur when a direct ion-selective electrode determines the sodium concentration, a technique that is increasingly used in clinical laboratories. In true hyponatremia, the *measured*

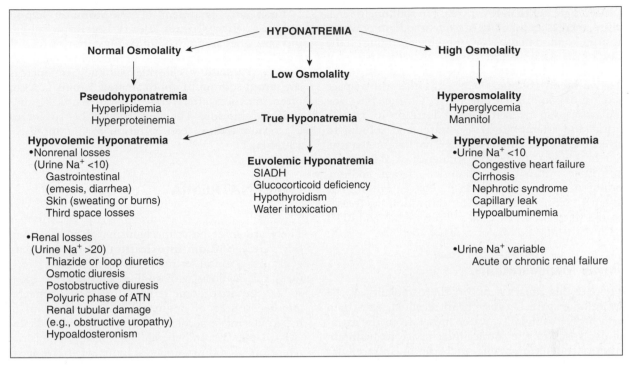

Figure 35–1

Differential diagnosis of hyponatremia. Assessment of hyponatremia is a three-step process: (1) Determine if the osmolality is low; if yes, the patient has true hyponatremia. (2) Evaluate the patient's volume status. (3) Determine the urine sodium concentration to help narrow the differential diagnosis. ATN, acute tubular necrosis; GI, gastrointestinal; SIADH, syndrome of inappropriate secretion of antidiuretic hormone.

osmolality is low, whereas it is normal in pseudohyponatremia. **Hyperosmolality**, resulting from mannitol infusion or hyperglycemia, causes a low serum sodium concentration because water moves down its osmotic gradient from the intracellular space into the extracellular space, diluting the sodium concentration. For every 100 mg/dL increment of the serum glucose, the serum sodium decreases by 1.6 mEq/L. Because the manifestations of hyponatremia are due to the low plasma osmolality, patients with hyponatremia owing to hyperosmolality do not have symptoms of hyponatremia.

Classification of true hyponatremia is based on the patient's volume status (see Fig. 35–1). In **hypovolemic hyponatremia**, the child has lost sodium from the body. Water balance may be positive or negative, but there has been a higher net sodium loss than water loss; this is due to oral or IV water intake, with water retention by the kidneys, to compensate for the intravascular volume depletion. If the sodium loss is due to a nonrenal disease, the urine sodium concentration is very low, as the kidneys attempt to preserve the intravascular volume by conserving sodium. In renal salt-wasting diseases, the urine sodium is inappropriately elevated.

Patients with hyponatremia and no evidence of volume overload or volume depletion have **euvolemic hyponatremia**. These patients typically have an excess of total body water and a slight decrease in total body sodium. Some of these patients have an increase in weight, implying that they are volume overloaded. Nevertheless, from a clinical standpoint, they usually appear normal or have subtle signs of fluid overload. In **SIADH**, there is secretion of ADH that is not inhibited by either low serum osmolality or expanded intravascular volume. Retention of water causes hyponatremia, and the expansion of the intravascular volume results in an increase in renal sodium excretion. Hyponatremia in hospitalized patients is due to inappropriately produced ADH secondary to stress in the presence of hypotonic fluids. SIADH is associated with pneumonia, mechanical ventilation, meningitis, and other CNS disorders (trauma). Ectopic (tumor) production of ADH is rare in children. Infants also can develop euvolemic hyponatremia as a result of consumption of large amounts of water or inappropriately diluted formula in the absence of dehydration.

In **hypervolemic hyponatremia**, there is an excess of total body water and sodium, although the increase in water is greater than the increase in sodium. In renal failure, there is an inability to excrete sodium or water; the urine sodium may be low or high, depending on the cause of the renal insufficiency. In the other causes of hypervolemic hyponatremia, there is a decrease in the effective blood volume, owing to either third space fluid loss or poor cardiac output (see Chapter 145). The regulatory systems sense this decrease in cardiac output and attempt to retain water and sodium to correct the problem. ADH causes renal water retention, and the kidneys, under the influence of aldosterone and other intrarenal mechanisms, retain sodium, leading to a low urine sodium concentration. The patient's serum sodium concentration decreases because water intake exceeds sodium intake, and ADH prevents the normal loss of excess water.

Clinical Manifestations

Hyponatremia causes a fall in the osmolality of the extracellular space. Because the intracellular space then has a higher osmolality, water moves from the extracellular space to the intracellular space to maintain osmotic equilibrium. The increase in intracellular water may cause cells to swell. **Brain cell swelling** is responsible for most of the symptoms of hyponatremia. Neurologic symptoms of hyponatremia include anorexia, nausea, emesis, malaise, lethargy, confusion, agitation, headache, seizures, coma, and decreased reflexes. Patients may develop hypothermia and Cheyne-Stokes respirations. Hyponatremia can cause muscle cramps and weakness. Symptoms are more severe when hyponatremia develops rapidly; chronic hyponatremia can be asymptomatic owing to a compensatory decrease in brain cell osmolality, which limits cerebral swelling.

Treatment

Rapid correction of hyponatremia can produce **central pontine myelinolysis**. Avoiding more than a 12 mEq/L increase in the serum sodium every 24 hours is prudent, especially if the hyponatremia developed gradually. Treatment of hypovolemic hyponatremia requires administration of IV fluids with sodium to provide maintenance requirements and deficit correction and to replace ongoing losses (see Chapter 33). For children with SIADH, water restriction is the cornerstone of the therapy. Children with hypothyroidism or cortisol deficiency need specific hormone replacement. Acute water intoxication rapidly self-corrects with transient restriction of water intake, which is followed by introduction of a normal diet. Treatment of hypervolemic hyponatremia centers on restriction of water and sodium intake, but disease-specific measures, such as dialysis in renal failure, also may be necessary.

Emergency treatment of **symptomatic hyponatremia**, such as seizures, uses IV hypertonic saline to increase the serum sodium concentration rapidly, which leads to a decrease in brain edema. Each milliliter of 3% sodium chloride per kilogram increases the serum sodium by approximately 1 mEq/L. A child often improves after receiving 4 to 6 mL/kg of 3% sodium chloride. The aim should be to increase the serum sodium concentration to not more than 130 mEq/L.

HYPERNATREMIA
Etiology

There are three basic mechanisms of hypernatremia (Fig. 35–2). **Sodium intoxication** is frequently iatrogenic in a hospital setting resulting from correction of metabolic acidosis with sodium bicarbonate. Baking soda, a putative home remedy for upset stomach, is another source of sodium bicarbonate in infants; hypernatremia is accompanied by a metabolic alkalosis (see Chapter 37). In hyperaldosteronism, there is renal retention of sodium and resultant hypertension; the hypernatremia is mild.

Hypernatremia resulting from water losses develops only if the patient does not have access to water or cannot drink adequately because of neurologic impairment, emesis, or anorexia. Infants are at high risk because of their inability to control their own water intake. Ineffective breastfeeding, often in a primiparous mother, can cause severe chronic hypernatremic dehydration with failure to thrive. Hereditary **nephrogenic diabetes insipidus** causes massive urinary water losses and dilute urine. Because it is most commonly an X-linked disorder, it usually occurs in boys, who may have episodes of severe hypernatremic dehydration and failure to thrive. The defect is in the gene for the ADH receptor in the X-linked form of nephrogenic diabetes insipidus.

Acquired nephrogenic diabetes insipidus may be secondary to interstitial nephritis, sickle cell disease, hypercalcemia, hypokalemia, or medications (lithium or amphotericin). High insensible losses of water are especially common in premature infants; the losses increase further as a result of radiant warmers or phototherapy for hyperbilirubinemia. Children with extrarenal causes of water loss have high levels of ADH and a very concentrated urine. In contrast, children with diabetes insipidus have inappropriately dilute urine. If the defect is due to *central diabetes insipidus*, the urine output decreases, and the urine osmolality increases in response to administration of an ADH analogue (central causes of ADH deficiency include tumor, infarction, or trauma). There is no response to an ADH analogue in a child with nephrogenic diabetes insipidus.

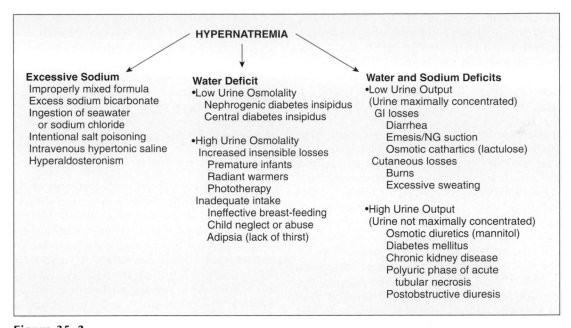

Figure 35-2

Differential diagnosis of hypernatremia by mechanism. GI, gastrointestinal; NG, nasogastric.

When hypernatremia occurs in conditions with deficits of sodium and water, the water deficit exceeds the sodium deficit; this occurs only if the patient is unable to ingest adequate water. Diarrhea results in sodium and water depletion. Most children with gastroenteritis do not develop hypernatremia because they drink enough hypotonic fluid to compensate at least partially for stool water losses. Hypernatremia is most likely in a child with diarrhea who has inadequate intake because of emesis, lack of access to water, or anorexia. Some renal diseases, including obstructive uropathy, renal dysplasia, and juvenile nephronophthisis, can cause losses of sodium and water, potentially producing hypernatremia if the patient consumes insufficient water.

In situations with combined sodium and water deficits, analysis of the urine differentiates renal and nonrenal etiologies. When the losses are extrarenal, the kidney responds to volume depletion with low urine volume, a concentrated urine, and sodium retention (urine sodium <10 mEq/L). With renal causes, the urine volume is not appropriately low, the urine is not maximally concentrated, and the urine sodium may be inappropriately elevated.

Clinical Manifestations

Most children with hypernatremia are dehydrated and have the typical signs and symptoms of dehydration (see Chapter 33). Children with hypernatremic dehydration tend to have better preservation of intravascular volume owing to the shift of water from the intracellular space to the extracellular space. Blood pressure and urine output are maintained, and hypernatremic infants are less symptomatic initially and potentially become more dehydrated before seeking medical attention. Breastfed infants with hypernatremia often are profoundly dehydrated and underweight from poor nutrition. Probably because of intracellular water loss, the pinched abdominal skin of a dehydrated, hypernatremic infant has a "doughy" feel.

Hypernatremia, even without dehydration, causes CNS symptoms that tend to parallel the degree of sodium elevation and the acuity of the increase. Patients are irritable, restless, weak, and lethargic. Some infants have a high-pitched cry and hyperpnea. Alert patients are very thirsty, although nausea may be present. Hypernatremia causes fever, although many patients have an underlying process that contributes to the fever. Hypernatremia is associated with hyperglycemia and mild hypocalcemia; the mechanisms are unknown.

Brain hemorrhage is the most devastating consequence of hypernatremia. As the extracellular osmolality increases, water moves out of brain cells, resulting in a decrease in brain volume. This decrease in volume can result in tearing of intracerebral veins and bridging blood vessels as the brain moves away from the skull and the meninges. Patients may have subarachnoid, subdural, and parenchymal hemorrhage. Seizures and coma are possible sequelae of the hemorrhage, although seizures are more common during treatment. The cerebrospinal fluid protein is often elevated in infants with significant hypernatremia, probably owing to leakage from damaged blood vessels.

Treatment

As hypernatremia develops, the brain generates idiogenic osmoles to increase the intracellular osmolality and prevent the loss of brain water. This mechanism is not instantaneous and is most prominent when hypernatremia has developed gradually. If the serum sodium concentration is lowered rapidly, there is movement of water from the serum into the brain cells to equalize the osmolality in the two compartments. The resultant brain swelling manifests as seizures or coma.

Because of the dangers of overly rapid correction, hypernatremia should not be corrected rapidly. The goal is to decrease the serum sodium by less than 12 mEq/L every 24 hours, a rate of 0.5 mEq/L/hr. The most important component of correcting moderate or severe hypernatremia is frequent monitoring of the serum sodium so that fluid therapy can be adjusted to provide adequate correction, neither too slow nor too fast. If a child develops seizures from brain edema secondary to rapid correction, administration of hypotonic fluid should be stopped, and an infusion of 3% saline can increase the serum sodium acutely, reversing the cerebral edema.

In a child with hypernatremic dehydration, as in any child with dehydration, the first priority is restoration of intravascular volume with isotonic fluid. Table 33–9 outlines a general approach for correcting hypernatremic dehydration secondary to gastroenteritis. If the hypernatremia and dehydration are secondary to water loss, as occurs with either form of diabetes insipidus, a more hypotonic IV fluid is appropriate. A child with central diabetes insipidus should receive an ADH analogue to prevent further excessive water loss. A child with nephrogenic diabetes insipidus requires a urine replacement solution to offset ongoing water losses. Chronically, reduced sodium intake, thiazide diuretics, and nonsteroidal anti-inflammatory drugs can decrease water losses in nephrogenic diabetes insipidus.

Acute, severe hypernatremia, usually secondary to sodium administration, can be corrected more rapidly because idiogenic osmoles have not had time to accumulate; this balances the high morbidity and mortality from severe, acute hypernatremia with the dangers of overly rapid correction. When hypernatremia is due to sodium intoxication, and the hypernatremia is severe, it may be impossible to administer enough water to correct the hypernatremia rapidly without worsening volume overload. Some patients require use of a loop diuretic or peritoneal dialysis. With sodium overload, hypernatremia is corrected with sodium-free IV fluid (D5 in water).

CHAPTER **36**
Disorders of Potassium

The kidneys are the principal regulator of potassium balance, adjusting excretion based on intake. Factors affecting renal potassium excretion include aldosterone, acid-base status, serum potassium concentration, and renal function. The intracellular potassium concentration is approximately 30 times the extracellular potassium concentration (see Fig. 32–2). A variety of conditions alter the distribution of potassium between the intracellular and extracellular compartments, potentially causing either hypokalemia or hyperkalemia. The plasma concentration does not always reflect the total body potassium content.

HYPOKALEMIA
Etiology

Hypokalemia is common in children, with most cases related to gastroenteritis. There are four basic mechanisms of hypokalemia (Table 36–1). Spurious hypokalemia occurs in patients with leukemia and elevated white blood cell counts if plasma for analysis is left at room temperature, permitting the white blood cells to take up potassium from the plasma. Low intake, nonrenal losses, and renal losses all are associated with total body potassium depletion. With a **transcellular shift**, there is no change in total body potassium, although there may be concomitant potassium depletion secondary to other factors.

The transcellular shift of potassium after initiation of insulin therapy in children with diabetic ketoacidosis (see Chapter 171) can be dramatic. These patients have reduced total body potassium owing to urinary losses, but they often have a normal serum potassium level before insulin therapy from a transcellular shift into the extracellular space secondary to insulin deficiency and metabolic acidosis. Children receiving aggressive doses of β-adrenergic agonists (albuterol) for asthma can have hypokalemia resulting from the intracellular movement of potassium. Poor intake is an unusual cause of hypokalemia, unless also associated with significant weight loss (anorexia nervosa).

Diarrhea has a high concentration of potassium, and the resulting hypokalemia usually is associated with a metabolic acidosis secondary to stool losses of

TABLE 36–1. Causes of Hypokalemia
Spurious
High white blood cell count
Transcellular shifts
Alkalemia
Insulin
β-Adrenergic agonists
Drugs/toxins (theophylline, barium, toluene)
Hypokalemic periodic paralysis
Decreased intake
Extrarenal losses
Diarrhea
Laxative abuse
Sweating
Renal losses
With metabolic acidosis
Distal RTA
Proximal RTA
Ureterosigmoidostomy
Diabetic ketoacidosis
Without specific acid-base disturbance
Tubular toxins (amphotericin, cisplatin,
aminoglycosides)
Interstitial nephritis
Diuretic phase of acute tubular necrosis
Postobstructive diuresis
Hypomagnesemia
High urine anions (e.g., penicillin or penicillin
derivatives)
With metabolic alkalosis
Low urine chloride
Emesis/nasogastric suction
Pyloric stenosis
Chloride-losing diarrhea
Cystic fibrosis
Low-chloride formula
Posthypercapnia
Previous loop or thiazide diuretic use
High urine chloride and normal blood pressure
Gitelman syndrome
Bartter syndrome
Loop and thiazide diuretics
High urine chloride and high blood pressure
Adrenal adenoma or hyperplasia
Glucocorticoid-remediable aldosteronism
Renovascular disease
Renin-secreting tumor
17α-Hydroxylase deficiency
11β-Hydroxylase deficiency
Cushing syndrome
11β-Hydroxysteroid dehydrogenase deficiency
Licorice ingestion
Liddle syndrome

RTA, renal tubular acidosis.

bicarbonate. Urinary potassium wasting may be accompanied by a metabolic acidosis (proximal or distal renal tubular acidosis [RTA] [see Chapter 37]). With emesis or nasogastric suction, there is gastric loss of potassium, but this is fairly minimal given the low potassium content of gastric fluid (approximately 10 mEq/L). More important is the gastric loss of hydrochloride, leading to a metabolic alkalosis and a state of volume depletion. Metabolic alkalosis and volume depletion increase urinary losses of potassium.

Loop and thiazide diuretics lead to hypokalemia and a metabolic alkalosis. **Bartter syndrome and Gitelman syndrome** are autosomal recessive disorders resulting from defects in tubular transporters. Both disorders are associated with hypokalemia and a metabolic alkalosis. Bartter syndrome usually is associated with hypercalciuria, often with nephrocalcinosis, whereas children with Gitelman syndrome have low urinary calcium losses, but hypomagnesemia secondary to urinary magnesium losses.

In the presence of a high aldosterone level, there is urinary loss of potassium, hypokalemia, and a metabolic alkalosis. There also is renal retention of sodium, leading to hypertension. A variety of genetic and acquired disorders can cause high aldosterone levels. **Liddle syndrome**, an autosomal dominant disorder caused by constitutively active sodium channels, has the same clinical features as hyperaldosteronism, but the serum aldosterone level is low.

Clinical Manifestations

The heart and skeletal muscle are especially vulnerable to hypokalemia. ECG changes include a flattened T wave, a depressed ST segment, and the appearance of a **U wave**, which is located between the T wave (if still visible) and P wave. Ventricular fibrillation and torsades de pointes may occur, although usually only in the context of underlying heart disease. Hypokalemia makes the heart especially susceptible to digitalis-induced arrhythmias, such as supraventricular tachycardia, ventricular tachycardia, and heart block.

The clinical consequences in skeletal muscle include muscle weakness and cramps. **Paralysis** is a possible complication (generally only at potassium levels <2.5 mEq/L). Paralysis usually starts with the legs, followed by the arms. Respiratory paralysis may require mechanical ventilation. Some patients develop rhabdomyolysis; the risk increases with exercise. Hypokalemia slows gastrointestinal motility; this manifests as constipation, or with levels less than 2.5 mEq/L, an ileus may occur. Hypokalemia impairs bladder function, potentially leading to urinary retention. Hypokalemia causes polyuria by producing secondary nephrogenic diabetes insipidus. Chronic hypokalemia may cause kidney damage, including interstitial nephritis and renal cysts. In children, chronic hypokalemia, as in Bartter syndrome, leads to poor linear growth.

Diagnosis

It is important to review the child's diet and history of gastrointestinal losses or medications. Emesis and diuretic use can be surreptitious. The presence of hypertension suggests excess mineralocorticoids. Concomitant electrolyte abnormalities are useful clues. The combination of hypokalemia and metabolic acidosis is characteristic of diarrhea, distal RTA, and proximal RTA. A concurrent metabolic alkalosis is characteristic of emesis or nasogastric losses, aldosterone excess, diuretics, and Bartter syndrome or Gitelman syndrome. Alkalosis also causes a transcellular shift of potassium intracellularly and increased urinary losses of potassium.

Treatment

Factors that influence the therapy of hypokalemia include the potassium level, clinical symptoms, renal function, presence of transcellular shifts of potassium, ongoing losses, and the patient's ability to tolerate oral potassium. Severe, symptomatic hypokalemia requires aggressive treatment. Supplementation is more cautious if renal function is decreased because of the kidney's limited ability to excrete excessive potassium. The plasma potassium level does not always provide an accurate estimation of the total body potassium deficit because there may be shifts of potassium from the intracellular space to the plasma. Clinically, this shift occurs most commonly with metabolic acidosis and as a result of the insulin deficiency of diabetic ketoacidosis; the plasma potassium underestimates the degree of total body potassium depletion. When these problems are corrected, potassium moves into the intracellular space, and these patients require more potassium supplementation to correct the hypokalemia. Likewise, the presence of a transcellular shift of potassium into cells indicates that the total body potassium depletion is less severe. Patients who have ongoing losses of potassium need correction of the deficit and replacement of the ongoing losses.

Because of the risk of hyperkalemia, IV potassium should be used cautiously. Oral potassium is safer, albeit not as rapid in urgent situations. The dose of IV potassium is 0.5 to 1 mEq/kg, usually given over 1 hour. The adult maximum dose is 40 mEq. Conservative dosing is generally preferred. For patients with excessive urinary losses, potassium-sparing diuretics are effective, but they need to be used cautiously in patients with renal insufficiency. If hypokalemia, metabolic alkalosis, and volume depletion are present (with gastric losses), restoration of intravascular volume with adequate sodium chloride decreases urinary potassium losses. Disease-specific therapy is effective in many of the genetic tubular disorders.

HYPERKALEMIA
Etiology

Three basic mechanisms cause hyperkalemia (Table 36-2). In the individual patient, the etiology is sometimes multifactorial. **Fictitious hyperkalemia** is common in children because of the difficulties in obtaining blood specimens. This hyperkalemia is usually due to hemolysis during phlebotomy, but it can be the result of prolonged tourniquet application or fist clinching, which causes local potassium release from muscle. Falsely elevated serum potassium levels can occur when serum levels are measured in patients with markedly elevated white blood cell counts; a promptly analyzed plasma sample usually provides an accurate result.

Because of the kidney's ability to excrete potassium, it is unusual for excessive intake, by itself, to cause hyperkalemia. This mechanism can occur in a patient who is receiving large quantities of IV or oral potassium for excessive losses that are no longer present. Frequent or rapid blood transfusions can increase the potassium level acutely secondary to the high potassium content of blood. Increased intake may precipitate hyperkalemia if there is an underlying defect in potassium excretion.

The intracellular space has a high potassium concentration, so a **shift of potassium from the intracellular space** to the extracellular space can have a significant impact on the plasma potassium. This shift occurs with acidosis, cell destruction (rhabdomyolysis or tumor lysis syndrome), insulin deficiency, medications (succinylcholine or β-blockers), malignant hyperthermia, and hyperkalemic periodic paralysis.

Hyperkalemia secondary to decreased excretion occurs with renal insufficiency. Aldosterone deficiency or unresponsiveness to aldosterone causes hyperkalemia, often with associated metabolic acidosis (see Chapter 37) and hyponatremia. A form of congenital adrenal hyperplasia, **21-hydroxylase deficiency**, is the most frequent cause of aldosterone deficiency in children. Male infants typically present with hyperkalemia, metabolic acidosis, hyponatremia, and volume depletion. Female infants with this disorder usually are diagnosed as newborns because of ambiguous genitalia; treatment prevents the development of electrolyte problems.

Renin, via angiotensin II, stimulates aldosterone production. A deficiency in renin, resulting from kidney damage, can lead to decreased aldosterone production. These patients typically have hyperkalemia

TABLE 36–2. Causes of Hyperkalemia

Spurious laboratory value
  Hemolysis
  Tissue ischemia during blood drawing
  Thrombocytosis
  Leukocytosis
Increased intake
  IV or PO
  Blood transfusions
Transcellular shifts
  Acidemia
  Rhabdomyolysis
  Tumor lysis syndrome
  Tissue necrosis
  Hemolysis/hematomas/gastrointestinal bleeding
  Succinylcholine
  Digitalis intoxication
  Fluoride intoxication
  β-Adrenergic blockers
  Exercise
  Hyperosmolality
  Insulin deficiency
  Malignant hyperthermia
  Hyperkalemic periodic paralysis
Decreased excretion
  Renal failure
  Primary adrenal disease
    Acquired Addison disease
    21-Hydroxylase deficiency
    3β-Hydroxysteroid-dehydrogenase deficiency
    Lipoid congenital adrenal hyperplasia
    Adrenal hypoplasia congenita
    Aldosterone synthase deficiency
    Adrenoleukodystrophy
  Hyporeninemic hypoaldosteronism
    Urinary tract obstruction
    Sickle cell disease
    Kidney transplant
    Lupus nephritis
  Renal tubular disease
    Pseudohypoaldosteronism type 1
    Pseudohypoaldosteronism type 2
    Urinary tract obstruction
    Sickle cell disease
    Kidney transplant
  Medications
    ACE inhibitors
    Angiotensin II blockers
    Potassium-sparing diuretics
    Cyclosporine
    NSAIDs
    Trimethoprim

ACE, angiotensin-converting enzyme; NSAIDs, nonsteroidal anti-inflammatory drugs.

and a metabolic acidosis, without hyponatremia. Some patients have impaired renal function, partially accounting for the hyperkalemia, but the impairment in potassium excretion is more extreme than expected for the degree of renal insufficiency.

Children with **pseudohypoaldosteronism type 1** have hyperkalemia, metabolic acidosis, and salt wasting leading to hyponatremia and volume depletion; aldosterone levels are elevated. In the autosomal recessive variant, there is a defect in the renal sodium channel that is normally activated by aldosterone. In the autosomal dominant form, patients have a defect in the aldosterone receptor, and the disease is milder, often remitting in adulthood. Pseudohypoaldosteronism type 2, also called **Gordon syndrome**, is an autosomal dominant disorder characterized by hypertension secondary to salt retention and impaired excretion of potassium and acid leading to hyperkalemia and metabolic acidosis. The risk of hyperkalemia secondary to medications that decrease renal potassium excretion is greatest in patients with underlying renal insufficiency.

Clinical Manifestations

The most import effects of hyperkalemia are due to the role of potassium in membrane polarization. The cardiac conduction system is usually the dominant concern. **ECG changes** begin with peaking of the T waves. As the potassium level increases, an increased P-R interval, flattening of the P wave, and widening of the QRS complex occur; this eventually can progress to ventricular fibrillation. Asystole also may occur. Some patients have paresthesias, weakness, and tingling, but cardiac toxicity usually precedes these clinical symptoms, emphasizing the danger of assuming that an absence of symptoms implies an absence of danger.

Diagnosis

The etiology of hyperkalemia is often readily apparent. Spurious hyperkalemia is common in children, so a repeat potassium level is often appropriate. If there is a significant elevation of the white blood cells, the repeat sample should be from plasma that is evaluated promptly. The history initially should focus on potassium intake, risk factors for transcellular shifts of potassium, medications that cause hyperkalemia, and the presence of signs of renal insufficiency, such as oliguria or an abnormal urinalysis. Initial laboratory evaluation should include creatinine and BUN levels and assessment of acid-base status. Many causes of hyperkalemia, such as renal insufficiency and aldosterone insufficiency or resistance, cause a metabolic acidosis, and a metabolic acidosis worsens hyperkalemia by the transcellular shift of potassium out of cells. Cell destruction, as seen in rhabdomyolysis or tumor lysis syndrome, can cause concomitant hyperphosphatemia, hyperuricemia, and an elevated serum lactate dehydrogenase.

Treatment

The plasma potassium level, the ECG, and the risk of the problem worsening determine the aggressiveness of the therapeutic approach. A high serum potassium level with ECG changes requires more vigorous treatment. An additional source of concern is a patient with increasing plasma potassium despite minimal intake. This situation can occur if there is cellular release of potassium (tumor lysis syndrome), especially in the setting of diminished excretion (renal failure).

The first action in a child with a concerning elevation of plasma potassium is to stop all sources of additional potassium (oral and IV). If the potassium level is greater than 6 to 6.5 mEq/L, an ECG should be obtained to help assess the urgency of the situation. Therapy of the hyperkalemia has two basic goals: (1) Prevent life-threatening arrhythmias, and (2) remove potassium from the body (Table 36–3). The treatments that acutely prevent arrhythmias all have the advantage of working quickly (within minutes), but do not remove potassium from the body. Because none of the measures that remove potassium from the body work quickly, it is important to start them as soon as possible.

Long-term management of hyperkalemia includes reducing intake via dietary changes and eliminating or reducing medications that cause hyperkalemia. Some patients require medications, such as sodium polystyrene sulfonate and loop or thiazide diuretics, to increase potassium losses. The disorders that are due to a deficiency in aldosterone respond to replacement therapy with fludrocortisone, a mineralocorticoid.

TABLE 36–3. Treatment of Hyperkalemia

Rapidly decrease the risk of life-threatening arrhythmias
  Shift potassium intracellularly
    Sodium bicarbonate administration (IV)
    Insulin + glucose (IV)
    β-Agonist (albuterol via nebulizer)
  Cardiac membrane stabilization
    IV calcium
Remove potassium from the body
  Loop diuretic (IV or PO)
  Sodium polystyrene (PO or rectal)
  Dialysis

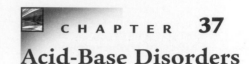

CHAPTER 37
Acid-Base Disorders

Close regulation of pH is necessary for cellular enzymes and other metabolic processes, which function optimally at a normal pH (7.35 to 7.45). Chronic, mild derangements in acid-base status may interfere with normal growth and development, whereas acute, severe changes in pH can be fatal. Control of acid-base balance depends on the kidneys, the lungs, and intracellular and extracellular buffers.

The lungs and the kidneys maintain a normal acid-base balance. Carbon dioxide (CO_2) generated during normal metabolism is a weak acid. The lungs prevent an increase in the partial pressure of CO_2 (PCO_2) in the blood by excreting the CO_2 that the body produces. CO_2 production varies depending on the body's metabolic needs. The rapid pulmonary response to changes in CO_2 concentration occurs via central sensing of the PCO_2 and a subsequent increase or decrease in ventilation to maintain a normal PCO_2 (35 to 45 mm Hg).

The kidneys must excrete endogenous acid production. An adult normally produces about 1 to 2 mEq/kg/day of hydrogen ions. Children normally produce 2 to 3 mEq/kg/day of hydrogen ions. The hydrogen ions from endogenous acid production are neutralized by bicarbonate, potentially causing the bicarbonate concentration to fall. The kidneys regenerate this bicarbonate by secreting hydrogen ions, maintaining the serum bicarbonate concentration in the normal range (20 to 28 mEq/L).

CLINICAL ASSESSMENT OF ACID-BASE DISORDERS

Acidemia is a pH below normal (<7.35), and **alkalemia** is a pH above normal (>7.45). An **acidosis** is a pathologic process that causes an increase in the hydrogen ion concentration, and an **alkalosis** is a pathologic process that causes a decrease in the hydrogen ion concentration. A **simple acid-base disorder** is a single primary disturbance. During a simple metabolic disorder, there is respiratory compensation; the PCO_2 decreases during a metabolic acidosis and increases during a metabolic alkalosis. With metabolic acidosis, the decrease in the pH increases the ventilatory drive, causing a decrease in the PCO_2. The fall in the CO_2 concentration leads to an increase in the pH. This **appropriate respiratory compensation** for a metabolic process happens quickly and is complete within 12 to 24 hours.

During a primary respiratory process, there is a slower metabolic compensation, mediated by the

TABLE 37–1. Appropriate Compensation During Simple Acid-Base Disorders

Disorder	Expected Compensation
Metabolic acidosis	$P_{CO_2} = 1.5 \times [HCO_3^-] + 8 \pm 2$
Metabolic alkalosis	P_{CO_2} increases by 7 mm Hg for each 10 mEq/L increase in the serum $[HCO_3^-]$
Respiratory acidosis	
Acute	$[HCO_3^-]$ increases by 1 for each 10 mm Hg increase in the P_{CO_2}
Chronic	$[HCO_3^-]$ increases by 3.5 for each 10 mm Hg increase in the P_{CO_2}
Respiratory alkalosis	
Acute	$[HCO_3^-]$ falls by 2 for each 10 mm Hg decrease in the P_{CO_2}
Chronic	$[HCO_3^-]$ falls by 4 for each 10 mm Hg decrease in the P_{CO_2}

kidneys. The kidneys respond to a respiratory acidosis by increasing hydrogen ion excretion, increasing bicarbonate generation, and raising the serum bicarbonate concentration. The kidneys increase bicarbonate excretion to compensate for a respiratory alkalosis; the serum bicarbonate concentration decreases. In contrast to a rapid respiratory compensation, it takes 3 to 4 days for the kidneys to complete **appropriate metabolic compensation**. There is, however, a small and rapid compensatory change in the bicarbonate concentration during a primary respiratory process. The expected appropriate metabolic compensation for a respiratory disorder depends on whether the process is acute or chronic.

A **mixed acid-base disorder** is present when there is more than one primary acid-base disturbance. An infant with bronchopulmonary dysplasia may have a respiratory acidosis from chronic lung disease and a metabolic alkalosis from furosemide-induced hypokalemia and hypochloremia used to treat the chronic lung disease. Formulas are available for calculating the appropriate metabolic or respiratory compensation for the six primary simple acid-base disorders (Table 37–1). The appropriate compensation is expected in a simple disorder; it is not optional. If a patient does not have the appropriate compensation, a mixed acid-base disorder is present.

METABOLIC ACIDOSIS

Metabolic acidosis occurs frequently in hospitalized children; diarrhea is the most common cause. For a patient with an unknown medical problem, the presence of a metabolic acidosis is often helpful diagnostically because it suggests a relatively narrow differential diagnosis (Table 37–2).

Etiology

Diarrhea causes a loss of bicarbonate from the body. The amount of bicarbonate lost in the stool depends on the volume of diarrhea and the bicarbonate concentration of the stool, which tends to increase with more severe diarrhea. Diarrhea often causes volume depletion owing to losses of sodium and water, potentially exacerbating the acidosis by causing hypoperfusion (shock) and a lactic acidosis.

There are three forms of **RTA**: distal (type I), proximal (type II), and hyperkalemic (type IV). In **distal RTA**, children may have accompanying hypokalemia, hypercalciuria, nephrolithiasis, and nephrocalcinosis; rickets is a less common finding. Failure to thrive, resulting from chronic metabolic acidosis, is the most common presenting complaint. Autosomal dominant and autosomal recessive forms of distal RTA exist. The autosomal dominant form is relatively mild; many patients do not present until adulthood. Autosomal recessive distal RTA is more severe and often associated with deafness secondary to a defect in the gene for a H^+-ATPase that is present in the kidney and the inner ear. Distal RTA also may be secondary to medications or congenital or acquired renal disease. Patients with distal RTA cannot acidify their urine and have a urine pH greater than 5.5, despite a metabolic acidosis.

Proximal RTA is rarely present in isolation. In most patients, proximal RTA is part of **Fanconi syndrome**, a generalized dysfunction of the proximal tubule. Along with renal wasting of bicarbonate, Fanconi syndrome causes glycosuria, aminoaciduria, and excessive urinary losses of phosphate and uric acid. The chronic hypophosphatemia is more clinically significant

TABLE 37–2. Causes of Metabolic Acidosis

Normal Anion Gap

Diarrhea
Renal tubular acidosis
Urinary tract diversions
Posthypocapnia
Ammonium chloride intake

Increased Anion Gap

Lactic acidosis
Ketoacidosis (diabetic, starvation, or alcoholic)
Kidney failure
Poisoning (e.g., ethylene glycol, methanol, or salicylates)
Inborn errors of metabolism

because it ultimately leads to rickets in children. Rickets or failure to thrive may be the presenting complaint. Fanconi syndrome is rarely an isolated genetic disorder, with pediatric cases usually secondary to an underlying genetic disorder, most commonly **cystinosis**. Toxic medications, such as ifosfamide or valproate, also may cause Fanconi syndrome. The ability to acidify the urine is intact in proximal RTA, and untreated patients have a urine pH less than 5.5. Bicarbonate therapy increases bicarbonate losses in the urine, however, and the urine pH increases.

In **hyperkalemic RTA**, renal excretion of acid and potassium is impaired. Hyperkalemic RTA is due to either an absence of aldosterone or an inability of the kidney to respond to aldosterone. In severe aldosterone deficiency, as occurs with congenital adrenal hyperplasia secondary to 21α-hydroxylase deficiency, the hyperkalemia and metabolic acidosis are accompanied by hyponatremia and volume depletion from renal salt wasting. Incomplete aldosterone deficiency causes less severe electrolyte disturbances; children may have isolated hyperkalemic RTA, hyperkalemia without acidosis, or isolated hyponatremia.

Lactic acidosis most commonly occurs when inadequate oxygen delivery to the tissues leads to anaerobic metabolism and excess production of lactic acid. Lactic acidosis may be secondary to shock, severe anemia, or hypoxemia. When the underlying cause of the lactic acidosis is alleviated, the liver is able to metabolize the accumulated lactate into bicarbonate, correcting the metabolic acidosis. Inborn errors of carbohydrate metabolism produce a severe lactic acidosis (see Chapter 52). In diabetes mellitus, inadequate insulin leads to hyperglycemia and diabetic ketoacidosis (see Chapter 171). Renal failure (see Chapter 165) causes a metabolic acidosis because the kidneys are unable to excrete the acid produced by normal metabolism.

A variety of **toxic ingestions** cause a metabolic acidosis. **Salicylate** intoxication is much less common because aspirin is no longer recommended for fever control in children. Acute salicylate intoxication occurs after a large overdose. Chronic salicylate intoxication is possible because of the gradual buildup of the drug. In addition to a metabolic acidosis, some patients may have a respiratory alkalosis. Other symptoms of salicylate intoxication include fever, seizures, lethargy, and coma. Hyperventilation may be particularly marked. Tinnitus, vertigo, and hearing impairment are more likely with chronic salicylate intoxication. **Ethylene glycol**, a component of antifreeze, is converted in the liver to glyoxylic and oxalic acids, causing a severe metabolic acidosis. Excessive oxalate excretion causes calcium oxalate crystals to appear in the urine, and calcium oxalate precipitation in the kidney tubules can cause renal failure. The toxicity of **methanol** ingestion also depends on liver metabolism; formic acid is the toxic end product that causes the metabolic acidosis and other sequelae, which include damage to the optic nerve and CNS.

There are many **inborn errors of metabolism** that may cause a metabolic acidosis (see Section X). The metabolic acidosis may be due to excessive production of ketoacids, lactic acid, or other organic anions. Some patients have accompanying hyperammonemia. In most patients, the acidosis occurs only episodically during acute decompensations, which may be precipitated by ingestion of specific dietary substrates (proteins), the stress of a mild illness (fasting, catabolism), or poor compliance with dietary or medical therapy.

Clinical Manifestations

The underlying disorder usually produces most of the signs and symptoms in children with a mild or moderate metabolic acidosis. The clinical manifestations of the acidosis are related to the degree of acidemia; patients with appropriate respiratory compensation and less severe acidemia have fewer manifestations than patients with a concomitant respiratory acidosis. At a serum pH less than 7.20, there is impaired cardiac contractility and an increased risk of arrhythmias, especially if underlying heart disease or other predisposing electrolyte disorders are present. With acidemia, there is a decrease in the cardiovascular response to catecholamines, potentially exacerbating hypotension in children with volume depletion or shock. Acidemia causes vasoconstriction of the pulmonary vasculature, which is especially problematic in newborns with persistent fetal circulation (see Chapter 61). The normal respiratory response to metabolic acidosis—compensatory hyperventilation—may be subtle with mild metabolic acidosis, but causes discernible increased respiratory effort with worsening acidemia. Chronic metabolic acidosis causes failure to thrive.

Diagnosis

The plasma anion gap is useful for evaluating patients with a metabolic acidosis. It divides patients into two diagnostic groups: normal anion gap and increased anion gap. The following formula determines the anion gap:

$$\text{Anion gap} = [Na^+] - [Cl^-] - [HCO_3^-]$$

A normal anion gap is 3 to 11. A decrease in the albumin concentration of 1 g/dL decreases the anion gap by roughly 4 mEq/L. Similarly, albeit less commonly, an increase in unmeasured cations, such as calcium, potassium, or magnesium, decreases the anion gap. Conversely, a decrease in unmeasured cations is a rare cause of an increased anion gap. Because of these variables, the broad range of a normal anion gap, and other factors, the presence of a normal or increased anion gap is not always reliable in differentiating the causes of a metabolic acidosis, especially when the metabolic acidosis is mild. Some patients have more than one explanation for their metabolic acidosis, such as a child with diarrhea and lactic acidosis secondary to hypoperfusion. The anion gap should not be interpreted in dogmatic isolation; consideration of other laboratory abnormalities and the clinical history improves its diagnostic utility.

Treatment

The most effective therapeutic approach for patients with a metabolic acidosis is repair of the underlying disorder, if possible. The administration of insulin in diabetic ketoacidosis or restoration of adequate perfusion in lactic acidosis eventually results in normalization of acid-base balance. The use of bicarbonate therapy is clearly indicated when the underlying disorder is irreparable; examples include RTA and chronic renal failure. In other disorders, the cause of the metabolic acidosis eventually resolves, but base therapy is necessary during the acute illness. In salicylate poisoning, alkali administration increases renal clearance of salicylate and decreases the amount of salicylate in brain cells. Short-term base therapy is often necessary in other poisonings and inborn errors of metabolism.

METABOLIC ALKALOSIS

Etiology

The causes of a metabolic alkalosis are divided into two categories based on the urinary chloride (Table 37–3). The alkalosis in patients with a low urinary chloride is maintained by volume depletion. They are called **chloride responsive** because volume repletion with fluid containing sodium chloride and potassium chloride is necessary to correct the metabolic alkalosis. Emesis, which causes loss of hydrochloride and volume depletion, is the most common cause of a metabolic alkalosis. Diuretic use increases chloride excretion in the urine. Consequently, while a patient is receiving diuretics, the urinary chloride is typically high (>20 mEq/L). After the diuretic effect has worn off, the urinary chloride is low (<15 mEq/L), owing to appropriate renal chloride retention in response to volume depletion. Categorization of diuretics based on urinary chloride depends on the timing of the measurement. The metabolic alkalosis from diuretics is clearly chloride responsive; it corrects only after adequate volume repletion. This is the rationale for including it among the chloride-responsive causes of a metabolic alkalosis.

The **chloride-resistant** causes of metabolic alkalosis can be subdivided based on blood pressure. Patients with the rare disorders that cause a metabolic alkalosis and hypertension either have increased aldosterone or act like they have increased aldosterone (owing to a genetic defect causing overproduction of another mineralocorticoid or a constitutively overactive sodium channel, as occurs in Liddle syndrome). Patients with Bartter syndrome or Gitelman syndrome (see Chapter 36) have metabolic alkalosis, hypokalemia, and normal blood pressure secondary to renal tubular defects that cause continuous urinary losses of chloride.

Clinical Manifestations

The symptoms in patients with a metabolic alkalosis often are related to the underlying disease and associated electrolyte disturbances. Hypokalemia is often present, and occasionally severe, in all the diseases that cause a metabolic alkalosis (see Chapter 36). Children with chloride-responsive causes of metabolic alkalosis often have symptoms related to volume depletion (see Chapter 33). In contrast, children with chloride-unresponsive causes may have symptoms related to hypertension. Alkalemia may cause arrhythmias, hypoxia secondary to hypoventilation, or decreased cardiac output.

TABLE 37–3.   Causes of Metabolic Alkalosis
Chloride Responsive (Urinary Chloride <15 mEq/L)
Gastric losses (emesis or nasogastric suction)
Pyloric stenosis
Diuretics (loop or thiazide)
Chloride-losing diarrhea
Chloride-deficient formula
Cystic fibrosis (sweat losses of chloride)
Posthypercapnia (chloride loss during metabolic acidosis)
Chloride Resistant (Urinary Chloride >20 mEq/L)
High blood pressure
Adrenal adenoma or hyperplasia
Glucocorticoid-remediable aldosteronism
Renovascular disease
Renin-secreting tumor
17α-Hydroxylase deficiency
11β-Hydroxylase deficiency
Cushing syndrome
11β-Hydroxysteroid dehydrogenase deficiency
Licorice ingestion
Liddle syndrome
Normal blood pressure
Gitelman syndrome
Bartter syndrome
Base administration

TABLE 37–4. Causes of Respiratory Acidosis

CNS depression (encephalitis or narcotic overdose)
Disorders of the spinal cord, peripheral nerves, or
  neuromuscular junction (botulism or Guillain-Barré
  syndrome)
Respiratory muscle weakness (muscular dystrophy)
Pulmonary disease (pneumonia or asthma)
Upper airway disease (laryngospasm)

Diagnosis

Measurement of the urinary chloride concentration is
the most helpful test in differentiating among the
causes of a metabolic alkalosis. The history usually suggests a diagnosis, although no obvious explanation
may be present in the patient with bulimia, surreptitious diuretic use, or an undiagnosed genetic disorder,
such as Bartter syndrome or Gitelman syndrome.

Treatment

The approach to therapy of metabolic alkalosis depends
on the severity of the alkalosis and the underlying
etiology. In children with a mild metabolic alkalosis
($[HCO_3^-]$ <32), intervention is often unnecessary.
Patients with chloride-responsive metabolic alkalosis
respond to correction of hypokalemia and volume
repletion with sodium and potassium chloride, but
aggressive volume repletion may be contraindicated if
mild volume repletion is medically necessary in the

child receiving diuretic therapy. In children with chloride-resistant causes of a metabolic alkalosis that are
associated with hypertension, volume repletion is contraindicated because it exacerbates the hypertension
and does not repair the metabolic alkalosis. Treatment
focuses on eliminating or blocking the action of the
excess mineralocorticoid. In children with Bartter syndrome or Gitelman syndrome, therapy includes oral
potassium supplementation and potassium-sparing
diuretics.

RESPIRATORY ACID-BASE DISTURBANCES

During a respiratory acidosis, there is a decrease in the
effectiveness of CO_2 removal by lungs. The causes of
a respiratory acidosis are either pulmonary or nonpulmonary (Table 37–4). A respiratory alkalosis is an
inappropriate reduction in the blood CO_2 concentration. A variety of stimuli can increase the ventilatory
drive and cause a respiratory alkalosis (Table 37–5).
Treatment of respiratory acid-base disorders focuses
on correction of the underlying disorder. Mechanical
ventilation may be necessary in a child with a refractory
respiratory acidosis.

SUGGESTED READING

Bockenhauer D: Ion channels in disease. Curr Opin Pediatr 13:142-
  149, 2001.
Chadha V, Alon U: Acid base and electrolyte disturbances. In Klieg-
  man RM, Greenbaum LA, Lye PS (eds): Practical Strategies in
  Pediatric Diagnosis and Therapy, 2nd ed. Philadelphia, WB
  Saunders, 2004, pp 447-464.
Chan JC, Scheinman JI, Roth KS: Consultation with the specialist:
  Renal tubular acidosis. Pediatr Rev 22:277-287, 2001.
Greenbaum LA: Pathophysiology of body fluids and fluid therapy.
  In Behrman RE, Kliegman RM, Jenson HB, (eds): Nelson Text-
  book of Pediatrics, 17th ed. Philadelphia, WB Saunders, 2004,
  pp 191-252.
Mascarenhas MR, Kerner JA, Stallings VA: Parenteral and enteral
  nutrition. In Walker WA, Durie PR, Hamilton JR, et al (eds): Pedi-
  atric Gastrointestinal Disease, 3rd ed. Toronto, BC Decker, 2000,
  pp 1705-1752.
Moritz ML, Ayus JC: Disorders of water metabolism in children:
  Hyponatremia and hypernatremia. Pediatr Rev 23:371-380, 2002.

TABLE 37–5. Causes of Respiratory Alkalosis

Hypoxemia or tissue hypoxia (carbon monoxide
  poisoning or cyanotic heart disease)
Lung receptor stimulation (pneumonia or pulmonary
  embolism)
Central stimulation (anxiety or brain tumor)
Mechanical ventilation

CHAPTER **38**

Assessment and Resuscitation

INITIAL ASSESSMENT

Initial assessment (the **ABCs—airway, breathing, and circulation**) of an acutely ill or injured child requires rapid identification of physiologic derangements in **tissue perfusion and oxygenation**. The goal is to identify a child already showing inadequate oxygen delivery and a child at risk for deterioration. Thereafter, immediate resuscitation must be implemented before pursuing the usual information needed to develop a differential diagnosis. Initial resuscitation measures are directed at improving and maintaining normal tissue perfusion and oxygenation. **Oxygen delivery** depends on cardiac output, hemoglobin concentration, and hemoglobin-oxygen saturation. The last-mentioned depends on respiratory effort, alveolar gas exchange, pulmonary blood flow, and oxygen-hemoglobin binding characteristics.

HISTORY

In the resuscitation phase, access to historical information may be limited. Characterization of onset of symptoms (acute versus insidious), details of events (e.g., time and nature of injury, mechanism of fluid loss), and a brief identification of underlying medical problems (e.g., known heart disease, sickle cell anemia, other chronic illness) may be sought by members of the team not actively involved in the resuscitation and relayed to team members at the bedside. Attempts at identifying historical issues that affect the ABCs are useful, but should not delay intervention if tissue oxygenation and perfusion are markedly impaired.

PHYSICAL EXAMINATION

Initial examination must focus rapidly on the **ABCs** (Table 38–1). This assessment systematically addresses the issues of oxygen delivery to tissues. Airway patency is the first to be addressed, including assessment of the neurologically injured child's ability to protect the airway. Protection of the cervical spine also should be initiated at this step in any child with traumatic injury or who presents with altered mental status of uncertain etiology. Assessment of breathing includes auscultation of air movement and application of a pulse oximeter (when available) to identify current oxygenation status. Then the examination must address the adequacy of the circulation. Palpation for pulses should focus on the presence of distal and central pulses and on the volume of the pulse. Bounding pulses and a wide pulse pressure are often the first sign of the vasodilatory phase of shock and require immediate resuscitation measures. Weak, thready, or absent pulses are indicators for fluid resuscitation, initiation of chest compression, or both. When assessment of the **ABCs** is complete and measures have been taken to achieve an acceptable level of tissue oxygenation, a more complete physical examination is performed. The sequence of this examination depends on whether the situation involves an acute medical illness or trauma. In trauma patients, the examination follows the **ABCDE pathway**. **D** stands for disability and prompts assessment of the neurologic system and evaluation for major traumatic injuries. **E** stands for exposure; the child is disrobed and searched for evidence of any life-threatening or limb-threatening problems. For the acutely ill and the injured child, the subsequent physical examination should identify evidence of organ

TABLE 38–1. Rapid Cardiopulmonary Assessment

Airway patency

Patent, able to be maintained independently
Maintainable with positioning, suctioning
Unmaintainable, requires assistance

Breathing

Rate
Mechanics
  Retractions
  Grunting
  Use of accessory muscles
  Nasal flaring
Air entry
  Chest expansion
  Breath sounds
  Stridor
  Wheezing
  Paradoxical chest motion
Color

Circulation

Heart rate
Peripheral pulses
  Present/absent
  Volume/strength
Skin perfusion
  Capillary refill time
  Skin temperature
  Color
  Mottling
Blood pressure
  Central pulse strength

CNS Perfusion

Responsiveness (AVPU)
Recognition of parents or caregivers
Muscle tone
Pupil size
Posturing

AVPU, *a*lert, responds to *v*oice, responds to *p*ain, *u*nresponsive.

dysfunction starting with areas suggested in the chief complaint and progressing to a thorough and systematic investigation of the entire patient.

COMMON MANIFESTATIONS

The physiologic responses to acute illness and injury are mechanisms that attempt to correct inadequacies of tissue oxygenation and perfusion. Changes in physiologic parameters, such as increasing heart and respiratory rates, are the initial attempts to maintain adequate tissue oxygenation. When these mechanisms fail to meet the body's needs, other manifestations of impending cardiopulmonary failure occur (Table 38–2). **Respiratory failure**, the most common cause of acute deterioration in children, may result in inadequate tissue oxygenation and in respiratory acidosis. Signs and symptoms of respiratory failure (tachypnea, tachycardia, increased work of breathing, abnormal mentation) progress as tissue oxygenation becomes more inadequate. Inadequate perfusion (shock) results in inadequate oxygen delivery and a resulting metabolic acidosis. **Shock** is characterized by signs of inadequate tissue perfusion (pallor, cool skin, poor pulses, delayed capillary refill, oliguria, and abnormal mentation). The presence of any of these symptoms demands careful assessment and intervention to correct the abnormality and to prevent further deterioration.

INITIAL DIAGNOSTIC EVALUATION

Screening Tests

During the initial phase of resuscitation, monitoring vital signs and physiologic status is the key screening activity (Table 38–3). Monitoring of heart and respiratory rates, blood pressure, pulse oximetry, and neurologic status must be continuous, with attention to changes that may indicate response to therapy or further deterioration requiring additional intervention. During the initial rapid assessment, diagnostic laboratory evaluation often is limited to pulse oximetry (an arterial blood gas may be obtained later) and bedside measurement of glucose levels. The latter is important in any child with altered mental status or at risk for inadequate glycogen stores (e.g., infants, malnourished patients). After resuscitation measures

TABLE 38–2. Warning Signs and Symptoms Suggesting the Potential Need for Resuscitative Intervention*

CNS	Lethargy, agitation, delirium obtundation, confusion
Respiratory	Apnea, grunting, nasal flaring, dyspnea retracting, tachypnea, poor air movement, stridor, wheezing
Cardiovascular	Arrhythmia, bradycardia, tachycardia, weak pulses, poor capillary refill, hypotension
Skin and mucous membranes	Mottling, pallor, cyanosis, diaphoresis, poor membrane turgor, dry mucous membranes

*Action would seldom be taken if only one or two of these signs and symptoms were present, but the occurrence of several in concert foreshadows grave consequences. Intervention should be directed at the primary disorder.

TABLE 38–3.   Elements of Acute Care
Examine
Perform an initial assessment followed by complete and systematic evaluation Focus examination on areas of chief complaints; determine life-threatening and organ-threatening conditions Synthesize findings to plan further evaluation
Monitor
Monitor vital signs Monitor the physiologic parameters required to 1. Make a diagnosis 2. Ascertain response to therapy or progression of disease Prospectively determine allowable limits for changes in monitored parameters; generate and record objective data to guide therapy
Intervene
Before initiating therapy, determine therapeutic goals and endpoints Prioritize life-threatening and organ-threatening conditions Initiate therapy based on recognized pathophysiologic derangements Adjust therapeutic strategies to individual patient needs Use objective data to guide changes in therapy
Anticipate
Anticipation requires understanding of the underlying pathophysiology Always plan for the "worst-case" scenario Use data obtained through examination and monitoring to update prognostic impressions continually

aimed at ensuring tissue oxygenation, further diagnostic tests and imaging are often necessary.

Diagnostic Tests and Imaging

The choice of appropriate diagnostic tests and imaging is determined by the mechanism of disease and results of evaluation after initial resuscitation. The initial evaluation of major trauma patients is focused on identifying evidence of hemorrhage and organ and tissue injury. For an acutely ill child with respiratory distress, a chest x-ray is important. Suspicion of sepsis should result in obtaining appropriate cultures. A complete blood count determines the hematocrit and platelet counts. The complete blood count is a potential screen for infection despite poor sensitivity and specificity of the white blood cell and band counts. Children with historical or physical evidence of inadequate intravascular volume should have serum electrolyte levels obtained, including bicarbonate, BUN, and creatinine.

RESUSCITATION

Resuscitation is focused on identifying abnormalities of oxygenation and perfusion. The goal is to correct these abnormalities and prevent further deterioration. After assessment of the ABCs, interventions are directed at the abnormalities identified. **Oxygen supplementation** may improve oxygen saturation, but may not completely correct inadequate tissue oxygenation. When oxygen supplementation is insufficient or air exchange is inadequate, intubation and mechanical ventilation must be initiated. Inadequate perfusion is best managed initially by providing a fluid bolus. **Isotonic crystalloids** (normal saline, lactated Ringer solution) are the initial fluid of choice. A bolus of 10 to 20 mL/kg should be delivered in monitored conditions. Unless renal function is appropriate, potassium-containing maintenance crystalloids should be avoided. Improvement, but not correction, after an initial bolus should prompt repeated boluses until circulation has been re-established. If hemorrhage is known or highly suspected, administration of packed red blood cells is appropriate. Because most children with shock have noncardiac causes, fluid administration of this magnitude is well tolerated. Monitoring for deteriorating physiologic status (increase in heart rate, decrease in blood pressure) identifies children who may have cardiogenic shock. Fluid resuscitation under these conditions results in an increased preload, which may worsen pulmonary edema and cardiac function. If increased preload occurs, fluid administration should be interrupted, and the focus of resuscitation measures should be aimed at improving cardiac function.

When respiratory support and fluid resuscitation are insufficient, introduction of **vasoactive substances** is the next step. The choice of which agent to use depends on the type of shock present. Hypovolemic shock (when further volume is contraindicated) and distributive shock benefit from drugs that increase systemic vascular resistance (drugs with α-agonist activity, such as epinephrine, norepinephrine, and, in some patients, dopamine). The treatment of cardiogenic shock is more complex. To improve cardiac output by increasing the heart rate, drugs with positive chronotropy are used (epinephrine, norepinephrine, and dopamine). Afterload reduction, using drugs such as dobutamine, nitroprusside, or milrinone, also may be needed. Measuring mixed venous saturation and regional oxygen saturations helps to monitor responses to therapy and adjust the use of vasoactive agents.

CARDIOPULMONARY ARREST

Each year, an estimated 16,000 U.S. children die after unexpected cardiopulmonary arrest; more than half are younger than 1 year of age. Children who need CPR usually have an isolated respiratory arrest. The outcome of cardiopulmonary arrest in children is poor; only 10% to 15% survive, and most survivors have permanent disability. The ability to anticipate or recognize pre–cardiopulmonary arrest conditions and initiate prompt and appropriate therapy not only is lifesaving, but also preserves the quality of life (see Table 38–2).

Hypoxia has a central role in most of the events leading to cardiopulmonary arrest in children. Hypoxia also produces organ dysfunction or damage (Table 38–4). The approach to cardiopulmonary arrest extends beyond CPR and includes efforts to preserve vital organ function. The goal in resuscitating a pediatric patient who has had a cardiopulmonary arrest should be to optimize **cardiac output** and tissue oxygen delivery, which may be accomplished by using artificial ventilation and chest compression and by the judicious administration of pharmacologic agents.

Airway

On recognizing that a clinical situation requiring resuscitation exists, the physician first should ensure that there is a **patent airway**. In children, airway patency often is compromised by a loss of muscle tone, allowing the mandibular block of tissue, including the tongue, the bony mandible, and the soft surrounding tissues, to rest against and obstruct the posterior pharyngeal wall. The use of a manual head tilt maneuver, which is often effective in adults, may result in excessive overextension of the neck and further narrowing of the tracheal airway in infants and young children. The jaw thrust maneuver is the most effective intervention in children.

TABLE 38–4. Target Organs for Hypoxic-Ischemic Damage

Organ	Effect
Brain	Seizures, cerebral edema, infarction, herniation, anoxic damage, SIADH, diabetes insipidus
Cardiovascular	Heart failure, myocardial infarct, mitral and tricuspid insufficiency, peripheral gangrene
Lung and pulmonary vasculature	Acute respiratory distress syndrome, pulmonary hypertension
Liver	Infarction, necrosis, cholestasis
Kidney	Acute tubular necrosis, acute cortical necrosis
GI tract	Gastric ulceration, mucosal damage
Hematologic	Disseminated intravascular coagulation

GI, gastrointestinal; SIADH, syndrome of inappropriate secretion of antidiuretic hormone.

Pediatric patients requiring resuscitation should be endotracheally intubated. Oral intubation is the preferred method in resuscitation and is technically easier than nasal intubation. Before intubation, the patient should be ventilated with 100% oxygen using a bag and mask. Cricoid pressure should be used to minimize inflation of the stomach. Many conscious patients may benefit from the use of induction medications (sedatives, analgesics, and paralytics) to assist intubation, but caution is necessary to prevent further cardiovascular compromise from vasodilating effects of many sedatives. The correct size of the tube may be estimated according to the size of the child's mid-fifth phalanx or the following formula: 4 + (patient age in years/4). Cuffed endotracheal tubes should not be used in children younger than 8 years old because of a narrow airway segment at the level of the cricoid ring.

When the endotracheal tube is in place, the adequacy of ventilation and the position of the tube must be assessed. Use of end-tidal carbon dioxide (CO_2) monitoring devices may assist with validation of endotracheal placement, but low levels of detected CO_2 may be secondary to lack of pulmonary circulation. Adequate chest wall movement and auscultation of the chest to detect bilateral and symmetric breath sounds provide information on adequacy of air entry. If air exchange is not heard or cyanosis continues, the position or patency of the tube must be re-evaluated through direct visualization of tube location via laryngoscopy or, in patients with sufficient circulation, indirectly through the use of end-tidal CO_2 measurement.

Breathing

The major role of endotracheal intubation is to protect or maintain the airway and ensure the delivery of adequate oxygen to the patient. Because hypoxemia is the final common pathway in pediatric cardiopulmonary arrests, providing oxygen is more important than correcting the respiratory acidosis. The clinician should deliver 100% oxygen at an initial rate of 20 breaths/min through the endotracheal tube using a tidal volume necessary to produce adequate chest rise and relieve cyanosis; this usually requires a tidal volume equal to 10 to 15 mL/kg of body weight.

Circulation

When a patent airway is established and oxygenation and ventilation are maintained, **cardiac output** is re-established in many children. Carefully reassessing the patient before proceeding with other mechanical and pharmacologic maneuvers is essential. This reassessment should include observation of the color of the skin and mucous membranes and palpation of central and peripheral pulses. If cyanosis persists or the brachial or femoral pulses remain weak or absent, adequate circulation has not been re-established.

Chest compressions should be initiated if a pulse cannot be palpated or if the heart rate is less than 60 beats/min with signs of poor systemic perfusion. For compressions to be optimal, the child should be supine on a hard, flat surface. In infants and children, the area for compression is the lower half of the sternum. Effective CPR in infants requires a compression depth between 0.5 and 1 inch. If two healthcare workers are available, encircling the chest with both hands to provide compressions is preferable for infants. A child age 1 to 8 years requires a compression depth of 1 to 1.5 inches. In both cases, the compression rate should be at least 100/min, coordinated with assisted ventila-

tion at a ratio of 5:1 compressions to breaths. The effectiveness of compressions should be assessed via palpation of the carotid, brachial, or femoral artery.

The availability of **automated external defibrillators** outside the hospital setting may be useful in the relatively small number of older children who are in ventricular fibrillation or pulseless ventricular tachycardia. Current recommendations include use in children older than age 8 years.

Drugs

When mechanical means fail to re-establish adequate circulation, pharmacologic intervention is essential (Table 38–5). Drug therapy is directed toward improv-

TABLE 38–5. Drug Doses for Cardiopulmonary Resuscitation

Drug	Indication	Dose
Adenosine	Supraventricular tachycardia	0.1-0.2 mg/kg (may repeat at 0.4 mg/kg); maximum 12 mg
Amiodarone	Pulseless VF/VT Perfusing tachyarrhythmias	5 mg/kg over 20-60 min Maximum dose is 15 mg/kg/day
Atropine	Supraventricular or junctional bradycardia Asystole?	0.02 mg/kg/dose (minimum dose 0.1 mg); up to 0.5 mg (child), 1 mg (adolescent); higher doses needed in anticholinesterase poisoning
Bicarbonate	Metabolic acidosis? Hyperkalemia	0.5-1 mEq/kg bolus, if metabolic acidosis present; ensure adequate ventilation; use 4.2% solution in neonates; monitor ABGs, can repeat q 10 min
Calcium	Hypocalcemia Hyperkalemia Wide QRS pattern?	25 mg/kg calcium chloride; stop if bradycardia occurs
Dobutamine	Inotropy	2-30 μg/kg/min
Dopamine	Inotropy	0.5-2 μg/kg/min splanchnic, renal dilation; 2-7 μg/kg/min inotrope; 7-20 μg/kg/min inotrope + pressor
Epinephrine	Chronotropy Inotropy Hypotension	0.01 mg/kg bolus q 5 min; 0.1 mg/kg as subsequent doses if 0.01 mg/kg is ineffective; 0.05-2 μg/kg/min drip, inotrope + pressor; may cause subendocardial ischemia and arrhythmias
Fluid	Hypovolemia Sepsis	Use crystalloid tailored to patient's physiologic needs
Glucose	Hypoglycemia	2 mL/kg 10% dextrose; follow Dextrostix
Isoproterenol	Chronotropy Inotropy	0.05-1 μg/kg/min inotrope + vasodilator effects; chronotropic response may limit dose; may cause subendocardial ischemia and arrhythmias
Lidocaine	Ventricular tachycardia	1 mg/kg/bolus followed by 20-50 μg/kg/min continuous infusion; monitor serum concentration and widening of QRS for toxicity
Nitroprusside	Reduce systemic vascular resistance Hypertensive crisis	0.05-10.0 μg/kg/min by continuous infusion
Oxygen	Hypoxia	100%, humidified
Phenytoin	Ventricular tachycardia, digitalis-induced arrhythmias	15-20 mg/kg slow loading dose; titrate maintenance therapy to serum concentrations of 15-30 μg/mL

?, Controversial, uncertain, or unproved efficacy; ABG, arterial blood gas; VF, ventricular fibrillation; VT, ventricular tachycardia.
Data from Pediatric Working Group of the International Liaison Committee on Resuscitation: Guidelines 2000 for Cardiopulmonary Resuscitation and Emergency Cardiovascular Care. Part 10. Pediatric advanced life support. The American Heart Association in collaboration with the International Liaison Committee on Resuscitation. Circulation 102(Suppl):1291-1342, 2000.

ing cardiac output and delivering oxygen to tissues. Administration of drugs through a central venous line is preferred, although this is difficult to achieve in cases of unanticipated cardiopulmonary arrest. The effectiveness of peripheral IV administration is limited by poor circulation. If intravascular access is not present or rapidly established, administration through an intraosseous route is recommended. Some drugs can be administered effectively through the endotracheal tube (e.g., epinephrine, lidocaine).

Perhaps the most important agent used during CPR is **oxygen**. Whenever possible, 100% oxygen should be administered through an endotracheal tube. Short periods of exposure to high oxygen tensions cause little pulmonary toxicity, and high oxygen tensions may be required to reverse some of the reactive pulmonary vascular responses to poor cardiac output.

Epinephrine constitutes the mainstay of drug therapy for CPR. It is a catecholamine with mixed α-agonist and β-agonist properties. The α-adrenergic effects are most important during the acute phases of resuscitation, causing an increase in systemic vascular resistance that results in a greater pressure gradient across the coronary bed and an improved coronary blood flow. Standard dose therapy is recommended (0.01 mg/kg) as a bolus, but high-dose therapy (0.1 to 0.2 mg/kg) may be considered if administered through an endotracheal tube or if there is no response to repeated standard doses. Caution is necessary in using high-dose epinephrine in children (and premature infants) at risk for intracranial hemorrhage. Vasopressin, an endogenous hormone, causes constriction of capillaries and small arterioles and may be useful. There are insufficient data to support its routine use, but vasopressin may be considered in children failing standard medication administration.

The use of buffers is currently not recommended as a first-line approach. In pediatric patients, acidosis is more often respiratory rather than metabolic. Oxygen delivery and elimination of CO_2 must be established first. The use of **sodium bicarbonate** is controversial because its risks may outweigh potential benefits. Sodium bicarbonate may be judiciously used to correct identified excessive intake of acids or losses of bases. The use of sodium bicarbonate in an attempt to correct what is primarily a respiratory problem can exacerbate respiratory acidosis, however, by inducing the production of more CO_2. Sodium bicarbonate may produce hypernatremia, hyperosmolality, hypokalemia, metabolic alkalosis (shifting the oxyhemoglobin curve to the left and impairing tissue oxygen delivery), reduced ionized calcium level, and impaired cardiac function.

Prompt electrical **defibrillation** is indicated when ventricular fibrillation is noted (Table 38–6). Bolus administration of lidocaine is recommended before defibrillation, but defibrillation should not be delayed

TABLE 38–6.　Recommendations for Defibrillation and Cardioversion in Children

Defibrillation

Pretreat with 0.01 mg/kg epinephrine (1:10,000) iv
Place saline gauze or conduction jellied pad at apex and upper right sternal border
Use 4.5-cm diameter paddles for infants and 8-10-cm diameter paddles for children
Notify all participating personnel before discharging paddles so that no one is in contact with patient or bed
Begin with 2 watts/sec/kg (2 J/kg)
If unsuccessful, double current (4 J/kg) and repeat rapidly ×3

Cardioversion

Determine mechanism of the predominant rhythm
Consider pretreatment with lidocaine, 1 mg/kg iv, for risk of inducing ventricular tachycardia and diazepam for sedation
For symptomatic supraventricular tachycardia* or ventricular tachycardia with a pulse, synchronize signal with ECG
Choose paddles, position pads, and notify personnel as above
Begin with 0.5-1 W/sec/kg (J/kg)
If unsuccessful, double the current

*Consider adenosine first (see Table 38–5).

if lidocaine cannot be administered immediately. Children failing two episodes of defibrillation may benefit from administration of amiodarone (5 mg/kg administered rapidly). Hypotension occurs in 10% to 20% of children receiving amiodarone. Defibrillation should be distinguished from **cardioversion** of supraventricular tachycardias, which also may compromise cardiac output. Cardioversion requires a lower starting dose and a synchronization of the discharge to the ECG to prevent discharging during a susceptible period, which may convert supraventricular tachycardia to ventricular tachycardia or fibrillation.

CHAPTER 39
Respiratory Failure

ETIOLOGY

Acute respiratory failure occurs when the pulmonary system is unable to maintain adequate gas exchange to meet metabolic demands. The resulting failure can be classified as hypercarbic ($PaCO_2$ >50 mm Hg in previously healthy children), hypoxemic (PaO_2 <60 mm Hg in previously healthy children without an intracardiac shunt), or both. **Hypoxemic respiratory failure** frequently is caused by ventilation-perfusion mismatch (perfusion of lung that is not adequately ventilated) and shunting (deoxygenated blood bypasses ventilated alveoli). **Hypercarbic respiratory failure** results from inadequate alveolar ventilation secondary to decreased minute ventilation (tidal volume × respiratory rate) or an increase in dead space ventilation (ventilation of areas receiving no perfusion).

Respiratory failure may occur with **acute respiratory distress syndrome (ARDS)**, which may occur in children with sepsis or children in shock or with burns or traumatic injury. The mechanism underlying this syndrome is an inflammatory process that affects the pulmonary capillary-alveolar unit. Increased vascular permeability (noncardiogenic pulmonary edema) is caused by the release of vasoactive mediators and results in the leakage of proteinaceous fluid into the interstitium and alveoli. Surfactant action also may be affected. Numerous mediators of inflammation (tumor necrosis factor, interferon-γ, nuclear factor κB, and adhesion molecules) may be involved in the development of ARDS.

EPIDEMIOLOGY

Respiratory failure frequently is caused by bronchiolitis, asthma, upper airway obstruction (croup, foreign body, tonsil hypertrophy), and sepsis/ARDS. Hospitalization for bronchiolitis, most often caused by respiratory syncytial virus, is most common in infants younger than 6 months during the winter. Respiratory failure develops in 3% to 10% of hospitalized respiratory syncytial virus patients.

Asthma is increasing in prevalence and is the most frequent reason for nonscheduled pediatric hospital admissions in the U.S. Environmental factors (exposure to cigarette smoke) and prior disease characteristics (severity of asthma, exercise intolerance, delayed start of therapy, and previous ICU admissions) affect hospitalization and near-fatal episodes. The mortality rate of asthma for children 5 to 14 years old increased more than threefold in the 1980s and 1990s; deaths are twice as common in African American children. More than half of asthma-related deaths occur outside the hospital.

Chronic respiratory failure (with acute exacerbations) is often due to chronic lung disease (bronchopulmonary dysplasia, cystic fibrosis), neurologic or neuromuscular abnormalities, and congenital anomalies.

Mortality rates vary with the cause of respiratory failure, but may reach 30% for children with ARDS. ARDS accounts for approximately 3% of all admissions to pediatric ICUs. ARDS is a diffuse localized inflammatory process that develops in association with such diverse etiologies as sepsis, shock, trauma, burns, and pneumonia.

CLINICAL MANIFESTATIONS

Signs and symptoms of hypoxic respiratory failure result from inadequate tissue oxygen delivery and the underlying disease process. Early signs of hypoxemia include **tachypnea and tachycardia** as attempts are made to improve minute ventilation and cardiac output and to maintain delivery of oxygenated blood to the tissues. Further progression of disease may result in dyspnea, nasal flaring, grunting, use of accessory muscles of respiration, and diaphoresis. Late signs of inadequate oxygen delivery include **cyanosis** and **altered mental status** (initially confusion and agitation). Caution must be taken in interpreting the absence of cyanosis. Visual detection of cyanosis requires 5 g/dL of deoxygenated hemoglobin, resulting in delayed visualization in children who are anemic. Signs and symptoms of hypercarbic respiratory failure include attempts to increase minute ventilation (tachypnea and increased depth of breathing), and altered mental status (somnolence). Hypercarbia may result in vasoconstriction causing hypertension.

LABORATORY AND IMAGING STUDIES

A chest radiograph may show evidence of the etiology of respiratory failure. The presence of atelectasis, hyperinflation, infiltrates, or pneumothoraces assists with ongoing management. Diffuse (or perihilar) infiltrates, redistribution of pulmonary vascular patterns, pleural effusions, and at times cardiomegalies provide support for ARDS. The chest radiograph may be normal when upper airway obstruction or impaired respiratory controls are the etiology. Patients presenting with evidence of upper airway obstruction (stridor) may benefit from radiographic studies, including a lateral neck film, and CT to delineate anatomic defects. Direct visualization through flexible bronchoscopy allows identification of dynamic abnormalities of the anatomic airway. Helical CT helps diagnose a pulmonary embolus.

Pulse oximetry allows noninvasive, continuous assessment of oxygenation, but is unable to provide information about ventilation abnormalities. Determination of CO_2 levels requires a blood gas measurement (arterial, venous, or capillary). An **arterial blood gas** allows measurement of CO_2 levels and analysis of the severity of oxygenation defect through calculation of an alveolar-arterial oxygen difference. A normal PCO_2 in a patient who is hyperventilating should heighten concern about the risk of further deterioration. A complete blood count provides detection of an elevated white blood cell count and identification of anemia, which further compromises oxygen delivery to tissues. A chemistry panel identifies abnormalities of renal or hepatic function as possible causes of the respiratory failure or as markers of the severity of hypoxemia (ischemic hepatitis).

DIFFERENTIAL DIAGNOSIS

Hypoxic respiratory failure resulting from impairment of the alveolar-capillary function is seen in ARDS; cardiogenic pulmonary edema; interstitial lung disease; aspiration pneumonia; bronchiolitis; bacterial, fungal, or viral pneumonia; and sepsis. Hypoxic respiratory failure also can be due to intrapulmonary or intracardiac shunting seen with atelectasis and embolism.

Hypercarbic respiratory failure occurs when the respiratory center fails owing to drugs (opioids, barbiturates, anesthetic agents), neurologic or neuromuscular junction abnormalities (cervical spine trauma, demyelinating diseases, anterior horn cell disease, Guillain-Barré syndrome, botulism), chest wall injuries, or diseases that cause increased resistance to expiratory airflow (croup, vocal cord paralysis, postextubation edema). Maintenance of ventilation requires adequate function of the chest wall. Disorders of the neuromuscular pathways, such as muscular dystrophy, myasthenia gravis, and botulism, result in inadequate chest wall movement, development of atelectasis, and respiratory failure. Scoliosis rarely may result in significant chest deformity that leads to restrictive pulmonary function. Similar impairments of gas exchange may result from distention of the abdomen (postoperatively or due to ascites, obstruction, or a mass) and thoracic trauma (flail chest).

Mixed forms of respiratory failure are common and occur when disease processes result in more than one pathophysiologic change. Increased secretions seen in asthma often lead to atelectasis and hypoxia, whereas restrictions of expiratory airflow may lead to hypercarbia. Progression to respiratory failure results from peripheral airway obstruction, extensive atelectasis, and resultant hypoxemia unresponsive to oxygen supplementation and retention of CO_2. The identification of respiratory failure for patients with asthma includes a PaO_2 less than 60 mm Hg (as in other forms), but includes a $PaCO_2$ greater than 45 mm Hg.

TREATMENT

Initial treatment of patients in respiratory distress includes addressing the ABCs (see Chapter 38). **Bag/mask ventilation** must be initiated for patients with apnea or with signs of respiratory fatigue. In other patients, oxygen therapy is administered using appropriate methods. Administration of oxygen by nasal cannula allows the patient to entrain room air and oxygen, making it an insufficient delivery method for most children in respiratory failure. Delivery methods, including intubation and mechanical ventilation, should be escalated if there is inability to increase oxygen saturations appropriately.

Patients presenting with hypercarbic respiratory failure are often hypoxic as well. When oxygenation is established, ventilation abnormalities should be addressed. Patients who are hypercarbic without signs of respiratory fatigue or somnolence may not require intubation based on the PCO_2 alone. Measures should be taken to address the underlying cause of hypercarbia (reversal of drug action, control of fever, or seizures causing increased CO_2 production). Failure of these interventions should result in intubation and mechanical ventilation for patients with marked increase in the work of breathing.

After identification of the etiology of respiratory failure, specific interventions and treatments should be tailored to the needs of the patient. External support of oxygenation and ventilation may be provided by **noninvasive ventilation** methods (continuous positive airway pressure, biphasic positive airway pressure, or negative pressure ventilation) or through invasive methods (traditional **mechanical ventilation**, high-frequency oscillatory ventilation, or extracorporeal membrane oxygenation). Elimination of CO_2 is achieved through manipulation of minute ventilation (tidal volume [difference between peak inspiratory and positive end-expiratory pressure (PEEP)] and respiratory rate). Oxygenation is improved by altering variables that affect oxygen delivery (fraction of inspired oxygen) or mean airway pressure (PEEP, peak inspiratory pressure, inspiratory time, gas flow).

COMPLICATIONS

Respiratory failure is the most frequent cause of cardiorespiratory arrest in children. The major complication of hypoxic respiratory failure is the development of organ dysfunction. **Multiple organ dysfunction** includes the development of two or more of the following: respiratory failure, cardiac failure, renal insufficiency/failure, gastrointestinal or hepatic insufficiency, disseminated intravascular coagulation, and hypoxic-ischemic brain injury. Mortality rates increase with increasing numbers of involved organs (see Table 38-4).

Complications associated with mechanical ventilation include pressure-related and volume-related lung injury. Overdistention and insufficient lung distention (loss of functional residual capacity) are associated with lung injury. Pneumomediastinum and pneumothorax are potential complications of the disease process and overdistention. Inflammatory mediators may play a role in the development of chronic fibrotic lung diseases in ventilated patients.

PROGNOSIS

Prognosis varies with the etiology of respiratory failure. Mortality rates due to bronchiolitis have decreased since the 1980s. Less than 1% of previously healthy children with bronchiolitis die, whereas 3.5% of children with underlying respiratory or cardiac disease who develop bronchiolitis die. Asthma mortality rates, although still low, have increased. Despite advances in support and understanding of the pathophysiology of ARDS, the mortality rate remains 30%. Respiratory failure is the cause of death for only 15% of ARDS patients, however.

PREVENTION

Prevention strategies are explicit to the etiology of respiratory failure. Some infectious causes can be prevented through active immunization against organisms causing primary respiratory disease (pertussis, pneumococcus, *Haemophilus influenzae* type b) and sepsis (pneumococcus, *H. influenzae* type b). Passive immunization with respiratory syncytial virus immunoglobulins prevents severe illness in highly susceptible patients (prematurity, bronchopulmonary dysplasia). Primary prevention of traumatic injuries may decrease the incidence of ARDS. Compliance with appropriate therapies for asthma may decrease the number of episodes of respiratory failure (see Chapter 78).

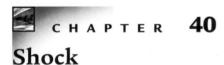

CHAPTER **40**
Shock

ETIOLOGY AND EPIDEMIOLOGY

Shock is the inability to provide sufficient perfusion of oxygenated blood to tissues to maintain organ function. **Oxygen delivery** is directly related to the arterial oxygen content (oxygen saturation and hemoglobin concentration) and to cardiac output (stroke volume, heart rate, and systemic vascular resistance). Changes in metabolic needs are met primarily by adjustments in cardiac output, which are determined by the amount of blood ejected from the left ventricle (stroke volume) and by the heart rate (Fig. 40-1). Stroke volume is related to myocardial end-diastolic fiber length (preload), myocardial contractility (inotropy), and resistance of blood ejection from the ventricle (after-

load) (see Chapter 138). In a young infant whose myocardium possesses relatively less contractile tissue, increased demand for cardiac output is met primarily by a neurally mediated increase in heart rate. In older children and adolescents, cardiac output is most efficiently augmented by increasing stroke volume through neurohormonally mediated changes in vascular tone, resulting in increased venous return to the heart (increased preload), decreased arterial resistance (decreased afterload), and increased myocardial contractility (Fig. 40-2).

HYPOVOLEMIC SHOCK

Acute hypovolemia is the most common cause of shock in children. It results from loss of fluid from the intravascular space through fluid and electrolyte depletion secondary to vomiting and diarrhea, blood loss, third space fluid losses caused by capillary leak syndromes, and pathologic renal fluid losses. Reduced blood volume causes a decreased preload, stroke volume, and cardiac output. Hypovolemic shock results in increased sympathoadrenal activity producing an increased heart rate and enhanced myocardial contractility. Neurohormonally mediated constriction of the arterioles and capacitance vessels maintains blood pressure, augments venous return to the heart to improve preload, and redistributes blood flow from nonvital to vital organs. If hypovolemic shock remains untreated, the increased heart rate may impair coronary blood flow and ventricular filling, while elevated systemic vascular resistance increases myocardial oxygen consumption, resulting in poorer myocardial function. Ultimately, intense systemic vasoconstriction and hypovolemia produce tissue ischemia, which impairs cell metabolism and releases potent vasoactive mediators from injured cells. Cytokines and other vasoactive peptides can change myocardial contractility and vascular tone and promote release of other inflammatory mediators that increase capillary permeability and impair organ function further (see Fig. 40-2).

DISTRIBUTIVE SHOCK

Abnormalities in the distribution of blood flow may result in profound inadequacies in tissue perfusion, even in the presence of a normal or high cardiac output. This maldistribution of flow usually results from abnormalities in vascular tone. Septic shock is the most common type of distributive shock in children. It is commonly a complication of sepsis caused by grampositive and gram-negative bacteria and by infection resulting from rickettsiae and viruses (Table 40-1 and Fig. 40-3).

The **systemic inflammatory response syndrome** is one form of distributive shock in which a wide variety

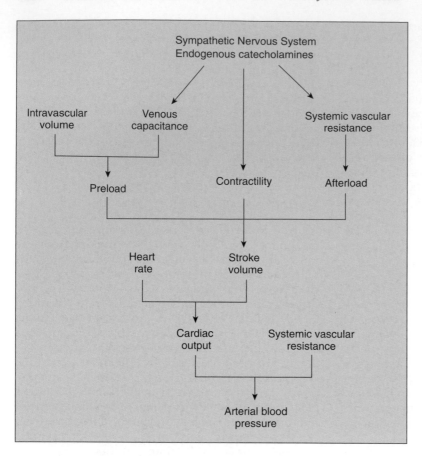

Figure 40–1

Determinants of cardiac output and arterial blood pressure. (From Witte MK, Hill JH, Blumer JL: Shock in the pediatric patient. Adv Pediatr 34:139-174, 1987.)

of vasoactive and inflammatory mediators are produced (or inhibited or both). Endotoxins, produced by bacteria, activate macrophage production of tumor necrosis factor and interleukin-1 in addition to the complement, kinin, fibrinolytic, and coagulation pathways. Endothelial injury causes release of cellular mediators of inflammation, such as cytokines (interleukin-6), bioactive lipids (platelet-activating factor and leukotrienes), interferons, and the products of primary and secondary leukocyte granules. Most secondary mediators decrease vascular tone and increase vascular permeability, resulting in maldistribution of blood flow. Arteriolar vasodilation (vasculopathy) results in reduced systemic vascular resistance, which serves to lower tissue perfusion pressure and impair coronary blood flow. The increased venous capacitance produced by venodilation results in venous stasis and decreased venous return to the heart (reduced preload). Mediator induced changes in vascular permeability cause capillary leaks and loss of intravascular volume, which impair ventricular filling and cardiac output. Activated complement components and arachidonic acid metabolites promote leukocyte and platelet aggregation in capillary beds, producing an obstruction to flow in the microcirculation. Vasculotoxins also directly depress cardiac output by decreasing intrinsic cardiac contractility or by inducing coronary vasospasm.

CARDIOGENIC SHOCK

Cardiogenic shock is caused by an abnormality in myocardial function and is expressed as depressed myocardial contractility and cardiac output with poor tissue perfusion. Compensatory mechanisms may contribute to the progression of shock by depressing cardiac function further. Neurohormonal vasoconstrictor responses increase afterload and add to the work of the failing ventricle. Tachycardia may impair coronary blood flow, which decreases myocardial oxygen delivery. Increased central blood volume caused by sodium and water retention and by incomplete emptying of the ventricles during systole results in elevated left ventricular volume and pressure, which impair subendocardial blood flow. As compensatory mechanisms are overcome, the failing left ventricle produces increased ventricular end-diastolic volume and pressure, which leads to increased left atrial pressure, resulting in pulmonary edema. This sequence also

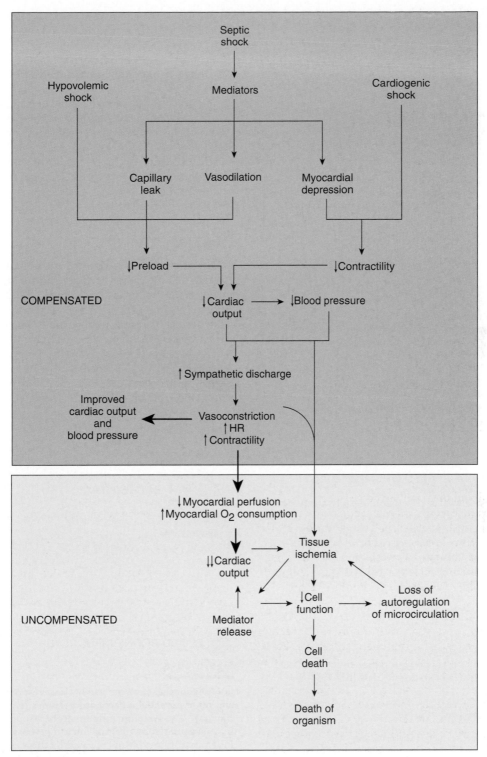

Figure 40-2

Sequence of pathophysiologic events in the clinical shock state. HR, heart rate. (From Witte MK, Hill JH, Blumer JL: Shock in the pediatric patient. Adv Pediatr 34:139-174, 1987.)

TABLE 40–1.   Definitions of Related Infectious and Shock States

Infection: Microbial phenomenon characterized by an inflammatory response to the presence of microorganisms or the invasion of normally sterile host tissue by those organisms

Bacteremia: The presence of viable bacteria in the blood

Systemic inflammatory response syndrome: The systemic inflammatory response to a variety of severe clinical insults. The response is manifested by two or more of the following conditions

   Temperature >38°C or <36°C
   Heart rate >90 beats/min*
   Respiratory rate >20 breaths/min* or PaCO₂
      <32 mm Hg
   WBC >12,000 cells/mm³, <4000 cells/mm³, or
      >10% immature (band) forms

Sepsis: The systemic response to infection. This systemic response is manifested by two or more of the following conditions as a result of infection

   Temperature >38°C or <36°C
   Heart rate >90 beats/min*
   Respiratory rate >20 breaths/min* or PaCO₂
      <32 mm Hg
   WBC >12,000 cells/mm³, <4000 cells/mm³, or
      >10% immature (band) forms

Severe sepsis: Sepsis associated with organ dysfunction, hypoperfusion, or hypotension. Hypoperfusion and perfusion abnormalities may include, but are not limited to, lactic acidosis, oliguria, or an acute alteration in mental status

Septic shock: Sepsis with hypotension, despite adequate fluid resuscitation, along with the presence of perfusion abnormalities that may include, but are not limited to, lactic acidosis, oliguria, or an acute alteration in mental status. Patients who are on inotropic or vasopressor agents may not be hypotensive at the time that perfusion abnormalities are measured

Hypotension: A systolic BP of <900 mm Hg* or a reduction of >40 mm Hg from baseline in the absence of other causes for hypotension.

Multiple organ dysfunction syndrome: Presence of altered organ function in an acutely ill patient such that homeostasis cannot be maintained without intervention

*Adults; must use age-appropriate norms.
BP, Blood pressure.
From American College of Chest Physicians/Society of Critical Care Medicine Consensus Conference: Definitions for sepsis and organ failure and guidelines for the use of innovative therapies in sepsis. Crit Care Med 20:864-874, 1992.

contributes to right ventricular failure because of increased pulmonary artery pressure and increased right ventricular afterload.

Primary cardiogenic shock may occur in children who have congenital heart disease. Heart failure precedes cardiogenic shock in most patients who have congenital heart disease (except hypoplastic left heart syndrome) and in patients who have circulatory obstruction (coarctation of the aorta or critical aortic stenosis [see Chapters 143 and 144]). Cardiogenic shock also may occur in previously healthy children secondary to viral myocarditis, dysrhythmias, or toxic or metabolic abnormalities or after hypoxic-ischemic injury (see Chapters 141, 142, 145, and 147).

OBSTRUCTIVE SHOCK

Obstructive shock results from the patient's inability to produce adequate cardiac output, despite normal intravascular volume and normal myocardial contractility. This inability occurs as a result of mechanical obstruction of ventricular outflow. The major cause is pericardial tamponade (see Chapter 148). Clinically, when trauma or previous heart surgery is involved, tamponade should be suspected when a patient has a narrow pulse pressure, a muffled heart tone, jugular vein distention, an enlarged heart as determined by per-

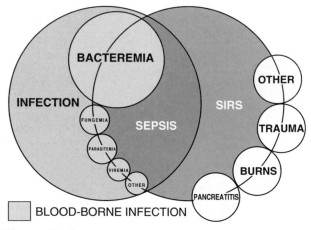

Figure 40–3

Interrelationship between various host responses to infections and other potential inflammatory injuries (e.g., burns or trauma). The systemic inflammatory response syndrome may be initiated by multiple inciting events; the inflammatory mediators released by these events initiate and perpetuate the systemic inflammatory response syndrome. (From American College of Chest Physicians/Society of Critical Care Medicine Consensus Conference: Definitions for sepsis and organ failure and guidelines for the use of innovative therapies in sepsis. Crit Care Med 20:864-874, 1992.)

cussion or radiograph, or pulseless electrical activity. Echocardiography may be diagnostic, but in symptomatic patients attempts at needle pericardiocentesis should not await confirmation by diagnostic studies.

DISSOCIATIVE SHOCK

Dissociative shock refers to conditions in which tissue perfusion is normal, but cells are unable to use oxygen because the hemoglobin has an abnormal affinity for oxygen, preventing its release to the tissues (Table 40–2).

CLINICAL MANIFESTATIONS

All forms of shock produce evidence that tissue perfusion and oxygenation are insufficient (increased heart rate, abnormal blood pressure, alterations of peripheral pulses). The etiology of shock may alter the initial presentation of these signs and symptoms.

Hypovolemic Shock

Hypovolemic shock is distinguished from other causes of shock by history and the absence of signs of heart failure (hepatomegaly, pulmonary crackles, edema, jugular venous distention, or a gallop) or sepsis (fever, leukocytosis, or focal infection). In addition to the signs of sympathoadrenal activity (tachycardia, vasoconstriction), clinical manifestations include signs of dehydration (dry mucous membranes, decreased urine output) or blood loss (pallor). Recovery depends on the degree of hypovolemia, the patient's preexisting status, and rapid diagnosis and treatment. The prognosis is good, with a low mortality (<10%) in uncomplicated cases.

Distributive Shock

Patients with distributive shock usually have tachycardia and alterations of peripheral perfusion. In early stages, when cytokine release results in vasodilation, pulses may be bounding, and vital organ function may be maintained (an alert patient, with rapid capillary refill and maintenance of some urine output in "warm shock"). Widespread cellular dysfunction, resulting from inadequate tissue perfusion in the early phases of shock, subsequently leads to diminishing organ function. As the disease progresses untreated, extremities become cool and mottled with a delayed capillary refill time. At this stage, the patient has hypotension and vasoconstriction. If the etiology of distributive shock is sepsis,

TABLE 40–2. Classification of Shock and Common Underlying Causes

Type	Primary Circulatory Derangement	Common Causes
Hypovolemic	Decreased circulating blood volume	Hemorrhage Diarrhea Diabetes insipidus Diabetes mellitus Burns Adrenogenital syndrome Capillary leak syndrome
Distributive	Vasodilation → venous pooling → decreased preload Maldistribution of regional blood flow	Sepsis Anaphylaxis CNS/spinal injury Drug intoxication
Cardiogenic	Decreased myocardial contractility	Congenital heart disease Severe heart failure Arrhythmia Hypoxic/ischemic injuries Cardiomyopathy Metabolic derangements Myocarditis Drug intoxication Kawasaki disease
Obstructive	Mechanical obstruction to ventricular outflow	Cardiac tamponade Massive pulmonary embolus Tension pneumothorax Cardiac tumor
Dissociative	Oxygen not released from hemoglobin	Carbon monoxide poisoning Methemoglobinemia

the patient often has fever, lethargy, petechiae, or purpura and may have an identifiable source of infection.

Cardiogenic Shock

Cardiogenic shock results when the myocardium is unable to supply the cardiac output required to support tissue perfusion and organ function. Because of this self-perpetuating cycle, congestive heart failure progressing to death may be rapid. Patients with cardiogenic shock have tachycardia and tachypnea. The liver is usually enlarged, a gallop is often present, and jugular venous distention may be noted. Because renal blood flow is poor, sodium and water are retained, resulting in oliguria and peripheral edema.

Obstructive Shock

Restriction of cardiac output results in an increase in heart rate and an alteration of stroke volume. The pulse pressure is narrow (making pulses harder to feel), and capillary refill is delayed. The liver is often enlarged, and jugular venous distention may be evident.

Dissociative Shock

The principal abnormality in dissociative shock is the inability to deliver oxygen to tissues. Symptoms include tachycardia, tachypnea, alterations in mental status, and ultimately cardiovascular collapse.

LABORATORY AND IMAGING STUDIES

Shock requires immediate resuscitation before obtaining laboratory or diagnostic studies. When initial stabilization has occurred (including a rapid blood glucose determination and treatment if hypoglycemia is present), the type of shock present dictates the necessary laboratory studies. All patients with shock may benefit from determination of a baseline arterial blood gas and blood lactate level to assess the impairment of tissue oxygenation. Measurement of **mixed venous oxygen saturation** aids in the assessment of the adequacy of oxygen delivery. In contrast to other forms of shock, patients with sepsis often have high mixed venous saturation values because of impairment of mitochondrial function and inability of tissues to extract oxygen. A complete blood count can potentially assess intravascular blood volume after equilibration following a hemorrhage. Electrolyte measurements in patients with hypovolemic shock may identify abnormalities from losses. Patients presenting in distributive shock require appropriate bacterial and viral cultures to identify a cause of infection. If cardiogenic or obstructive shock is suspected, an echocardiogram assists with the diagnosis and, in the case of tampon-

ade, assists with placement of a pericardial drain to relieve the fluid. Patients with dissociative shock require detection of the causative agent (carbon monoxide, methemoglobin). The management of shock also requires monitoring of arterial blood gases for oxygenation, ventilation (CO_2), and acidosis and frequently assessing the levels of serum electrolytes, calcium, magnesium, phosphorus, and BUN.

DIFFERENTIAL DIAGNOSIS

▶ SEE TABLE 40-2.

TREATMENT
General Principles

The key to therapy is the recognition of shock in its early, partially compensated state, when many of the hemodynamic and metabolic alterations may be reversible. Initial therapy for shock is directed largely at treating the signs and symptoms as they appear, rather than directly addressing the primary cause or mechanisms involved. Therapy should minimize cardiopulmonary work, while ensuring cardiac output, blood pressure, and gas exchange. Intubation combined with mechanical ventilation with 100% oxygen improves oxygenation and decreases or eliminates the work of breathing, but may impede venous return if distending airway pressures (PEEP or peak inspiratory pressure) (see Chapter 61) are excessive. Blood pressure support is crucial because the vasodilation in sepsis may reduce perfusion despite supranormal cardiac output.

Monitoring a critically ill child in shock requires maintaining access to the arterial and central venous circulation to record pressure measurements, perform blood sampling, and measure systemic blood pressure continuously. These measurements facilitate the estimation of preload and afterload. When knowing the patient's left atrial pressure is crucial, the pressure can be measured through a left atrial catheter connected to a pressure monitor or more often estimated by measuring pulmonary capillary wedge pressure with a flow-directed balloon-tip catheter. Directly measuring the cardiac index by thermodilution, injection of indocyanine green, or a Fick procedure also may be helpful.

Organ-Directed Therapeutics
Cardiovascular Support

In general, shock states are characterized by primary or secondary impairment of myocardial function. Efforts to improve cardiac output are a basic component of shock therapy. Cardiovascular therapy should be targeted at fluid resuscitation and at improvement of

TABLE 40–3. Intravenous Fluids Available for Pediatric Volume Resuscitation

Crystalloids

0.9% sodium chloride
Ringer's lactate
Hypertonic saline (3%)

Colloids

5% human serum albumin in 0.9% sodium chloride*
25% human serum albumin in 0.9% sodium chloride*
6% hydroxyethyl starch in 0.9% sodium chloride
10% dextran 40 in 5% dextrose in water
Fresh frozen plasma
Whole blood

*Albumin-containing solutions are being used less frequently because of concerns of infection and poor overall outcomes.

cardiac output, heart rate and rhythm, preload, afterload, and contractility.

Fluid Resuscitation

Alterations in preload have a dramatic effect on cardiac output. In hypovolemic and distributive shock, decreased preload significantly impairs cardiac output. In cardiogenic shock, an elevated preload contributes to pulmonary edema. Plasma volume may be restored successfully with the use of crystalloid solutions, provided that sufficient volumes are used, but edema fluid may accumulate (as a result of capillary leakage) if excessive amounts are infused (Table 40–3). This accumulation may be unavoidable and usually is associated with a good outcome. Colloids contain larger molecules that theoretically may stay in the intravascular space longer than crystalloid solutions and exert oncotic pressure and draw fluid out of the tissues into the vascular compartment.

Selection of fluids for resuscitation and ongoing use is dictated by clinical circumstances. Crystalloid volume expanders generally are recommended as initial choices because they are effective and inexpensive. Most acutely ill children with signs of shock may receive safely, and usually benefit greatly from, a 20-mL/kg bolus of an isotonic crystalloid over 15 to 30 minutes. This dose may need to be repeated until a response is noted. Care must be exercised, however, in treating cardiogenic shock with volume expansion because the ventricular filling pressures may rise without improvement of the cardiac performance. Carefully monitoring cardiac output or central venous pressure helps guide safe volume replacement. In patients with significant cerebral edema, the need to improve cardiac output by fluid replacement and the need to maintain an acceptable **cerebral perfusion pressure** (mean blood pressure – intracranial pressure) should be balanced by the requirement to reduce intracranial pressure; excessive fluid resuscitation may increase intracranial pressure, exacerbating cerebral edema. The restoration of blood pressure and cardiac output has the highest priority, however.

Cardiotonic and Vasodilator Therapy

In an effort to improve cardiac output after volume resuscitation or when further volume replacement may be dangerous, a variety of cardiotonic and vasodilator drugs may be useful (Table 40–4). Therapy is directed first at increasing myocardial contractility, then at decreasing left ventricular afterload. The hemodynamic status of the patient dictates the choice of the agent.

Therapy usually is initiated with dopamine at 3 to 15 µg/kg/min. The chronotropic and vasoconstrictor effects of dopamine often limit further dosing. In children who fail to respond to several increments of an initial pressor, a more potent cardiotonic agent, such as epinephrine or norepinephrine, may be indicated. In addition to improving contractility, certain catecholamines may cause an increase in systemic vascular resistance. The addition of a vasodilator drug may improve cardiac performance by decreasing the resistance against which the heart must pump (afterload). Afterload reduction may be achieved with dobutamine,

TABLE 40–4. Catecholamines Used for Cardiopulmonary Resuscitation and in Shock

	Positive Inotrope	Positive Chronotrope	Direct Pressor	Indirect Pressor	Vasodilator
Dopamine	++	+	±	++	++*
Dobutamine	++	±	–	–	+
Epinephrine	+++	+++	+++	–	–
Isoproterenol	+++	+++	–	–	+++
Norepinephrine	+++	+++	+++	–	–

*Primarily splanchnic and renal in low doses (3-5 µg/kg/min).

milrinone, isoproterenol, amrinone, nitroprusside, nitroglycerin, and angiotensin-converting enzyme inhibitors. The use of these drugs may be particularly important in late shock, when vasoconstriction is prominent.

Respiratory Support

The lung is a target organ for inflammatory mediators in shock and the systemic inflammatory response syndrome. Respiratory failure may develop rapidly and become progressive. Intervention requires endotracheal intubation and mechanical ventilation accompanied by the use of supplemental oxygen and PEEP. Severe cardiopulmonary failure may be managed with inhaled nitric oxide and, if needed, extracorporeal membrane oxygenation (see Chapter 61).

Renal Salvage

Poor cardiac output accompanied by decreased renal blood flow may cause prerenal azotemia and oliguria/anuria. Severe hypotension may produce **acute tubular necrosis** and **acute renal failure**. Prerenal azotemia is corrected when blood volume deficits are replaced or myocardial contractility is improved, but acute tubular necrosis does not improve immediately when shock is corrected. Prerenal azotemia is associated with a serum BUN-to-creatinine ratio of greater than 10 : 1 and a urine sodium level less than 20 mEq/L; acute tubular necrosis has a ratio of 10 : 1 and a urine sodium level between 40 and 60 mEq/L (see Chapter 165). Aggressive fluid replacement is often necessary to improve oliguria associated with prerenal azotemia. Because the management of shock requires administering large volumes of fluid (often >50 mL/kg during resuscitation), maintaining urine output greatly facilitates patient management.

Preventing acute tubular necrosis and the subsequent complications associated with acute renal failure (e.g., hyperkalemia, acidosis, hypocalcemia, edema) is an important goal. Using pharmacologic agents to augment urine output is indicated when the intravascular volume has been replaced. The use of loop diuretics, such as furosemide, or combinations of a loop diuretic and a thiazide agent may enhance urine output. Infusion of low-dose dopamine, which produces renal artery vasodilation, also may improve urine output. Nevertheless, if hyperkalemia, refractory acidosis, hypervolemia, or altered mental status associated with uremia occurs, dialysis or hemofiltration should be initiated.

COMPLICATIONS

Shock results in impairment of tissue perfusion and oxygenation and activation of inflammation and cytokine pathways. The major complication of shock is multiple organ system failure, defined as the dysfunction of more than one organ, including respiratory failure, renal failure, liver dysfunction, coagulation abnormalities, or cerebral dysfunction. Patients with shock and multiple organ failure have a higher mortality rate and, for survivors, a longer hospital stay.

PROGNOSIS

Early recognition and **goal-directed intervention** in patients with shock improve survival. Mortality rates for septic shock in children have decreased from greater than 90% in the 1960s to 8% to 9%. Specific mortality rates for other forms of shock are not readily available. Delays in treatment of hypotension increase the incidence of multiple organ failure and mortality, however. Goal-directed therapy focused on maintaining mixed venous oxygen saturation may improve survival.

PREVENTION

Prevention strategies for shock are focused for the most part on shock associated with sepsis and hypovolemia. Some forms of septic shock can be prevented through use of immunizations (*H. influenzae* type b, meningococcal, pneumococcal vaccines). Decreasing the risk of sepsis in a critically ill patient can be addressed through adherence to strict hand washing and isolation practices, minimizing the duration of indwelling catheters and the use of antibiotic-coated catheters. The appropriate use of prophylactic antibiotics (perioperative antibiotics) also may decrease the incidence of sepsis. Measures to decrease pediatric trauma do much to minimize hemorrhage-induced shock.

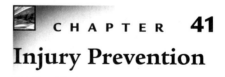

CHAPTER **41**

Injury Prevention

EPIDEMIOLOGY AND ETIOLOGY

Injury is the leading cause of death in children 1 to 18 years old. Approximately 50% of these deaths are caused by motor vehicle crashes. Most remaining injury-related deaths are the result of homicide/suicide (23%) and drowning (10%). Geography, climate, population density (access to care), and population traits vary by region and affect the frequency, etiology, and severity of injuries.

Injury prevention requires evaluation of factors that affect the **host** (e.g., child), the **agent** (e.g., drivers), and the **environment** (e.g., roadways, weather). The age and gender of the child often determine the exposure to various agents and environments. Most injuries in infants and toddlers occur in the home as the result of exposure to agents found there (e.g., hot water heaters, bathtubs, medications). As children expand their activities and environments, exposure to other agents and environments results in increased frequency in injuries secondary to motor vehicle crashes and drowning. Changes in the host, agent, and environment are in part responsible for homicides by firearms becoming the second most frequent cause of injury in adolescents. Boys are 10 times more likely to be injured in falls, motor vehicle crashes, and firearm injuries.

More than 50% of trauma fatalities occur at the scene of the injury rather than at a secondary site to which the victim may be transported. These scene deaths occur in patients who receive injuries to the brainstem, head, aorta, heart, and upper cervical spine. The next substantial group of deaths occurs within several hours of arrival in the emergency department; survival depends on the severity of shock at the time of arrival and the length of time shock has been present. If the patient is taken to a center at which definitive care can be provided and is stabilized within 1 hour of the time of the injury, the outcome is likely to be optimal. A final peak in mortality occurs days to weeks after the initial injury and results from multisystem organ failure or other severe, life-threatening complications that have not responded to medical and surgical management.

EDUCATION FOR PREVENTING INJURIES

The recognition that much morbidity and mortality are determined at the scene of an injury has stimulated the development of prevention measures. The **Haddon matrix** combines the epidemiologic components (host, agent, physical and social environments) with time factors (before, during, or after the event) to identify effective interventions focused on different aspects of the injury event. Primary strategies (preventing the event), secondary strategies (minimizing the severity of injury), and tertiary strategies (interventions that are effective in minimizing long-term impact) can be targeted for each epidemiologic component. Such strategies typically fall into one of three areas: education, enforcement, and environment (including engineering). Education is often the first strategy considered, but requires behavioral change and actions on the part of people. Most educational strategies (requiring action or behavioral change) are not well evaluated. Despite the reliance on an action by the individuals involved, some active strategies benefit from enforce-

ment and result in decreased injuries. Children wearing bicycle helmets experience a significantly lower incidence of traumatic brain injury and death. Enforcement of seatbelt laws increases seatbelt use and may decrease injuries. Automatic strategies require no action on the part of the population and are most often found in strategies that change the environment (speed bumps) or engineering (child-resistant pill bottles, air bags). Automatic strategies have more consistently resulted in a significant reduction in injuries (modifications of automobiles and highways to reduce injuries in motor vehicle crashes). The most successful approaches to preventing injury have combined strategies (education, environmental changes, and engineering changes focused on the host, agent, and environment in all three time phases).

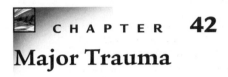

CHAPTER 42
Major Trauma

ASSESSMENT AND RESUSCITATION

Trauma care begins at the scene of the injury with a rapid assessment of the ABCs and initiation of basic or advanced life support interventions. The scope of care provided in the field is determined by the nature of the injured child's physiologic state and associated injuries, the anticipated transit time to the hospital, and the skill level or scope of practice of the prehospital care providers. The general goal of **prehospital trauma care** is rapid assessment, support of the ABCs, immobilization, and transportation. Prehospital care providers, with the assistance of protocols and on-line medical direction, must also determine which injured children require transport to a trauma center (Table 42–1). Numerous **trauma triage scoring** tools have been developed to assist the evaluation of injury severity, trauma center triage decision making, and patient prognosis (Table 42–2).

On arrival to the emergency department, the trauma team must initiate an organized and synchronized response. The initial assessment of a seriously injured child should involve a systematic approach including a primary survey, resuscitation, secondary survey, postresuscitation monitoring, and definitive care. The **primary survey** focuses on the **ABCDEs** of emergency care, as modified for trauma from the ABCs of cardiopulmonary resuscitation (see Chapter 38). The assessment of the airway and breathing components should include meticulous control of the cervical spine (especially if the patient has an altered mental status), evaluation for anatomic injuries that would impair air

TABLE 42–1. Children Requiring Pediatric Trauma Center Care

Patients with serious injury to more than one organ or system

Patients with one-system injury who require critical care or monitoring in an intensive care unit

Patients with signs of shock who require more than one transfusion

Patients with fracture complicated by suspected neurovascular or compartment injury

Patients with fracture of axial skeleton

Patients with two or more long-bone fractures

Patients with potential replantation of an extremity

Patients with suspected or actual spinal cord or column injuries

Patients with head injury with any one of the following:
  Orbital or facial bone fracture
  CSF leaks
  Altered state of consciousness
  Changing neural signs
  Open head injuries
  Depressed skull fracture
  Requiring intracranial pressure monitoring

Patients suspected of requiring ventilator support

entry or gas exchange, and consideration of the likelihood of a full stomach (risk of aspiration pneumonia). Circulation can be assessed via observation (heart rate, skin color, mental status) and palpation (pulse quality, capillary refill, skin temperature) and restored while control of bleeding is accomplished through the use of direct pressure or careful use of extremity tourniquets. Assessment for **disabilities** (D), including neurologic status, includes two components: (1) examination of pupil size and reactivity and (2) a brief mental status assessment (*AVPU—a*lert; responds to *v*oice; responds to *p*ain; *u*nresponsive). The **Glasgow Coma Scales** can

direct decisions regarding the initiation of cerebral resuscitation (hyperventilation or osmolar therapy for increased intracranial pressure) in patients with suspected closed head injuries (Table 42–3). Head injury is present in 80% of all patients with multiple traumas, and in 60% of pediatric cases the head is the most severely affected part of the body. **E,** for *exposure,* reminds the team to perform a full assessment of the patient, by completely disrobing the child so that the entire body can be examined in detail. The examiner should ensure a neutral thermal environment to prevent hypothermia.

On completion of the primary survey, a more detailed head-to-toe examination (the **secondary survey**) should ensue. The purpose of this careful re-examination is to identify life-threatening and limb-threatening injuries and less serious injuries. Coincident with the secondary survey and depending, in part, on the assessed physiologic status of the patient, certain procedures and resuscitative measures (large-bore vascular access, fluid therapy) are initiated. The prioritization of definitive care needs is determined by the injury findings collected from the primary and secondary surveys, the child's physiologic response to resuscitative care, and data from continuous monitoring.

ETIOLOGY AND EPIDEMIOLOGY

▶ SEE CHAPTER 41.

LABORATORY AND IMAGING STUDIES

Screening laboratory studies during initial resuscitation often include the tests found in Table 42–4. Obtaining an arterial blood gas, serum lactate, base deficit, and mixed venous oxygen saturation assists in determining adequacy of resuscitation in many

TABLE 42–2. Pediatric Trauma Score*

Category Component	+2	+1	−1
Size	>20 kg	10-20 kg	<10 kg
Airway	Normal	Maintainable	Unmaintainable
Systolic BP†	>90 mm Hg	50-90 mm Hg	<50 mm Hg
CNS	Awake	Obtunded/LOC	Coma/decerebrate
Skeletal	None	Closed fracture	Open/multiple fractures
Cutaneous/wounds	None	Minor	Major/penetrating

*If score <8, refer to Pediatric Trauma Center.
†If proper size BP cuff is not available
+2, palpable pulse at wrist; +1, palpable pulse at groin; −1, no palpable pulse; BP, blood pressure; LOC, loss of consciousness.
Modified from Tepas JJ 3rd, Mollitt DL, Talbert JL, Bryant M: The pediatric trauma score as a predictor of injury severity in the injured child. J Pediatr Surg 22:14-18, 1987.

TABLE 42–3. Glasgow Coma Scales

Glasgow Coma Scale			Modified Coma Scale for Infants		
Activity	Best Response	Score	Activity	Best Response	Score
Eye opening	Spontaneous	4	Eye opening	Spontaneous	4
	To verbal stimuli	3		To speech	3
	To pain	2		To pain	2
	None	1		None	1
Verbal	Oriented	5	Verbal	Coos, babbles	5
	Confused	4		Irritable, cries	4
	Inappropriate words	3		Cries to pain	3
	Nonspecific sounds	2		Moans to pain	2
	None	1		None	1
Motor	Follows commands	6	Motor	Spontaneous movements	6
	Localizes pain	5		Withdraws to touch	5
	Withdraws to pain	4		Withdraws to pain	4
	Flexion to pain	3		Abnormal flexion	3
	Extension to pain	2		Abnormal extension	2
	None	1		None	1

patients. Radiographic studies are determined by the pattern of injuries. Patients with obvious injury to the thorax or abdomen or who have pulmonary or abdominal symptoms may benefit from a CT scan. A spiral enhanced CT scan should be performed if there is concern about aortic injuries.

TABLE 42–4. Initial Laboratory Evaluation of the Major Trauma Patient

Hematology

Complete blood count
Platelet count
Type and cross-match

Urinalysis

Gross
Microscopic

Clinical Chemistry

Amylase
AST/ALT

Radiology

Cervical spine films
Anteroposterior chest radiograph
Radiographs of all apparent fractures
CT scans where indicated for head, chest, and abdominal trauma

AST/ALT, aspartate aminotransferase/alanine aminotransferase.

CLINICAL MANIFESTATIONS AND TREATMENT
Specific Organ Injuries

After the initial evaluation and stabilization, the team focuses on the involved organ systems. Head injuries and injuries to the limbs are the most common and may require immediate intervention to avoid long-term disability. Isolated injuries to most organ systems (e.g., thorax, abdomen) are associated with low mortality rates, but when present in combination, especially with head injuries, the mortality rate increases. Trauma requiring immediate surgical intervention includes injuries to the chest and mediastinum (with the exception of pulmonary contusion) and limb-threatening injuries. Fractures contribute most to the long-term morbidity associated with multiple trauma and, if inappropriately assessed, may lead to loss of limb or life. The failure rate in the diagnosis of significant fractures is approximately 12% at the time of injury.

Head Trauma

▶ SEE CHAPTER 184.

Abdominal Trauma

Injury to the abdomen occurs in approximately 8% of pediatric trauma patients. The relative size and closer proximity of intra-abdominal organs in children increase their risk of significant injury after blunt

TABLE 42–5. Criteria for a Positive Paracentesis
Free aspiration ≥10 mL gross blood
Turbid or bloody fluid that prevents reading newsprint
Free egress through indwelling urinary catheter or chest tube
Presence of >500 WBC/mL or >100,000 RBC/mL
Amylase >175 U/mL
Presence of gross stool or food debris

trauma. Penetrating trauma, which accounts for less than 10% of pediatric abdominal trauma, may result in a child who is asymptomatic or who presents in hypovolemic shock. Gunshot wounds to the abdomen involve multiple organs in 80% of cases.

Performing serial physical examinations is the primary method of obtaining information on which to base decisions regarding operative intervention. Operative intervention may be required in patients whose vital signs are persistently unstable in the face of aggressive fluid resuscitation, even in the absence of extravascular volume loss or an enlarging abdomen. The presence of peritoneal irritation or abdominal wall discoloration, together with signs of intravascular volume loss, indicates the need for laparotomy.

Abdominal CT is invaluable for assessing hemodynamically stable children with intra-abdominal trauma. Operative exploration is based on CT and physical findings and may be indicated when peritoneal irritation, hypovolemia, free air on plain film, or positive results of paracentesis (Table 42–5) are present.

Injury to the Spleen

The most frequently injured abdominal organ in children is the spleen. A positive *Kehr sign* (pressure on the left upper quadrant eliciting left shoulder pain) is due to diaphragmatic irritation by the ruptured spleen and strongly suggests splenic injury. Suspicion of a splenic injury should be heightened if there are left upper quadrant abrasions or tenderness. CT scans are used to grade splenic injury from 1 to 5 (grade 1, capsular tear or nonexpanding subcapsular hemorrhage, to grade 5, completely ruptured spleen).

Nonoperative management is the treatment of choice for most serious splenic injuries. Surgery may be indicated for patients who have an estimated blood loss greater than 40 mL/kg of transfused blood in 24 to 36 hours or evidence of hemodynamic instability. The operative approach often involves repair of the lesion rather than removal of the spleen. If a splenectomy is performed, patients should receive penicillin prophylaxis and should receive pneumococcal and

H. influenzae vaccines to lower the increased risk of overwhelming sepsis in asplenic patients.

Liver Trauma

Major trauma to the liver is a serious cause of morbidity and accounts for 40% of all deaths associated with blunt abdominal trauma in children. The right lobe of the liver is injured more frequently than the left, and the clinical diagnosis usually is based on the presence of pain in the right shoulder or right upper quadrant (Kehr sign). Severe hemorrhage is more common in patients with liver injury than with other abdominal injuries because of its dual blood supply. The site of the traumatic lesion may determine its severity. Subcapsular hematomas are less serious than capsular tears, which are less serious than minor or deep lacerations. Burst injuries, with or without major vascular injury, are the most severe of all traumatic injuries to the liver and almost invariably are fatal. For most children who have liver trauma, conservative management is recommended. This management involves admission to an ICU and the monitoring of ongoing blood loss, hepatic function, and liver structure with serial CT scans or ultrasound examinations. Operative management should be reserved for life-threatening situations.

Renal Injury

The kidney commonly is injured by blunt abdominal trauma, and more than 40% of children with injured kidneys have other internal injuries. A young child's kidney is more vulnerable to trauma than an adult's because of its anterior position in the peritoneal cavity, a more compliant rib cage, and relatively immature abdominal muscle development. The diagnosis of renal injury is based on history and physical examination, coupled with urinalysis showing blood and increased protein levels. An intravenous pyelogram may be diagnostic; however, CT scans with renal contrast also are useful. In more than 80% of children with positive intravenous pyelogram results, simple monitoring only is required. In the remaining patients, surgery usually is indicated for falling hemoglobin levels, refractory shock, or urinary obstruction caused by clots.

Injuries of the Pancreas and Duodenum

Injuries of the pancreas are less common in children than in adults but are seen in bicycle handlebar injuries, motor vehicle crashes, and nonaccidental trauma. The diagnosis is difficult unless there is obvious injury to overlying structures, such as the stomach or duodenum. Diffuse abdominal tenderness, pain, and vomiting may be accompanied by elevations of amylase and lipase, but may not occur until several days after the injury. Hemodynamic instability secondary to retro-peritoneal hemorrhage may be the presenting sign. In the management of these patients, nasogastric suction and parenteral nutrition are indicated. Nonoperative management is appropriate for contusions, but surgical intervention may be required in patients with distal transection. Drainage of pseudocysts in patients who develop them may be required if they are unresponsive to bowel rest and parenteral nutrition.

Duodenal injuries include hematomas and perforation. Duodenal hematomas result from blunt injury to the abdomen and often present with persistent pain and bilious emesis. Most hematomas respond to non-operative management with gastric decompression and parenteral nutrition. Perforations are difficult to diagnose. Amylase and lipase elevations or persistent abdominal pain may suggest perforation of a viscus. Perforation is not always obvious on CT. A high index of suspicion and CT findings of free fluid without evidence of other solid organ injury support an exploratory laparotomy for investigation.

Intestinal Injury

Injury to the intestine occurs less frequently than injury to solid intra-abdominal organs. The risk of intestinal injury varies with the amount of intestinal contents. A full bowel is likely to shear more easily than an empty bowel, and the shearing occurs at points of fixation (the ligament of Treitz, the ileocecal valve, and the ascending and descending peritoneal reflections). Use of a lap belt or seatbelt in motor vehicle crashes results in a sudden deceleration and increase in intra-luminal pressure and can result in perforation or transection of the intestine. The diagnosis should be pursued in patients with contusions over the seatbelt area and pain in the abdomen or back or both. Pneumo-peritoneum that exists in association with intestinal perforation occurs in only 20% of patients. This diagnosis can be missed by CT and often is established by paracentesis that is positive for bowel contents. Prompt surgical intervention is required.

COMPLICATIONS

Patients requiring hospitalization for multiple trauma are at risk for a variety of complications based on the type and severity of injury. Sepsis and multiple organ failure may occur in children with multiple trauma. Delays in enteral nutrition because of an ileus may increase further the risk of sepsis secondary to trans-location of bacteria across the intestinal mucosa.

Renal failure secondary to myoglobinuria may be seen in children who sustain crushing or electrical injuries and burns. Deep venous thrombosis is unusual in the pediatric population, but prophylaxis for older

children (>14 years old) who will be immobilized because of injury is often provided.

PROGNOSIS

Injuries are the largest cause of morbidity and mortality in children, accounting for more than 60% of deaths in children 1 to 19 years old. Mortality rates for head-injured patients range from 6% to 16%, with younger children with head injuries having higher mortality rates. Isolated thoracic injury has a mortality rate of 5%, which increases to 25% if there is a concurrent head or abdominal injury. Penetrating trauma accounts for 5% to 15% of trauma seen in an emergency department. Firearm penetrating injuries have significant mortality, with 30% of victims dying in the field and another 12% in the emergency department. Morbidities are numerous and include hypoxic-ischemic brain injury, loss of limbs, and psychological dysfunction.

PREVENTION

▶ SEE CHAPTER 41.

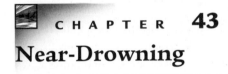

CHAPTER 43
Near-Drowning

ETIOLOGY

Drowning, by definition, is fatal; near-drowning is sometimes fatal. Drowning has been defined as a death resulting from suffocation within 24 hours of submersion in water; victims of near-drowning survive for at least 24 hours. Submersion of a child results in panic and aspiration of small amounts of fluid into the larynx triggering breath holding or laryngospasm. After relief of laryngospasm, the child aspirates large volumes of water into the lungs, destroying surfactant and causing alveolitis and dysfunction of the alveolar-capillary gas exchange. The resulting hypoxemia leads to hypoxic brain injury that is exacerbated by ischemic injury after circulatory collapse.

EPIDEMIOLOGY

Drowning is the third leading cause of death for children 1 to 18 years old. Boys are 10 times as likely as girls to die from drowning. Boys younger than age 4 and age 15 and 19 have the highest rate of drowning (>3/100,000). Most drowning in the U.S. occurs in freshwater; most infants drown in bathtubs. It is estimated that for every child who drowns, four children are hospitalized for near-drowning. Near-drowning victims who are coma-tose on admission but survive often develop significant neurologic impairment.

CLINICAL MANIFESTATIONS

Hypoxemia is the result of laryngospasm and aspiration during drowning. Victims may also develop respiratory distress secondary to **pulmonary endothelial injury**, **increased capillary permeability**, and **destruction of surfactant**. This respiratory distress results in further atelectasis and increases ventilation-perfusion mismatch. Clinical manifestations include tachypnea, tachycardia, increased work of breathing, and decreased breath sounds with or without crackles. The hypoxic-ischemic injury that may occur can lead to depressed myocardial function, resulting in tachycardia, impaired perfusion, and potentially cardiovascular collapse. After resuscitation, ARDS is common. Depression of cerebral function occurs when circulation to the brain is impaired. Altered mental status may be present and requires frequent monitoring of neurologic status. Hypothermia may coincide with drowning that occurs in cold bodies of water. Hypothermia may result in relative bradycardia and hypotension and place the child at risk for cardiac dysrhythmias.

LABORATORY AND IMAGING STUDIES

After resuscitation, an arterial blood gas assists in assessing pulmonary gas exchange. Serial blood gases should be obtained for victims with compromised respiratory or neurologic function. A chemistry profile may reveal elevated liver functions if hypoxemia and ischemia were of long duration and provide baseline renal functions. Electrolytes are often obtained, although alterations of serum electrolytes are minimal, even in freshwater drowning.

TREATMENT

Resuscitation of a near-drowning victim includes the basic ABCs. Emesis is common during resuscitation, requiring careful attention to prevent further aspiration. Victims of unwitnessed submersions require stabilization of the cervical spine because of the possibility of a fall or diving injury. Optimizing oxygenation and maintaining cerebral perfusion are two of the major foci of treatment. Rewarming the hypothermic patient requires careful attention to detail, including acid-base and cardiac status. Further treatment is based on the patient response to initial resuscitation. Some children begin breathing spontaneously and awaken before arrival at an emergency department. If submersion was significant, these children still require careful observation for pulmonary complications over the subsequent 6 to 12 hours. Children who have evidence of lung

injury, cardiovascular compromise, or neurologic compromise must be admitted to an ICU. Pulmonary dysfunction often results in hypoxemia. Oxygen supplementation should be implemented to maintain normal oxygen saturations. Mechanical ventilation may be needed to maintain oxygenation and ventilation in patients with significant pulmonary or neurologic dysfunction. Cardiovascular compromise is often the result of impaired contractility owing to hypoxic-ischemic injury. Fluid resuscitation and use of vasoactive pressors are useful in the maintenance of adequate tissue perfusion. The use of intracranial pressure monitoring devices and medical management with hypothermia and sedation is controversial; data to support improved outcomes are lacking. Use of ventilator strategies and cardiac support aimed at minimizing secondary brain injury may be beneficial. Prophylactic antibiotics have not been shown to be beneficial and may increase the selection of resistant organisms.

PROGNOSIS

The outcome of a near-drowning event is determined by the severity of the **hypoxic-ischemic injury** to the brain. Unfavorable prognostic markers for victims of near-drowning episodes include three or more of the following: age younger than 3 years, submersion time of more than 5 minutes, greater than 10-minute delay in resuscitation efforts, coma on admission to emergency department, and pH less than 7.10.

PREVENTION

Despite the decreased incidence of drowning since the 1990s, few prevention strategies have been shown to be effective. Exceptions include implementation of mandatory four-sided fencing around pools (decreased the number of children <5 years old who drown) and immediate provision of CPR to children who are submerged. The use of safety flotation devices in older children during water sport activities may be beneficial. Enhanced supervision is required to reduce the incidence of infants drowning in bathtubs.

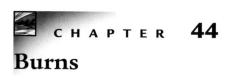

CHAPTER 44

Burns

ETIOLOGY

The pathophysiology of burn injury is caused by disruption of the three key functions of the skin: regulation of heat loss, preservation of body fluids, and barrier to infection. Burn injury releases inflammatory and vasoactive mediators and promotes many hemo-dynamic changes, including increased capillary per-meability, decreased plasma volume, and decreased cardiac output. Shock is common in children with burns that involve more than 10% to 12% of the total body surface area. For treatment of severe burns, admission to a qualified burn center is necessary. Burns usually are classified on the basis of four criteria:

1. Depth of injury
2. Percent of body surface area involved
3. Location of the burn
4. Association with other injuries

EPIDEMIOLOGY

Nearly 1% (>400,000) of all children sustain a burn injury each year. More than 25,000 require hospitaliza-tion, and more than 800 children 1 to 14 years old die each year. Boys are more likely to sustain a burn injury, with the highest rate of injury in boys younger than 5 years old. African American, Native American, and Hispanic children are at greater risk than white children.

Most fire-related childhood deaths and injuries occur in homes without working smoke detectors. Mortality is primarily associated with burn severity (extent of body surface area and depth), although the presence of inhalation injury and young age also predict mortality. The upper extremities are the areas most frequently involved in burns (71% of cases), fol-lowed by the head and neck (52%). Scalding injuries are most common and inhalation injuries least common in pediatric patients.

CLINICAL MANIFESTATIONS

The depth of injury should be assessed by the clinical appearance. **First-degree burns** are red, painful, and dry. These burns are superficial, with damage limited to the epidermis. They are commonly seen with sun exposure or with mild, hot solid or scald injuries. They heal in 3 to 6 days without scarring. First-degree burns are not included in burn surface area calculations. **Second-degree**, or partial-thickness, burns may be superficial (red, painful, mottled, blistered) and heal in 10 to 21 days with little or no scarring or deep dermal (pale, painful, and yellow), taking 3 weeks to heal and possibly resulting in scarring. They may result from immersion or flames. **Third-degree burns** are full thickness and require grafts if they are more than 1 cm in diameter. They are avascular and are characterized by coagulation necrosis. **Fourth-degree burns** involve underlying fascia, muscle, or bone.

A severe burn covers greater than 15% of the body surface area or involves the face or perineum. Second-

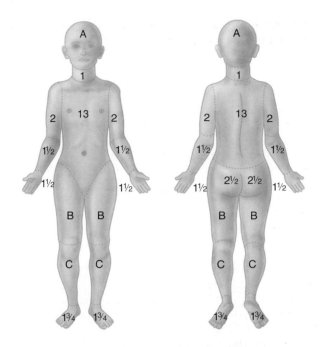

PERCENTAGE OF SURFACE AREA OF HEAD AND LEGS AT VARIOUS AGES

	AGE IN YEARS				
AREA IN DIAGRAM	0	1	5	10	15
A = ½ of head	9½	8½	6½	5½	4½
B = ½ of one thigh	2¾	3¼	4	4¼	4½
C = ½ of one lower leg	2½	2½	2¾	3	3¼

Figure 44–1

This chart of body areas, together with the table inserted in the figure showing the percentage of surface area of head and legs at various ages, can be used to estimate the surface area burned in a child. (From Solomon JR: Pediatric burns. Crit Care Clin 1:159-174, 1985.)

degree and third-degree burns of the hands or feet and circumferential burns of the extremities also are classi-fied as severe. **Inhalation injuries** resulting in bron-chospasm and impaired pulmonary function also must be considered severe burns. A method for estimating the percentage of skin surface area involved in burns in children of various ages is presented in Figure 44–1. The extent of skin involvement of older adolescent and adult patients is estimated as follows: each upper extremity, 9%; each lower extremity, 18%; anterior trunk, 18%; posterior trunk, 18%; head, 9%; and per-ineum, 1%.

The location of the burn is important in assessing the risk for disability. The risk is greatest when the face, eyes, ears, feet, perineum, or hands are involved. With partial-thickness burns, generally no disability results; however, full-thickness burns usually result in per-manent impairment. Inhalation injuries not only cause respiratory compromise, but also may result in difficulty in eating and drinking. Inhalation injuries also may be associated with burns of the face and neck.

LABORATORY AND IMAGING STUDIES

Most burn patients do not require immediate routine laboratory testing or imaging. A **carboxyhemoglobin** assessment should be performed for any suspected inhalation exposure (a house or closed-space fire or a burn victim who requires CPR). Cyanide levels should be considered in children who sustain smoke inhalation and have altered mental status. Unusual patterns of burns may increase suspicion of child abuse and result in appropriate evaluation to rule out nonaccidental trauma to the skeleton or CNS.

TREATMENT

The triage decision is based on (1) extent of the burn, (2) body surface area involved, (3) type of burn, (4) associated injuries, (5) any complicating medical or social problems, and (6) availability of ambulatory management (Fig. 44–2). The goal of initial treatment is to stop the burning process; this includes removing the patient from the site of injury, cleansing away any chemical or injurious contactants, and removing the clothing. The next priority is airway management; the upper airway is susceptible to burn injury, whereas the subglottic space seems to be protected. Few signs of injury may be present initially, although facial burns, singed nasal hairs or eyebrows, and acute inflammation of the oropharynx suggest inhalation injury. Smoke inhalation may be associated with carbon monoxide toxicity; 100% humidified oxygen should be given if hypoxia or inhalation is suspected. Hoarseness on vocalization also is consistent with a supraglottic injury. Some children with inhalation burns require endoscopy, an artificial airway, and mechanical ventilation.

The **systemic capillary leak** that occurs after a serious burn makes initial fluid and electrolyte support of a burned child crucial. The first priority is to support the circulating blood volume, which requires the administration of IV fluids to provide maintenance fluid and electrolyte requirements and to replace ongoing burn-related losses. No formula accurately predicts the fluid needs of every burn patient. Children with a significant burn should receive a rapid bolus of 20 mL/kg of lactated Ringer solution. The resuscitation formula for fluid therapy must provide replacement fluid and maintenance fluid and is determined by the percent of body surface burned. Total fluids are 2 to 4 mL/kg/percent burn/24 hr with half the estimated burn requirement administered during the first 8 hours. (If resuscitation is delayed, half of the fluid replacement should be completed by the end of the 8th hour postinjury). The goal of this fluid replacement is maintenance of equal to or greater than 1 mL/kg/hr of urine output. Fluids should be titrated to accomplish this goal. During the second 24 hours, dextrose in 0.25 normal saline is substituted for this regimen. Controversy exists over whether and when to administer colloid during fluid resuscitation. Colloid therapy may be needed for burns covering more than 30% of body surface area and may be provided after 24 hours of successful resuscitation with crystalloids.

Because burn injury produces a **hypermetabolic** response, children with significant burns require immediate nutritional support. Although enteral feeding may be resumed on day 2 or 3 of therapy, children with critical burn injury may require parenteral nutrition if unable to tolerate full enteral feeds. The hypermetabolic state can be modulated to a degree through the effective management of anxiety and pain (with sedation and analgesia) and the prevention of hypothermia by maintenance of a neutral thermal environment.

Wound care requires careful surgical management. Initial management includes relief of any pressure on peripheral circulation caused by eschar and débridement to allow classification of burns. Coverage with topical agents aids pain control and decreases insensible losses. Burns generally are covered with silver sulfadiazine (1%) applied to fine-mesh gauze or, if the burn is shallow, with polymyxin B/bacitracin/ neomycin (Neosporin) ointment. Silver nitrate (0.5%) and 11.1% mafenide acetate (which is painful, produces metabolic acidosis, and penetrates eschar) are alternative antimicrobial agents. These agents inhibit but do not prevent bacterial growth. Various grafts, such as cadaver allografts, porcine xenografts, artificial bilaminate (cross-linked chondroitin-6-sulfate and silicone) skin substitute, and cultured patient's keratinocytes, have been used initially to cover wounds. For full-thickness burns, skin autografting and artificial skin substitutes are required for eventual closure. Burn management and rehabilitation are highly specialized skills, involving the recognition of many complications of burns (Table 44-1) and evaluation of the wound and its cause for suspected child abuse or neglect. Tetanus toxoid should be provided for patients with incomplete immunization status; immune globulin is indicated in the nonimmunized patient.

COMPLICATIONS

▶ SEE TABLE 44—1.

PROGNOSIS

Most children who sustain burns recover without significant disability; however, 1300 to 1500 children die from burn injuries, making deaths from burns the

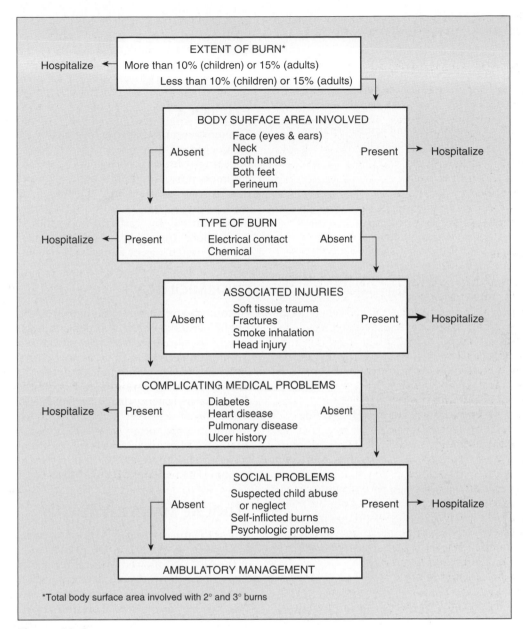

Figure 44–2

Triage of the burned patient. Additional considerations for hospitalization include involvement of major joints, third-degree burns of greater than 5%, and poor guardianship at home regarding wound care. (From Wachtel TL: Epidemiology, classification, initial care, and administrative considerations for critically burned patients. Crit Care Clin 1:3-26, 1985.)

TABLE 44–1. Complications of Burns

Problem	Treatment
Sepsis	Monitor for infection, avoid prophylactic antibiotics
Hypovolemia	Fluid replacement
Hypothermia	Adjust ambient temperature: dry blankets in field
Laryngeal edema	Endotracheal intubation, tracheostomy
Carbon monoxide poisoning	100% oxygen, hyperbaric O_2
Cyanide poisoning	100% O_2 plus amyl nitrate, sodium nitrate, and sodium thiosulfate
Cardiac dysfunction	Inotropic agents, diuretics
Gastric ulcers	H_2-receptor antagonist, antacids
Compartment syndrome	Escharotomy incision
Contractures	Physical therapy
Hypermetabolic state	Enteral and parenteral nutritional support
Renal failure	Supportive care, dialysis
Transient antidiuresis	Expectant management
Anemia	Transfusions as indicated
Psychological trauma	Psychological rehabilitation
Pulmonary infiltrates	PEEP, ventilation, O_2
Pulmonary edema	Avoid overhydration, give diuretics
Pneumonia	Antibiotics
Bronchospasm	β-agonist aerosols

PEEP, positive end-expiratory pressure.

third leading cause of injury-related pediatric deaths. Estimation of morbidity from burns is difficult to ascertain from databases. Physical scarring and emotional impact of disfiguring burns are long-term consequences of burn injuries.

PREVENTION

More than 600,000 children sustain burns each year; 92% occur in the home. Prevention is possible by using smoke and fire alarms, having identifiable escape routes and a fire extinguisher, and reducing hot water temperature to 49°C (120°F). Immersion full-thickness burns develop after 1 second at 70°C (158°F), after 5 seconds at 60°C (140°F), after 30 seconds at 54.5°C (130°F), after 60 seconds at 53°C (127°F), after 5 minutes at 50°C (122°F), and after 10 minutes at 49°C (120°F).

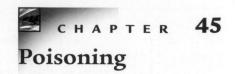

CHAPTER 45

Poisoning

ETIOLOGY

The most common agents ingested by young children include family members' medications, cleaning or polishing solutions, plants, and cosmetics. The most common poisonings that lead to hospitalization are due to acetaminophen, lead, and antidepressant medications. Fatal childhood poisonings are commonly caused by carbon monoxide, hydrocarbons, medications (iron, cardiovascular drugs, cyclic antidepressants), drugs of abuse, and caustic ingestions.

EPIDEMIOLOGY

Poisoning and ingestions account for more than 130,000 visits to emergency departments and approximately 1% of all pediatric hospitalizations each year. Unintentional ingestions are most common in the 1- to 5-year-old age group, an incidence that reveals the inquisitiveness of young children and the carelessness of adults in leaving drugs and household chemicals within reach. In older children, drug overdoses (poisonings) most often are associated with suicide attempts. Most ingestions are unintentional (88%), occur in the home (92%), and produce no (82%) or minor (17%) toxicity; 0.01% are fatal.

CLINICAL MANIFESTATIONS

Unless the ingested drug is revealed, poisoning is often a diagnosis of exclusion. On presentation, assessment of the ABCs is followed by careful examination for evidence of ingestion. A comatose child should be considered to have ingested a poison until proved otherwise. The history and physical examination by someone who understands the signs and symptoms of various ingestions often provide sufficient clues to distinguish between toxic ingestion and organic disease (Table 45–1). Because the comatose patient's history and physical examination may be unrevealing, using the toxicology laboratory to obtain information is often helpful.

HISTORY

A thorough and thoughtful history is a key component in the evaluation of a child with possible poisoning. Determination of all substances that the child was exposed to, type of medication, amount of medication, and time of exposure is crucial in directing interventions. Available data often are incomplete or

TABLE 45–1. Historical and Physical Findings in Poisoning

Odor

Bitter almonds	Cyanide
Acetone	Isopropyl alcohol, methanol, paraldehyde, salicylate
Alcohol	Ethanol
Wintergreen	Methyl salicylate
Garlic	Arsenic, thallium, organophosphates
Violets	Turpentine

Ocular Signs

Miosis	Narcotics (except meperidine), organophosphates, muscarinic mushrooms, clonidine, phenothiazines, chloral hydrate, barbiturates (late), PCP
Mydriasis	Atropine, alcohol, cocaine, amphetamines, antihistamines, cyclic antidepressants, cyanide, carbon monoxide
Nystagmus	Phenytoin, barbiturates, ethanol, carbon monoxide
Lacrimation	Organophosphates, irritant gas or vapors
Retinal hyperemia	Methanol
Poor vision	Methanol, botulism, carbon monoxide

Cutaneous Signs

Needle tracks	Heroin, PCP, amphetamine
Bullae	Carbon monoxide, barbiturates
Dry, hot skin	Anticholinergic agents, botulism
Diaphoresis	Organophosphates, nitrates, muscarinic mushrooms, aspirin, cocaine
Alopecia	Thallium, arsenic, lead, mercury
Erythema	Boric acid, mercury, cyanide, anticholinergics

Oral Signs

Salivation	Organophosphates, salicylate, corrosives, strychnine
Dry mouth	Amphetamine, anticholinergics, antihistamine
Burns	Corrosives, oxalate-containing plants
Gum lines	Lead, mercury, arsenic
Dysphagia	Corrosives, botulism

Intestinal Signs

Cramps	Arsenic, lead, thallium, organophosphates
Diarrhea	Antimicrobials, arsenic, iron, boric acid
Constipation	Lead, narcotics, botulism
Hematemesis	Aminophylline, corrosives, iron, salicylates

Cardiac Signs

Tachycardia	Atropine, aspirin, amphetamine, cocaine, cyclic antidepressants, theophylline
Bradycardia	Digitalis, narcotics, mushrooms, clonidine, organophosphates, β-blockers, calcium channel blockers
Hypertension	Amphetamine, LSD, cocaine, PCP
Hypotension	Phenothiazines, barbiturates, cyclic antidepressants, iron, β-blockers, calcium channel blockers

Respiratory Signs

Depressed respiration	Alcohol, narcotics, barbiturates
Increased respiration	Amphetamines, aspirin, ethylene glycol, carbon monoxide, cyanide
Pulmonary edema	Hydrocarbons, heroin, organophosphates, aspirin

CNS Signs

Ataxia	Alcohol, antidepressants, barbiturates, anticholinergics, phenytoin, narcotics
Coma	Sedatives, narcotics, barbiturates, PCP, organophosphates, salicylate, cyanide, carbon monoxide, cyclic antidepressants, lead
Hyperpyrexia	Anticholinergics, quinine, salicylates, LSD, phenothiazines, amphetamine, cocaine
Muscle fasciculation	Organophosphates, theophylline
Muscle rigidity	Cyclic antidepressants, PCP, phenothiazines, haloperidol
Paresthesia	Cocaine, camphor, PCP, MSG
Peripheral neuropathy	Lead, arsenic, mercury, organophosphates
Altered behavior	LSD, PCP, amphetamines, cocaine, alcohol, anticholinergics, camphor

LSD, lysergic acid diethylamide; MSG, monosodium glutamate; PCP, phencyclidine.

inaccurate, requiring a careful physical examination and laboratory approach.

PHYSICAL EXAMINATION

A complete physical examination including vital signs is necessary. For many agents, the level of consciousness, pupillary size, presence of muscle fasciculations, bowel and bladder activity, cardiac arrhythmias, seizures, or hypothermia may assist with the identification of the causative agent. The recognition of additional clinical manifestations is helpful in determining poisoning involving a particular agent. Certain complexes of symptoms and signs are relatively specific to a given class of drugs (toxidrome) (Table 45–2). Evaluation of the lungs may reveal pulmonary edema, which can be caused by cyclic antidepressants, organophosphates, or methaqualone. The patient's breath odor may provide valuable clues to potential ingestions.

COMPLICATIONS

A poisoned child can exhibit any one of six basic clinical patterns: coma, toxicity, metabolic acidosis, heart rhythm aberrations, gastrointestinal symptoms, and seizures.

Coma

Coma is perhaps the most striking symptom of a poison ingestion, but also may be seen as a result of trauma,

a cerebrovascular accident, asphyxia, or meningitis. A careful history and clinical examination are needed to distinguish among these alternatives. Pinpoint pupils suggest either a pontine lesion or toxic ingestion of opiates, organophosphates, phenothiazines, or chloral hydrate. Dilated pupils often are associated with cyclic antidepressants or atropine-like agents.

Systemic and Pulmonary Toxicity

Hydrocarbon ingestion occasionally may result in systemic toxicity, but more often in pulmonary toxicity (Table 45–3). Halogenated hydrocarbons or hydrocarbons with toxic additives have the greatest systemic toxicities and should be removed by lavage. Hydrocarbons with low viscosity, low surface tension, and high volatility pose the greatest risk for producing aspiration pneumonia; when swallowed, however, they pose no risk unless emesis is induced. Emesis or lavage should *not* be initiated in a child who has ingested volatile hydrocarbons.

Caustic ingestions may cause dysphagia, epigastric pain, oral mucosal burns, and low-grade fever. Patients with esophageal lesions may have no oral burns or may have significant signs and symptoms. Treatment depends on the agent ingested and the presence or absence of esophageal injury. Alkali agents may be solid, granular, or liquid (e.g., Liquid Drano, 9.5% sodium hydroxide, or Liquid Plumer, 8% potassium hydroxide). These liquid agents are tasteless and

---

TABLE 45–2. Toxic Syndromes

Agent	Manifestations
Acetaminophen	Nausea, vomiting, pallor, delayed jaundice–hepatic failure (72–96 hr)
Amphetamine, cocaine, and sympathomimetics	Tachycardia, hypertension, hyperthermia, psychosis and paranoia, seizures, mydriasis, diaphoresis, piloerection, aggressive behavior
Anticholinergics	Mania, delirium, fever, red dry skin, dry mouth, tachycardia, mydriasis, urinary retention
Carbon monoxide	Headache, dizziness, coma, skin bullae, other systems affected
Cyanide	Coma, convulsions, hyperpnea, bitter almond odor
Ethylene glycol (antifreeze)	Metabolic acidosis, hyperosmolarity, hypocalcemia, oxalate crystalluria
Iron	Vomiting (bloody), diarrhea, hypotension, hepatic failure, leukocytosis, hyperglycemia, radiopaque pills on KUB, late intestinal stricture, *Yersinia* sepsis
Narcotics	Coma, respiratory depression, hypotension, pinpoint pupils, hyporeflexia
Cholinergics (organophosphates, nicotine)	Miosis, salivation, urination, diaphoresis, lacrimation, bronchospasm (bronchorrhea), muscle weakness and fasciculations, emesis, defecation, coma, confusion, pulmonary edema, bradycardia, reduced erythrocyte and serum cholinesterase, late peripheral neuropathy
Phenothiazines	Tachycardia, hypotension, muscle rigidity, coma, ataxia, oculogyric crisis, miosis, radiopaque pills on KUB
Salicylates	Tachypnea, fever, lethargy, coma, vomiting, diaphoresis, alkalosis (early), acidosis (late)
Cyclic antidepressants	Coma, convulsions, mydriasis, hyperreflexia, arrhythmia (prolonged Q-T interval), cardiac arrest, shock

KUB, kidney-ureter-bladder radiograph.

TABLE 45–3.   Acute Hydrocarbon Risk Assessments

Systemic Toxicity Common*

Trichloroethane (spot remover), trichloroethylene, carbon tetrachloride, methylene chloride, benzene, hydrocarbon additives (camphor, heavy metals, insecticides, aniline), toluene

Local Toxicity by Aspiration Common,† Systemic Toxicity Uncommon

Mineral seal oil, signal oil, furniture polish, turpentine, gasoline, kerosene, charcoal lighter fluid

Nontoxic in 95% of Cases

Asphalt, tar, motor oil, mineral or liquid petroleum, lubricants, baby oil

*Chronic abuse of volatile hydrocarbons (e.g., sniffing) may cause ataxia, tremor, seizures, coma, myopathy, peripheral neuropathy, and renal tubular defects. Lead poisoning also is noted with abuse of lead-containing gasoline.
†Hydrocarbons of low viscosity (30-60 standard Saybolt Universal Seconds [SUS]), low surface tension, and high volatility have the greatest risk for inducing aspiration pneumonia.

produce full-thickness liquefaction necrosis of the esophagus or oropharynx. When the esophageal lesions heal, strictures form. Ingestion of these agents also creates a long-term risk of esophageal carcinoma. Many clinicians do not recommend the routine use of diluents as a first aid measure because of the lack of proven efficacy and the potential risk of induced vomiting. Subsequent treatment includes antibiotics if there are signs of infection and dilation of late-forming (2 to 3 weeks later) strictures.

Ingested button batteries also may produce a caustic mucosal injury from sodium hydroxide, potassium hydroxide, or mercuric oxide. If the batteries pass to the stomach, no further therapy is needed because they are likely to be passed in the stool within 1 week. Batteries that remain in the esophagus may cause esophageal burns and erosion and should be removed with an endoscope. Acid agents, such as Lysol Toilet Bowl Cleaner (8.5% hydrochloric acid) or Vanish Toilet Bowl Cleaner (65% sodium acid sulfate), can injure the lungs (with hydrochloric acid fumes), oral mucosa, esophagus, and stomach. Because acids taste sour, children usually stop drinking the solution, limiting the injury. Acids produce a coagulation necrosis, which limits the chemical from penetrating into deeper layers of the mucosa and damages tissue less severely than alkali. The signs and symptoms and initial therapeutic measures (dilution and no emesis or neutralization) are similar to those for alkali ingestion.

Metabolic Acidosis

A poisoned child also may have metabolic acidosis (mnemonic *MUDPIES*) (Table 45–4), which is assessed easily by measuring arterial blood gases, serum electrolyte levels, and urine pH. Determining serum sodium, potassium, chloride, glucose, urea nitrogen, and CO_2 levels permits the calculation of the serum anion gap (see Chapter 37) and osmolality:

$$Osm = 2 \times Na + (glucose/18) + (BUN/2.8)$$

which may be compared with measured osmolality. A difference of more than 10 between the measured and

TABLE 45–4.   Screening Laboratory Clues in Toxicologic Diagnosis

Metabolic Acidosis (Mnemonic = mudpies)

Methanol,* carbon monoxide
Uremia*
Diabetes mellitus*
Paraldehyde,* phenformin
Isoniazid, iron
Ethanol,* ethylene glycol*
Salicylates, starvation, seizures

Hypoglycemia

Ethanol
Isoniazid
Insulin
Propranolol
Oral hypoglycemic agents

Hyperglycemia

Salicylates
Isoniazid
Iron
Phenothiazines
Sympathomimetics

Hypocalcemia

Oxalate
Ethylene glycol
Fluoride

Radiopaque Substance on KUB (Mnemonic = chipped)

Chloral hydrate, calcium carbonate
Heavy metals (lead, zinc, barium, arsenic, lithium, bismuth as in Pepto-Bismol)
Iron
Phenothiazines
Play-Doh, potassium chloride
Enteric-coated pills
Dental amalgam

*Indicates hyperosmolar condition.
KUB, kidney-ureter-bladder radiograph.

calculated osmolality strongly suggests the presence of an unmeasured component, such as methanol or ethylene glycol. These ingestions require thorough assessment and prompt intervention; the approach described here allows a tentative diagnosis to be made pending access to the toxicology laboratory.

Dysrhythmias

Dysrhythmias may be prominent signs of a variety of toxic ingestions, although ventricular arrhythmias are rare. Prolonged Q-T intervals may suggest phenothiazine or antihistamine ingestion, and widened QRS complexes are seen with ingestions of cyclic antidepressants and quinidine. Because many drug and chemical overdoses may lead to sinus tachycardia, it is not a useful or discriminating sign; however, sinus bradycardia suggests digoxin, cyanide, a cholinergic agent, or β-blocker ingestion (Table 45–5).

Gastrointestinal Symptoms

Gastrointestinal symptoms of poisoning include emesis, nausea, abdominal cramps, and diarrhea. These symptoms may be the result of direct toxic effects on the intestinal mucosa or of systemic toxicity after absorption.

Seizures

Seizures are the sixth major mode of presentation for children with toxic ingestions, but poisoning is an uncommon cause of afebrile seizures. When seizures do occur with intoxication, they may be life-threatening and require aggressive therapeutic intervention.

LABORATORY AND IMAGING STUDIES

Laboratory studies helpful in initial management include specific toxin-drug assays; measurement of arterial blood gases and electrolytes, osmoles, and glucose; and calculation of the anion or osmolar gap. A full 12-lead ECG should be part of the initial evaluation in all patients suspected of ingesting toxic substances. Urine screens for drugs of abuse or to confirm suspected ingestion of medications in the home may be revealing.

Quantitative toxicology assays are important for some agents (Table 45–6) not only for identifying the specific drug, but also for providing guidance for therapy, anticipating complications, and estimating the prognosis. The timing of the physician's testing of the plasma level relative to the time of the patient's ingestion of the drug also is useful in predicting the severity of illness for acetaminophen (Fig. 45–1) and salicylate (Fig. 45–2). Patients with drug levels (related to the time after ingestion) in the serious zone require immediate treatment.

TABLE 45–5. Drugs Associated with Major Modes of Presentation

Common Toxic Causes of Cardiac Arrhythmia

Amphetamine
Antiarrhythmics
Anticholinergics
Antihistamines
Arsenic
Carbon monoxide
Chloral hydrate
Cocaine
Cyanide
Cyclic antidepressants
Digitalis
Freon
Phenothiazines
Physostigmine
Propranolol
Quinine, quinidine
Theophylline

Causes of Coma

Alcohol
Anticholinergics
Antihistamines
Barbiturates
Carbon monoxide
Clonidine
Cyanide
Cyclic antidepressants
Hypoglycemic agents
Lead
Lithium
Methemoglobinemia*
Methyldopa
Narcotics
Phencyclidine
Phenothiazines
Salicylates

Common Agents Causing Seizures (Mnemonic = caps)

Camphor
Carbamazepine
Carbon monoxide
Cocaine
Cyanide
Aminophylline
Amphetamine
Anticholinergics
Antidepressants (cyclic)
Pb (lead) (also lithium)
Pesticide (organophosphate)
Phencyclidine
Phenol
Phenothiazines
Propoxyphene
Salicylates
Strychnine

*Causes of methemoglobinemia: amyl nitrite, aniline dyes, benzocaine, bismuth subnitrate, dapsone, primaquone, quinones, spinach, sulfonamides.

TREATMENT

Supportive Care

Prompt attention must be given to protecting and maintaining the airway, establishing effective breathing, and supporting the circulation. This management sequence takes precedence over other diagnostic or therapeutic procedures. If the level of consciousness is depressed, and a toxic substance is suspected, glucose (1 g/kg IV), 100% oxygen, and naloxone should be administered.

Gastric Decontamination

The intent of gastrointestinal decontamination is to prevent the absorption of a potentially toxic ingested substance and, in theory, to prevent the poisoning. There has been great controversy about which methods are the safest and most efficacious. Gastric emptying, through administration of syrup of ipecac or orogastric lavage, is used when life-threatening ingestions present early (≤60 minutes), and the airway is

TABLE 45–6. Drugs Amenable to Therapeutic Monitoring for Drug Toxicity
Antibiotics
Aminoglycosides—gentamicin, tobramycin, and amikacin Chloramphenicol Vancomycin
Immunosuppression
Methotrexate Cyclosporine
Antipyretics
Acetaminophen Salicylate
Other
Digoxin Lithium Theophylline Anticonvulsant drugs Serotonin uptake inhibitor agent

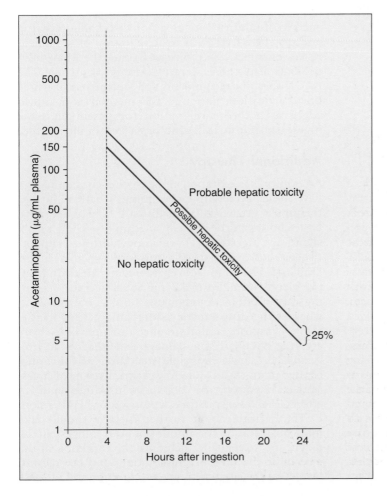

Figure 45–1

Semilogarithmic plot of plasma acetaminophen levels versus time. Rumack-Matthews nomogram for acetaminophen poisoning. Cautions for use of this chart are as follows: (1) The time coordinates refer to time of ingestion; (2) serum levels drawn before 4 hours may not represent peak levels; (3) the graph should be used only in relation to a single, acute ingestion; and (4) the lower solid line, 25% below the standard nomogram, is included to allow for possible errors in acetaminophen plasma assays and estimated time from ingestion of an overdose. (Adapted from Rumack BH, Matthew H: Acetaminophen poisoning and toxicity. Pediatrics 55:871-876, 1975.)

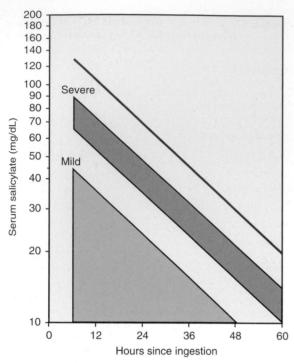

Figure 45–2

Nomogram relating serum salicylate concentration and expected severity of intoxication at various intervals after ingestion of a single dose of salicylate. (From Done AK: Salicylate intoxication. Significance of measurements of salicylate in blood in cases of acute ingestion. Pediatrics 26:800, 1960.)

protected. It is contraindicated if the ingestion is minimally toxic, there has been prior vomiting, the airway is unprotected, or the ingested substance is caustic, a hydrocarbon, or foreign body. The American Academy of Clinical Toxicology (AACT) has recommended that ipecac should not be administered routinely to poisoned patients because there is no evidence that ipecac improves the outcome of poisoned patients. The AACT also noted that lavage is associated with varying success in removal of the ingested agent and associated with potential complications (aspiration, laryngospasm, esophageal perforation) without evidence of improved clinical outcomes.

Activated charcoal is the mainstay for decontamination. Activated charcoal is prepared by pyrolyzing organic materials, then activating them by exposure to oxidizing gas flows at high temperatures. A substance with a large relative surface area and an affinity to bind with certain compounds is created. By binding with toxins, charcoal may prevent the toxin from being absorbed by the intestinal tract. Historically, charcoal has been used as a single-dose (25 to 50 g for small children; 50 to 100 g for children >12 years old or 1 g/kg)

and multiple-dose intervention for poisonings. Multiple-dose therapy was advocated as a means to enhance enterohepatic circulation. Charcoal is known to be ineffective against caustic or corrosive agents, hydrocarbons, heavy metals (arsenic, lead, mercury, iron, lithium), glycols, and water-insoluble compounds.

The greatest benefit with activated charcoal is likely achieved within 1 hour of the ingestion. The AACT has recommended that single-dose activated charcoal be administered only in situations in which it can be given within 1 hour of the ingestion of a potentially lethal agent that is known to be adsorbed by charcoal.

Cathartics

The administration of a cathartic (sorbitol or magnesium citrate) alone has no role in the management of the poisoned patient. The AACT has stated that based on available data, the use of a cathartic in combination with activated charcoal is not recommended.

Whole Bowel Irrigation

Whole bowel irrigation is advocated for gastrointestinal decontamination. It involves the use of polyethylene glycol (GoLYTELY) as a nonabsorbable cathartic and may be effective for toxic ingestion of sustained-release or enteric-coated drugs. To date, there have been no controlled studies showing improved outcome. The AACT does not recommend the routine use of whole bowel irrigation, although the method is acknowledged as a theoretical option for potentially toxic ingestions of iron, lead, zinc, or packets of illicit drugs.

Additional Therapy

After initial resuscitation and gastric decontamination have been achieved, determining whether further therapy is needed is often difficult. There are three basic choices in the subsequent care of a child with a significant ingestion: (1) providing continued supportive care, (2) using specific antidotes where available (Table 45–7), and (3) actively removing the toxin from the bloodstream. To make a rational decision regarding these options, a judgment should be made as to whether the drug causes tissue damage (e.g., methyl alcohol, aspirin, acetaminophen, theophylline, iron, ethylene glycol). Tissue damage is defined as an irreversible or slowly reversible structural or functional change in an organ system as a direct result of ingestion of a poison; this definition precludes indirect effects, such as respiratory depression or hypotension.

The decision about further therapy should take into consideration the amount of poison ingested; the diagnostic assessment, including the condition of the patient at the time of presentation; and the natural history of the suspected type of ingestion. All of these

TABLE 45–7. Emergency Antidotes

Poison	Antidote	Dosage	Comments
Acetaminophen	N-Acetyl cysteine	140 mg/kg PO initial dose, then 70 mg/kg PO q4h × 17 doses	Most effective within 16 hr of ingestion
Atropine	Physostigmine	Initial dose 0.01-0.03 mg/kg IV	Can produce convulsions, bradycardia; reserve for life-threatening situations only
Benzodiazepine	Flumazenil	0.01-0.02 mg/kg IV; 0.2 mg max	Possible seizures, arrhythmias
β-blocking agents	Atropine	0.01-0.10 mg/kg IV	Minimum dose 0.1 mg
	Isoproterenol	0.05-1.5 µg/kg/min IV infusion	
	Glucagon	0.05-0.1 mg/kg IV	
Calcium channel blockers	Glucagon	0.05-0.1 mg/kg IV	Increases cAMP, resulting in positive inotropy and chronotropy
Carbon monoxide	Oxygen	100%; hyperbaric O_2	Half-life of carboxyhemoglobin is 5 hr in room air but 1.5 hr in 100% O_2
Coumarin	Vitamin K	2-5 mg IV/SC	Monitor PT; fresh frozen plasma or plasma for acute bleeding; repeated vitamin K for super-warfarin
Cyanide	Amyl nitrite, then	1-2 pearls every 2 min	Methemoglobin-cyanide complex
	Sodium nitrite, then	4.5-10 mg/kg (0.15-0.33 mL/kg 3% solution)	Causes hypotension; dosage assumes normal hemoglobin
	Sodium thiosulfate	50 mg/kg IV	Forms harmless sodium thiocyanate
Cyclic antidepressants	Sodium bicarbonate	0.5-1.0 mEq/kg IV, titrated to produce pH 7.5-7.55	—
Digoxin, digitoxin	Digoxin-specific Fab antibody fragments	Dose based on serum digoxin concentration and body weight; 1 vial (40 mg) neutralizes 0.6 mg digoxin	With acute life-threatening ingestion, dose and serum concentration are unknown; give contents of 20 vials
Iron	Deferoxamine	Initial dose 10-15 mg/kg/hr IV	Deferoxamine mesylate—forms excretable ferrioxamine complex; hypotension
Isoniazid	Pyridoxine	Give dose equal to the amount of isoniazid ingested, up to 250 mg/kg	For treatment of seizures or coma
Lead	Edetate calcium (calcium disodium versenate [EDTA])	1500 mg/m²/day × 5 days; divided q6h or by continuous infusion	May lower to 1000 mg/m²/day if given with BAL; nephrotoxic
	BAL (British anti-Lewisite [dimercaprol])	3-5 mg/kg/dose q4h × 3-7 days	May cause hypertension and sterile abscesses
	Penicillamine	20-30 mg/kg/day PO divided q8h	Requires weekly monitoring for hepatic and bone marrow toxicity; should not be used in the presence of ongoing ingestion
	Succimer (2,3-dimercaptosuccinic acid ([DMSA])	10 mg/kg/day PO tid × 5 days then 10 mg/kg/day PO bid × 14 days	Few toxic effects, requires lead-free home plus compliant family

Continued

TABLE 45–7.   Emergency Antidotes—cont'd

Poison	Antidote	Dosage	Comments
Mercury, arsenic, gold	BAL	5 mg/kg IM as soon as possible	Each 1 mL BAL in oil has dimercaprol, 100 mg in 210 mL (21%) benzyl benzoate, and 680 mL peanut oil—forms stable nontoxic excretable cyclic compound
Methyl alcohol (ethylene glycol)	Fomepizole	15 mg/kg loading dose followed by 10 mg/kg q12h × 4 doses	May be a better alternative to ethanol therapy
	Ethyl alcohol in conjunction with dialysis	1 mL/kg of 100% ethanol initially in glucose solution; maintain blood level of 100 mg/dL	Competes for alcohol dehydrogenase; prevents formation of formic acid and oxalates
Nitrites/ methemoglobinemia*	Methylene blue	1-2 mg/kg, repeat in 1-4 hr if needed; treat for levels >30%	Exchange transfusion may be needed for severe methemoglobinemia; methylene blue overdose also causes methemoglobinemia
Opiates, Darvon, Lomotil	Naloxone	0.10 mg/kg IV, ET, SC, IM for children, up to 2 mg	Naloxone causes no respiratory depression (0.4 mg/1 mL ampule)
Organophosphates	Atropine	Initial dose 0.02-0.05 mg/kg IV	Physiologic: blocks acetylcholine; up to 5 mg IV every 15 min may be necessary in the critically ill adult patient
	Pralidoxime (2 PAM; Protopam)	Initial dose 20-50 mg/kg IV	Specific: disrupts phosphate-cholinesterase bond; up to 500 mg/hr may be necessary in the critically ill adult patient
Sympathomimetic agents	Blocking agents: phentolamine; β-blocking agents; other antihypertensives		Must be used in a setting in which vital signs can be monitored effectively

*See Table 45–5 for causes of methemoglobinemia.
ET, endotracheal.
Data from Kulig K: Initial management of ingestions of toxic substances. N Engl J Med 326:1677-1681, 1992; Liebelt EL: Newer antidotal therapies for pediatric poisonings. Clin Pediatr Emerg Med 1:234-243, 2000; Leikin JB, Paloucek EP, editors: Poisoning and Toxicology Compendium. Cleveland, Lexi-Comp, 1998.

variables may be influenced by the child's prior clinical status or underlying medical problems. In a patient with underlying severe hepatic or renal impairment, a more aggressive approach involving active removal might be selected, even though the ingestion ordinarily would require only simple supportive care. In the presence of a chronic ingestion, an acute overdose may cause significant clinical toxicity with a lower dose of the drug.

For most common ingestions, continued supportive care and treatment directed toward specific complications are appropriate for otherwise healthy individuals. Specific antidotes should be used according to prescribed guidelines (see Table 45–7). Active removal (hemoperfusion or dialysis) should be undertaken only for toxins that may cause tissue damage, for toxins that have been ingested by a patient already exhibiting confounding medical problems, or to avoid prolonged supportive care.

PROGNOSIS

Mortality from poisoning is rare (0.002%). The most common exposures resulting in death include carbon monoxide, hydrocarbons, and opioids (all of which interfere with oxygen delivery to tissues). Medications that affect cardiac function (calcium channel antagonists, β-adrenergic sustained-release medications, tricyclic antidepressants and adrenergic ingestions) also are in the top 10 causes of death from poisoning.

PREVENTION

Most ingestions occur in the home, and the toxins involved are common household medications, household cleaning and work solutions, or vitamins. Unintentional poisonings are more frequent in children younger than 5 years old, in boys, in families of low socioeconomic status, and during times of family disorganization. These poisonings occur most frequently in the kitchen, bathroom, or garage. Properly educating parents to use childproof medication containers, to store toxic substances in locked cabinets, and to label toxic chemicals properly is necessary for preventing ingestions. Kerosene and other toxic liquids should not be stored in soda pop bottles, and children should not come in contact with clothing exposed to pesticides. Old or unused medications should be discarded, and currently used medications should not be left on tabletops or in the mother's purse. If a child has ingested poison, the poison control center should be called.

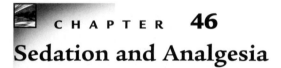

CHAPTER 46
Sedation and Analgesia

An acutely ill pediatric patient may have pain, discomfort, and anxiety resulting from injury, surgery, and invasive procedures (intubation, bone marrow aspiration, venous access placement) or during life-sustaining mechanical ventilation. The physician has a commitment to relieve discomfort and treat pain. Clear goals should be identified to allow provision of optimal analgesia or sedation without compromising the physiologic status of the patient. Anxiolysis, cooperation, amnesia, immobility, and lack of awareness all are goals of sedation and can be accomplished with various drugs (Table 46-1). Many of these goals are behavioral and may benefit from behavioral techniques (preprocedural teaching), but sedation is often a necessary adjunct for painful procedures. Pain may be expressed by verbal or visible discomfort, crying, agitation, tachycardia, hypertension, and tachypnea. A variety of scales have been developed in an attempt to quantify pain and allow more directed therapy. Few of these scales are well validated, especially in populations of acutely ill children with physiologic derangements secondary to the underlying pathology. Pain caused by procedural interventions should always be treated with analgesics in addition to sedation (Table 46-2).

ASSESSMENT
Procedural Sedation

A medical evaluation must be performed for any patient receiving procedural sedation. The goal is to identify underlying medical conditions that may affect the choice of sedative agents. Specific attention must be paid to assessment of the airway (for ability to maintain a patent airway) and respiratory system (asthma, recent respiratory illness, loose teeth), cardiovascular status (especially adequacy of volume status), factors affecting drug metabolism (renal or liver disease), and risk for aspiration (adequate nothing-by-mouth status, gastroesophageal reflux). During the administration

---

TABLE 46-1. Agents That Produce Sedation

Sedative-Hypnotics	Effect	Concerns
Midazolam	Anxiolysis, sedation, muscle relaxation, amnesia	Tolerance is possible; apnea, hypotension, depressed myocardial function; short action
Lorazepam	Anxiolysis, sedation, muscle relaxation, amnesia	Same as midazolam; long action
Ketamine	Anesthesia, analgesia, amnesia	Dissociative reactions, tachycardia, hypertension, increased bronchial secretions, emergent delirium, hallucinations; increases intracranial pressure
Chloral hydrate	Sedative	Emesis, hypotension, arrhythmias, hepatic dysfunction, possible carcinogen
Propofol	Rapid-onset sedative for induction and maintenance of anesthesia	Metabolic acidosis in children, may depress cardiac function

TABLE 46–2. Agents That Produce Analgesia

Analgesic	Effect	Complications
Acetaminophen and NSAIDs	Moderate analgesia, antipyresis	Ceiling effect, requires PO administration; NSAIDs—gastrointestinal bleed, ulceration
Opioids		**No ceiling effect, respiratory depression, sedation, pruritus, nausea/vomiting, decreased gastric motility, urinary retention, tolerance with abuse potential**
Morphine	Analgesia	May cause myocardial depression
Codeine	Analgesia	Nausea/vomiting
Fentanyl, alfentanil, sufentanil	Analgesia, sedation	No adverse effects on cardiovascular system; stiff chest syndrome
Partial agonists/ agonist-antagonist		**Dysphoria, withdrawal symptoms**
Propoxyphene	Analgesia	Dizziness, sedation
Meperidine	Analgesia, sedation	May increase intracranial pressure, respiratory depressant, hypotension
Methadone	Analgesia	

NSAIDs, nonsteroidal anti-inflammatory drugs.

of procedural sedation, assessment of status must include monitoring of oxygen saturation, heart rate, and respiratory rate and some assessment of effectiveness of ventilation. This assessment must be performed by someone who is not involved in the procedure; this person is also responsible for recording vital signs and drugs administered on a time-based graph. Monitoring must be continued until the child has returned to baseline. Patients who are receiving long-term sedation (to maintain endotracheal tube placement) may need only local anesthetic for painful procedures, but may benefit from additional sedation or analgesia as well.

Nonprocedural Sedation

Many ventilated pediatric patients require sedation and some analgesia while intubated. The initial assessment of a child who requires nonprocedural sedation is unchanged. The most common choice is a combination of a longer acting benzodiazepine and an opioid. Avoidance of oversedation is important. Use of appropriate pain and sedation scores allows for titration of medications to achieve goals of the sedation plan. Long-term use of benzodiazepines and opioids leads to tolerance, a problematic occurrence that must be considered as medications are added and weaned. True addiction is a rare occurrence, especially when medications are provided at the minimum level needed to achieve adequate sedation and pain control.

PAIN AND ANALGESIA

The subjective aspect of pain requires that self-reporting be used for assessment. Visual analogue scales, developed for adult patients (allowing patients to rate pain on a scale of 1 to 10), have been used for older children. Pain scales for younger children often incorporate behavioral and physiologic parameters, despite the imprecision of physiologic responses.

Local anesthetics, such as lidocaine, can be used for minor procedures. Lidocaine requires SC or intradermal injection, however. The use of EMLA, a cream containing lidocaine and prilocaine, is less effective than intradermal lidocaine, but is preferred by many patients.

Patient-controlled analgesia is an effective method for providing balanced analgesia care in older children and adolescents. Children using patient-controlled analgesia have better pain relief and experience less sedation than patients receiving intermittent, nurse-controlled, bolus analgesics. Analgesics can be administered through the patient-controlled analgesia pump with continuous basal infusions, bolus administration, or both. Morphine is the most frequent opioid used for patient-controlled analgesia. Monitoring of oxygen saturations and respiratory rate are crucial with continuous opioid infusions owing to the shift in CO_2 response curve and potential to decrease ventilatory response to hypoxia.

Epidural analgesia decreases the need for inhalation anesthetics during surgery and can provide significant analgesia without sedation in the postoperative period. Decreased costs and length of stay also may be benefits of epidural analgesic approaches. Medications used in epidurals include bupivacaine and morphine. Adverse effects include nausea and vomiting, motor blockade, and technical problems requiring catheter removal. Infection and permanent neurologic deficits are rare.

SUGGESTED READING

Behrman RE, Kliegman RM, Jenson HB (eds): Nelson Textbook of Pediatrics, 17th ed. Philadelphia, WB Saunders, 2004, pp 253-366.

Kliegman RM, Greenbaum LA, Lye PS (eds): Practical Strategies in Pediatric Diagnosis and Therapy, 2nd ed. Philadelphia, WB Saunders, 2004.

HUMAN GENETICS AND DYSMORPHOLOGY

Paul A. Levy and Robert W. Marion

CHAPTER **47**

Patterns of Inheritance

TYPES OF GENETIC DISORDERS

Among infants born in the U.S., 2% to 4% have **congenital malformations,** abnormalities of form or function identifiable at birth. At 1 year of age, the number approaches 7% because some anomalies, such as ventriculoseptal defects, may not be identifiable until after the neonatal period. The incidence of congenital malformations is much greater in inpatient pediatric populations; 30% to 50% of hospitalized children have congenital anomalies or genetic disorders.

The clinical geneticist attempts to identify the etiology, the mode of inheritance, and the risk that this or a similar disorder might occur in the affected child's siblings. In evaluating children with congenital malformations, the clinical geneticist attempts to classify the patient's condition into one of five different categories:

1. Single gene mutations, accounting for 6% of children with congenital anomalies
2. Chromosomal disorders, accounting for approximately 7.5%
3. Multifactorially inherited conditions, accounting for 20%
4. Disorders that show an unusual pattern of inheritance, accounting for 2% to 3%
5. Teratogenically caused conditions, accounting for 6%

INTRODUCTION TO GENETICS AND GENOMICS

DNA is composed of four nucleotide building blocks. Each nucleotide comprises a five-carbon sugar (deoxyribose) linked to a nitrogen base and a phosphate group. The nucleotides forming DNA are adenine (A), guanine (G), cytosine (C), and thymine (T). Each nucleotide is linked to other nucleotides via phosphodiester bonds, forming a chain. The DNA molecule consists of two chains of the nucleotides held together by hydrogen bonds. The purine nucleotides, adenine and guanine, cross-link by hydrogen bonds to the pyrimidines, thymine and cytosine. Because of cross-linking (A-to-T and C-to-G), the nucleotide sequence of one strand sets the other strand's sequence. Separating the two strands permits complementary nucleotides to bind to each DNA strand; this copies the DNA and replicates the sequence.

DNA exists not as one long molecule, but as multiple fragments that together with a protein skeleton (chromatin) form chromosomes. Every human cell has 23 pairs of chromosomes. One copy of each chromosome is inherited from each parent. Twenty-two pairs of chromosomes are **autosomes**; the remaining pair is called the **sex chromosomes**. Females have two X chromosomes; males have one X and one Y.

Spread along the chromosomes, similar to beads on a string, DNA sequences form **genes**, the basic units of heredity. A typical gene contains a promoter sequence, an untranslated region, and an open reading frame, all arrayed from the 5′ to the 3′ end of the DNA. In the open reading frame, every three nucleotides represent a single **codon**, which codes for a particular amino acid. In this way, the sequence of bases in the DNA dictates the sequence of the amino acids in the corresponding protein. Some of the codons, rather than coding for a specific amino acid, act as a start signal, whereas others act as stop signals. Between the start and stop codons, genes consist of two major portions: **exons**, which are regions containing the code that ultimately corresponds to a sequence of amino acids, and **introns** (intervening sequence), which do not become part of the amino acid sequence.

Genes are **transcribed** into messenger RNA (mRNA), then **translated** into proteins. During transcription, the RNA is processed to remove the introns. The mRNA is used as a template to construct the protein.

Human genetic material is composed of 3.1 gigabases (3.1 billion). Less than 2% of DNA codes for proteins, composing the approximately 25,000 genes in the genome. Through a mechanism called **alternative splicing**, these 25,000 genes may represent more than 100,000 proteins. Greater than 50% of DNA appears as repeat sequences, in which two or three bases are repeated. The purpose of these repeat sequences and of the remainder of DNA is unknown.

Disease may be caused by changes or **mutations** in the DNA sequence. Mutations can be classified by causative mechanism or functional effect. When using a classification system involving causative mechanism, point mutations are the most common type. A change in a single DNA base is called a **point mutation**. A point mutation that changes a codon and the resulting amino acid that goes into the protein is referred to as a **missense mutation**. A **nonsense mutation** is a point mutation that changes the codon to a stop codon so that transcription stops prematurely. A **frameshift mutation** often stems from the loss or addition of one or more DNA bases; this causes a shift in how the DNA is transcribed. Frameshift mutations generally lead to premature stop codons.

These mutations are referred to as **single gene mutations.** There are autosomal dominant (AD), autosomal recessive (AR), or X-linked single gene mutations. If a mutation in only one of the two copies of a gene is sufficient to cause disease, that disorder is considered **AD** (Table 47–1); if two copies of the gene must have the mutation for disease to result, the condition is termed **AR** (Table 47–2). If a condition results from a mutation in a gene on the X chromosome, it causes disease in males, but generally not in females. This pattern of inheritance is termed **X-linked** (Table 47–3).

TABLE 47–1.   Autosomal Dominant Diseases

Disease	Frequency	Comments
Achondroplasia Thanatophoric dysplasia Crouzon syndrome with acanthosis nigricans Nonsyndromic craniosynostosis	~1:12,000	Mutations are in the gene for *fibroblast growth factor receptor-3* on chromosome 4p16.3 40% of cases are new mutations (different mutations in the same gene cause achondroplasia, thanatophoric dysplasia, Crouzon syndrome with acanthosis, and nonsyndromic craniosynostosis)
Neurofibromatosis I	1:3500	About 50% of cases result from new mutations in the gene for neurofibromin, a tumor suppressor gene located at 17q11.2. Expression is quite variable
Neurofibromatosis II (NF II, bilateral acoustic neuromas, Merlin)	Genotype at birth 1:33,000 Phenotype prevalence 1:200,000	The NF II gene is a tumor suppressor gene located at 22q12.2. The protein is called "Merlin"
Huntington disease (HD)	Variable in populations, 1:5000-1:20,000	The disease is caused by a (CAG) repeat expansion in the "Huntington" protein gene on chromosome 4p16.3
Myotonic dystrophy (DM, Steinert disease)	1:500 in Quebec 1:25,000 Europeans	The disease is caused by a (CTG) repeat expansion in the DM kinase gene at chromosome 19q13.2. The condition shows genetic anticipation with successive generations
Marfan syndrome (FBN-1)	1:10,000	The syndrome is caused by mutations in the fibrillin 1 (FBN 1) gene on chromosome 15q21.1; there is variable expression
Hereditary angioneurotic edema (HANE) (C-1 esterase inhibitor that regulates the C-1 component of complement)	1:10,000	The gene is located on chromosome 11q11-q13.2. The phenotype of episodic and variable subcutaneous and submucosal swelling and pain is caused by diminished or altered esterase inhibitor protein, which can result from any one of many mutations in the gene

TABLE 47–2. Autosomal Recessive Diseases

Disease	Frequency	Comments
Adrenal hyperplasia, congenital (CAH, 21-hydroxylase deficiency, CA21H, CYP21, cytochrome P450, subfamily XXI)	1:5000	Phenotype variation corresponds roughly to allelic variation. A deficiency causes virilization in females. The gene is located at 6p21.3 within the HLA complex and within 0.005 centimorgans (cM) of HLA B
Phenylketonuria (PKU, phenylalanine hydroxylase deficiency, PAH)	1:12,000-1:17,000	There are hundreds of disease-causing mutations in the PAH gene located on chromosome 12q22-q24.1. The first population-based newborn screening was a test for PKU because the disease is treatable by diet. Women with elevated phenylalanine have infants with damage to the CNS because high phenylalanine is neurotoxic and teratogenic
Cystic fibrosis (CF)	1:2500 whites	The gene *CF transmembrane conductance regulator* (CFTR) is on chromosome 7q31.2
Friedreich ataxia (FA, frataxin)	1:25,000	Frataxin is a mitochondrial protein involved with iron metabolism and respiration. The gene is on chromosome 9q13-q21, and the common mutation is a GAA expanded triplet repeat located in the first *intron* of the gene. FA does not show anticipation
Gaucher disease, all types (glucocerebrosidase deficiency, acid β-glucosidase deficiency) (a lysosomal storage disease)	1:2500 Ashkenazi Jews	The gene is located on chromosome 1q21. There are many mutations; some mutations lead to neuropathic disease, but most are milder in expression. The phenotypes correspond to the genotypes, but the latter are difficult to analyze
Sickle cell disease (hemoglobin beta locus, beta 6 glu→val mutation)	1:625 African Americans	This is the first condition with a defined molecular defect (1959). A single base change results in an amino acid substitution of valine for glutamic acid at position 6 of the beta chain of hemoglobin with resulting hemolytic anemia. The gene is on chromosome 11p15.5. Penicillin prophylaxis reduces death from pneumococcal infections in affected persons, especially in infants

Occasionally, as a result of skewing of inactivation (a phenomenon known as **lyonization**) of the X chromosome, an X-linked disorder may manifest symptoms of a disease in a heterozygous female. Genetic disorders also may result from abnormalities in the amount of genetic material present (termed *chromosomal disorders*), from interplay between genetic factors and environmental factors (called *multifactorial inheritance*), from unusual modes of inheritance, and as the result of exposure to certain drugs and chemicals known to cause birth defects (called *teratogens*).

Pedigree Drawing

To appreciate specific patterns of inheritance, geneticists construct and analyze pedigrees. A pedigree is a pictorial representation of a family; males are represented by squares and females are represented by circles. Matings are connected with a solid line between each partner's symbols. Unmarried couples are often connected by a dashed line. Children from a couple are represented below their parents and are the next generation.

Grandparents, uncles, and aunts are added in similar fashion. Children of aunts and uncles also may be included. Ages or birthdays may be written next to or underneath each person. The proband, the patient who is the initial contact, is indicated with an arrow. Affected individuals are indicated by shading, or some other technique, which should be explained in a key. Carriers for a disorder (e.g., sickle cell disease) usually are indicated by a dot in the center of their symbol (Fig. 47–1).

Autosomal Dominant Disorders

If a single copy of a gene bearing a mutation is sufficient to cause disease, that condition is autosomal

TABLE 47-3.   X-Linked Recessive Diseases

Disease	Frequency	Comments
Fragile X syndrome (FRAXA, and numerous other names)	1 : 4000 males	The gene is located at Xq27.3 The condition is attributable to a CGG triplet expansion that is associated with localized methylation (inactivation) of distal genes. Females may have some expression. Instability of the site may lead to tissue mosaicism; lymphocyte genotype and phenotype may not correlate
Duchenne muscular dystrophy (DMD, pseudohypertrophic progressive MD, dystrophin, Becker variants)	1 : 4000 males	The gene is located at Xp21 The gene is relatively large, with 79 exons, and mutations and deletions may occur anywhere. The gene product is called *dystrophin*. Dystrophin is absent in DMD but abnormal in Becker MD
Hemophilia A (factor VIII deficiency, classic hemophilia)	1 : 5000-1 : 10,000 males	The gene is located at Xq28 Factor VIII is essential for normal blood clotting. Phenotype depends on genotype and the presence of any residual factor VIII activity
Rett syndrome (RTT, RTS autism, dementia, ataxia, and loss of purposeful hand use); gene MECP2 (methyl-CpG-binding protein 2)	1 : 10,000-1 : 15,000 girls	The gene is located at locus Xq28 These diseases are a subset of autism. There is a loss of regulation (repression) for other genes, including those in *trans* positions. The disease is lethal in males. Cases represent new mutations or parental gonadal mosaicism
Color blindness (partial deutan series, green color blindness [75%]; partial protan series, red color blindness [25%])	1 : 12 males	The gene is located at Xq28 (proximal) for deutan color blindness and at Xq28 (distal) for protan color blindness
Adrenoleukodystrophy (ALD, XL-ALD, Addison disease, and cerebral sclerosis)	Uncommon	The gene is located at Xq28 The disease involves a defect in peroxisome function relating to *very long chain fatty acid CoA synthetase* with accumulation of C-26 fatty acids. Phenotype is variable, from rapid childhood progression to later onset and slow progression
Glucose-6-phosphate dehydrogenase deficiency (G6PD)	1 : 10 African Americans 1 : 5 Kurdish Jews A heteromorphism in these and other populations	The gene is located at Xq28 There are numerous variants in which oxidants cause hemolysis. Variants can confer partial resistance to severe malaria

dominantly inherited (see Table 47-1). In AD disorders, an affected parent may have one or more children who are affected with the same disorder. The parent, who has a mutation in one gene (the other copy is "normal"), has a 50% chance of passing the mutated gene and the disorder to the child (Fig. 47-2). Possessing one "normal" gene and one gene with a mutation that causes disease occurs is termed **heterozygous.** If both copies or alleles are the same, they are referred to as **homozygous** (Table 47-4).

Some people who are obligate carriers of a mutation known to cause an AD disorder may not show clinical signs of the disorder, whereas other such individuals manifest symptoms. This phenomenon is referred to as **penetrance**. If all individuals who carry a mutation for an AD disorder show signs of having that disorder, the gene is said to have complete or 100% penetrance. Many AD disorders show decreased penetrance.

Often, AD disorders show variability in the symptoms expressed in different individuals carrying the same mutated gene. Some individuals may have only mild clinical symptoms, whereas others have much more severe disease. This phenomenon is referred to as **variable expressivity**. To illustrate the differences between penetrance and expressivity, consider the condition neurofibromatosis type 1 (NF1). Caused

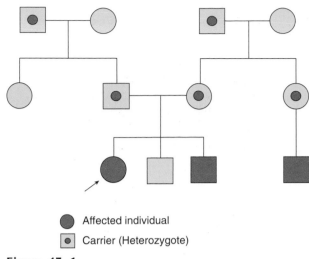

Affected individual

Carrier (Heterozygote)

Figure 47–1

Pedigree showing affected individuals and carriers.

TABLE 47–4. Rules of Autosomal Dominant Inheritance

Trait appears in every generation
Each child of an affected parent has a 1 in 2 chance of being affected
Males and females are equally affected
Male-to-male transmission occurs
Traits generally involve mutations in genes that code for regulatory or structural proteins (collagen)

Sometimes, seemingly unrelated clinical findings may be caused by a mutation in a single gene or gene pair. The café au lait spots and neurofibromas of NF1 are an example of this. Known as **pleiotropy**, this phenomenon occurs in numerous single gene disorders.

AD disorders sometimes appear in a child of unaffected parents because of a **spontaneous mutation**. Known in some cases to be associated with advanced paternal age (>35 years old), spontaneous mutations may account for most individuals with some disorders. Approximately 80% of patients with achondroplasia are believed to have experienced a mutation in the fibroblast growth factor receptor type 3 (*FGFR3*) gene.

by a mutation in the neurofibromin gene on chromosome 17p11.2, NF1 is an AD disorder that causes café au lait macules, neurofibromas, and an assortment of other findings. Although 100% penetrant, NF1 has marked variability in expression. Some affected individuals have only café au lait spots, whereas others in the same family may experience life-threatening complications.

Examples of Some Autosomal Dominant Disorders

Achondroplasia (Online Mendelian Inheritance in Man Catalog [OMIM] #100800)

An AD disorder caused by a defect in cartilage-derived bone, achondroplasia is the most common skeletal dysplasia in humans. The bony abnormalities in achondroplasia lead to short stature, macrocephaly, a flat midface with a prominent forehead, and rhizomelic shortening of the limbs. This disorder occurs in approximately 1 in 12,000 births.

Achondroplasia is caused by a mutation in the *FGFR3* gene, which is located on chromosome 4p16. Early in development, the *FGFR3* gene is expressed during endochondral bone formation of the long bones. More than 95% of cases of achondroplasia are caused by one of two mutations in the same base pair (site 1138). This site is extremely active for mutations. As such, it is often referred to as a mutational **"hot spot."**

Children with achondroplasia often develop associated medical and psychological problems as they grow. Hydrocephalus and central apnea may occur secondary to narrowing of the foramen magnum and compression of the brainstem. Bowing of the legs may occur later in childhood because of unequal growth of the tibia and fibula. Dental malocclusion and hearing loss

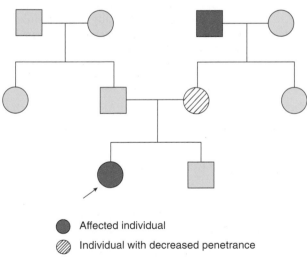

Affected individual

Individual with decreased penetrance

Figure 47–2

Pedigree showing decreased penetrance for an autosomal dominant disorder. Proband (with *arrow*) is affected. Maternal grandfather also is affected. The individual's mother is presumed to be the carrier of the gene even though she may show only slight symptoms of disease.

secondary to middle ear dysfunction are common in later childhood. During later childhood and adolescence, the psychological effects of the child's extreme short stature may manifest. In adulthood, further complications include compression of nerve roots and sciatica. People with achondroplasia have normal life spans and normal intelligence.

The diagnosis of achondroplasia is made on the basis of the clinical and radiologic findings. Characteristic x-ray abnormalities confirm the diagnosis. Molecular testing can be performed, but usually is reserved for cases that are difficult to diagnose by physical features and x-rays or for cases for which prenatal diagnosis for future progeny is requested. Prenatal diagnosis is possible by molecular testing, using fetal cells obtained through amniocentesis or chorionic villus sampling.

Neurofibromatosis Type 1 (OMIM #162200)

NF1 is one of the most commonly occurring AD disorders. Estimated to be present in 1 in 3500 individuals, NF1 is caused by a mutation in the gene neurofibromin, located on chromosome 17q11.2 (see Chapter 186).

Although the penetrance of NF1 is 100%, the expression is extremely variable. Many individuals who have a mutation in the gene have features so mild that they are never diagnosed. These individuals may manifest only café au lait spots, axillary or inguinal freckling (smaller and darker than the café au lait spots and always found in clusters), Lisch nodules (pigmented hamartomas of the iris, best seen on slit-lamp examination), and neurofibromas (Schwann cell tumors). Ten percent to 20% of individuals have more severe symptoms, including brain tumors (optic gliomas, astrocytomas, or other brain tumors), hypertension, skeletal involvement (scoliosis, pseudarthrosis of the tibia), and craniofacial disfigurement. Because of the large size of the NF1 gene and the fact that most individuals or families have a different mutation, molecular diagnosis is generally not possible in this condition. Diagnosis is based on clinical features (Table 47–5).

Marfan Syndrome (OMIM #154700)

A condition that occurs in approximately 1 in 10,000 individuals, Marfan syndrome shows pleiotropy. Clinical symptoms mostly involve three systems: **cardiac**, **musculoskeletal**, and **ophthalmologic**. Musculoskeletal findings include dolichostenomelia (a tall, thin body habitus), arachnodactyly (spider-like fingers and toes), abnormalities of the sternum (pectus excavatum or carinatum), kyphoscoliosis, pes planus, and joint laxity. Eye findings include high myopia, which eventually can lead to vitreoretinal degeneration; an abnormal suspensory ligament of the lens, which can lead to

TABLE 47–5. Diagnostic Criteria for Neurofibromatosis Type 1*

Café au lait spots
   Prepubertal: ≥5 (>0.5 cm in diameter)
   Postpubertal: ≥5 (>1.5 cm in diameter)
Axillary or inguinal "freckling"
Two or more **neurofibromas** (Schwann cell tumors)
Presence of **plexiform neuroma**
Lisch nodules
Optic glioma
Skeletal manifestations
   Scoliosis (often rapidly progressing)
   Pseudarthrosis
   Bony rarefaction or overgrowth due to presence of
     plexiform neuroma
   Sphenoid wing dysplasia (5%)
Family history of neurofibromatosis type 1 in parent

*Patients must fulfill at least two criteria.

ectopia lentis (dislocation of the lens; in Marfan syndrome, the lens usually dislocates upward and outward); and cataracts. Cardiac findings include a weakened aortic wall, which leads to progressive dilation of the aortic root. Aortic insufficiency followed ultimately by aortic dissection is a common complication of this disorder. Other clinical features of Marfan syndrome include dural ectasia and striae. Diagnostic criteria for Marfan syndrome are summarized in Table 47–6.

New mutations in *FBN-1* account for approximately 25% of cases of Marfan syndrome. Marfan syndrome is caused by many mutations. Virtually every family in which a member is affected with Marfan syndrome has a different mutation in this large gene.

Autosomal Recessive Disorders

Disorders that are inherited in an AR manner manifest only when *both* copies of a gene pair have a mutation (Table 47–7). Affected children usually are born to unaffected parents, each of whom, by definition, carries one copy of the mutation. If both members of a couple are carriers, or heterozygotes, for this mutation, each of their offspring has a 25% chance of being affected (Fig. 47–3).

Sickle Cell Disease (OMIM #603903)

▶ SEE CHAPTER 150.

Tay-Sachs Disease (OMIM # 272800)

▶ SEE CHAPTERS 55 AND 185.

TABLE 47-6. Diagnostic Criteria for Marfan Syndrome*

System	Major Criteria	Minor Criteria

Skeletal	*Presence of at least 4 of the following manifestations:*
	  Pectus carinatum
	  Pectus excavatum requiring surgery
	  Reduced upper-to-lower segment ratio or arm span–to-height ratio >1.05
	  Wrist and thumb signs
	  Scoliosis >20° or spondylolisthesis present
	  Reduced extension at the elbows (<170°)
	  Medial displacement of medial malleolus causing pes planus
	  Protrusio acetabuli of any degree (as ascertained on radiographs)
		Pectus excavatum of moderate severity
		Joint hypermobility
		Highly arched palate with crowding of teeth
		Facial appearance (dolichocephaly, malar hypoplasia, enophthalmos, retrognathia, down-slanting palpebral fissures)

Ocular	Ectopia lentis (dislocated lens)	Abnormally flat cornea (as measured by keratometry) Increased axial length of globe (as measured by ultrasound)
Cardiac	Dilation of the ascending aorta with or without aortic regurgitation and involving at least the sinuses of Valsalva, *or* Dissection of the ascending aorta	Mitral valve prolapse with or without mitral valve regurgitation Dilation of the main pulmonary artery, in the absence of valvular or peripheral pulmonic stenosis or any other obvious cause (<40 years old) Calcification of the mitral annulus (<40 years old) Dilation or dissection of the descending thoracic or abdominal aorta (<50 years old)
Pulmonary	None	Spontaneous pneumothorax Apical blebs (ascertained by chest x-ray)
Skin	None	Stretch marks not associated with marked weight changes, pregnancy, or repetitive stress Recurrent incisional hernias
Dura	Lumbosacral dural ectasia by CT or MRI	None
Family genetic history	Having a parent, child, or sibling who meets these diagnostic criteria independently Presence of a haplotype around *FBN1*, inherited by descent, known to be associated with unequivocally diagnosed Marfan syndrome in the family	None

*If there is an affected family member, only one major criterion is necessary for diagnosis. If no family history, two major criteria (organ systems) and one minor criterion (involvement of a third organ system) are necessary.

X-Linked Disorders

More than 500 genes have been identified on the X chromosome, whereas only about 50 are believed to be present on the Y chromosome. Females, whose cells have two copies of an X chromosome, possess two copies of each of the genes on the X chromosome, whereas males, who have one X chromosome and a Y chromosome, have only one copy of these genes. Early in female embryonic development, one X chromosome is randomly inactivated in each cell (the **Lyon hypothesis**). There are many X-linked disorders (colorblindness, Duchenne muscular dystrophy, hemophilia A) in which heterozygous females show some manifestations of the disorder. Selective (skewed) inactivation of the normal gene produces symptoms in "carrier" women.

X-Linked Recessive Inheritance

Most disorders involving the X chromosome are recessive. Males, with only one copy of the X chromosome, are more likely to manifest these diseases than females, who have two copies of the chromosome. Each son born to a female carrier of an X-linked recessive trait has a 50% chance of inheriting the trait, but none of this woman's daughters would be affected (each daughter has a 50%

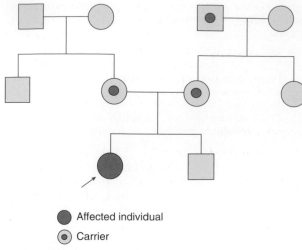

● Affected individual

◉ Carrier

Figure 47–3

Pedigree of family showing autosomal recessive inheritance.

chance of being a carrier). An affected father transmits the mutation to all of his daughters, who become carriers, but his sons, having received their father's Y chromosome, would not be affected (as such, there is no male-to-male transmission) (Table 47–8 and Fig. 47–4).

DUCHENNE MUSCULAR DYSTROPHY (OMIM #310200)

▶ SEE CHAPTER 182.

HEMOPHILIA A (OMIM #306700)

▶ SEE CHAPTER 151.

TABLE 47–7. Rules of Autosomal Recessive Inheritance
Trait appears in siblings, not in their parents or their offspring
On average, 25% of siblings of the proband are affected (at the time of conception, each sibling has a 25% chance of being affected)
A "normal" sibling of an affected individual has a two thirds chance of being a carrier (heterozygote)
Males and females are likely to be affected equally
Rare traits are likely to be associated with parental consanguinity
Traits generally involve mutations in genes that code for enzymes (e.g., phenylalanine hydroxylase–deficient in PKU) and are associated with serious illness and shortened life span

TABLE 47–8. Rules of X-Linked Recessive Inheritance
Incidence of the trait is higher in males than in females
Trait is passed from carrier females, who may show mild expression of the gene, to half of their sons, who are more severely affected
Each son of a carrier female has a 1 in 2 chance of being affected
Trait is transmitted from affected males to all of their daughters; it is never transmitted father to son
Because the trait can be passed through multiple carrier females, it may "skip" generations

X-Linked Dominant Inheritance

Only a few X-linked dominant disorders have been described. For some of these disorders, it would be expected that males and females would be equally affected, with females being less severely affected than males, the result of lyonization. This is the case for **X-linked vitamin D–resistant rickets** (hypophosphatemic rickets). This is a disorder in which the kidney's ability to reabsorb phosphate is impaired. Phosphate levels and resulting rickets are not as severe in females as in males.

Another group of X-linked dominant disorders are lethal in males. Affected mothers can have affected or normal daughters and normal sons. Affected sons die in utero. **Incontinentia pigmenti** (OMIM #308300) involves a characteristic swirling skin pattern of hyperpigmentation that develops after a perinatal skin rash with blistering. Affected females also have variable

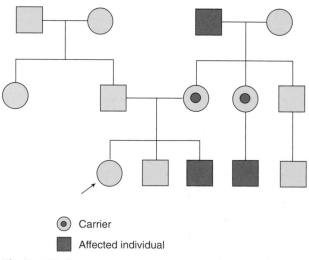

◉ Carrier

■ Affected individual

Figure 47–4

Pedigree showing X-linked recessive inheritance.

involvement of the CNS, hair, nails, teeth, and eyes. In **Rett syndrome** (OMIM #312750), females are normal at birth, but then after a period of normal development (6 to 18 months) develop microcephaly and regression of developmental milestones followed by developmental arrest. About 50% of patients develop seizures. Patients often appear autistic and by age 2 years lose all purposeful hand movements.

OTHER TYPES OF GENETIC DISORDERS

Most congenital malformations and inherited conditions are not associated with a single gene mutation or an abnormality in the amount of chromosomal material. The largest group of these conditions shows multifactorial inheritance. Some conditions show unusual patterns of inheritance. Some disorders are due largely to the exposure of the fetus to drugs or chemicals known as teratogens.

Multifactorial Disorders

Often described as **polygenic inheritance**, multifactorially inherited disorders result from interplay of genetic and environmental factors. In addition to 20% of all congenital malformations, including cleft lip and palate, spina bifida, and hypertrophic pyloric stenosis, most common disorders of childhood and adult life, such as asthma, atherosclerosis, diabetes, and cancer, result from such an interaction between genes and the environment. These disorders do not follow simple mendelian modes of inheritance; rather, affected individuals seem to cluster in families: The disorders occur more commonly in first-degree and second-degree relatives than would be expected by chance, and they are more likely to be concordant (although not 100%) in monozygotic twins than in dizygotic twins.

Hypertrophic Pyloric Stenosis

Occurring in approximately 1 in 300 children, hypertrophic pyloric stenosis is five times more likely to occur in males than in females. When a child with hypertrophic pyloric stenosis is born in a family, the recurrence risk for future progeny is 5% to 10% for males and 1.5% to 2% for females. In adulthood, the risk that an affected male would have an affected child is markedly increased over the general population: 4% of sons and 1% of daughters of such men would be likely to be affected. Even more striking is the risk to children born to an affected female: 17% to 20% of sons and 7% of daughters are affected.

The thickness of the pyloric muscle may be distributed across a bell-shaped curve; one's position on the bell-shaped curve is determined by many factors, including the expression of multiple, unknown genes. Hypertrophic pyloric stenosis may result when an individual's genetic and environmental influences cause him or her to fall to an extreme position on this curve, past a certain point, which is called a **threshold**. In hypertrophic pyloric stenosis, this threshold is farther to the left for males than it is for females.

Neural Tube Defects

Myelomeningocele affects 1 in 1000 live-born infants in the U.S. Anencephaly occurs with a similar frequency, although most of these infants are either stillborn or die in the neonatal period. Multiple genetic and nongenetic factors dictate the speed with which the neural tube closes, as follows:

1. The frequency of neural tube defects (NTDs) varies greatly in different ethnic groups. NTDs are far more common in the British Isles, where, in 1990, they occurred in 1 in 250 live births, and are much less common in Asia, where the frequency was 1 in 4000. These ethnic differences suggest a genetic component.
2. Couples from the British Isles who come to the U.S. have a risk intermediate between the risks in the United Kingdom and the U.S., suggesting an environmental component.
3. The occurrence of NTDs exhibits seasonality. Affected infants are more likely to be born during the late fall and early winter, again suggesting an environmental component.
4. Periconceptual supplementation with folic acid significantly decreases the risk of having an infant with an NTD. This nutritional influence suggests an environmental component and a folate-susceptible gene or enzyme.
5. Parents who have one child with an NTD are 20 to 40 times more likely to have a second affected child; this provides further evidence of a genetic component.

Disorders with Unusual Patterns of Inheritance

Mitochondrial Inheritance

Human cells contain non-nuclear DNA; a single chromosome exists in each mitochondrion, and mutations within this DNA are associated with a few related diseases. Mitochondrial DNA (mtDNA), which is circular and 16.5 kb in length, replicates independently of nuclear DNA. Involved in the production of energy used to run the cell, mtDNA codes for a few respiratory chain proteins (however, most mitochondrial proteins are coded on nuclear DNA) and for a set of transfer RNAs that are unique to mitochondrial protein synthesis. Virtually all of the mitochondria are supplied to the developing zygote by the oocyte. A woman with a mutation in mtDNA passes this mutation to all of her children. More than one population of mitochondria may be present in the oocyte, a phenomenon called **heteroplasmy**. mtDNA mutation may be present in a few or in many of these mitochondria. When the fertilized egg divides, the mitochondria are distributed randomly to the developing zygote. It is possible that the mutant mitochondria end up in tissues that support the developing embryo (placenta), rather than the embryo itself. The presence of symptoms and signs in the offspring and the severity of the symptoms and signs depend on the ratio of mutant to wild-type mtDNA present in that tissue. If an abundance of mutant mitochondria exists in tissue that has high energy requirements, such as brain, muscle, liver, and kidney, clinical symptoms occur. If fewer mutant mitochondria are present in this tissue, few clinical symptoms may be seen.

An example of this type of mitochondrial disorder is **MELAS** (**m**itochondrial **e**ncephalomyopathy with **l**actic **a**cidosis and **s**trokelike episodes). Individuals affected with MELAS are normal in early childhood. Then, between the ages of 5 and 15 years, they develop episodic vomiting, seizures, and recurrent cerebral insults that resemble strokes. In 80% of cases, analysis of the mtDNA reveals a specific mutation (A3243G) in the *MTTL1* gene (a gene that codes for a mitochondrial transfer RNA).

In families in which MELAS occurs, a wide range of neurologic symptoms and signs may be seen in first-degree relatives, including **progressive external ophthalmoplegia**, hearing loss, cardiomyopathy, and diabetes mellitus. Although all offspring of a woman who carries the mutation would be affected, because of heteroplasmy, the severity of clinical disease varies, depending on the percentage of mitochondria bearing the mutation that are present.

Uniparental Disomy

Evaluation of a child with uniparental disomy (UPD) reveals a normal karyotype. Chromosomal markers are identical to the markers found on the chromosomes of the patient's mother or father (but not both). In UPD, the patient inherits two copies of the mother's or father's chromosome and no copy from the other parent.

UPD probably occurs as the result of a spontaneous rescue mechanism. At the time of conception, through nondisjunction, the fertilized egg is trisomic for a particular chromosome, with two copies of one parent's chromosome and one copy of the other parent's chromosome; conceptuses with trisomy often miscarry early in development. Patients with UPD survive

because they spontaneously lose one of three copies of the affected chromosome. If the single chromosome from one parent is lost, the patient has UPD.

An alternate explanation involves monosomy for a chromosome rather than trisomy. Had the patient, at the time of conception, inherited only a single copy of a chromosome, spontaneous duplication of the single chromosome would lead to UPD.

Prader-Willi Syndrome (OMIM #176270) and Angelman Syndrome (OMIM #105830)

Occurring in approximately 1 in 10,000 live-born infants, **Prader-Willi syndrome** is characterized by hypotonia of prenatal onset, postnatal growth delay, a characteristic appearance including almond-shaped eyes and small hands and feet, developmental disability, hypogonadotropic hypogonadism, and obesity after infancy. Early in life, affected infants are so hypotonic that they cannot take in enough calories to maintain their weight. Nasogastric feeding is invariably necessary for some time, and failure to thrive is a common problem. During the first year of life, muscle tone improves, and children develop a voracious appetite. Some patients with Prader-Willi syndrome have a small deletion of chromosome 15 (15q11). In patients without a deletion, 20% have UPD of chromosome 15.

Angelman syndrome is a condition with a characteristic facial appearance, moderate to severe mental retardation, absence of speech, ataxic movements of the arms and legs, a characteristic craniofacial appearance, and a seizure disorder that is characterized by laughter. Angelman syndrome also has a deletion in the 15q11 region. The 15q11 deletion is identifiable in 70% of children with Angelman syndrome; some patients (approximately 10%) have UPD of chromosome 15.

If the deletion occurs in the paternal chromosome 15, the affected individual has Prader-Willi syndrome, whereas Angelman syndrome results from deletions occurring only in the maternal chromosome 15. When UPD is responsible, maternal UPD results in Prader-Willi syndrome, whereas paternal UPD results in Angelman syndrome. If the patient has two copies of the *maternal* chromosome 15 (and no copy of paternal chromosome 15), the patient has Prader-Willi syndrome. If there is *paternal* UPD (two copies of the father's chromosome 15), features of Angelman syndrome are manifested.

This phenomenon is explained by **genomic imprinting**. Imprinting is an epigenetic phenomenon, a nonheritable change in the DNA that causes an alteration in gene expression. Prader-Willi syndrome is caused by deficiency of the protein product of the gene *SNRPN* (small nuclear ribonucleoprotein). Although

SNRPN is present on the maternally derived and the paternally derived chromosome 15, it is normally expressed only in the paternally derived chromosome. Expression is normally blocked in the maternal chromosome because the bases of the open reading frame are methylated; this physical change in the DNA prevents gene expression. Prader-Willi syndrome results whenever a paternal chromosome 15 is missing, either through deletion or through UPD.

In Angelman syndrome, in the same region of chromosome 15, a second gene, ubiquitin-protein ligase E3A (*UBE3A*), exists and is normally expressed only in the maternally derived chromosome 15. Although the gene is present in the paternal chromosome 15, *UBE3A* is methylated, and gene expression is blocked. Angelman syndrome, a deficiency of the gene product of *UBE3A*, results either from deletion of the critical region of maternal chromosome 15 or from paternal UPD.

Expansion of a Triplet Repeat

More than 50% of human DNA appears as repeat sequences. Disorders caused by expansions of triplet repeats include **fragile X syndrome**, **Huntington disease**, **myotonic dystrophy**, **Friedreich ataxia**, and the **spinocerebellar ataxias**. Although an increase in the number of the three bases that are repeated is at the heart of each disorder, the molecular mechanism differs.

Fragile X Syndrome. Occurring with a frequency of approximately 1 in 2000 children, fragile X syndrome is the most common cause of inherited mental retardation. The **phenotype** includes characteristic craniofacial findings (large head; prominent forehead, jaw, and ears); macro-orchidism with testicular volume twice that expected in adulthood; a mild connective tissue disorder including joint laxity, patulous eustachian tubes, and mitral valve prolapse; and a characteristic neurobehavioral profile, including mental retardation (ranging from mild to profound), autistic-spectrum disordes, and pervasive developmental disorder.

In fragile X syndrome, it appears that the distal region of the X chromosome is breaking off—hence the term *fragile X*. In the Xq27 region, there is a triplet repeat composed of a cytosine and two guanines (–CGG–). Occurring in the CpG island, a part of the promoter region of a gene that has been called *FMR-1* (fragile X mental retardation-1), in unaffected individuals who have no family history of fragile X, the number of –CGG– repeats ranges from 0 to 45, with most people having between 25 and 35. In individuals with fragile X syndrome, the number of these repeats is always greater than 230; such people are said to carry the "full mutation." Between these two categories, there is a third group of people, who have between 57 and 230 –CGG– repeats. Always phenotypically normal, these individuals are said to be **premutation carriers**.

The molecular mechanism involved in fragile X syndrome seems to be due to failure to express the protein product of the *FMR-1* gene, which has been called *fragile X mental retardation protein* (FMRP). FMRP is a carrier protein that shuttles mRNA between the nucleus and cytoplasm in the CNS and other areas (e.g., the developing testis) during early embryonic development and is produced in unaffected individuals and premutation carriers. In individuals with the full mutation, FMRP is not produced, transcription being blocked because of methylation (an epigenetic phenomenon) of the large number of –CGG– repeats in the CpG island. Fragile X syndrome seems to result as a consequence of a **loss-of-function mutation**, the failure of expression of FMRP because of methylation of the promoter sequence.

Most children with fragile X syndrome are born to couples in which mental retardation did not previously occur. In women who are premutation carriers, an expansion in the number of –CGG– repeats occurs during gametogenesis. The cause of this expansion, which can be quite dramatic, increasing the number of repeats from 100 in the mother to 500 or more in the child, is not understood.

TERATOGENIC AGENTS

Approximately 6.5% of all birth defects are attributed to teratogens, chemical, physical, or biologic agents that have the potential to damage embryonic tissue, resulting in one or more congenital malformations. Agents known to be teratogenic include certain drugs (prescription and nonprescription); intrauterine infections (rubella); maternal diseases, such as diabetes mellitus and hyperthermia; and substances found in the environment, such as heavy metals. Knowledge of which agents are potential teratogens and their effect on the developing fetus is important because limiting exposure to teratogens is an effective way to prevent birth defects. (See Chapters 58, 59, and 60.)

Maternal Infections

Rubella was the first maternal infection known to cause a pattern of malformations in fetuses affected in utero. Cytomegalovirus, *Toxoplasma gondii*, herpes simplex, and varicella are additional potentially teratogenic in utero infections. (See Chapter 66.)

Maternal Disease

Maternal diabetes mellitus and maternal PKU can result in congenital anomalies in the fetus. Strict control of these disorders before and during pregnancy protects the developing child. (See Chapter 59.)

Medications and Chemicals

Fetal alcohol syndrome may be the most common teratogenic syndrome, occurring in 3 to 5 per 1000 children. Features include prenatal and postnatal growth deficiency, microcephaly, developmental delay, skeletal and cardiac anomalies, and a characteristic facial appearance. Pregnant women must drink at least 6 oz of alcohol each day during the pregnancy to cause the full fetal alcohol syndrome. If alcohol consumption begins after the first trimester, when organogenesis has completed, the child is unlikely to have physical features consistent with fetal alcohol syndrome, but remains at risk for the developmental and behavioral abnormalities of the syndrome. This latter condition is called **fetal alcohol effect** and is much more common than the full fetal alcohol syndrome; fetal alcohol effect affects 20% to 30% of children born to alcoholic women. Warfarin, retinoic acid, phenytoin, and thalidomide are additional teratogenic agents (see Chapter 59).

Hyperthermia

Hyperthermia in humans has not been conclusively associated with birth defects. Studies in rats suggest a potential teratogenic effect, which resulted in microphthalmia, encephalocele, facial clefting, and maxillary hypoplasia. Current recommendations include avoiding conditions (e.g., hot tubs) that might increase core temperatures during the first trimester.

Radiation

High-dose radiation exposure during pregnancy in Hiroshima, Japan, and Nagasaki, Japan, was shown to increase the rate of spontaneous abortion and result in children born with microcephaly, mental retardation, and skeletal malformations. Estimates of exposure to cause these effects were approximately 25 rad. The dose from routine radiologic diagnostic examinations is in the millirad range.

Methyl Mercury

An inadvertent spill of methyl mercury into the water supply of Minamata, Japan, led to an outbreak of congenital malformations. Children were born with neurologic abnormalities, including mental retardation, cerebral palsy–like movement disorders, and, in a few cases, blindness. This incident raised concern about exposure of fetuses to heavy metals (especially mercury) from contaminated fish in the diets of pregnant women.

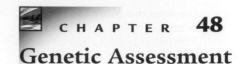

CHAPTER 48

Genetic Assessment

Individuals referred to a geneticist because of the suspicion that they have a genetic disorder are called **probands**; individuals who come for genetic counseling are called **consultands**. Referral for genetic evaluation may be made for a wide variety of reasons and at different stages of life (fetus, neonate, pregnancy, adolescence).

PRECONCEPTION AND PRENATAL COUNSELING

Familial Factors

Families with affected relatives with genetic disorders may have questions about how the disorder is inherited. In consultation with a geneticist, the inheritance pattern and the risk for having an affected child would be discussed.

In some cultures, it is common for relatives to mate. **Consanguinity** does not increase the likelihood of offspring having any particular known genetic disorder, but may increase the chance that a child will be born with a rare autosomal recessively inherited condition, the mutated gene for which segregates through that family. Generally the closer the relation between the partners, the greater the number of genes the individuals share in common, and the greater the risk that offspring would have some problem. The risk of first cousins producing a child with an AR disorder is 1 in 64. In evaluating such couples, it is important to determine to which ethnic group the couple belongs, and to test for conditions commonly found in that group.

Screening

It is common for couples to be screened for disorders that may occur in their ethnic group. People of Ashkenazi Jewish background may choose to be screened for heterozygosity for a panel of autosomal recessively inherited disorders, including Tay-Sachs disease, Niemann-Pick disease, Bloom syndrome, Canavan disease, Gaucher syndrome, cystic fibrosis, Fanconi anemia, and familial dysautonomia. People of African American ancestry may choose to be screened for sickle cell anemia and people whose ancestors originated in the Mediterranean basin may be screened for thalassemia.

Maternal serum screening is offered to most pregnant women at 16 weeks' gestation (see Chapter 58). This test is used to assess the risk for NTDs, as well as to assess pregnancies at increased risk for a chromosomal abnormality (e.g., Down syndrome, trisomy 18). **Alpha-fetoprotein (AFP)** is a major protein secreted by the fetal liver, gastrointestinal tract, and yolk sac. If there is an open NTD, such as encephalocele, anencephaly, or myelomeningocele, or any other defect in which the fetus' skin is disrupted, such as an omphalocele, abnormal amounts of AFP can be found in the amniotic fluid. Some of the AFP crosses the placenta and enters the maternal circulation. Levels of AFP are highest during 14 to 18 weeks of gestation, but some level of AFP generally can be detected in maternal blood samples at almost any time during the pregnancy. If the fetus has an NTD, high levels of AFP generally are detected in the maternal serum, but there is overlap between normal levels and levels detected in fetuses with NTDs. About 80% of fetuses with NTDs can be detected in this manner.

Some women with lower than normal AFP levels have fetuses with chromosomal defects. Approximately 50% of fetuses with chromosomal abnormalities (Down syndrome, trisomy 18, trisomy 13) can be detected by low AFP levels. Three other proteins—unconjugated estriol (uE3), inhibin A, and human chorionic gonadotropin (HCG)—are added to the maternal serum screening to give what is often referred to as the **quadruple screen**. The addition of these compounds increases the detection rate to about 80%. There is an increased risk for Down syndrome (trisomy 21) when levels of uE3 and AFP are both low and there is an increased level of HCG. The risk for trisomy 18 is greatly increased when AFP, uE3, and HCG are low. Women with an abnormal maternal serum screening test result are offered genetic counseling, fetal ultrasonography, and an amniocentesis. A negative screening test does not eliminate the chance of having a child with an NTD or chromosomal abnormality.

It is common for a pregnant woman to have a "screening" ultrasound done at 18 weeks' gestation. An anatomy scan is generally done to look for congenital anomalies. Brain, heart, kidneys, lungs, and spine are examined.

Maternal Factors

The presence of either acute or chronic maternal illness during pregnancy may lead to complications in the developing fetus. Chronic conditions often lead to exposure of the fetus to medications used to treat the mother that are potentially teratogenic. Acute illnesses such as varicella, Lyme disease, West Nile virus, and cytomegalovirus expose the fetus to infectious agents that may cause birth defects. Other factors, such as maternal smoking, alcohol use, and maternal exposure to radiation or chemicals, also may necessitate genetic counseling. Advanced maternal age is defined as a mother who is 35 years old or older at the time of delivery. These women have an increased risk for a nondisjunctional event and are at risk for having an infant born with a trisomy.

Amniocentesis may be recommended for reasons other than advanced maternal age. Known chromosomal problems in the family, a family history of an NTD, a past history of multiple pregnancy losses, and a history of one or more family members with a known genetic disorder that requires biochemical or DNA testing for prenatal diagnosis are common reasons for referral to a geneticist for amniocentesis. The procedure typically is performed in the midtrimester, between 15 and 18 weeks of gestation. Under ultrasound guidance, a needle is inserted transabdominally into the amniotic cavity, and approximately 20 mL of amniotic fluid is withdrawn for diagnostic studies. Generally, cytogenetic studies are done on the amniotic cells, but biochemical or DNA testing also may be performed.

An alternative to amniocentesis is **chorionic villus sampling**. Also performed under ultrasound guidance, chorionic villus sampling can be performed either transabdominally or transcervically. A small sample of the chorionic villi is taken by needle biopsy. The advantage of chorionic villus sampling is that it can be performed earlier than amniocentesis, usually between 10 and 12 weeks of gestation; its disadvantage is that the procedure introduces a greater risk of pregnancy loss than amniocentesis. Chorionic villus sampling is associated with an approximately 1% risk of spontaneous pregnancy loss, whereas the risk inherent in amniocentesis is approximately 1 in 300.

Postnatal—Newborn and Infant

Two percent to 4% of newborns have a genetic abnormality or birth defect. This broad definition of a birth defect is meant to include not only a visible malformation, but also functional defects that might not be apparent at birth.

Birth defects have a significant impact on childhood morbidity and mortality. Birth defects have a more significant impact on childhood mortality because death from infectious diseases has decreased. Almost 11% of childhood deaths can be traced to a genetic cause. If contributing genetic factors related to childhood deaths are considered, this increases to almost 25%. Consultation with a geneticist for a newborn or infant may be prompted by many different findings, including the presence of a birth defect or malformation, abnormal results on a routine newborn screening test, abnormalities in growth (e.g., failure to gain weight, increase in length, or abnormal head growth), developmental delay, blindness or deafness, and the knowledge of a family history of a genetic disorder or chromosomal abnormality or (owing to prenatal testing) the presence of genetic disorder or chromosomal abnormality in the infant.

Adolescent and Adult

Adolescents and adults may be seen by a geneticist for evaluation for a genetic disorder with later onset. Some neurodegenerative disorders, such as Huntington disease, adult-onset spinal muscular atrophy, and the Charcot-Marie-Tooth peripheral neuropathies, present later in life. Some forms of hereditary blindness (retinal degenerative diseases) and deafness (Usher syndrome, neurofibromatosis type 2) may not show significant symptoms until adolescence or early adulthood. Genetic consultation also may be prompted for a known family history of a **hereditary cancer syndrome** (multiple endocrine neoplasia type 2, breast and ovarian cancer, hereditary nonpolyposis colon cancer). Individuals may wish to have testing done to determine if they carry a mutation for these syndromes and would be at risk for developing certain types of cancers. A known family history or personal history of a genetic disorder or chromosomal abnormality might prompt testing in anticipation of pregnancy planning.

GENERAL APPROACH TO PATIENTS

Family History

A pedigree usually is drawn to help visualize various inheritance patterns. Answers to questions about the family help to determine if there is an AD, AR, X-linked, or sporadic disorder. It may be necessary to examine the parents closely when a child apparently has a new onset of an AD disorder. The recurrence risk for AD disorders is different if a parent is found to be affected, even if there is decreased penetrance, than if the parent is unaffected. If the parents are unaffected, the child is most likely a new mutation. The recurrence risk would be low, but is complicated by the need to consider gonadal mosaicism. When the parent is affected (even mildly so), the recurrence risk is 50%. With X-linked disorders, such as fragile X syndrome, the focus is on the maternal family history to determine if there is a significant enough risk to warrant testing.

Questions about the couple's age are important to ascertain the risk related to advanced maternal age for nondisjunction and increased paternal age for new mutations leading to AD and X-linked disorders. If there have been more than two spontaneous abortions, there is an increased risk that one of the parents has a balanced translocation and that the spontaneous abortions are due to chromosomal abnormalities in the fetus.

Pregnancy

For prenatal counseling and genetics consultations for newborns and children, it is often important to gather information about the pregnancy (see Chapters 58, 59, and 60). A maternal history of a chronic medical condition, such as a seizure disorder or diabetes, has known complications in a fetus. Medication used in pregnancy can be teratogenic to the developing fetus. The pregnant woman's exposure to toxic chemicals (work related) or use of alcohol, cigarettes, or drugs of abuse can have serious effects on the developing fetus. Maternal infection during pregnancy with varicella, *Toxoplasma,* cytomegalovirus, and parvovirus B19, among others, has been found to cause malformations in the fetus.

Sometimes previous testing has been performed, such as amniocentesis or chorionic villus sampling, and there are abnormal results. A fetal ultrasound may have detected a malformation that needs follow-up when the infant is born. Often hydronephrosis is detected prenatally. These infants need a repeat ultrasound soon after birth.

Delivery and Birth

An infant born prematurely is likely to have more complications than a term infant. It should be determined whether the infant is premature, full term, or post term. An infant can be small for gestational age, appropriate for gestational age, or large for gestational age. Each of these has implications for the child (see Chapters 58, 59, and 60). Large for gestational age infants are often born to mothers with gestational diabetes, and the increased size is due to the exposure of the infant to high glucose levels and the resulting high insulin levels. These infants are at risk for hypoglycemia in the newborn period because of the persistently elevated levels of insulin and the decreased postnatal supply of glucose.

It is important to establish if there were problems with the labor or delivery. Prolonged labor may stress the fetus. Hypoxia or anoxia usually does not occur with most deliveries, but can have devastating consequences on the infant. Seizures in the newborn period are often an ominous sign and are a consequence of severe hypoxia or are secondary to metabolic causes. Asking if the parents noted any complications at the delivery may reveal important information.

Past Medical History

Children with inborn errors of metabolism who have intermittent symptoms often have a history of multiple hospitalizations for dehydration or vomiting. Neuromuscular disorders may have a normal period followed by increasing weakness or ataxia. Children with lysosomal storage diseases, such as the mucopolysaccharidoses, often have recurrent ear infections and can develop sleep apnea.

Development

Many disorders may start to have symptoms after a period of normal development, and others have symptoms from birth (see Chapters 7 and 8). Some adult-onset disorders have no symptoms until the teens or later. Assessing school problems is important. The type of learning problem, age of onset, and whether there is improvement with intervention or continued decline all are important for proper assessment.

Physical Examination

A careful and thorough physical examination is necessary for all patients with signs or symptoms of genetic disease and patients suspected to have a genetic disease. Sometimes subtle clues may lead to an unsuspected diagnosis. Features suggestive of a syndrome are discussed in more detail in Chapter 50.

Laboratory Evaluation

Chromosome Analysis

An individual's chromosomal material, known as the *karyotype,* can be analyzed using cells capable of dividing. In pediatrics, lymphocytes obtained from peripheral blood are the usual source for such cells, but cells obtained from bone marrow aspiration, skin biopsy (fibroblasts), or prenatally from amniotic fluid or chorionic villi also can be used. Cells are placed in culture medium and stimulated to grow, their division is arrested in either metaphase or prophase, slides are made, the chromosomes are stained with Giemsa or other dyes, and the chromosomes are analyzed.

In metaphase, chromosomes are short, squat, and easy to count. Metaphase analysis should be ordered in children whose features suggest a known aneuploidy syndrome, such as a trisomy or monosomy. Chromosomes analyzed in prophase are long, thin, and drawn out; analysis gives far more details than are seen in metaphase preparations. Prophase analysis is ordered in individuals with multiple congenital anomalies in whom an obvious disorder is not evident.

Fluorescent In Situ Hybridization

Fluorescent in situ hybridization allows the identification of the presence or absence of a specific region of DNA. A probe of complementary DNA that is specific for the region in question is generated in the laboratory, and a fluorescent marker is attached. The probe is incubated with cells from the subject and viewed under a microscope. The bound probe fluoresces, allowing the number of copies of DNA segment in question to be counted. This technique is useful in Prader-Willi syndrome and Angelman syndrome, in which a deletion in a segment of 15q11.2 occurs, and in velocardiofacial syndrome, which is associated with a deletion of 22.q11.2.

Direct DNA Analysis

Direct DNA analysis allows identification of mutations in a growing number of genetic disorders. Using **polymerase chain reaction**, the specific gene in question can be amplified and analyzed. The website www.genetests.org lists disorders in which direct DNA analysis is available and identifies laboratories performing such testing.

CHAPTER 49
Chromosomal Disorders

Errors that occur in meiosis, during the production of the gametes, can lead to abnormalities of chromosome structure or number. Chromosomal abnormalities cause disorders such as Down syndrome, trisomy 13, trisomy 18, Turner syndrome, and Klinefelter syndrome and rarer chromosomal duplications, deletions, or inversions.

Chromosomal abnormalities occur in approximately 8% of fertilized ova, but only in 0.6% of live-born infants. Fifty percent of spontaneous abortuses have chromosomal abnormalities. The most common aneuploidy chromosomal abnormality found in fetuses is Turner syndrome (45,X). It is estimated that 99% of 45,X fetuses are spontaneously aborted. The fetal loss rate for Down syndrome, the most viable of the autosomal aneuploidies, approaches 80%. Most other chromosomal abnormalities also severely affect fetal viability. In newborns and in older children, many features suggest the presence of chromosome anomalies, including low birth weight (small for gestational age), failure to thrive, developmental delay, and the presence of three or more congenital malformations.

ABNORMALITIES IN NUMBER (ANEUPLOIDY)

During meiosis or mitosis, failure of a chromosomal pair to separate properly results in nondisjunction. **Aneuploidy** is a change in the number of chromosomes that occurs as a result of nondisjunction. A cell may have one (**monosomy**) or three (**trisomy**) copies of a particular chromosome.

Trisomies

Down Syndrome

Down syndrome is the most common of all the abnormalities of chromosomal number. Occurring in 1 of every 800 births, most cases (92.5%) of Down syndrome are due to nondisjunction; in 80%, the nondisjunctional event occurs in maternal meiosis phase I. As a result of nondisjunction, there are three copies of chromosome 21 (trisomy 21); using standard cytogenetic nomenclature, trisomy 21 is designated 47,XX,+21 or 47,XY,+21. In 4.5% of cases, the extra chromosome 21 is part of a robertsonian translocation, which occurs when the long arms (q) of two acrocentric chromosomes (chromosomes 13, 14, 15, 21, or 22) fuse at the centromeres, and the short arms (p), containing copies of ribosomal RNA, are lost. The most common robertsonian translocation leading to Down syndrome is between chromosomes 14 and 21; standard nomenclature is 46,XX,t (14q21q) or 46,XY,t (14q21q).

In approximately 3% of cases of Down syndrome, mosaicism occurs. In these individuals, there are two populations of cells: one with trisomy 21 and one with a normal complement of chromosomes. This mosaicism occurs because of a nondisjunction event that occurs after fertilization and after a few cell divisions or from what is referred to as **trisomic rescue**. The loss of this aneuploidy returns the cell to 46,XX or 46,XY, and "rescues" this cell. This is a rescue not of the entire organism, but of some of the cell lines. The person is referred to as a mosaic for these two populations of cells and according to standard nomenclature is designated 47,XX,+21/46XX or 47,XY,+21/ 46,XY. Although it is widely believed that these individuals are more mildly affected, there are wide variations in the clinical findings of these individuals.

Children with Down syndrome are most likely to be diagnosed in the newborn period. Although these infants have normal birth weight and length, they have hypotonia. The characteristic facial appearance, with brachycephaly, flattened occiput, hypoplastic midface, flattened nasal bridge, upward slanting palpebral fissures, epicanthal folds, and large protruding tongue, is apparent at birth. Infants also have short broad hands often with a transverse palmar crease and a wide gap between the first and second toes. The severe hypotonia may cause feeding problems and decreased activity (Table 49–1).

Approximately 40% have **congenital heart disease**. Mostly caused by endocardial cushion defects, these anomalies include atrioventricular canal, ventriculoseptal or atrioseptal defects, and valvular disease. Approximately 10% of newborns with Down syndrome have **gastrointestinal tract anomalies**. The three most common defects are duodenal atresia, annular pancreas, and imperforate anus.

One percent of infants with Down syndrome are found to have congenital hypothyroidism, which is identified as part of the newborn screening program. Acquired hypothyroidism is a more common problem. Thyroid function testing must be monitored periodically during the child's life.

Polycythemia at birth (hematocrit levels >70%) is common and may require treatment. Some infants with Down syndrome show a leukemoid reaction, with white blood cell counts of 100,000/mm³. Although this reaction resembles congenital leukemia, it usually is a

---

TABLE 49–1.   Clinical Findings That May Be Present with Trisomy 21*

Stature smaller than peer age group Developmental delays Congenital heart disease (e.g., endocardial cushion defect and ventricular septal defect) Structural abnormalities of the bowel (e.g., tracheoesophageal fistula, duodenal atresia, annular pancreas, duodenal web, and Hirschsprung disease) Central hypotonia Brachycephaly Delayed closure of fontanels Small midface, hypoplastic frontal sinuses, myopia, and small (short) ears	Lax joints, including laxity of the atlantoaxial articulation (the latter predisposing the patient to C1-2 dislocation) Short, broad hands, feet, and digits; single palmar crease, clinodactyly Exaggerated space between first and second toe Velvety, loosely adhering mottled skin (cutis marmorata) in infancy; coarse, dry skin in adolescence Statistically increased risk for leukemia, Alzheimer disease, hypothyroidism

*An individual may exhibit any combination of these findings. There is no correlation between the number of physical findings and eventual level of mental performance. The increased risk for leukemia is significant, but probably no greater than 1% for any individual. Alzheimer disease is relatively common in persons with trisomy 21 who die in middle adult life, but the frequency in all adults with Down syndrome is not known.

self-limited condition, resolving on its own over the first month of life. Nonetheless, there is an increased risk for **leukemia** for children with Down syndrome. This increased risk is estimated to be 10 to 18 times the risk of individuals without Down syndrome. In children with Down syndrome younger than 1 year of age, congenital and infantile leukemia is generally acute nonlymphoblastic leukemia. In individuals with trisomy 21 older than 3 years, the types of leukemia are similar to children without Down syndrome, with the predominant type being acute lymphoblastic leukemia.

Down syndrome patients also are more susceptible to infection. They are more likely to develop cataracts. Also, approximately 10% have atlantoaxial instability, an increased distance between the first and second cervical vertebrae, which may predispose to spinal cord injury. Most individuals older than 35 years of age develop Alzheimer-like features.

Seventy-five percent of affected infants are born to women younger than 35 years old. Because only 5% of all infants are born to women older than 35, but 25% of Down syndrome infants are born to women older than 35, the risk for a child with Down syndrome increases strikingly with increasing maternal age. Four pregnancy-related markers (maternal serum AFP, uE3, inhibin A, and HCG) are studied to develop a risk profile for a woman's chance for having an infant with Down syndrome. This is a screening test; it is able only to identify women who are at increased risk for having an infant with Down syndrome and other trisomies, essentially indicating which women should be referred for more definitive testing. Amniocentesis should be offered to women who are identified by the screening test to be at increased risk.

The recurrence risk for parents who have had a child with Down syndrome depends on the child's cytogenetic findings. If the finding was 47,XX,+21 or 47,XY,+21 (i.e., trisomy 21), the recurrence risk based on empirical observation is approximately 1% (added to the age-specific risk for women <35 years old; use just the age-specific risk for women >35 years old) for subsequent pregnancies. If a translocation occurred to cause Down syndrome, chromosomal analysis of both parents must be performed. In approximately 65% of cases, the translocation is found to have arisen de novo (i.e., spontaneously, with both parents having normal karyotypes), but in 35% of cases, one of the parents has a balanced translocation. The recurrence risk depends on which parent is the carrier: if the mother is the carrier, the risk of recurrence is 10% to 15%; if the father is the carrier, the recurrence risk is 2% to 5%.

Trisomy 18

Trisomy 18 (47,XX,+18 or 47,XY,+18) is the second most common autosomal trisomy, occurring in approximately 1 in 7500 live births. It is more common among conceptuses, but greater than 95% of trisomy 18 conceptuses are spontaneously aborted in the first trimester. Trisomy 18 is usually lethal; less than 10% of affected infants survive until their first birthday. As a result of this poor prognosis, many clinicians favor limited medical intervention for the prolongation of life. Most infants with trisomy 18 are small for gestational age. Clinical features include hypertonia, prominent occiput, receding jaw, low-set and malformed ears, short sternum, rocker-bottom feet, hypoplastic nails, and characteristic clenching of fists—the second and fifth digits overlap the third and fourth digits (Table 49–2).

Trisomy 13

The third of the "common trisomies," trisomy 13 (47,XX,+13 or 47,XY,+13) is not as frequent as either trisomy 21 or trisomy 18, occurring in 1 in 12,000 live births. It is usually fatal in the first year of life; only 8.6% of infants survive beyond their first birthday.

Infants with trisomy 13 have numerous malformations (see Table 49–2). These infants are small for gestational age and microcephalic. Midline facial defects, such as cyclopia (single orbit), cebocephaly (single nostril), and cleft lip and palate are common, as are midline CNS anomalies, such as alobar holoprosencephaly. The forehead is generally sloping, ears are often small and malformed, and microphthalmia or anophthalmia may occur. Postaxial polydactyly of the hands is common, as is clubfeet or rocker-bottom feet. Hypospadias and cryptorchidism are common in boys, whereas girls generally have hypoplasia of the labia minora. Most infants with trisomy 13 also have congenital heart disease. Many infants with this condition have a punched-out scalp lesion over the left or right occiput called **aplasia cutis congenita**; when seen in conjunction with polydactyly and some or all of the above-mentioned facial findings, this finding is essentially pathognomonic for the diagnosis of trisomy 13.

Klinefelter Syndrome

Klinefelter syndrome, which occurs in 1 in 1000 male births, is the most common genetic cause of hypogonadism and infertility in men and is caused by the presence of an extra X chromosome (47,XXY) (see Chapter 174). The extra X chromosome arises from a nondisjunction in either the sperm or the egg. About 15% of boys with Klinefelter syndrome are found to be mosaic. These mosaic patterns are generally 46,XY/47,XXY, but 48,XXYY, 48,XXXY, and 49,XXXXY have been observed. The increasing number of X chromosomes is associated with increasing risk of mental retardation

TABLE 49–2. Findings That May Be Present in Trisomy 13 and Trisomy 18

	Trisomy 13	Trisomy 18
Head and face	Scalp defects (e.g., cutis aplasia)	Small and premature appearance
	Microphthalmia, corneal abnormalities	Tight palpebral fissures
	Cleft lip and palate in 60%-80% of cases	Narrow nose and hypoplastic nasal alae
	Microcephaly	Narrow bifrontal diameter
	Sloping forehead	Prominent occiput
	Holoprosencephaly (arrhinencephaly)	Micrognathia
	Capillary hemangiomas	Cleft lip or palate
	Deafness	
Chest	Congenital heart disease (e.g., VSD, PDA, and ASD) in 80% of cases	Congenital heart disease (e.g., VSD, PDA, and ASD)
	Thin posterior ribs (missing ribs)	Short sternum, small nipples
Extremities	Overlapping of fingers and toes (clinodactyly)	Limited hip abduction
	Polydactyly	Clinodactyly and overlapping fingers; index over third, fifth over fourth
	Hypoplastic nails, hyperconvex nails	Rocker-bottom feet
		Hypoplastic nails
General	Severe developmental delays and prenatal and postnatal growth retardation	Severe developmental delays and prenatal and postnatal growth retardation
	Renal abnormalities	Premature birth, polyhydramnios
	Nuclear projections in neutrophils	Inguinal or abdominal hernias
	Only 5% live >6 mo	Only 5% live >1 yr

ASD, Atrial septal defect; PDA, patent ductus arteriosus; VSD, ventricular septal defect.

and more dysmorphic features. Prepubertal boys with Klinefelter syndrome appear normal.

The diagnosis is most often made when the boy is 15 or 16 years old. At that point, the finding of the progressive development of pubic and axillary hair in the presence of testicular volume that remains at infantile levels should alert the clinician to this disorder. Adolescents and young adults with Klinefelter syndrome tend to be tall, with long arms and legs. During adolescence or adulthood, gynecomastia occurs.

Because of failure of growth and maturation of the testes, males with Klinefelter syndrome have testosterone deficiency and failure to produce viable sperm. Production of testosterone is low; this results in failure to develop later secondary sexual characteristics, such as development of facial hair, deepening of the voice, and libido. In adulthood, osteopenia and osteoporosis develop. Because of these findings, testosterone supplementation is indicated.

Most men with Klinefelter syndrome are infertile because they produce few viable sperm. Through the use of isolation of viable sperm through testicular biopsy, coupled with in vitro fertilization and intracytoplasmic sperm injection, it is now possible for men with Klinefelter syndrome to father children; all children born to these men using this technology have had a normal chromosome complement.

Monosomies

Turner Syndrome

Turner syndrome is the only condition in which a monosomic conceptus survives to term; however, 99% of embryos with a 45,X karyotype are spontaneously aborted. The most common aneuploidy found in studies of conceptuses (accounting for 1.4%, whereas Down syndrome accounts 0.5% of conceptions), 45,X fetuses account for 13% of first-trimester pregnancy losses. Occurring in 1 in 3200 live female births, Turner syndrome is notable for its lack of significant physical or developmental disabilities. Women with Turner syndrome tend to have normal intelligence and normal life expectancy.

Females with Turner syndrome typically have a characteristic facial appearance with low-set, mildly malformed ears; a triangular-appearing face; flattened nasal bridge; and epicanthal folds. There is webbing of the neck, with or without cystic hygroma, a shieldlike chest with widened internipple distance, and puffiness of the hands and feet. Internal malformations may include congenital heart defect in 45% (coarctation of the aorta is most common, followed by bicuspid aortic valve; later in life, poststenotic aortic dilation with aneurysm may develop). Renal anomalies, including horseshoe kidney and duplication of the collecting system, are seen in more than half of patients. Short stature is a cardinal feature of this condition, and hypothyroidism is estimated to occur five times more frequently in women with Turner syndrome than in the general population.

The presence of streak gonads (gonadal dysgenesis) instead of well-developed ovaries leads to estrogen deficiency, which prevents these women from developing secondary sexual characteristics and leads to amenorrhea. Although 10% of women with Turner syndrome may have normal pubertal development and are even fertile, most affected women require estrogen replacement to complete secondary sexual development.

The infertility in these women is not corrected by estrogen replacement. Assisted fertilization technology, using donor ova, has allowed women with Turner syndrome to bear children. During pregnancy, however, these women must be followed carefully: An adverse effect of pregnancy on the aorta may hasten the development of an aortic aneurysm and the resulting dissection.

Many girls with Turner syndrome may escape detection during the newborn period because phenotypic features may be subtle. About 33% of children with Turner syndrome are diagnosed soon after birth, usually because of congenital heart disease and physical features, such as a webbed neck and puffy hands and feet; another 33% are diagnosed in childhood, often during a workup for short stature; the final 33% are diagnosed during adolescence, when they fail to develop secondary sexual characteristics.

The karyotypic spectrum in girls with Turner syndrome is wide. Only 50% have a 45,X karyotype; 15% have an isochromosome Xq, designated 46,X,i(Xq), in which one X chromosome is represented by two copies of the long arm (leading to a trisomy of Xq and a monosomy of Xp); approximately 25% are mosaic, 45,X/46,XX or 45,X/46,XY; deletions involving the short (p) arm of the X chromosome (Xp22) can produce the short stature and congenital malformations, and deletions involving Xq often produce only gonadal dysgenesis.

Although monosomy X is caused by nondisjunction, Turner syndrome is not associated with advanced maternal or paternal age. Rather, it is believed that 45,X results from a loss of either an X or a Y chromosome that occurs after conception. It is a mitotic (rather than meiotic) nondisjunction.

SYNDROMES INVOLVING CHROMOSOMAL DELETIONS

Cri du Chat Syndrome

A deletion of the short arm of chromosome 5 is responsible for cri du chat syndrome, with its characteristic catlike cry during early infancy, which is the result of tracheal hypoplasia. Other clinical features include low birth weight and postnatal failure to thrive, hypotonia, developmental delay, microcephaly, and craniofacial dysmorphism, including ocular hypertelorism, epicanthal folds, downward obliquity of the palpebral fissures, and low-set malformed ears. Clefts of the lip and plate, congenital heart disease, and other malformations may be seen.

The clinical severity of cri du chat syndrome seems to depend on the size of the chromosomal deletion. Larger deletions are associated with more severe expression. Most cases arise de novo. The deletion is usually in the chromosome 5 inherited from the father. This phenomenon is believed to be due to imprinting. Other names for this syndrome are *deletion 5p syndrome, 46,XY,del(5p),* or *46,XX,del(5p).*

Wolf-Hirschhorn Syndrome

Marked prenatal and postnatal growth retardation, severe mental retardation, and abnormal facies (often described as "Greek helmet"—frontal bossing, high anterior hairline, hypertelorism, ptosis, epicanthal folds) are found in Wolf-Hirschhorn syndrome with partial deletion of chromosome 4p. A critical region for this disorder has been identified in 4p16.3. Other features include microcephaly; upward slanted palpebral fissures; large, low-set ears often with preauricular pits or tags; and coloboma of the iris. Genital abnormalities, such as cryptorchidism, scrotal hypoplasia, and hypospadias, are common. Seizures are common, occurring in most, if not all, Wolf-Hirschhorn syndrome patients, often beginning in the first 2 years of life. Additional names for this syndrome are *deletion 4p syndrome, 46,XX,del(4p)* or *46,XY,del(4p).*

Williams Syndrome

Williams syndrome, which is generally easily recognized, is due to a small deletion of chromosome 7q11. Congenital heart disease is seen in 80% of affected children, with supravalvar aortic and pulmonic stenosis and peripheral pulmonic stenosis being the most common anomalies. Although they have a normal birth weight, these children have poor growth, manifesting short stature. They have an unusual facial appearance (erroneously described as "an elfin facies"), with median flare of the eyebrows, fullness of the perioral and periorbital region, blue irides with a stellate pattern of pigment, and depressed nasal bridge with anteversion of the nares. Moderate mental retardation (average IQ in the 50 to 60 range) is common, but developmental testing reveals strength in personal social skills and deficiencies in cognitive areas.

Individuals with Williams syndrome have a striking personality. Loquacious and gregarious, they are frequently described as having a "cocktail party" personality; however, approximately 10% of children with Williams syndrome have classic features of autism. Patients often have remarkable musical ability. Most children with Williams syndrome have a de novo deletion, which includes the genes for elastin. A few cases are inherited from parent to child in an AD-like pattern.

Aniridia Wilms Tumor Association (WAGR Syndrome)

WAGR syndrome (**W**ilms tumor, **a**niridia, **g**enitourinary anomalies, and mental **r**etardation) is caused by a deletion of 11p13 and is generally a de novo deletion. Genitourinary abnormalities include cryptorchidism and hypospadias. Patients often have short stature, and half may have microcephaly. Wilms tumor develops in 50% of patients with aniridia, genitourinary abnormalities, and mental retardation (see Chapter 159).

Prader-Willi Syndrome

▶ SEE CHAPTER 47.

Angelman Syndrome

▶ SEE CHAPTER 47.

Miller-Dieker Syndrome

Children with Miller-Dieker syndrome have brain abnormalities and dysmorphic facial features. The brain abnormality consists of a smooth surface and lack of gyri (lissencephaly). Facial features may include bitemporal narrowing, high forehead, occasional vertical ridging of the forehead, small upturned nose, upward slanting palpebral fissures, protuberant upper lip with a thin vermilion border, and low-set and posteriorly rotated ears. A deletion of 17p13.3 has been documented in most individuals with Miller-Dieker syndrome. A fluorescent in situ hybridization probe is available for the *LIS-1* gene (within 17p13.3) that is believed to be responsible for the lissencephaly seen in Miller-Dieker syndrome. Other features of Miller-Dieker syndrome are most likely due to deletions of other genes within 17p13.3.

Chromosome 22 Deletions

Velocardiofacial syndrome, conotruncal anomaly face syndrome, and DiGeorge syndrome all are due to deletions of chromosome 22q11. There are overlapping clinical findings, and it may be that there is one 22q11.2 syndrome with variant phenotypes rather than three relatively distinct syndromes.

Velocardiofacial Syndrome

An AD disorder, common clinical features of velocardiofacial syndrome include clefting of the palate with velopharyngeal insufficiency, conotruncal cardiac defects, and a characteristic facial appearance, including a large prominent nose and a broad nasal root. Speech and language difficulties are common, as is mild intellectual impairment. More than 200 additional abnormalities have been identified in individuals with velocardiofacial syndrome. Some 70% have immunodeficiencies, largely related to T cell dysfunction. A wide spectrum of psychiatric disturbances, including schizophrenia and bipolar disorder, has been seen in more than 33% of affected adults.

In 75% of individuals affected with velocardiofacial syndrome, fluorescent in situ hybridization has revealed a deletion of 22q11.2. This deletion usually is not identifiable using metaphase chromosome analysis, but may be seen in high-resolution (prophase) preparations. Although most cases are sporadic, resulting from a de novo deletion, AD inheritance is seen sometimes.

DiGeorge Syndrome

Although there is significant overlap with velocardiofacial syndrome, DiGeorge syndrome generally describes neonatal onset of symptoms with conotruncal cardiac abnormalities and hypocalcemia often as the presenting features. Patients have hypoplasia of thymus and parathyroid glands, which results in immunodeficiency and in hypocalcemia. Dysmorphic features may include micrognathia, cleft palate, velopalatal insufficiency, low-set ears, and hypertelorism. Patients generally have mild to moderate mental retardation. Most cases of DiGeorge syndrome are found to have a deletion of 22q11. There are reports of a similar clinical picture with a deletion of 10p13 or exposure to alcohol or isotretinoin (Accutane).

Conotruncal Anomaly Face Syndrome

Conotruncal anomaly face syndrome, which was initially described in the Japanese literature, seems to represent velocardiofacial syndrome.

SYNDROMES INVOLVING CHROMOSOME DUPLICATION

Duplications and deletions occur secondary to misalignment and unequal crossing over during meiosis. Small extra chromosomes are found in a small percentage of the population (0.06%). These "marker" chromosomes sometimes are associated with mental retardation and other abnormalities, and other times they have no apparent phenotypic effects.

Inverted Duplication Chromosome 15

Chromosome 15 is the most common of all marker chromosomes, and its inverted duplication accounts for almost 40% of this group of chromosomal abnormalities. The features seen in children with 47,XX, +inv dup (15q) or 47,XY, inv dup (15q) largely depend on the size of the extra chromosomal material present: The larger the region, the worse the prognosis. Typically, children with this disorder have a variable degree of developmental delay; seizures are common, as are behavior problems. The phenotype shows minimal dysmorphic features, with a sloping forehead, short and downward slanting palpebral fissures, a prominent nose with a broad nasal bridge, a long and well-defined philtrum, a midline crease in the lower lip, and micrognathia.

Cat Eye Syndrome

Named for the iris coloboma that gives patients' eyes a catlike appearance, cat eye syndrome is due to a marker chromosome with an interstitial duplication of 22q11. Although the colobomas name the syndrome, they occur in less than 50% of patients with the marker chromosome. Other clinical features include mild mental retardation or normal intelligence with emotional retardation, mild hypertelorism, downward slanting palpebral fissures, micrognathia, auricular pits or tags or both, anal atresia with rectovestibular fistula, and renal agenesis.

CHAPTER 50

The Approach to the Dysmorphic Child

Dysmorphology is the recognition of the pattern of congenital malformations (often multiple congenital malformations) and dysmorphic features that characterize a particular syndrome. **Syndromes** are collections of abnormalities, including **malformations**, **deformations**, dysmorphic features, and abnormal behaviors that have a unifying, identifiable etiology. This etiology may be the presence of a mutation in a single gene, as is the case in **Rett syndrome**, a disorder that affects females and is characterized by developmental arrest, acquired microcephaly, and loss of purposeful hand movements and is caused by a mutation in the *MECP2* gene on Xq28; deletion or duplication of chromosomal material, such as is the case in Prader-Willi syndrome, which is caused by the deletion of the paternal copies of the imprinted *SNRPN* gene,

the *Necdin* gene, and possibly other genes on chromosome 15q11; or exposure to a teratogenic substance during embryonic development, as in fetal alcohol syndrome.

DEFINITIONS

Congenital **malformations** are defined as clinically significant abnormalities in either form or function. They result from localized **intrinsic** defects in morphogenesis as a result of an event that occurred in embryonic or early fetal life. This event may be a disturbance of development from some unknown cause, but it is often due to mutations in developmental genes. **Extrinsic** factors may cause **disruptions** of development by disturbing the development of apparently normal tissues. These disruptions may include amniotic bands, interruption or disruption of blood supply to developing tissues, or exposure to teratogens. A **malformation sequence** is the end result of a malformation that has secondary effects on later developmental events. An example is the **Pierre Robin sequence**. The primary malformation, the failure of the growth of the mandible during the first weeks of gestation, results in micrognathia. Micrognathia forces the tongue, which is normal in size, into an unusual position. The abnormally placed tongue blocks the fusion of the palatal shelves, which normally come together in the midline to produce the hard and soft palate; this leads to the presence of a U-shaped cleft palate in the infant. After delivery, the normal-sized tongue in the smaller than normal oral cavity leads to airway obstruction and obstructive apnea, a potentially life-threatening complication.

Deformations arise as a result of environmental forces acting on normal structures. They occur later in pregnancy or after delivery. Oligohydramnios may inhibit lung growth and cause compression of fetal structures, producing clubfoot, dislocated hips, and flattened facies (see Chapter 196). Deformations often resolve with minimal intervention, but malformations often require aggressive surgical and medical management.

Minor malformations are variants of normal that occur in less than 3% of the population and include findings such as transverse palmar creases, low-set ears, or hypertelorism; when isolated they have no clinical significance. A **multiple malformation syndrome** is the recognizable pattern of anomalies that results from a single identifiable underlying cause. It may involve a series of malformations, malformation sequences, and deformations. These syndromes often prompt a consultation with a clinical geneticist. **Dysmorphology** is the art of recognizing the pattern of multiple congenital anomalies that occurs with various malformation syndromes (Table 50–1).

TABLE 50–1. Glossary of Selected Terms Used in Dysmorphology

Terms Pertaining to the Face and Head

Brachycephaly: Condition in which head shape is shortened from front to back along the sagittal plane; the skull is rounder than normal

Canthus: The lateral or medial angle of the eye formed by the junction of the upper and lower lids

Columella: The fleshy tissue of the nose that separates the nostrils

Glabella: Bony midline prominence of the brows

Nasal alae: The lateral flaring of the nostrils

Nasolabial fold: Groove that extends from the margin of the nasal alae to the lateral aspects of the lips

Ocular hypertelorism: Increased distance between the pupils of the two eyes

Palpebral fissure: The shape of the eyes based on the outline of the eyelids

Philtrum: The vertical groove in the midline of the face between the nose and the upper lip

Plagiocephaly: Condition in which head shape is asymmetric in the sagittal or coronal planes; can result from asymmetry in suture closure or from asymmetry of brain growth

Scaphocephaly: Condition in which the head is elongated from front to back in the sagittal plane; most normal skulls are scaphocephalic

Synophrys: Eyebrows that meet in the midline

Telecanthus: A wide space between the medial canthi

Terms Pertaining to the Extremities

Brachydactyly: Condition of having short digits

Camptodactyly: Condition in which a digit is bent or fixed in the direction of flexion (a "trigger finger"-type appearance)

Clinodactyly: Condition in which a digit is crooked and curves toward or away from adjacent digits

Hypoplastic nail: An unusually small nail on a digit

Melia: Suffix meaning "limb" (e.g., amelia—missing limb; brachymelia—short limb)

Polydactyly: The condition of having six or more digits on an extremity

Syndactyly: The condition of having two or more digits at least partially fused (can involve any degree of fusion, from webbing of skin to full bony fusion of adjacent digits)

An **association** differs from a syndrome in that in the former, no single underlying etiology has been identified to explain a recognizable pattern of anomalies that occur together more than would be expected by chance alone. The **VACTERL** association (**v**ertebral anomalies, **a**nal atresia, **c**ardiac defects, **t**racheo-**e**sophageal fistula, **r**enal anomalies, and **l**imb anomalies) is an example of a group of malformations that occur more commonly together than might be expected by chance. No single unifying etiology explains this condition, however, so it is considered an association.

In approximately half of children noted to have one or more congenital malformations, only a single malformation is identifiable; in the other half, multiple malformations are present. About 6% of infants with congenital malformations have chromosomal defects, 7.5% have a single gene disorder, 20% are multifactorial, and approximately 7% are due to exposure to a teratogen. In more than 50% of cases, no cause can be identified.

HISTORY AND PHYSICAL EXAMINATION

The first important skill for a clinical geneticist is observation.

Pregnancy History

- What was the birth weight? Small for gestational age infants may have a chromosome anomaly or may have been exposed to a teratogen. Large for gestational age infants may be infants of diabetic mothers or have an overgrowth syndrome, such as Beckwith-Wiedemann syndrome. Infants who are appropriate for gestational age may have a single gene mutation, a multifactorial condition, or, most likely, no genetic disease.

- Was the infant full term, premature, or postmature? When evaluating an older child with developmental disabilities, complications of extreme prematurity may be responsible for the patient's problems. Postmaturity also is associated with some chromosome anomalies (e.g., trisomy 18) and anencephaly.

- Was the infant born by vaginal delivery or caesarean section? If the latter, what was the cause? Infants born from breech presentation are more likely to have congenital malformations.

- How old were the parents at the time of the child's delivery? Advanced maternal age is associated with an increased risk of nondisjunction leading to trisomies. Advanced paternal age may be associated with an increased risk of a new mutation leading to an AD trait.

- Were there complications during the pregnancy? Does the mother have any underlying medical problems? Does she take any medications? Did she smoke cigarettes, drink alcohol, or take any drugs? (See Chapters 47 and 48.)

- When did the mother feel quickening? Were fetal movements active? Neonatal hypotonia may have manifested prenatally; answers to these questions may provide information.

- Was there a normal amount of amniotic fluid? An increased amount of fluid may be associated with intestinal obstruction or a CNS anomaly that leads to poor swallowing. A decreased amount of fluid may point to a urinary tract abnormality leading to failure to produce urine or a chronic amniotic fluid leak.

Family History

A pedigree should be constructed, searching for similar or dissimilar abnormalities in first-degree and second-degree relatives. Also, a history of pregnancy or neonatal losses should be documented. For a complete discussion of pedigrees, see Chapter 47.

Physical Examination

When examining children with dysmorphic features, the following approach should be used.

Growth

The height (length), weight, and head circumference should be measured carefully and plotted on appropriate growth curves. Growth appropriate for age is consistent with the presence of a single gene disorder, a multifactorially inherited condition, or, most commonly, no genetic disease. Small size or growth restriction may be secondary to a chromosomal abnormality, skeletal dysplasia, or exposure to toxic or teratogenic agents. Larger than expected size suggests an overgrowth syndrome (Sotos or Beckwith-Wiedemann syndrome), or if in the newborn period, it might suggest a diabetic mother.

The clinician should check if the child is proportionate. If the limbs are too short for the head and trunk, this implies the presence of a short-limbed bone dysplasia, such as achondroplasia. If the trunk and head are too short for the extremities, it may suggest a disorder affecting the vertebrae, such as spondyloepiphyseal dysplasia.

Craniofacial

Careful examination of the craniofacial region is crucial for the diagnosis of many congenital malformation syndromes. Head shape should be assessed carefully. If the head is not normal in size and shape (normocephalic), it may be long and thin (dolichocephalic), short and wide (brachycephalic), or asymmetric or lopsided (plagiocephalic).

Facial features should be assessed next. Any asymmetry should be noted; asymmetry may be due to either a deformation related to the intrauterine position or a malformation of one side of the face. The face should be divided into four regions, which should be evaluated separately. The **forehead** may show overt prominence (achondroplasia) or deficiency (often described as a sloping appearance, which occurs in children with primary microcephaly). The **midface**, which extends from the eyebrows to the upper lip and from the outer canthi of the eyes to the commissures of the mouth, is especially important. Careful assessment of the distance between the eyes (inner canthal distance) and the pupils (interpupillary distance) may confirm the impression of hypotelorism (eyes that are too close together), which suggests a defect in midline brain formation, or **hypertelorism** (eyes that are too far apart), which suggests Aarskog syndrome (hypertelorism, brachydactyly [short digits], and shawl scrotum). The length of the palpebral fissure should be noted and may help define whether the opening for the eye is short, as is found with fetal alcohol syndrome, or excessively long, as in Kabuki makeup syndrome (short stature, mental retardation, long palpebral fissures with eversion of lateral portion of lower lid).

Other features of the eyes should be noted. The obliquity (slant) of the palpebral fissures may be upward (as seen with Down syndrome) or downward (as in Treacher Collins syndrome). The presence of epicanthal folds (Down syndrome and fetal alcohol syndrome) is also important. Features of the nose—especially the nasal bridge, which can be flattened in Down syndrome, fetal alcohol syndrome, and many other syndromes, or prominent as in velocardiofacial syndrome—should be noted.

The **malar** region of the face is examined next. It extends from the ear to the midface. The ears should be checked for size (measured and checked against "growth" charts that record length for age), shape (noting thinning of the pinnae, unusual folding), position (low-set ears are below a line drawn from the outer canthus to the occiput), and orientation (posterior rotation is where the ear appears turned toward the rear of the head). Ears may be low set because they are small (or microtic) or because of a malformation of the mandibular region.

The **mandibular region** is the area from the lower portion of the ears bounded out to the chin by the mandible. In most newborns, the chin is often slightly retruded (that is slightly behind the vertical line extending from the forehead to the philtrum). If this retrusion is pronounced, the child may have the Pierre Robin malformation sequence.

Neck

Examination of the neck may reveal webbing, a common feature in Turner syndrome and Noonan syndrome, or shortening, as is seen occasionally in some skeletal dysplasias and in conditions in which anomalies of the cervical spine occur, such as Klippel-Feil syndrome. The position of the posterior hairline also should be evaluated. The size of the thyroid gland should be assessed.

Trunk

The chest may be examined for shape (a shieldlike chest is found in Noonan syndrome and Turner syndrome) and symmetry. The presence of a pectus deformity should be noted and is common in Marfan syndrome. The presence of scoliosis should be assessed; it is common in Marfan syndrome and many other syndromes.

Extremities

Many congenital malformation syndromes have anomalies of the extremities. All joints should be examined for range of motion. The presence of single or multiple joint contractures suggests either intrinsic neuromuscular dysfunction, as in the case of some forms of muscular dystrophy, or external deforming forces that limited motion of the joint in utero. Multiple contractures also are found with arthrogryposis multiplex congenita and are due to a variety of causes. Radioulnar synostosis, an inability to pronate or supinate the elbow, occurs in fetal alcohol syndrome and in some X chromosome aneuploidy syndromes.

Examination of the hands is important. **Polydactyly** (the presence of extra digits) usually occurs as an isolated AD trait, but also can be seen in trisomy 13. **Oligodactyly** (a deficiency in the number of digits) is seen in Fanconi syndrome (anemia, leukopenia, thrombocytopenia, and associated heart, renal, and limb anomalies—usually radial aplasia and thumb malformation or aplasia), in which it is generally part of a more severe limb reduction defect, or secondary to intrauterine amputation, which may occur with amniotic band disruption sequence. **Syndactyly** (a joining of two or more digits) is common to many syndromes, including Smith-Lemli-Opitz syndrome (see Chapters 199 and 201).

Dermatoglyphics include palmar crease patterns. A transverse palmar crease, indicative of hypotonia during early fetal life, is seen in approximately 50% of children with Down syndrome (and 10% of individuals in the general population). A characteristic palmar crease pattern is seen in fetal alcohol syndrome.

Genitalia

Genitalia should be examined closely for abnormalities in structure. In boys, if the penis appears short, it should be measured and compared with known age-related data. Ambiguous genitalia often are associated with endocrinologic disorders, such as congenital adrenal hyperplasia (girls have masculinized external genitalia, but male genitalia may be unaffected), or chromosomal disorders such as 45,X/46,XY mosaicism or possibly secondary to a multiple congenital anomaly syndrome (see Chapters 174 and 177). Although hypospadias, which occurs in 1 in 300 newborn boys, is a common congenital malformation that often occurs as an isolated defect, if it is associated with other anomalies, especially cryptorchidism, there is a strong possibility of a syndrome.

LABORATORY EVALUATION

Chromosome analysis, either metaphase or prophase, should be ordered for children with multiple congenital anomalies, the involvement of one major organ system and the presence of multiple dysmorphic features, or the presence of mental retardation. For a complete discussion of chromosome analysis, see Chapter 49.

Fluorescent in situ hybridization should be requested when a syndrome with a known chromosomal defect in which probes are available is suspected. Disorders such as velocardiofacial syndrome, Williams syndrome, and Prader-Willi syndrome are included in this group.

Direct DNA analysis can be performed to identify specific mutations. It is necessary to use Web-based resources to keep up-to-date. An extremely helpful website is www.genetests.org, which provides information about the availability of testing for specific conditions and identifies laboratories performing the testing.

Radiologic imaging plays an important role in the evaluation of children with dysmorphic features. Individuals found to have multiple external malformations should have a careful evaluation to search for the presence of internal malformations. Testing might include **ultrasound evaluations** of the head and abdomen, the latter to look for anomalies in the kidney, bladder, liver, and spleen. **Skeletal radiographs** should be performed if there is concern about a possible skeletal dysplasia. The presence of a heart murmur should trigger a cardiology consultation, and an **ECG** and **echocardiogram** may be indicated. **MRI** may be indicated in children with neurologic abnormalities or a spinal defect. The presence of craniosynostosis may indicate a **CT scan** of the head.

DIAGNOSIS

Although the presence of characteristic findings sometimes may make the definitive diagnosis of a malformation syndrome simple, in most cases no specific diagnosis is immediately evident. Some constellations of findings are rare, and finding a "match" may prove difficult. In many cases, all laboratory tests are normal, and confirmation relies on subjective findings. Clinical geneticists have attempted to resolve this difficulty by developing scoring systems, cross-referenced tables of anomalies that help in the development of a differential diagnosis, and computerized diagnostic programs. An accurate diagnosis is important for the following reasons:

1. It offers an explanation to the family why their child was born with congenital anomalies. This may help to allay guilt because parents often believe that they are responsible for their child's problem.
2. The natural history of many disorders is well described, so a diagnosis allows the physician to anticipate medical problems associated with a particular syndrome and perform appropriate screening. It also provides reassurance that other medical problems are no more likely to occur than they might with other children who do not have the diagnosis.
3. It permits genetic counseling to be done so that the parents can understand the risk to future children. An accurate diagnosis also permits prenatal testing to be done for the disorders for which it is available.

Diagnosis enables the clinician to provide the family with educational materials about the diagnosis and for contact with support groups for particular disorders. The Internet has become an important source for such information, but care should be exercised because information on the Internet is not subject to editorial control, and some of the information may be inaccurate. A good site is the National Organization for Rare Disorders (www.rarediseases.org), which acts as a clearinghouse for information about rare diseases and their support groups. Genetic testing information is available at the Genetests website (www.genetests.org). This site provides information on available clinical and research testing for many diseases.

SUGGESTED READING

Baldini A: DiGeorge's syndrome: A gene at last. Lancet 362:1342-1343, 2003.

Behrman RE, Kliegman RM, Jenson HB (eds): Nelson Textbook of Pediatrics, 17th ed. Philadelphia, WB Saunders, 2003.

Burke W: Genetic testing. N Engl J Med 347:1867-1875, 2002.

Guttmacher AE, Collins FS: Genomic medicine—a primer. N Engl J Med 347:1512-1520, 2002.

Hobbs CA, Cleves MA, Simmons CJ: Genetic epidemiology and congenital malformations. Arch Pediatr Adolesc Med 156:315-320, 2002.

Holland A, Whittington J, Hinton E: The paradox of Prader-Willi syndrome: A genetic model of starvation. Lancet 362:989-991, 2003.

Jacquemont S, Hagerman RJ, Leehey MA, et al: Penetrance of the fragile X–associated tremor/ataxia syndrome in a premutation carrier population. JAMA 291:460-468, 2004.

Kliegman RM, Greenbaum LA, Lye PS (eds): Practical Strategies in Pediatric Diagnosis and Therapy, 2nd ed. Philadelphia, WB Saunders, 2004.

Langranco F, Kamischke A, Zitzmann M, Nieschlag E: Klinefelter's syndrome. Lancet 364:273-283, 2004.

McCandless SE, Brunger JW, Cassidy SB: The burden of genetic disease on inpatient care in a children's hospital. Am J Hum Genet 74:121-127, 2004.

Meyerson M: Human genetic variation and disease. Lancet 362:259-260, 2003.

Roizen NJ, Patterson D: Down's syndrome. Lancet 361:1281-1288, 2003.

Wapner R, Thom E, Simpson JL, et al: First-trimester screening for trisomies 21 and 18. N Engl J Med 349:1405-1412, 2003.

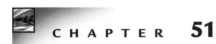

CHAPTER 51

Assessment

Although each inborn error of metabolism is rare, in the aggregate they make a significant contribution to the causes of mental retardation, seizures, sudden infant death, and neurologic impairment. Inborn errors of metabolism are a cause of acute neonatal illness in which prompt diagnosis and treatment make a difference in outcome and even survival. They affect all age groups. Prompt recognition of the possibility of an inborn error is the responsibility of primary care physicians, who then need the expertise of metabolic teams that specialize in the diagnosis and management of these disorders.

Inborn errors of metabolism result from a genetic deficiency in a metabolic pathway; signs and symptoms result from the accumulation of metabolites related to the pathway. These metabolites may be toxic or may destroy cells because of storage in organelles. Deficiency of metabolites downstream of the block also plays a role in pathogenesis. The process can involve one or multiple systems (Fig. 51–1). All mechanisms of inheritance occur.

The approach to diagnosis and management requires knowledge of the pathophysiology of these disorders, the typical presentations in each age group, and the clinical consequences in body organs and systems. Evaluation begins with clinical assessment and proceeds to clinical laboratory assessment and specific specialty laboratory testing. **Management strategies** depend on understanding the pathophysiology and what laboratory analyses provide the best measure of clinical control.

SIGNS AND SYMPTOMS THAT SHOULD SUGGEST AN INBORN ERROR OF METABOLISM

The **signs and symptoms of an inborn error are protean**. Because any organ or system can be involved, the assessment of the child should lead to the appropriate diagnosis. Presentation varies among different age groups. Inborn errors of metabolism usually do not present immediately after birth. There is an interval that may last a few weeks during which the infant appears well. In infants who survive the neonatal period without developing recognized symptoms, the history is often marked by intermittent illness separated by periods of being entirely well. Family history may be helpful if positive. A history of early infant deaths is particularly suggestive. A negative family history does not exclude an inborn error of metabolism because this may be the first affected child in the family. The presentations may include toxicity, specific organ involvement, energy deficiency, dysmorphic findings, and appearance of organ storage.

TYPES OF CLINICAL PRESENTATION OF INBORN ERRORS

Toxic Presentation

Although some aspects of the clinical scenario are specific to the abnormal pathway, many features are nonspecific and occur in a wide range of disorders. The toxic presentation often presents as an **encephalopathy**. The patient may have periods of being well that are punctuated by an acute illness. Fever, infection, fasting, or other catabolic stress may precipitate the symptom complex. A **metabolic acidosis**, vomiting, lethargy, and other neurologic findings may be present. During the acute

TABLE 51–1.   Inborn Errors of Metabolism Presenting with Neurologic Signs in Infants <3 Months Old

Generalized Seizures	Encephalopathic Coma with or without Seizures
All disorders that cause hypoglycemia	Maple syrup urine disease
Most hepatic glycogen storage diseases	Nonketotic hyperglycinemia
Galactosemia, hereditary fructose intolerance	Diseases producing extreme hyperammonemia
Fructose-1,6-bisphosphatase deficiency	Disorders of the urea cycle
Disorders of the propionate pathway	Disorders of the propionate pathway
HMG-lyase deficiency	Disorders of beta oxidation
Disorders of beta oxidation	Congenital lactic acidosis (PCD)
Pyruvate carboxylase deficiency (PCD)	
Maple syrup urine disease	
Seizures and/or Posturing	
Nonketotic hyperglycinemia	
Maple syrup urine disease	

presentation, diagnostic testing is most effective when diagnostic metabolites are present in highest concentration in blood and urine during this time. Abnormal metabolism of amino acids, organic acids, ammonia, or carbohydrates may be at fault. Hyperammonemia is an important diagnostic possibility if an infant or child presents with features of toxic encephalopathy. Symptoms and signs depend on the underlying cause of the hyperammonemia, the age at which it develops, and its degree. The severity of hyperammonemia may provide a clue to the etiology (Tables 51–1 and 51–2).

Severe Neonatal Hyperammonemia

Infants with genetic defects in urea synthesis, transient neonatal hyperammonemia, and impaired synthesis of urea and glutamine secondary to genetic disorders of organic acid metabolism can have levels of blood ammonia 100 times normal (>1000 μmol/L) in the neonatal period. Poor feeding, hypotonia, apnea, hypothermia, and vomiting rapidly give way to **coma** and occasionally to intractable seizures. Death occurs within days if the condition remains untreated.

Moderate Neonatal Hyperammonemia

Moderate neonatal hyperammonemia (range 200 to 400 μmol/L) is associated with depression of the CNS, poor feeding, and vomiting. Seizures are not characteristic. This type of hyperammonemia may be

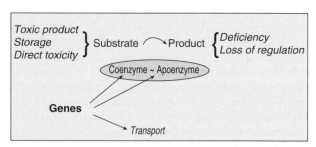

Figure 51–1

Depiction of the basic paradigm in inherited disorders of metabolism. Deficiency of an enzyme complex results in accumulation of metabolites proximal to the blocked metabolism and deficiency of the product of the reaction. Sites of genetic control are indicated.

TABLE 51–2.   Etiologies of Hyperammonemia in Infants

Etiology of Hyperammonemia	Comments
Disorders of the urea cycle	Lethal hyperammonemia is common
Disorders of the propionate pathway	Severe hyperammonemia may precede acidosis
Disorders of fatty acid catabolism and of ketogenesis	Reye-like syndrome possible
Transient neonatal hyperammonemia	Idiopathic, self-limited
Portal-systemic shunting	Thrombosis of portal vein, cirrhosis, hepatitis
Idiopathic Reye syndrome	Uncommon
Drug intoxication: salicylate, valproic acid, acetaminophen	Obtain drug levels
Hyperinsulinism/hyperammonemia syndrome	Clinical hypoglycemia, subclinical hyperammonemia

caused by partial blocks in urea synthesis and commonly is caused by disorders of organic acid metabolism that secondarily interfere with the elimination of nitrogen.

Clinical Hyperammonemia in Later Infancy and Childhood

Infants who are affected by defects in the urea cycle and who are not ill in the neonatal period may continue to do well while receiving the low-protein intake of breast milk, only to develop clinical hyperammonemia when dietary protein is increased or when catabolic stress occurs. The clinical presentation is dominated by vomiting and lethargy, which frequently progresses to coma. As protein intake is restricted by anorexia and vomiting or if IV glucose is given, the sensorium clears, and the infant recovers, but the infant may develop symptoms again when metabolically stressed or ingesting an increased protein intake. Seizures are not typical. During a crisis, the plasma ammonia level is usually 200 to 500 μmol/L, but when dietary protein is restricted, the ammonia level decreases and may become normal. If the CNS symptoms are not prominent, the condition may go unrecognized for years. When a crisis occurs during an epidemic of influenza, the child mistakenly may be thought to have **Reye syndrome**. Older children may have neuropsychiatric or behavioral abnormalities (Fig. 51-2).

Specific Organ Presentation

Any organ or system can be injured by toxic accumulation of any of the kinds of metabolites involved in inborn errors. Symptoms relate to organ-specific or system-specific toxicity and injury. Examples include nervous system (seizures, coma, ataxia), liver (hepatocellular damage), eye (cataracts, dislocated lenses), renal (tubular dysfunction, cysts), and heart (cardiomyopathy, pericardial effusion) (Table 51-3; see Table 51-1).

Energy Deficiency

Disorders whose pathophysiology results in energy deficiency may manifest myopathy, CNS dysfunction including mental retardation and seizures, cardiomyopathy, vomiting, or renal tubular acidosis. Examples include disorders of fatty acid oxidation, disorders of mitochondrial function/oxidative phosphorylation, and disorders of carbohydrate metabolism.

Ketosis and Ketotic Hypoglycemia

Acidosis is often found in children with fasting associated with anorexia, vomiting, and diarrhea in the course of a viral illness. The clinical manifestations are those of the causative illness; the acidosis is mild, ketonuria occurs, and administration of carbohydrate restores balance. In this normal response to fasting, the blood glucose level is relatively low. Severe ketosis may also be the result of ketothiolase deficiency (see Fig. 54-1) and other disorders of ketone utilization or glycogen synthase deficiency, a disorder of glycogen synthesis. In these conditions, hypoglycemia is significant, and the ketosis clears slowly, requiring significant amounts of carbohydrate. These disorders frequently present in the context of fasting, infection with fever, or decreased intake secondary to vomiting and diarrhea. **Ketotic hypoglycemia** is a common condition in which tolerance for fasting is impaired to the extent that symptomatic hypoglycemia with seizures or coma occurs when the child encounters a ketotic stress. The stress may be significant (viral infection with vomiting) or minor (a prolongation by several hours of the normal overnight fast). Ketotic hypoglycemia first appears in the second year of life and occurs in otherwise healthy children. It is treated by frequent snacks and the provision of glucose during periods of stress. The pathophysiology is poorly understood (see Chapter 172). In older infants and children, ketonuria is a normal response to fasting but not to a normal overnight fast. In neonates, ketonuria indicates meta-

TABLE 51-3. **Inborn Errors of Metabolism Presenting with Hepatomegaly or Hepatic Dysfunction in Infants**

Hepatomegaly	Hepatic Failure	Jaundice
GSD I	Galactosemia	Galactosemia
GSD III	Hereditary fructose intolerance	Hereditary fructose intolerance
Mucopolysaccharidosis I and II	Infantile tyrosinemia (fumarylacetoacetate hydrolase deficiency)	Infantile tyrosinemia (fumarylacetoacetate hydrolase deficiency)
Gaucher and Niemann-Pick diseases	GSD IV (slowly evolving)	Crigler-Najjar disease
		Rotor, Dubin-Johnson syndromes

GSD, glycogen storage disease.

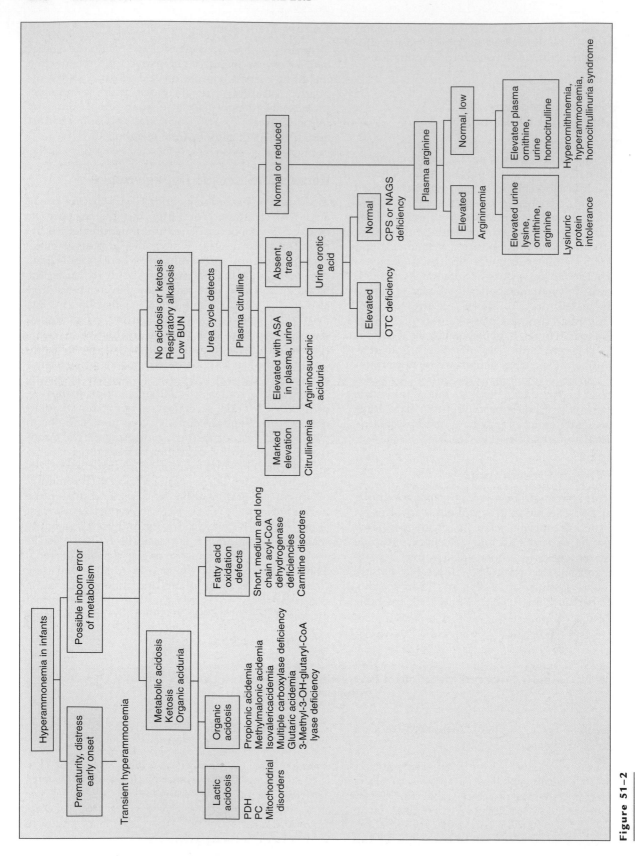

Figure 51–2

Algorithm for the approach to hyperammonemia in infants. ASA, argininosuccinic acid; CPS, carbamylphosphate synthase; NAGS, *N*-acetylglutamate synthase; OTC, ornithine transcarbamylase; PC, pyruvate carboxylase deficiency; PDH, pyruvate dehydrogenase deficiency.

TABLE 51–4. Etiologies of Metabolic Acidosis Caused by Inborn Errors of Metabolism in Infants

Disorder	Comment
Methylmalonic acidemia (MMA)	Hyperammonemia, ketosis, neutropenia, thrombocytopenia
Propionic acidemia	Similar to MMA
Isovaleric acidemia	Similar to MMA
Pyruvate dehydrogenase deficiency	Lactic acidosis, hyperammonemia
Pyruvate carboxylase deficiency	Lactic acidosis, hypoglycemia, and ketosis
Respiratory chain (mitochondrial) disorders	Lactic acidosis, ketosis
Medium-chain acyl-CoA dehydrogenase deficiency (MCAD)	Moderate acidosis, hypoglycemia, absent ketosis, possible hyperammonemia
Other fatty acid oxidation defects	Similar to MCAD
Galactosemia	Renal tubular acidosis, *Escherichia coli* sepsis, hypoglycemia
3-Hydroxy-3-methyl-glutaryl-CoA lyase deficiency	Severe lactic acidosis, hyperammonemia, hypoglycemia
3-Methylcrotonyl-CoA carboxylase deficiency	Severe lactic acidosis, hyperammonemia, hypoglycemia, ketosis
Multiple acyl-CoA dehydrogenase deficiency (glutaric aciduria 2)	Lactic acidosis, hypoglycemia

bolic disease. **A high anion gap metabolic acidosis with or without ketosis suggests a metabolic disorder** (Table 51–4).

Disorders Associated with Dysmorphic Findings

Congenital malformations or dysmorphic features are not intuitively thought of as symptoms and signs of inborn errors. Conditions that cause congenital malformations include carbohydrate-deficient glycoprotein syndrome, disorders of cholesterol biosynthesis (Smith-Lemli-Opitz syndrome), disorders of copper transport (Menkes syndrome, occipital horn syndrome), maternal PKU syndrome, glutaric aciduria II (also called multiple acyl-coenzyme A [CoA] dehydrogenase deficiency), and several storage diseases.

Storage Disorders

Storage disorders are caused by accumulation of incompletely metabolized large molecules. This storage often occurs in subcellular organelles, such as lysosomes. The glycogen storage diseases and mucopolysaccharide disorders are other examples of storage disorders.

Different Age Groups and Differing Clinical Phenotypes

A neonate no longer has the protective functions of the placenta to detoxify metabolites that accumulate because of an inborn error; in addition, maternal metabolism no longer provides nutrition to the neonate who cannot metabolize substrates such as glycogen and fatty acids. Introduction of new foods in older infancy and

frequency of metabolic stress with fasting and fever in that age group make the infant vulnerable. Increased protein intake associated with growth in older children and adolescents may stress deficient pathways that previously were compensated. Hormonal factors in adolescence influence intermediary metabolism in unpredictable ways. Examples include:

1. **Neonatal**
   Galactosemia: introduction of milk
   Fatty acid disorders: fasting/breastfeeding
   Loss of maternal detoxification: organic acid disorders: urea cycle
2. **Infancy**
   Hereditary fructose intolerance: introduction of fructose (sucrose)
   Disorders of fatty acid oxidation: fasting, infectious illness, fever
3. **Childhood**
   Disorders of ammonia detoxification, females with X-linked ornithine carbamoyltransferase (OTC) deficiency: increased protein intake
4. **Adolescence**
   Cobalamin C methylmalonic aciduria (cblC MMA) neurologic deterioration: unknown triggers, possible hormonal changes

CLINICAL ASSESSMENT AND CLINICAL LABORATORY TESTING

The assessment begins with a careful history and clinical evaluation. Clinical laboratory testing is targeted to define the metabolic derangement (Table 51–5). The results of this evaluation generate a differential diagnosis and a list of more specific laboratory testing to help confirm the diagnosis.

TABLE 51–5. Initial Diagnostic Evaluation for a Suspected Inborn Error of Metabolism*

Blood and Plasma	Urine
Arterial blood gas	Glucose
Electrolytes—anion gap	pH
Glucose	Ketones
Ammonia	Reducing substances
Liver enzymes	Organic acids
Complete blood count, differential,† and platelet count	Acylcarnitine
	Orotic acid
Lactate, pyruvate	
Organic acids	
Amino acids	
Carnitine	

*Organ-specific evaluation is indicated for specific symptoms (e.g., cranial MRI for coma or seizures; echocardiography for cardiomyopathy; CSF amino acids by column chromatography if nonketotic hyperglycemia is suspected).
†Thrombocytopenia and neutropenia are seen in organic acidurias; vacuolated lymphocytes and metachromatic granules are seen in lysosomal disorders.

A metabolic disorder should be considered when a pattern of nonspecific and nonpathognomonic symptoms is recognized. The combination of symptoms and abnormal clinical laboratory findings demands urgent metabolic evaluation. Features in the history that may reflect a metabolic emergency include vomiting, acidosis, hypoglycemia, ketosis (*or lack of appropriate ketosis*), intercurrent infection, anorexia/failure to feed, lethargy proceeding to coma, and hyperventilation or hypoventilation. Clinical evaluation should focus particularly on the cardiac, renal, neurologic, and developmental assessment and look for change in mental status, seizures, abnormal tone, visual symptoms, poor developmental progress, global developmental delay, loss of milestones, cardiomyopathy, cardiac failure, cystic renal malformation, and renal tubular dysfunction.

Clinical laboratory testing should begin with tests that are available in most hospital clinical laboratories. Care in the collection and handling of laboratory specimens is crucial to obtaining accurate results. Plasma measurements of lactate and ammonia are particularly subject to spurious results if not handled correctly. Significant ketosis in the neonate is unusual and suggests an organic acid disorder. Ketosis out of proportion to fasting status in an older child occurs in disorders of ketone usage. Lack of ketosis in an older child under conditions of metabolic stress is a feature of fatty acid oxidation disorders.

GENETIC ASPECTS OF INBORN ERRORS

Mechanisms of Inheritance

Although all of the classic mechanisms of inheritance are represented in the inborn errors of metabolism, most of them are autosomal recessive (Table 51–6). In some populations, because of isolation or founder effect, a specific recessive condition may be common; an example is the high frequency of maple syrup urine disease (MSUD) in the Old Order Mennonite population in Pennsylvania. Conditions that are inherited in an X-linked manner exhibit the usual increased prevalence in males. Carriers of recessive genes or X-linked genes (females) are usually asymptomatic except in a few conditions. Females who carry a mutation on the X chromosome have two populations of cells: one with normal activity of the enzyme and one with deficient activity. In OTC deficiency, females can be symptomatic if they have a significant distribution of abnormal cells in the liver. These girls often present with symptoms of hyperammonemia in childhood beyond infancy and often give a history of several episodes before the cause is recognized. Mitochondrial inheritance, caused by a mutation in 1 of 13 mitochondrial genes coding for proteins involved in oxidative phosphorylation, shows a maternal pattern of inheritance. The clinical disorders produced by abnormalities of these maternal genes depend on the specific defects and the tissue distribution of affected and normal mitochondria over time. Dominantly inherited diseases may be sporadic or evident in the family; inborn errors of metabolism that present in childhood rarely show autosomal dominant inheritance. When parents are closely related (*consanguineous*), there is a significant chance that a child has inherited two copies of the same abnormal allele that the parents acquired from a common ancestor. This child would be affected with a recessive condition.

Identification of Molecular Pathology

If the molecular basis of an inborn error of metabolism is known (i.e., the gene [or genes] has been mapped and cloned and mutations are defined), specific molecular testing may be clinically available. A defined set of mutations comprises most of the mutations in the population for many disorders. In other conditions, there may be many hundreds of different mutations. In recessive disorders, it is common for a patient to be doubly heterozygous for two different mutations at the gene locus involved. There is a good correlation between specific mutations and clinical outcome for some disorders; the result of this testing can be an additional guide to treatment. The ability to perform genetic testing in other at-risk family members can

TABLE 51–6.   Inheritance Patterns: Genotypes and Phenotypes

	Examples	Phenotypes	Clinical Problems
Autosomal Genes			
Dominant inheritance	Familial hypercholesterolemia	Heterozygous—affected	Xanthomas and heart disease in adult life
		Homozygous—affected markedly by "gene dose effect"	Xanthomas and heart disease in childhood
Recessive inheritance	Phenylketonuria	Heterozygous—normal	Normal
		Homozygous—affected	Severe developmental delay
	Galactosemia	Heterozygous—risk factors	? Ovarian failure (adult) ? Cataracts (adult)
		Homozygous—affected	Neonatal liver failure, cataracts
X-Linked Genes	Ornithine transcarbamylase deficiency	Male—affected	Severe infantile hyperammonemia
		Female—variably affected depending on X-chromosome inactivation	Normal phenotype, postpartum hyperammonemia, recurrent Reye syndrome, neonatal hyperammonemia
Mitochondrial Genes	Mutant leucine transfer RNA (A3243G)	Both sexes affected equally, but clinical manifestations variable among family members	Lactic acidosis, skeletal myopathy, cardiomyopathy, seizures, mental retardation, ataxia, deafness in various syndromic combinations

provide important genetic information for them, enabling decision making throughout the rest of the family, when desired.

Identifying Other Family Members at Risk

The risk to other family members depends on mechanism of inheritance. If the family history is positive, the pattern of inheritance provides clues to other family members at risk. If the condition is known to be autosomal recessive, unless there is consanguinity or the disease is common, it is unlikely that family members more distant than first-degree relatives carry the mutant gene. When the condition is known to be X-linked, maternal relatives are at risk. Genetic testing is helpful if it is available. In recessive conditions, heterozygote carriers usually never have biochemical abnormalities that can be measured. For some X-linked conditions, people who carry a mutation show biochemical abnormalities; in OTC deficiency, carrier females may show abnormalities in the plasma amino acid profile or may respond to challenge testing with increased orotic acid in urine. A normal result does not exclude the carrier state. Dominant disorders are notoriously variable, and a normal examination does not exclude the diagnosis.

If the gene location is known and linkage markers are identified, linkage testing can be performed to identify family members who carry the mutation. If the molecular pathology is understood and the mutation (or mutations) in the affected family member is known, molecular testing may be available.

IDENTIFICATION OF INBORN ERRORS BY NEONATAL SCREENING

Disorders Identified by Neonatal Screening

Most states screen for at least eight or nine disorders. In states where tandem mass spectrometry (MS/MS) is the method used, 30 metabolic disorders may be identifiable (Table 51–7). The **disorders of amino acid metabolism**, PKU, homocystinuria, MSUD, and tyrosinemia all need to be treated early in infancy for treatment to be effective. In MSUD, severe ketoacidosis may supervene in the first 2 weeks of life. The disorders of **organic acid metabolism**, propionic acidemia, methylmalonic acidemia, and isovaleric acidemia may result in vomiting and ketoacidosis early in life; some forms of methylmalonic acidemia present later, but CNS damage already may have occurred. **Galactosemia** is the disorder of carbohydrate metabolism screened for. Initial presentation of galactosemia not identified by screening includes jaundice, bleeding, cataract, and liver failure. Presymptomatic treatment affects outcome in all of these conditions; in some it is lifesaving.

TABLE 51–7.   Disorders Identified in Newborn Screening Programs in the U.S.

Disorder	Methods	Optimal Age of Treatment	Confirmatory Testing
Amino Acid			
PKU	Guthrie, MS/MS	First weeks of life	Plasma phenylalanine, mutation testing
Tyrosinemia	Guthrie, MS/MS	First week of life	Plasma amino acid profile, urine succinylacetone
MSUD	Guthrie, MS/MS	First week of life	Plasma amino acid profile, look for alloisoleucine
Organic Acid			
Propionic acidemia	MS/MS	First week of life	Urine organic acid profile
Methylmalonic acidemia	MS/MS	First weeks of life	Urine organic acid profile, plasma amino acid profile, plasma homocysteine
Isovaleric acidemia	MS/MS	First weeks of life	Urine organic acid profile
Biotinidase deficiency	Enzyme measurement	First weeks of life	Quantitative biotinidase measurement, DNA mutations
Fatty Acid			
MCAD	MS/MS	First weeks of life	Urine organic acid profile, urine acylglycine profile, plasma acylcarnitine profile
LCHAD	MS/MS	First weeks of life	Urine organic acid profile, urine acylglycine profile, plasma acylcarnitine profile
VLCAD	MS/MS	First weeks of life	Urine organic acid profile, urine acylglycine profile, plasma acylcarnitine profile
Carbohydrate			
Galactosemia	GALT enzyme measurement	First few days of life	GALT enzyme measurement, DNA mutations, galactose-1-P measurement
Urea Cycle	MS/MS	First few days of life	Plasma amino acid profile, DNA mutations

GALT, galactose-1-p-uridyltransferase; LCHAD, long chain 3-hydroxyacyl coenzyme A dehydrogenase; MCAD, medium-chain acyl-coenzyme A dehydrogenase; MS/MS, tandem mass spectrometry; MSUD, maple syrup urine disease; VLCAD; very long chain acyl-coenzyme A dehydrogenase.

Strategy of Neonatal Screening

The purpose of neonatal screening is the **early detection** and **rapid treatment** of disorders before onset of symptoms and early enough to prevent the morbidity and mortality of the disorders. The screening tests for inborn errors of metabolism traditionally have used microbiologic (Guthrie) assays for single analytes or semiquantitative fluorometric methods. The adaptation of MS/MS of blood specimens to neonatal screening is being adopted in many states. The advantage of MS/MS is that it allows rapid neonatal diagnosis of numerous metabolic diseases with a single blood specimen.

In most states, infants are tested just before discharge or by 7 days of age if the infant remains hospitalized (see Chapter 58). A positive test demands prompt evaluation, in keeping with the purpose of early identification and treatment before symptoms. Specific follow-up testing and treatment of an affected child depends on the disorder. Many infants who have a positive neonatal screening test do not always have a metabolic disorder. Parents may need to be reassured that this "false-positive" test in no way reflects the infant's health and is the result of establishing cutoff values for the screening test to ensure that no affected infant is missed.

Confirmatory Testing Principles

Neonatal screening is designed not to miss affected infants. Cutoff values for each analyte are established carefully to identify all infants with an elevated concentration of the analyte without having an unacceptable number of false-positive results. Screening tests are not diagnostic tests. A positive screening test must be followed by specific clinical evaluation and laboratory testing to confirm the disorder. In each category of disorders, protocols for the evaluation of an infant with an abnormal screening result clarify which infants need to be treated and which have had a false-positive test.

A positive screening test result causes anxiety for new parents who were expecting a healthy infant.

Definitive testing must be carried out promptly and accurately. Parents need to be educated and reassured while testing proceeds. If the diagnosis is confirmed, treatment must be begun immediately. If an inborn error of metabolism is excluded, parents need a thorough explanation and reassurance that the infant is well.

Specialized Laboratory and Clinical Testing

Specialized testing for inherited disorders of metabolism are effective in confirming a diagnosis suspected on the basis of an abnormal newborn screening result or on the basis of clinical suspicion. The analytes that are helpful and examples of diagnoses made using these measurements depend on the pathway that is deficient in the disorder under consideration (Table 51–8).

Amino acid analysis is performed in plasma, urine, and CSF. The plasma amino acid profile is most useful in identifying disorders of amino acid catabolism. Amino acids in the deficient pathway of the organic acid disorders may be abnormal, but often they are normal.

The urine amino acid profile is helpful in diagnosing primary disorders of renal tubular function, such as **Lowe syndrome** and **cystinuria**, and secondary disorders of renal tubular function, such as **cystinosis** and **Fanconi syndrome** of any cause. The urine amino acid profile is not the test of choice for diagnosing disorders of amino acid or organic acid metabolism.

Markers of disordered fatty acid oxidation are measured in urine and plasma. Intermediates of fatty acid oxidation and organic acid catabolism are conjugated with glycine and carnitine when they accumulate in excess. The **urine acylglycine** profile and the **plasma acylcarnitine** profile reflect this accumulation. In organic acid disorders and fatty acid oxidation disorders, carnitine depletion may occur, and measurement of plasma carnitines reveals the secondary deficiency of carnitine and the distribution of free and acylated carnitine. The plasma free **fatty acid profile** is helpful in diagnosis of disorders of fatty acid oxidation. Excess 3-OH-butyrate in plasma suggests a disorder of ketone metabolism, and absence of ketones or decreased amounts of 3-OH-butyrate suggest a fatty acid oxidation disorder.

The **urine organic acid profile** is a useful test. Disorders of organic acid metabolism, such as propionic acidemia and methylmalonic acidemia, have typical urine organic acid profiles. Clinical laboratory studies usually reveal the presence of acidosis; ketosis and hyperammonemia are frequently present. Although the analytes in blood and urine usually suggest the specific diagnosis, further, more targeted testing may be needed, in which enzymatic activity in the pathway is measured, or molecular abnormalities in the gene are sought.

Disorders of **creatine biosynthesis** are reflected by an increase in guanidinoacetic acid in blood and urine. Disorders of **purine** and **pyrimidine** metabolism are suggested by the presence of an abnormal profile of purines, such as xanthine, hypoxanthine, inosine,

---

TABLE 51–8. Specialized Metabolic Testing

Test	Analytes Measured	Test Helpful in Identifying Disorders
Plasma amino acid profile	Amino acids, including alloisoleucine	PKU, tyrosinemias, MSUD, homocystinuria
Plasma total homocysteine	Protein-bound and free homocysteine	Homocystinuria, some forms of methylmalonic acidemia
Urine amino acid profile	Amino acids	Disorders of amino acid renal transport
Plasma acylcarnitine profile	Acylcarnitine derivatives of organic and fatty acid catabolism	Organic acid disorders, fatty acid oxidation disorders
Urine acylglycine profile	Acylglycine derivatives of organic and fatty acid catabolism	Organic acid disorders, fatty acid oxidation disorders
Plasma carnitines	Free, total, and acylated carnitine	Primary and secondary carnitine deficiency; abnormal in many organic acid and fatty acid disorders
Urine organic acid profile	Organic acids	Organic acid, mitochondrial and fatty acid disorders
Urine succinylacetone	Succinylacetone	Tyrosinemia I
Urine oligosaccharide chromatography	Glycosaminoglycans, mucopolysaccharides	Lysosomal storage disorders

MSUD, maple syrup urine disease.

guanosine, adenosine, adenine, and succinyladenosine, in urine. Similarly, disorders of pyrimidine metabolism are identified by an abnormal profile of pyrimidines, including uracil, uridine, thymine, thymidine, orotic acid, orotidine, dihydrouracil, dihydrothymine, pseudo-uridine, N-carbamoyl-β-alanine, and N-carbamoyl-β-amino-isobutyrate, in the urine.

Storage disorders show abnormalities in urine mucopolysaccharides (glycosaminoglycans, glycoproteins), sialic acid, heparan sulfate, dermatan sulfate, and chondroitin sulfate. Specific enzymology depends on the disorder; tissue can be either white blood cells or cultured skin fibroblasts, depending on assay. In several disorders, **CSF** is the most helpful specimen, including glycine encephalopathy (amino acid profile), disorders of neurotransmitter synthesis (biogenic amine profile), glucose transporter (GLUT1) deficiency (plasma-to-CSF glucose ratio), and serine synthesis defect (amino acid profile).

In many disorders, an abnormal metabolic profile is consistently present during illness and when the child is well. In some cases, during an episode of illness is the time when metabolic profiles are most likely to be diagnostic.

Metabolic Challenge Testing

After extensive prior testing has failed to reveal a diagnosis and in a unit experienced in metabolic challenge testing, such challenges can play a role in elucidating an inborn error of metabolism. Fasting studies can be dangerous in children who have a disorder of fatty acid oxidation. For that reason, first exclude a disorder of fatty acid oxidation before performing a fasting test. Loading tests sometimes can be helpful when other studies have not provided an answer. Glucose loading can be informative in disorders of lactate and mitochondrial energy metabolism, but must not be performed if plasma lactate is elevated. Although fructose loading can be done, the risk of hypoglycemia is high, and fructose loading should not be done except under controlled circumstances in expert hands and only if testing for hereditary fructose intolerance, including mutation testing, has failed to confirm a diagnosis. Fat loading tests for disorders of fat catabolism have been largely superseded by metabolic profiling of acylglycines in urine and acylcarnitines in plasma.

OVERVIEW OF TREATMENT

There are several basic principles to treatment of inborn errors of metabolism. In the syndromes that have toxicity, often with encephalopathy as their major pathophysiology, the **removal of toxic compounds is the first goal of therapy**. These strategies include

hemodialysis, hemovenovenous filtration, and compounds that serve as ammonia trapping agents (see Chapter 53). A second strategy is to enhance deficient enzyme activity; this involves administration of enzyme cofactors. In cases in which deficiency of a product of a pathway plays an important role, providing missing products is helpful; this is exemplified by the provision of tyrosine in the treatment of PKU. A major principle is to decrease flux through deficient pathway by restricting precursors in the diet. Examples include the restriction of phenylalanine in PKU, of protein in disorders of ammonia detoxification, and of amino acid precursors in the organic acid disorders.

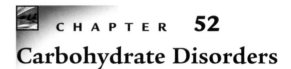

CHAPTER 52
Carbohydrate Disorders

GLYCOGEN STORAGE DISEASES

The glycogen storage diseases enter into the differential diagnoses of **hypoglycemia and hepatomegaly** (Table 52–1). Glycogen is the storage form of glucose and is found most abundantly in the liver, where it modulates blood glucose, and in muscles, where it facilitates anaerobic work. Glycogen is synthesized from uridine diphosphoglucose through the concerted action of glycogen synthetase and brancher enzyme (Fig. 52–1). The accumulation of glycogen is stimulated by insulin. Glycogenolysis occurs through a cascade phenomenon that is initiated by epinephrine or glucagon and results in rapid phosphorolysis of glycogen to yield glucose-1-phosphate, accompanied by a lesser degree of hydrolysis of glucose residues from the branch points in glycogen molecules. In the liver and kidneys, glucose-1-phosphate can produce glucose through the actions of phosphoglucomutase and glucose-6-phosphatase. The latter enzyme is not present in muscles. Glycogen storage diseases fall into the following four categories:

1. Diseases that predominantly affect the liver and have a direct influence on blood glucose (types I, VI, and VIII)
2. Diseases that predominantly involve muscles and affect the ability to do anaerobic work (types V and VII)
3. Diseases that can affect the liver and muscles and directly influence blood glucose and muscle metabolism (type III)
4. Diseases that affect various tissues but have no direct effect on blood glucose or on the ability to do anaerobic work (types II and IV)

TABLE 52–1.   Glycogen Storage Diseases

Disease	Affected Enzyme	Organs Affected	Clinical Syndrome	Neonatal Manifestations	Prognosis
Type I: von Gierke	Glucose-6-phosphatase	Liver, kidney, GI tract, platelets	Hypoglycemia, lactic acidosis, ketosis, hepatomegaly, hypotonia, slow growth, diarrhea, bleeding disorder, gout, hypertriglyceridemia, xanthomas	Hypoglycemia, lactic acidemia, liver may not be enlarged	Early death from hypoglycemia, lactic acidosis; may do well with supportive management; hepatomas occur in late childhood
Type II: Pompe	Lysosomal α-glucosidase	All, notably striated muscle, nerve cells	Symmetric profound muscle weakness, cardiomegaly, heart failure, shortened P-R interval	May have muscle weakness, cardiomegaly, or both	Very poor; death in the first year of life is usual; variants exist; therapy with recombinant human α-glucosidase is promising
Type III: Forbes	Debranching enzyme	Liver, muscles	Early in course hypoglycemia, ketonuria, hepatomegaly that resolves with age; may show muscle fatigue	Usually none	Very good for hepatic disorder; if myopathy present, it tends to be like that of type V
Type IV: Andersen	Branching enzyme	Liver, other tissues	Hepatic cirrhosis beginning at several months of age; early liver failure	Usually none	Very poor; death from hepatic failure before age of 4 years
Type V: McArdle	Muscle phosphorylase	Muscle	Muscle fatigue beginning in adolescence	None	Good, with sedentary lifestyle
Type VI: Hers	Liver phosphorylase	Liver	Mild hypoglycemia with hepatomegaly, ketonuria	Usually none	Probably good
Type VII: Tarui	Muscle phosphofructokinase	Muscle	Clinical findings similar to type V	None	Similar to that of type V
Type VIII	Phosphorylase kinase	Liver	Clinical findings similar to type III, without myopathy	None	Good

GI, gastrointestinal.
Except for one form of hepatic phosphorylase kinase, which is X-linked, these disorders are autosomal recessive.

The **diagnosis** of glycogen storage disease can often be confirmed by DNA mutation testing in blood cells. When this is feasible, invasive procedures, such as muscle and liver biopsy, can be avoided. When mutation testing is not available, enzyme measurements in the tissue suspected to be affected (either liver or muscle) confirm the diagnosis. If the diagnosis cannot be established, metabolic challenge and exercise testing may be needed. **Treatment** of hepatic glycogen storage disease is aimed at maintaining satisfactory blood glucose levels or supplying alternative energy sources to muscle. In glucose-6-phosphatase deficiency (type I), the treatment usually requires nocturnal intragastric feedings of glucose during the first 1 or 2 years of life. Thereafter, snacks or nocturnal intragastric feedings of uncooked cornstarch may be satisfactory, but hepatic

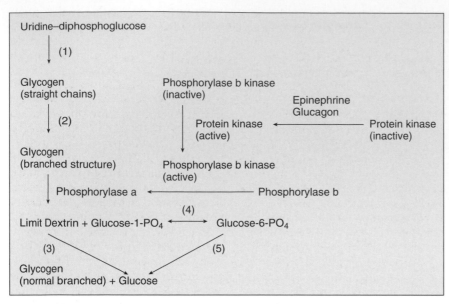

Figure 52-1

Glycogen synthesis and degradation. (1) Glycogen synthetase, (2) brancher enzyme, (3) debrancher enzyme, (4) phosphoglucomutase, (5) glucose-6-phosphatase.

tumors (sometimes malignant) are a threat in adolescence and adult life. No specific treatment exists for the diseases of muscle that impair skeletal muscle ischemic exercise. Enzyme replacement is effective in Pompe disease (type II), which involves cardiac and skeletal muscle.

GALACTOSEMIA

Galactosemia is an autosomal recessive disease caused by deficiency of the enzyme galactose-1-phosphate uridyltransferase (Fig. 52–2). Clinical manifestations are most striking in a neonate who when fed milk generally exhibits evidence of **liver failure** (hyperbilirubinemia, disorders of coagulation, and hypoglycemia), disordered **renal tubular function** (acidosis, glycosuria, and aminoaciduria), and **cataracts**. The neonatal screening test must have a rapid turnaround time because affected infants may die in the first week of life. Infants with galactosemia are at increased risk for severe neonatal *Escherichia coli* sepsis. Major effects on liver and kidney function and the development of cataracts are limited to the first few years of life, but older children have learning disorders. Girls may develop premature ovarian failure, which occurs despite treatment.

Laboratory manifestations of galactosemia depend on dietary galactose intake. When galactose is ingested (as lactose), levels of plasma galactose and erythrocyte galactose-1-phosphate are elevated. Hypoglycemia is frequent, and albuminuria is present. Galactose frequently is present in the urine and can be detected by a positive reaction for reducing substances (Clinitest tablets) and no reaction with glucose oxidase

on urine strip tests. The absence of urinary reducing substance cannot be relied on to exclude the diagnosis. Renal tubular dysfunction may be evidenced by a normal anion gap hyperchloremic metabolic acidosis. The diagnosis is made by showing extreme reduction in erythrocyte galactose-1-phosphate uridyltransferase. The concentration of galactose-1-phosphate rarely returns to normal even after treatment is begun. DNA testing for the mutations in galactose-1-phosphate uridyltransferase confirms the diagnosis. **Treatment** by the elimination of dietary galactose results in rapid correction of abnormalities, but infants who are extremely ill before treatment may die before therapy is effective.

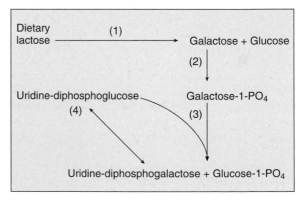

Figure 52-2

Pathway of galactose metabolism. (1) Lactase (intestinal), (2) galactokinase, (3) galactose-1-phosphate uridyltransferase, (4) uridine diphosphoglucose 4-epimerase.

Galactokinase deficiency, an autosomal recessive disorder, also leads to the accumulation of galactose in body fluids (see Fig. 52–2), which results in the formation of galactitol (dulcitol) through the action of aldose reductase. Galactitol, acting as an osmotic agent, can be responsible for cataract formation and, rarely, for increased intracranial pressure. These are the only clinical manifestations. Persons homozygous for galactokinase deficiency develop cataracts in the neonatal period, whereas heterozygous individuals may be at risk for cataracts as adults. *Treatment* consists of lifelong elimination of galactose from the diet.

Hereditary fructose intolerance in many ways is analogous to galactosemia. When fructose is ingested, deficiency of fructose-1-phosphate aldolase leads to the intracellular accumulation of fructose-1-phosphate with resultant emesis, hypoglycemia, and severe liver and kidney disease. Elimination of fructose and sucrose from the diet cures the clinical disease. Affected patients spontaneously avoid fructose-containing foods and have no dental caries. **Fructosuria** is analogous to galactokinase deficiency in that it is caused by fructokinase deficiency, but the defect in fructosuria is harmless.

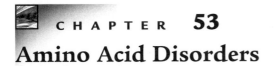

C H A P T E R   53
Amino Acid Disorders

DISORDERS OF AMINO ACID METABOLISM

Disorders of amino acid metabolism are the result of the inability to catabolize specific amino acids derived from protein. Usually a single amino acid pathway is involved. This amino acid accumulates in excess and is toxic to various organs, such as the brain, eye, skin, or liver. Treatment is directed at the specific pathway, and usually involves dietary restriction of the offending amino acid and supplementation with special medical foods (formulas) that provide the other amino acids and other nutrients. Confirmatory testing includes quantitative specific plasma amino acid profiles along with specific mutation testing and sometimes enzymology.

PHENYLKETONURIA

PKU, an autosomal recessive disease, primarily affects the brain. It occurs in 1:10,000 persons. Classic PKU is the result from a defect in the hydroxylation of phenylalanine to form tyrosine (Fig. 53–1); the activity of phenylalanine hydroxylase in the liver is absent or

greatly reduced. Affected infants are normal at birth, but severe mental retardation (IQ 30) develops in the first year of life. The clinical syndrome classically described of blond hair, blue eyes, eczema, and mousy odor of the urine is rarely seen because of neonatal screening for PKU. A positive newborn screening test must be followed up by performing quantitative plasma amino acid analysis, measuring phenylalanine and tyrosine. A plasma phenylalanine value of greater than 360 μM (6 mg/dL) is consistent with the diagnosis of one of the hyperphenylalaninemias and demands prompt evaluation and treatment. Untreated, classic PKU has blood phenylalanine concentrations greater than 600 μM. Milder forms of hyperphenylalaninemia show values of plasma phenylalanine lower than this but greater than 360 μM. A significant percentage of premature infants and a few full-term infants have transient elevations in phenylalanine. Short-term follow-up usually identifies these infants promptly. Mutation testing of the *PAH* gene reveals more than 400 mutations. For some mutations, such as R408W, clinical correlation is almost always reliable; classic PKU is seen if the patient has two copies of that allele. Some mutations are usually associated with mild hyperphenylalaninemia. There is enough variability, however, that prediction is not possible.

Clinical care should be designed to maintain plasma phenylalanine values in the therapeutic range of 120 to 360 μM, at least for the first 10 years of life. Most centers have difficulty achieving this level of control consistently, however, particularly as the child grows older.

A small percentage of infants diagnosed with PKU (≤2% in the U.S.) have a defect in the synthesis or metabolism of tetrahydrobiopterin, the cofactor for phenylalanine hydroxylase and for other enzymes involved in the intermediary metabolism of aromatic amino acids. In these infants, a progressive, lethal CNS disease develops, reflecting abnormalities in other neurotransmitter metabolism for which tetrahydrobiopterin is necessary. Disorders in **biopterin metabolism** are diagnosed by measuring dihydrobiopterin reductase in erythrocytes and by analyzing biopterin metabolites in urine. This testing is carried out in all hyperphenylalaninemic infants.

Outcome of treatment in classic PKU is excellent. Most infants with classic PKU who are treated using a diet specifically restricted in phenylalanine and begun within the first 10 days of life achieve normal intelligence. Learning problems and problems with executive function are reported; early and consistent dietary control provides the best chance for optimal outcome. In the disorders of biopterin biosynthesis, restriction of dietary phenylalanine reduces plasma phenylalanine, but does not ameliorate the clinical symptoms. This condition must be treated by replace-

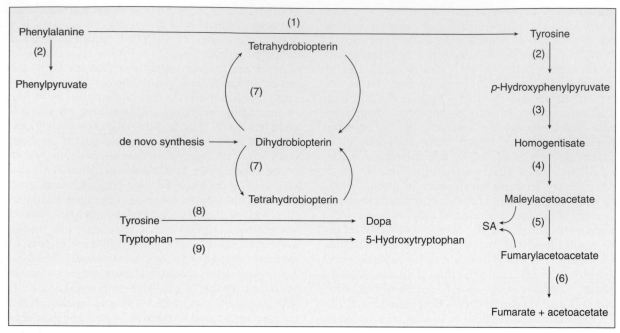

Figure 53–1

Metabolism of aromatic amino acids. (1) Phenylalanine hydroxylase, (2) transaminase, (3), p-hydroxyphenylpyruvate oxidase, (4) homogentisate oxidase, (5) maleylacetoacetate isomerase, (6) fumarylacetoacetate hydrolase, (7) dihydrobiopterin reductase, (8) tyrosine hydroxylase, (9) tryptophan hydroxylase. SA, succinylacetone.

ment of the cofactor or by neuropharmacologic agents. Outcome is less predictable than in classic PKU.

Sustained control is difficult to achieve after the first 10 years of life. The safe concentration of phenylalanine in older children and adults with PKU has not been clearly established. Reversible cognitive dysfunction is associated with acute elevations of plasma phenylalanine in treated adults and children with PKU. If the elevated level has been sustained, the dysfunction may be permanent. **Maternal hyperphenylalaninemia** is a major problem requiring rigorous management before conception and throughout pregnancy to prevent fetal brain damage, congenital heart disease, and microcephaly in the fetus.

TYROSINEMIAS

Tyrosinemia is identified in neonatal screening programs using MS/MS methods. Elevated tyrosine levels also can occur as a nonspecific consequence of severe liver disease. In addition, transient tyrosinemia of the newborn, which responds to ascorbic acid treatment, may be the cause. The inherited disorders of tyrosine metabolism are the target of neonatal screening. **Tyrosinemia I**, which is due to fumarylacetoacetate hydrolase deficiency (see Fig. 53–1), is a rare disease in

which accumulated metabolites produce severe liver disease associated with bleeding disorder, hypoglycemia, hypoalbuminemia, elevated transaminases, and defects in renal tubular function. Hepatocellular carcinoma may occur eventually. Quantitative measurement of plasma amino acids to look for excess tyrosine or the pattern of liver disease is the next step after a positive neonatal screening test for hypertyrosinemia. The **diagnosis** of tyrosinemia I is confirmed by measuring succinylacetone in urine. DNA testing is available for some mutations in tyrosinemia I. **Treatment** with NTBC (an inhibitor of the oxidation of parahydroxyphenylpyruvic acid) effectively eliminates the production of the toxic succinylacetone. A low-phenylalanine, low-tyrosine diet may also play a role. These treatments have supplanted liver transplantation in many children identified by neonatal screening. Whether or not they completely eliminate the occurrence of hepatocellular carcinoma is unknown.

Tyrosinemia II and **III** are more benign forms of hereditary tyrosinemia. Blocked metabolism of tyrosine at earlier steps in the pathway is responsible, and succinylacetone is not produced. The clinical features include hyperkeratosis of palms and soles and keratitis, which can cause severe visual disturbance. Treatment with a phenylalanine-restricted and tyrosine-restricted diet is effective.

HOMOCYSTINURIA

Homocystinuria, an autosomal recessive disease (1:200,000 live births) involving connective tissue, the brain, and the vascular system, is caused by a deficiency of cystathionine β-synthase. In the normal metabolism of the sulfur amino acids, methionine gives rise to cystine; homocysteine is a pivotal intermediate (Fig. 53–2). When cystathionine β-synthase is deficient, homocysteine accumulates in the blood and appears in the urine. Another result is enhanced reconversion of homocysteine to methionine, resulting in an increase in the concentration of methionine in the blood. The neonatal screening test most commonly used measures methionine in whole blood. Through mechanisms not clearly understood, an excess of homocysteine produces a slowly evolving **clinical syndrome** that includes dislocated ocular lenses; long, slender extremities; malar flushing; and livedo reticularis. Arachnodactyly, scoliosis, pectus excavatum or carinatum, and genu valgum are skeletal features. Mental retardation, psychiatric illness, or both may be present. Major arterial or venous thromboses are a constant threat.

Homocystinuria has no neonatal manifestations. Confirmation of the **diagnosis** requires demonstration of elevated total homocysteine in the blood. A plasma amino acid profile reveals hypermethioninemia.

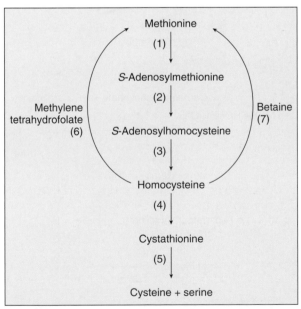

Figure 53–2

Metabolism of methionine and homocysteine. (1) Methionine adenosyltransferase, (2) S-methyltransferase, (3) S-adenosylhomocysteine hydrolase, (4) cystathionine β-synthase, (5) cystathionase, (6) homocysteine methyltransferase, (7) betaine-homocysteine methyltransferase.

Measurement of cystathionine β-synthase can be performed, but is not clinically available. Numerous mutations in the cystathionine β-synthase gene are known and can be tested.

There are two clinical forms of homocystinuria. In one form, activity of the deficient enzyme can be enhanced by the administration of large doses of pyridoxine (100 to 1000 mg/day); folate supplementation is added to overcome folate deficiency if folate is trapped in the process of remethylation of homocysteine to methionine. The pyridoxine-responsive form comprises about 50% of the cases and is the more likely form to be missed by neonatal screening because the methionine concentrations are not always above the screening cutoff. The second form is not responsive to pyridoxine therapy, and the accumulation of homocysteine is controlled with a methionine-restricted diet and cystine and folate supplementation. The use of supplemental betaine (trimethylglycine) as a donor of methyl groups for remethylation of homocysteine to methionine also has a role in the management of pyridoxine-unresponsive patients. Sometimes diet and betaine are required to control plasma homocysteine even in pyridoxine-responsive patients. The prognosis is good for infants whose plasma homocysteine concentration is controlled.

MAPLE SYRUP URINE DISEASE

MSUD is an autosomal recessive disease, more properly named **branched chain ketoaciduria**. MSUD is caused by deficiency of the decarboxylase that initiates the degradation of the ketoacid analogues of the three branched chain amino acids—leucine, isoleucine, and valine (Fig. 53–3). MSUD is rare (1:250,000) in the general population but much more common in some population isolates (among Pennsylvania Mennonites 1:150). Neonatal screening programs commonly include MSUD.

Although MSUD does have intermittent-onset and late-onset forms, **clinical manifestations** of the classic form typically begin within 1 to 4 weeks of birth. Poor feeding, vomiting, and tachypnea commonly are noted, but the hallmark of the disease is profound depression of the CNS, associated with alternating hypotonia and hypertonia (extensor spasms), opisthotonos, and seizures. The urine has the odor of maple syrup.

Laboratory manifestations of MSUD include hypoglycemia and a variable presence of metabolic acidosis, with elevation of the undetermined anions; the acidosis is caused in part by plasma branched chain organic acids and in part by the usual "ketone bodies," β-hydroxybutyrate and acetoacetate. The branched chain ketoacids (but not the β-hydroxybutyrate or the acetoacetate) react immediately with 2,4-dinitrophenylhydrazine to form a copious, white precipitate.

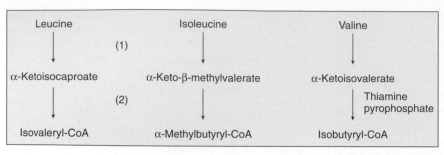

Figure 53–3

Metabolism of the branched chain amino acids. (1) Aminotransferases, (2) α-ketoacid dehydrogenase complex.

The **definitive diagnosis** of MSUD generally is made by showing large increases in plasma leucine, isoleucine, and valine concentrations and by the identification of alloisoleucine in the plasma in excess. The urinary organic acid profile also is usually abnormal and shows the ketoacid derivatives of the branched chain amino acids.

Treatment of MSUD consists of restricting the intake of branched chain amino acids (all three are essential amino acids) to the amounts required for growth in severely affected infants. Hemodialysis, hemofiltration, or peritoneal dialysis can be lifesaving during acidotic crises. Treatment with special diets must be continued for life. Ordinary catabolic stresses, such as moderate infections or labor and delivery in a pregnant mother with MSUD, can precipitate clinical crises. Liver transplantation effectively treats MSUD.

DISORDERS OF AMMONIA DISPOSAL

Inherited enzymatic deficiencies have been described for each of the steps of urea synthesis (Fig. 53-4). Neonatal screening does not currently detect all of the disorders of ammonia disposal.

Ornithine Carbamoyltransferase Deficiency

OTC deficiency is unique among the defects in the urea cycle in that it is X-linked. The number of known gene mutations is quite large with deletions and point mutations described. If the enzyme is nonfunctional, there is no OTC activity in the affected male, who is likely to die in the neonatal period. Affected females are heterozygous and, because of lyonization, may have a significant degree of enzyme deficiency and may be clinically affected. **Clinical manifestations** range through lethal disease in the male (coma, encephalopathy) to clinical normalcy in a high percentage of females. Manifestations in clinically affected females include recurrent emesis, lethargy, seizures, developmental delay, and mental retardation. Affected females may spontaneously limit their protein intake.

Confirmatory testing includes a plasma amino acid profile, which may show deficient citrulline and arginine concentrations. A urine organic acid profile shows increased excretion of orotic acid. Mutation testing and sequencing of the entire coding region are available as clinical tests.

Argininosuccinic Aciduria

Argininosuccinic acid lyase deficiency results in accumulation of argininosuccinic acid in tissues and blood;

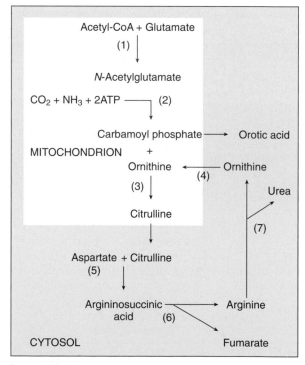

Figure 53–4

The urea cycle. (1) *N*-acetylglutamate synthase, (2) carbamoylphosphate synthetase, (3) ornithine carbamoyltransferase (OCT), (4) ornithine translocator, (5) argininosuccinic acid synthetase, (6) argininosuccinic acid lyase, (7) arginase.

however, because the kidney readily clears the acid, it is best identified in the urine, where it is found in gram quantities. Plasma citrulline concentration is increased. Hyperammonemia is not present at all times in all patients. The defect disrupts the urea cycle, however, and hyperammonemia does occur. Death in the neonatal period has been reported, as has symptomatic hyperammonemia in later infancy and childhood. Failure to thrive, hepatomegaly, friable hair (**trichorrhexis nodosa**), slow motor and mental development, and seizures are characteristic features of the disease, with or without clinical hyperammonemia. Argininosuccinic aciduria is an autosomal recessive disease. Mutation testing and gene sequencing are clinically available.

Treatment of Hyperammonemia

During episodes of symptomatic hyperammonemia, protein intake is eliminated, and IV glucose is given in sufficient quantity to suppress catabolism of endogenous protein. Ammonia can be eliminated by use of the **ammonia scavenger** agents, **sodium benzoate** and **sodium phenylacetate**, which are excreted in the urine as conjugates of glycine and glutamine. Arginine, which is usually deficient, is also supplied. Sterilization of the intestine and treatment with lactulose can provide brief benefit during acute episodes of hyperammonemia. When hyperammonemia is extreme, direct removal of ammonia, usually using hemodialysis or hemofiltration, is more effective than exchange transfusion or peritoneal dialysis. Despite successful management of hyperammonemic crises, the long-term outcome for males with severe neonatal hyperammonemia is poor. Early liver transplantation has increased survival, especially in males with OTC deficiency.

A reduction of dietary protein intake is the mainstay of ongoing treatment for hyperammonemia. Crystalline essential amino acids can be supplied in amounts just sufficient to support new protein synthesis in OTC deficiency. Arginine is an essential amino acid when arginine synthesis via the urea cycle is grossly impaired, and arginine must be supplied. Citrulline needs to be supplied for some urea cycle disorders. For OTC deficiency and carbamoyl phosphate synthase deficiency, treatment with phenylbutyrate (which is metabolized to phenylacetate) prevents accumulation of ammonia.

DISORDERS OF AMINO ACID TRANSPORT THAT AFFECT SPECIFIC TRANSPORT MECHANISMS IN THE KIDNEY AND INTESTINE

Cystinuria is a disorder of renal tubular transport of cystine, lysine, arginine, and ornithine. Although intestinal transport is affected in some of the genetic forms,

the symptoms are largely due to the renal transport abnormality. The concentration of cystine exceeds its solubility product and results in significant renal stones. Evaluation and diagnosis is based on the pattern of amino acid excretion in the urine. Mutation testing can be done. **Treatment** is based on increasing the solubility of cystine by complexing it with compounds such as penicillamine.

Intestinal transport of tryptophan is impaired in **Hartnup syndrome**, and symptoms result from this deficiency. Diagnosis is based on the amino acid pattern in urine, and treatment with tryptophan is successful.

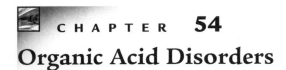

CHAPTER 54

Organic Acid Disorders

DISORDERS OF ORGANIC ACID METABOLISM

Organic acid disorders result from a metabolic block in the pathways of catabolism of amino acids. Occurring at the end of the pathways of catabolism of amino acids after the amino moiety has been removed, they result in the accumulation of specific organic acids in the blood and urine. Treatment is directed at the specific abnormality, with restriction in precursor substrates and administration of enzyme cofactors when available. Outcome is influenced by frequency and severity of ketoacidotic crises and is optimal when diagnosis is made before the onset of the first episode. Liver transplantation has been employed in some patients and can be successful, but long-term outcome after liver transplantation has not been well studied. Confirmatory testing begins with a urine organic acid profile and plasma amino acid profile. When abnormal results confirm the specific organic acid disorder, DNA testing may identify the mutations involved. More specific testing if a mutation is not found requires enzyme measurements in appropriate tissues.

PROPIONIC ACIDEMIA AND METHYLMALONIC ACIDEMIA

Propionic acidemia and methylmalonic acidemia result from defects in a series of reactions called the *propionate pathway* (Fig. 54-1). Defects in these steps produce **ketosis** and **hyperglycinemia**. Propionic acidemia and methylmalonic acidemia are identified by neonatal screening when MS/MS methods are used. The **clinical manifestations** of both of these disorders in the neonatal period consist of tachypnea, vomiting, lethargy, coma, intermittent ketoacidosis, hyperglycin-

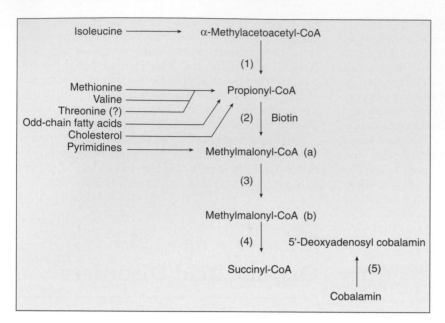

Figure 54–1

The propionate pathway. (1) β-Ketothiolase, (2) propionyl-CoA carboxylase, (3) methylmalonyl-CoA isomerase, (4) methylmalonyl-CoA mutase, (5) cobalamin metabolic pathway. CoA, coenzyme A.

emia, neutropenia, thrombocytopenia, hyperammonemia, and hypoglycemia. If these disorders are not identified by neonatal screening, intermittent episodes of metabolic acidosis occur. Crises occur during periods of catabolic stress, such as fever, vomiting, and diarrhea; they also may occur without an apparent precipitating event. During periods of neutropenia, the risk of serious bacterial infection is increased. Failure to thrive and impaired development are common.

Propionic acidemia results from deficiency in propionyl CoA-carboxylase, an enzyme that has two pairs of identical subunits. All forms of propionic acidemia are inherited in an autosomal recessive manner and are due to mutations in one or the other of those subunits. **Methylmalonic acidemia** results from deficiency in methylmalonyl mutase; this may be caused by mutations in the gene for the mutase protein itself or in one of the steps of the synthesis of the cobalamin cofactors for the enzyme. A complex set of defects in cobalamin metabolism results in other forms of methylmalonic acidemia, some of which are associated with hyperhomocystinemia. **Treatment** with massive doses of hydroxycobalamin (the active form of vitamin B_{12}) is helpful in some cases of methylmalonic acidemia.

For propionic acidemia and the vitamin B_{12}–unresponsive forms of methylmalonic acidemia, management includes the restriction of dietary protein and addition of a medical food deficient in the specific amino acid precursors of propionyl-CoA (isoleucine, valine, methionine, and threonine). Carnitine supplementation often is needed because carnitine is lost in the urine as acylcarnitines. Because intestinal bacteria produce a significant quantity of propionate, antibacterial treatment to reduce the population of bacteria in the gut has some beneficial effect in propionic acidemia and vitamin B_{12}–unresponsive methylmalonic acidemia.

ISOVALERIC ACIDEMIA

Isovaleric acidemia results from a block in the catabolism of leucine. Its clinical manifestations are similar to those of defects in the propionate pathway. Because isovaleric acid has a strong odor, infants with isovaleric acidemia have a **"sweaty feet" odor** when untreated. In addition to a diet restricted in the intake of leucine, glycine therapy is beneficial through enhancement of the formation of isovalerylglycine, a relatively harmless conjugate of isovaleric acid (Fig. 54–2), which is excreted in the urine.

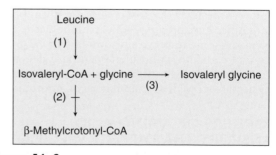

Figure 54–2

Metabolism in isovaleric acidemia. (1) Leucine catabolic pathway (transamination and decarboxylation), (2) isovaleryl-CoA dehydrogenase, (3) glycine acyltransferase. CoA, coenzyme A.

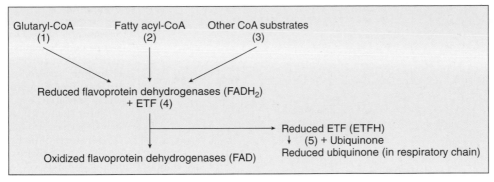

Figure 54–3

Scheme of flavoprotein metabolism with reference to glutaric aciduria types I and II.
(1) Glutaryl-CoA dehydrogenase (deficient in glutaric aciduria type I), (2) fatty acyl-CoA dehydrogenases, (3) other flavoprotein dehydrogenases, (4) ETF (deficiency results in glutaric aciduria type II), (5) ETF–ubiquinone oxidoreductase (deficiency results in glutaric aciduria type II). CoA, coenzyme A; ETF, electron transfer flavoprotein.

GLUTARIC ACIDEMIA I

Glutaric acidemia I results from a deficiency at the end of the lysine catabolic pathway. It is an autosomal recessive disease produced by deficiency of glutaryl-CoA dehydrogenase activity (Fig. 54–3). **Clinical manifestations** include **macrocephaly**, which may be present at birth, and **dystonia**, which characteristically develops after the first 18 months of life, after an episode of intercurrent illness associated with fever and metabolic distress. Clinical features include "metabolic" strokelike episodes associated with infarction of the basal ganglia. **Treatment** includes a protein-restricted diet accompanied by a medical food deficient in lysine. Some investigators report improved outcome when episodes of metabolic distress are managed aggressively to prevent the strokelike episodes.

BIOTINIDASE DEFICIENCY AND HOLOCARBOXYLASE DEFICIENCY

Biotin is a ubiquitous vitamin that is covalently linked to many carboxylases, including propionyl CoA carboxylase, by holocarboxylase synthetase in a variety of tissues. Inherited biotinidase deficiency greatly increases the dietary requirement for biotin because biotin cannot be recycled from its attachment to the carboxylases. Affected individuals become biotin deficient while consuming normal diets. Clinical disease can appear in the neonatal period or be delayed until later infancy, depending on the degree of deficiency.

The **clinical manifestations** of biotin deficiency vary greatly (seizures, hypotonia, alopecia, skin rash, metabolic acidosis, and immune deficits) and undoubtedly depend on which enzymes in which tissues have the most biotin depletion. Carboxylation is a crucial reaction in the metabolism of organic acids; most patients with biotinidase deficiency excrete abnormal amounts of several organic acids, among which β-methylcrotonylglycine is prominent. In addition to biotinidase deficiency, an inherited deficiency of holocarboxylase synthetase gives rise to severe disease and to similar patterns of organic aciduria. Both conditions respond well to **treatment** with large (10 to 40 mg/day) doses of biotin. Confirmatory testing is accomplished with quantitative measurement of biotinidase activity.

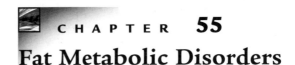

CHAPTER 55
Fat Metabolic Disorders

DISORDERS OF FATTY ACID OXIDATION

Fatty acids are derived from hydrolysis of triglycerides and catabolism of fat. The fatty acids important in human biology range in chain length from 18 carbons to 6 carbons. The catabolism of fatty acids (Fig. 55–1) proceeds through the serial, oxidative removal of two carbons at a time as acetyl groups (each as acetyl-CoA). The reactions are catalyzed by a group of enzymes that exhibit specificities related to the chain length and other properties of the fatty acids: very long chain acyl-CoA dehydrogenase, long chain hydroxyacyl-CoA dehydrogenase (trifunctional protein), medium chain acyl-CoA dehydrogenase (MCAD), and short chain

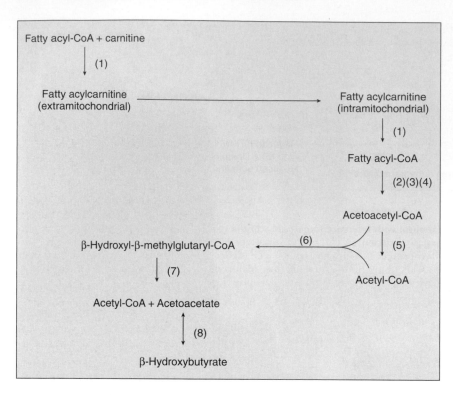

Within the figure:

Fatty acyl-CoA + carnitine

(1)

Fatty acylcarnitine (extramitochondrial) → Fatty acylcarnitine (intramitochondrial)

(1)

Fatty acyl-CoA

(2)(3)(4)

Acetoacetyl-CoA

β-Hydroxyl-β-methylglutaryl-CoA ← (6)   (5)

(7)   Acetyl-CoA

Acetyl-CoA + Acetoacetate

(8)

β-Hydroxybutyrate

Figure 55–1

Scheme of fatty acid catabolism and ketone body formation. (1) Carnitine acyl-CoA dehydrogenases, (2) long chain fatty acyl-CoA dehydrogenase (trifunctional protein), (3) medium chain fatty acyl-CoA dehydrogenase, (4) short chain fatty acyl-CoA dehydrogenase, (5) β-ketothiolase, (6) β-hydroxy-β-methlyglutaryl-CoA synthase, (7) β-hydroxy-β-methylglutaryl-CoA lyase, (8) β-hydroxybutyrate dehydrogenase. CoA, coenzyme A.

acyl-CoA dehydrogenase. MCAD deficiency is the most common inborn error of β-oxidation. Hypoketotic hypoglycemia is a common manifestation, as is **Reye syndrome–like** illness with hypoglycemia and elevated liver enzymes. Fatty infiltration of the liver also occurs. True hepatic failure is rare. Reye syndrome–like illnesses may be recurrent in the patient or the family. **Sudden infant death syndrome** may occur in infants with MCAD deficiency. Most of the other rarer disorders of fatty acid oxidation involve skeletal and cardiac muscle more than does MCAD. In all of the disorders of β-oxidation, carnitine depletion can occur through excessive urinary excretion of carnitine esters of incompletely oxidized fatty acids.

Hydroxymethylglutaryl-CoA lyase deficiency, although not a disorder of β-oxidation, interferes profoundly with hepatic adaptation to fasting by impairing ketogenesis (see Fig. 55–1). The *clinical manifestations* are those of MCAD deficiency except that carnitine depletion is less prominent than in MCAD deficiency because hydroxymethylglutaric acid does not form an ester with carnitine.

The **diagnosis** of disorders involving a deficiency of β-oxidation is suggested by the clinical picture and by hypoketotic hypoglycemia. The diagnosis is confirmed by analysis of urinary organic acid and acylglycine profiles, along with plasma acylcarnitine and free fatty acid profiles. Enzyme measurements and DNA testing complete the confirmatory testing. The profile of acylcar-

nitines in cultured skin fibroblasts also may be helpful if other testing is not conclusive. In MCAD deficiency, a single mutation, 985A-G, accounts for most cases. **Treatment** consists of a high-carbohydrate diet, carnitine supplements, avoidance of fasting, and aggressive administration of dextrose during intercurrent stresses.

GLUTARIC ACIDURIA TYPE II

Glutaric aciduria type II (multiple acyl-CoA dehydrogenase deficiency) is a clinical disease produced by a defect in the transfer of electrons from flavine adenine nucleotides to the electron transport chain; this defect is caused by a deficiency of either electron transport flavoprotein or electron transfer flavoprotein–ubiquinone oxidoreductase (see Fig. 54–2). When the enzyme essentially is nonfunctional, congenital anomalies are common, including renal cysts, facial abnormalities, rocker-bottom feet, and hypospadias. Severely affected infants have hypoglycemia without ketosis, metabolic acidosis, and the odor of sweaty feet soon after birth; these infants may die within the neonatal period. Less severely affected infants may have a more episodic, Reye syndrome–like illness. Skeletal and cardiac myopathy can be prominent in this complex, pansystemic disease. Onset in later childhood may be marked mainly by recurrent hypoglycemia and myopathy. **Treatment** has not been effective in infants with complete deficiency. Milder forms respond to avoidance of fasting and caloric support during metabolic stress. Glutaric aciduria type II exhibits autosomal recessive inheritance. Confirmatory testing is similar to the other fatty acid oxidation disorders.

CARNITINE DEFICIENCY

Carnitine is a crucial cofactor in the transport of long chain fatty acids across the mitochondrial inner membrane (see Fig. 55–1). It is synthesized from lysine by humans and is present in dietary red meat and dairy products. Carnitine deficiency is either primary (caused by failure of intake, synthesis, or transport to tissues of carnitine) or secondary (caused by the excretion of excessive amounts of carnitine as carnityl esters in patients with other inborn errors of metabolism or treatment with drugs that complex carnitine, such as valproic acid). Primary systemic carnitine deficiency is rare and results from inadequate renal reabsorption of carnitine secondary to a mutation in the sodium-dependent carnitine transporter. It responds well to carnitine supplementation. There are numerous examples of secondary carnitine deficiency among the organic acidurias, most prominently in disorders of the propionate pathway and in disorders of the β-oxidation of long chain and medium chain fatty acids. Clinical manifestations of carnitine deficiency include failure to produce acetoacetic and β-hydroxybutyric acids, hypoglycemia, lethargy, lassitude, muscle weakness, and cardiomyopathy.

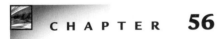

CHAPTER 56

Lysosomal and Peroxisomal Disorders

PEROXISOMAL DISORDERS

Peroxisomes are subcellular organelles that are involved in complex lipid metabolism, such as metabolism and biosynthesis of bile acids, membrane phospholipids, and some β-oxidation of long chain fatty acids. Disorders include conditions caused by abnormal peroxisomal enzyme function and abnormal peroxisomal biogenesis. **Clinical symptoms are protean** and nearly always include **developmental delay** and **mental retardation** and **dysmorphic features** that can involve the skeleton and the head. Zellweger syndrome, neonatal adrenoleukodystrophy, and infantile Refsum disease are examples of disorders of peroxisome biogenesis. **Zellweger syndrome**, an autosomal recessive disease (1:100,000 births), is also called *cerebrohepatorenal syndrome*. Peroxisomes are virtually absent, as are normal peroxisomal functions, which include the oxidation of very long chain fatty acids. Affected infants have high foreheads, flat orbital ridges, widely open fontanels, hepatomegaly, and hypotonia. Other anomalies are common. Failure to thrive, seizures, and nystagmus develop early, and death occurs within the first year. Refsum disease, neonatal adrenoleukodystrophy, and malonic aciduria are examples of peroxisomal single enzyme disorders. **Diagnostic testing** includes measurement of very long chain fatty acids in plasma and pipecolic acid in urine. Specific molecular testing, particularly for the disorders involving one in the series of *PEX* genes, is available for some disorders. Most of these conditions are untreatable; bone marrow transplant can be helpful in X-linked adrenoleukodystrophy.

LYSOSOMAL STORAGE DISORDERS

Lysosomes are subcellular organelles that contain degradative enzymes for complex **glycosaminoglycans**, also called **mucopolysaccharides**. Genetic disorders can result from the formation of the lysosome itself or from deficiency in specific hydrolytic enzymes, in the mechanisms that protect intralysosomal enzymes from hydrolytic destruction, and in the transport of materials into the lysosome and of metabolites out of the lysosome. These materials are stored in cells and ultimately result in their destruction, especially in the nervous system. The clinical disorders are diverse, reflecting tissue specificity of lysosomal function and the intrinsic turnover rates of the compounds whose cycling is affected (Table 56–1). Some disorders affect many tissues but spare the brain, whereas others are apparent only during adult life. Storage in solid organs results in organomegaly. Developmental delay, corneal clouding, and limitation of joint mobility are common features. Nonimmune hydrops fetalis occurs in several lysosomal disorders. Diagnostic testing includes measurement of glycosaminoglycans in urine and enzyme assay in white blood cells. The disorders caused by deficient α-L-iduronidase (Hurler syndrome, Scheie syndrome, and their variants) respond to treatment with IV human recombinant α-L-iduronidase (laronidase). CNS manifestations are not helped.

Treatment is now available for some lysosomal disorders. For some individuals, bone marrow transplantation can restore lysosomal function. For others, replacement of the missing hydrolytic enzyme by systemic administration of the enzyme allows degradation of stored material. The diseases that are treatable should be treated before clinical signs appear. Screening tests for this group of lysosomal disorders are being investigated.

The number of genetic errors is large. Most of these are inherited in an autosomal recessive fashion. Hunter syndrome is X-linked.

TABLE 56–1. Lysosomal Storage Diseases

Disease (Eponym)	Enzyme Deficiency	Clinical Onset	Dysostosis Multiplex	Cornea	Retina
Mucopolysaccharidoses (MPS)					
MSP I (Hurler)	α-L-Iduronidase	~1 yr	Yes	Cloudy	—
MSP II (Hunter)	Iduronate-2-sulfatase	1-2 yr	Yes	Clear	Retinitis, papilledema
MSP III (Sanfilippo)	One of several degrading heparan SO$_4$s	2-6 yr	Mild	Clear	—
MSP IV (Morquiro)	Galactose-6-sulfatase or β-galactosidase	2 yr	No, dwarfism deformities	Faint clouding	—
MSP VI (Maroteaux-Lamy)	N-Acetylgalactosamine-4-sulfatase	2 yr	Yes	Cloudy	—
MPS VII (Sly)	β-glucuronidase	Variable neonatal	Yes	± Cloudy	—
Lipidoses					
Glucosylceramide lipidosis 1 (Gaucher 1)	Glucocerebrosidase	Any age	No	Clear	Normal
Glucosylceramide lipidosis 2 (Gaucher 2)	Glucocerebrosidase	Fetal life to 2nd year	No	Clear	Normal
Sphingomyelin lipidosis A (Niemann-Pick A)	Sphingomyelinase	1st mo	No	Clear	Cherry-red spots (50%)
Sphingomyelin lipidosis B (Niemann-Pick B)	Sphingomyelinase	1st mo or later	No	Clear	Normal
Niemann-Pick C	Unknown	Fetal life to adolescence	No	Clear	Normal
GM$_2$ gangliosidosis (Tay-Sachs)	Hexosaminidase A	3-6 mo	No	Clear	Cherry-red spots
Generalized gangliosidosis (infantile) (GM$_1$)	β-galactosidase	Neonatal to 1st mo	Yes	Clear	Cherry-red spots (50%)
Metachromatic leukodystrophy	Arylsulfatase A	1-2 yr	No	Clear	Normal
Febry disease	α-galactosidase A (cerebrosidase)	Childhood, adolescence	No	Cloudy by slit lamp	—
Galactosyl ceramide lipidosis (Krabbe)	Galactocerebroside β-galactosidase	Early months	No	Clear	Optic atropy
Wolman disease	Acid lipase	Neonatal	No	Clear	Normal
Farber lipogranulomatosis	Acid ceramidase	1st 4 mo	No	Usually clear	Cherry-red spots (12%)

TABLE 56–1. Lysosomal Storage Diseases—cont'd

Liver, Spleen	CNS Findings	Stored Material in Urine	WBC/Bone Marrow	Comment	Multiple Forms
Both enlarged	Profound loss of function	Acid mucopolysaccharide	Alder-Reilly bodies (WBC)	Kyphosis	Yes—Scheie and compounds
Both enlarged	Slow loss of function	Acid mucopolysaccharide	Alder-Reilly bodies (WBC)	X-linked	Yes
Liver ± enlarged	Rapid loss of function	Acid mucopolysaccharide	Alder-Reilly bodies (WBC)	—	Several types biochemically
—	Normal	Acid mucopolysaccharide	Alder-Reilly bodies (WBC)	—	Yes
Normal in size	Normal	Acid mucopolysaccharide	Alder-Reilly bodies (WBC)	—	Yes
Both enlarged	± Affected	Acid mucopolysaccharide	Alder-Reilly bodies (WBC)	Nonimmune hydrops	Yes
Both enlarged	Normal	No	Gaucher cells in marrow	Bone pain fractures	Variability is the rule
Both enlarged	Profound loss of function	No	Gaucher cells in marrow	—	Yes
Both enlarged	Profound loss of function	No	Foam cells in marrow	—	No
Both enlarged	Normal	No	Foam cells in marrow	—	Yes
Enlarged	Vertical ophthalmoplegia, dystonia, cataplexy, seizures	No	Foam cells and sea-blue histiocytes in marrow	Pathogenesis not as for NP-A and NP-B	Lethal neonatal to adolescent onset
Normal	Profound loss of function	No	Normal	Sandhoff disease related	Yes
Both enlarged	Profound loss of function	No	Inclusion in WBC	—	Yes
Normal	Profound loss of function	No	Normal	—	Yes
Liver may be enlarged	Normal	No	Normal	X-linked	No
Normal	Profound loss of function	No	Normal	Storage not lysosomal	Yes
Both enlarged	Profound loss of function	No	Inclusion in WBC	—	Yes
May be enlarged	Normal or impaired	Usually not	—	Arthritis, nodules, hoarseness	Yes

Continued

TABLE 56–1. Lysosomal Storage Diseases—cont'd

Disease (Eponym)	Enzyme Deficiency	Clinical Onset	Dysostosis Multiplex	Cornea	Retina
Mucolipidoses (ML) and Clinically Related Disease					
Sialidosis II (formerly ML I)	Neuraminidase	Neonatal	Yes	Cloudy	Cherry-red spot
Sialidosis I (formerly ML I)	Neuraminidase	Usually second decade	No	Fine opacities	Cherry-red spot
Galactosialidosis	Absence of PP/CathA causes loss of neuraminidase and β-galactosidase	Usually second decade	Frequent	Clouding	Cherry-red spot
ML II (I-cell disease)	Mannosyl phosphotransferase	Neonatal	Yes	Clouding	—
ML III (pseudo-Hurler polydystrophy)	Mannosyl phosphotransferase	2-4 yr	Yes	Late clouding	Normal
Multiple sulfatase deficiency	Many sulfatases	1-2 yr	Yes	Usually clear	Usually normal
Aspartylglycosaminuria	Aspartylglucosaminidase	6 mo	Mild	Clear	Normal
Mannosidosis	α-Mannosidase	1st mo	Yes	Cloudy	—
Fucosidosis	α-L-Fucosidase	1st mo	Yes	Clear	May be pigmented
Storage Diseases Caused by Defects in Lysosomal Proteolysis					
Neuronal ceroid lipofuscinosis (NCL), Batten disease	Impaired lysosomal proteolysis—various specific etiologies	6 mo-10 yr, adult form	No	Normal	May have brown pigment
Storage Diseases Caused by Defective Synthesis of the Lysosomal Membrane					
Cardiomyopathy, myopathy, mental retardation, Danon disease	Lamp-2, a structural protein of lysosomes, is deficient	Usually 5-6 yr	No	Normal	Normal
Storage Diseases Caused by Dysfunction of Lysosomal Transport Proteins					
Nephropathic cystinosis	Defect in cystine transport from lysosome to cytoplasm	6 mo-1 yr	No	Cystine crystals	Pigmentary retinopathy
Salla disease	Defect in sialic acid transport from lysosome to cytoplasm	6-9 mo	No	Normal	Normal

TABLE 56–1.   Lysosomal Storage Diseases—cont'd

Liver, Spleen	CNS Findings	Stored Material in Urine	WBC/Bone Marrow	Comment	Multiple Forms
Both enlarged	Yes	Oligosaccharides	Vacuolated lymphocytes	—	Yes (also see galactosialidosis)
Normal	Myoclonus, seizures	Oligosaccharides	Usually none	Cherry-red spot/ myoclonus syndrome	Severity varies
Occasionally enlarged	Myoclonus, seizures Mental retardation	Oligosaccharides	Foamy lymphocytes	Onset from 1-40 yr	Congenital and infantile forms such as sialidosis 2
Liver often enlarged	Profound loss of function	Oligosaccharides	No	Gingival hyperplasia	No
Normal in size?	Modest loss of function	Oligosaccharides	No	—	No
Both enlarged	Profound loss of function	Acid mucopolysaccharide	Alder-Reilly bodies (WBC)	Ichthyosis	Yes
Early, not late	Profound loss of function	Aspartylglucosamine	Inclusions in lymphocytes	Develop cataracts	No
Liver enlarged	Profound loss of function	Generally no	Inclusions in lymphocytes	Cataracts	Yes
Both enlarged commonly	Profound loss of function	Oligosaccharides	Inclusions in lymphocytes	—	Yes
Normal	Optic atrophy, seizures, dementia			Clinical picture consistent, time course variable	Etiologies distinct for age-related forms
Hepatomegaly	Delayed development, seizures			X-linked; pediatric disease in males only	Variability in time course of signs
Hepatomegaly common	Normal CNS function	Generalized aminoaciduria	Elevated cystine in WBCs	Treatment with cysteamine is effective	Yes
Normal	Delayed development, ataxia, nystagmus, exotropia	Sialic aciduria	Vacuolated lymphocytes may be found	Growth retarded in some	Lethal infantile form

CHAPTER 57

Mitochondrial Disorders

LACTIC ACIDOSIS

Metabolism of glucose to carbon dioxide and water, with pyruvate as an intermediate (Fig. 57–1), occurs as part of the energy cycle in many tissues. Interference with mitochondrial oxidative metabolism results in the accumulation of pyruvate. Because lactate dehydrogenase is ubiquitous, and because the equilibrium catalyzed by this enzyme greatly favors lactate over pyruvate, the accumulation of pyruvate results in lactic acidosis. The most common cause of such lactic acidosis is oxygen deficiency caused by anoxia or poor perfusion, as seen in cardiac arrest, shock, severe cyanosis, and profound heart failure. Poisons, such as cyanide, sulfide, and carbon monoxide, which, similar to anoxia, block the terminal reaction of the mitochondrial respiratory chain, also produce lactic acidosis (see Chapter 45).

Lactic acidosis also occurs when specific reactions of pyruvate are impaired. Pyruvate has three major fates. In muscle, it is transaminated to form alanine, which can be used for protein synthesis or transported to the liver and may appear in blood in the presence of intermittent lactic acidosis. In the liver, it undergoes carboxylation to form oxaloacetate using the enzyme pyruvate carboxylase; deficiency in this enzyme causes severe lactic acidosis. In many tissues, lactate is catabolized to form acetyl CoA. The reaction is catalyzed by the pyruvate dehydrogenase complex; deficiency in pyruvate dehydrogenase also can cause lactic acidosis. Because these reactions also play a role in gluconeogenesis, hypoglycemia can be a feature of these disorders. The clinical spectrum in this group

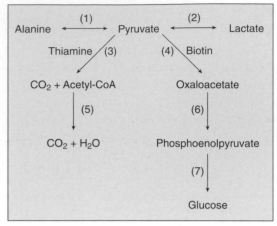

Figure 57–1

Metabolism of pyruvate and lactate. (1) Alanine aminotransferase, (2) lactate dehydrogenase, (3) pyruvate dehydrogenase, (4) pyruvate carboxylase, (5) Krebs cycle, (6) phosphoenolpyruvate carboxykinase, (7) reverse glycosis. CoA, coenzyme A.

of disorders ranges from metabolic acidosis and mental retardation to intractable, lethal acidosis in the first months of life or the CNS phenotype of **Leigh syndrome**.

Defects of the **mitochondrial respiratory chain** itself also can produce lactic acidosis. Given the complexity of the respiratory chain, it is not surprising that the defects described are varied as to cause, intensity, and tissues affected. Some defects show autosomal recessive inheritance; others show mitochondrial (maternal mtDNA) inheritance; some, particularly the mtDNA deletions, are sporadic. Myopathy is common, frequently showing ragged red fibers on muscle biopsy (Table 57–1). **Alper disease** (cerebral degeneration and

---

TABLE 57–1.   Some Disorders of the Respiratory Chain that Cause Lactic Acidosis

Disease	Inheritance	Clinical Picture
Myoclonic epilepsy with ragged red fibers (MERRF)	Maternal mtDNA	Lactic acidosis may be severe; variable clinical picture
Myopathy, encephalopathy, lactic acidosis, strokelike episodes (MELAS)	Maternal mtDNA	Highly variable clinical picture, including type 2 diabetes mellitus
Pearson syndrome	Maternal mtDNA	Macrocytic anemia, sideroblasts, pancreatic insufficiency
Alpers syndrome	Unclear	Cerebral degeneration and liver disease
Leigh disease	Autosomal recessive in some and maternal mtDNA in others	Degenerative disease of thalamus, basal ganglia, and spinal cord

liver disease) and **Leigh disease** (subacute necrotizing encephalomyelopathy) show similar brain lesions, but in distinctly different areas of the brain. **Treatment** is limited for most mitochondrial defects. Vitamin cofactors for the respiratory chain and coenzyme Q are often employed.

SUGGESTED READING

Behrman RE, Kliegman RM, Jenson HB (eds): Nelson Textbook of Pediatrics, 17th ed. Philadelphia, WB Saunders, 2004.

Carreiro-Lewandowski E: Newborn screening: An overview. Clin Lab Sci 15:229-238, 2002.

Gregersen N, Bross P, Andresen BS: Genetic defects in fatty acid beta-oxidation and acyl-CoA dehydrogenases: Molecular pathogenesis and genotype-phenotype relationships. Eur J Biochem 271:470-482, 2004.

Ogier de Baulny H: Management and emergency treatments of neonates with a suspicion of inborn errors of metabolism. Semin Neonatol 7:17-26, 2002.

Scriver C, et al: The Metabolic Basis of Inherited Disease, 8th ed. New York, McGraw-Hill, 2001.

Seashore MR: Organic acidemias: An overview. 2004, updated 12/2003. In: GeneReviews at GeneTests: Medical Genetics Information Resource (database online). Seattle, University of Washington, 1997-2004. http://www.genetests.org. Accessed March 13, 2004.

FETAL AND NEONATAL MEDICINE

Clarence W. Gowen, Jr.

CHAPTER **58**

Assessment of the Mother, Fetus, and Newborn

ASSESSMENT OF THE MOTHER

The optimal care of low-risk and high-risk newborns requires knowledge of the family history, history of prior and current pregnancies, and events of labor and delivery. Neonatal medicine requires a comprehensive understanding of the physiology of normal pregnancy; placental and fetal growth, function, and maturity; and any extrauterine or intrauterine pathologic events that affect the mother, placenta, or fetus. These latter adverse effects may result in an unfavorable neonatal outcome and include such significant influences as poor maternal nutrition, maternal cigarette smoking, maternal poverty, maternal physical or psychological stresses, extremes of maternal age (<16 years, >35 years), maternal race, maternal medical illness present before pregnancy, maternal medications, obstetric complications during the antepartum and intrapartum periods, perinatal infections, exposure to toxins and illicit drugs, and the inherent genetic predisposition of the fetus.

Pregnancies associated with perinatal morbidity or mortality are considered high risk. Identification of high-risk pregnancies is essential to the care of the infant. High-risk pregnancies may result in intrauterine fetal death, intrauterine growth retardation (IUGR), congenital anomalies, excessive fetal growth, birth asphyxia and trauma, prematurity (birth at <38 weeks) or postmaturity (birth at ≥42 weeks), neonatal disease, or long-term risks of cerebral palsy, mental retardation, and chronic sequelae of neonatal ICU stays (Table 58–1). Ten percent to 20% of women can be considered at high risk at some time during their pregnancy. Although some obstetric complications are first seen during labor and delivery and cannot be predicted before parturition, many problems are present before labor and delivery. Overall, 50% of perinatal mortality and morbidity results from pregnancies identified before delivery as high risk. After a high-risk pregnancy is identified, measures can be instituted to prevent complications, provide intensive fetal surveillance, and initiate appropriate treatments of the mother and fetus.

Additional maternal factors may be identified from past pregnancies. A history of previous premature birth, intrauterine fetal death, multiple gestation, IUGR, congenital malformation, explained or unexplained neonatal death (e.g., group B streptococcal sepsis), birth trauma, preeclampsia, gestational diabetes, grand multipara status (five or more pregnancies), or cesarean section is associated with additional risk for the subsequent pregnancy.

Pregnancy complications during the current gestation that increase the risk of a poor outcome can be secondary to maternal or fetal causes or both (Table 58–2). Complications include placenta previa; abruptio placentae; preeclampsia; diabetes; oligohydramnios or polyhydramnios; multiple gestation; blood group sensitization; abnormal levels of unconjugated estriols, chorionic gonadotropin, or alpha-fetoprotein; abnormal fetal ultrasound; hydrops fetalis; maternal trauma or surgery; abnormal fetal presentation (breech); exposure to prescribed or illicit drugs; prolonged labor; cephalopelvic disproportion; prolapsed cord; fetal distress; prolonged or premature rupture of membranes; short cervical length (<25 mm) and the presence of fetal fibronectin in cervical secretions at less than 35

TABLE 58–1. Morbidities and Sequelae of Perinatal and Neonatal Illness

Morbidities	Examples
CNS	
Spastic diplegic-quadriplegic cerebral palsy	Hypoxic-ischemic encephalopathy, periventricular leukomalacia, undetermined antenatal factors
Choreoathetotic cerebral palsy	Bilirubin encephalopathy (kernicterus)
Microcephaly	Hypoxic-ischemic encephalopathy, intrauterine infection (rubella, CMV)
Communicating hydrocephalus	Intraventricular hemorrhage, meningitis
Seizures	Hypoxic-ischemic encephalopathy, hypoglycemia
Encephalopathy	Congenital infections (rubella, CMV, HIV, toxoplasmosis)
Educational failure	Prematurity, hypoxia, low socioeconomic status
Mental retardation	Hypoxia, hypoglycemia, cerebral palsy, intraventricular hemorrhage
Sensation-Peripheral Nerves	
Reduced visual acuity (blindness)	Retinopathy of prematurity
Strabismus	Undetermined
Hearing impairment (deafness)	Drug toxicity (furosemide, aminoglycosides), bilirubin encephalopathy, hypoxia ± hyperventilation
Poor speech	Immaturity, chronic illness, hypoxia, prolonged endotracheal intubation, hearing deficit
Paralysis-paresis	Birth trauma—brachial plexus, phrenic nerve, spinal cord
Respiratory	
BPD	Oxygen toxicity, ventilator barotrauma
Subglottic stenosis	Endotracheal tube injury
Sudden infant death syndrome	Prematurity, BPD, infant of illicit drug user
Choanal stenosis, nasal septum destruction	Nasotracheal intubation
Cardiovascular	
Cyanosis	Precorrective palliative care of congenital cyanotic heart disease, cor pulmonale from BPD, reactive airway disease
Heart failure	Precorrective palliative care of complex congenital heart disease, BPD, ventricular septal defect
Gastrointestinal	
Short gut syndrome	Necrotizing enterocolitis, gastroschisis, malrotation-volvulus, cystic fibrosis, intestinal atresias
Cholestatic liver disease (cirrhosis, hepatic failure)	Hyperalimentation toxicity, sepsis, short gut syndrome
Failure to thrive	Short gut syndrome, cholestasis, BPD, cerebral palsy, severe congenital heart disease
Inguinal hernia	Unknown
Miscellaneous	
Cutaneous scars	Chest tube or IV placement; hyperalimentation subcutaneous infiltration; fetal puncture; intrauterine varicella; aplasia cutis
Absent radial artery pulse	Frequent arterial punctures
Hypertension	Renal thrombi: repair of coarctation of aorta

BPD, bronchopulmonary dysplasia; CMV, cytomegalovirus.
From Stoll BJ, Kliegman RM: The newborn infant. In Behrman RE, Kliegman RM, Jenson HB (eds): Nelson Textbook of Pediatrics, 16th ed. Philadelphia, WB Saunders, 2000.

TABLE 58–2. Major Causes of Perinatal and Neonatal Mortality

Fetus

Abruptio placentae
Chromosomal anomalies
Congenital malformations (heart, CNS, renal)
Hydrops fetalis
Intrauterine asphyxia*
Intrauterine infection*
Maternal underlying disease (chronic hypertension, autoimmune disease, diabetes mellitus)
Multiple gestation*
Placental insufficiency*
Umbilical cord accident

Preterm Infant

Congenital anomalies
Infection
Intraventricular hemorrhage*
Necrotizing enterocolitis
Respiratory distress syndrome/bronchopulmonary dysplasia (chronic lung disease)*
Severe immaturity*

Full-Term Infant

Birth asphyxia*
Birth trauma
Congenital anomalies*
Infection*
Macrosomia
Meconium aspiration pneumonia
Persistent pulmonary hypertension

*Common.

weeks' gestation (a predictor of preterm labor); cervical infections and vaginosis; and congenital infections, including rubella, cytomegalovirus (CMV), herpes simplex, HIV, toxoplasmosis, syphilis, and gonorrhea.

Maternal medical complications associated with increased risk of maternal and fetal morbidity and mortality include diabetes, chronic hypertension, congenital heart disease (especially with right-to-left shunting and Eisenmenger complex), glomerulonephritis, collagen vascular disease (especially systemic lupus erythematosus with or without antiphospholipid antibodies), lung disease (cystic fibrosis), severe anemia (sickle cell anemia), hyperthyroidism, myasthenia gravis, idiopathic thrombocytopenic purpura, inborn errors of metabolism (maternal PKU), and malignancy. Inheritance of maternal autosomal recessive genes (cystic fibrosis, galactosemia, sickle cell anemia) places the newborn at increased risk for complications of these diseases. Complications may become manifested in utero, in the newborn, or in the older infant.

Obstetric complications often are associated with increased fetal or neonatal risk. Vaginal bleeding in the first trimester or early second trimester may be caused by a threatened or actual spontaneous abortion. If pregnancy continues, the fetus may be at increased risk for congenital malformations or chromosomal disorders. Vaginal bleeding that is painless, is not associated with labor, and occurs in the late second or (more likely) the third trimester often is the result of **placenta previa**. Bleeding develops when the placental mass overlies the internal cervical os; this may produce maternal hemorrhagic shock, necessitating transfusions. Bleeding also may result in premature delivery. Painful vaginal bleeding is often the result of retroplacental hemorrhage or **placental abruption**. Associated findings may be advanced maternal age and parity, maternal chronic hypertension, maternal cocaine use, preterm rupture of membranes, polyhydramnios, twin gestation, and preeclampsia. Fetal asphyxia ensues as the retroplacental hematoma causes placental separation that interferes with fetal oxygenation. Both types of bleeding are associated with fetal blood loss. Neonatal anemia may be more common with placenta previa.

Abnormalities in the volume of amniotic fluid, resulting in oligohydramnios or polyhydramnios, are associated with increased fetal and neonatal risk. **Oligohydramnios** (amniotic ultrasound fluid index ≤2 cm) is associated with IUGR and major congenital anomalies, particularly of the fetal kidneys. It also is associated with chromosomal syndromes. Bilateral renal agenesis results in diminished production of amniotic fluid. It also results in a specific deformation syndrome (**Potter syndrome**), which is indicated by clubfeet, characteristic compressed facies, low-set ears, scaphoid abdomen, and diminished chest wall size that is accompanied by pulmonary hypoplasia and often pneumothorax. Uterine compression in the absence of amniotic fluid retards lung growth, and patients with this condition die of respiratory failure rather than renal insufficiency. Twin-to-twin transfusion syndrome (donor) and complications from amniotic fluid leakage also are associated with oligohydramnios. Oligohydramnios increases the risk of fetal distress during labor (because of meconium-stained fluid and variable decelerations); the risk may be reduced by saline amnioinfusion during labor.

Polyhydramnios may be acute and may be associated with premature labor, maternal discomfort, and respiratory compromise. More often, polyhydramnios is chronic and is associated with diabetes, immune or nonimmune hydrops fetalis, multiple gestation, trisomy 18 or 21, and major congenital anomalies. Anencephaly, hydrocephaly, and meningomyelocele are neurologic problems associated with reduced fetal swallowing. Esophageal and duodenal atresia and cleft palate interfere with swallowing and gastrointestinal fluid dynamics. Additional causes of polyhydramnios include Werdnig-Hoffmann and Beckwith-Wiedemann syndromes, conjoined twins, chylothorax, cystic adenomatoid lung malformation, diaphragmatic hernia, gastroschisis, sacral teratoma, placental chorioangioma, and myotonic dystrophy. **Hydrops fetalis** may be a result of Rh or other blood group incompatibilities and anemia caused by intrauterine hemolysis of fetal erythrocytes by maternal IgG-sensitized antibodies crossing the placenta. Hydrops is characterized by fetal edema, ascites, hypoalbuminemia, and congestive heart failure. Causes of nonimmune hydrops include fetal arrhythmias (supraventricular tachycardia, congenital heart block), fetal anemia (bone marrow suppression, nonimmune hemolysis, or twin-to-twin transfusion), severe congenital malformation, intrauterine infections, congenital neuroblastoma, inborn errors of metabolism (storage diseases), fetal hepatitis, nephrotic syndrome, and pulmonary lymphangiectasia. Twin-to-twin transfusion syndrome (recipient) also may be associated with polyhydramnios. Polyhydramnios is often the result of unknown causes. If severe, polyhydramnios may be managed with bed rest, indomethacin, or serial amniocenteses.

Premature rupture of the membranes, which occurs in the absence of labor, and **prolonged rupture of the membranes** (>24 hours) are associated with an increased risk of maternal or fetal infection (chorioamnionitis) and preterm birth. Typically, group B streptococci, *Escherichia coli,* and *Listeria monocytogenes* are associated with fetal infection, although *Mycoplasma hominis, Ureaplasma urealyticum, Chlamydia trachomatis,* and anaerobic bacteria of the vaginal flora also have been implicated in infection of the amniotic fluid. The risk of serious fetal infection increases as the length of time between rupture and labor (latent period) increases, especially if the period is greater than 24 hours. Intrapartum antibiotic therapy decreases the risks of neonatal sepsis.

Multiple gestations are associated with increased risk resulting from polyhydramnios, premature birth, IUGR, abnormal presentation (breech), congenital anomalies (intestinal atresia, porencephaly, and single umbilical artery), intrauterine fetal demise, birth asphyxia, and twin-to-twin transfusion syndrome. **Twin-to-twin transfusion syndrome** is associated with a high mortality and is seen only in monozygotic twins who share a common placenta and show an arteriovenous connection between their circulations. The fetus on the arterial side of the shunt serves as the blood donor, which results in fetal anemia, growth retardation, and oligohydramnios for this fetus. The recipient, or venous-side twin, is larger or discordant in size, is plethoric and polycythemic, and may show polyhydramnios. Weight differences of 20% and hemoglobin differences of 5 g/dL suggest the diagnosis.

Ultrasonography in the second trimester reveals discordant amniotic fluid volume with oliguria/oligohydramnios ("stuck twin" syndrome, against the uterine wall) and hypervolemia/polyuria/polyhydramnios with a distended bladder, with or without hydrops and heart failure. Mortality is high if presentation occurs in the second trimester; however, most monochorionic twins have bidirectional balanced shunts and are not affected. Treatment includes amniocentesis and attempts to ablate the arteriovenous connection (using a laser). The birth order of twins also affects morbidity by increasing the risk of the second-born twin for breech position, birth asphyxia, birth trauma, and respiratory distress syndrome (RDS).

Overall, twinning is observed in 1:80 pregnancies, and 80% of all twin gestations are dizygotic twins. The diagnosis of the type of twins can be determined by placentation, sex, fetal membrane structure, and, if necessary, tissue and blood group typing or DNA analysis.

Toxemia of pregnancy, or **preeclampsia/eclampsia**, is a disorder of unknown but probably vascular etiology that may lead to maternal hypertension, uteroplacental insufficiency, IUGR, intrauterine asphyxia, maternal seizures, and maternal death. Toxemia is more common in nulliparous women and in women with twin gestation, chronic hypertension, obesity, renal disease, positive family history of toxemia, or diabetes mellitus. A subcategory of preeclampsia, the *HELLP* syndrome (*h*emolysis, *e*levated *l*iver enzyme levels, *l*ow *p*latelets), is more severe and is often associated with a fetal inborn error of fatty acid oxidation (long chain hydroxyacyl–coenzyme A dehydrogenase of the trifunctional protein complex).

FETUS AND NEWBORN

The late fetal–early neonatal period is the time of life with the highest mortality rate of any age interval. **Perinatal mortality** refers to fetal deaths occurring from the 20th week of gestation until the 7th to 28th day after birth and is expressed as number of deaths per 1000 live births. Intrauterine fetal death accounts for 40% to 50% of the perinatal mortality rate. Such infants, defined as **stillborn**, are born without a heart rate and are apneic, limp, pale, and cyanotic. Many stillborn infants exhibit evidence of maceration; pale, peeling skin; corneal opacification; and soft cranial contents.

The **neonatal mortality rate** includes all infants dying during the period from after birth to the first 28 days of life and is expressed as number of deaths per 1000 live births. Modern neonatal intensive care has delayed the mortality of many newborns with life-threatening diseases so that they survive the neonatal period, only to die of their original diseases or of complications of therapy after 28 days of life. This delayed mortality and mortality caused by acquired illnesses occur during the **postneonatal period**, which begins after 28 days of life and extends to the end of the first year of life.

The **infant mortality rate** encompasses the neonatal and the postneonatal periods; it is expressed as the number of deaths per 1000 live births. The infant mortality rate in the U.S. declined in 2001 to 6.8:1000; the rate for African American infants was approximately 14:1000. The most common causes of perinatal and neonatal death are listed in Table 58-2. Overall, congenital anomalies and diseases of the premature infant are the most significant causes of neonatal mortality.

Low birth weight (LBW) infants, defined as infants having birth weights of less than 2500 g, represent a disproportionately large component of the neonatal and infant mortality rates. Although births of LBW infants make up only about 6% to 7% of all births, they account for greater than 70% of neonatal deaths. IUGR is the most common cause of LBW in developing countries, whereas most LBW in infants in developed countries is secondary to prematurity.

Very low birth weight (VLBW) infants, weighing less than 1500 g at birth, represent about 1% of all births, but account for 50% of neonatal deaths. Compared with infants weighing 2500 g or more, LBW infants are 40 times more likely to die in the neonatal period; VLBW infants have a 200-fold higher risk of neonatal death. The LBW rate has not improved in recent years. The LBW rate is one of the major reasons that the infant mortality rate in the U.S. is high compared with that of other large, modern, industrialized countries. If birth weight–specific mortality rates are calculated, the U.S. has one of the highest survival rates; because of the large number of LBW infants, the total infant mortality rate remains relatively high.

Maternal factors associated with a LBW caused by premature birth or IUGR include a previous LBW birth, low socioeconomic status, low level of maternal education, no antenatal care, maternal age younger than 16 years or older than 35 years, short interval between pregnancies, cigarette smoking, alcohol and illicit drug use, physical (excessive standing or walking) or psychological (little social support) stresses, unmarried status, low prepregnancy weight (<45 kg [<100 lb]) and poor weight gain during pregnancy (<10 lb), and African American race. Race is especially significant because LBW and VLBW rates for African American women are twice the rates for white women. The neonatal and infant mortality rates are twofold higher among African American infants. These racial differences are only partly explained by poverty.

In addition to the sociodemographic variables associated with LBW, specific, identifiable medical causes of preterm birth exist (Table 58-3). Factors such as

uterine anomalies, hydrops fetalis, and most medical illnesses are not seen more frequently in African Americans or in patients of lower socioeconomic status. Prematurity may be caused by spontaneous labor (50% of cases), spontaneous rupture of membranes (25%), or premature delivery for maternal or fetal indications (25%).

ASSESSMENT OF THE FETUS

Fetal growth can be assessed clinically by determining the fundal height of the uterus through bimanual examination of the gravid abdomen. Ultrasound measurements of the fetal biparietal diameter, femur length, and abdominal circumference are used to estimate fetal growth. A combination of these measurements pre-

TABLE 58-3. Identifiable Causes of Preterm Birth

Fetal

Fetal distress
Multiple gestation
Erythroblastosis
Nonimmune hydrops fetalis
Congenital anomalies

Placental

Placenta previa
Abruptio placentae

Uterine

Bicornuate uterus
Incompetent cervix (premature dilation)
Short cervix

Maternal

Preeclampsia
Chronic medical illness (chronic hypertension or cyanotic heart disease)
Infection (group B streptococcus, herpes simplex, syphilis, bacterial vaginosis, genital mycoplasma, and chorioamnionitis*)
Drug use (cocaine)

Other

Premature rupture of membranes
Polyhydramnios
Iatrogenic (cesarean section)
Trauma/surgery

*Chorioamnionitis is probably a fetal infection too. It is associated with increased risk of neonatal sepsis, respiratory distress syndrome, seizures, intraventricular hemorrhage, periventricular leukomalacia, and cerebral palsy.

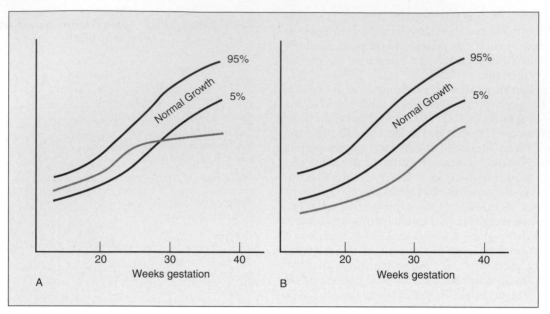

Figure 58–1

Hypothetical fetal growth curves depicting two patterns of intrauterine growth retardation. A, In this pattern, there is normal fetal growth during weeks 20 to 30 of gestation. Thereafter, fetal growth stops, and the fetal growth parameter (biparietal diameter, abdominal circumference, and femur length) declines to less than 5%. In contrast to weight, head growth is usually spared and less severely affected. This "late flattening" pattern is noted in the donor twin involved in a twin-to-twin transfusion syndrome, in a fetus supplied by poor maternal nutrition, and in fetuses growing within an environment of maternal preeclampsia. Catch-up growth is common after delivery from the adverse in utero environment. **B,** Fetal growth parameters are persistently less than 5%. These fetuses show continued growth, albeit at a reduced rate. Fetuses with this "low-profile" pattern may have reduced growth potential, as noted in fetuses with intrauterine viral infections, chromosome disorders, or malformation syndromes. Fetuses born to mothers who themselves were small for gestational age and who show reduced pregnancy weight often have this characteristic growth profile. Some of these fetuses are normal in all other parameters except that they exhibit reduced intrauterine growth.

dicts fetal weight. Deviations from the normal fetal growth curve are associated with high-risk conditions.

IUGR is present when fetal growth stops and over time declines to less than the 5th percentile of growth for gestational age or when growth proceeds slowly, but absolute size remains less than the 5th percentile (Fig. 58-1). Growth restriction may result from fetal conditions that reduce the innate growth potential, such as fetal rubella infection, primordial dwarfing syndromes, chromosomal abnormalities, and congenital malformation syndromes. Reduced fetal production of insulin and insulin-like growth factor I is associated with fetal growth restriction. Placental causes of IUGR include villitis (congenital infections), placental tumors, chronic abruptio placentae, twin-to-twin transfusion syndrome, and placental insufficiency. Maternal causes include severe peripheral vascular diseases that reduce uterine blood flow, such as chronic hypertension, diabetic vasculopathy, and preeclampsia/eclampsia. Addi-

tional maternal causes include reduced nutritional intake, alcohol or drug abuse, cigarette smoking, and uterine constraint, noted predominantly in mothers of small stature with a low prepregnancy weight and reduced weight gain during pregnancy. The outcome of IUGR depends on the cause of the reduced fetal growth and the associated complications after birth (Table 58-4). Fetuses subjected to chronic intrauterine hypoxia as a result of uteroplacental insufficiency are at an increased risk for the comorbidities of birth asphyxia, polycythemia, and hypoglycemia. Fetuses with reduced tissue mass resulting from chromosomal, metabolic, or multiple congenital anomaly syndromes have poor outcomes based on the prognosis for the particular syndrome. Fetuses born to small mothers and fetuses with poor nutritional intake usually do well and show catch-up growth after birth.

Fetal size can be determined accurately by ultrasound techniques. Fetal size does not always correlate

TABLE 58–4.   Problems of Intrauterine Growth Retardation and Small for Gestational Age

Problem*	Pathogenesis
Intrauterine fetal demise	Placental insufficiency, hypoxia, acidosis, infection, lethal anomaly
Temperature instability	Cold stress, ↓ fat stores, hypoxia, hypoglycemia
Perinatal asphyxia	↓ Uteroplacental perfusion during labor with or without chronic fetal hypoxia-acidosis, meconium aspiration syndrome
Hypoglycemia	↓ Tissue glycogen stores; ↓ gluconeogenesis, hyperinsulinism, ↑ glucose needs of hypoxia, hypothermia, relatively large brain
Polycythemia-hyperviscosity	Fetal hypoxia with ↑ erythropoietin production
Reduced oxygen consumption/ hypothermia	Hypoxia, hypoglycemia, starvation effect, poor subcutaneous fat stores
Dysmorphology	Syndrome anomalads, chromosomal-genetic disorders, oligohydramnios-induced deformations
Pulmonary hemorrhage	Hypothermia, polycythemia, hypoxia

*Other problems are common to the gestational age–related risks of prematurity if born before 37 weeks.
Modified from Stoll BJ, Kliegman RM: The high-risk infant. In Behrman RE, Kliegman RM, Jenson HB (eds): Nelson Textbook of Pediatrics, 16th ed. Philadelphia, WB Saunders, 2000.

with functional or structural maturity. Determining **fetal maturity** is crucial when a decision has been made to deliver a fetus because of fetal or maternal disease. Fetal gestational age may be determined accurately on the basis of a correct estimate of the last menstrual period. Clinically relevant landmark dates can be used to determine gestational age; the first audible heart tones by fetoscope are detected at 18 to 20 weeks (12 to 14 weeks by Doppler methods), and quickening of fetal movements usually is perceived at 18 to 20 weeks. It is not always possible, however, to determine fetal maturity by such dating, especially in a high-risk situation, such as preterm labor or a diabetic pregnancy.

Fetal pulmonary maturity may be determined through examination of the profile of phospholipids present in the amniotic fluid. **Surfactant**, a combination of surface-active phospholipids and proteins, is produced by the maturing fetal lung and eventually is secreted into the amniotic fluid. The amount of surfactant in amniotic fluid is a direct reflection of surface-active material in the fetal lung and can be used to predict the presence or absence of pulmonary maturity. Because phosphatidylcholine, or lecithin, is a principal component of surfactant, the determination of lecithin in amniotic fluid is used to predict a mature fetus. Lecithin concentration increases with increasing gestational age, beginning at 32 to 34 weeks.

Methods used to assess fetal well-being before the onset of labor are focused on identifying a fetus at risk for asphyxia or a fetus who has hypoxia and already is compromised by uteroplacental insufficiency. The **oxytocin challenge test** simulates uterine contractions through an infusion of oxytocin sufficient to produce three contractions in a 10-minute period. The development of periodic fetal bradycardia out of phase with uterine contractions (late deceleration) is a positive test result and predicts an at-risk fetus.

The **nonstress test** examines the heart rate response to fetal body movements. Heart rate increments of greater than 15 beats/min, lasting 15 seconds, are reassuring. If two such episodes occur in 30 minutes, the test result is considered reactive (versus nonreactive), and the fetus is not at risk. Additional signs of fetal well-being are fetal breathing movements, gross body movements, fetal tone, and the presence of amniotic fluid pockets of greater than 2 cm, as noted by ultrasound. The **biophysical profile** combines the nonstress test with these four parameters and offers the most accurate fetal assessment.

Doppler examination of the fetal aorta or umbilical arteries can permit identification of decreased or reversed diastolic blood flow, which is associated with increased peripheral vascular resistance, fetal hypoxia with acidosis, and placental insufficiency. **Cordocentesis** (percutaneous umbilical blood sampling) can provide fetal blood for PO_2, pH, lactate, and hemoglobin measurements. These values can be used to identify a hypoxic, acidotic, or anemic fetus who is at risk for intrauterine fetal demise or birth asphyxia. Cordocentesis also can be used to determine fetal blood type, platelet count, microbial culture, antibody titer, and rapid karyotype.

In a high-risk pregnancy, the fetal heart rate should be monitored continuously, as should uterine contractions during labor. Fetal heart rate abnormalities may indicate baseline tachycardia (>160 beats/min as a result of anemia, β-sympathomimetic drugs, maternal fever, hyperthyroidism, arrhythmia, or fetal distress), baseline **bradycardia** (<120 beats/min as a result of fetal distress, complete heart block, or local anesthetics), or reduced beat-to-beat variability (flattened tracing resulting from fetal sleep, tachycardia, atropine, sedatives, prematurity, or fetal distress). Periodic changes of the heart rate relative to the tracing of uterine pressure help determine the presence of hypoxia and acidosis caused by uteroplacental insufficiency or maternal hypotension (late or type II decelerations) or by umbilical cord compression (variable decelerations). In the presence of severe decelerations (any late or repeated prolonged variable), a fetal scalp blood gas level should be obtained to assess **fetal acidosis**. A scalp pH of less than 7.20 indicates fetal hypoxic compromise. A pH between 7.20 and 7.25 is in a borderline zone and warrants repeating the test.

Fetal anomalies may be detected by ultrasonography; emphasis should be placed on visualization of the genitourinary tract; the head (for anencephaly or hydrocephaly), neck (for thickened nuchal translucency), and back (for spina bifida); the skeleton; the gastrointestinal tract; and the heart. Four-chamber and great artery views are required for detection of heart anomalies. **Chromosomal anomaly syndromes** may reveal choroid cysts, hypoplasia of the middle phalanx of the fifth digit, nuchal fluid, retrognathism, and low-set ears. In addition, chromosomal syndromes often are associated with an abnormal "triple test" (low estriols, low maternal serum alpha-fetoprotein levels, and elevated placental chorionic gonadotropin levels). If a fetal abnormality is detected, fetal therapy (Table 58–5) or delivery with therapy in the neonatal ICU may be lifesaving.

ASSESSMENT OF THE NEWBORN

The approach to the birth of an infant, similar to the approach to any other medical situation, requires a detailed history (Table 58–6). Knowing the mother's risk factors enables the delivery room team to anticipate problems that may occur after birth. The history of a woman's labor and delivery can reveal events that might lead to complications adversely affecting either the mother or the neonate, even when the pregnancy was previously considered low risk. Anticipating the need to resuscitate a newborn as a result of fetal distress increases the likelihood of successful resuscitation.

At birth the transition from fetal to neonatal physiology occurs. Oxygen transport across the human placenta results in a gradient between the maternal and the fetal PaO_2. Although fetal oxygenated blood has a low PaO_2 level compared with that of adults and infants, the fetus is not anaerobic. Fetal oxygen uptake and consumption are similar to neonatal rates of oxygen use, even though the thermal environments and activity levels of fetuses and neonates differ. The oxygen content of fetal blood is almost equal to the oxygen content in older infants and children because fetal blood has a much higher concentration of hemoglobin.

Fetal hemoglobin (two alpha and two gamma chains) has a higher affinity for oxygen than adult hemoglobin, facilitating oxygen transfer across the placenta. The fetal hemoglobin-oxygen dissociation curve is shifted to the left of the adult curve (Fig. 58–2); at the same PaO_2 level, fetal hemoglobin is more saturated than adult hemoglobin. Because fetal hemoglobin functions on the steep, lower end of the oxygen saturation curve (PaO_2 20 to 30 mm Hg), however, oxygen unloading to the tissue is not deficient. In contrast, at the higher oxygen concentrations present in the placenta, oxygen loading is enhanced. In the last trimester, fetal hemoglobin production begins to decrease, and adult hemoglobin production begins to increase, becoming the only hemoglobin available to the infant by 3 to 6 months of life. At this time, the fetal hemoglobin dissociation curve has shifted to the adult position (see Fig. 58–2).

A portion of the well-oxygenated umbilical venous blood returning to the heart from the placenta perfuses the liver. The remainder bypasses the liver through a shunt (the **ductus venosus**) and enters the inferior vena cava. This oxygenated blood in the vena cava constitutes 65% to 70% of venous return to the right atrium. The crista dividens in the right atrium directs one third of this vena caval blood across the patent foramen ovale to the left atrium, where it subsequently is pumped to the coronary, cerebral, and upper extremity circulations by the left ventricle. Venous return from the upper body combines with the remaining two thirds of the vena caval blood in the right atrium and is directed to the right ventricle. This mixture of venous low-oxygenated blood from the upper and lower body enters the pulmonary artery, from which only 8% to 10% of it is pumped to the pulmonary circuit. The remaining 80% to 92% of the right ventricular output bypasses the lungs through a **patent ductus arteriosus (PDA)** and enters the descending aorta. The amount of blood (8% to 10%) flowing to the pulmonary system is low because vasoconstriction produced by medial muscle hypertrophy of the small pulmonary arterioles and fluid in the fetal lung increases vascular resistance to blood flow. Pulmonary artery tone also responds to hypoxia, hypercapnia, and acidosis with vasoconstriction, a response that may increase pulmonary vascular resistance further. The ductus arteriosus remains patent in the fetus because of low PaO_2 levels and dilating prostaglandins. In utero, the right ventricle is the dominant ventricle, pumping 65% of the combined ventricular output, which is a high volume (450 mL/kg/

TABLE 58–5. Fetal Therapy

Disorder	Possible Treatment
Hematology	
Anemia with hydrops (erythroblastosis fetalis)	Umbilical vein packed red blood cell transfusion
Thalassemia	Fetal stem cell transplantation
Thrombocytopenia	
Isoimmune	Umbilical vein platelet transfusion, maternal IV immunoglobulin
Autoimmune (ITP)	Maternal steroids and IV immunoglobulin
Metabolic-Endocrine	
Maternal PKU	Phenylaline restriction
Fetal galactosemia	Galactose-free diet (?)
Multiple carboxylase deficiency	Biotin if responsive
Methylmalonic acidemia	Vitamin B_{12} if responsive
21-Hydroxylase deficiency	Dexamethasone
Maternal diabetes mellitus	Tight insulin control during pregnancy, labor, and delivery
Fetal goiter	Maternal hyperthyroidism—maternal propylthiouracil
	Fetal hypothyroidism—intra-amniotic T_4
Fetal Distress	
Hypoxia	Maternal oxygen, position
Intrauterine growth restriction	Maternal oxygen, position, improve nutrition if deficient
Oligohydramnios, premature rupture of membranes with variable deceleration	Amnioinfusion (antepartum and intrapartum)
Polyhydramnios	Amnioreduction (serial), indomethacin (if due to ↑ urine output) if indicated
Supraventricular tachycardia	Maternal digoxin,* flecainide, procainamide, amiodarone, quinidine
Lupus anticoagulant	Maternal aspirin, prednisone
Meconium-stained fluid	Amnioinfusion
Congenital heart block	Dexamethasone, pacemaker (with hydrops)
Premature labor	Sympathomimetics, magnesium sulfate, antibiotics
Respiratory	
Pulmonary immaturity	Betamethasone
Bilateral chylothorax–pleural effusions	Thoracentesis, pleuroamniotic shunt
Congenital Abnormalities†	
Neural tube defects	Folate, vitamins (preventions), surgery
Obstructive uropathy (with oligohydramnios without renal dysplasia)	>24 wk <32 wk, vesicoamniotic shunt plus amniofusion, ablation of posterior urethral valve
Cystic adenomatoid malformation (with hydrops)	Pleuroamniotic shunt or resection
Infectious Disease	
Group B streptococcus	Ampicillin, penicillin
Chorioamnionitis	Antibiotics
Toxoplasmosis	Spiramycin, pyrimethamine, sulfadiazine, and folic acid
Syphilis	Penicillin
Tuberculosis	Antituberculosis drugs
Lyme disease	Penicillin, ceftriaxone
Parvovirus	Intrauterine red blood cell transfusion for hydrops, severe anemia
Chlamydia trachomatis	Erythromycin
HIV-AIDS	Zidovudine plus protease inhibitors
Cytomegalovirus	Ganciclovir by umbilical vein

Continued

TABLE 58–5.   Fetal Therapy—cont'd

Disorder	Possible Treatment
Other	
Nonimmune hydrops (anemia)	Umbilical vein packed red blood cell transfusion
Narcotic abstinence (withdrawal)	Maternal low-dose methadone
Severe combined immunodeficiency disease	Fetal stem cell transplantation
Sacrococcygeal teratoma (with hydrops)	In utero resection, or vessel obliteration
Twin-twin transfusion syndrome	Repeated amniocentesis, YAG-laser photocoagulation of shared vessels
Twin reversed arterial perfusion syndrome	Digoxin, indomethacin, cord occlusion
Multifetal gestation	Selective reduction

(?) denotes possible but not proved efficacy.

*Drug of choice (may require percutaneous umbilical cord sampling and umbilical vein administration if hydrops is present). Most drug therapy is given to the mother, with subsequent placental passage to the fetus.

†Detailed fetal ultrasonography is needed to detect other anomalies; karyotype is also indicated.

ITP, idiopathic thrombocytopenic purpura; T_4, thyroxine.

From Stoll BJ, Kliegman RM: The fetus. In Berhman RE, Kliegman RM, Jenson HB (eds): Nelson Textbook of Pediatrics, 16th ed. Philadelphia, WB Saunders, 2000.

TABLE 58–6.   Components of the Perinatal History

Demographic Social Information

Age
Race
Sexually transmitted diseases, hepatitis, AIDS
Illicit drugs, cigarettes, ethanol, cocaine, abuse
Immune status (syphilis, rubella, hepatitis B, blood group)
Occupational exposure

Past Medical Diseases

Chronic hypertension
Heart disease
Diabetes mellitus
Thyroid disorders
Hematologic/malignancy
Collagen-vascular disease (SLE)
Genetic history—inborn errors of metabolism, bleeding, jaundice
Drug therapy

Prior Pregnancy

Abortion
Intrauterine fetal demise
Congenital malformation
Incompetent cervix
Birth weight
Prematurity
Twins
Blood group sensitization/neonatal jaundice
Hydrops
Infertility

Present Pregnancy

Current gestational age
Method of assessing gestational age
Fetal surveillance (OCT, NST, biophysical profile)
Ultrasonography (anomalies, hydrops)
Amniotic fluid analysis (L/S ratio)
Oligohydramnios-polyhydramnios
Vaginal bleeding
Preterm labor
Premature (prolonged) rupture of membranes (duration)
Preeclampsia
Urinary tract infection
Colonization status (herpes simplex, group B streptococcus)
Medications/drugs
Acute medical illness/exposure to infectious agents
Fetal therapy

Labor and Delivery

Duration of labor
Presentation—vertex, breech
Vaginal versus cesarean section
Spontaneous labor versus augmented or induced with oxytocin (Pitocin)
Forceps delivery
Presence of meconium-stained fluid
Maternal fever/amnionitis
Fetal heart rate patterns (distress)
Scalp pH
Maternal analgesia, anesthesia
Nuchal cord
Apgar score/methods of resuscitation
Gestational age assessment
Growth status (AGA, LGA, SGA)

AGA, average for gestational age; LGA, large for gestational age; L/S, lecithin/sphingomyelin ratio; NST, nonstress test; OCT, oxytocin challenge test; SGA, small for gestational age; SLE, systemic lupus erythematosus.

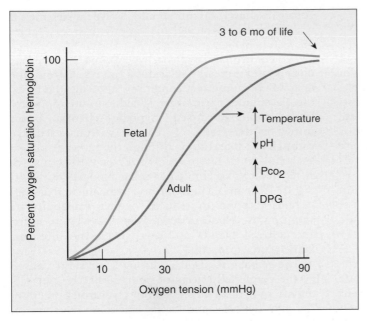

Figure 58-2

Hemoglobin-oxygen dissociation curves. The position of the adult curve depends on the binding of adult hemoglobin to 2,3-diphosphoglycerate (DPG), temperature, P_{CO_2}, and hydrogen ion concentration (pH).

min) compared with that pumped by an older infant's right ventricle (200 mL/kg/min).

The transition of the circulation occurring between the fetal and neonatal periods involves the removal of the low-resistance circulation of the placenta, the onset of air respiration and reduction of the pulmonary arterial resistance, and the closure of in utero shunts. When the umbilical cord is clamped, the low-pressure system of the placenta is eliminated, increasing systemic blood pressure. Venous return from the placenta is reduced, also decreasing right atrial pressure. When breathing begins, air replaces lung fluid, maintaining the functional residual capacity. Fluid leaves the lung in part through the trachea and is either swallowed or squeezed out during vaginal delivery. The pulmonary lymphatic and venous systems reabsorb the remaining fluid.

Most normal infants require little pressure to "open" the lungs after birth (5 to 10 cm H_2O). A few infants require greater opening pressures (20 to 30 cm H_2O). With the onset of breathing, pulmonary vascular resistance decreases, partly a result of the mechanics of breathing and partly a result of the elevated arterial oxygen tensions. The increased blood flow to the lungs results in a greater quantity of pulmonary venous blood returning to the left atrium; left atrial pressure now exceeds right atrial pressure, and the foramen ovale closes. As the flow through the pulmonary circulation increases, and the arterial oxygen tensions become elevated, the ductus arteriosus begins to constrict. In a term infant, this constriction functionally closes the ductus arteriosus within 1 day after birth. A permanent closure requires thrombosis and

fibrosis, a process that may take several weeks. In a premature infant, the ductus arteriosus is less sensitive to the effects of oxygen; if circulating levels of vasodilating prostaglandins are elevated, the ductus arteriosus may remain patent. This patency is a common problem in a premature infant with RDS.

Ventilation, oxygenation, and normal pH and P_{CO_2} levels immediately reduce pulmonary artery vasoconstriction by causing smooth muscle relaxation. Remodeling of the medial muscle hypertrophy begins at birth and continues for the next 3 months, resulting in a further reduction of pulmonary vascular resistance and a further increase of pulmonary blood flow. In infants with a ventricular septal defect (VSD), significant left-to-right shunt and heart failure usually do not develop until pulmonary vascular resistance declines. Term infants with a VSD may become ill at 2 to 3 months of age. A full complement of pulmonary arteriole medial muscle has not developed in premature infants, and these infants have a more rapid decline of pulmonary vascular resistance. Because of a more rapid decline of pulmonary artery pressure, a preterm infant with a VSD has left-to-right shunting and symptoms sooner than a term infant does, often before discharge from the nursery. Persistence or aggravation of pulmonary vasoconstriction caused by acidosis, hypoxia, hypercapnia, hypothermia, polycythemia, asphyxia, shunting of blood from the lungs, or pulmonary parenchymal hypoplasia results in **persistent pulmonary hypertension of the newborn (PPHN)**. Failure to replace pulmonary alveolar fluid completely with air can lead to respiratory distress (**transient tachypnea of the newborn**).

Routine Delivery Room Care and Resuscitation

Silver nitrate (1%) instilled into both eyes without being washed out is an indicated effective therapy for the prevention of neonatal gonococcal ophthalmia, which can result in severe panophthalmitis and subsequent blindness. Silver nitrate may produce a chemical conjunctivitis with a mucopurulent discharge and is not effective against *C. trachomatis.* Many hospitals use erythromycin drops to prevent neonatal gonococcal and chlamydial eye disease.

Bacterial colonization of a newborn may begin in utero if the fetal membranes have been ruptured. Most infants undergo colonization after birth and acquire the bacteria present in the mother's genitourinary system, such as group B streptococci, staphylococci, *E. coli,* and clostridia. Colonization is common at the umbilicus, skin, nasopharynx, and intestine. Antiseptic skin or cord care is routine in most nurseries to prevent the spread of pathologic bacteria from one infant to another and to prevent disease in the individual infant. Staphylococcal bullous impetigo, omphalitis, diarrhea, and systemic disease may result from colonization with virulent *Staphylococcus aureus.* For term infants, washing of the skin with 3% hexachlorophene is not routinely recommended, but may prevent serious staphylococcal disease; preterm infants may absorb hexachlorophene, and neurotoxicity may develop. Triple Antibiotic ointment (polymyxin B, neomycin, and bacitracin) or bacitracin may be applied to the umbilical cord effectively to reduce its colonization with gram-positive bacteria. Epidemics of *S. aureus* nursery infections are managed with strict infectious disease control measures (cohorting, hand washing, and monitoring for colonization).

Vitamin K prophylaxis (IM) should be given to all infants to prevent hemorrhagic disease of the newborn.

Before discharge, infants should receive the hepatitis B vaccine and be screened for various diseases (Tables 58–7 and 58–8).

Fetal or neonatal hypoxia, hypercapnia, poor cardiac output, and a metabolic acidosis can result from one or many of numerous conditions affecting the fetus, the placenta, or the mother. Whether in utero or after birth, **asphyxia-caused hypoxic-ischemic brain injury** is the result of reduced gaseous exchange through the placenta or through the lungs. Asphyxia associated with severe bradycardia or cardiac insufficiency reduces or eliminates tissue blood flow, resulting in ischemia. The fetal and neonatal circulatory systems respond to reduced oxygen availability by shunting the blood preferentially to the brain, heart, and adrenal glands and away from the intestine, kidney, lung, and skin.

The metabolic acidosis during asphyxia is caused by the combined effects of poor cardiac output secondary to hypoxic depression of myocardial function, systemic hypoxia, and tissue anaerobic metabolism. With severe or prolonged intrauterine or neonatal asphyxia, multiple vital organs are affected (Table 58–9).

Many conditions that contribute to fetal or neonatal asphyxia are the same medical or obstetric problems associated with high-risk pregnancy (Table 58–10). Maternal diseases that interfere with uteroplacental perfusion, such as chronic hypertension, preeclampsia, and diabetes mellitus, place the fetus at risk for intrauterine asphyxia. Maternal epidural anesthesia and the development of the vena caval compression syndrome may produce maternal hypotension, which decreases uterine perfusion. Maternal medications given to relieve pain during labor may cross the placenta and depress the infant's respiratory center, resulting in apnea at the time of birth.

TABLE 58–7. Approximate Frequencies in the U.S. of Disorders Included in or Considered for Newborn Screening

Disorder	Estimated Frequency	Disorder	Estimated Frequency
Congenital hypothyroidism	1:4000	Sickle cell disease	1:4000
PKU	1:12,000	Cystic fibrosis	1:4000
Medium chain acyl-CoA dehydrogenase	1:10,000	Duchenne muscular dystrophy	1:8000*
Galactosemia	1:60,000	Congenital toxoplasmosis	1:10,000
Maple syrup urine disease	1:200,000	Hyperlipidemia	1:500
Homocystinuria	1:200,000	α_1-Antitrypsin deficiency	1:8000
Biotinidase deficiency	1:70,000		
Congenital adrenal hyperplasia	1:19,000		

*For males, 1:4000.

From Kim SZ, Levy HL: Newborn screening. In Taeusch HW, Ballard RA (eds): Avery's Diseases of the Newborn, 7th ed. Philadelphia, WB Saunders, 1998.

TABLE 58–8. Abnormal Newborn Screening Results: Possible Implications and Initial Action to Be Taken

Newborn Screening Finding	Differential Diagnosis	Initial Action
↑ Phenylalanine	PKU, non-PKU hyperphenylalaninemia, pterin defect, galactosemia, transient hyperphenylalaninemia	Repeat blood specimen
↓ T_4, ↑ TSH	Congenital hypothyroidism, iodine exposure	Repeat blood specimen or thyroid function testing, begin thyroxine treatment
↓ T_4, normal TSH	Maternal hyperthyroidism, thyroxine-binding globulin deficiency, secondary hypothyroidism, congenital hypothyroidism with delayed TSH elevation	Repeat blood specimen
↑ Galactose (1-P)	Galactosemia, liver disease, portosystemic shunt, transferase deficiency variant (Duarte), transient	Clinical evaluation, urine for reducing substance, repeat blood specimen. If reducing substance positive, begin lactose-free formula
↓ Galactose-1-phosphate uridyltransferase	Galactosemia, transferase deficiency variant (Duarte), transient	Clinical evaluation, urine for reducing substance, repeat blood specimen. If reducing substance positive, begin lactose-free formula
↑ Methionine	Homocystinuria, isolated hypermethioninemia, liver dysfunction, tyrosinemia type I, transient hypermethioninemia	Repeat blood and urine specimen
↑ Leucine	Maple syrup urine disease, transient elevation	Clinical evaluation including urine for ketones, acid-base status, amino acid studies, immediate neonatal ICU care if urine ketones positive
↑ Tyrosine	Tyrosinemia type I or type II, transient tyrosinemia, liver disease	Repeat blood specimen
↑ 17α-Hydroxyprogesterone	Congenital adrenal hyperplasia, prematurity, transient (residual fetal adrenal cortex), stress in neonatal period, early specimen collection	Clinical evaluation including genital examination, serum electrolytes, repeat blood specimen
S-hemoglobin	Sickle cell disease, sickle cell trait	Hemoglobin electrophoresis
↑ Trypsinogen	Cystic fibrosis, transient, intestinal anomalies, perinatal stress, trisomies 13 and 18, renal failure	Repeat blood specimen, possible sweat test and DNA testing
↑ Creatinine phosphokinase	Duchenne muscular dystrophy, other type of muscular dystrophy, birth trauma, invasive procedure	Repeat blood test
↓ Biotinidase	Biotinidase deficiency	Serum biotinidase assay, biotin therapy
↓ G6PD	G6PD deficiency	Complete blood count, bilirubin determination
↓ α₁-Antitrypsin	α₁-Antitrypsin deficiency	Confirmatory test
Toxoplasma antibody (IgM)	Congenital toxoplasmosis	Infectious disease consultation
HIV antibody (IgG)	Maternally transmitted HIV, possible AIDS	Infectious disease consultation
↑ Organic acids	Fatty acid oxidation defects (medium chain acyl-CoA dehydrogenase deficiency)	Perform specific assay (tandem mass spectroscopy); frequent feeds

G6PD, glucose-6-phosphate dehydrogenase; T_4, thyroxine; TSH, thyroid-stimulating hormone.
From Kim SZ, Levy HL: Newborn screening. In Taeusch HW, Ballard RA (eds): Avery's Diseases of the Newborn, 7th ed. Philadelphia, WB Saunders, 1998.

TABLE 58–9.   Effects of Asphyxia

System	Effect
CNS	Hypoxic-ischemic encephalopathy, IVH, PVL, cerebral edema, serizures, hypotonia, hypertonia
Cardiovascular	Myocardial ischemia, poor contractility, tricuspid insufficiency, hypotension
Pulmonary	Persistent pulmonary hypertension, respiratory distress syndrome
Renal	Acute tubular or cortical necrosis
Adrenal	Adrenal hemorrhage
Gastrointestinal	Perforation, ulceration, necrosis
Metabolic	Inappropriate ADH, hyponatremia, hypoglycemia, hypocalcemia, myoglobinuria
Integument	Subcutaneous fat necrosis
Hematology	Disseminated intravascular coagulation

ADH, antidiuretic hormone; IVH, intraventricular hemorrhage; PVL, periventricular leukomalacia.

Fetal conditions associated with asphyxia usually do not become manifested until delivery, when the infant must initiate and sustain ventilation, which requires an intact respiratory drive from the centers for respiration in the medulla. In addition, the upper and lower airways must be patent and unobstructed. The alveolus must be free from foreign material, such as meconium, amniotic fluid debris, and infectious exudates, which increases airway resistance, reduces lung compliance, and leads to respiratory distress and hypoxia (see Table 58–10). Some extremely immature infants weighing less than 1000 g at birth may be unable to expand their lungs, even in the absence of pneumonia or other obvious signs of CNS dysfunction. The compliant chest wall and surfactant deficiency may result in poor air exchange at birth, retractions, hypoxia, and apnea. Usually, more mature newborns do not manifest apnea in the delivery room as a sign of RDS.

Any condition leading to hypoxia in the delivery room may cause apnea because a newborn (particularly a preterm infant) responds paradoxically to hypoxia with apnea rather than tachypnea as occurs in adults. Episodes of intrauterine asphyxia also may depress the neonatal CNS. If recovery of the fetal heart rate occurs as a result of improved uteroplacental perfusion, fetal hypoxia and acidosis may resolve. Nonetheless, if the effect on the respiratory center is more severe, a newborn may not initiate an adequate ventilatory response at birth and may undergo another episode of asphyxia.

The **Apgar examination**, a rapid scoring system based on physiologic responses to the birth process, is a good method for assessing the need to resuscitate a newborn (Table 58–11). At intervals of 1 minute and 5 minutes after birth, each of the five physiologic parameters is observed or elicited by a qualified examiner. Full-term infants with a normal cardiopulmonary adaptation should score 8 to 9 at 1 and 5 minutes. Apgar scores of 4 to 7 warrant close attention to determine whether the infant's status will improve and to ascertain whether any pathologic condition resulting from labor or delivery or residing within the newborn is contributing to the low Apgar score.

By definition, an Apgar score of 0 to 3 represents either a cardiopulmonary arrest or a condition caused by severe bradycardia, hypoventilation, or CNS depres-

TABLE 58–10.   Etiology of Birth Asphyxia

Type	Example
Intrauterine	
Hypoxia-ischemia	Uteroplacental insufficiency, abruptio placentae, prolapsed cord, maternal hypotension, unknown
Anemia-shock	Vasa previa, placenta previa, fetomaternal hemorrhage, erythroblastosis
Intrapartum	
Birth trauma	Cephalopelvic disproportion, shoulder dystocia, breech presentation, spinal cord transection
Hypoxia-ischemia	Umbilical cord compression, tetanic contraction, abruptio placentae
Postpartum	
CNS	Maternal medication, trauma, previous episodes of fetal hypoxia–acidosis
Congenital neuromuscular disease	Congenital myasthenia gravis, myopathy, myotonic dystrophy
Infection	Consolidated pneumonia, shock
Airway disorder	Choanal atresia, severe obstructing goiter, laryngeal webs
Pulmonary disorder	Severe immaturity, pneumothorax, pleural effusion, diaphragmatic hernia, pulmonary hypoplasia
Renal disorder	Pulmonary hypoplasia, pneumothorax

TABLE 58–11. Apgar Score

Signs	Points		
	0	*1*	*2*
Heart rate	0	<100/min	>100/min
Respiration	None	Weak cry	Vigorous cry
Muscle tone	None	Some extremity flexion	Arms, legs well flexed
Reflex irritability	None	Some motion	Cry, withdrawal
Color of body	Blue	Pink body, blue extremities	Pink all over

sion. Most low Apgar scores are caused by difficulty in establishing adequate ventilation and not by primary cardiac pathology. In addition to an Apgar score of 0 to 3, most infants with asphyxia severe enough to cause neurologic injury also manifest fetal acidosis (pH <7); seizures, coma, or hypotonia; and multiorgan dysfunction. Low Apgar scores may be caused by fetal hypoxia or other factors listed in Table 58–10. Most infants with low Apgar scores respond to assisted ventilation by facemask or by endotracheal intubation and usually do not need emergency medication.

Resuscitation of a newborn with a low Apgar score follows the same systematic sequence as that for resuscitation of older patients, but in the newborn period this simplified *ABCD* approach requires some qualification (Fig. 58–3). In the ABCD approach, **A** stands for securing a patent airway by clearing amniotic fluid or meconium by suctioning; "A" should also remind us about "anticipation" and the need for knowing the events of pregnancy, labor, and delivery. Evidence of a diaphragmatic hernia and a low Apgar score indicate that immediate endotracheal intubation is required. If a mask and bag are used, gas enters the lung and the stomach, and the latter may act as an expanding mass in the chest that compromises respiration. Knowing the blood group sensitization and that fetal hydrops has occurred with pleural effusions may indicate the need for bilateral thoracentesis to evacuate the pleural effusions so that adequate ventilation can be established.

B represents breathing. If the patient is apneic or hypoventilates and remains cyanotic, artificial ventilation should be initiated. Ventilation should be performed with a well-fitted mask that is attached to an anesthesia bag and a manometer to prevent extremely high pressures from being given to the newborn; 100% oxygen should be given through the mask. If the infant does not revive, an endotracheal tube should be placed through the vocal cords, then attached to the anesthesia bag and manometer, and 100% oxygen should be administered. The pressure generated should begin at 20 to 25 cm H_2O, with a rate of 40 to 60 breaths/min.

An adequate response to ventilation is indicated by good chest rise, return of breath sounds, well-oxygenated color, heart rate returning to the normal range (120 to 160 beats/min), normal end-tidal carbon dioxide, and later increased muscle activity and wakefulness. The usual recovery after a cardiac arrest first involves a return to a normal heart rate. After that, cyanosis disappears, and the infant appears well perfused. An infant may remain limp and may be apneic for a prolonged time after return of cardiac output and correction of acidosis.

For an asphyxiated newborn, breathing initially should be briefly delayed if meconium-stained amniotic fluid is present. If the meconium is not cleared from the oropharyngeal and tracheal airways, it may be disseminated into the lungs, producing severe aspiration pneumonia. If meconium is noted in the amniotic fluid, the oropharynx should be suctioned when the head is delivered. After the birth of a **depressed infant**, the oral cavity should be suctioned again; the vocal cords should be visualized with a laryngoscope and the infant intubated, with suction applied while the tube is below the vocal cords. If meconium is noted below the cords, intubation should be repeated quickly to clear the remaining meconium. During this time, the infant should not be stimulated to breathe, and positive-pressure ventilation should not be applied.

C represents circulation and external cardiac massage. If artificial ventilation does not improve the bradycardia, if asystole is present, or if peripheral pulses cannot be palpated, external cardiac massage should be performed at a rate of 90 compressions/min with intervening 30 breaths/min. External cardiac massage usually is not needed because most infants in the delivery room respond to ventilation.

D represents the administration of drugs. If bradycardia that is unresponsive to ventilation persists or if asystole is present, drugs should be added to the process of resuscitation. IV epinephrine (1:10,000), 0.1 to 0.3 mL/kg, should be given through an umbilical venous line or injected into the endotracheal tube. Additional medications for resuscitation include

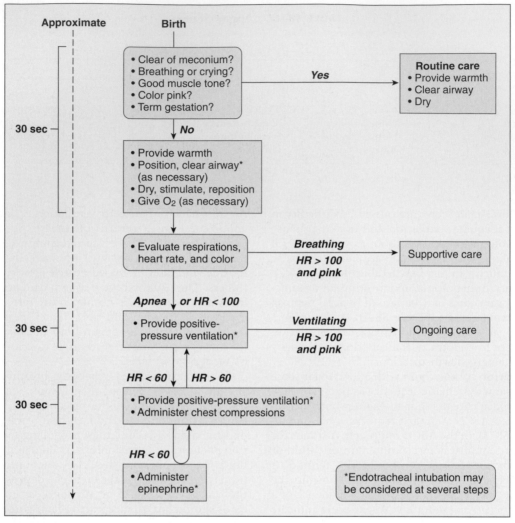

Figure 58–3

Algorithm for resuscitation of the newborn infant. HR, heart rate. (From National guidelines for neonatal resuscitation. Pediatrics 106:E29, 2000.)

2 mEq/kg of IV sodium bicarbonate (0.5 mEq/mL) if acidosis is prolonged and a rapid infusion of fluids (normal saline or O-negative red blood cells [RBCs] if anemia is present) if poor perfusion suggests hypovolemia. Sodium bicarbonate should be given only if severe metabolic acidosis is suspected or is proven by blood gas analysis. Sodium bicarbonate should not be given unless the lungs are being adequately ventilated. Before medications are administered in the presence of electrical cardiac activity with poor pulses, it is important to determine whether there is a **pneumothorax**. Transillumination of the thorax, involving the use of a bright light through each of the two sides of the thorax and over the sternum, may suggest pneumothorax if

one side transmits more light than the other. Breath sounds also are decreased over a pneumothorax. There is a shift of the heart tones away from the side of a tension pneumothorax.

If CNS depression in the infant might be caused by a narcotic medication that was given to the mother, 0.1 mg/kg of naloxone (Narcan) can be given to the infant intravenously or endotracheally as a specific antidote. Before this drug is administered, however, the ABCs should be followed carefully. Naloxone should not be given to a newborn of a mother who is suspected of being addicted to narcotics or is on methadone maintenance because the newborn may experience severe seizures.

TABLE 58–12.   Life-Threatening Congenital Anomalies

Name	Manifestations
Choanal atresia (stenosis)	Respiratory distress in delivery room, apnea, unable to pass nasogastric tube through nares
Pierre Robin syndrome	Micrognathia, cleft palate, airway obstruction
Diaphragmatic hernia	Scaphoid abdomen, bowel sounds present in left chest, heart shifted to right, respiratory distress, polyhydramnios
Tracheoesophageal fistula	Polyhydramnios, aspiration pneumonia, excessive salivation, unable to place nasogastric tube in stomach
Intestinal obstruction: volvulus, duodenal atresia, ileal atresia	Polyhydramnios, bile-stained emesis, abdominal distention
Gastroschisis/omphalocele	Polyhydramnios; intestinal obstruction
Renal agenesis/Potter syndrome	Oligohydramnios, anuria, pulmonary hypoplasia, pneumothorax
Hydronephrosis	Bilateral abdominal masses
Neural tube defects: anencephalus, meningomyelocele	Polyhydramnios, elevated α-fetoprotein; decreased fetal activity
Down syndrome (trisomy 21)	Hypotonia, congenital heart disease, duodenal atresia
Ductal-dependent congenital heart disease	Cyanosis, murmur, shock

Physical Examination and Gestational Age Assessment

The first physical examination of a newborn may be a general physical examination of a well infant or an examination to confirm fetal diagnoses or to determine the cause of various manifestations of neonatal diseases. Problems in the transition from fetal to neonatal life may be detectable immediately in the delivery room or during the first day of life. Physical examination also may reveal effects of the labor and delivery resulting from asphyxia, drugs, or birth trauma. The first newborn examination is an important way to detect congenital malformations or deformations (Table 58–12). Congenital malformations are the result of chromosomal trisomies, teratogens, or recognizable syndromes without identifiable causes. Significant congenital malformations may be present in 1% to 3% of all births.

Appearance

The general appearance of the infant should be evaluated first. Signs such as cyanosis, nasal flaring, intercostal retractions, and grunting suggest pulmonary disease. Meconium staining of the umbilical cord, nails, and skin suggests fetal distress and the possibility of aspiration pneumonia (discussed subsequently). The level of spontaneous activity, passive muscle tone, quality of the cry, and apnea are useful screening signs to evaluate the state of the nervous system initially.

Vital Signs

After the general appearance of the infant is evaluated, the examination should proceed with an assessment of vital signs, particularly heart rate (normal rate 120 to 160 beats/min), respiratory rate (normal rate 30 to 60 breaths/min), temperature (usually done initially per rectum and later as an axillary measurement), and blood pressure (often reserved for sick infants). Length, weight, and head circumference should be measured and plotted on growth curves to determine whether growth is normal, accelerated, or retarded for the specific gestational age.

Gestational Age

Gestational age is determined by an assessment of various physical signs (Fig. 58–4) and neuromuscular characteristics (Fig. 58–5) that vary according to fetal age and maturity. Physical criteria are features that mature with advancing fetal age, including increasing firmness of the pinna of the ear; increasing size of the breast tissue; decreasing fine, immature lanugo hair over the back; and decreasing opacity of the skin. Neurologic criteria are features that mature with gestational age, including increasing flexion of the legs, hips, and arms; increasing tone of the flexor muscles of the neck; and decreasing laxity of the joints. These signs are determined during the first day of life and are assigned scores. The cumulative score is correlated with a gestational age, which is usually accurate to within 2 weeks (Fig. 58–6).

Physical maturity	−1	0	1	2	3	4	5
Skin	Sticky, friable, transparent	Gelatinous, red, translucent	Smooth, pink, visible veins	Superficial peeling or rash, few veins	Cracking, pale areas, rare veins	Parchment, deep cracking, no vessels	Leathery, cracked, wrinkled
Lanugo	None	Sparse	Abundant	Thinning	Bald areas	Mostly bald	
Plantar surface	Heel–toe 40-50 mm: −1 Less than 40 mm: −2	<50 mm, no crease	Faint red marks	Anterior transverse crease only	Creases on anterior 2/3	Creases over entire sole	
Breast	Imperceptible	Barely perceptible	Flat areola– no bud	Stripped areola, 1-2 mm bud	Raised areola, 3-4 mm bud	Full areola, 5-10 mm bud	
Eye/ear	Lids fused, loosely (−1), tightly (−2)	Lids open, pinna flat, stays folded	Slightly curved pinna; soft, slow recoil	Well-curved pinna, soft but ready recoil	Formed and firm; instant recoil	Thick cartilage, ear stiff	
Genitals male	Scrotum flat, smooth	Scrotum empty, faint rugae	Testes in upper canal, rare rugae	Testes descending, few rugae	Testes down, good rugae	Testes pendulous, deep rugae	
Genitals female	Clitoris prominent, labia flat	Prominent clitoris, small labia minora	Prominent clitoris, enlarging minora	Majora and minora equally prominent	Majora large, minora small	Majora cover clitoris and minora	

Figure 58–4

Physical criteria for assessment of maturity and gestational age. Expanded New Ballard Score (NBS) includes extremely premature infants and has been refined to improve accuracy in more mature infants. (From Ballard JL, et al: New Ballard Score, expanded to include extremely premature infants. J Pediatr 119:417, 1991.)

Gestational age assessment permits the detection of abnormal fetal growth patterns, aiding in predicting the neonatal complications of largeness or smallness for gestational age (Fig. 58–7). Infants born at a weight greater than the 90th percentile for their age are considered **large for gestational age (LGA)**. Among the risks associated with being LGA are all the risks of the infant of a diabetic mother and risks associated with postmaturity. Infants born at a weight less than the 10th percentile for their age (some growth curves use <2 SD or the 5th percentile) are **small for gestational age (SGA)** and have IUGR. Problems associated with SGA infants include congenital malformations, in addition to the problems listed in Table 58–4.

Skin

The skin should be evaluated for pallor, plethora, jaundice, cyanosis, meconium staining, petechiae, ecchymoses, congenital nevi, and neonatal rashes. Vasomotor instability with cutis marmorata, telangiectasia, phlebectasia (intermittent mottling with venous prominence), and acrocyanosis (feet and hands) is normal in a premature infant. Acrocyanosis also may be noted in a healthy term infant in the first days after birth. The harlequin color change is a striking, transient, but normal sign of vasomotor instability and divides the body from head to pubis, through the midline, into equal halves of pink and pale color.

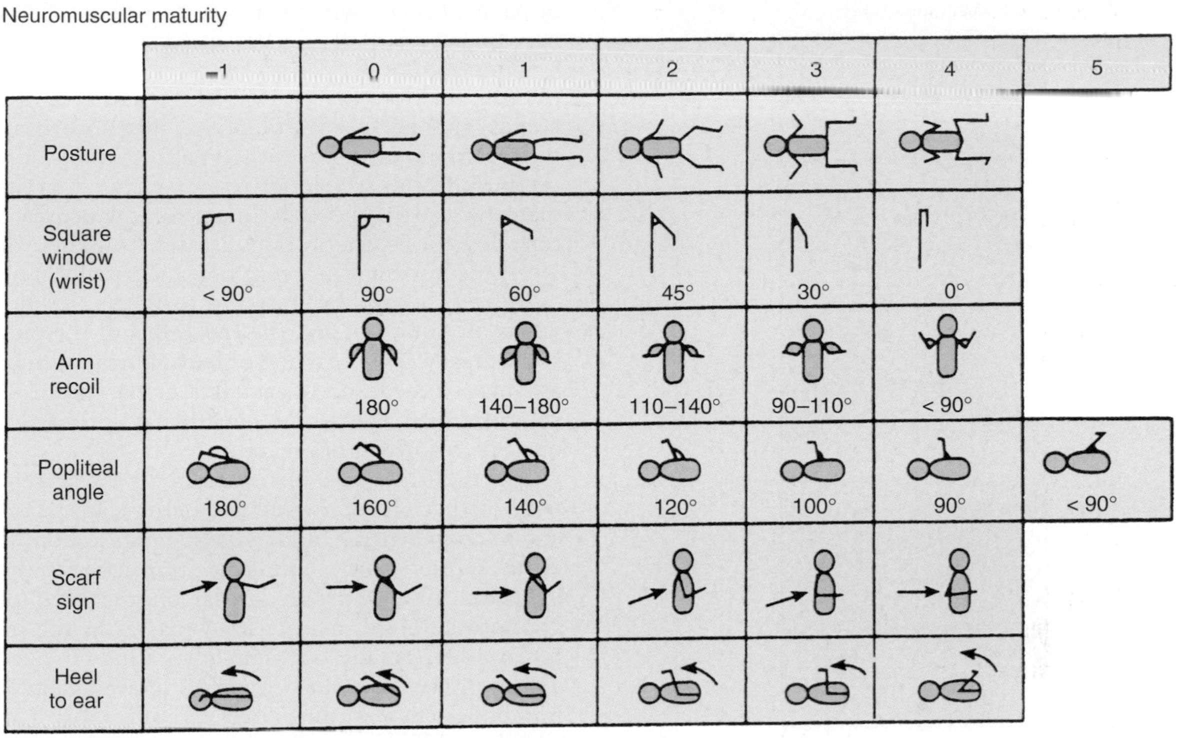

Neuromuscular maturity

	−1	0	1	2	3	4	5
Posture							
Square window (wrist)	< 90°	90°	60°	45°	30°	0°	
Arm recoil		180°	140–180°	110–140°	90–110°	< 90°	
Popliteal angle	180°	160°	140°	120°	100°	90°	< 90°
Scarf sign							
Heel to ear							

Figure 58–5

Neuromuscular criteria for assessment of maturity and gestational age. Expanded New Ballard Score (NBS) includes extremely premature infants and has been refined to improve accuracy in more mature infants. (From Ballard JL, et al: New Ballard Score, expanded to include extremely premature infants. J Pediatr 119:417, 1991.)

The skin is covered with lanugo hair, which disappears by term gestation. **Hair tufts** over the lumbosacral spine suggest a spinal cord defect. **Vernix caseosa**, a soft, white, creamy layer covering the skin in preterm infants, disappears by term. Post-term infants often have peeling, parchment-like skin. **Mongolian spots** are transient, dark blue to black pigmented macules seen over the lower back and buttocks in 90% of African American, Indian, and Asian infants. **Nevus simplex** ("salmon patch"), or pink macular hemangiomas, is common, usually transient, and noted on the back of the neck, eyelids, and forehead. **Nevus flammeus**, or **port-wine stain**, commonly is seen on the face and should cause the examiner to consider Sturge-Weber syndrome (trigeminal angiomatosis, convulsions, and ipsilateral intracranial "tram-line" calcifications).

Congenital melanocytic nevi are pigmented lesions of varying size noted in 1% of neonates. **Giant pigmented nevi** are uncommon but have malignant potential. **Capillary hemangiomas** are raised, red lesions, whereas **cavernous hemangiomas** are deeper, blue masses. Both lesions increase in size after birth,

only to resolve when the child is 1 to 4 years old. When enlarged, these hemangiomas may produce high-output heart failure or platelet trapping and hemorrhage. **Erythema toxicum** is an erythematous, papular-vesicular rash common in neonates that develops after birth and involves eosinophils in the vesicular fluid. **Pustular melanosis**, more common in African American infants, may be seen at birth and consists of a small, dry vesicle on a pigmented brown macular base. Erythema toxicum and pustular melanosis are benign lesions, but may mimic more serious conditions, such as the vesicular rash of disseminated herpes simplex or the bullous eruption of *S. aureus* impetigo. Tzanck smear, Gram stain, Wright stain, direct fluorescent antibody stain, polymerase chain reaction (PCR) for herpes DNA, and appropriate cultures may be needed to distinguish these rashes. Other common characteristic rashes are **milia** (yellow-white epidermal cysts of the pilosebaceous follicles that are noted on the nose) and **miliaria** (prickly heat), which is caused by obstructed sweat glands. **Edema** may be present in preterm infants, but also suggests hydrops fetalis, sepsis, hypoalbuminemia, or lymphatic disorders.

Maturity rating

Score	Weeks
−10	20
−5	22
0	24
5	26
10	28
15	30
20	32
25	34
30	36
35	38
40	40
45	42
50	44

Figure 58–6

Maturity rating as calculated by adding the physical and neurologic scores, calculating the gestational age. (From Ballard JL, et al: New Ballard Score, expanded to include extremely premature infants. J Pediatr 119:417, 1991.)

Skull

The skull may be elongated and molded after a prolonged labor, but this resolves 2 to 3 days after birth. The sutures should be palpated to determine the width and the presence of premature fusion or cranial synostosis. The anterior and posterior fontanels should be soft and nonbulging, with the anterior larger than the posterior. A large fontanel is associated with hydrocephalus, hypothyroidism, rickets, and other disorders. Soft areas away from the fontanel are **craniotabes**; these lesions feel like a Ping-Pong ball when they are palpated. They may be a result of in utero compression. The skull should be examined carefully for signs of trauma or lacerations from internal fetal electrode sites or fetal scalp pH sampling; abscess formation may develop in these areas.

Face, Eyes, and Mouth

The face should be inspected for dysmorphic features, such as epicanthal folds, hypertelorism, preauricular tags or sinuses, low-set ears, long philtrum, and cleft lip or palate. Facial asymmetry may be a result of seventh nerve palsy; head tilt may be caused by torticollis.

The eyes should open spontaneously, especially in an upright position. Before 28 weeks' gestational age, the eyelids may be fused. Coloboma, megalocornea, and microphthalmia suggest other malformations or intrauterine infections. A cloudy cornea greater than 1 cm in diameter also may be seen in congenital glaucoma, uveal tract dysgenesis, and storage diseases. Conjunctival and retinal hemorrhages are common and usually of no significance. The pupillary response to light is present at 28 weeks of gestation, and the **red reflex** of the retina is shown easily. A white reflex, or **leukokoria**, is abnormal and may be the result of cataracts, ocular tumor, severe chorioretinitis, persistent hyperplastic primary vitreous, or retinopathy of prematurity.

The mouth should be inspected for the presence of natal teeth, clefts of the soft and hard palate and uvula, and micrognathia. A bifid uvula suggests a submucosal cleft. White, shiny, multiple transient epidermal inclusion cysts (Epstein pearls) on the hard palate are normal. Hard, marble-sized masses in the buccal mucosa are usually transient idiopathic fat necrosis. The *tympanic membranes* are dull, gray, opaque, and immobile. These findings may persist for 1 to 4 weeks and should not be confused with otitis media.

Neck and Chest

The neck appears short and symmetric. Abnormalities include midline clefts or masses caused by thyroglossal duct cysts or by goiter and lateral neck masses (or sinuses), which are the result of branchial clefts. Cystic hygromas and hemangiomas are other masses that may be present. Shortening of the sternocleidomastoid muscle with a fibrous "tumor" over the muscle produces head tilt and asymmetric facies (neonatal torticollis). Arnold-Chiari malformation and cervical spine lesions also produce torticollis. Edema and webbing of the neck suggest Turner syndrome. Both clavicles should be palpated for fractures.

Examination of the *chest* includes inspection of the chest wall to identify asymmetry resulting from absence of the pectoralis muscle and inspection of the breast tissue to determine gestational age and detect a breast abscess. Boys and girls may have breast engorgement and produce milk; milk expression should not be attempted. **Supernumerary nipples** may be bilateral and occasionally are associated with renal anomalies.

Lungs

Examination of the lungs includes observations of the rate, depth, and nature of intercostal or sternal retractions. Breath sounds should be equal on both sides of the chest, and rales should not be heard after the first

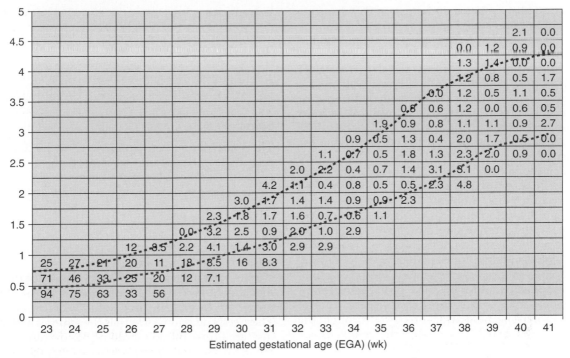

Figure 58–7

Birth weight–specific and estimated gestational age–specific mortality rates. The dashed lines of the figure represent the 10th and 90th percentile weights. The grid lines are plotted by each gestational age and in 250-g weight increments. Each number in the box is the percent mortality rate for the grid defined by gestational age and birth weight range. (From Thomas P, Peabody J, Turnier V, et al: A new look at intrauterine growth and impact of race, attitude, and gender. Pediatrics 106:E21, 2000.)

1 to 2 hours of life. Diminished or absent breath sounds on one side suggest pneumothorax, collapsed lung, pleural effusion, or diaphragmatic hernia. Shift of the cardiac impulse away from a tension pneumothorax and diaphragmatic hernia and toward the collapsed lung is a helpful physical finding for differentiating these disorders. Subcutaneous emphysema of the neck or chest also suggests a pneumothorax or pneumomediastinum, whereas bowel sounds auscultated in the chest in the presence of a scaphoid abdomen suggest a diaphragmatic hernia.

Heart

The position of the heart in infants is more midline than in older children. The first heart sound is normal, whereas the second heart sound may not be split in the first day of life. Decreased splitting of the second heart sound is noted in PPHN (also known as *persistent fetal circulation*), transposition of the great vessels, and pulmonary atresia. Heart murmurs in newborns are common in the delivery room and during the first day of life. Most of these murmurs are transient and are a result of closure of the ductus arteriosus, peripheral pulmonary artery stenosis, or a small VSD. Pulses should be palpated in the upper and lower extremities, usually over the brachial and femoral arteries. Blood pressure in the upper and lower extremities should be measured in all patients with a murmur or heart failure. An upper-to-lower extremity gradient of more than 10 to 20 mm Hg suggests coarctation of the aorta.

Abdomen

In the abdomen, the liver may be palpable 2 cm below the right costal margin. The spleen tip is less likely to be palpable. A left-sided liver suggests situs inversus and asplenia syndrome. Both kidneys should be palpable in the first day of life with gentle, deep palpation. The first urination occurs during the first day of life in greater than 95% of normal term infants.

Abdominal masses usually represent hydronephrosis or dysplastic-multicystic kidney disease. Less often, masses indicate ovarian cysts, intestinal duplication, neuroblastoma, or mesoblastic nephroma. Masses should be evaluated immediately with ultrasound. Abdominal distention may be caused by intestinal obstructions, such as ileal atresia, meconium ileus, midgut volvulus, imperforate anus, or Hirschsprung disease. Meconium stool is passed normally within 48 hours of birth in 99% of term infants. The anus should be patent. An imperforate anus is not always visible; the first temperature taken with a rectal thermometer should be taken carefully. The abdominal wall musculature may be absent, as in prune-belly syndrome, or weak, resulting in diastasis recti. **Umbilical hernias** are common among African American infants. The umbilical cord should be inspected to determine the presence of two arteries and one vein and the absence of a urachus or a herniation of abdominal contents, as occurs with an **omphalocele**. The latter is associated with extraintestinal problems, such as genetic trisomies and hypoglycemia (Beckwith-Wiedemann syndrome). Bleeding from the cord suggests a coagulation disorder, and a chronic discharge may be a granuloma of the umbilical stump or, less frequently, a draining omphalomesenteric cyst. Erythema around the umbilicus is **omphalitis** and may cause portal vein thrombophlebitis and subsequent extrahepatic portal hypertension. The herniation of bowel through the abdominal wall 2 to 3 cm lateral to the umbilicus is a **gastroschisis**.

Genitalia

The appearance of the genitalia varies with gestational age. At term, the testes should be descended into a well-formed pigmented and rugated scrotum. The testes occasionally are in the inguinal canal; this is more common among preterm infants, as is cryptorchidism. Scrotal swelling may represent a hernia, transient hydrocele, in utero torsion of the testes, or, rarely, dissected meconium from meconium ileus and peritonitis. Hydroceles are clear and readily seen by transillumination, whereas testicular torsion in the newborn may present as a painless, dark swelling. The urethral opening should be at the end of the penis. Epispadias or hypospadias alone should not raise concern about pseudohermaphroditism. If no testes are present in the scrotum and hypospadias is present, however, problems of sexual development should be suspected (see Chapter 177). Circumcision should be deferred with hypospadias because the foreskin is needed for the repair. The normal prepuce is often too tight to retract in the neonatal period.

The female genitalia normally may reveal a milky white or blood-streaked vaginal discharge as a result of maternal hormone withdrawal. Mucosal tags of the labia majora are common. Distention of an imperforate hymen may produce hydrometrocolpos and a lower midline abdominal mass as a result of an enlarged uterus. Clitoral enlargement with fusion of the labial-scrotal folds (labia majora) suggests adrenogenital syndrome or exposure to masculinizing maternal hormones.

Extremities

Examination of the extremities should involve assessment of length, symmetry, and presence of hemihypertrophy, atrophy, polydactyly, syndactyly, simian creases, absent fingers, overlapping fingers, rocker-bottom feet, clubfoot, congenital bands, fractures, and amputations.

Spine

The spine should be examined for evidence of sacral hair tufts, a dermal sinus tract above the gluteal folds, congenital scoliosis (a result of hemivertebra), and soft tissue masses such as lipomas or meningomyeloceles.

Hips

The hips should be examined for congenital dysplasia (dislocation). Gluteal fold asymmetry or leg length discrepancy is a suggestive sign of dysplasia, but the examiner should perform the Barlow test and the Ortolani maneuver to evaluate the stability of the hip joint. These tests determine whether the femoral head can be displaced from the acetabulum (Barlow test) and then replaced (Ortolani maneuver) (see Chapter 198). The examiner's long finger is placed over the greater trochanter, and the thumb is placed medially, just distal to the long finger. With the thighs held in midabduction, the examiner attempts to pull the femoral head gently out of the acetabulum with lateral pressure of the thumb and by rocking the knee medially. The reverse maneuver is performed by pressing the long finger on the greater trochanter and rocking the knee laterally. A "clunking" sensation is palpated when the femoral head leaves and returns to the acetabulum.

Neurologic Assessment

The neurologic examination should include assessment of active and passive tone, level of alertness, primary neonatal (primitive) reflexes, deep tendon reflexes, spontaneous motor activity, and cranial nerves (involving retinal examination, extraocular muscle movement, masseter power as in sucking, facial motility, hearing, and tongue function). The Moro reflex is one of the primary newborn reflexes. This reflex is present at birth and gone in 3 to 6 months. It is elicited by sudden, slight dropping of the supported head from a slightly raised supine position. This slight drop should elicit opening of the hands and extension and abduction of the arms, followed by upper extremity flexion and a cry. The palmar grasp is present by 28 weeks of age and gone by 4 months of age. Deep tendon reflexes may be brisk in a normal newborn; 5 to 10 beats of ankle clonus are normal. The Babinski sign is extensor or upgoing. The sensory examination can be evaluated by withdrawal of an extremity, grimace, and cry in response to painful stimuli. The rooting reflex, or the turning of the head toward light tactile stimulation of the perioral area, is present by 32 weeks of age.

Special Conditions Requiring Resuscitation in the Delivery Room

Cyanosis

Acrocyanosis (blue color of the hands and feet with pink color of the rest of the body) is common in the delivery room and is usually normal. *Central cyanosis* of the trunk, mucosal membranes, and tongue can occur in the delivery room or at any time after birth and is always a manifestation of a serious underlying condition. Cyanosis is noted with 4 to 5 g/dL of deoxygenated hemoglobin. Central cyanosis can be caused by problems in many different organ systems, although cardiopulmonary diseases are the most common (Table 58–13). RDS, sepsis, and cyanotic heart disease are the three most common causes of cyanosis in infants admitted to a neonatal ICU. A systematic evaluation of these and other causes of cyanosis is required for every cyanotic infant after prompt administration of oxygen, with or without assisted ventilation.

Life-Threatening Congenital Malformations

Various congenital anomalies can interfere with vital organ function after birth (see Table 58–12). Some malformations, such as choanal atresia and other lesions obstructing the airway, may complicate ventilation.

TABLE 58–13. Differential Diagnosis of Neonatal Cyanosis

System/Disease	Mechanism
Pulmonary	
Respiratory distress syndrome	Surfactant deficiency
Sepsis, pneumonia	Inflammation, pulmonary hypertension, ARDS
Meconium aspiration pneumonia	Mechanical obstruction, inflammation, pulmonary hypertension
Persistent pulmonary hypertension of the newborn	Pulmonary hypertension
Diaphragmatic hernia	Pulmonary hypoplasia, pulmonary hypertension
Transient tachypnea	Retained lung fluid
Cardiovascular	
Cyanotic heart disease with decreased pulmonary blood flow	Right-to-left shunt as in pulmonary atresia, tetralogy of Fallot
Cyanotic heart disease with increased pulmonary blood flow	Mixing lesion as in single ventricle or truncus arteriosus
Cyanotic heart disease with congestive heart failure	Right-to-left shunt with pulmonary edema and poor cardiac output as in hypoplastic left heart and coarctation of aorta
Heart failure alone	Pulmonary edema and poor cardiac contractility as in sepsis, myocarditis, supraventricular tachycardia, or complete heart block; high-output failure as in PDA or vein of Galen or other arteriovenous malformations
CNS	
Maternal sedative drugs	Hypoventilation, apnea
Asphyxia	CNS depression
Intracranial hemorrhage	CNS depression, seizure
Neuromuscular disease	Hypotonia, hypoventilation, pulmonary hypoplasia
Hematologic	
Acute blood loss	Shock
Chronic blood loss	Congestive heart failure
Polycythemia	Pulmonary hypertension
Methemoglobinemia	Low-affinity hemoglobin or red blood cell enzyme defect
Metabolic	
Hypoglycemia	CNS depression, congestive heart failure
Adrenogenital syndrome	Shock (salt-losing)

ARDS, acute respiratory distress syndrome; PDA, patent ductus arteriosus.

Intrathoracic lesions, such as cysts or bowel that has herniated into the chest (diaphragmatic hernia), interfere with respiration. Other malformations that obstruct the gastrointestinal system at the level of the esophagus, duodenum, ileum, or colon may lead to aspiration pneumonia, intestinal perforation, or gangrene. Gastroschisis and omphalocele are associated with exposed bowel on the abdominal wall. Omphalocele also is often associated with other malformations, whereas intestinal necrosis is more common in gastroschisis.

Many congenital malformations are obvious in the delivery room. Using fetal ultrasound, the obstetrician can detect many serious congenital anomalies in utero. Immediate palliative medical or surgical treatment or corrective surgery must be planned for most infants with major congenital malformations. Prompt stabilization, as noted for the asphyxiated infant, is essential.

Shock

Shock in the delivery room is manifested by pallor, poor capillary refill time, unpalpable pulses, hypotonia, cyanosis, and eventually cardiopulmonary arrest. Blood loss before or during labor and delivery is a common cause of shock in the delivery room. Blood loss may be caused by fetal-maternal hemorrhage, placenta previa, vasa previa, twin-to-twin transfusion syndrome, or displacement of blood from the fetus to the placenta as during asphyxia (*asphyxia pallida*). Hemorrhage into a viscus, such as the liver or spleen, may be noted in macrosomic infants, and hemorrhage into the cerebral ventricles may produce shock and apnea in preterm infants. Anemia, hypoalbuminemia, hypovolemia, and shock at birth are common manifestations of Rh immune hydrops.

Severe intrauterine bacterial sepsis may present with septicemic shock in the delivery room or immediately after the infant is transferred to the nursery. Typically these infants are mottled, hypotonic, and cyanotic and have diminished peripheral pulses. They have a normal hemoglobin concentration but may manifest neutropenia, thrombocytopenia, and disseminated intravascular coagulation (DIC). Peripheral symmetric gangrene (purpuric rash) often is a sign of hypotensive shock among infants with severe congenital bacterial infections. Congenital left ventricular cardiac obstruction (critical aortic stenosis or hypoplastic left heart syndrome) also produces shock, although not usually in the delivery room.

Treatment of newborn infants with shock should involve the management approaches used for the sick infant. Problems may be anticipated through knowledge of the infant's immune status, evidence of hydrops, or suspicion of intrauterine infection or anomalies. Stabilization of the airway and institution of respiratory support are essential. Hypovolemic shock should be managed with repeated boluses of 10 to 15 mL/kg of normal saline or lactated Ringer solution. If severe immune hemolysis is predicted, blood typed against the mother's blood should be available in the delivery room and should be given to the newborn if signs of anemia and shock are present. Thereafter, all blood should be crossmatched with the infant's and mother's blood before transfusion. Drugs such as dopamine, dobutamine, epinephrine, or cortisol may improve cardiac output and tissue perfusion.

Birth Injury

Birth injury refers to avoidable and unavoidable injury to the fetus during the birth process. **Caput succedaneum** is a diffuse, edematous, often dark swelling of the soft tissue of the scalp that extends across the midline and suture lines. In infants delivered from a face presentation, soft tissue edema of the eyelids and face is an equivalent phenomenon. Caput succedaneum may be seen after prolonged labor in full-term and preterm infants. Molding of the head often is associated with caput succedaneum and is the result of pressure that is induced from overriding the parietal and frontal bones against their respective sutures.

A *cephalhematoma* is a subperiosteal hemorrhage that does not cross the suture lines surrounding the respective bones. A linear skull fracture rarely may be seen underlying a cephalhematoma. With time, the cephalhematoma may organize, calcify, and form a central depression.

Infants with cephalhematoma and caput succedaneum require no specific treatment. Occasionally a premature infant may develop a massive scalp hemorrhage. This *subgaleal bleeding* and the bleeding noted from a cephalhematoma may cause indirect hyperbilirubinemia that requires treatment with phototherapy. *Retinal* and *subconjunctival hemorrhages* are common but usually are small and insignificant. No treatment is necessary.

Spinal cord or **spine injuries** may occur in the fetus as a result of the hyperextended "star gazing" posture. Injuries also may occur in infants after excessive rotational (at C3-4) or longitudinal (at C7-T1) force is transmitted to the neck during vertex or breech delivery. Fractures of vertebrae are rarer and may cause direct damage to the spinal cord, leading to transection and permanent sequelae or hemorrhage, edema, and neurologic signs. Rarely a snapping sound indicating cord transection rather than vertebral displacement is heard at the time of delivery. Neurologic dysfunction usually involves complete flaccid paralysis, absence of deep tendon reflexes, and absence of responses to painful stimuli below the lesion. Painful stimuli may elicit reflex flexion of the legs. Infants with spinal cord injury often are flaccid, apneic, and asphyxiated, all of which may mask the underlying spinal cord transection. With time, these infants experience bowel and bladder problems, spasticity, and hyperreflexia.

Injury to the nerves of the *brachial plexus* may result from excessive traction on the neck, producing paresis or complete paralysis. The mildest injury (neurapraxia) is edema; axonotmesis is more severe and consists of disrupted nerve fibers with an intact myelin sheath; neurotmesis, or complete nerve disruption or root avulsion, is most severe. **Erb-Duchenne paralysis** involves the fifth and sixth cervical nerves and is the most common and usually mildest injury. The infant cannot abduct the arm at the shoulder, externally rotate the arm, or supinate the forearm. The usual picture is one of painless adduction, internal rotation of the arm, and pronation of the forearm. The **Moro reflex** is absent on the involved side, and the hand grasp is intact. A **phrenic nerve palsy** (C3, C4, and C5) may lead to diaphragmatic paralysis and respiratory distress. Elevation of the diaphragm caused by nerve injury must be differentiated from elevation caused by eventration resulting from congenital weakness or absence of diaphragm muscle. **Klumpke paralysis** is caused by injury to the seventh and eighth cervical nerves and the first thoracic nerve, resulting in a paralyzed hand and, if the sympathetic nerves are injured, an ipsilateral *Horner syndrome* (ptosis, miosis). Complete arm and hand paralysis is noted with the most severe form of damage to C5, C6, C7, C8, and T1. *Treatment* of brachial plexus injury is supportive and includes positioning to avoid contractures. Active and passive range of motion exercises also may be beneficial. If the deficit persists, nerve grafting may be beneficial.

Facial nerve injury may be the result of compression of the seventh nerve between the facial bone and the mother's pelvic bones or the physician's forceps. This peripheral nerve injury is characterized by an asymmetric, crying face whose normal side, including the forehead, moves in a regular manner. The affected side is flaccid, the eye does not close, the nasolabial fold is absent, and the side of the mouth droops at rest. If there is a central injury to the facial nerve, only the lower two thirds of the face (not the forehead) are involved. Complete agenesis of the facial nucleus results in a central facial paralysis; when this is bilateral, as in **Möbius syndrome**, the face appears expressionless.

Fractures of the cranium are rare, are usually linear, and require no treatment other than observation for very rare, delayed (1 to 3 months) complications (e.g., leptomeningeal cyst). Depressed **skull** fractures are unusual, but may be seen with complicated forceps delivery; they may need surgical elevation. Fractures of the **clavicle** usually are unilateral and are noted in macrosomic infants after shoulder dystocia. Often a snap is heard after a difficult delivery, and the infant exhibits an asymmetric Moro response and decreased movement of the affected side. The prognosis is excel-lent; many infants require no treatment or a **simple figure of eight bandage to immobilize the bone**.

Extremity fractures are less common than fractures of the clavicle and involve the humerus more often than the femur. *Treatment* involves immobilization and a triangular splint bandage for the humerus and traction suspension of the legs for femoral fractures. The *prognosis* is excellent.

Fractures of the **facial bones** are rare, but dislocation of the cartilaginous part of the nasal septum out of the vomeral groove and columella is common. *Clinical manifestations* include feeding difficulty, respiratory distress, asymmetric nares, and a flattened, laterally displaced nose. *Treatment* reduces the dislocation by elevating the cartilage back into the vomeral groove.

Visceral trauma to the liver, spleen, or adrenal gland is noted in macrosomic infants and in extremely premature infants, with or without breech or vaginal delivery. Rupture of the liver with subcapsular hematoma formation may lead to anemia, hypovolemia, shock, hemoperitoneum, and DIC. Infants with anemia and shock who are suspected to have an intraventricular hemorrhage (IVH) but who have normal findings with head ultrasound examination should be evaluated for hepatic or splenic rupture. Adrenal hemorrhage may be asymptomatic, as noted by a high incidence of normal infants with calcified adrenal glands. Infants with severe adrenal hemorrhage may exhibit a flank mass, jaundice, and hematuria, with or without shock.

Temperature Regulation

In utero thermoregulation of the fetus is performed by the placenta, which acts as an efficient heat exchanger. Fetal temperature is nonetheless higher than the mother's temperature. If maternal temperature becomes elevated during a febrile illness or on exposure to environmental heat, fetal temperature increases further. The immediate temperature at birth of an infant born to a febrile mother with chorioamnionitis is elevated regardless of the presence of infection in the infant, unless the infant has cooled in the delivery room.

After birth, a newborn begins life covered by amniotic fluid and situated in a cold environment (20°C to 25°C). An infant's skin temperature may decrease 0.3°C/min, and the core temperature may decrease 0.1°C/min in the delivery room. In the absence of an external heat source, the infant must increase metabolism substantially to maintain body temperature.

Heat loss occurs through four basic mechanisms. In the cold delivery room, the wet infant loses heat predominantly by **evaporation** (cutaneous and respiratory loss when wet or in low humidity), *radiation* (loss to nearby cold, solid surfaces), and **convection** (loss to air current). When the infant is dry, radiation, convection, and **conduction** (loss to object in direct contact with infant) are important causes of heat loss. After birth, all high-risk infants should be dried immediately to eliminate evaporative heat losses (Table 58–14). A radiant or convective heat source should be provided for these high-risk infants. Normal term infants should be dried and wrapped in a blanket.

The ideal environmental temperature is the **neutral thermal environment**, the ambient temperature that results in the lowest rate of heat being produced by the infant and maintains normal body temperature. The neutral thermal environmental temperature decreases with increasing gestational age and increasing postnatal age. Ambient temperatures less than the neutral thermal environment first result in increasing rates of oxygen consumption for heat production, which is designed to maintain normal body temperature. If the ambient temperature decreases further or if oxygen consumption cannot increase sufficiently (owing to hypoxia, hypoglycemia, or drugs), the core body temperature decreases.

Heat production by a newborn is created predominantly by *nonshivering thermogenesis* from chemical reactions of ATP hydrolysis in specialized areas of tissue containing brown adipose tissue. Brown fat is highly vascular, contains many mitochondria per cell, and is situated around large blood vessels, resulting in rapid heat transfer to the circulation. The vessels of the neck, thorax, and interscapular region are common locations of brown fat. These tissues also are innervated by the sympathetic nervous system, which serves as a primary stimulus for heat production by brown adipose cells. Shivering does not occur in newborns.

TABLE 58–14.   General Management Strategies for Sick Newborns

Procedure	Rationale
Warmth in a neutral thermal environment	Avoids cold stress, minimizes oxygen consumption
Humidification	Reduces insensible water losses
Intravenous fluids and glucose	Maintains fluid balance, avoids dehydration, prevents hyperbilirubinemia, prevents prerenal azotemia, prevents hypoglycemia, provides supplemental calories to support oxygen consumption
Oxygen	Treats hypoxia, supports oxygen consumption, prevents cell injury and death
Monitor blood gases and arterial oxygen saturation	Avoids hyperoxic retinal injury and hypoxic brain injury, guides treatment with mechanical ventilation

---

Severe *cold injury* in an infant is manifested by acidosis, hypoxia, hypoglycemia, apnea, bradycardia, pulmonary hemorrhage, and a pink skin color. The color is caused not by adequate oxygenation, but rather by trapping of oxygenated hemoglobin in the cutaneous capillaries. Many of these infants appear dead, but most respond to treatment and recover. Milder degrees of cold injury in the delivery room may contribute to metabolic acidosis and hypoxia after birth. Conversely, hypoxia delays heat generation in cold-stressed infants.

Treatment of severe hypothermia should involve resuscitation and rapid warming of core (e.g., lung and stomach) and external surfaces. Fluid resuscitation also is needed to treat the hypovolemia seen in many of these infants. Reduced core temperature (32°C to 35°C) in the immediate newborn period often requires only external warming with a radiant warmer, incubator, or both.

Elevated Temperature

Exposure to ambient temperatures above the neutral thermal environment results in *heat stress* and an elevated core temperature. Sweating is uncommon in newborns and may be noted only on the forehead. In response to moderate heat stress, however, infants may increase their respiratory rate to dissipate heat. Excessive environmental temperatures may result in heatstroke or in hemorrhagic shock encephalopathy syndrome.

MISCELLANEOUS DISORDERS

Hypocalcemia

Hypocalcemia is common in sick and premature newborns. Most infants are born with calcium levels that are higher in cord blood than in maternal blood because of active placental transfer of calcium to the fetus. Fetal calcium accretion in the third trimester approaches 150 mg/kg/24 hr, and fetal bone mineral content doubles between 30 and 40 weeks of gestation. All infants show a slight decline of serum calcium levels after birth; the decline reaches trough levels at 24 to 48 hours, the point at which hypocalcemia usually occurs. Total serum calcium levels of less than 7 mg/dL and ionized calcium levels of less than 3 to 3.5 mg/dL are considered hypocalcemic.

The *etiology* of hypocalcemia varies with the time of onset and the associated illnesses of the child. **Early neonatal hypocalcemia** occurs in the first 3 days of life and is often asymptomatic. Transient hypoparathyroidism and a reduced parathyroid response to the usual postnatal decline of serum calcium levels may be responsible for hypocalcemia in premature infants and infants of diabetic mothers. Congenital absences of the parathyroid gland and DiGeorge syndrome also have been associated with hypocalcemia. *Hypomagnesemia*

(<1.5 mg/dL) may be seen simultaneously with hypocalcemia, especially in infants of diabetic mothers. Treatment with calcium alone does not relieve symptoms or increase serum calcium levels; for this to occur, the hypomagnesemia also must be treated. Sodium bicarbonate therapy, phosphate release from cell necrosis, transient hypoparathyroidism, and hypercalcitoninemia may be responsible for early neonatal hypocalcemia associated with asphyxia. Early-onset hypocalcemia associated with asphyxia often occurs with seizures as a result of hypoxic-ischemic encephalopathy or hypocalcemia. **Late neonatal hypocalcemia**, or **neonatal tetany**, often is the result of ingestion of high phosphate–containing milk or of the inability to excrete the usual phosphorus in commercial infant formula. Hyperphosphatemia (>8 mg/dL) usually occurs in infants with hypocalcemia after the first week of life. Vitamin D deficiency states and malabsorption also have been associated with late-onset hypocalcemia.

The *clinical manifestations* of hypocalcemia and hypomagnesemia include apnea, muscle twitching, seizures, laryngospasm, **Chvostek sign** (facial muscle spasm when the side of the face over the seventh nerve is tapped), and **Trousseau sign** (carpopedal spasm induced by partial inflation of a blood pressure cuff). The latter two signs are rare in the immediate newborn period. Occasionally, heart failure has been associated with hypocalcemia.

Neonatal hypocalcemia may be *prevented* by administration of IV or oral calcium supplementation at a rate of 25 to 75 mg/kg/24 hr. Early asymptomatic hypocalcemia of preterm infants and infants of diabetic mothers often resolves spontaneously. Symptomatic hypocalcemia should be treated with 2 to 4 mL/kg of 10% calcium gluconate given intravenously and slowly over 10 to 15 minutes, followed by a continuous infusion of 75 mg/kg/24 hr of elemental calcium. If hypomagnesemia is associated with hypocalcemia, 50% magnesium sulfate, 0.1 mL/kg, should be given by IM injection and repeated every 8 to 12 hours.

The *treatment* of late hypocalcemia includes immediate management, as in early hypocalcemia, plus the initiation of feedings with formula containing low phosphate levels. Subcutaneous infiltration of IV calcium salts can cause tissue necrosis; oral supplements are hypertonic and may irritate the intestinal mucosa.

Neonatal Drug Addiction and Withdrawal

Infants may become passively and physiologically addicted to medications or to drugs of abuse (heroin, methadone, barbiturates, tranquilizers, amphetamines) taken chronically by the mother during pregnancy; these infants subsequently may have signs and symptoms of drug withdrawal. Many of these pregnancies are at high risk for other complications related to IV drug abuse, such as hepatitis, AIDS, and syphilis. In addition, the LBW rate and the long-term risk for sudden infant death syndrome are higher in the infants of these high-risk women.

Opiates

Neonatal withdrawal signs and symptoms usually begin at 1 to 5 days of life with maternal heroin use and at 1 to 4 weeks with maternal methadone addiction. *Clinical manifestations* of withdrawal include sneezing, yawning, ravenous appetite, emesis, diarrhea, fever, diaphoresis, tachypnea, high-pitched cry, tremors, jitteriness, poor sleep, poor feeding, and seizures. The illness tends to be more severe during methadone withdrawal. The initial *treatment* includes swaddling in blankets in a quiet, dark room. When hyperactivity is constant, and irritability interferes with sleeping and feeding, or when diarrhea or seizures are present, pharmacologic treatment is indicated. Seizures usually are treated with phenobarbital. The other symptoms may be managed with replacement doses of a narcotic (usually tincture of opium) to calm the infant; weaning from narcotics may be prolonged over 1 to 2 months.

Cocaine

Cocaine use during pregnancy is associated with preterm labor, abruptio placentae, neonatal irritability, and decreased attentiveness. Infants may be SGA and have small head circumferences. Usually no treatment is needed.

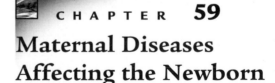

CHAPTER 59

Maternal Diseases Affecting the Newborn

Maternal diseases presenting during pregnancy can affect the fetus directly or indirectly (Table 59–1). Autoantibody-mediated diseases can have direct consequences on the fetus and neonate because the antibodies are usually of the IgG type and can cross the placenta to the fetal circulation.

ANTIPHOSPHOLIPID SYNDROME

Antiphospholipid syndrome is associated with thrombophilia and recurrent pregnancy loss. Antiphospholipid antibodies are found in 2% to 5% of the general healthy

TABLE 59–1.   Maternal Disease Affecting the Fetus or Neonate

Disorder	Effects	Mechanism
Cyanotic heart disease	Intrauterine growth restriction	Low fetal oxygen delivery
Diabetes mellitus		
Mild	Large for gestational age, hypoglycemia	Fetal hyperglycemia—produces hyperinsulinemia; insulin promotes growth
Severe	Growth retardation	Vascular disease, placental insufficiency
Drug addiction	Intrauterine growth restriction, neonatal withdrawal	Direct drug effect, plus poor diet
Endemic goiter	Hypothyroidism	Iodine deficiency
Graves disease	Transient thyrotoxicosis	Placental immunoglobulin passage of thyrotropin receptor antibody
Hyperparathyroidism	Hypocalcemia	Maternal calcium crosses to fetus and suppresses fetal parathyroid gland
Hypertension	Intrauterine growth restriction, intrauterine fetal demise	Placental insufficiency, fetal hypoxia
Idiopathic thrombocytopenia	Thrombocytopenia	Nonspecific platelet antibodies cross placenta
Infection	Neonatal sepsis (see Chapter 66)	Transplacental or ascending infection
Isoimmune neutropenia or thrombocytopenia	Neutropenia or thrombocytopenia	Specific antifetal neutrophil or platelet antibody crosses placenta after sensitization of mother
Malignant melanoma	Placental or fetal tumor	Metastasis
Myasthenia gravis	Transient neonatal myasthenia	Immunoglobulin to acetylcholine receptor crosses the placenta
Myotonic dystrophy	Neonatal myotonic dystrophy	Autosomal dominant with genetic anticipation
PKU	Microcephaly, retardation, ventricular septal defect	Elevated fetal phenylalanine levels
Rh or other blood group sensitization	Fetal anemia, hypoalbuminemia, hydrops, neonatal jaundice	Antibody crosses placenta directed at fetal cells with antigen
Systemic lupus erythematosus	Congenital heart block, rash, anemia, thrombocytopenia, neutropenia, cardiomyopathy, stillbirth	Antibody directed at fetal heart, red and white blood cells, and platelets; lupus anticoagulant

From Stoll BJ, Kliegman RM: The fetus and neonatal infant. In Behrman RE, Kliegman RM, Jenson HB (eds): Nelson Textbook of Pediatrics, 16th ed. Philadelphia, WB Saunders, 2000.

population, but also may be associated with systemic lupus erythematosus and other rheumatic diseases. Obstetric complications arise from the prothrombotic effects of the antiphospholipid antibodies on placental function. Vasculopathy, infarction, and thrombosis have been identified in mothers with antiphospholipid syndrome. Antiphospholipid syndrome can include fetal growth impairment, placental insufficiency, maternal preeclampsia, and premature birth. Cases of neonatal thrombosis have been reported, but are rare.

IDIOPATHIC THROMBOCYTOPENIA

Idiopathic thrombocytopenia (ITP) is seen in approximately 1 to 2 per 1000 live births and is an immune process in which antibodies are directed against platelets. Platelet-associated IgG antibodies can cross the placenta and cause thrombocytopenia in the fetus and newborn. The severely thrombocytopenic fetus is at increased risk of intracranial hemorrhage. ITP during pregnancy requires close maternal and fetal management, which is aimed at reducing the risks of life-threatening maternal hemorrhage and trauma to the fetus at delivery. Postnatal management involves observation of the infant's platelet count. For infants who have evidence of hemorrhage, single-donor irradiated platelets may be administered to control the bleeding. The infant may benefit from an infusion of IV immunoglobulin. Neonatal thrombocytopenia usually resolves within 4 to 6 weeks.

SYSTEMIC LUPUS ERYTHEMATOSUS

Immune abnormalities in systemic lupus erythematosus can lead to the production of anti-Ro (SS-A) and anti-La (SS-B) antibodies that can cross the placenta and injure fetal tissue. The most serious complication is damage to the cardiac conducting system, which results in congenital heart block. The heart block observed in association with maternal systemic lupus erythematosus tends to be complete (third degree), although less advanced blocks have been observed. The mortality rate is approximately 20%, and most surviving infants require pacing. Neonatal lupus may occur and is characterized by skin lesions (sharply demarcated erythematous plaques or central atrophic macules with peripheral scaling with predilection for the eyes, face, and scalp), thrombocytopenia, autoimmune hemolysis, and hepatic involvement.

NEONATAL HYPERTHYROIDISM

Graves disease is associated with thyroid-stimulating antibodies. The prevalence of clinical hyperthyroidism in pregnancy has been reported to be about 0.1% to 0.4% and is the most common endocrine disorder during pregnancy after diabetes. Neonatal hyperthyroidism is due to the transplacental passage of thyroid-stimulating antibodies; hyperthyroidism can appear

rapidly within the first 12 to 48 hours. Symptoms may include IUGR, prematurity, goiter (may be cause of tracheal obstruction), exophthalmos, stare, craniosynostosis (usually coronal), flushing, congestive heart failure, tachycardia, arrhythmias, hypertension, hypoglycemia, thrombocytopenia, and hepatosplenomegaly. Treatment includes propylthiouracil, iodine drops, and propranolol. Autoimmune neonatal hyperthyroidism usually resolves in 2 to 4 months.

DIABETES MELLITUS

Diabetes mellitus that develops during pregnancy (*gestational diabetes* is noted in about 5% of women) or diabetes that is present before pregnancy adversely influences fetal and neonatal well-being (Fig. 59–1). The effect of diabetes on the fetus depends in part on the severity of the diabetic state: age of onset of diabetes, duration of treatment with insulin, and presence of vascular disease. Poorly controlled maternal diabetes leads to maternal and fetal hyperglycemia that

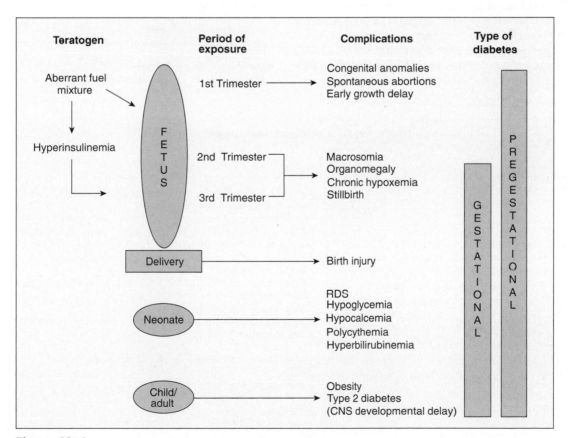

Figure 59–1

Diagrammatic representation of the multiple deleterious effects of the pregnancy of a diabetic patient on the offspring, during various periods of fetal and postnatal life. RDS, respiratory distress syndrome. (From Inzucchi SE: Diabetes in pregnancy. In Burrow GN, Duffy TP [eds]: Medical Complications During Pregnancy, 5th ed. Philadelphia, WB Saunders, 1999.)

stimulates the fetal pancreas, resulting in hyperplasia of the islets of Langerhans. Fetal hyperinsulinemia, which acts as a fetal growth hormone in the last trimester, results in increased fat and protein synthesis and fetal macrosomia, producing a fetus who is LGA. After birth, hyperinsulinemia persists, resulting in fasting neonatal hypoglycemia. Strictly controlling maternal diabetes during pregnancy and preventing hyperglycemia during labor and delivery prevent macrosomic fetal growth and neonatal hypoglycemia. Additional problems of the diabetic mother and her fetus and newborn are summarized in Table 59-2.

OTHER CONDITIONS

Other maternal illnesses, such as severe pulmonary disease (cystic fibrosis), cyanotic heart disease, and sickle cell anemia, may reduce oxygen availability to the fetus. Severe hypertensive or diabetic vasculopathy can result in uteroplacental insufficiency. In addition to the fact that the fetus is directly affected by maternal illnesses, the fetus and the newborn may be adversely affected by the medications used to treat the maternal illnesses. These effects may appear as teratogenesis (Table 59-3) or as an adverse metabolic, neurologic, or cardiopulmonary adaptation to extrauterine life (Table 59-4). Acquired infectious diseases of the mother also may affect the fetus or newborn adversely.

TABLE 59-2. Problems of Diabetic Pregnancy

Maternal

Ketoacidosis
Hyperglycemia/hypoglycemia
Nephritis
Preeclampsia
Polyhydramnios
Retinopathy

Neonatal

Birth asphyxia
Birth injury (macrosomia, shoulder dystocia)
Congenital anomalies (lumbosacral dysgenesis—caudal regression)
Congenital heart disease (ventricular and atrial septal defects, transposition of the great arteries, truncus arteriosus, double-outlet right ventricle, coarctation of the aorta)
Hyperbilirubinemia (unconjugated)
Hypocalcemia
Hypoglycemia
Hypomagnesemia
Neurologic disorders (neural tube defects, holoprosencephaly)
Organomegaly
Polycythemia (hyperviscosity)
Renal disorders (double ureter, renal vein thrombosis, hydronephrosis, renal agenesis)
Respiratory distress syndrome
Small left colon syndrome
Transient tachypnea of the newborn

TABLE 59-3. Common Teratogenic Drugs

Drug	Results
Alcohol	Fetal alcohol syndrome, microcephaly, congenital heart disease
Aminopterin	Mesomelia, cranial dysplasia
Coumarin	Hypoplastic nasal bridge, chondrodysplasia punctata
Fluoxetine	Minor malformations, low birth weight, poor neonatal adaptation
Folic acid antagonists*	Neural tube, cardiovascular, renal, and oral cleft defects
Isotretinoin (Accutane) and vitamin A	Facial and ear anomalies, congenital heart disease
Lithium	Ebstein anomaly
Methyl mercury	Microcephaly, blindness, deafness, retardation (Minimata disease)
Misoprostol	Arthrogryposis
Penicillamine	Cutis laxa syndrome
Phenytoin (Dilantin)	Hypoplastic nails, intrauterine growth retardation, typical facies
Radioactive iodine	Fetal hypothyroidism
Radiation	Microcephaly
Stilbestrol (DES)	Vaginal adenocarcinoma during adolescence
Streptomycin	Deafness
Testosterone-like drugs	Virilization of female
Tetracycline	Enamel hypoplasia
Thalidomide	Phocomelia
Toluene (solvent abuse)	Fetal alcohol–like syndrome, preterm labor
Trimethadione	Congenital anomalies, typical facies
Valproate	Spina bifida
Vitamin D	Supravalvular aortic stenosis

*Trimethoprim, triamterene, phenytoin, primidone, phenobarbital, carbamazepine.

TABLE 59–4. Agents Acting on Pregnant Women That May Adversely Affect the Newborn Infant

Agent	Potential Condition(s)
Acebutolol	IUGR, hypotension, bradycardia
Acetazolamide	Metabolic acidosis
Adrenal corticosteroids	Adrenocortical failure (rare)
Amiodarone	Bradycardia, hypothyroidism
Anesthetic agents (volatile)	CNS depression
Aspirin	Neonatal bleeding, prolonged gestation
Atenolol	IUGR, hypoglycemia
Blue cohosh herbal tea	Neonatal heart failure
Bromides	Rash, CNS depression, IUGR
Captopril, enalapril	Transient anuric renal failure, oligohydramnios
Caudal-paracervical anesthesia with mepivacaine (accidental introduction of anesthetic into scalp of infant)	Bradypnea, apnea, bradycardia, convulsions
Cholinergic agents (edrophonium, pyridostigmine)	Transient muscle weakness
CNS depressants (narcotics, barbiturates, benzodiazepines) during labor	CNS depression, hypotonia
Cephalothin	Positive direct Coombs test reaction
Fluoxetine	Possible transient neonatal withdrawal, hypertonicity, minor anomalies
Haloperidol	Withdrawal
Hexamethonium bromide	Paralytic ileus
Ibuprofen	Oligohydramnios, PPHN
Imipramine	Withdrawal
Indomethacin	Oliguria, oligohydramnios, intestinal perforation, PPHN
IV fluids during labor (e.g., salt-free solutions)	Electrolyte disturbances, hyponatremia, hypoglycemia
Iodide (radioactive)	Goiter
Iodides	Neonatal goiter
Lead	Reduced intellectual function
Magnesium sulfate	Respiratory depression, meconium plug, hypotonia
Methimazole	Goiter, hypothyroidism
Morphine and its derivatives (addiction)	Withdrawal symptoms (poor feeding, vomiting, diarrhea, restlessness, yawning and stretching, dyspnea and cyanosis, fever and sweating, pallor, tremors, convulsions)
Naphthalene	Hemolytic anemia (in G6PD-deficient infants)
Nitrofurantoin	Hemolytic anemia (in G6PD-deficient infants)
Oxytocin	Hyperbilirubinemia, hyponatremia
Phenobarbital	Bleeding diathesis (vitamin K deficiency), possible long-term reduction in IQ, sedation
Primaquine	Hemolytic anemia (in G6PD-deficient infants)
Propranolol	Hypoglycemia, bradycardia, apnea
Propylthiouracil	Goiter, hypothyroidism
Pyridoxine	Seizures
Reserpine	Drowsiness, nasal congestion, poor temperature stability
Sulfonamides	Interfere with protein binding of bilirubin; kernicterus at low levels of serum bilirubin, hemolysis with G6PD deficiency
Sulfonylurea	Refractory hypoglycemia
Sympathomimetic (tocolytic-β agonist) agents	Tachycardia
Thiazides	Neonatal thrombocytopenia (rare)

G6PD, glucose-6-phosphate dehydrogenase; IUGR, intrauterine growth retardation; PPHN, persistent pulmonary hypertension of the newborn.
From Stoll BJ, Kliegman RM: The fetus and neonatal infant. In Behrman RE, Kliegman RM, Jenson HB (eds): Nelson Textbook of Pediatrics, 16th ed. Philadelphia, WB Saunders, 2000.

CHAPTER 60

Diseases of the Fetus

The principal determinants of fetal disease include the fetal genotype and the maternal in utero environment. Variation in environmental factors rather than the fetal genetics plays a more significant role in determining overall fetal well-being, although a genetically abnormal fetus may not thrive as well or survive. The ability to assess a fetus genetically, biochemically, and physically is greatly enhanced through the development of amniocentesis, fetoscopy, chorionic villus sampling, fetal blood sampling, and real-time ultrasonography. These techniques permit the early diagnosis and recognition of many fetal disorders and the development of therapeutic interventions (see Table 58–5).

INTRAUTERINE GROWTH RETARDATION AND SMALL FOR GESTATIONAL AGE

Fetuses subjected to abnormal maternal, placental, or fetal conditions that restrain growth are a high-risk group and traditionally classified as having IUGR. SGA is used as a synonym for IUGR; however, the terms *IUGR* and *SGA* are not synonymous. IUGR represents a deviation from expected growth patterns. The decreased fetal growth associated with IUGR is an adaptation to unfavorable intrauterine conditions that result in permanent alterations in metabolism, growth, and development. IUGR most frequently occurs with a variety of maternal conditions that are associated with preterm delivery. SGA describes an infant whose birth weight is statistically less than the 10th percentile or 2 SD below the mean birth weight for gestational age. The cause of SGA may be pathologic, as in an infant with IUGR, or nonpathologic, as in an infant who is small but otherwise healthy (Table 60–1).

Only about 50% of IUGR infants are identified before delivery. Measurement and recording of maternal fundal height in conjunction with serial ultrasound assessment of the fetus (growth rate, amniotic fluid volume, malformations, anomalies, and Doppler velocimetry of uterine, placental, and fetal blood flow) can aid detection. When suspected and identified, IUGR and SGA fetuses must be monitored for fetal well-being, and appropriate maternal care needs to be instituted (see Chapter 58).

At birth, infants who are mildly to moderately SGA appear smaller than normal with decreased subcutaneous fat. More severely affected infants may present with a "wasted appearance" with asymmetric findings

TABLE 60–1. Etiologies for Intrauterine Growth Retardation and Small for Gestational Age at Birth

Maternal Factors

Age (young and advanced)
Cigarette smoking
Genetics (short stature, weight)
Illnesses during pregnancy (preeclampsia, severe diabetes, chronic hypertension, connective tissue disease)
Infections (intrauterine)
Lack of good prenatal care
Oligohydramnios
Poor nutrition
Race (African American)

Fetal Factors

Chromosomal abnormality and nonchromosomal syndrome
Congenital infections
Inborn errors of metabolism
Multiple gestations

Maternal Medications

Antimetabolites (methotrexate)
Heavy metals (mercury, lead)
Hydantoin
Narcotics (morphine, methadone)
Steroids (prednisone)
Substance and illicit drug use (alcohol, cocaine)
Warfarin

Placental and Uterine Abnormalities

Abruptio placentae
Abnormal implantation
Abnormal placental vessels
Chorioangioma
Circumvallate placenta
Fetal vessel thrombosis
Ischemic villous necrosis
Multiple gestations
True knots in umbilical cord
Villitis (congenital infection)

including larger heads for the size of the body (CNS sparing), widened anterior fontanels, small abdomen, thin arms and legs, decreased subcutaneous fat, dry and redundant skin, decreased muscle mass, and thin (often meconium-stained) umbilical cord. Gestational age is often difficult to assess when based on physical appearance and perceived advanced neurologic maturity. Physical examination should detail the presence of dysmorphic features, abnormal extremities, or gross anomalies that might suggest underlying congenital malformations, chromosomal defects, or exposure to teratogens. Hepatosplenomegaly, jaundice, and skin rashes in addition to ocular disorders, such as chorioretinitis, cataracts, glaucoma, and cloudy cornea, suggest the presence of a congenital infection or inborn error of metabolism.

Infants with severe IUGR or SGA, particularly in conjunction with fetal distress, may have problems at birth that include respiratory acidosis, metabolic acidosis, asphyxia, hypoxemia, hypotension, hypoglycemia, polycythemia, meconium aspiration syndrome, and PPHN (see Table 58–4).

Management of IUGR and SGA infants is usually symptomatic and supportive. The diagnostic evaluation at birth should be directed at identifying the cause of the IUGR and SGA if possible. The consequences of IUGR and SGA depend on the etiology, severity, and duration of growth retardation. Mortality rates of infants severely affected are 5 to 20 times the mortality rates of infants who are appropriate for gestational age. Postnatal growth and development depend in part on the etiology, the postnatal nutritional intake, and the social environment. Infants who have IUGR and SGA secondary to congenital infection, chromosomal abnormalities, or constitutional syndromes remain small throughout life. Infants who have growth inhibited late in gestation because of uterine contraints, placental insufficiency, or poor nutrition have catch-up growth and approach their inherited growth and development potential under optimal environmental conditions.

HYDROPS FETALIS

Hydrops fetalis is a condition caused by immune and nonimmune conditions. Hydrops fetalis is a fetal clinical condition of excessive fluid accumulation in the skin and one or more other body compartments, including the pleural space, peritoneal cavity, pericardial sac, or placenta with resultant high morbidity and mortality. Hydrops initially was described in association with Rhesus blood group isoimmunization. With the advent of Rho (D) immune globulin, there has been a decline in the incidence of isoimmune fetal hydrops. Concurrently the incidence of nonimmune hydrops has increased as a cause of this severe clinical condition.

The pathophysiology for the formation of fetal hydrops is an imbalance of interstitial fluid accumulation and decreased removal of fluid by the capillaries and lymphatic system. Fluid accumulation can be secondary to congestive heart failure, obstructed lymphatic flow, or decreased plasma oncotic pressure (hypoproteinemic states). Edema formation is the final common pathway for many disease processes that affect the fetus (Table 60–2).

The diagnostic workup of the hydropic fetus should focus on discovering the underlying cause. Clinical,

TABLE 60–2. Causes for Nonimmune Hydrops

Fetal **Cardiac Conditions**	Right heart failure (pulmonary valve atresia/incompetence, Ebstein anomaly) Left heart failure (aortic valve stenosis/atresia, hypoplastic left heart, coarctation of the aorta, truncus arteriosus, endocardial fibroelastosis) Arrhythmia (supraventricular tachyarrhythmia, congenital heart block) Cardiomyopathy
Genetic Abnormalities	Chromosomal abnormalities (Turner syndrome; trisomy 13, 15, 16, 18, 21; Noonan syndrome, tuberous sclerosis; myotonic dystrophy; inborn errors of metabolism)
Malformations	Congenital diaphragmatic hernia, congenital cystic adenomatoid malformation, congenital pulmonary lymphangiectasis, bronchopulmonary sequestration, fetal tumors (cystic hygroma), arteriovenous malformations, chylothorax
Hematologic Conditions	Parvovirus, anemia (fetomaternal and intracranial hemorrhage, hemoglobinopathy, G6PD)
Infectious Conditions	Congenital infection
Endocrine Conditions	Thyrotoxicosis
Maternal	Diabetes mellitus
Placental	Placental chorioangioma and choriocarcinoma, twin-to-twin transfusion
Idiopathic	

G6PD, glucose-6-phosphate dehydrogenase.

laboratory, and ultrasound findings may include *maternal* hypertension, anemia, multiple gestation, thickened placenta, and polyhydramnios, whereas *fetal* findings may include tachycardia, ascites, scalp and body wall edema, and pleural and pericardial effusion. Invasive fetal testing may be indicated. Amniocentesis provides amniotic fluid samples for karyotype, culture, alpha-fetoprotein, and metabolic and enzyme analysis. Percutaneous umbilical cord blood sampling can provide fetal blood for chromosomal analysis and hematologic and metabolic studies and provide a source for intervention (fetal transfusion for profound anemia).

Management depends on the underlying cause of the hydrops and the gestational age of the fetus. Resuscitative efforts at delivery are often required. It is often necessary to remove ascitic fluid from the abdomen or pleural fluid to improve ventilation. Profound anemia necessitates immediate transfusion with packed RBCs.

The overall mortality for infants with nonimmune hydrops is approximately 50%. If the diagnosis is made before 24 weeks of gestation with subsequent premature delivery, the survival rate is approximately 4% to 6%.

CHAPTER 61

Respiratory Diseases of the Newborn

Respiratory distress that becomes manifested by tachypnea, intercostal retractions, reduced air exchange, cyanosis, expiratory grunting, and nasal flaring is a nonspecific response to serious illness. Not all of the disorders producing neonatal respiratory distress are primary diseases of the lungs. The differential diagnosis of respiratory distress includes pulmonary, cardiac, hematologic, infectious, anatomic, and metabolic disorders that may involve the lungs directly or indirectly. Surfactant deficiency causes **RDS**, resulting in cyanosis and tachypnea; *infection* produces pneumonia, shown by interstitial or lobar infiltrates; *meconium aspiration* results in a chemical pneumonitis with hypoxia and pulmonary hypertension; *hydrops fetalis* causes anemia and hypoalbuminemia with high-output heart failure and pulmonary edema; and congenital or acquired *pulmonary hypoplasia* causes pulmonary hypertension and pulmonary insufficiency. It also is clinically useful to differentiate the common causes of respiratory distress according to gestational age (Table 61–1).

In addition to the specific therapy for the individual disorder, the supportive care and evaluation of the infant with respiratory distress can be applied to all the problems mentioned earlier (Table 61–2; see also Table 58–14). Blood gas monitoring and interpretation are key components of general respiratory care.

Treatment of hypoxemia requires knowledge of normal values. In term infants, the arterial PaO_2 level is 55 to 60 mm Hg at 30 minutes of life, 75 mm Hg at 4 hours, and 90 mm Hg at 24 hours. Preterm infants have slightly lower values. $PaCO_2$ levels should be 35 to 40 mm Hg, and the pH should be 7.35 to 7.40. It is imperative that arterial blood gas analysis be performed in all infants with significant respiratory distress, whether or not cyanosis is perceived. Cyanosis becomes

TABLE 61–1. Etiology of Respiratory Distress
Preterm Infant
Respiratory distress syndrome (RDS)*
Erythroblastosis fetalis
Nonimmune hydrops
Pulmonary hemorrhage
Full-Term Infant
Primary pulmonary hypertension of the neonate*
Meconium aspiration pneumonia*
Polycythemia
Amniotic fluid aspiration
Preterm and Full-Term Infant
Bacterial sepsis (GBS)*
Transient tachypnea*
Spontaneous pneumothorax
Congenital anomalies (e.g., congenital lobar emphysema, cystic adenomatoid malformation, diphragmatic hernia)
Congenital heart disease
Pulmonary hypoplasia
Viral infection (e.g., herpes simplex, CMV)
Inborn metabolic errors

*Common.
CMV, cytomegalovirus; GBS, group B streptococcus.

evident when there is 5 g of unsaturated hemoglobin; anemia may interfere with the perception of cyanosis. Jaundice also may interfere with the appearance of cyanosis. Capillary blood gas determinations are useful in determining blood pH and the $PaCO_2$ level. Because of the nature of the heel-stick capillary blood gas technique, venous blood may mix with arterial blood, resulting in falsely low blood PaO_2 readings. Serial blood gas levels may be monitored by an indwelling arterial catheter placed in a peripheral artery or through the umbilical artery to the aorta at the level of the T6-10 or the L4-5 vertebrae. This placement avoids catheter occlusion of the celiac (T12), superior mesenteric (T12-L1), renal (L1-2), and inferior mesenteric (L2-3) arteries. Another method for monitoring blood gas levels is to combine capillary blood gas techniques with noninvasive methods used to monitor oxygen (pulse oximetry or transcutaneous oxygen diffusion).

Metabolic acidosis, defined as a reduced pH (<7.25) and bicarbonate concentration (<18 mEq/L) accompanied by a normal or low PCO_2 level, may be caused by hypoxia or by insufficient tissue perfusion; the origin of the disorder may be pulmonary, cardiac, infectious, renal, hematologic, nutritional, metabolic, or iatrogenic. The initial approach to metabolic acidosis is to determine the cause and treat the pathophysiologic problem. This approach may include, as in the

TABLE 61–2. Initial Laboratory Evaluation of Respiratory Distress

Test	Rationale
Chest radiograph	To determine reticular granular pattern of RDS; to determine presence of pneumothorax, cardiomegaly, life-threatening congenital anomalies
Arterial blood gas	To determine severity of respiratory compromise, hypoxemia, and hypercapnia and type of acidosis; the severity determines treatment strategy
Complete blood count	Hemoglobin/hematocrit to determine anemia and polycythemia; white blood cell count to determine neutropenia/sepsis; platelet count and smear to determine DIC
Blood culture	To recover potential pathogen
Blood glucose	To determine presence of hypoglycemia, which may produce or occur simultaneously with respiratory distress; to determine stress hyperglycemia
Echocardiogram, ECG	In the presence of a murmur, cardiomegaly, or refractory hypoxia; to determine structural heart disease or PPHN

DIC, disseminated intravascular coagulation; PPHN, primary pulmonary hypertension of the newborn; RDS, respiratory distress syndrome.

sequence of therapy for hypoxia, increasing the inspired oxygen concentration; applying continuous positive airway pressure nasally, using oxygen as the gas; or initiating mechanical ventilation using positive end-expiratory pressure and oxygen. Patients with hypotension produced by hypovolemia require fluids and may need inotropic or vasoactive drug support. If metabolic acidosis persists despite specific therapy, sodium bicarbonate (1 mEq/kg/dose) may be given by slow IV infusion. Near-normal or low PCO_2 levels should be documented before sodium bicarbonate infusion. The buffering effect of sodium bicarbonate results in increased PCO_2 levels, unless adequate ventilation is maintained.

Respiratory acidosis, defined as an elevated PCO_2 level and reduced pH without a reduction in the bicarbonate concentration, may be caused by pulmonary insufficiency or central hypoventilation. Most disorders producing respiratory distress can lead to hypercapnia. Treatment involves assisted ventilation but not sodium bicarbonate. If CNS depression of respirations is caused by placental passage of narcotic analgesics, assisted ventilation is instituted first, then the CNS depression is reversed by naloxone.

RESPIRATORY DISTRESS SYNDROME (HYALINE MEMBRANE DISEASE)

RDS occurs after the onset of breathing and is associated with an insufficiency of pulmonary surfactant.

Lung Development

The lining of the alveolus consists of 90% type I cells and 10% type II cells. After 20 weeks of gestation, the type II cells contain vacuolated, osmophilic, lamellar inclusion bodies, which are packages of surface-active material (Fig. 61–1). This lipoprotein surfactant is 90% lipid and is composed predominantly of saturated phosphatidylcholine (lecithin), but also contains phosphatidylglycerol, other phospholipids, and neutral lipids. The surfactant proteins SP-A, SP-B, SP-C, and SP-D are packaged into the lamellar body and contribute to surface-active properties and recycling of surfactant. Surfactant prevents atelectasis by reducing surface tension at low lung volumes when it is concentrated at end expiration as the alveolar radius decreases; surfactant contributes to lung recoil by increasing surface tension at larger lung volumes when it is diluted during inspiration as the alveolar radius increases. Without surfactant, surface tension forces are not reduced, and atelectasis develops during end expiration as the alveolus collapses.

The timing of surfactant (lecithin) production in quantities sufficient to prevent atelectasis depends on an increase in fetal cortisol levels that begins between 32 and 34 weeks of gestation. By 34 to 36 weeks, sufficient surface-active material is produced by the type II cells in the lung, is secreted into the alveolar lumen, and is excreted into the amniotic fluid. The concentration of lecithin in amniotic fluid indicates fetal pulmonary maturity. Because the amount of lecithin is difficult to quantify, the ratio of lecithin (which increases with maturity) to sphingomyelin (which remains constant during gestation) (L/S ratio) is determined. L/S ratio of 2:1 usually indicates pulmonary maturity. The presence of minor phospholipids, such as phosphatidylglycerol, also is indicative of fetal lung maturity and may be useful in situations in which the L/S ratio is borderline or possibly affected by maternal diabetes, which reduces lung maturity. The absence of phosphatidylglycerol suggests that surfactant might not be mature.

Clinical Manifestations

A deficiency of pulmonary surfactant results in atelectasis, decreased functional residual capacity, arterial

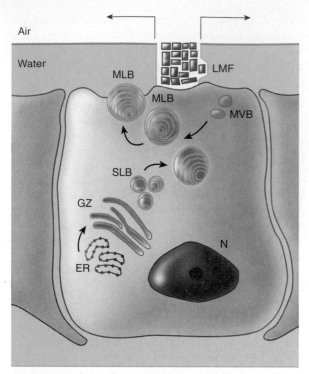

Figure 61–1

Proposed pathway of synthesis, transport, secretion, and reuptake of surfactant in the type II alveolar cell.
Phospholipids are synthesized in the smooth endoplasmic reticulum (ER). The glucose/glycerol precursor may be derived from lung glycogen or circulating glucose. Phospholipids and surfactant proteins are packaged in the Golgi apparatus (GZ), emerge as small lamellar bodies (SLB), coalesce to mature lamellar bodies (MLB), migrate to the apical membrane, and are released by exocytosis into the liquid hypophase below the air-liquid interface. The tightly coiled lamellar body unravels to form the lattice (tubular) myelin figure (LMF), the immediate precursor to the phospholipid monolayer at the alveolar surface. Reuptake by endocytosis forms multivesicular bodies (MVB) that recycle surfactant. The enzymes, receptors, transporters, and surfactant proteins are controlled by regulatory processes at the transcriptional level in the nucleus (N). Corticosteroid and thyroid hormones are regulatory ligands that may accelerate surfactant synthesis. (From Hansen T, Corbet A: Lung development and function. In Taeusch HW, Ballard R, Avery ME [eds]: Diseases of the Newborn, 6th ed. Philadelphia, WB Saunders, 1991, p 465.)

hypoxemia, and respiratory distress. Surfactant synthesis may be reduced as a result of hypovolemia, hypothermia, acidosis, hypoxemia, and rare genetic disorders of surfactant synthesis. These factors also produce pulmonary artery vasospasm, which may contribute to RDS in larger premature infants who have developed sufficient pulmonary arteriole smooth muscle to produce vasoconstriction. Surfactant deficiency–induced atelectasis causes alveoli to be perfused but not ventilated, which results in a pulmonary shunt and hypoxemia. As atelectasis increases, the lungs become increasingly difficult to expand, and lung compliance decreases. Because the chest wall of the premature infant is very compliant, the infant attempts to overcome decreased lung compliance with increasing inspiratory pressures, resulting in retractions of the chest wall. The sequence of decreased lung compliance and chest wall retractions leads to poor air exchange, an increased physiologic dead space, alveolar hypoventilation, and hypercapnia. A cycle of hypoxia, hypercapnia, and acidosis acts on type II cells to reduce surfactant synthesis and, in some infants, on the pulmonary arterioles to produce pulmonary hypertension.

Infants at greatest risk for RDS are premature and have an immature L/S ratio. The incidence of RDS increases with decreasing gestational age. RDS develops in 30% to 60% of infants between 28 and 32 weeks of gestation. Other risk factors include delivery of a previous preterm infant with RDS, maternal diabetes, hypothermia, fetal distress, asphyxia, male sex, white race, being the second born of twins, and delivery by cesarean section without labor.

RDS may develop immediately in the delivery room in extremely immature infants at 26 to 30 weeks of gestation. Some more mature infants (34 weeks' gestation) may not show signs of RDS until 3 to 4 hours after birth, correlating with the initial release of stored surfactant at the onset of breathing accompanied by the ongoing inability to replace the surfactant owing to inadequate stores. *Manifestations* of RDS include cyanosis, tachypnea, nasal flaring, intercostal and sternal retractions, and grunting. **Grunting** is caused by closure of the glottis during expiration, the effect of which is to maintain lung volume (decreasing atelectasis) and gas exchange during exhalation. Atelectasis is well documented by radiographic examination of the chest, which shows a ground-glass haze in the lung surrounding air-filled bronchi (the air bronchogram) (Fig. 61–2). Severe RDS may show an airless lung field or a "whiteout" on a radiograph, even obliterating the distinction between the atelectatic lungs and the heart.

During the first 72 hours, infants with RDS have increasing distress and hypoxemia. In infants with severe RDS, the development of edema, apnea, and respiratory failure necessitates assisted ventilation. Thereafter, uncomplicated cases show a spontaneous improvement that often is heralded by diuresis and a marked resolution of edema. Complications include the development of a pneumothorax, a PDA, and bronchopulmonary dysplasia (BPD). The differential diagnosis of RDS includes diseases associated with cyanosis and respiratory distress (see Table 58–13).

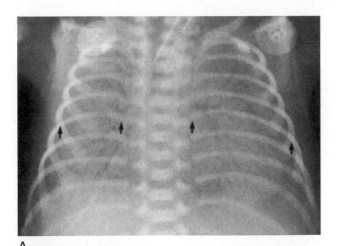

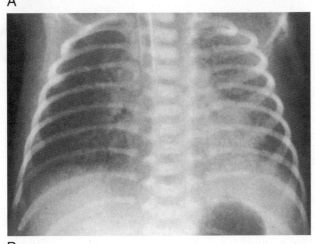

Figure 61–2

Respiratory distress syndrome. The infant is intubated, and the lungs show a dense reticulonodular pattern with air bronchograms **(A)**. To evaluate rotation on the frontal chest, the lengths of the posterior ribs are compared from left to right *(arrows)*. Because the infant is supine, the side of the longer ribs indicates to which side the thorax is rotated. In this case, the left ribs are longer, and this radiograph is a left posterior oblique view. Surfactant was administered, resulting in significant improvement in the density of the lung **(B)**. The right lung is slightly better aerated than the left. Uneven distribution of clearing is common. (From Hilton S, Edwards D: Practical Pediatric Radiology, 2nd ed. Philadelphia, WB Saunders, 1994.)

Prevention and Treatment

Strategies to prevent preterm birth include maternal cervical cerclage, bed rest, treatment of infections, and administration of tocolytic medications. Additionally, prevention of neonatal cold stress, birth asphyxia, and hypovolemia reduces the risk of RDS. If premature delivery is unavoidable, the antenatal administration of corticosteroids (e.g., betamethasone) to the mother (and thus to the fetus) stimulates fetal lung production of surfactant; this approach requires multiple doses for at least 48 hours.

After birth, RDS may be prevented or its severity reduced by intratracheal administration of exogenous surfactant immediately after birth in the delivery room or within a few hours of birth. A mammalian-derived surfactant is currently preferred. Exogenous surfactant can be administered repeatedly during the course of RDS in patients receiving endotracheal intubation, mechanical ventilation, and oxygen therapy. Additional management includes the general supportive and ventilation care presented in Tables 58–14, 61–2, and 61–3.

The PaO_2 level should be maintained between 60 and 70 mm Hg (oxygen saturation 90%), and the pH should be maintained greater than 7.25. An increased concentration of warm and humidified inspired oxygen administered by an oxygen hood or nasal cannula may be all that is needed for larger premature infants. If hypoxemia (PaO_2 <50 mm Hg) is present, and the needed inspired oxygen concentration is 70% to 100%, nasal continuous positive airway pressure should be added at a distending pressure of 8 to 10 cm H_2O. If respiratory failure ensues (PCO_2 >60 mm Hg, pH <7.20, and PaO_2 <50 mm Hg with 100% oxygen), assisted ventilation using a respirator is indicated. Conventional rate (25 to 60 breaths/min), high-frequency jet (150 to 600 breaths/min), and oscillator (900 to 3000 breaths/min) ventilators all have been successful in managing respiratory failure caused by severe RDS. Suggested starting settings on a conventional ventilator are fraction of inspired oxygen, 60% to 100%; peak inspiratory pressure, 20 to 25 cm H_2O; positive end-expiratory pressure, +5 cm H_2O; and respiratory rate, 30 to 50 breaths/min.

In response to persistent hypercapnia, alveolar ventilation (tidal volume – dead space × rate) must be increased. Ventilation can be increased by an increase in the ventilator's rate or an increase in the tidal volume, which is the gradient between peak inspiratory pressure and positive end-expiratory pressure. In response to hypoxia, the inspired oxygen content may be increased. Alternatively, the degree of oxygenation depends on the mean airway pressure. Mean airway pressure is directly related to peak inspiratory pressure, positive end-expiratory pressure, flow, and inspiratory-to-expiratory ratio. Increased mean airway pressure may improve oxygenation by improving lung volume, enhancing ventilation-perfusion matching. Because of the difficulty in distinguishing sepsis and pneumonia from RDS, broad-spectrum parenteral antibiotics (ampicillin and gentamicin) are administered for 48 to 72 hours, pending the recovery of an organism from a previously obtained blood culture.

TABLE 61–3. Ventilator Management of Respiratory Distress Syndrome			
Setting	**Result**	**Rationale**	**Risks**
↑ FIO_2	↑ PO_2	↑ Alveolar O_2	Oxygen toxicity
↑ PIP	↑ PO_2	↑ Paw	Pneumothorax, barotrauma, ↓ cardiac output?
	↓ PCO_2	↑ Tidal volume	
↑ PEEP	↑ PO_2	↑ Paw	↑ PCO_2 by ↓ tidal volume
			↓ Cardiac output?
↑ Rate	↓ PCO_2	↑ Alveolar ventilation	↓ Expiratory time causes gas trapping
↑ I : E ratio	↑ PO_2	↑ Paw	↓ Expiratory time causes gas trapping

FIO_2, fraction of inspired oxygen; I : E, inspiratory-to-expiratory time ratio; Paw, mean airway pressure; PEEP, positive end-expiratory pressure; PIP, peak inspiratory pressure.

COMPLICATIONS OF RESPIRATORY DISTRESS SYNDROME

Complications of RDS include clinical conditions associated with prematurity in general and conditions that arise as complications of therapy.

Patent Ductus Arteriosus

PDA is a common complication that occurs in many LBW infants who have RDS. The incidence of PDA is inversely related to the maturity of the infant. In term newborns, the ductus closes within 24 to 48 hours after birth. In preterm newborns, the ductus frequently fails to close, however, requiring medical or surgical closure. The ductus arteriosus in a preterm infant is less responsive to vasoconstrictive stimuli, which when complicated with hypoxemia during RDS, may lead to a persistent PDA that creates a shunt between the pulmonary and systemic circulations.

During the acute phase of RDS, hypoxia, hypercapnia, and acidosis lead to pulmonary arterial vasoconstriction and increased pressure. The pulmonary and systemic pressures may be equal, and flow through the ductus may be small or bidirectional. When RDS improves and pulmonary vascular resistance declines, flow through the ductus arteriosus increases in a left-to-right direction. Significant systemic-to-pulmonary shunting may lead to heart failure and pulmonary edema. Excessive IV fluid administration may increase the incidence of symptomatic PDA. The infant's respiratory status deteriorates because of increased lung fluid, hypercapnia, and hypoxemia. In response to poor blood gas levels, the infant is subjected to higher inspired oxygen concentrations and higher peak inspiratory ventilator pressures, both of which can damage the lung and cause chronic lung disease.

Clinical manifestations of a PDA usually become apparent on day 2 to 4 of life. Because the left-to-right shunt directs flow to a low-pressure circulation from one of high pressure, the pulse pressure widens; a previously inactive precordium now shows an extremely active precordial impulse, and the peripheral pulses become easily palpable and bounding. The murmur of a PDA may be continuous in systole and diastole, but usually only the systolic component is auscultated. Heart failure and pulmonary edema result in rales and hepatomegaly. A chest radiograph shows cardiomegaly and pulmonary edema; a two-dimensional echocardiogram shows patency, whereas Doppler studies show markedly increased left-to-right flow through the ductus.

Treatment of a PDA during RDS involves an initial period of fluid restriction and diuretic administration. If there is no improvement after 24 to 48 hours, indomethacin, a prostaglandin synthetase inhibitor, is administered (0.2 mg/kg) intravenously every 12 to 24 hours for three doses. Contraindications to using indomethacin include thrombocytopenia (platelets <50,000/mm³), bleeding, serum creatinine measuring more than 1.8 mg/dL, and oliguria. Because 20% to 30% of infants do not respond initially to indomethacin and because the PDA reopens in 10% to 20% of infants who do, a repeat course of indomethacin or surgical ligation is required in some patients.

Pulmonary Air Leaks

Assisted ventilation with high peak inspiratory pressures and positive end-expiratory pressures may cause overdistention of alveoli in localized areas of the lung. Rupture of the alveolar epithelial lining may produce pulmonary interstitial emphysema as gas dissects along the interstitial space and the peribronchial lymphatics. Extravasation of gas into the parenchyma reduces lung compliance and worsens respiratory failure. Gas dissection into the mediastinal space produces a pneumomediastinum, occasionally with gas

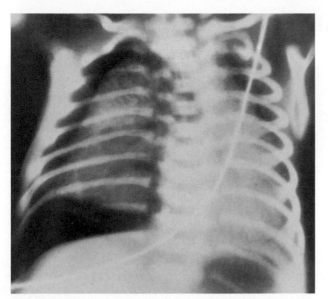

Figure 61–3

Pneumothorax. Right-sided hyperlucent pleural air is obvious. The findings of linear interstitial air and the resultant noncompliant but collapsed right lung are noted. (From Heller R, Kirchner S: Advanced Exercises in Diagnostic Radiology: The Newborn, Philadelphia, WB Saunders, 1979.)

dissecting into the subcutaneous tissues around the neck, causing subcutaneous emphysema.

Alveolar rupture adjacent to the pleural space produces a pneumothorax. If the gas is under tension, the pneumothorax shifts the mediastinum to the opposite side of the chest, producing hypotension, hypoxia, and hypercapnia. The diagnosis of a pneumothorax may be based on unequal transillumination of the chest and may be confirmed by chest radiograph (Fig. 61–3). Treatment of a symptomatic pneumothorax requires insertion of a pleural chest tube connected to negative pressure or to an underwater drain. Prophylactic or therapeutic use of exogenous surfactant has reduced the incidence of pulmonary air leaks.

Pneumothorax also is observed after vigorous resuscitation, meconium aspiration pneumonia, pulmonary hypoplasia, and diaphragmatic hernia. Spontaneous pneumothorax is seen in less than 1% of deliveries and may be associated with renal malformations.

Bronchopulmonary Dysplasia (Chronic Lung Disease)

BPD is a clinical diagnosis defined by oxygen dependence at 36 weeks' postconceptual age and accompanied by characteristic clinical and radiographic findings that correspond to anatomic abnormalities. Oxygen concentrations greater than 40% are toxic to the neonatal lung. Oxygen-mediated lung injury results from the generation of superoxides, hydrogen peroxide, and oxygen free radicals, which disrupt membrane lipids. Assisted ventilation with high peak pressures produces barotrauma, compounding the damaging effects of highly inspired oxygen levels. In most patients, BPD develops after ventilation for RDS that may have been complicated by PDA or pulmonary interstitial emphysema. Inflammation from prolonged assisted ventilation and repeated systemic and pulmonary infections may play a major role. Failure of RDS to improve after 2 weeks, the need for prolonged mechanical ventilation, and oxygen therapy required at 36 weeks' postconception age are characteristic of patients with RDS in whom BPD develops. BPD also may develop in infants weighing less than 1000 g who require mechanical ventilation for poor respiratory drive in the absence of RDS. Fifty percent of infants of 24 to 26 weeks' gestational age require oxygen at 36 weeks' corrected age.

The **radiographic appearance** of BPD may involve phases that are characterized initially by lung opacification and subsequently by development of cysts accompanied by areas of overdistention and atelectasis, giving the lung a spongelike appearance. The histopathology of BPD reveals interstitial edema, atelectasis, mucosal metaplasia, interstitial fibrosis, necrotizing obliterative bronchiolitis, and overdistended alveoli.

The **clinical manifestations** of BPD are oxygen dependence, hypercapnia, compensatory metabolic alkalosis, pulmonary hypertension, poor growth, and development of right-sided heart failure. Increased airway resistance with reactive airway bronchoconstriction also is noted and is treated with bronchodilating agents. Severe chest retractions produce negative interstitial pressure that draws fluid into the interstitial space. Together with cor pulmonale, these chest retractions cause fluid retention, necessitating fluid restriction and the administration of diuretics.

Patients with severe BPD may need treatment with mechanical ventilation for many months. To reduce the risk of subglottic stenosis, a tracheotomy may be indicated. To reduce oxygen toxicity and barotrauma, ventilator settings are reduced to maintain blood gases with slightly lower PaO_2 (50 mm Hg) and higher $PaCO_2$ (50 to 75 mm Hg) levels than for infants during the acute phase of RDS. Dexamethasone therapy may reduce inflammation, improve pulmonary function, and enhance weaning of patients from assisted ventilation. Dexamethasone may increase the risk, however, of cerebral palsy or abnormal neuromotor developmental outcome. Older survivors of BPD have hyperinflation, reactive airways, and developmental delay. They are at risk for severe respiratory syncytial virus pneumonia and as infants should receive prophylaxis against respiratory syncytial virus.

Retinopathy of Prematurity (Retrolental Fibroplasia)

Retinopathy of prematurity (ROP) is caused by the acute and chronic effects of oxygen toxicity on the developing blood vessels of the premature infant's retina. The completely vascularized retina of the term infant is not susceptible to ROP. ROP is a leading cause of blindness for VLBW infants (<1500 g). Excessive arterial oxygen tensions produce vasoconstriction of the immature retinal vasculature in the first stage of this disease. The vasoconstriction is followed by vaso-obliteration if the duration and extent of hyperoxia are prolonged beyond the time when vasoconstriction is reversible. Hypercarbia and hypoxia may contribute to ROP. The subsequent proliferative stages are characterized by extraretinal fibrovascular proliferation, forming a ridge between the vascular and avascular portions of the retina, and by the development of neovascular tufts. In mild cases, vasoproliferation is noted at the periphery of the retina. Severe cases may have neovascularization involving the entire retina, retinal detachment resulting from traction on vessels as they leave the optic disc, fibrous proliferation behind the lens producing leukokoria, and synechiae displacing the lens forward and leading to glaucoma. Both eyes usually are involved, but severity may be asymmetric.

The incidence of ROP may be reduced by careful monitoring of arterial blood gas levels in all patients receiving oxygen. Although there is no absolutely safe PaO_2 level, it is wise to keep the arterial oxygen level between 50 and 70 mm Hg in premature infants. Infants who weigh less than 1500 g or who are born before 28 weeks' gestational age (some authors say 32 weeks) should be screened when they are 4 weeks old or more than 34 weeks' corrected gestational age, whichever comes first. Laser therapy or (less often) cryotherapy may be used for vitreous hemorrhage or for severe, progressive vasoproliferation. Surgery is indicated for retinal detachment. Less severe stages of ROP resolve spontaneously and without visual impairment in most patients.

Transient Tachypnea of the Newborn

Transient tachypnea of the newborn is a self-limited condition characterized by tachypnea, mild retractions, hypoxia, and occasional grunting, usually without signs of severe respiratory distress. Cyanosis, when present, usually requires treatment with supplemental oxygen in the range of 30% to 40%. Transient tachypnea of the newborn usually is noted in larger premature infants and in term infants born by precipitious delivery or cesarean section without prior labor. Infants of diabetic mothers and infants with poor respiratory drive as a result of placental passage of analgesic drugs are at risk. Chest radiographs show prominent central vascular markings, fluid in the lung fissures, overaeration, and occasionally a small pleural effusion. Air bronchograms and a reticulogranular pattern are not seen in transient tachypnea of the newborn, and their presence suggests another pulmonary process, such as RDS or pneumonia. Transient tachypnea of the newborn may be caused by retained lung fluid or slow resorption of lung fluid.

Meconium Aspiration Syndrome

Meconium-stained amniotic fluid is seen in 15% of predominantly term and post-term deliveries. Although the passage of meconium into amniotic fluid is common in infants born in the breech presentation, meconium-stained fluid should be considered clinically as a sign of fetal distress for all infants. The presence of meconium in the amniotic fluid suggests in utero distress with asphyxia, hypoxia, and acidosis.

Aspiration of amniotic fluid contaminated with particulate meconium may occur in utero in a distressed, gasping fetus; more often, meconium is aspirated into the lung immediately after delivery. Affected infants have abnormal chest radiographs, showing a high incidence of pneumonia and pneumothoraces.

Meconium aspiration pneumonia is characterized by tachypnea, hypoxia, hypercapnia, and small airway obstruction causing a ball-valve effect, leading to air trapping, overdistention, and extra-alveolar air leaks. Complete small airway obstruction produces atelectasis. Within 24 to 48 hours, a chemical pneumonia develops in addition to the mechanical effects of airway obstruction. Abnormal pulmonary function may be caused by the meconium in part through inactivation of surfactant. PPHN frequesntly accompanies meconium aspiration with right-to-left shunting caused by increased pulmonary vascular resistance. The chest radiograph reveals patchy infiltrates, overdistention, flattening of the diaphragm, increased anteroposterior diameter, and a high incidence of pneumomediastinum and pneumothoraces. Comorbid diseases include those associated with in utero asphyxia that initiated the passage of meconium.

Treatment of meconium aspiration includes general supportive care and assisted ventilation. Infants with a PPHN-like presentation should be treated for PPHN.

If severe hypoxia does not subside with conventional or high-frequency ventilation, surfactant therapy, and inhaled nitric oxide, extracorporeal membrane oxygenation (ECMO) may be beneficial.

Prevention of meconium aspiration syndrome involves careful in utero monitoring to prevent asphyxia. When meconium-stained fluid is observed, the obstetrician should suction the infant's oropharynx before delivering the rest of the infant's body. If the infant is depressed with poor tone, minimal respiratory effort, and cyanosis, the infant's oropharynx should be suctioned, the vocal cords visualized, and the area below the vocal cords suctioned to remove any meconium from the trachea. This procedure can be repeated two to three times as long as meconium is present, before either stimulating the infant to breathe or initiating assisted ventilation. Saline intrauterine amnioinfusion during labor may reduce the incidence of aspiration and pneumonia.

Primary Pulmonary Hypertension of the Newborn (Persistent Fetal Circulation)

PPHN occurs in post-term, term, or near-term infants. PPHN is characterized by severe hypoxemia, without evidence of parenchymal lung or structural heart disease that also may cause right-to-left shunting. PPHN is often seen with asphyxia or meconium-stained fluid. The chest radiograph usually reveals normal lung fields rather than the expected infiltrates and hyperinflation that may accompany meconium aspiration. Additional problems that may lead to PPHN are congenital pneumonia, hyperviscosity-polycythemia, congenital diaphragmatic hernia, pulmonary hypoplasia, congenital cyanotic heart disease, hypoglycemia, and hypothermia. Total anomalous venous return associated with obstruction of blood flow may produce a clinical picture that involves severe hypoxia and that is indistinguishable from PPHN; however, a chest radiograph reveals severe pulmonary venous engorgement and a small heart. Echocardiography or cardiac catheterization confirms the diagnosis.

Significant right-to-left shunting through a patent foramen ovale, through a PDA, and through intrapulmonary channels is characteristic of PPHN. The pulmonary vasculature often shows hypertrophied arterial wall smooth muscle, suggesting that the process of or predisposition to PPHN began in utero as a result of previous periods of fetal hypoxia. After birth, hypoxia, hypercapnia, and acidosis exacerbate pulmonary artery vasoconstriction, leading to further hypoxia and acidosis. Some infants with PPHN have extrapulmonary manifestations as a result of asphyxia. Myocardial injuries include heart failure, transient mitral insufficiency, and papillary muscle or myocardial infarction. Thrombocytopenia, right atrial thrombi, and pulmonary embolism also may be noted.

The **diagnosis** is confirmed by echocardiographic examination, which shows elevated pulmonary artery pressures and sites of right-to-left shunting. Echocardiography also rules out structural congenital heart disease and transient myocardial dysfunction.

Treatment involves general supportive care; correction of hypotension, anemia, and acidosis; and management of complications associated with asphyxia. If myocardial dysfunction is present, dopamine or dobutamine is needed. The most important therapy for PPHN is assisted ventilation. Reversible mild pulmonary hypertension may respond to conventional assisted ventilation. Patients with severe PPHN do not always respond to conventional therapy, however; some clinicians try hyperventilation to reverse pulmonary vasoconstriction by reducing PCO_2 levels and increasing pH to 7.5 to 7.6. Paralysis with pancuronium may be needed to assist such vigorous ventilation. Surfactant replacement seems to have no effect when PPHN is the primary diagnosis. If mechanical ventilation and supportive care are unsuccessful in improving oxygenation, inhaled nitric oxide, a selective pulmonary artery vasodilating agent, should be administered. If hypoxia persists, the patient may be a candidate for ECMO. Infants who require extremely high ventilator settings, marked by an alveolar-to-arterial oxygen gradient greater than 620 mm Hg, have a high mortality rate and benefit from ECMO if they do not respond to nitric oxide. In addition, the oxygenation index (OI) is used to assess the severity of hypoxemia and to guide the timing of interventions such as inhaled nitric oxide and ECMO. The OI is calculated using the equation: OI = [(mean airway pressure × fraction of inspired oxygen)/PaO_2] × 100. A high OI indicates severe hypoxemic respiratory failure.

Apnea of Prematurity

Although apnea typically is associated with immaturity of the respiratory control system, it also may be the presenting sign of other diseases or pathophysiologic states that affect preterm infants (Table 61–4). A thorough consideration of possible causes is always warranted, especially with the onset or unexpected increase in the frequency of episodes of apnea (or bradycardia).

Apnea is defined as the cessation of pulmonary airflow for a specific time interval, usually longer than 10 to 20 seconds. Bradycardia often accompanies prolonged apnea. Central apnea refers to a complete cessation of airflow and respiratory efforts with no chest wall movement; in obstructive apnea, no airflow is exhibited, but chest wall movements continue. A

TABLE 61–4. Potential Causes of Neonatal Apnea

CNS	IVH, drugs, seizures, hypoxic injury
Respiratory	Pneumonia, obstructive airway lesions, atelectasis, extreme prematurity (<1000 g), laryngeal reflex, phrenic nerve paralysis, severe RDS, pneumothorax
Infectious	Sepsis, necrotizing enterocolitis, meningitis (bacterial, fungal, viral)
Gastrointestinal	Oral feeding, bowel movement, gastroesophageal reflux, esophagitis, intestinal perforation
Metabolic	↓ Glucose, ↓ calcium, ↓ PO_2, ↓↑ sodium, ↑ ammonia, ↑ organic acids, ↑ ambient temperature, hypothermia
Cardiovascular	Hypotension, hypertension, heart failure, anemia, hypovolemia, change in vagal tone
Idiopathic	Immaturity of respiratory center, sleep state, upper airway collapse

IVH, intraventricular hemorrhage; RDS, respiratory distress syndrome.

combination of these two events, mixed apnea, is the most frequent type. It may begin as a brief episode of obstruction followed by a central apnea. Alternatively, central apnea may produce upper airway closure (passive pharyngeal hypotonia), resulting in mixed apnea.

A careful evaluation to determine the cause of apnea should be performed immediately in any infant with apnea. The incidence of apnea increases as gestational age decreases. Idiopathic apnea, a disease of premature infants, appears in the absence of any other identifiable disease states during the first week of life and usually resolves by 36 to 40 weeks of postconceptional age (gestational age at birth + postnatal age). The premature infant's process of regulating respiration is especially vulnerable to apnea. Preterm infants respond paradoxically to hypoxia by developing apnea rather than by increasing respirations as do mature infants. Poor tone of the laryngeal muscles also may lead to collapse of the upper airway, causing obstruction. Isolated obstructive apnea also may occur as a result of flexion or extreme lateral positioning of the premature infant's head, which obstructs the soft trachea.

Treatment of apnea of prematurity involves administration of oxygen to hypoxic infants, transfusion of anemic infants, and physical cutaneous stimulation for infants with mild apnea. Methylxanthines (caffeine or theophylline) are the mainstay of pharmacologic treatment of apnea. Xanthine therapy increases minute ventilation, improves the carbon dioxide sensitivity, decreases hypoxic depression of breathing, enhances diaphragmatic activity, and decreases periodic breathing. Treatment usually is initiated with a loading dose followed by maintenance therapy. High-flow nasal cannula therapy and nasal continuous positive airway pressure of 4 to 6 cm H_2O also are effective and relatively safe methods of treating obstructive or mixed apneas; they may work by stimulating the infant and splinting the upper airway. Continuous positive airway pressure also probably increases functional residual capacity, improving oxygenation.

MISCELLANEOUS RESPIRATORY DISORDERS

Pulmonary hypoplasia becomes manifested in the delivery room as severe respiratory distress that progresses rapidly to pulmonary insufficiency. The lungs, which are very small, develop pneumothoraces with normal resuscitative efforts. A small chest size radiographically, joint contractures, and early onset of pneumothoraces (often bilateral) are early clues to the diagnosis. Pulmonary hypertension results from the decreased lung mass and hypertrophy of pulmonary arteriole muscle.

Pulmonary hypoplasia may be a result of asphyxiating thoracic dystrophies (a small chest wall) or of decreased amniotic fluid volume that causes uterine compression of the developing chest wall, inhibiting lung growth. The latter failure of lung development may be associated with renal agenesis (Potter syndrome) or with a chronic leak of amniotic fluid from ruptured membranes. Isolated agenesis of one lung (usually the left lung) often is asymptomatic and familial. In contrast, serious pulmonary hypoplasia is noted in patients with a diaphragmatic hernia. Herniated bowel interferes with lung growth and leads to hypertrophy of the muscle layers of small pulmonary arteries, producing pulmonary hypertension. Pneumothoraces are common.

Treatment of congenital diaphragmatic hernia involves surgical evacuation of the chest and repair of the diaphragmatic defect after the pulmonary hypertension is treated. Respiratory care is similar to that for patients with PPHN.

Neuromuscular diseases that interfere with fetal breathing movements also may produce pulmonary hypoplasia (e.g., congenital anterior horn cell disease [Werdnig-Hoffmann syndrome]). Another cause of bilateral pulmonary hypoplasia is hydrops fetalis (see Chapter 60). Hydrops from any cause is characterized by anasarca, ascites, and pleural and pericardial effusions. Bilateral pleural effusions act as space-occupying masses that interfere with lung growth, resulting in pulmonary hypoplasia.

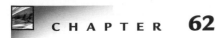

C H A P T E R 62

Anemia and Hyperbilirubinemia

ANEMIA

Embryonic hematopoiesis begins by the 20th day of gestation and is evidenced as blood islands in the yolk sac. In midgestation, erythropoiesis occurs in the liver and spleen; the bone marrow becomes the predominant site in the last trimester. Hemoglobin concentration increases from 8 to 10 g/dL at 12 weeks to 16.5 to 18 g/dL at 40 weeks. Fetal RBC production is responsive to erythropoietin, and the concentration of this hormone increases with fetal hypoxia and anemia.

After birth, hemoglobin levels increase transiently at 6 to 12 hours, then decline to 11 to 12 g/dL at 3 to 6 months. A premature infant (<32 weeks' gestational age) has a lower hemoglobin concentration and a more rapid postnatal decline of hemoglobin level, which achieves a nadir 1 to 2 months after birth. Fetal and neonatal RBCs have a shorter life span (70 to 90 days) and a higher mean corpuscular volume (110 to 120 fL) than adult cells. In the fetus, hemoglobin synthesis in the last two trimesters of pregnancy produces fetal hemoglobin (hemoglobin F), composed of two alpha chains and two gamma chains. Immediately before term, the infant begins to synthesize beta-hemoglobin chains; the term infant should have some adult hemoglobin (two alpha chains and two beta chains). Fetal hemoglobin represents 60% to 90% of hemoglobin at birth, and the levels decline to adult levels of less than 5% by 4 months of age.

The time of presentation of hemoglobinopathy depends on the timing of chain synthesis. α-Thalassemia caused by a four-gene defect produces no alpha chains and presents as severe anemia and hydrops (Bart hemoglobin, composed of four gamma chains) (see Chapter 150). Hemoglobin H is caused by a thalassemia three-gene defect resulting in four beta chains and appears with hemolysis and anemia in infants. In contrast, infants with beta-chain abnormalities, such as Cooley anemia (β-thalassemia major) and sickle cell anemia, do not manifest anemia in the neonatal period (see Chapter 150).

The blood volume of a term infant is 72 to 93 mL/kg; for a preterm infant, blood volume is 90 to 100 mL/kg. The placenta and umbilical vessels contain approximately 20 to 30 mL/kg of additional blood that can increase neonatal blood volume and hemoglobin levels transiently for the first 3 days of life if clamping or milking ("stripping") of the umbilical cord is delayed at birth. Delayed clamping increases the risk for polycythemia, increased pulmonary vascular resistance, hypoxia, and jaundice, but improves glomerular filtration. Early clamping may lead to anemia, a cardiac murmur, poor peripheral perfusion but lower pulmonary vascular pressures, and less tachypnea. To prevent both situations, the cord should be clamped at approximately 30 to 45 seconds after birth. Hydrostatic pressure affects blood transfer between the placenta and the infant at birth, and an undesired fetal-to-placental transfusion occurs if the infant is situated above the level of the placenta.

The physiologic anemia noted at 2 to 3 months of age in term infants and at 1 to 2 months of age in preterm infants is a normal process that does not result in signs of illness and does not require any treatment. It is a physiologic condition believed to be related to several factors, including increased tissue oxygenation experienced at birth, shortened RBC life span, and low erythropoietin levels.

Etiology

Symptomatic anemia in the newborn period (Fig. 62–1) may be caused by the following:

1. Decreased RBC production
2. Increased RBC destruction
3. Blood loss

Decreased Red Blood Cell Production

Anemia caused by decreased production of RBCs appears at birth with pallor, a low reticulocyte count, and absence of erythroid precursors in the bone marrow. Potential causes of neonatal decreased RBC production include bone marrow failure syndromes (congenital RBC aplasia [Diamond-Blackfan anemia]), infection (congenital viral infections [parvovirus, rubella], acquired bacterial or viral sepsis), nutritional deficiencies (protein, iron, folate, vitamin B_{12}), and congenital leukemia.

Increased Red Blood Cell Destruction

Immunologically mediated hemolysis in utero may lead to **erythroblastosis fetalis**, or the fetus may be spared, and **hemolytic disease** may appear in the newborn. Hemolysis of fetal erythrocytes is a result of blood group differences between the sensitized mother and fetus, which causes production of maternal IgG antibodies directed against an antigen on fetal cells.

ABO blood group incompatibility with neonatal hemolysis develops only if the mother has IgG antibodies from a previous exposure to A or B antigens. These IgG antibodies cross the placenta by active transport and affect the fetus or newborn. Sensitization of

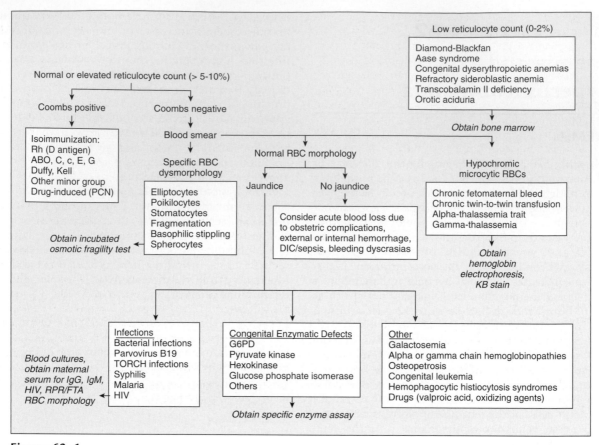

Figure 62-1

Differential diagnosis of neonatal anemia. The physician obtains information from the family, maternal and labor and delivery histories, and laboratory tests, including hemoglobin, reticulocyte count, blood type, direct Coombs test, peripheral smear, red blood cell (RBC) indices, and bilirubin concentration. DIC, disseminated intravascular coagulation; FTA, fluorescent treponemal antibody test; G6PD, glucose-6-phosphate dehydrogenase; KB, Kleihauer-Betke; PCN, penicillin; RPR, rapid plasma reagin tests. (From Ohls RK: Anemia in the neonate. In Christensen RD [ed]: Hematologic Problems of the Neonate. Philadelphia, WB Saunders, 2000, p 162.)

the mother to fetal antigens may have occurred by previous transfusions or by conditions of pregnancy that result in transfer of fetal erythrocytes into the maternal circulation, such as first trimester abortion, ectopic pregnancy, amniocentesis, or normal pregnancy. The risk of fetal-maternal transfusion is increased by manual extraction of the placenta and by version (external or internal) procedures.

ABO incompatibility with sensitization usually does not cause fetal disease other than extremely mild anemia. It may produce **hemolytic disease of the newborn**, however, which is manifested as significant anemia and hyperbilirubinemia. Because many mothers who have blood group O have IgG antibodies to A and B before pregnancy, the firstborn infant of A or B blood type may be affected. In contrast to Rh disease, ABO hemolytic disease does not become more

severe with subsequent pregnancies. Hemolysis with ABO incompatibility is less severe than hemolysis in Rh-sensitized pregnancy, either because the anti-A or anti-B antibody may bind to nonerythrocytic cells that contain A or B antigen or because fetal erythrocytes have fewer A or B antigenic determinants than they have Rh sites. With the declining incidence of Rh hemolytic disease, ABO incompatibility has become the most common cause of neonatal hyperbilirubinemia requiring therapy—currently accounting for approximately 20% of clinically significant jaundice in the newborn.

Erythroblastosis fetalis classically is caused by Rh blood group incompatibility. Most Rh-negative women have no anti-Rh antibodies at the time of their first pregnancy. The Rh antigen system consists of five antigens: C, D, E, c, and e; the d type is not antigenic. In most Rh-sensitized cases, the D antigen of the fetus sensitizes the Rh-negative (d) mother, resulting in IgG antibody production during the first pregnancy.

Because most mothers are not sensitized to Rh antigens at the start of pregnancy, Rh erythroblastosis fetalis is usually a disease of the second and subsequent pregnancies. The first affected pregnancy results in an antibody response in the mother, which may be detected during antenatal screening with the Coombs test and determined to be anti-D antibody. The first affected newborn may show no serious fetal disease and may manifest hemolytic disease of the newborn only by the development of anemia and hyperbilirubinemia (discussed later). Subsequent pregnancies result in an increasing severity of response because of an earlier onset of hemolysis in utero. Fetal anemia, heart failure, elevated venous pressure, portal vein obstruction, and hypoalbuminemia result in **fetal hydrops**, which is characterized by ascites, pleural and pericardial effusions, and anasarca (see Chapter 60). The risk of fetal death is high.

The *management* of a pregnancy complicated by Rh sensitization depends on the severity of hemolysis, its effects on the fetus, and the maturity of the fetus at the time it becomes affected. The severity of the hemolysis can be assessed by the quantity of bilirubin transferred from the fetus to the amniotic fluid, quantified by spectrophotometric analysis of the optical density (at 450 nm) of amniotic fluid.

Three zones of optical densities with decreasing slopes toward term gestation have been developed to predict the severity of the illness. The high optical density zone 3 is associated with severe hemolysis; fetuses in the lower zones probably are not affected. If a fetus' optical density measurement for bilirubin falls into zone 3, and the fetus has pulmonary maturity as determined by the L/S ratio, the infant should be delivered and treated in the neonatal ICU. If the lungs are immature and the fetus is between 22 and 33 weeks of gestational age, an ultrasound-guided intrauterine transfusion with O-negative blood into the umbilical vein is indicated and may have to be repeated until pulmonary maturity is reached or fetal distress is detected. Indications for fetal intravascular transfusion in sensitized fetuses between 22 and 32 weeks of gestational age include a fetal hematocrit of less than 25% to 30%, fetal hydrops, and fetal distress too early in gestation for delivery. Intravascular intrauterine transfusion corrects fetal anemia, improves the outcome of severe hydrops, and reduces the need for postnatal exchange transfusion, but is associated with neonatal anemia as a result of continued hemolysis plus suppressed erythropoiesis.

Prevention of sensitization of the mother carrying an Rh-positive fetus is possible by treating the mother during gestation (>28 weeks' gestational age) and within 72 hours after birth with anti-Rh-positive immune globulin (RhoGAM). The dose of RhoGAM (300 μg) is based on the ability of this amount of anti-Rh-positive antibody to bind all the possible fetal Rh-positive erythrocytes entering the maternal circulation during the fetal-to-maternal transfusion at birth (approximately 30 mL). RhoGAM may bind Rh-positive fetal erythrocytes or interfere with maternal anti-Rh-positive antibody production by another, unknown mechanism. RhoGAM is effective only in preventing sensitization to the D antigen. Other blood group antigens that can cause immune hydrops and erythroblastosis include Rh C, E, Kell, and Duffy. Anti-Kell alloimmunity produces lower amniotic bilirubin levels and a lower reticulocyte count because in addition to hemolysis it inhibits erythropoiesis.

Nonimmune causes of hemolysis in the newborn include RBC enzyme deficiencies of the Embden-Meyerhof pathway, such as pyruvate kinase or glucose-6-phosphate dehydrogenase deficiency. RBC membrane disorders are another cause of nonimmune hemolysis. Hereditary spherocytosis is inherited as a severe autosomal recessive form or less severe autosomal dominant form and is the result of a deficiency of spectrin, a protein of the RBC membrane. Hemoglobinopathies, such as thalassemia, are another cause of nonimmunologically mediated hemolysis.

Blood Loss

Anemia from blood loss at birth is manifested by two patterns of presentation, depending on the rapidity of blood loss. Acute blood loss after fetal-maternal hemorrhage, rupture of the umbilical cord, placenta previa, or internal hemorrhage (hepatic or splenic hematoma; retroperitoneal) is characterized by pallor, diminished peripheral pulses, and shock. There are no signs of extramedullary hematopoiesis and no hepatosplenomegaly. The hemoglobin content and serum iron levels initially are normal, but the hemoglobin levels decline during the subsequent 24 hours. Newborns with chronic blood loss caused by chronic fetal-maternal hemorrhage or a twin-to-twin transfusion present with marked pallor, heart failure, hepatosplenomegaly with or without hydrops, a low hemoglobin level at birth, a hypochromic microcytic blood smear, and decreased serum iron stores. Fetal-maternal bleeding occurs in 50% to 75% of all pregnancies, with fetal blood losses ranging from 1 to 50 mL; most blood losses are 1 mL or less, 1 in 400 are approximately 30 mL, and 1 in 2000 are approximately 100 mL.

The diagnosis of fetal-maternal hemorrhage is confirmed by the Kleihauer-Betke acid elution test; pink fetal RBCs are observed and counted in the mother's peripheral blood smear because fetal hemoglobin is resistant to acid elution; adult hemoglobin is eluted, leaving discolored maternal cells (patients with sickle cell anemia or hereditary persistence of fetal hemoglobin may have a false-positive result, and ABO incompatibility may produce a false-negative result).

Diagnosis and Management

Hemolysis in utero resulting from any cause may produce a spectrum of *clinical manifestations* at birth. Severe hydrops with anasarca, heart failure, and pulmonary edema may prevent adequate ventilation at birth, resulting in asphyxia. Infants affected with hemolysis in utero have hepatosplenomegaly and pallor and become jaundiced within the first 24 hours after birth. Less severely affected infants manifest pallor and hepatosplenomegaly at birth and become jaundiced subsequently. Patients with ABO incompatibility often are asymptomatic and show no physical signs at birth; mild anemia with jaundice develops during the first 24 to 72 hours of life.

Because hydrops, anemia, or jaundice is secondary to many diverse causes of hemolysis, a laboratory evaluation is needed in all patients with suspected hemolysis. A complete blood count, blood smear, reticulocyte count, blood type, and direct Coombs test (to determine the presence of antibody-coated RBCs) should be performed in the initial evaluation of all infants with hemolysis. Reduced hemoglobin levels, reticulocytosis, and a blood smear characterized by polychromasia and anisocytosis are expected with isoimmune hemolysis. Spherocytes commonly are observed in ABO incompatibility. The determination of the blood type and the Coombs test identify the responsible antigen and antibody in immunologically mediated hemolysis.

In the absence of a positive Coombs test and blood group differences between the mother and fetus, other causes of nonimmune hemolysis must be considered. RBC enzyme assays, hemoglobin electrophoresis, or RBC membrane tests (osmotic fragility, spectrin assay) should be performed. Internal hemorrhage also may be associated with anemia, reticulocytosis, and jaundice when the hemorrhage reabsorbs; ultrasound evaluation of the brain, liver, spleen, or adrenal gland may be indicated when nonimmune hemolysis is suspected. Shock is more typical in patients with internal hemorrhage, whereas in hemolytic diseases heart failure may be seen with severe anemia. Evaluation of a possible fetal-maternal hemorrhage should include the Kleihauer-Betke test.

The **treatment** of *symptomatic* neonatal anemia is transfusion of crossmatched packed RBCs. If immune hemolysis is present, the cells to be transfused must be crossmatched against maternal and neonatal plasma. Acute volume loss may necessitate resuscitation with nonblood products, such as saline if blood is not available; packed RBCs can be given subsequently. To correct anemia and any remaining blood volume deficit, 10 to 15 mL/kg of packed RBCs should be sufficient. CMV-seronegative blood should be given to CMV-seronegative infants, and all blood products should be irradiated to reduce the risk of graft-versus-host disease; blood should be screened for HIV, hepatitis B and C, and syphilis. Recombinant erythropoietin may improve the hematocrit in infants with a hyporegenerative anemia after in utero transfusion.

HYPERBILIRUBINEMIA

Hemolytic disease of the newborn is a common cause of neonatal jaundice. Nonetheless, because of the immaturity of the pathways of bilirubin metabolism, many newborn infants without evidence of hemolysis become jaundiced.

Bilirubin is produced by the catabolism of hemoglobin in the reticuloendothelial system. The tetrapyrrole ring of heme is cleaved by heme oxygenase to form equivalent quantities of biliverdin and carbon monoxide. Because no other biologic source of carbon monoxide exists, the excretion of this gas is stoichiometrically identical to the production of bilirubin. Biliverdin is converted to bilirubin by biliverdin reductase. One gram of hemoglobin produces 35 mg of bilirubin. Sources of bilirubin other than circulating hemoglobin represent 20% of bilirubin production; these sources include inefficient (shunt) hemoglobin production and lysis of precursor cells in bone marrow. Compared with adults, newborns have a twofold to threefold greater rate of bilirubin production (6 to 10 mg/kg/24 hr versus 3 mg/kg/24 hr). This increased production is caused in part by an increased RBC mass (higher hematocrit) and a shortened erythrocyte life span of 70 to 90 days compared with the 120-day erythrocyte life span in adults.

Bilirubin produced after hemoglobin catabolism is lipid soluble and unconjugated and reacts as an indirect reagent in the van den Bergh test. Indirect-reacting, unconjugated bilirubin is toxic to the CNS and is insoluble in water, limiting its excretion. Unconjugated bilirubin binds to albumin on specific bilirubin binding sites; 1 g of albumin binds 8.5 mg of bilirubin in a newborn. If the binding sites become saturated or if a competitive compound binds at the site, displacing bound bilirubin, free bilirubin becomes available to enter the CNS. Organic acids such as free fatty acids and drugs such as sulfisoxazole can displace bilirubin from its binding site on albumin.

Bilirubin dissociates from albumin at the hepatocyte and becomes bound to a cytoplasmic liver protein "Y" (ligandin). Hepatic conjugation results in the production of bilirubin diglucuronide, which is water soluble and capable of biliary and renal excretion. The enzyme glucuronosyltransferase represents the rate-limiting step of bilirubin conjugation. The concentrations of ligandin and glucuronosyltransferase are lower in newborns, particularly in premature infants, than in older children.

Conjugated bilirubin gives a direct reaction in the van den Bergh test. Most conjugated bilirubin is excreted through the bile into the small intestine and eliminated in the stool. Some bilirubin may undergo hydrolysis back to the unconjugated fraction by intestinal glucuronidase, however, and may be reabsorbed (enterohepatic recirculation). In addition, bacteria in the neonatal intestine convert bilirubin to urobilinogen and stercobilinogen, which are excreted in urine and stool and usually limit bilirubin reabsorption. Delayed passage of meconium, which contains bilirubin, also may contribute to the enterohepatic recirculation of bilirubin.

Bilirubin is produced in utero by the normal fetus and by the fetus affected by erythroblastosis fetalis. Indirect, unconjugated, lipid-soluble fetal bilirubin is transferred across the placenta and subsequently becomes conjugated by maternal hepatic enzymes. The placenta is impermeable to conjugated water-soluble bilirubin. Fetal bilirubin levels become only mildly elevated in the presence of severe hemolysis, but may increase when hemolysis produces fetal hepatic inspissated bile stasis and conjugated hyperbilirubinemia. Maternal indirect (but not direct) hyperbilirubinemia also may increase fetal bilirubin levels.

Etiology of Indirect Unconjugated Hyperbilirubinemia

Physiologic jaundice is a common cause of hyperbilirubinemia among newborns. It is a diagnosis of exclusion, made after careful evaluation has ruled out more serious causes of jaundice, such as hemolysis, infection, and metabolic diseases. Physiologic jaundice is the result of many factors that are normal physiologic characteristics of newborns: increased bilirubin production resulting from an increased RBC mass, shortened RBC life span, and hepatic immaturity of ligandin and glucuronosyltransferase. Physiologic jaundice may be exaggerated among infants of Greek and Asian ancestry.

The clinical pattern of physiologic jaundice in term infants includes a peak indirect-reacting bilirubin level of no more than 12 mg/dL on day 3 of life. In premature infants, the peak is higher (15 mg/dL) and occurs later (fifth day). The peak level of indirect bilirubin during physiologic jaundice may be higher in breast milk–fed infants than in formula-fed infants (15 to 17 mg/dL versus 12 mg/dL). This higher level may be partly a result of the decreased fluid intake of infants fed breast milk. Jaundice is unphysiologic or pathologic if it is clinically evident on the first day of life, if the bilirubin level increases more than 0.5 mg/dL/hr, if the peak bilirubin is greater than 13 mg/dL in term infants, if the direct bilirubin fraction is greater than 1.5 mg/dL, or if hepatosplenomegaly and anemia are present.

Crigler-Najjar syndrome is a serious, rare, permanent deficiency of glucuronosyltransferase that results in severe indirect hyperbilirubinemia. The autosomal dominant variety responds to enzyme induction by phenobarbital, producing an increase in enzyme activity and a reduction of bilirubin levels. The autosomal recessive form does not respond to phenobarbital and manifests as persistent indirect hyperbilirubinemia, often leading to kernicterus. Gilbert disease is caused by a mutation of the promoter region of glucuronosyltransferase and results in a mild indirect hyperbilirubinemia. In the presence of another icterogenic factor (hemolysis), more severe jaundice may develop.

Breast milk jaundice may be associated with unconjugated hyperbilirubinemia without evidence of hemolysis during the first to second week of life. Bilirubin levels rarely increase to greater than 20 mg/dL. Interruption of breastfeeding for 1 to 2 days results in a rapid decline of bilirubin levels, which do not increase significantly after breastfeeding resumes. Breast milk may contain an inhibitor of bilirubin conjugation or may increase the enterohepatic recirculation of bilirubin because of breast milk glucuronidase.

Jaundice on the first day of life is always pathologic, and immediate attention is needed to establish the cause. Early onset often is a result of hemolysis, internal hemorrhage (cephalhematoma, hepatic or splenic hematoma), or infection (Table 62-1). Infection also is often associated with direct-reacting bilirubin resulting from perinatal congenital infections or from bacterial sepsis.

Physical evidence of jaundice is observed in infants when bilirubin levels reach 5 to 10 mg/dL (versus 2 mg/dL in adults). When jaundice is observed, the laboratory evaluation for hyperbilirubinemia should include a total bilirubin measurement to determine the magnitude of hyperbilirubinemia. Bilirubin levels greater than 5 mg/dL on the first day of life or greater than 13 mg/dL thereafter in term infants should be evaluated further with measurement of indirect and direct bilirubin levels, blood typing, Coombs test, complete blood count, blood smear, and reticulocyte count. These tests must be performed before treatment of hyperbilirubinemia with phototherapy or exchange transfusion. In the absence of hemolysis or evidence for either the common or the rare causes of nonhemolytic indirect hyperbilirubinemia, the diagnosis is either physiologic or breast milk jaundice. Jaundice present after 2 weeks of age is pathologic and suggests a direct-reacting hyperbilirubinemia.

TABLE 62–1.   Etiology of Unconjugated Hyperbilirubinemia

	Hemolysis Present	Hemolysis Absent
Common	*Blood group incompatibility:* ABO, Rh, Kell, Duffy *Infection*	Physiologic jaundice, breast milk jaundice, internal hemorrhage, polycythemia, infant of diabetic mother
Rare	*Red blood cell enzyme defects:* glucose-6-phosphate dehydrogenase, pyruvate kinase *Red blood cell membrane disorders:* spherocytosis, ovalocytosis *Hemoglobinopathy:* thalassemia	Mutations of glucuronyl transferase enzyme (Crigler-Najjar syndrome, Gilbert disease), pyloric stenosis, hypothyroidism, immune thrombocytopenia

Etiology of Direct Conjugated Hyperbilirubinemia

Direct-reacting hyperbilirubinemia (defined as a direct bilirubin level >2 mg/dL or >20% of the total bilirubin) is never physiologic and should always be evaluated thoroughly according to the diagnostic categories noted in Table 62–2. Direct-reacting bilirubin (composed mostly of conjugated bilirubin) is not neurotoxic to the infant, but signifies a serious underlying disorder involving cholestasis or hepatocellular injury. The diagnostic evaluation of patients with direct-reacting hyperbilirubinemia involves the determination of the levels of liver enzymes (aspartate aminotransferase, alkaline phosphatase, alanine aminotransferase, and γ-glutamyl transpeptidase), bacterial and viral cultures, metabolic screening tests, hepatic ultrasound, sweat chloride test, and occasionally liver biopsy. Additionally, the presence of dark urine and gray-white (acholic) stools with jaundice after the second week of life strongly suggests biliary atresia. The treatment of disorders manifested by direct bilirubinemia is specific for the diseases that are listed in Table 62–2. These diseases do not respond to phototherapy or exchange transfusion.

Kernicterus (Bilirubin Encephalopathy)

Lipid-soluble, unconjugated, indirect bilirubin fraction is toxic to the developing CNS, especially when indirect bilirubin concentrations are high and exceed the binding capacity of albumin. Kernicterus results when indirect bilirubin is deposited in brain cells and disrupts neuronal metabolism and function, especially in the basal ganglia. Indirect bilirubin may cross the blood-brain barrier because of its lipid solubility; other theories propose that a disruption of the blood-brain barrier permits entry of a bilirubin-albumin or free bilirubin–fatty acid complex.

Kernicterus usually is noted when the biliribin level is excessively high for gestational age. Kernicterus

usually does not develop in term infants when bilirubin levels are less than 20 to 25 mg/dL. The incidence of kernicterus increases as serum bilirubin levels increase to greater than 25 mg/dL. Kernicterus may be noted at bilirubin levels less than 20 mg/dL in the presence of sepsis, meningitis, hemolysis, asphyxia, hypoxia, hypothermia, hypoglycemia, bilirubin-displacing drugs (sulfa drugs), and prematurity. Other risks for kernicterus in term infants are hemolysis, jaundice noted within 24 hours of birth, and delayed diagnosis of hyperbilirubinemia. Kernicterus has developed in extremely immature infants weighing less than 1000 g when bilirubin levels are less than 10 mg/dL

TABLE 62–2.   Etiology of Conjugated Hyperbilirubinemia

Common

Hyperalimentation cholestasis
CMV infection
Other perinatal congenital infections (TORCH)
Inspissated bile from prolonged hemolysis
Neonatal hepatitis
Sepsis

Uncommon

Hepatic infarction
Inborn errors of metabolism (galactosemia, tyrosinosis)
Cystic fibrosis
Biliary atresia
Choledochal cyst
α₁-Antitrypsin deficiency
Neonatal iron storage disease
Alagille syndrome (arteriohepatic dysplasia)
Byler disease

CMV, cytomegalovirus; TORCH, *t*oxoplasmosis, *o*ther, *r*ubella, *c*ytomegalovirus, *h*erpes simplex.

because of a more permeable blood-brain barrier associated with prematurity.

The earliest *clinical manifestations* of kernicterus are lethargy, hypotonia, irritability, poor Moro response, and poor feeding. A high-pitched cry and emesis also may be present. Early signs are noted after day 4 of life. Later signs include bulging fontanel, opisthotonic posturing, pulmonary hemorrhage, fever, hypertonicity, paralysis of upward gaze, and seizures. Infants with severe cases of kernicterus die in the neonatal period. Spasticity resolves in surviving infants, who may manifest later nerve deafness, choreoathetoid cerebral palsy, mental retardation, enamel dysplasia, and discoloration of teeth as permanent sequelae. Kernicterus may be *prevented* by avoiding excessively high indirect bilirubin levels and by avoiding conditions or drugs that may displace bilirubin from albumin. Early signs of kernicterus occasionally may be reversed by immediately instituting an exchange transfusion (see later).

Therapy of Indirect Hyperbilirubinemia

Phototherapy is an effective and safe method for reducing indirect bilirubin levels, particularly when initiated before serum bilirubin increases to levels associated with kernicterus. In term infants, phototherapy is begun when indirect bilirubin levels are between 16 and 18 mg/dL. Phototherapy is initiated in premature infants when bilirubin is at lower levels, to prevent bilirubin from reaching the high concentrations necessitating exchange transfusion. Blue lights and white lights are effective in reducing bilirubin levels.

Under the effects of phototherapy light with maximal irradiance in the 425- to 475-nm wavelength band, bilirubin is transformed into isomers that are water soluble and easily excreted. Unconjugated bilirubin (IX) is in the 4Z, 15Z configuration. Phototherapy causes a photochemical reaction producing the reversible, more water-soluble isomer 4Z, 15E bilirubin IX. This isomer can be excreted easily, bypassing the liver's conjugation system. Another photochemical reaction results in the rapid production of lumirubin, a more water-soluble isomer than the aforementioned isomer, which does not spontaneously revert to unconjugated native bilirubin and can be excreted in urine.

Complications of phototherapy include an increased insensible water loss, diarrhea, and dehydration. Additional problems are macular-papular red skin rash, lethargy, masking of cyanosis, nasal obstruction by eye pads, and potential for retinal damage. Skin bronzing may be noted in infants with direct-reacting hyperbilirubinemia. Infants with mild hemolytic disease of the newborn occasionally may be managed successfully with phototherapy for hyperbilirubinemia, but care must be taken to follow these infants for the late occurrence of anemia from continued hemolysis.

Exchange transfusion usually is reserved for infants with dangerously high indirect bilirubin levels who are at risk for kernicterus. As a rule of thumb, a level of 20 mg/dL for indirect-reacting bilirubin is the "exchange number" for infants *with hemolysis* who weigh more than 2000 g. Asymptomatic infants with physiologic or breast milk jaundice may not require exchange transfusion, unless the indirect bilirubin level exceeds 25 mg/dL. The exchangeable level of indirect bilirubin for other infants may be estimated by calculating 10% of the birth weight in grams: the level in an infant weighing 1500 g would be 15 mg/dL. Infants weighing less than 1000 g usually do not require an exchange transfusion until the bilirubin level exceeds 10 mg/dL.

Small infusions of whole blood crossmatched with that of the mother and infant are alternated with withdrawals of an equivalent quantity of the infant's blood, which is discarded. Depending on the size of the infant, aliquots of 5 to 20 mL per cycle are withdrawn and infused, with the total procedure lasting 45 to 90 minutes. The total amount of blood exchanged is equal to twice the infant's blood volume, calculated as:

$$\text{Weight (kg)} \times 85 \text{ mL/kg} \times 2$$

This volume should remove 85% of the infant's RBCs (the source of bilirubin), maternal antibodies, and exchangeable tissue indirect bilirubin. The exchange transfusion usually is performed through an umbilical venous catheter placed in the inferior vena cava or, if free flow is obtained, at the confluence of the umbilical vein and the portal system. The level of serum bilirubin immediately after the exchange transfusion declines to levels that are about half of those before the exchange; levels rebound 6 to 8 hours later as a result of continued hemolysis and redistribution of bilirubin from tissue stores.

Complications of exchange transfusion include problems related to the blood (transfusion reaction, metabolic instability, or infection), the catheter (vessel perforation or hemorrhage), or the procedure (hypotension or necrotizing enterocolitis). Unusual complications include thrombocytopenia and graft-versus-host disease. Continuation of phototherapy may reduce the necessity for subsequent exchange transfusions.

Polycythemia (Hyperviscosity Syndrome)

Polycythemia is an excessively high hematocrit (≥65%) and leads to hyperviscosity that produces symptoms related to vascular stasis, hypoperfusion, and ischemia. As the hematocrit increases from 40% to 60%, there is a small increase in blood viscosity. When the central hematocrit increases to greater than 65%, the blood viscosity begins to increase markedly, and symptoms may appear. Neonatal erythrocytes are less filterable or deformable than adult erythrocytes, which further contributes to hyperviscosity. A central venous hematocrit of 65% or greater is noted in 3% to 5% of infants. Infants at special risk for polycythemia are term and post-term SGA infants, infants of diabetic mothers, infants with delayed cord clamping, and infants with neonatal hyperthyroidism, adrenogenital syndrome, trisomy 13, trisomy 18, trisomy 21, twin-to-twin transfusion syndrome (recipient), and Beckwith-Wiedemann syndrome. In some infants, polycythemia may reflect a compensation for prolonged periods of fetal hypoxia caused by placental insufficiency; these infants have increased erythropoietin levels at birth.

Polycythemic patients appear plethoric or ruddy and may develop acrocyanosis. Symptoms are a result of the increased RBC mass and of vascular compromise. Seizures, lethargy, and irritability reflect abnormalities of microcirculation of the brain, whereas hyperbilirubinemia may reflect the poor hepatic circulation or the increased amount of hemoglobin that is being broken down into bilirubin. Additional problems include respiratory distress and PPHN that result in part from elevated pulmonary vascular resistance. The chest radiograph often reveals cardiomegaly, increased vascular markings, pleural effusions, and interstitial edema. Other problems are necrotizing enterocolitis, hypoglycemia, thrombocytopenia, priapism, testicular infarction, hemiplegic stroke, and feeding intolerance. Many of these complications also are related to the primary condition associated with polycythemia (SGA infants are at risk for hypoglycemia and PPHN after periods of hypoxia in utero).

Long-term sequelae of neonatal polycythemia relate to neurodevelopmental abnormalities that may be prevented by treatment of symptomatic infants with partial exchange transfusion after birth. A partial exchange transfusion removes whole blood and replaces it with normal saline. The equation used to calculate the volume exchanged is based on the central venous hematocrit because peripheral hematocrits may be falsely elevated:

Volume to exchange (mL) = [blood volume × (observed hematocrit − desired hematocrit)]/ observed hematocrit

The desired hematocrit is 50%, and the blood volume 85 mL/kg.

COAGULATION DISORDERS

Disorders of coagulation are common in the neonatal period. Hemorrhage during this time may be a result of trauma, inherited permanent deficiency of coagulation factors, transient deficiencies of vitamin K–dependent factors, disorders of platelets, and DIC seen in sick newborns with shock or hypoxia. Thrombosis also is a potential problem in the newborn because of developmentally lower circulating levels of antithrombin III, protein C (a vitamin K–dependent protein that inhibits factors VIII and V), and the fibrinolytic system.

Coagulation factors do not pass through the placenta to the fetus, and newborn infants have relatively low levels of the vitamin K–dependent factors II, VII, IX, and X. Contact factors XI and XII, prekallikrein, and kininogen also are lower in newborns than in adults. Fibrinogen (factor I); plasma levels of factors V, VIII, and XIII; and platelet counts are within the adult normal range.

Because of the transient, relative deficiencies of the contact and the vitamin K–dependent factors, the *partial thromboplastin time* (PTT), which is dependent on factors XII, IX, VIII, X, V, II, and I, is prolonged in the newborn period. Preterm infants have the most marked prolongation of the PTT (50 to 80 seconds) compared with term infants (35 to 50 seconds) and older, more mature infants (25 to 35 seconds). The administration of heparin and the presence of DIC, hemophilia, and severe vitamin K deficiency prolong the PTT.

The *prothrombin time* (PT), which is dependent on factors VII, X, V, II, and I, is a more sensitive test for vitamin K deficiency. The PT is only slightly prolonged in term infants (13 to 20 seconds) compared with preterm infants (13 to 21 seconds) and more mature patients (12 to 14 seconds). Abnormal prolongations of the PT occur with vitamin K deficiency, hepatic injury, and DIC. Levels of *fibrinogen* and *fibrin degradation products* are similar in infants and adults. The *bleeding time*, which reflects platelet function and number, is normal during the newborn period in the absence of maternal salicylate therapy.

Vitamin K is a necessary cofactor for the carboxylation of glutamate on precursor proteins, converting them into the more active coagulation factors II, VII, IX, and X; γ-carboxyglutamic acid binds calcium, which is required for the immediate activation of factors during hemorrhage. There is no congenital deficiency of hepatic synthesis of these precursor proteins, but in the absence of vitamin K their conversion to the active factor is not possible. Levels of *protein induced by vitamin K absence* increase in vitamin K deficiency and are helpful diagnostic markers; vitamin K administration rapidly corrects the coagulation defects, reducing protein induced by vitamin K absence to undetectable levels.

Although most newborns are born with reduced levels of vitamin K–dependent factors, hemorrhagic complications develop only rarely. Infants at risk for **hemorrhagic disease of the newborn** have the most profound deficiency of vitamin K–dependent factors, and these factors decline further after birth. Because breast milk is a poor source of vitamin K, breastfed infants are at increased risk for hemorrhage that usually occurs between days 3 and 7 of life. Bleeding usually ensues from the umbilical cord, circumcision site, intestines, scalp, mucosa, and skin, but internal hemorrhage places the infant at risk for fatal complications, such as intracranial bleeding.

Hemorrhage on the first day of life resulting from a deficiency of the vitamin K–dependent factors often is associated with administration to the mother of drugs that affect vitamin K metabolism in the infant. This early pattern of hemorrhage has been seen with maternal warfarin or antibiotic (e.g., isoniazid or rifampin) therapy and in infants of mothers receiving phenobarbital and phenytoin. Bleeding also may occur 1 to 3 months after birth, particularly among breastfed infants. Vitamin K deficiency in breastfed infants also should raise suspicion about the possibility of vitamin K malabsorption resulting from cystic fibrosis, biliary atresia, hepatitis, or antibiotic suppression of the colonic bacteria that produce vitamin K.

Bleeding associated with vitamin K deficiency may be **prevented** by administration of vitamin K to all infants at birth. Before routine administration of vitamin K, 1% to 2% of all newborns have hemorrhagic disease of the newborn. One IM dose (1 mg) of vitamin K prevents vitamin K–deficiency bleeding. **Treatment** of bleeding resulting from vitamin K deficiency involves IV administration of 1 mg of vitamin K. If severe, life-threatening hemorrhage is present, fresh frozen plasma also should be given. Unusually high doses of vitamin K may be needed for hepatic disease and for maternal warfarin or anticonvulsant therapy.

Clinical Manifestations and Differential Diagnoses of Bleeding Disorders

Bleeding disorders in a newborn may be associated with cutaneous bleeding, such as cephalhematoma, subgaleal hemorrhage, ecchymosis, and petechiae. Facial petechiae are common in infants born by vertex presentation, with or without a nuchal cord, and usually are insignificant. Mucosal bleeding may appear as hematemesis, melena, or epistaxis. Internal hemorrhage results in organ-specific dysfunction, such as seizures accompanied by intracranial hemorrhage. Bleeding from venipuncture or heel-stick sites, circumcision sites, or the umbilical cord also is common.

The *differential diagnosis* depends partly on the clinical circumstances associated with the hemorrhage. In a **sick newborn**, the differential diagnosis should include DIC, hepatic failure, and thrombocytopenia. Thrombocytopenia in an ill neonate may be secondary to consumption by trapping of platelets in a hemangioma (**Kasabach-Merritt syndrome**) or may be

associated with perinatal, congenital, or bacterial infections; necrotizing enterocolitis (NEC); thrombotic endocarditis; PPHN; organic acidemia; maternal preeclampsia; or asphyxia. Thrombocytopenia also may be due to peripheral washout of platelets after an exchange transfusion. *Treatment* of a sick infant with thrombocytopenia should be directed at the underlying disorder, supplemented by infusions of platelets, blood, or both.

The etiology of DIC in a newborn includes hypoxia, hypotension, asphyxia, bacterial or viral sepsis, NEC, death of a twin while in utero, cavernous hemangioma, nonimmune hydrops, neonatal cold injury, neonatal neoplasm, and hepatic disease. The *treatment* of DIC should be focused primarily on therapy for the initiating or underlying disorder. Supportive management of consumptive coagulopathy involves platelet transfusions and factor replacement with fresh frozen plasma. Heparin and factor C concentrate should be reserved for infants with DIC who also have thrombosis.

Disorders of hemostasis in a well child are not associated with systemic disease in a newborn, but reflect coagulation factor or platelet deficiency. *Hemophilia* initially is associated with cutaneous or mucosal bleeding and no systemic illness. If bleeding continues, hypovolemic shock may develop. Bleeding into the brain, liver, or spleen may result in organ-specific signs and shock.

In a **well child**, *thrombocytopenia* may be part of a syndrome such as Fanconi anemia syndrome (involving hypoplasia and aplasia of the thumb), radial aplasia-thrombocytopenia syndrome (thumbs present), or Wiskott-Aldrich syndrome. Various maternal drugs also may reduce the neonatal platelet count without producing other adverse effects. These drugs include sulfonamides, quinidine, quinine, and thiazide diuretics.

The most common causes of thrombocytopenia in well newborns are transient isoimmune thrombocytopenia and transient neonatal thrombocytopenia in well infants born to mothers with idiopathic thrombocytopenic purpura (ITP). **Isoimmune thrombocytopenia** is caused by antiplatelet antibodies produced by the HPLA1-negative mother after her sensitization to specific paternal platelet antigen (HPA-1a and HPA-5b represent 85% and 10% of cases) expressed on the fetal platelet. The incidence is 1:1000 to 1:2000 births. This response to maternal-sensitized antibodies that produce isoimmune thrombocytopenia is analogous to the response that produces erythroblastosis fetalis. The maternal antiplatelet antibody does not produce maternal thrombocytopenia, but after crossing the placenta this IgG antibody binds to fetal platelets that are trapped by the reticuloendothelial tissue, resulting in thrombocytopenia. Infants with thrombocytopenia produced in this manner are at risk for development of petechiae, purpura, and intracranial hemorrhage (an incidence of 10% to 15%) before or after birth. Vaginal delivery may increase the risk for neonatal bleeding; cesarean section may be indicated.

Specific *treatment* for severe thrombocytopenia (<20,000 platelets/mm³) or significant bleeding is transfusion of ABO-compatible and RhD-compatible, HPA-1a-negative and HPA-5b-negative maternal platelets. Because the antibody in isoimmune thrombocytopenia is directed against the fetal rather than the maternal platelet, plateletpheresis of the mother yields sufficient platelets for performing a platelet transfusion to treat the affected infant. After one platelet transfusion, the infant's platelet count dramatically increases and usually remains in a safe range. Without treatment, thrombocytopenia resolves during the first month of life as the maternal antibody level declines. *Treatment* of the mother with IV immunoglobulin or the thrombocytopenic fetus with intravascular platelet transfusion (cordocentesis) is also effective. Cesarean section reduces the risk of intracranial hemorrhage.

Neonatal thrombocytopenia in infants born to women with ITP also is a result of placental transfer of maternal IgG antibodies. In ITP, these autoantibodies are directed against all platelet antigens, and mother and newborn may have low platelet counts. The risks of hemorrhage in an infant born to a mother with ITP may be lessened by cesarean section and by treatment of the mother with corticosteroids.

Treatment of an affected infant born to a mother with ITP may involve prednisone and IV immunoglobulin. In an emergency, random donor platelets may be used and may produce a transient increase in the infant's platelet count. Thrombocytopenia resolves spontaneously during the first month of life as maternal-derived antibody levels decline. Elevated levels of platelet-associated antibodies also have been noted in thrombocytopenic infants with sepsis and thrombocytopenia of unknown cause who were born to mothers without demonstrable platelet antibodies.

The *laboratory evaluation* of an infant (well or sick) with bleeding must include a platelet count, blood smear, and evaluation of PTT and PT. Isolated thrombocytopenia in a well infant suggests immune thrombocytopenia. Laboratory evidence of DIC includes a markedly prolonged PTT and PT (minutes rather than seconds), thrombocytopenia, and a blood smear suggesting a microangiopathic hemolytic anemia (burr or fragmented blood cells). Further evaluation reveals low levels of fibrinogen (<100 mg/dL) and elevated levels of fibrin degradation products. Vitamin K deficiency prolongs the PT more than the PTT, whereas hemophilia resulting from factors VIII and IX deficiency prolongs only the PTT. Specific factor levels confirm the *diagnosis* of hemophilia.

CHAPTER **63**
Necrotizing Enterocolitis

NEC is a syndrome of intestinal injury and is the most common intestinal emergency occurring in preterm infants admitted to the neonatal ICU. NEC occurs in 1 to 3 per 1000 live births and 1% to 7% of admissions to the neonatal ICU. Prematurity is the most consistent and significant factor associated with neonatal NEC. The disease occurs in 10% of infants who weigh less than 1500 g at birth. NEC is infrequent among term infants (<10% of affected infants).

Most cases of NEC occur in premature infants born before 34 weeks' gestation who have been fed enterally. Prematurity is associated with immaturity of the gastrointestinal tract, including decreased integrity of the intestinal mucosal barrier, depressed mucosal enzymes, suppressed gastrointestinal hormones, suppressed intestinal host defense system, decreased coordination of intestinal motility, and differences in blood flow autoregulation, which is thought to play a significant role in the pathogenesis of NEC. More than 90% of infants diagnosed with NEC have been fed enterally; however, NEC has been reported in infants who have never been fed. Feeding hypotheses have considered formula osmolality and strength, rate and route of feeding administration, bolus versus continuous feeds, and formula versus human milk. Only human milk has shown a beneficial role in reducing the incidence of NEC.

It also is theorized that compromised intestinal blood flow contributes to NEC. The pathogenesis of NEC also has been attributed to an ischemic insult to the gastrointestinal tract, although most infants with NEC have not had an obvious hypoxic-ischemic event.

Preterm infants in a neonatal ICU exhibit a different intestinal microflora than healthy infants. Primary invasion of the gut by bacteria is an alternative mechanism in the pathogenesis of NEC. Approximately 20% to 30% of infants with NEC have associated bacteremia with enteric organisms.

Early clinical signs of NEC include abdominal distention, feeding intolerance/increased gastric residuals, emesis, rectal bleeding, and occasional diarrhea. As the disease progresses, patients may develop marked abdominal distention, bilious emesis, ascites, abdominal wall erythema, lethargy, temperature instability, increased episodes of apnea/bradycardia, disseminated intravascular coagulation, and shock. With abdominal perforation, the abdomen may develop a bluish discoloration.

The white blood cell count can be elevated, but often it is depressed. Thrombocytopenia is common. In addition, infants may develop coagulation abnormalities along with metabolic derangements, including metabolic acidosis, electrolyte imbalance, and hypoglycemia and hyperglycemia. No unique infectious agent has been associated with NEC; bacteriologic and fungal cultures may prove helpful but not conclusive.

Radiographic imaging is essential to the diagnosis of NEC. The earliest radiographic finding is intestinal ileus, often associated with thickening of the bowel loops and air-fluid levels. The pathognomonic radiographic finding is **pneumatosis intestinalis** caused by hydrogen gas production from pathogenic bacteria present between the subserosal and muscularis layers of the bowel wall. Radiographic findings also may include a fixed or persistent dilated loop of bowel, intrahepatic venous gas, and *pneumoperitoneum* seen with bowel perforation.

The **differential diagnosis** of NEC includes sepsis with intestinal ileus or a volvulus. Both conditions can present with systemic signs of sepsis and abdominal distention. The absence of pneumatosis on abdominal radiographs does not rule out the diagnosis of NEC; however, other causes of abdominal distention and perforation (gastric or ileal perforation) should be considered and investigated. Patients diagnosed with Hirschsprung enterocolitis or severe gastroenteritis may present with pneumatosis intestinalis.

The **management** of NEC includes the discontinuation of enteral feedings, gastrointestinal decompression with nasogastric suction, fluid and electrolyte replacement, total parenteral nutrition, and systemic broad-spectrum antibiotics. When the diagnosis of NEC is made, consultation with a pediatric surgeon should be obtained. Even with aggressive and appropriate medical management, 25% to 50% of infants with NEC require surgical intervention. The decision to perform surgery is obvious when the presence of a pneumoperitoneum is observed on abdominal radiograph. Other, not so obvious indications for surgical intervention include rapid clinical deterioration despite medical therapy, rapid onset and progression of pneumatosis, abdominal mass, and intestinal obstruction. The surgical procedure of choice is laparotomy with removal of the frankly necrotic and nonviable bowel. Many extremely small infants are managed initially with primary peritoneal drainage followed by surgical intervention as needed later when the infant is stable, and a laparotomy can be performed safely. The long-term outcome includes intestinal strictures requiring further surgical intervention, short bowel syndrome with poor absorption of enteral fluids and nutrients, associated cholestasis with resultant cirrhosis and liver failure from prolonged parenteral nutrition, and neurodevelopmental delay from prolonged hospitalization.

CHAPTER 64

Hypoxic-Ischemic Encephalopathy, Intracranial Hemorrhage, and Seizures

The neonatal CNS is anatomically and functionally immature. Although division of cerebral cortical neuronal cells stops during the second trimester of pregnancy, glial cell growth, dendritic arborization, myelination, and cerebellar neuronal cell number continue to increase beyond term gestation and into infancy. At birth, the human newborn spends more time asleep (predominantly in rapid eye movement or active sleep) than in a wakeful state and is totally dependent on adults. Primitive reflexes, such as the Moro, grasp, stepping, rooting, sucking, and crossed extensor reflexes, are readily elicited and are normal for this age. In addition, the newborn has a wealth of cortical functions that are less easily shown (e.g., the ability to extinguish repetitive or painful stimuli and to show visual preference for new or novel objects). The newborn also has the capacity for attentive eye fixation and differential responses to the mother's voice. During the perinatal period, many pathophysiologic mechanisms can adversely and permanently affect the developing brain, including prenatal events, such as hypoxia, ischemia, infections, inflammation, malformations, maternal drugs, and coagulation disorders, and postnatal events, such as birth trauma, hypoxia-ischemia, inborn errors of metabolism, hypoglycemia, hypothyroidism, hyperthyroidism, polycythemia, hemorrhage, and meningitis.

NEONATAL SEIZURES

Seizures during the neonatal period may be the result of multiple causes, with characteristic **historical and clinical manifestations**. **Seizures caused by hypoxic-ischemic encephalopathy** (postasphyxial seizures), a common cause of seizures in the full-term infant, usually occur 12 to 24 hours after a history of birth asphyxia and often are refractory to conventional doses of anticonvulsant medications. Postasphyxial seizures also may be caused by metabolic disorders associated with neonatal asphyxia, such as hypoglycemia and hypocalcemia. **IVH** is a common cause of seizures in premature infants and often occurs between 1 and 3 days of age. Seizures with IVH are associated with a bulging fontanel, hemorrhagic spinal fluid, anemia, lethargy, and coma. Seizures caused by **hypoglycemia** often occur when blood glucose levels decline to the lowest postnatal value (at 1 to 2 hours of age or after 24 to 48 hours of poor nutritional intake). Seizures caused by **hypocalcemia** and **hypomagnesemia** develop in high-risk infants and respond well to therapy with calcium, magnesium, or both.

Seizures noted in the delivery room often are caused by direct *injection of local anesthetic agents* into the fetal scalp (associated with transient bradycardia and fixed dilated pupils), severe *anoxia,* or *congenital brain malformation.* Seizures after the first 5 days of life may be the result of *infection* or *drug withdrawal.* Seizures associated with lethargy, acidosis, and a family history of infant deaths may be the result of an *inborn error of metabolism.* An infant whose parent has a history of a neonatal seizure also is at risk for *benign familial seizures.* In an infant who appears well, a sudden onset on day 1 to 3 of life of seizures that are of short duration and that do not recur may be the result of a *subarachnoid hemorrhage.* Focal seizures often are the result of local cerebral infarction.

Seizures may be difficult to differentiate from benign jitteriness or from tremulousness in infants of diabetic mothers, in infants with narcotic withdrawal syndrome, and in any infants after an episode of asphyxia. In contrast to seizures, jitteriness and tremors are sensory dependent, elicited by stimuli, and interrupted by holding the extremity. Seizure activity becomes manifested as coarse, fast and slow clonic activity, whereas jitteriness is characterized by fine, rapid movement. Seizures may be associated with abnormal eye movements, such as tonic deviation to one side. The electroencephalogram often shows seizure activity when the clinical diagnosis is uncertain. Identifying seizures in the newborn period is often difficult because the infant, especially the LBW infant, usually does not show the tonic-clonic major motor activity typical of the older child (Table 64–1). Subtle seizures are a common manifestation among newborns. The subtle signs of seizure activity include apnea, eye deviation, tongue thrusting, eye blinking, fluctuation of vital signs, and staring. Continuous bedside electroencephalogram monitoring can help identify subtle seizures.

The *diagnostic evaluation* of infants with seizures should involve an immediate determination of capillary blood glucose levels with a Chemstrip. In addition, blood concentrations of sodium, calcium, glucose, and bilirubin should be determined. When infection is suspected, CSF and blood specimens should be obtained for culture. After the seizure has stopped, a careful examination should be done to identify signs of increased intracranial pressure, congenital malformations, and systemic illness. If signs of elevated intracranial pressure are absent, a lumbar puncture should be

performed. If the diagnosis is not apparent at this point, further evaluation should involve MRI, CT, or cerebral ultrasound and tests to determine the presence of an inborn error of metabolism. Determinations of inborn errors of metabolism are especially important in infants with unexplained lethargy, coma, acidosis, ketonuria, or respiratory alkalosis (see Section X).

TABLE 64–1. Clinical Characteristics of Neonatal Seizures

Designation	Characterization
Focal clonic	Repetitive, rhythmic contractions of muscle groups of the limbs, face, or trunk
	May be unilateral or multifocal
	May appear synchronously or asynchronously in various body regions
	Cannot be suppressed by restraint
Focal tonic	Sustained posturing of single limbs
	Sustained asymmetric posturing of the trunk
	Sustained eye deviation
	Cannot be provoked by stimulation or suppressed by restraint
Myoclonic	Arrhythmic contractions of muscle groups of the limbs, face, or trunk
	Typically not repetitive or may recur at a slow rate
	May be generalized, focal, or fragmentary
	May be provoked by stimulation
Generalized tonic	Sustained symmetric posturing of limbs, trunk, and neck
	May be flexor, extensor, or mixed extensor/flexor
	May be provoked by stimulation
	May be suppressed by restraint or repositioning
Ocular signs	Random and roving eye movements or nystagmus
	Distinct from tonic eye deviation
Orobuccolingual movements	Sucking, chewing, tongue protrusions
	May be provoked by stimulation
Progression movements	Rowing or swimming movements of the arms
	Pedaling or bicycling movements of the legs
	May be provoked by stimulation
	May be suppressed by restraint or repositioning

From Mizrahi EM: Neonatal seizures. In Shinnar S, Branski D (eds): Pediatric and Adolescent Medicine, Vol 6. Childhood Seizures. Basel, S. Karger, 1995.

The *treatment* of neonatal seizures may be specific, such as treatment of meningitis or the correction of **hypoglycemia, hypocalcemia, hypomagnesemia, hyponatremia, or vitamin B$_6$** deficiency or dependency. In the absence of an identifiable cause, therapy should involve an anticonvulsant agent, such as 20 to 40 mg/kg of phenobarbital, 10 to 20 mg/kg of phenytoin (Dilantin), or 0.1 to 0.3 mg/kg of diazepam (Valium), followed by one of the two longer acting drugs. Treatment of status epilepticus requires repeated doses of phenobarbital and may require diazepam or midazolam, titrated to clinical signs. The long-term outcome for neonatal seizures usually is related to the underlying cause and to the primary pathology, such as hypoxic-ischemic encephalopathy, meningitis, drug withdrawal, stroke, or hemorrhage.

INTRACRANIAL HEMORRHAGE

Intracranial hemorrhage may be confined to one anatomic area of the brain, such as the subdural, subarachnoid, periventricular, intraventricular, intraparenchymal, or cerebellar region. **Subdural hemorrhages** are seen in association with birth trauma, cephalopelvic disproportion, forceps delivery, LGA infants, skull fractures, and postnatal head trauma. The subdural hematoma does not always cause symptoms immediately after birth; with time, however, the RBCs undergo hemolysis, and water is drawn into the hemorrhage because of the high oncotic pressure of protein, resulting in an expanding symptomatic lesion. Anemia, vomiting, seizures, and macrocephaly may occur in an infant who is 1 to 2 months old and has a subdural hematoma. *Child abuse* also must be suspected, and appropriate diagnostic evaluation must be undertaken to identify other possible signs of skeletal, ocular, or soft tissue injury. Occasionally a massive subdural hemorrhage in the neonatal period is caused by rupture of the vein of Galen or by an inherited coagulation disorder, such as hemophilia. Infants with these conditions exhibit shock, seizures, and coma. The **treatment** of all symptomatic subdural hematomas is surgical evacuation.

Subarachnoid hemorrhages may be spontaneous, associated with hypoxia, or caused by bleeding from a cerebral arteriovenous malformation. Seizures are a common presenting manifestation, and the *prognosis* depends on the underlying injury. *Treatment* is directed at the seizure and the rare occurrence of posthemorrhagic hydrocephalus.

Periventricular hemorrhage and **IVH** are common in VLBW infants, and the risk decreases with increasing gestational age. Fifty percent of infants weighing less than 1500 g have evidence of intracranial bleeding. The *pathogenesis* for these hemorrhages is unknown (they usually are not caused by coagulation disorders), but the initial site of bleeding may be the weak blood vessels in the periventricular germinal matrix. The vessels in this area have poor structural support. These vessels may rupture and hemorrhage because of passive changes in cerebral blood flow occurring with the variations of blood pressure that sick premature infants often exhibit (failure of autoregulation). In some sick infants, these blood pressure variations are the only identifiable etiologic factors. In others, the disorders that may cause the elevation or depression of blood pressure or that interfere with venous return from the head (venous stasis) increase the risk of IVH; these disorders include asphyxia, pneumothorax, mechanical ventilation, hypercapnia, hypoxemia, prolonged labor, breech delivery, PDA, heart failure, and therapy with hypertonic solutions such as sodium bicarbonate.

Most periventricular hemorrhages and IVHs occur in the first 3 days of life. It is unusual for IVH to occur after day 5 of life. The *clinical manifestations* of IVH include seizures, apnea, bradycardia, lethargy, coma, hypotension, metabolic acidosis, anemia not corrected by blood transfusion, bulging fontanel, and cutaneous mottling. Many infants with small hemorrhages (grade 1 or 2) are asymptomatic; infants with larger hemorrhages (grade 4) often have a catastrophic event that rapidly progresses to shock and coma.

The *diagnosis* of IVH is confirmed and the severity graded by ultrasound or CT examination through the anterior fontanel. Grade 1 IVH is confined to the germinal matrix; grade 2 is an extension of grade 1, with blood noted in the ventricle without ventricular enlargement; grade 3 is an extension of grade 2 with ventricular dilation; and grade 4 has blood in dilated ventricles and in the cerebral cortex, either contiguous with or distant from the ventricle. Grade 4 hemorrhage has a poor prognosis, as does the development of periventricular, small, echolucent cystic lesions, with or without porencephalic cysts and posthemorrhagic hydrocephalus. Periventricular cysts often are noted after the resolution of echodense areas in the periventricular white matter. The cysts may correspond to the development of **periventricular leukomalacia**, which may be a precursor to cerebral palsy. Extensive intraparenchymal echodensities represent hemorrhagic necrosis. They are associated with a high mortality rate and have a poor neurodevelopmental prognosis for survivors.

Treatment of an acute hemorrhage involves standard supportive care, including ventilation for apnea and blood transfusion for shock. Posthemorrhagic hydrocephalus may be managed with serial daily lumbar punctures, an external ventriculostomy tube, or a permanent ventricular-peritoneal shunt. Implementation of the shunt often is delayed because of the high protein content of the hemorrhagic ventricular fluid.

TABLE 64–2. Hypoxic-Ischemic Encephalopathy in Term Infants

Signs	Stage 1	Stage 2	Stage 3
Level of consciousness	Hyperalert	Lethargic	Stuporous
Muscle tone	Normal	Hypotonic	Flaccid
Tendon reflexes/clonus	Hyperactive	Hyperactive	Absent
Moro reflex	Strong	Weak	Absent
Pupils	Mydriasis	Miosis	Unequal, poor light reflex
Seizures	None	Common	Decerebration
Electroencephalographic	Normal	Low voltage changing to seizure activity	Burst suppression to isoelectric
Duration	>24 hr if progresses, otherwise may remain normal	24 hr to 14 days	Days to weeks

Modified from Sarnat HB, Sarnat MS: Neonatal encephalopathy following fetal distress. Arch Neurol 33:696, 1976.

HYPOXIC-ISCHEMIC ENCEPHALOPATHY

Conditions known to reduce uteroplacental blood flow or to interfere with spontaneous respiration lead to perinatal hypoxia, to lactic acidosis and, if severe enough to reduce cardiac output or cause cardiac arrest, to ischemia. The combination of the reduced availability of oxygen for the brain that is a result of hypoxia and the diminished or absent blood flow to the brain that is a result of ischemia leads to reduced glucose for metabolism and to an accumulation of lactate that produces local tissue acidosis. After reperfusion, hypoxic-ischemic injury also may be complicated by cell necrosis and vascular endothelial edema, reducing blood flow distal to the involved vessel. Typically, hypoxic-ischemic encephalopathy in the term infant is characterized by cerebral edema, cortical necrosis, and involvement of the basal ganglia, whereas in the preterm infant, it is characterized by periventricular leukomalacia. Both lesions may result in cortical atrophy, mental retardation, and spastic quadriplegia or diplegia.

The *clinical manifestations* and characteristic course of hypoxic-ischemic encephalopathy vary according to the severity of the injury (Table 64–2). Infants with severe stage 3 hypoxic-ischemic encephalopathy are usually hypotonic, although occasionally they initially appear hypertonic and hyperalert at birth. As cerebral edema develops, brain functions are affected in a descending order; cortical depression produces coma, and brainstem depression results in apnea. As cerebral edema progresses, refractory seizures begin 12 to 24 hours after birth. Concurrently the infant has no signs of spontaneous respirations, is hypotonic, and has diminished or absent deep tendon reflexes.

Survivors of stage 3 hypoxic-ischemic encephalopathy have a high incidence of seizures and serious neurodevelopmental handicaps. The prognosis of severe asphyxia also depends on other organ system injury (see Table 58–9). Another indicator of poor prognosis is time of onset of spontaneous respiration as estimated by Apgar score. Infants with Apgar scores of 0 to 3 at 10 minutes have a 20% mortality and a 5% incidence of cerebral palsy; if the score remains this low by 20 minutes, the mortality increases to 60%, and the incidence of cerebral palsy increases to 57%.

CHAPTER 65

Sepsis and Meningitis

Systemic and local infections (lung, cutaneous, ocular, umbilical, kidney, bone-joint, and meningeal) are common in the newborn period. Infection may be acquired in utero through the transplacental or transcervical routes and during or after birth. Ascending infection through the cervix, with or without rupture of the amniotic fluid membranes, may result in amnionitis, funisitis (infection of the umbilical cord), congenital pneumonia, and sepsis. The bacteria responsible for ascending infection of the fetus are common bacterial organisms of the maternal genitourinary tract, such as group B streptococci, *E. coli, Haemophilus influenzae,* and *Klebsiella.* Herpes simplex virus (HSV)-1 or more often HSV-2 also causes ascending infection that at times may be indistinguishable from bacterial sepsis. Syphilis and *Listeria monocytogenes* are acquired by transplacental infection.

Maternal humoral immunity may protect the fetus against some neonatal pathogens, such as group B streptococci and HSV. Nonetheless, various deficiencies of the neonatal antimicrobial defense mechanism probably are more important than maternal immune status as a contributing factor for neonatal infection, especially in the LBW infant. The incidence of sepsis is approximately 1:1500 in full-term infants and 1:250 in preterm infants. The sixfold-higher rate of sepsis among preterm infants compared with term infants relates to the more immature immunologic systems of preterm infants and to their prolonged periods of hospitalization, which increase risk of nosocomially acquired infectious diseases.

Preterm infants before 32 weeks of gestational age have not received the full complement of maternal antibodies (IgG), which cross the placenta by active transport predominantly in the latter half of the third trimester. In addition, although LBW infants may generate IgM antibodies, their own IgG response to infection is reduced. These infants also have deficiencies of the alternate and, to a smaller degree, the classic complement activation pathways, which results in diminished complement-mediated opsonization. Newborn infants also show a deficit in phagocytic migration to the site of infection (to the lung) and in the bone marrow reserve pool of leukocytes. In addition, in the presence of suboptimal activation of complement, neonatal neutrophils ingest and kill bacteria less effectively than adult neutrophils do. Neutrophils from sick infants seem to have an even greater deficit in bacterial killing capacity compared with phagocytic cells from normal neonates.

Defense mechanisms against viral pathogens also may be deficient in a newborn. Neonatal antibody-dependent, cell-mediated immunity by the natural killer lymphocytes is deficient in the absence of maternal antibodies and in the presence of reduced interferon production; reduced antibody levels occur in premature infants and in infants born during a primary viral infection of the mother, such as with enteroviruses, HSV-2, or CMV. In addition, antibody-independent cytotoxicity may be reduced in lymphocytes of newborns.

Bacterial sepsis and meningitis often are linked closely in neonates. Despite this association, the incidence of meningitis relative to neonatal sepsis has been on a steady decline. The incidence of meningitis is approximately 1 in 20 cases of sepsis. The causative organisms isolated most frequently are the same as for neonatal sepsis: group B streptococci, *E. coli*, and *L. monocytogenes*. Gram-negative organisms, such as *Klebsiella* and *Serratia marcescens*, are more common in less developed countries, and coagulase-negative

staphylococci need to be considered in VLBW infants. Male infants seem to be more susceptible to neonatal infection than female infants. Severely premature infants are at even greater risk secondary to less effective defense mechanisms and deficient transfer of antibodies from the mother to the fetus (which occurs mostly after 32 weeks' gestation). Neonates in the neonatal ICU live in a hostile environment, with exposure to endotracheal tubes, central arterial and venous catheters, and blood draws all predisposing to bacteremia and meningitis. Genetic factors have been implicated in the ability of bacteria to cross the blood-brain barrier. This penetration has been noted for group B streptococci, *E. coli*, *Listeria*, *Citrobacter*, and *Streptococcus pneumoniae*.

Neonatal sepsis presents during three periods. **Early-onset sepsis** often begins in utero and usually is a result of infection caused by the bacteria in the mother's genitourinary tract. Organisms related to this sepsis include group B streptococci, *E. coli*, *Klebsiella*, *L. monocytogenes*, and nontypable *H. influenzae*. Most infected infants are premature and show nonspecific cardiorespiratory signs, such as grunting, tachypnea, and cyanosis at birth. Risk factors for early-onset sepsis include vaginal colonization with group B streptococci, prolonged rupture of the membranes (>24 hours), amnionitis, maternal fever or leukocytosis, fetal tachycardia, and preterm birth. African American race and male sex are unexplained additional risk factors for neonatal sepsis.

Early-onset sepsis (birth to 7 days) is an overwhelming multiorgan system disease frequently manifested as respiratory failure, shock, meningitis (in 30% of cases), DIC, acute tubular necrosis, and symmetric peripheral gangrene. Early manifestations—grunting, poor feeding, pallor, apnea, lethargy, hypothermia, or an abnormal cry—may be nonspecific. Profound neutropenia, hypoxia, and hypotension may be refractory to treatment with broad-spectrum antibiotics, mechanical ventilation, and vasopressors such as dopamine and dobutamine. In the initial stages of early-onset septicemia in a preterm infant, it is often difficult to differentiate sepsis from RDS. Because of this difficulty, premature infants with RDS receive broad-spectrum antibiotics.

The clinical manifestations of sepsis are difficult to separate from the manifestations of meningitis in the neonate. Infants with early-onset sepsis should be *evaluated* by blood and CSF cultures, CSF Gram stain, cell count, and protein and glucose levels. Normal newborns generally have an elevated CSF protein content (100 to 150 mg/dL) and may have 25 to 30/mm^3 white blood cells (mean 9/mm^3), which are 75% lymphocytes in the absence of infection. Some infants with neonatal meningitis caused by group B streptococci do not have an elevated CSF leukocyte count but are seen to have microorganisms in the CSF on Gram stain. In addition to culture, other methods of identifying the pathogenic bacteria are the determination of bacterial antigen in samples of blood, urine, or CSF. In cases of neonatal meningitis, the ratio of CSF glucose to blood glucose usually is less than 50%. The PCR test primarily is used to identify viral infections. Serial complete blood counts should be performed to identify neutropenia, an increased number of immature neutrophils (bands), and thrombocytopenia. C-reactive protein levels are often elevated in neonatal patients with bacterial sepsis.

A chest radiograph also should be obtained to determine the presence of pneumonia. In addition to the traditional neonatal pathogens, pneumonia in VLBW infants may be the result of acquisition of maternal genital mycoplasmal agent (e.g., *U. urealyticum* or *M. hominis*). Arterial blood gases should be monitored to detect hypoxemia and metabolic acidosis that may be caused by hypoxia, shock, or both. Blood pressure, urine output, and peripheral perfusion should be monitored to determine the need to treat septic shock with fluids and vasopressor agents.

The mainstay of treatment for sepsis and meningitis is antibiotic therapy. Antibiotics are used to suppress bacterial growth, allowing the infant's defense mechanisms time to respond. In addition, support measures, such as assisted ventilation and cardiovascular support, are equally important to the management of the infant. A combination of ampicillin and an aminoglycoside (usually gentamicin) for 10 to 14 days is effective *treatment* against most organisms responsible for early-onset sepsis. The combination of ampicillin and cefotaxime also is proposed as an alternative method of treatment. If meningitis is present, the treatment should be extended to 21 days or 14 days after a negative result from a CSF culture. Persistently positive results from CSF cultures are common with neonatal meningitis caused by gram-negative organisms, even with appropriate antibiotic treatment, and may be present for 2 to 3 days after antibiotic therapy. If gram-negative meningitis is present, some authorities continue to treat with an effective penicillin derivative combined with an aminoglycoside, whereas most change to a third-generation cephalosporin. High-dose penicillin (250,000 to 450,000 U/kg/24 hr) is appropriate for group B streptococcal meningitis. Inhaled nitric oxide, ECMO (in term infants), or both may improve the outcome of sepsis-related pulmonary hypertension. Intratracheal surfactant may reverse respiratory failure. Intrapartum penicillin empirical prophylaxis for group B streptococcal colonized mothers or mothers with risk factors (e.g., fever, preterm labor, previous infant with group B streptococci, and amnionitis) has reduced the rate of early-onset infection. The approach to the infant after prophylaxis is summarized in Figure 65–1.

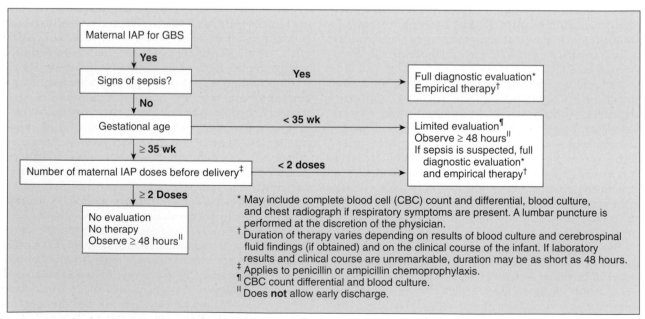

Figure 65–1

Suggested empirical management of a neonate after maternal intrapartum antimicrobial prophylaxis (IAP) for prevention of early-onset group B streptococcal (GBS) disease. This is not an exclusive approach to management. (From American Academy of Pediatrics: Red Book 2000, 25th ed. Chicago, The Academy, 2000, p 542.)

Late-onset sepsis (8 to 28 days) usually occurs in a healthy full-term infant who was discharged in good health from the normal newborn nursery. *Clinical manifestations* may include lethargy, poor feeding, hypotonia, apathy, seizures, bulging fontanel, fever, and direct-reacting hyperbilirubinemia. In addition to bacteremia, hematogenous seeding may result in focal infections, such as meningitis (in 75% of cases), osteomyelitis (group B streptococci, *S. aureus*), arthritis (gonococcus, *S. aureus, Candida albicans,* gram-negative bacteria), and urinary tract infection (gram-negative bacteria).

The *evaluation* of infants with late-onset sepsis is similar to that for infants with early-onset sepsis, with special attention given to a careful physical examination of the bones (infants with osteomyelitis may exhibit pseudoparalysis) and to the laboratory examination and culture of urine obtained by sterile suprapubic aspiration or urethral catheterization. Late-onset sepsis may be caused by the same pathogens as early-onset sepsis, but infants exhibiting sepsis late in the neonatal period also may have infections caused by the pathogens usually found in older infants (*H. influenzae, S. pneumoniae,* and *Neisseria meningitidis*). In addition, viral agents (HSV, CMV, or enteroviruses) may manifest with a late-onset, sepsis-like picture.

Because of the increased rate of resistance of *H. influenzae* and pneumococcus to ampicillin, some centers begin treatment with ampicillin and a third-generation cephalosporin (and vancomycin if meningitis is present) when sepsis occurs in the last week of the first month of life. The treatment of late-onset neonatal sepsis and meningitis is the same as that for early-onset sepsis.

Nosocomially acquired sepsis (8 days to discharge) occurs predominantly in premature infants in the neonatal ICU; many of these infants have been colonized with the multidrug-resistant bacteria indigenous to the neonatal ICU. The risk of such serious bacterial infection is increased by frequent treatment with broad-spectrum antibiotics for sepsis and by the presence of central venous indwelling catheters, endotracheal tubes, umbilical vessel catheters, and electronic monitoring devices. Epidemics of bacterial (coagulase-negative staphylococci, fungi, enteric bacteria) or viral sepsis, bacterial or aseptic meningitis, staphylococcal bullous skin infections, cellulitis, pneumonia (bacterial or caused by adenovirus or respiratory syncytial virus), omphalitis (caused by *S. aureus* or gram-negative bacilli), and diarrhea (staphylococcal, enteroviral, or caused by rotavirus or enteropathogenic *E. coli*) are common in the neonatal ICU and in the nursery for well infants.

The initial *clinical manifestations* of nosocomial infection in a premature infant may be subtle and include apnea and bradycardia, temperature instability, abdominal distention, and poor feeding. In the later stages, signs of infection are shock, DIC, worsening respiratory status, and local reactions, such as omphalitis, eye discharge, diarrhea, and bullous impetigo.

The *treatment* of nosocomially acquired sepsis depends on the indigenous microbiologic flora of the particular hospital and the antibiotic sensitivities. Because *S. aureus* (occasionally methicillin-resistant), *Staphylococcus epidermidis* (methicillin-resistant), and gram-negative pathogens are common nosocomial bacterial agents in many nurseries, a combination of vancomycin or oxacillin/nafcillin (some use ampicillin) with an aminoglycoside (gentamicin or tobramycin) is appropriate. The dose and interval for administering all aminoglycosides, such as gentamicin, vary with postnatal age and birth weight. In addition, treatment with aminoglycosides for more than 3 days necessitates monitoring of the serum peak and trough concentrations to optimize therapy and to avoid ototoxicity and nephrotoxicity. Persistent signs of infection despite antibacterial treatment suggest candidal or viral sepsis.

CHAPTER 66
Congenital Infections

An infection acquired transplacentally during gestation is a *congenital infection.* Numerous pathogens that produce mild or subclinical disease in older infants and children can cause severe disease in neonates who acquire such infections prenatally or perinatally. Sepsis, meningitis, pneumonia, and other infections caused by numerous perinatally acquired pathogens are the cause of significant neonatal morbidity and mortality. Congenital infections include a well-known group of fungal, bacterial, and viral pathogens: toxoplasmosis, rubella, CMV, HSV, varicella-zoster virus, congenital syphilis, parvovirus, HIV, hepatitis B, *Neisseria gonorrhoeae, Chlamydia,* and *Mycobacterium tuberculosis.*

Many of the clinical manifestations of congenital infections are similar, including IUGR, nonimmune hydrops, anemia, thrombocytopenia, jaundice, hepatosplenomegaly, chorioretinitis, and congenital malformations. Some unique manifestations and epidemiologic characteristics of these infections are listed in Table 66-1. Evaluation of patients thought to have a congenital infection should include attempts to isolate the organism by culture (for rubella, CMV, HSV, gonorrhea, and *M. tuberculosis*), to identify the antigen of the pathogen (for hepatitis B and *C. trachomatis*), to identify the pathogen's genome with PCR, and to identify specific fetal production of antibodies (IgM or

TABLE 66–1. Perinatal Congenital Infections (TORCH)

Agent	Maternal Epidemiology	Neonatal Features
Toxoplasma gondii	Heterophil-negative mononucleosis Exposure to cats or raw meat or immunosuppression High-risk exposure at 10-24 wk gestation	Hydrocephalus, abnormal spinal fluid, intracranial calcifications, chorioretinitis, jaundice, hepatosplenomegaly, fever Many infants asymptomatic at birth *Treatment:* pyrimethamine plus sulfadiazine

Rubella virus	Unimmunized seronegative mother; fever ± rash
	Detectable defects with infection:
	  by 8 wk, 85%
	  9-12 wk, 50%
	  13-20 wk, 16%
	Virus may be present in infant's throat for 1 yr
	Prevention: vaccine
		Intrauterine growth retardation, microcephaly, microphthalmia, cataracts, glaucoma, "salt and pepper" chorioretinitis, hepatosplenomegaly, jaundice, PDA, deafness, blueberry muffin rash, anemia, thrombocytopenia, leukopenia, metaphyseal lucencies, B cell and T cell deficiency
		Infant may be asymptomatic at birth

CMV	Sexually transmitted disease: primary genital infection may be asymptomatic Heterophil-negative mononucleosis; infant may have viruria for 1-6 yr	Sepsis, intrauterine growth retardation, chorioretinitis, microcephaly, periventricular calcifications, blueberry muffin rash, anemia, thrombocytopenia, neutropenia, hepatosplenomegaly, jaundice, deafness, pneumonia Many asymptomatic at birth *Prevention:* CMV-negative blood products *Possible treatment:* ganciclovir?
Herpes simplex type 2 or 1 virus	Sexually transmitted disease: primary genital infection may be asymptomatic; intrauterine infection rare, acquisition at time of birth more common	*Intrauterine infection:* chorioretinitis, skin lesions, microcephaly *Postnatal:* encephalitis, localized or disseminated disease, skin vesicles, keratoconjunctivitis *Treatment:* acyclovir
Varicella-zoster virus	Intrauterine infection with chickenpox during first trimester Infant develops severe neonatal varicella with maternal illness 5 days before or 2 days after delivery	Microphthalmia, cataracts, chorioretinitis, cutaneous and bony aplasia/hypoplasia/atrophy, cutaneous scars Zoster as in older child *Prevention of neonatal* condition with VZIG *Treatment of ill neonate:* acyclovir
Treponema pallidum (syphilis)	Sexually transmitted disease Maternal primary asymptomatic: painless "hidden" chancre Penicillin, not erythromycin, prevents fetal infection	Presentation *at birth* as nonimmune hydrops, prematurity, anemia, neutropenia, thrombocytopenia, pneumonia, hepatosplenomegaly *Late neonatal* as snuffles (rhinitis), rash, hepatosplenomegaly, condylomata lata, metaphysitis, cerebrospinal fluid pleocytosis, keratitis, periosteal new bone, lymphocytosis, hepatitis *Late onset:* teeth, eye, bone, skin, CNS, ear *Treatment:* penicillin
Parvovirus	Etiology of fifth disease; fever, rash, arthralgia in adults	Nonimmune hydrops, fetal anemia *Treatment:* in utero transfusion
HIV	AIDS; most mothers are asymptomatic and HIV positive; high-risk history; prostitute, drug abuse, married to bisexual, or hemophiliac	AIDS symptoms develop between 3 and 6 mo of age in 10-25%; failure to thrive, recurrent infection, hepatosplenomegaly, neurologic abnormalities *Management:* trimethoprim/sulfamethoxazole, AZT, other antiretroviral agents *Prevention:* prenatal, intrapartum, postpartum AZT; avoid breastfeeding
Hepatitis B virus	Vertical transmission common; may result in cirrhosis, hepatocellular carcinoma	Acute neonatal hepatitis; many become asymptomatic carriers *Prevention:* HBIG, vaccine

TABLE 66–1. Perinatal Congenital Infections (TORCH)—cont'd

Agent	Maternal Epidemiology	Neonatal Features
Neisseria gonorrhoeae	Sexually transmitted disease, infant acquires at birth *Treatment:* cefotaxime, ceftriaxone	Gonococcal ophthalmia, sepsis, meningitis *Prevention:* silver nitrate, erythromycin eye drops *Treatment:* intravenous ceftriaxone
Chlamydia trachomatis	Sexually transmitted disease, infant acquires at birth *Treatment:* oral erythromycin	Conjunctivitis, pneumonia *Prevention:* erythromycin eye drops *Treatment:* oral erythromycin
Mycobacterium tuberculosis	Positive PPD skin test, recent converter, positive chest radiograph, positive family member *Treatment:* INH and rifampin ± ethambutol	Congenital rare septic pneumonia; acquired primary pulmonary TB; asymptomatic, follow PPD *Prevention:* INH, BCG, separation *Treatment:* INH, rifampin, pyrazinamide
Trypanosoma cruzi (Chagas disease)	Central South American native, immigrant, travel Chronic disease in mother	Failure to thrive, heart failure, achalasia *Treatment:* nifurtimox

AZT, zidovudine (azidothymidine); BCG, bacille Calmette-Guérin; CMV, cytomegalovirus; HBIG, hepatitis B immune globulin; INH, isoniazid; PDA, patent ductus arteriosus; PPD, purified protein derivative; TB, tuberculosis; VZIG, varicella-zoster immune globulin.

increasing titer of IgG for *Toxoplasma,* syphilis, parvovirus, HIV, or *Borrelia*).

Treatment is not always available, specific, or effective. Nonetheless, some encouraging results have been reported for preventing the disease and for specifically treating the infant when the correct diagnosis is made (see Table 66–1).

TOXOPLASMOSIS

Vertical transmission of *Toxoplasma gondii* occurs by transplacental transfer of the organism from the mother to the fetus after an acute maternal infection. Fetal infection rarely can occur after reactivation of disease in an immunocompromised pregnant mother. Transmission from an acutely infected mother to her fetus occurs in about 30% to 40% of cases, but the rate varies directly with gestational age. Transmission rates and the timing of fetal infection correlate directly with placental blood flow; the risk of infection increases throughout gestation to 90% or greater near term, and the time interval between maternal and fetal infection decreases.

The severity of fetal disease varies inversely with the gestational age at which maternal infection occurs. Most infants have subclinical infection with no overt disease at birth; however, specific ophthalmologic and CNS evaluations may reveal abnormalities. The classic findings of hydrocephalus, chorioretinitis, and intracerebral calcifications suggest the diagnosis of congenital toxoplasmosis. Affected infants tend to be SGA, develop early-onset jaundice, have hepatosplenomegaly, and present with a generalized maculopapular rash. Seizures are common, and skull films may reveal diffuse cortical calcifications in contrast to the periventricular pattern observed with CMV. These infants are at increased risk for long-term neurologic and neurodevelopmental complications.

Serologic tests are the primary means of diagnosis. IgG-specific antibodies achieve a peak concentration 1 to 2 months after infection and remain positive indefinitely. For infants with seroconversion or a fourfold increase in IgG titers, specific IgM antibody determinations should be performed in patients to confirm disease. Especially for congenital infections, measurement of IgA and IgE antibodies can be useful to confirm the disease. Thorough ophthalmologic, auditory, and neurologic evaluations (head CT and CSF examination) are indicated.

For symptomatic and asymptomatic congenital infection, initial therapy should include pyrimethamine (supplemented with folic acid) combined with sulfadiazine. Duration of therapy is often prolonged even up to 1 year. Optimal dosages of medications and duration of therapy should be determined in consultation with appropriate specialists.

RUBELLA

With the widespread use of vaccination, congenital rubella is rare in developed countries. Acquired in utero during early gestation, rubella can cause severe neonatal consequences. The occurrence of congenital defects approaches 85% if infection is acquired during the first

4 weeks of gestation; close to 40% spontaneously abort or are stillborn. If infection occurs during weeks 13 to 16, 35% of infants can have abnormalities. Infection after 4 months' gestation does not seem to cause disease.

The most common characteristic abnormalities associated with congenital rubella include ophthalmologic (cataracts, retinopathy, and glaucoma), cardiac (PDA and peripheral pulmonary artery stenosis), auditory (sensorineural hearing loss), and neurologic (behavioral disorders, meningoencephalitis, and mental retardation) conditions. Additionally, infants can present with growth retardation, hepatosplenomegaly, early-onset jaundice, thrombocytopenia, radiolucent bone disease, and purpuric skin lesions ("blueberry muffin" appearance from dermal erythropoiesis).

Detection of rubella-specific IgM antibody usually indicates recent infection. Additionally, measurement of rubella-specific IgG over several months can be confirmatory. Rubella virus can be isolated from blood, urine, CSF, and throat swab specimens. Infants with congenital rubella are chronically and persistently infected and tend to shed live virus in urine, stools, and respiratory secretions for 1 year. Infants should be isolated while in the hospital and kept away from susceptible pregnant women when sent home.

CYTOMEGALOVIRUS

CMV is the most common congenital infection and the leading cause of sensorineural hearing loss, mental retardation, retinal disease, and cerebral palsy. Congenital CMV occurs in about 0.5% to 1.5% of births. When primary infection occurs in mothers during a pregnancy, the virus is transmitted to the fetus in approximately 35% of cases. Rates of CMV infection are three to seven times greater among infants born to adolescent mothers. The risk for transmission of CMV to the fetus is independent of gestational age at the time of maternal infection. The earlier in gestation that the primary maternal infection occurs, the more symptomatic the infant will be at birth. The most common sources of CMV for primary infections occurring in mothers during pregnancy are sexual contacts and contact with young children. It is well known that CMV can be transmitted to the fetus even when maternal infection occurred long before conception. This transmission can occur as the result of virus reactivation, chronic infection, or reinfection with a new strain.

More than 90% of infants who have congenital CMV infection exhibit no clinical evidence of disease at birth. Approximately 10% of infected infants have symptoms at birth. Findings include SGA, microcephaly, thrombocytopenia, hepatosplenomegaly, hepatitis, intracranial calcifications, chorioretinitis, and hearing abnormalities. Some infants can present with a blueberry muffin appearance as the result of dermal erythropoiesis. Skull films may reveal periventricular calcifications. An additional 10% of infected infants may not present until later in infancy or early childhood, when they are found to have sensorineural hearing loss and developmental delays. Mortality is 10% to 15% among symptomatic newborns. Perinatal CMV infection acquired during birth or from mother's milk is not associated with newborn illness or CNS sequelae.

Congenital CMV infection is diagnosed by detection of virus in the urine or saliva. Detection is often accomplished by traditional virus culture methods, but can take several weeks to obtain a result. Rapid culture methods using centrifugation to enhance infectivity and monoclonal antibody to detect early antigens in infected tissue culture can give results in 24 hours. PCR also can be used to detect small amounts of CMV DNA in the urine. Detection of CMV within the first 3 weeks after birth is considered proof of congenital CMV infection.

There are no antiviral agents currently approved for the treatment of congenital CMV infection. Trial studies in severely symptomatic newborns of the antiviral agent, ganciclovir, have shown a lack of progression of hearing loss.

HERPES SIMPLEX VIRUS

HSV-2 accounts for 90% of primary genital herpes. About 70% to 85% of neonatal herpes simplex infections are caused by HSV-2. Most commonly, neonatal infections are acquired from the mother shortly before (ascending infection) or during passage through the birth canal at delivery. The incidence of neonatal HSV is estimated to range from 1 in 3000 to 20,000 live births. Infants with HSV infections are more likely to be born prematurely (40% of affected infants are <36 weeks' gestation). The risk of infection at delivery in an infant born vaginally to a mother with primary genital herpes is about 33% to 50%. The risk to an infant born to a mother with a reactivated infection is less than 5%. More than 75% of infants who acquire HSV infection are born to mothers who have no previous history or clinical findings consistent with HSV infection.

Most infants are normal at birth, and symptoms of infection develop at 5 to 10 days of life. Symptoms of neonatal HSV infection include disseminated disease involving multiple organ systems, most notably the liver and lungs; localized infection to the CNS; or localized infection to the skin, eyes, and mouth. Symptoms may overlap, and in many cases of disseminated disease, skin lesions are a late finding. Disseminated infection should be considered in any infant with symptoms of sepsis, liver dysfunction, and negative bacteriologic cultures. HSV infection also should be suspected in any neonate who presents with fever, irritability, abnormal CSF findings, and seizures. Initial symptoms can occur anytime between birth and 4 weeks of age, although disseminated disease usually occurs during the first week of life. HSV infections are often severe, and a delay in treatment can result in significant morbidity and mortality.

For the diagnosis of neonatal HSV infection, specimens for culture should be obtained from any skin vesicle, nasopharynx, eyes, urine, blood, CSF, stool, or rectum. Positive cultures obtained from these sites more than 48 hours after birth indicate intrapartum exposure. PCR is a sensitive method for detecting HSV DNA in blood, urine, and CSF.

Parenteral acyclovir is the treatment of choice for neonatal HSV infections. Acyclovir should be administered to all infants suspected to have infection or diagnosed with HSV. The most benign outcome with regard to morbidity and mortality is observed in infants with disease limited to the skin, eyes, and mouth.

VARICELLA-ZOSTER VIRUS

The incidence of congenital infection among infants born to mothers who have varicella is about 2% when infection occurs within the first 20 weeks of gestation. Fetal infection after maternal varicella can result in varicella embryopathy, which is characterized by "zigzag" skin scarring and limb atrophy. CNS manifestations (hydrocephalus and microcephaly) and eye abnormalities (cataracts and chorioretinitis) also may occur.

Varicella infection can be fatal for the infant of a mother who develops varicella 5 days before to 2 days after delivery. Clinical features include severe rash, pneumonia, hepatitis, and death in 20% to 30% of cases. Infants born to mothers who are infected before 5 days prior to delivery have less severe disease secondary to the placental transfer of varicella-specific IgG antibody.

Varicella-zoster virus can be isolated from scrapings of a vesicle base during the first 3 to 4 days of the eruptions, but rarely from secretions from other sites, such as the respiratory tract. A significant increase in serum varicella IgG antibody can confirm the diagnosis. PCR is a sensitive method for detecting varicella DNA in any body fluid or tissue.

CONGENITAL SYPHILIS

Congenital syphilis most commonly results from transplacental infection of the fetus, although the fetus can acquire infection by contact with a chancre at birth. Additionally, hematogenous infection can occur throughout pregnancy. The longer the time elapsed between the mother's infection and pregnancy, the least likely she is to transmit the disease to the fetus.

Intrauterine infection can result in stillbirth, hydrops fetalis, or prematurity. Clinical symptoms vary but include hepatosplenomegaly, snuffles, lymphadenopathy, mucocutaneous lesions, osteochondritis, rash, hemolytic anemia, and thrombocytopenia. Untreated infants, regardless of whether they manifest symptoms at birth, may develop late symptoms, which usually appear after 2 years of age and involve the CNS, bones, joints, teeth, eyes, and skin. Some manifestations of disease may not become apparent until many years after birth, such as interstitial keratitis, eighth cranial nerve deafness, Hutchinson teeth, bowing of the skins, frontal bossing, mulberry molars, saddle nose, rhagades, and Clutton joints. The combination of interstitial keratitis, eighth cranial nerve deafness, and Hutchinson teeth is commonly referred to as the *Hutchinson triad*.

Many infants are asymptomatic at the time of diagnosis. If untreated, most infants develop symptoms within the first 5 weeks of life. The most striking lesions affect the mucocutaneous tissues and bones. Early signs of infection may be poor feeding and snuffles (syphilitic rhinitis). Snuffles are more severe and persistent than the common cold and are often bloody. A maculopapular desquamative rash develops over the palms and soles and around the mouth and anus. The rash may progress to become vesicular with bullae. Severely ill infants may be born with hydrops and have profound anemia. Severe consolidated pneumonia may be present at birth, and there may be laboratory findings consistent with a glomerulonephritis. CSF evaluation may reveal a pleocytosis and elevated protein. More than 90% of symptomatic infants exhibit radiographic abnormalities of the long bones consistent with osteochondritis and perichondritis.

No newborn should be discharged from the hospital without knowledge or determination of the mother's serologic status for syphilis. All infants born to seropositive mothers require a careful examination and a quantitative nontreponemal syphilis test. Dark-field examination of direct fluorescent antibody staining of organisms obtained by scraping a skin or mucous membrane lesion is the quickest and most direct method of diagnosis. More commonly, serologic testing is used. The nontreponemal reaginic antibody assays—the Venereal Disease Research Laboratory (VDRL) and the rapid plasma reagin—are helpful as indicators of disease. All infants born to seropositive mothers require a careful examination and a quantitative nontreponemal syphilis test. The test performed on the infant should be the same as that performed on the mother to enable comparison of results. An infant should be evaluated further if the maternal titer has increased fourfold, if the infant's titer is fourfold greater than the mother's titer, if the infant is symptomatic, or if the mother has inadequately treated syphilis. A mother infected later in pregnancy may deliver an infant who is incubating active disease. The mother and infant may have negative serologic testing at birth. When clinical or serologic tests suggest congenital syphilis, CSF should be examined microscopically, and a CSF VDRL test should be performed. An increased CSF white blood cell count and protein concentration suggests neurosyphilis; a positive CSF VDRL is diagnostic.

Parenteral penicillin is the preferred drug of choice for treatment of syphilis. Penicillin G for 10 to 14 days is the only documented effective therapy for infants who have congenital syphilis and neurosyphilis. Infants should have repeat nontreponemal antibody titers repeated at 3, 6, and 12 months to document falling titers. Infants with neurosyphilis must be followed carefully with serologic testing and CSF determinations every 6 months for at least 3 years or until CSF findings are normal.

HUMAN PARVOVIRUS B19

Infection with parvovirus B19 is recognized most often as erythema infectiosum, which is characterized by mild systemic symptoms, fever, and commonly a distinctive "slapped cheek" facial rash. Approximately 30% to 60% of adults are seropositive for human parvovirus B19. A significant proportion of childbearing women is potentially susceptible to infection.

Parvovirus B19 selectively infects erythropoietic precursors and inhibits their growth by inducing cell cycle arrest and apoptosis. Parvovirus infections often are associated with mild neutropenia and thrombocytopenia, but instances of transient pancytopenia also have been reported. Although the actual risk is probably low, the virus can infect the fetus, leading to fetal anemia, nonimmune hydrops, and fetal demise. Pathologic studies of parvovirus B19 human fetuses also have suggested that myocardial inflammation and subendocardial fibroelastosis may contribute to fetal hydrops.

Detection of serum parvovirus B19–specific IgM antibody is the preferred diagnostic test. A positive IgM test result indicates that infection probably occurred within the past 2 to 4 months. Antenatal treatment of parvovirus B19–infected fetuses with hydrops has included serial maternal ultrasound, fetal intrauterine blood transfusion, and maternal digitalization. Spontaneous resolution of fetal hydrops with normal outcome has been reported. Treatment for the infant after birth is mainly supportive and centered on the management of hydrops. Infants with aplastic crisis may require transfusions of blood products.

HUMAN IMMUNODEFICIENCY VIRUS

▶ (SEE CHAPTER 125.)

HEPATITIS B

▶ (SEE CHAPTER 113.)

NEISSERIA GONORRHOEAE

N. gonorrhoeae infection in a newborn usually involves the eyes (ophthalmia neonatorum). Other sites of infection include scalp abscesses (often associated with fetal monitoring with scalp electrodes), vaginitis, and disseminated disease with bacteremia, arthritis, or meningitis. Transmission to the infant usually occurs during passage through the birth canal when mucous membranes come in contact with infected secretions.

Infection usually is present within the first 5 days of life and is characterized initially by a clear, watery discharge, which rapidly becomes purulent. There is marked conjunctival hyperemia and chemosis. Infection tends to be bilateral; however, one eye may be clinically worse than the other. Untreated infections can spread to the cornea (keratitis) and anterior chamber of the eye. This extension can result in corneal perforation and blindness.

Recommended treatment for isolated infection, such as ophthalmia neonatorum, is one IM dose of ceftriaxone. Infants with gonococcal ophthalmia should receive eye irrigations with saline solution at frequent intervals before discharge. Topical antibiotic therapy alone is inadequate and is unnecessary when recommended systemic antimicrobial therapy is given. Infants with gonococcal ophthalmia should be hospitalized and evaluated for disseminated disease (sepsis, arthritis, meningitis). Disseminated disease should be treated with antimicrobial therapy (ceftriaxone or cefotaxime) for 7 days. Cefotaxime can be used in infants with hyperbilirubinemia. If documented, infants with meningitis should be treated for 10 to 14 days.

Tests for concomitant infection with *C. trachomatis,* congenital syphilis, and HIV should be performed. Results of the maternal test for hepatitis B surface antigen should be confirmed. Topical prophylaxis with silver nitrate, erythromycin, or tetracycline is recommended for all newborns for the prevention of gonococcal ophthalmia.

CHLAMYDIA

C. trachomatis is the most common reportable sexually transmitted infection, with a high rate of infection among sexually active adolescents and young adults. Prevalence of the organism in pregnant women ranges from 6% to 12% and can be 40% in adolescents. *Chlamydia* can be transmitted from the genital tract of infected mothers to their newborns. Acquisition occurs in about 50% of infants born vaginally to infected mothers. Transmission also has been reported in some infants delivered by cesarean section with intact membranes. In infected infants, the risk of conjunctivitis is 25% to 50%, and the risk of pneumonia is 5% to 20%. The nasopharynx is the most commonly infected anatomic site.

Neonatal chlamydial conjunctivitis is characterized by ocular congestion, edema, and discharge developing 5 to 14 days to several weeks after birth and lasting for 1 to 2 weeks. Clinical manifestations vary from mild conjunctivitis to intense inflammation and swelling. Both eyes are almost always involved; however, one eye may appear to be more swollen and infected than the other. The cornea is rarely involved and preauricular adenopathy is rare.

Pneumonia in a young infant can occur between 2 and 19 weeks of age and is characterized by an afebrile illness with a repetitive staccato cough, tachypnea, and rales. Wheezing is uncommon. Hyperinflation with diffuse infiltrates can be seen on chest radiograph. Nasal stuffiness and otitis media can occur.

Diagnosis can be made by scraping the conjunctiva and culturing the material. Giemsa staining of the conjunctival scrapings revealing the presence of blue-stained intracytoplasmic inclusions within the epithelial cells is diagnostic. PCR is also available. Infants with conjunctivitis and pneumonia are treated with oral erythromycin for 14 days. Topical treatment of conjunctivitis is ineffective and unnecessary. The recommended topical prophylaxis with silver nitrate, erythromycin, or tetracycline for all newborns for the prevention of gonococcal ophthalmia does not prevent neonatal chlamydial conjunctivitis.

MYCOBACTERIUM TUBERCULOSIS

▶ (SEE CHAPTER 124.)

SUGGESTED READING

Baird TM, Martin RL, Abu-Shaweesh: Clinical associations, treatment, and outcome of apnea of prematurity. NeoReviews 3:c66-c69, 2002.

Buyon JP, Nugent D, Mellins E, Sandborg C: Maternal immunologic diseases and neonatal disorders. NeoReviews 3:c3-c9, 2002.

Caplan MS, Jilling T: The pathophysiology of necrotizing enterocolitis. NeoReviews 2:e103-e108, 2001.

Christou H, Van Marter LJ, Wessel DL, et al: Inhaled nitric oxide reduces the need for extracorporeal membrane oxygenation in infants with persistent pulmonary hypertension of the newborn. Crit Care Med 28:3722, 2000.

Committee on Fetus and Newborn, American Academy of Pediatrics, and Committee on Obstetric Practice, American College of Obstetricians and Gynecologists: Use and abuse of Apgar score. Pediatrics 98:141-142, 1996.

Cowett RM: The infant of the diabetic mother. NeoReviews 3:e173-e189, 2002.

Darville T: Syphilis. Pediatr Rev 20:160-164, 1999.

Davis PJ, Shekerdemian LS: Meconium aspiration syndrome and extracorporeal membrane oxygenation. Arch Dis Child Fetal Neonatal Educ 84:F1, 2001.

Dimmitt RA, Moss RL: Clinical management of necrotizing enterocolitis. NeoReviews 2:e110-e116, 2001.

English R: Varicella. Pediatr Rev 24:372-378, 2003.

Gluckman PD, Pinal CS, Gunn AJ: Hypoxic-ischemic brain injury in the newborn: Pathophysiology and potential strategies for intervention. Semin Neonatol 6:109-120, 2001.

Hay WM, Thureen PJ, Anderson MS: Intrauterine growth restriction. NeoReviews 2:c129-c137, 2001.

Hill A: Neonatal seizures. Pediatr Rev 21:117-121, 2000.

Mulligan MJ, Stiehm ER: Neonatal hepatitis B infection: Clinical and immunologic considerations. J Perinatol 14:2, 1994.

Murphy JH: Nonimmune hydrops fetalis. NeoReviews 5:e5-e14, 2004.

Nuss R, Manco-Johnson M: Bleeding disorders in the neonate. NeoReviews 1:e196-e199, 2000.

Palmer RH, Clanton M, Ezhuthachan S, et al: Applying the "10 simple rules" of medicine to management of hyperbilirubinemia in newborns. Pediatrics 112:1388-1393, 2003.

Pass RF: Cytomegalovirus infection. Pediatr Rev 23:163-169, 2002.

Phelps DL: Retinopathy of prematurity: History, classification, and pathophysiology. NeoReviews 2:c153-c166, 2001.

Phillip AGS: Neonatal meningitis in the new millennium. NeoReviews 4:c73-c80, 2003.

Polin RA, Harris MC: Neonatal bacterial meningitis. Semin Neonatol 6:157-172, 2001.

Regnault TR, Limesand SW, Hay WM: Factors influencing fetal growth. NeoReviews 2:c119-c127, 2001.

Tumbaga PF, Phillip AGS: Perinatal group B streptococcal infections: Past, present, and future. NeoReviews 4:c65-c71, 2003.

Vaucher YE: Bronchopulmonary dysplasia: An enduring challenge. Pediatr Rev 23:349-357, 2002.

Widness JA: Pathophysiology, diagnosis, and prevention of neonatal anemia. NeoReviews 1:e61-e67, 2000.

ADOLESCENT MEDICINE

Kim Blake and Victoria Davis

CHAPTER 67

Overview and Assessment of Adolescents

The leading causes of **mortality** (Table 67–1) and **morbidity** (Table 67–2) among adolescents in the U.S. are behavioral in origin. Motor vehicle injuries and other unintentional or intentional injuries account for more than 75% of all deaths. Unhealthy dietary behaviors and inadequate physical activity result in adolescent obesity with associated health complications (diabetes, hypertension).

Adolescents can present with chronic medical illnesses. Nonetheless, physical symptoms in adolescents are often related to psychosocial problems. Adolescents infrequently present to physicians with acute medical illnesses (sprained ankle, sore throat). It is the physician's responsibility to use this opportunity to inquire about risk-taking behaviors (Fig. 67–1).

INTERVIEWING ADOLESCENTS

The adolescent interview differs from the pediatric interview. There is a shift of information gathering from the parent to the adolescent. Interviewing an adolescent alone and discussing confidentiality are the cornerstones of obtaining information regarding adolescent risk-taking behaviors and anticipatory guidance (see Chapters 7 and 9).

The physical surroundings of the office and waiting room should make the adolescent feel comfortable and welcome (e.g., adolescent-targeted information and magazines). The interview should take into account the developmental age of the adolescent (Table 67–3). General conversations about sports, friends, movies, and activities outside school can be useful for all ages and act as ice breakers throughout the interview to develop a rapport with an adolescent patient (Fig. 67–2 and Table 67–4).

Confidentiality is a key element when interviewing an adolescent (Table 67–5). When discussing confidentiality at the beginning of the interview, parents may be uneasy with this approach, usually because the idea of interviewing their son or daughter alone may not have been addressed by a previous healthcare worker. The physician should reassure parents that this is common practice when interviewing adolescents. Parents can be offered their own time alone with the physician for a confidential discussion at this or another date. It is vital

	TABLE 67–1. Leading Causes of Death in Adolescents	
Rank	**Cause**	**Rate (per 100,000)**
1	Accidents and adverse effects	35.5
	Motor vehicle accidents	27
	All other	8.5
2	Homicide and legal intervention	12.5
3	Suicide	10.1
4	Malignant neoplasms	4.3
5	Diseases of the heart	2.4
6	Congenital anomalies	1.1
7	HIV infection	0.5
All others	Pulmonary disease, pneumonia, cerebrovascular disease	12.8

From Centers for Disease Control, National Center for Health Statistics: Nat Vital Stat Rep 49(12), 2001.

TABLE 67–2. Prevalence of Common Chronic Illnesses of Children and Adolescents

Illness	Prevalence
Pulmonary	
Asthma	3-5%
Cystic fibrosis	1:2500 white, 1:17,000 black
Neuromuscular	
Cerebral palsy	2:1000
Mental retardation	3%
Seizure disorder	3:1000
Auditory-visual defects	10-30%
Traumatic paralysis	2:1000
Scoliosis	5% males, 10% females
Migraine	10%
Endocrine/Nutrition	
Diabetes mellitus	2:1000
Obesity	10%-25%
Anorexia nervosa	0.5%-1%
Bulimia	1% (young adolescence), 5%-10% (19-20 yr)
Dysmenorrhea	10%
Acne	80%

Modified from Gortmaker S, Sappenfield W: Chronic childhood disorders: Prevalence and impact. Pediatr Clin North Am 31:3-18, 1984.

TABLE 67–4. Interviewing the Adolescent Alone: Discussion of HEADDSS Topics*

HOME/FRIENDS	Family, relationships, and activities. "What do you do for fun?" "When you are not in school . . . ?"
EDUCATION/ EMPLOYMENT	"What do you like best at school?" "How's school going?"
ALCOHOL	"Are any of your friends drinking?" "Are you drinking?"
DRUGS	Cigarettes, marijuana, street drugs. "Have you ever smoked?" "Many adolescents experiment with different drugs and substances . . . have you tried anything?"
DIET	Weight, diet/eating habits. "Many adolescents worry about their weight and try dieting. Have you ever done this?"
SEX	Sexual activity, contraception. "Are you dating anybody?" "Do you know what to use if you were going to have sex?"
SUICIDE/ DEPRESSION	Mood swings, depression, suicide attempts or thoughts, self-image. "Feeling down or depressed is common for everyone. Have you ever felt so bad that you wanted to kill yourself?"

*Also see Figure 67–1.

to engage the adolescent in an open discussion about risk-taking behavior, and this is more likely to happen when the adolescent is alone. Some issues cannot be kept confidential, such as suicidal intent, a positive HIV test (a duty to warn third parties), and disclosure of sexual or physical abuse. If there is an ambiguous situation, it is wise to obtain legal, ethical, or social worker consultation. When caring for a young adolescent, the healthcare provider should encourage open discussions with a parent, guardian, or other adult.

Adolescents seek health care intermittently and often for minor reasons. It is important for all healthcare professionals to take these opportunities to interview adolescents alone and discuss risk-taking issues and provide anticipatory guidance to avoid esca-

TABLE 67–3. Adolescent Psychological Development

Stage	Age	Thinking	Characteristics
Early teens	10-14	Concrete	Appearance—"Am I normal?" Invincible Peer group No tomorrow
Middle teens	15-17		Risk-taking increased Limit testing "Who am I?" Experiment with ideas
Late teens	18-21	Formal Operational	Future Planning Partner Separation

TABLE 67–5. Guidelines for Confidentiality

Prepare the preadolescent and parent for confidentiality and being interviewed alone
Discuss confidentiality at start of the interview
Conversations with parents/guardians/adolescent are confidential (with exceptions*)
Reaffirm confidentiality when alone with adolescent

*Exceptions to confidentiality include major or impending harm to any person (i.e., abuse, suicide, homicide).

Structured Communication Adolescent Guide
(SCAG)

Instructions for scoring this form

After your check-up, please score your doctor (or medical student) using this form.

Examples:

0 = Did Not

Dr. didn't ask at all.

1 = Did

Dr. asked as if reading a list.
Dr. asked as if embarrassed.
I felt judged.
I felt a bit uncomfortable.

2 = Did Well

Dr. established a relationship.
Dr. comfortable with questions.
Dr. did not judge.
I felt comfortable.

General Rating: Give a general impression of each section.

A = Excellent, B = Good, C = Average, D = Poor, F = Fail

	Did Not 0	Did 1	Did Well 2	Give examples of things that stood out in your interview, one positive and one negative.
A. GETTING STARTED				*Example: I liked that you talked to me and not just my mom.*
1. Greeted me.	0	1	2	
2. Introduced self.	0	1	2	
3. Discussed confidentiality.	0	1	2	
GENERAL RATING A B C D F				

	Did Not 0	Did 1	Did Well 2	Give examples of things that stood out in your interview, one positive and one negative.
B. GATHERING INFORMATION				*Examples: I felt bad when you asked about smoking with my mom in the room.*
4. Good body language.	0	1	2	
5. Encouraged me to speak by asking questions other than ones with a yes/no answer.	0	1	2	
6. Encouraged parent to speak *(leave out if no parent present).*	0	1	2	
7. Listened and did not judge me.	0	1	2	
8. Established relationship with me by appropriate choice of words.	0	1	2	
GENERAL RATING A B C D F				

Figure 67–1

Structured Communication Adolescent Guide (SCAG). SCAG is an interviewing tool developed for use with adolescent patients. It organizes the adolescent interview in a simple, practical format incorporating the four major interview components: confidentiality, separation of the adolescent from the adult, psychosocial data gathering (using the HEADDSS mnemonic), and a nonjudgmental approach. SCAG is at a grade 5 reading level and has demonstrated reliability and validity when used by trained adolescents to assess interviewing abilities of medical students and physicians. It offers a chance to obtain written feedback from an adolescent.

Continued

	Did Not 0	Did 1	Did Well 2	Give examples of things that stood out in your interview, one positive and one negative.
C. TEEN ALONE				*Example: I was glad you talked about confidentiality. I need lots of reassurance that you won't tell my mom.*
9. Separated me and parent. (*Leave out if no parent present.*)	0	1	2	
10. Discussed confidentiality.	0	1	2	
11. Gave me a chance to talk about things other than what I came in to discuss.	0	1	2	
12. Reflected on my feelings or concerns (example: You seem…)	0	1	2	
LIFESTYLES: Physician asks or talks about the following:				
13. **Home:** Family	0	1	2	
14. **Education:** School	0	1	2	
15. Friends	0	1	2	
16. Activities				
17. **Alcohol:** beer and hard liquor	0	1	2	
18. **Drugs:** Cigarettes	0	1	2	
19. Marijuana	0	1	2	
20. Street drugs	0	1	2	
21. **Diet:** weight/diet/eating habits	0	1	2	
22. **Sex:** Boyfriend/girlfriend	0	1	2	
23. Sexual activity	0	1	2	
24. Safe sex/contraception	0	1	2	
25. **Self:** Body image, self-esteem	0	1	2	*Example: You weren't embarrassed to talk about sex. OR You seemed embarrassed to talk about sex.*
26. Moods/depression/suicide	0	1	2	
GENERAL RATING A B C D F				
	Did Not 0	Did 1	Did Well 2	Comments: Please give examples of things that stood out in your interview.
D. WRAP UP				*Example: I wasn't sure what the next step would be.*
27. Summary, recapped issues	0	1	2	
28. Kept the confidentiality	0	1	2	
29. Asked if there were any questions	0	1	2	
30. Talked about what to do next (plan and follow-up)	0	1	2	
GENERAL RATING A B C D F				

Figure 67–1, cont'd

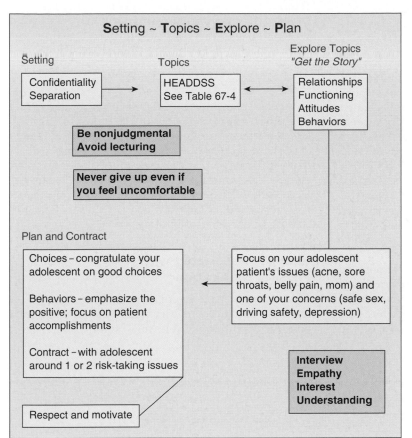

Figure 67–2

STEP guide for adolescent interviewing.

lation of risks (see Table 67–4). Time should not be a limiting factor, and leaving this discussion and guidance to another healthcare professional means disregarding the known mortality and morbidity for this population.

Adolescent healthcare providers should know the laws of the state and the policies of the institution that are relevant to adolescents. The law confers certain rights on adolescents, depending on the health condition and personal characteristics, allowing them to receive health services without parental permission (Table 67–6). Usually adolescents can seek health care without parental consent for reproductive, mental, and emergency health services. In addition, emancipated adolescents and "mature minors" may be treated without parental consent; such status should be documented in the record. The key characteristics of mature minors are their competence and capacity to understand, not their chronologic age. There should be documentation, however, that the healthcare provider discussed the importance of involving parents in health decisions. There must be a reasonable judgment that the health intervention is in the best interests of the minor.

During the physical examination, early adolescents may want a parent present, but middle and late adolescents usually prefer to be seen alone or with a chaperone of the same sex. A choice always should be offered.

TABLE 67–6.   **Legal Rights of Minors**
Age of majority (≥18 years old in most states)
*Exceptions in which healthcare services can be provided to a minor**   Emergency care (e.g., life-threatening condition or condition in which a delay in treatment would increase significantly the likelihood of morbidity)   Diagnosis and treatment of sexuality-related health care   Diagnosis and treatment of drug-related health care   Emancipated minors (physically and financially independent of family; Armed Forces; married; childbirth)   Mature minors (able to comprehend the risks and benefits of evaluation and treatment)   All exceptions should be documented clearly in health record.
*Determined by individual state laws.

PHYSICAL GROWTH AND DEVELOPMENT OF ADOLESCENTS
Girls

Breast budding under the areola (**thelarche**) and pubertal fine straight pubic hair over the mons pubis (**adrenarche** or **pubarche**) are early pubertal changes occurring around 11 years of age (range 8 to 13 years) (see Chapter 174). These changes mark the sexual maturity rating (SMR), or Tanner stage, II of pubertal development (Figs. 67–3 and 67–4). Completion of the Tanner stages should take approximately 4 to 5 years. The peak growth spurt usually occurs approximately 1 year after thelarche at SMR stage III to IV breast development and before the onset of menstruation (**menarche**). Menarche is a relatively late pubertal event. Females grow only 2 to 5 cm in height after menarche (see Chapter 174).

The mean ages of thelarche and adrenarche are approximately 9 and 10 years for African American and white girls, respectively. The mean ages of menarche are 12.2 and 12.9 years for African American and white girls, respectively. The interval from the initiation of thelarche to the onset of menses (**menarche**) is 2.3 ± 1 years. Pubertal changes before age 6 years in African American and 7 years in white girls is considered precocious.

Boys

Testicular enlargement (>2.5 cm) corresponds to SMR, or Tanner, stage I to II (Figs. 67–5 and 67–6). Testicular enlargement is followed by pubic hair development at the base of the penis (**adrenarche**), and then axillary hair within the year. The growth spurt is a relatively late event; it can occur from 10.5 years old to 16 years old. Deepening of the voice, facial hair, and acne indicate the early stages of puberty. See Chapter 174 for discussion of disorders of puberty.

Changes Associated with Physical Maturation

Tanner stages mark biologic maturation that can be related to specific laboratory value changes and certain physical conditions (Tables 67–7 and 67–8). Higher

---

TABLE 67–7. Correlates of Female Pubertal Maturation

	Sexual Maturity Rating (Tanner Stage)				
	1	*2*	*3*	*4*	*5*
Hematocrit (%)					
White *mean*	39.1	39.2	39.6	39.2	39.2
White *range*	36.1-42.1	37.1-41.3	37.0-42.2	36.9-41.6	36.2-42.2
Black *mean*	37.3	38.9	39.0	38.4	38.7
Black *range*	34.6-39.9	35.7-42.1	35.2-42.6	34.9-42.8	35.9-41.5
Alkaline phosphatase (IU/L) (serum)					
White *mean*	70	89	76	33	38
White *range*	51-90	49-134	36-108	16-60	23-76
Black *mean*	84	95	86	44	31
Black *range*	69-108	65-138	26-148	18-144	13-70
Short female with growth potential		+		+	++
Short female with limited growth potential					
Slipped capital femoral epiphysis		+	++		
Acute worsening of scoliosis		+	+++		
Osgood-Schlatter disease		+	+		
Oral contraceptive prescription				+	++
Diaphragm prescription					+
Acute worsening of straight back syndrome		+	++	+	
Acne vulgaris		+	++	++	
Physiologic leukorrhea			+		
Gonococcal vaginitis	+				
Gonococcal cervicitis		+	+	+	+
Regression of virginal breast hypertrophy					+
Timing of breast reduction or rhinoplasty					+

+, possible; ++, more likely than +; +++, most likely.

Data from Copeland KC, Brookman RR, Rauh JL: Assessment of Pubertal Development. Columbus, Ohio, Ross Laboratories, 1986; and Daniel WA: Semin Adolesc Med 1:15-24, 1985.

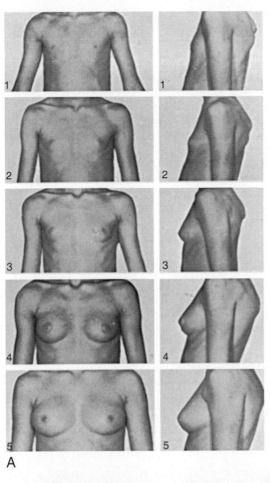

Stage 1 The breasts are preadolescent. There is elevation of the papilla only.

Stage 2 Breast bud stage. A small mound is formed by the elevation of the breast and papilla. The areolar diameter enlarges.

Stage 3 There is further enlargement of breast and areola with no separation of their contours.

Stage 4 There is a projection of the areola and papilla to form a secondary mound above the level of the breast.

Stage 5 The breasts resemble those of a mature female as the areola has recessed to the general contour of the breast.

A

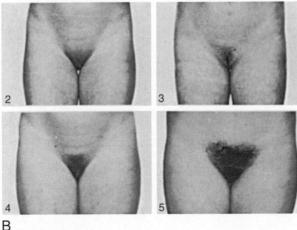

Stage 2 There is sparse growth of long, slightly pigmented, downy hair, straight or only slightly curled, primarily along the labia.

Stage 3 The hair is considerably darker, coarser, and more curled. The hair spreads sparsely over the junction of the pubes.

Stage 4 The hair, now adult in type, covers a smaller area than in the adult and does not extend onto the thighs.

Stage 5 The hair is adult in quantity and type, with extension onto the thighs.

B

Figure 67–3

Typical progression of female pubertal development, stages 1 to 5. A, Pubertal development in size of female breasts. **B,** Pubertal development of female pubic hair. Note that in Stage 1 (not shown) there is no pubic hair. (Courtesy of J.M. Tanner, MD, Institute of Child Health, Department of Growth and Development, University of London, London, England.)

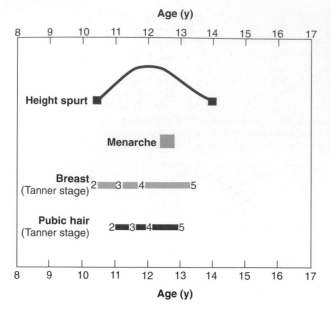

Age (y)

Figure 67–4

Sequence of pubertal events in the average American female. More recent studies suggest that onset of breast development may be 9 years old for African-American girls and 10 years old for white girls. (Adapted from Brookman RR, Rauh JL, Morrison JA, et al: The Princeton maturation study. 1976, unpublished data for adolescents in Cincinnati, Ohio. Reprinted from Assessment of Pubertal Development. Columbus, Ohio, Ross Laboratories, 1986.)

TABLE 67–8. Correlates of Male Pubertal Maturation

	Sexual Maturity Rating (Tanner Stage)				
	1	*2*	*3*	*4*	*5*
Hematocrit (%)					
White *mean*	39.5	39.8	40.9	42.3	43.8
White *range*	37.1-41.8	36.7-42.8	38.2-43.5	39.7-44.8	41.1-46.4
Black *mean*	37.7	38.4	39.7	41.1	42.7
Black *range*	35.2-40.2	36.0-40.9	37.3-42.0	38.3-43.8	39.6-45.9
Alkaline phosphatase (IU/L) (serum)					
White *mean*	72	77	101	75	58
White *range*	54-110	42-106	53-141	41-158	21-120
Black *mean*	77	94	122	116	75
Black *range*	43-130	53-204	46-240	32-228	23-228
Short male with growth potential		+			
Short male with limited growth potential				+	++
Slipped capital femoral epiphysis		+	++		
Acute worsening of scoliosis		+	+++		
Osgood-Schlatter disease		+	+		
Acute worsening of straight back syndrome		+	++	+	
Gynecomastia		+	++		
Acne vulgaris		+	++	++	
Orchiopexy timing	+				
Timing of rhinoplasty					+

+, possible; ++, more likely than +; +++, most likely.
Data from Copeland KC, Brookman RR, Rauh JL: Assessment of Pubertal Development. Columbus, Ohio, Ross Laboratories, 1986; and Daniel WA: Semin Adolesc Med 1:15-24, 1985.

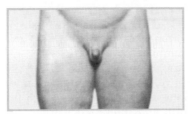

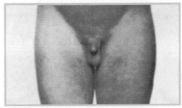

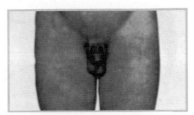

Stage 1 The penis, testes, and scrotum are of childhood size.

Stage 2 There is enlargement of the scrotum and testes, but the penis usually does not enlarge. The scrotal skin reddens.

Stage 3 There is further growth of the testes and scrotum and enlargement of the penis, mainly in length.

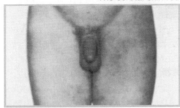

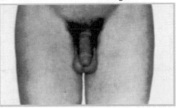

Stage 4 There is still further growth of the testes and scrotum and increased size of the penis, especially in breadth.

Stage 5 The genitalia are adult in size and shape.

A

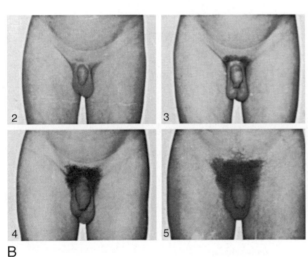

Stage 2 There is sparse growth of long, slightly pigmented, downy hair, straight or only slightly curled, primarily at the base of the penis.

Stage 3 The hair is considerably darker, coarser, and more curled. The hair spreads sparsely over the junction of the pubes.

Stage 4 The hair, now adult in type, covers a smaller area than in the adult and does not extend onto the thighs.

Stage 5 The hair is adult in quantity and type, with extension onto the thighs.

B

Figure 67–5

Typical progression of male pubertal development. **A,** Pubertal development in size of male genitalia. **B,** Pubertal development of male pubic hair. Note that in Stage 1 (not shown) there is no pubic hair. (Courtesy of J.M. Tanner, MD, Institute of Child Health, Department of Growth and Development, University of London, London, England.)

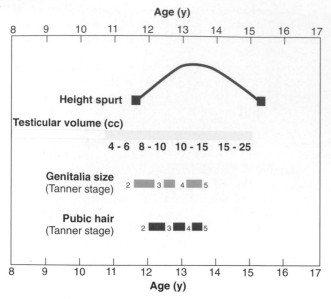

Figure 67-6

Sequence of pubertal events in the average American male. Testicular volume less than 4 mL using orchidometer (Prader Beads) represents prepubertal stage. (Adapted from Brookman RR, Rauh JL, Morrison JA, et al: The Princeton maturation study. 1976, unpublished data for adolescents in Cincinnati, Ohio. Reprinted from Assessment of Pubertal Development. Columbus, Ohio, Ross Laboratories, 1986.)

hematocrit values in adolescent boys than in adolescent girls are the result of greater androgenic stimulation of the bone marrow, not the result of loss through menstruation. Alkaline phosphatase levels in boys and girls increase during puberty because of rapid bone turnover, especially during the growth spurt. Worsening of mild scoliosis is common in adolescents during their growth spurt.

PSYCHOLOGICAL GROWTH AND DEVELOPMENT OF ADOLESCENTS

▶ SEE TABLE 67-3 AND CHAPTERS 7 AND 9.

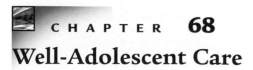

CHAPTER 68
Well-Adolescent Care

A nonjudgmental approach when history taking and collection of information in a friendly, open-minded manner produce a more accurate assessment of the adolescent. The HEADDSS mnemonic can be used to remember the risk-taking elements of the history (see Table 67-4). Adolescents who experiment in one area of risk taking often have multiple other areas that they either contemplate or have tried. The physician should not ask too many questions at one time. The physician should find some common ground to get adolescents talking about themselves. The physician should be truthful and interested in the adolescent. It is important to collect the information before embarking on advice. When all the risk-taking information has been gathered, the physician should choose a healthcare issue to discuss with the adolescent. Throughout the interview, the physician should make it clear that the information is confidential, and that he or she is there to help the adolescent in a partnership way. Although the focus in adolescent care is on psychosocial issues, a general examination also needs to be performed (Table 68-1). General pediatric issues, such as immunization (see Chapter 94) and health screening, should be included (see Table 9-5).

TABLE 68-1. Examination of the Adolescent

Physical Examination—Checklist

Explain what you are going to do
Explain how you are going to do it
Ask if the adolescent prefers to be alone or with the parent
Be sensitive to the adolescent's needs
Always use a sheet or blanket to provide privacy
Let the adolescent remain in his or her underwear with or without other clothes and work around clothing
Ask some questions as you go through the physical to keep the adolescent at ease. Give reassurance that elements of the physical are normal for this age

Assessment

Examination can be used to offer reassurance about normalcy*
Assess
  Height/weight/BMI and plot on percentile charts
  Skin for acne
  Mouth for periodontal disease
  Tanner staging
  Breasts and testicles
  Thyroid (palpation)
  Back for scoliosis
  Mental status for depression
  Signs of substance abuse, risk-taking behaviors, and trauma

*For example, 70% of boys can have breast enlargement (gynecomastia), and girls often have one breast larger than the other.

EARLY ADOLESCENCE (AGE 10 TO 14)

Rapid changes in physical appearance and behavior are the major characteristics of early adolescence. The early adolescent has a great deal of self-consciousness and need for privacy. The history focuses on an overall appraisal of the early adolescent's physical and psychosocial health.

MIDDLE ADOLESCENCE (AGE 15 TO 17)

Autonomy and a global sense of identity are the major characteristics of middle adolescence. The history focuses on the middle adolescent's interactions with family, school, and peers. High-risk behaviors as a result of experimentation are common.

LATE ADOLESCENCE (AGE 18 TO 21)

Individuality and planning for the future are the major characteristics of late adolescence. Greater emphasis is placed on the late adolescent's responsibility for his or her health.

PELVIC EXAMINATION

A full pelvic examination is rarely required in a virginal adolescent girl. Occasionally, palpation of the pelvic organs is essential for diagnosis or management, when imaging has been inconclusive. In a virgin, bimanual rectal-abdominal examination (all midline internal genitalia are immediately anterior to the rectal wall) is as efficient as a vaginal-abdominal examination. In some girls, especially virginal, anesthesia may be required for a full pelvic examination.

Before a pelvic examination, the patient should be informed about the importance of the assessment and what maneuvers will take place; she should be encouraged to ask questions before, during, or after the examination. In addition, a chaperone should be offered when a family caregiver is not present. The patient should be told that she has complete control over the examination and be supported to participate by using a mirror or to help guide the examiner. The patient can choose a supine or partially sitting position, and the examiner should maintain eye contact during the examination. Before all maneuvers, the patient must be informed of what to expect and the sensations.

A padded examination table with the patient in a frog-leg position maximizes comfort of a pelvic examination. Stirrups can be used but are less comfortable. The examination room, lubricants, and instruments should be warm, and the examination should be conducted in an unhurried, but efficient manner.

Inspection of the genitalia includes evaluation of the pubic hair, labia majora and minora, clitoris, urethra, and hymenal ring. When a **speculum examination** is required, it must be performed before bimanual palpation of internal genitalia because lubricants used interfere with the evaluation of microscopic and microbiologic samples. The speculum allows visualization of the vaginal walls and cervical os for collection of appropriate specimens, such as cultures or Papanicolaou (Pap) smears. A Pap smear does not need to be performed until the adolescent is sexually active, unless there is a history of sexual abuse or vulvar infection with human papillomavirus. In the rare circumstance that a vaginal examination is necessary in a virginal girl, a Huffman (0.5 inch × 4.5 inches) or Pedersen (0.9 inch × 4.5 inches) speculum should be used. A nonvirginal introitus frequently admits a small to medium-sized adult speculum.

NORMAL VARIANTS OF PUBERTY

Breast Asymmetry and Masses

It is not unusual for one breast to begin growth before, or to grow more rapidly than, the other with resulting asymmetry. This situation can be distressing for some girls, who need to be reassured that after full maturation the asymmetry will be less obvious, and that all women have some degree of asymmetry. The breast bud is a pea-sized mass below the nipple that is often tender. Occasionally, young women present with a breast mass; usually these are **benign fibroadenomas** or cysts (Table 68–2). It is important to explain that breast cancer is extremely rare in this age group. Ultrasound evaluation is better for evaluation of young, dense, breasts and avoids the radiation exposure of mammography.

TABLE 68–2. Etiology of Breast Masses in Adolescents
Classic or juvenile fibroadenoma (70%)
Fibrocystic disease
Breast cyst
Abscess/mastitis
Intraductal papilloma
Fat necrosis/lipoma
Cystosarcoma phyllodes (low-grade malignancy)
Adenomatous hyperplasia
Hemangioma, lymphangioma, lymphoma (rare)
Carcinoma (<1%)

Physiologic Leukorrhea

Peripubertal girls (SMR stage III) often complain of vaginal discharge. If the discharge is clear, without symptoms of pruritus or odor, it is most likely physiologic leukorrhea. This condition is due to ovarian estrogen stimulation of the uterus and vagina. On physical examination, there should be evidence of an estrogenized vulva and hymen without erythema or excoriation. The physician should always be alert to signs of abuse. If there are symptoms, cultures should be obtained. In these circumstances, vaginal cultures can be obtained without a speculum because **sexually transmitted infections (STIs)** are vaginal until menarche, when cervical infections are the rule. Inspection of physiologic leukorrhea shows few white blood cells, estrogen maturation of vaginal epithelial cells, and no pathogens on culture.

Irregular Menses

Menarche typically occurs approximately 2 years after thelarche at the average age of 12.6 years. The initial menses are anovulatory and tend to be irregular in duration. This irregularity may persist for 2 to 5 years, so reassurance may be required if the patient or parents are seeking advice. During this phase, estrogen feedback on the hypothalamus decreases gonadotropin secretion, which reduces estrogen production and induces an estrogen withdrawal bleed that can be prolonged and heavy. In addition, anovulatory bleeding is usually painless. As the hypothalamic-pituitary-gonadal axis matures, the cycle becomes ovulatory, and menses are secondary to progesterone withdrawal. When ovulation is established, the average cycle length is 21 to 45 days. Some adolescents ovulate with their first cycle, as indicated by pregnancy before menarche.

Gynecomastia

Breast enlargement in boys is usually a benign, self-limited condition. Gynecomastia is noted in 50% to 60% of boys during early adolescence. It is often idiopathic, but may be noted in various conditions (Table 68–3). Typical findings include the appearance of a 1- to 3-cm, round, freely mobile, often tender, and firm mass immediately beneath the areola during SMR stage III. Large, hard, or fixed enlargements and masses associated with any nipple discharge warrant further investigation. Reassurance that the condition is self-limited is usually the only treatment required. If the condition worsens and is associated with psychological morbidity, it may be treated with bromocriptine. Surgical treatment with reduction mammoplasty can be helpful with massive hypertrophy.

TABLE 68–3. Etiology of Gynecomastia
Idiopathic
Hypogonadism (primary or secondary)
Liver disease
Renal disease
Hyperthyroidism
Neoplasms
Adrenal
Ectopic human chorionic gonadotropin secreting
Testicular
Drugs
Antiandrogens
Antibiotics (isoniazid, ketoconazole, metronidazole)
Antacids (H₂ blockers)
Cancer chemotherapy (especially alkylating agents)
Cardiovascular drugs
Drugs of abuse
Alcohol
Amphetamines
Heroin
Marijuana
Hormones (for female sex)
Psychoactive agents (e.g., diazepam, phenothiazines, tricyclics)

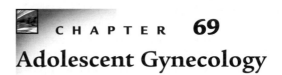

CHAPTER 69

Adolescent Gynecology

MENSTRUAL DISORDERS

Irregular menses is the most common complaint of early adolescent girls. As regular, ovulatory cycles become established, pain with menstruation (**dysmenorrhea**) is a frequent complaint.

Amenorrhea

Primary amenorrhea is the complete absence of menstruation by age 16 in the presence of breast development or by age 14 in the absence of breast development. **Secondary amenorrhea** refers to the cessation of menses for more than 3 consecutive months, any time after menarche, although irregular menses are the norm in the first 2 years after menarche.

Primary amenorrhea may be a result of functional or anatomic abnormalities of the hypothalamus, pituitary gland, ovaries, or uterus (Table 69–1). Physiologic immaturity, stress, excessive exercise, and abnormal dietary patterns (anorexia/bulimia) are the most common causes of amenorrhea. Pregnancy should be

TABLE 69–1.   Causes of Primary and Secondary Amenorrhea

Primary Amenorrhea—Secondary Sexual Characteristics Absent

Gonadal dysgenesis—Turner syndrome, triple X
Gonadal agenesis
Enzyme deficiency—17α-hydroxylase, 17,20-lyase
Gonadotropin hormone deficiency—idiopathic, Kallmann syndrome, hypothalamic disorder

Primary Amenorrhea—Secondary Sexual Characteristics Present

Outflow tract obstruction—imperforate hymen, müllerian agenesis, transverse vaginal septum, androgen insensitivity
Hypothalamic-pituitary disorder (normal prolactin)—stressors (low weight, chronic disease, excessive exercise)
Premature ovarian failure—idiopathic, Turner mosaic, autoimmune, infection, chemotherapy, radiation therapy

Secondary Amenorrhea

Hypothalamic-pituitary disorder (normal prolactin)—stressors
Hypothalamic-pituitary disorder (elevated prolactin)—hypothyroid, drugs, tumor, trauma, renal failure
Premature ovarian failure—idiopathic, Turner mosaic, autoimmune, infection, chemotherapy, radiation therapy
With androgen excess—polycystic ovarian syndrome, congenital adrenal hyperplasia, ovarian tumor, adrenal disorder

considered in all cases of secondary amenorrhea, even if the patient denies sexual activity.

The **history** and **physical examination** usually point to a diagnosis and should guide the investigation. In adolescents with primary amenorrhea, abdominal pain, and secondary sexual characteristics, an outflow tract obstruction should be ruled out by ultrasound. There also may be an abdominal mass resulting from accumulated blood; imperforate hymen is visible on physical examination. For girls with primary amenorrhea without secondary sexual characteristics and an unremarkable history and physical examination, an endocrine evaluation is indicated. Follicle-stimulating hormone (FSH) and luteinizing hormone (LH) provide information about the origin of amenorrhea. A prolactinoma, although rare, also must be ruled out. Elevated FSH and LH indicate primary ovarian failure, ovarian dysgenesis, or ovarian agenesis that warrants a karyotype. **Turner syndrome** is a common cause, but other chromosomal anomalies should be ruled out. Low levels of FSH and LH suggest hypothalamic

dysfunction, which may be due to physiologic immaturity (often familial), isolated gonadotropin deficiency, or hypogonadotropic hypogonadism (chronic illness, low body weight, stressful life events). Additional hormone evaluation includes thyroid hormone, thyroid-stimulating hormone, and prolactin because hypothyroidism is a common cause of menstrual dysfunction.

Girls with secondary amenorrhea have secondary sexual characteristics. The most common causes of secondary amenorrhea are pregnancy, anorexia/stress (low LH, FSH, and estradiol), and **polycystic ovary syndrome**. In polycystic ovary syndrome, there may be symptoms of androgen excess, such as acne and hirsutism, and recent weight gain. If hirsutism or virilization is present, free and total testosterone, androstenedione, and dihydroepiandrosterone sulfate should be measured to rule out ovarian or adrenal tumors. 17-Hydroxyprogesterone rules out late-onset **congenital adrenal hyperplasia**. In polycystic ovary syndrome, the LH-to-FSH ratio is 2:1 or more; estradiol may be normal or low; and androgens, including dihydroepiandrosterone sulfate, are elevated, although not to the extent a tumor produces.

In a patient with amenorrhea (primary or secondary), normal secondary sex characteristics, negative pregnancy test, normal prolactin and thyroid-stimulating hormone, and no evidence of outflow tract obstruction, the total effect of estrogen on the uterus (rather than a single point estradiol level) can be determined by a **progesterone withdrawal test**. To achieve this, 5 to 10 mg of medroxyprogesterone (depending on body weight) is given daily for 5 days. If the uterus is normal and primed by estrogen (an intact hypothalamic-pituitary-gonadal axis) with no outflow tract obstruction, there should be bleeding within 1 week after the last progesterone tablet. If there is bleeding, the amenorrhea is secondary to anovulation, and cyclic progesterone withdrawal is recommended to induce uniform shedding to prevent endometrial hyperplasia and prolonged heavy bleeding secondary to asynchronous endometrial shedding. If there is no progesterone withdrawal bleeding, the uterus has been insufficiently exposed to estrogen, and there is systemic estrogen deficiency.

Therapy for the amenorrhea should be directed at the cause. Anovulation can be managed with either progesterone withdrawal or combined oral contraceptives (COC). In hypothalamic amenorrhea and ovarian failure, there is an associated hypoestrogenism; therapy needs to be directed at replacing estrogen and progesterone, usually with a COC. Polycystic ovary syndrome usually can be treated effectively with weight loss, exercise, progesterone withdrawal, or COC. If there is evidence of androgen excess, the COC reduces androgen production from the ovaries and increases sex hormone-binding globulin to reduce the amount of available androgen. Spironolactone helps treat hirsutism, and when there is evidence of insulin insensitivity, metformin can restore ovulatory cycles.

Abnormal Uterine Bleeding

Normal, ovulatory menses can occur 21 to 45 days apart, measuring from the first day of menstruation to the first day of the next menstruation. The average duration of flow is 3 to 7 days, with more than 7 days considered prolonged. More than 8 well-soaked pads or 12 tampons per day may be considered excessive, although classically blood loss is difficult to estimate because the frequency of pad change varies greatly among women. Table 69–2 defines menstrual disorders. If the menstrual problem is unclear and nonacute, observation and charting on a menstrual calendar are warranted (Fig. 69–1). Excessively heavy, prolonged, or infrequent bleeding in the first year after menarche is often physiologic but should be investigated, especially if there is associated iron deficiency anemia.

TABLE 69–2. Definition of Menstrual Disorders

Amenorrhea—no menstruation
Oligomenorrhea—too few (episodes of bleeding)
Menorrhagia—too much (blood loss)
Metrorrhagia—too many (episodes of bleeding)
Menometrorrhagia—too much and too many

In adolescents with heavy or prolonged menses, especially presenting in early menarche, approximately 20% have a coagulation disorder, and 10% have another pathology. If an underlying pathology is discovered (**functional uterine bleeding**), treatment should be directed at the primary disorder and the secondary menstrual dysfunction.

Dysfunctional uterine bleeding is any abnormal pattern of endometrial shedding not caused by an underlying pathologic process and is one of the few

YOUR MENSTRUAL CALENDAR NAME ____________

	1	2	3	4	5	6	7	8	9	10	11	12	13	14	15	16	17	18	19	20	21	22	23	24	25	26	27	28	29	30	31
JAN																															
FEB																															
MAR																															
APR																															
MAY																															
JUNE																															
JULY																															
AUG																															
SEPT																															
OCT																															
NOV																															
DEC																															

PATIENT INSTRUCTIONS

Record your MENSTRUAL BLOOD FLOW or any INTERMENSTRUAL BLEEDING by marking one of the following notations in the appropriate day (square) on your Menstrual Calendar:

For Heavy Flow	■	Fill in the square
For Normal Flow	☒	Mark an X
For Scant Flow	◪	Mark a Diagonal
For Spotting	⊡	Mark a Dot
Oral Contraceptive Pill	P	Mark a P

PHYSICIAN'S COMMENTS

____
____
____
____
____
____

Figure 69–1

Menstrual calendar for patient completion.

TABLE 69–3. Differential Diagnosis of Abnormal Vaginal Bleeding*

Pregnancy, including ectopic pregnancy
Infection—usually sexually transmitted
Endocrine disorder—thyroid disorder, PCO, pituitary
  disorder
Systemic disease
Trauma
Medications
Blood dyscrasia
Vaginal, cervical, or uterine disorders
Ovarian tumor/cyst
Contraception
Foreign body

*When all excluded, the diagnosis of dysfunctional uterine bleeding can be made.
PCO, polycystic ovaries.

conditions in adolescent health care that is a diagnosis of exclusion (Table 69–3). **Anovulation** occurs in most of these cases. Without progesterone from the corpus luteum, unopposed estrogen causes endometrial hyperplasia and irregular endometrial shedding, which can be prolonged and heavy, sometimes life-threatening. Progesterone induces a secretory endometrium. When progesterone is withdrawn, the endometrium sheds in a synchronous fashion with myometrial and vascular contractions (causing dysmenorrhea but limiting blood loss). After 1 year of regular cycles, irregular bleeding usually indicates an organic abnormality.

A thorough history with a menstrual calendar indicating the amount of flow and associated symptoms is followed by physical examination, including a pelvic examination in a nonvirginal adolescent or an ultrasound in a virginal adolescent. A complete blood count, pregnancy test, thyroid function tests, and coagulation screen should be performed. In sexually active adolescents, **STIs** should be ruled out.

Unpredictable, heavy, and prolonged menses may impair school attendance and social functioning; iron deficiency anemia is associated with lower academic scores. **Treatment** is indicated for heavy menses. Chronic and acute bleeding can be managed with COCs; multiple daily doses may be required until blood loss is controlled. Occasionally, uncontrollable bleeding requires hospitalization for IV fluids and high-dose estrogen. Uterine curettage is rarely indicated in adolescents. Iron therapy also is important. Use of COCs to regulate menstruation and allow the hypothalamic-pituitary-gonadal axis to mature is appropriate; only 6 to 12 months of therapy may be required. COCs are paramount in the management of menorrhagia in individuals with **bleeding disorders** (von Willebrand disease), although adjuvant therapy with tranexamic acid may be needed if the COC is given cyclically. Parents are often concerned that COC use will cause their daughter to become sexually active, but literature and experience do not support this.

Menstrual Suppression

The most common medical indication for menstrual suppression is for an adolescent who cannot cope with menstruation where hygiene is an issue. If the individual is mobile, continuous COC can be given indefinitely. In adolescents confined to a wheelchair, medroxyprogesterone acetate (Depo-Provera) is preferable because of the risk of venous thrombosis associated with estrogen. Other indications for menstrual suppression are continued heavy bleeding or dysmenorrhea on cyclic COC, menstrual-associated symptoms such as migraines or seizure exacerbation, and "designer menses." The last-mentioned refers to purposeful menstrual manipulation, using COCs, to avoid bleeding at certain times in a woman's life (e.g., while camping, traveling).

Dysmenorrhea

The most common gynecologic complaint of young women is painful menstruation, or dysmenorrhea, during the first 1 to 3 days of bleeding. **Primary dysmenorrhea** is defined as pelvic pain during menstruation in the absence of pelvic pathology and is a feature of ovulation, typically developing 1 to 3 years after menarche, with an increasing incidence to the age of 24 as ovulatory cycles are established. The etiology is the release of prostaglandins and leukotrienes from the degenerating endometrium after progesterone levels decline from the ovulatory follicle (corpus luteum). This release causes increased uterine tone, with a greater frequency and dysrhythmia of uterine contractions creating excessive uterine pressures and ischemia, which heightens the sensitivity of pain fibers to bradykinin and other physical stimuli.

Pain occurring at menarche should be investigated by ultrasound to rule out an underlying structural problem, such as an obstructive müllerian anomaly. Primary dysmenorrhea is the most common form of painful menses and is experienced by most adolescent girls and is a leading cause of short-term school absenteeism.

Secondary dysmenorrhea is menstrual pain associated with pelvic pathology and is caused most frequently by **endometriosis** or **pelvic inflammatory disease**. Adolescents with endometriosis usually have mild to moderate disease, but girls with obstructed outflow tracts tend to have severe endometriosis soon

TABLE 69–4. Treatment of Dysmenorrhea

NSAIDs
Over-the-counter ibuprofen or naproxen sodium taken
  every 4 hr
Prescription ibuprofen 400 mg po qid,
  naproxen 550 mg PO stat then 250 PO qid,
  mefenamic acid 500 mg PO stat then 250 mg qid,
  valdecoxib 40 mg PO od
Combined oral contraceptives—cyclic or continuous
Progesterone-only pill
Depo-Provera—150 mg IM every 13 wk

NSAIDs, nonsteroidal anti-inflammatory drugs.

after menarche. Intrauterine device use and benign tumors of the uterus (leiomyomas or polyps) are a rare cause of acquired dysmenorrhea in adolescents. The types of dysmenorrhea usually can be distinguished by history and physical examination. Ultrasound is preferred to define obstructing genital tract lesions. MRI may be useful in complex reproductive tract anomalies. Laparoscopy is required to diagnose endometriosis and pelvic inflammatory disease with certainty, although it usually is reserved for patients who fail medical therapy.

Treatment of primary dysmenorrhea should be considered with symptoms causing significant distress. First-line therapy is with nonsteroidal anti-inflammatory drugs (NSAIDs), either prescription or nonprescription, to inhibit the synthesis of prostaglandins (Table 69–4). To maximize pain relief, NSAIDs should be taken before or as soon as menstruation begins, and the dosing schedule should be followed closely. NSAIDs also decrease blood flow, but they do not regulate menstrual cycles. Typically, NSAIDs are needed for 2 to 3 days. If NSAIDs fail to provide adequate relief, COCs may be added.

If dysmenorrhea persists despite an adequate trial of COCs (≥4 months), an alternative diagnosis, such as endometriosis, should be considered. Endometriosis can usually be managed with COCs. When they fail, a laparoscopy should be performed before advancing therapy to confirm the diagnosis and excise endometriotic lesions. Continuous COC therapy (84 days of active COC followed by a 5- to 7-day hormone-free interval) may control symptoms. An alternative is depot medroxyprogesterone acetate (150 mg) every 2 months until symptoms are controlled, then every 3 months. Because treatment for endometriosis is long-term, medications used in older women, such as danazol (a weak synthetic male hormone) or gonadotropin-releasing hormone agonists (nafarelin or leuprolide), are a last resort for symptom relief.

PREGNANCY

The median age of first intercourse in the U.S. is 16 years; this is similar to other industrial countries. Although the age of coital initiation is similar among different socioeconomic groups, the prevalence of adolescent childbearing outside of marriage is greatest in the lower socioeconomic strata. Approximately 1 million females age 12 to 19 years become pregnant per year. In women younger than 20 years old, there are 97 pregnancies, 54 births, and 29 abortions per 1000. The reduction in adolescent pregnancy since the peak year of 1990 is due to increased use of contraceptives. Adolescents who choose to continue their pregnancy have an increased incidence of premature births, small for gestational age infants, postneonatal mortality, child abuse, subsequent maternal unemployment, and poor maternal educational achievement. These risks are primarily due to behavior rather than inherent biologic risks within adolescents. With good prenatal care, nutrition, and social support, a pregnant adolescent has the same chance of delivering a healthy term infant as an adult of similar sociodemographic background.

Diagnosis

Pregnancy should be considered and ruled out in any adolescent presenting with secondary amenorrhea. Frequently, pregnant adolescents delay seeking a diagnosis until several periods have been missed and initially may deny having intercourse. Pregnant females in early adolescence often present with other symptoms, such as vomiting, vague pains, or deteriorating behavior and may report normal periods. Because of the varied presentations of adolescent pregnancy, a thorough menstrual history should be obtained in all menstruating adolescents. Urine pregnancy tests are sensitive approximately 7 to 10 days after conception. Rape or incest should be ruled out in all cases of adolescent pregnancy.

When pregnancy is confirmed, immediate gestational dating is important to assist in planning. Options are to continue or terminate the pregnancy (if not beyond 20 to 24 weeks' gestation). With the former, the adolescent may choose to parent the child or have the child adopted. Healthcare professionals should encourage pregnant adolescents to involve their families because the adolescent may not be mature enough to make the decision alone; parents may be more understanding than the adolescent expects.

Continuation of the Pregnancy

Adolescents who choose to continue the pregnancy need early, consistent, and comprehensive prenatal care by a team of healthcare providers. All aspects of the adolescent's socioeconomic situation should be evaluated in an effort to optimize the infant's health and development. Although fewer than 5% of adolescents have their infants adopted, this option should be discussed. Pregnancy is the most common cause for females to drop out of school, so special attention should be given to keeping the adolescent in school during and after pregnancy.

Termination

If a pregnant adolescent chooses to terminate her pregnancy, she should be referred immediately to a nonjudgmental abortion service. The options for pregnancy termination depend on the gestational age; there is increasing morbidity and mortality with increasing gestational age. Surgical procedures include manual vacuum aspiration (≤8 weeks' gestational age), suction curettage (≤12 to 14 weeks' gestational age depending on the provider), and dilation and evacuation (14 to 20 weeks' gestational age). Dilation and evacuation requires considerable experience. Early pregnancy (<8 weeks' gestational age) can be terminated medically with oral mifepristone (RU-486) in combination with misoprostol, methotrexate with misoprostol, or misoprostol alone. Adolescents rarely present early enough to explore this option. In the second trimester (>12 weeks' gestational age), labor induction and delivery can be effected by vaginal misoprostol or the intra-amniotic instillation of prostaglandins or hypertonic saline. Psychosocial support and subsequent contraceptive counseling and implementation should be available for adolescents who choose abortion.

CONTRACEPTION

Adolescents often begin intercourse without adequate birth control, and knowledge about sexuality and contraception is crucial. Because unintended pregnancy can be associated with significant psychosocial morbidity for the mother, father, and child, prevention should be a primary goal. All methods of contraception significantly reduce the risk of pregnancy when used in a consistent and correct fashion. The best form of contraception is the one an individual will use.

Abstinence

Abstaining from sexual intercourse is the most commonly used and most effective form of adolescent birth control. A degree of self-control, self-assuredness, and self-esteem is necessary; these qualities are not found in all adolescents. Adolescents who choose to be sexually active should be offered birth control because there is a 70% chance of pregnancy in 1 year of regular, unprotected intercourse.

Steroidal Contraception

It is important to remind young women that steroidal contraception does not provide any protection from STIs, and condoms should be used to reduce the risk of infection.

Combined Oral Contraceptives

COCs contain a synthetic estrogen and progesterone that suppress gonadotropin secretion and ovarian follicle development and ovulation. COCs also produce an atrophic endometrium (inhospitable for blastocyst implantation) and thicken cervical mucus to inhibit sperm penetration. COCs are 99% effective if taken regularly and have numerous noncontraceptive benefits (Table 69–5). After a history and physical examination, COCs can be started on the first day of the patient's next menstrual period. Contraindications and relative contraindications to COCs are listed in Tables 69–6 and 69–7. The only recommended part of a physical examination before prescribing a COC is blood pressure measurement to rule out preexisting hypertension. In many countries, COCs are sold over-the-counter.

Pap smear and STI screening should be suggested as part of wellness care of adolescent females. They are not mandatory for the initiation of contraception because birth control and health screenings are separate issues. If the healthcare provider has established a good rapport with the adolescent, she will agree to screening tests, which can be left to the next visit. Initially the adolescent should be seen monthly to reinforce good contraceptive use and safer sex (condom use to reduce STI). Counseling is the key to good contraceptive use and continuation. Until adolescents show the ability to take a pill daily, contraception with COCs should be

TABLE 69–5. Noncontraceptive Benefits of Combined Oral Contraceptives

Cycle regulation
Decreased menstrual flow
Increased bone mineral density
Decreased dysmenorrhea
Decreased perimenopausal symptoms
Decreased acne
Decreased hirsutism
Decreased endometrial cancer
Decreased ovarian cancer
Decreased risk of fibroids
Possibly fewer ovarian cysts
Possibly less benign breast disease
Possibly less colorectal carcinoma
Decreased incidence of salpingitis
Decreased incidence or severity of moliminal symptoms

TABLE 69–6. Absolute Contraindications to Combined Oral Contraceptives

<6 wk postpartum
Smoking and age >35 yr
Hypertension (systolic ≥160 mm Hg or diastolic ≥100 mm Hg)
Current or past history of venous thromboembolism
Ischemic heart disease
History of cerebrovascular accident
Complicated valvular heart disease (pulmonary hypertension, atrial fibrillation, history of subacute bacterial endocarditis)
Migraine with focal neurologic symptoms
Breast cancer (current)
Diabetes with retinopathy/nephropathy/neuropathy
Severe cirrhosis
Liver tumor (adenoma or hepatoma)

avoided. When COCs are prescribed, 20 μg or less low-dose ethinyl estradiol pills in 28-day packets are recommended because they encourage a daily routine without the need to remember when to start the next packet. One novel contraceptive regimen called *Seasonale* has packaged 84 active tablets to be taken sequentially followed by a 7-day hormone-free interval and the next package. Any COC can be used in such a fashion to induce long intervals between withdrawal bleeding.

Initially, **side effects**, such as nausea (pills should be taken at night to reduce this), breast tenderness, and breakthrough bleeding (especially if pills are missed), are common. The adolescent should be counseled that these symptoms are usually transient and not to discontinue COC use until discussion with a healthcare professional. In addition, adolescents should be informed that COCs do not generally cause weight gain, but rather as women mature weight gain is normal. Usually 3 to 4 months on one COC is needed to determine acceptability. If there is breakthrough bleeding, before changing pills, the physician should determine how often pills are forgotten. If **a single pill**

TABLE 69–7. Relative Contraindications to Combined Oral Contraceptives

Adequately controlled hypertension
Hypertension (systolic 140-159 mm Hg, diastolic 90-99 mm Hg)
Migraine and age >35 yr
Currently symptomatic gallbladder disease
Mild cirrhosis
History of combined oral contraceptive–related cholestasis

is forgotten, two pills should be taken on the subsequent day. **If 2 days were missed**, two pills may be taken on the 2 subsequent days. **If 3 or more days are missed**, the adolescent should consider emergency contraception, if at risk for pregnancy, and take a total of 7 days off, while using another form of birth control, then start a new cycle. If taken properly, COCs are effective in the first month of use, but healthcare providers usually suggest use of additional contraception in the first month.

Progesterone-Only Pill or Minipill

Although not as well known or widely used as COCs, the progestin-only pill, *norethindrone (Micronor),* is a safe and effective form of contraception when used consistently. It is supplied in packages of 28 tablets, each containing 0.35 mg of norethindrone with no hormone-free interval. The mechanisms of action in preventing pregnancy are through reduced volume, increased viscosity, and altered molecular structure of cervical mucus, resulting in little or no sperm penetration. In addition, endometrial changes reduce the potential for implantation, and ovulation is partially or completely suppressed. Approximately 40% of women using progestin-only contraceptives continue to ovulate. Progesterone-only contraception is indicated for women who have a contraindication to estrogen-based contraceptives (see Table 69–6) or have estrogen-related side effects.

Contraceptive Vaginal Ring

The vaginal contraceptive ring (*NuvaRing*) is a flexible, Silastic ring with an outer diameter of 54 mm and a cross-sectional diameter of 4 mm. The ring releases a constant rate of 15 μg of ethinyl estradiol and 0.120 mg of etonogestrel per day. Each ring is used continuously for 3 weeks, then removed with a new ring inserted 7 days later. Because the need for daily or coital use is circumvented, failure secondary to missed dosing is reduced. The contraindications and side effects are the same as with COCs.

Contraceptive Patch

The contraceptive patch (*norelgestromin [Evra]*) is a 25-cm^2 pink patch that is applied, usually on the buttocks, for 1 week followed by removal and application of a new patch with the process repeated in 1 week for a total of 3 weeks of patch use, then a patch-free week for a withdrawal bleed, followed by the next patch cycle. The daily dose is equivalent to a 35-μg ethinyl estradiol COC. Because the need for daily or coital use is circumvented, failure secondary to missed dosing is reduced. In women weighing 90 kg or more, the contraceptive patch is less efficacious, however. Contraindications and side effects are the same as COCs.

Hormonal Injections and Implants

IM injection of 150 mg of medroxyprogesterone acetate (*Depo-Provera*) every 13 weeks is an effective form of birth control. Progesterone-only contraception is associated with menstrual irregularities (70% amenorrhea and 30% metrorrhagia). This problem is ameliorated by *Lunelle,* a preparation that contains 25 mg of medroxyprogesterone acetate and 5 mg of estradiol cypionate given as an IM injection monthly. There are no implants currently available in North America, although some young women still may be using a 5-year, six-rod subdermal implant system (*Norplant*). These forms of contraception are user and coital independent and reduce failure secondary to missed doses.

Emergency Postcoital Contraception

Emergency postcoital contraception should be discussed at every visit and a prescription given in advance of need in areas where no over-the-counter access is available. This practice encourages appropriate and early use with the potential to decrease the incidence of unintended pregnancies. Emergency contraception reduces the risk of pregnancy after unprotected intercourse if used within 72 hours, although efficacy is greatest when used as early as possible. There is some efficacy, although reduced, for up to 5 days. Other indications and contraindications to emergency postcoital contraception are listed in Table 69–8. There are two forms of emergency contraception: the **Yuzpe Regimen** consisting of 2 Ovral tablets (50 µg of ethinyl estradiol and 250 µg of norgestrel each) repeated in 12 hours (a total of four pills) and **Plan B** (0.75 mg of levonorgestrel), 1 pill taken twice 12 hours apart or two tablets given once. If 100 women have unprotected

TABLE 69–8.   Emergency Contraception

Indications

No method of contraception being used
Condom breaks
Diaphragm dislodged/removed <6 hr
Missed birth control pills
>1 wk late for Depo-Provera
Ejaculation on external genitalia
Sexual assault

Contraindications

Known pregnancy
If strong contraindications to estrogens, use progestin

sex in the second or third week of the menstrual cycle (most fertile time), 8 will become pregnant without emergency contraception, 1 will become pregnant using Plan B (89% reduction), and 2 will become pregnant using the Yuzpe Regimen (75% reduction). Plan B also is associated with significantly less nausea and vomiting than the Yuzpe Regimen. Mifepristone is also an effective postcoital contraceptive; it is not approved for this use in the U.S.

Postcoital Copper Intrauterine Device

A copper intrauterine device (IUD) can be inserted 7 days from the act of unprotected intercourse and has an efficacy of greater than 99%. Among 879 women who had a postcoital IUD, 1 became pregnant, and 1 had a possible miscarriage.

Barrier Methods
Condoms and Foam

When condoms and spermicide (foam, gel, film, sponge) are used together in a consistent (each and every act of intercourse) and correct (film must be placed 10 minutes before intercourse) fashion, they are almost as effective as COCs in the prevention of pregnancy, especially in individuals who have infrequent intercourse. Advantages of this method are they are available over-the-counter without the need for a physician visit or prescription, and they reduce the risk of STIs, including HIV (latex and polyurethane condoms). The female condom (*Reality*) is an additional barrier method made of polyurethane that affords females more control, but it is usually considered aesthetically unpleasing by adolescents.

Sponge, Caps, and Diaphragm

The vaginal sponge (*Protectaid*) is a spermicide-impregnated synthetic sponge that is effective for 24 hours of intercourse. The *Femcap* is a silicone cap fitted by a healthcare provider, then placed on the cervix by the user before intercourse. This method is technically difficult, especially for an adolescent. The *diaphragm* is fitted by a healthcare provider but is technically simpler to use than the cap because the edges go into the vaginal fornices. To be effective, the diaphragm should be used with spermicide applied to the cervical side and along the rim. The diaphragm needs additional spermicide with each act of intercourse. The *Leashield* is a silicone device, similar to a diaphragm, that covers the cervix and adheres to the vaginal vault by a mild vacuum generated by its design. All of these methods need to be left in place for 6 hours after the last act of intercourse for optimal efficacy.

Coitus Interruptus

Withdrawal is a common method of birth control used by sexually active adolescents, but it is ineffective because sperm are released into the vagina before ejaculation, and withdrawal may occur after ejaculation has begun.

Rhythm Method (Periodic Coital Abstinence)

The rhythm method is the practice of periodic abstinence just before, during, and just after ovulation. This method requires the user to have an accurate knowledge of her cycle, awareness of clues indicating ovulation, and discipline, usually a rarity in adolescents. Adolescents tend to have unpredictable cycles and consequently less predictable ovulation, so it is difficult to determine with any accuracy a time of the month that can be considered completely safe.

Oral and Anal Sex

Some adolescents engage in oral or anal sex because they believe that it eliminates the need for contraception. Many do not consider this activity to mean "having sex." Condoms generally are not used during oral or anal sex, but the risk of acquiring an STI is still present. Heterosexual adolescents who deny being sexually active should be asked specifically about non-vaginal forms of sexual activity, and adolescents who engage in oral and anal sex require STI and HIV counseling and screening.

RAPE

Rape is a legal term for nonconsensual intercourse. Almost half of rape victims are adolescents, and the perpetrator is known in 50% of cases. Although gathering historical and physical evidence for a criminal investigation is important, the physician's primary responsibility is to perform these functions in a supportive, nonjudgmental manner. The history should include details of the sexual assault, time from the assault until presentation, whether the victim cleaned herself, date of last menstrual period, and previous sexual activity, if any.

For optimal results, forensic material should be collected within 72 hours of the assault. Clothes, especially undergarments, need to be placed in a paper bag for drying (plastic holds humidity, which allows organisms to grow, destroying forensic evidence). The patient should be inspected for bruising, bites, and oral, genital, and anal trauma. Photographs are the best record to document injuries. Specimens should be obtained from the fingernails, mouth, vagina, pubic

hair, and anus. The sexual assault kit provides materials to obtain DNA from semen, saliva, blood, fingernail scrapings, and pubic hair. A wet mount of vaginal fluids shows the presence or absence of sperm under the microscope. Cultures for STIs should be taken, but are often negative (unless previously infected) because 72 hours are needed for the bacterial load to be sufficient for culture. Blood should be drawn for baseline HIV and syphilis (Venereal Disease Research Laboratories test). All materials must be maintained in a "chain of evidence" that cannot be called into question in court.

Therapy after a rape includes prophylaxis for emergency contraception and STI and, if indicated, hepatitis immune globulin and hepatitis vaccine. A single oral dose of cefixime, 400 mg, and azithromycin, 1 g, treats *Chlamydia,* gonorrhea, and syphilis. An alternative regimen is a single IM dose of ceftriaxone, 125 mg, with a single oral dose of azithromycin, 1 g. For prophylaxis against bacterial vaginosis and *Trichomonas,* a single oral dose of metronidazole, 2 g, is recommended. Repeat cultures, wet mounts, and a pregnancy test should be performed 3 weeks after the assault, followed by serology for syphilis, hepatitis, and HIV at 12 weeks. Long-term sequelae are common; patients should be offered immediate and ongoing psychological support, such as that offered by local rape crisis services.

SEXUAL ORIENTATION

▶ SEE CHAPTER 23.

CHAPTER **70**

Eating Disorders

Eating disorders are common chronic diseases in adolescents, especially in females. The *Diagnostic and Statistical Manual of Mental Disorders, fourth edition (DSM-IV),* classifies these psychiatric illnesses as *anorexia nervosa, bulimia nervosa, binge eating disorder (compulsive eating),* and *eating disorder not otherwise specified.* The diagnosis in young adolescents (pre–growth spurt and premenstrual) may not follow the classic DSM IV–diagnostic criteria. The normal developmental milestones of adolescence may be triggers for eating disorders (Table 70–1).

ANOREXIA NERVOSA

The prevalence of anorexia nervosa is 1.5% in teenage girls. The female-to-male ratio is approximately 20:1, and the condition shows a familial pattern. The cause

TABLE 70–1. Normal Adolescent Milestones

Psychological Stages	Issues That Can Trigger Eating Disorders
Early adolescence—increased body awareness	Fear of growing up
Middle adolescence—increased self-awareness	Rebelliousness
	Competition and achievement
Late adolescence—identity	Anxiety and worry for the future
	Need for control

of anorexia nervosa is unknown, but it involves a complex interaction between social, environmental, psychological, and biologic events (Fig. 70–1). Risk factors have been identified (Fig. 70–2).

Clinical Manifestations and Diagnosis

It is important to screen early for eating disorders. This screening is best done as a part of the larger psychosocial screen for risk-taking factors (see Fig. 67–1). It is recommended that the adolescent be interviewed

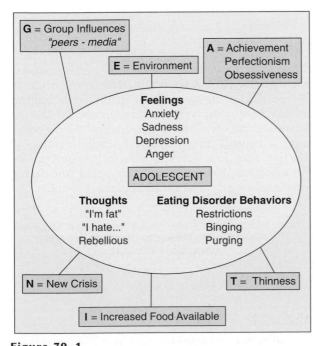

Figure 70–1

The EATING disorder cycle.

alone; an adolescent with an eating disorder may minimize the problem. It is important to interview the patient alone because this may provide more accurate information. The first event that a patient with anorexia or bulimia usually describes is a behavioral change in eating or exercise (food obsession, food-related ruminations, mood changes). The patient has an unrealistic body image and feels too fat despite appearing excessively thin. Parents' response to this situation can be anger, self-blame, focusing attention on the child, ignoring the disorder, or approving of the behavior.

The physician should be nonjudgmental, collect information, and work on a differential diagnosis. The **differential diagnosis** of weight loss includes gastroesophageal reflux, peptic ulcer, malignancy, chronic diarrhea, malabsorption, inflammatory bowel disease, increased energy demands, hypothalamic lesions, hyperthyroidism, diabetes mellitus, and Addison disease. Psychiatric disorders also need to be considered (drug abuse, depression, obsessive-compulsive disorders).

The **clinical features** of anorexia include the patient wearing oversized layered clothing to hide skeletal appearance, fine hair on the face and trunk (lanugo-like hair), rough and scaly skin, bradycardia, hypothermia, decreased body mass index, erosion of enamel of teeth (acid from emesis), and acrocyanosis of hands and feet. Signs of hyperthyroidism should not be present (see Chapter 175). The diagnostic criteria for anorexia nervosa are listed in Table 70–2.

Treatment and Prognosis

Treatment requires a multidisciplinary approach consisting of a feeding program and individual and family therapy. Feeding is accomplished through voluntary intake of regular foods or of a nutritional formula ingested orally or by nasogastric tube. When vital signs are stable, discussion and negotiation of a detailed treatment contract with the patient and the parents are essential. The first step is to restore body weight. Hospitalization may be necessary (Table 70–3). When 80% of normal weight is achieved, the patient is given freedom to gain weight at a personal pace. The *prognosis* includes a 3% to 5% mortality (suicide, malnutrition) rate, the development of bulimic symptoms (30% of individuals), and persistent anorexia nervosa syndrome (20% of individuals).

BULIMIA NERVOSA

Table 70–4 presents the diagnostic criteria for bulimia nervosa. The prevalence of bulimia nervosa is 5% in female college students. The female-to-male ratio is 10:1. Binge-eating episodes consist of large quantities of often forbidden foods or leftovers or both, con-

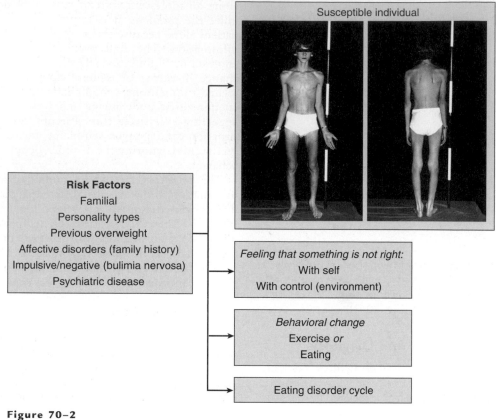

Figure 70–2

The slippery slope to eating disorders.

sumed rapidly, followed by vomiting. Metabolic abnormalities result from the excessive vomiting or laxative and diuretic intake. Binge-eating episodes and the loss of control over eating often occur in young women who are slightly overweight with a history of dieting.

Nutritional, educational, and self-monitoring techniques are used to increase awareness of the maladaptive behavior, following which efforts are made to change the eating behavior. Patients with bulimia nervosa may respond to antidepressant therapy because they often have personality disturbances, impulse control difficulties, and family histories of affective disorders. Patients feel embarrassed, guilty, and ashamed of their actions. Attempted suicide and completed suicide (5%) are an important concern.

TABLE 70–2.   Diagnostic Criteria for Anorexia Nervosa

Refusal to maintain body weight at or above a minimally normal weight for age and height (e.g., weight loss leading to body weight <85% of ideal)*

Intense fear of gaining weight or becoming fat, even though underweight

Denial of the seriousness of the low body weight—a disturbance in the way in which one's body weight or shape is experienced

Amenorrhea in postmenarche females*

*The diagnostic criteria may be difficult to meet in a young adolescent. Allow for a wide spectrum of clinical features.

TABLE 70–3.   When to Hospitalize an Anorexic Patient

Weight loss >25% ideal body weight*

Risk of suicide

Bradycardia, hypothermia

Dehydration, hypokalemia, dysrhythmias

Outpatient treatment fails

*Less weight loss accepted in young adolescent.

TABLE 70–4. Diagnostic Criteria for Bulimia Nervosa

Recurrent episodes of binge eating characterized by the following:

Eating in a discrete period an amount of food that is definitely larger than most people would eat during a similar period

A sense of lack of control over eating during the episode (e.g., a feeling that one cannot stop eating or control what or how much one is eating)

Compensatory behavior to prevent weight gain (i.e., self-induced vomiting, misuse of laxatives or diuretics, excessive exercise)

Binge eating and compensatory behaviors at least twice a week for 3 mo

Self-evaluation unduly influenced by body shape and weight

Disturbance does not occur exclusively during episodes of anorexia nervosa

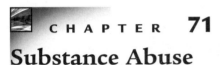

CHAPTER 71

Substance Abuse

There is a wide geographic and sociocultural variability in substance use. The age at which street drugs are first used is decreasing (<12 years old), with many adolescents abusing multiple substances. The Youth Risk Behavior Surveillance survey in 1997 found that 70% of high school students had tried smoking cigarettes, and of these, 36% went on to smoke daily. Ninety percent of adult smokers began their habit during their teenage years. Trends in alcohol use have not changed since the 1980s. Trends in marijuana and stimulant drug use declined during the 1980s, but are showing an upward trend. Inhalant use (glue solvents, aerosol products) continues a downward trend except in the aboriginal population. The use of "club drugs" by adolescents from upper income groups at rave parties (3,4-methylenedioxymethamphetamine [Ecstasy]) and so-called date-rape drugs (gamma-hydroxybutyrate or flunitrazepam [Rohypnol]) has risen sharply. Anabolic steroid use has increased in adolescent boys seeking enhanced athletic performance.

A history of drug use should be taken in a nonjudgmental and supportive manner. The history should include the types of substances, frequency, timing, circumstances, and outcomes of substance use. Table 71–1 is a helpful screening tool. There are few positive physical findings even with chronic adolescent substance use. An adolescent may present in an overdose or intoxicated state, or in a psychosis triggered by a hallucinogen, such as phencyclidine ("angel dust"). Club drugs have direct (coma and seizures) and indirect (sexual assault and dehydration) adverse effects. Anabolic steroids also have direct (gynecomastia and testicular atrophy) and indirect (mood swings and violence) adverse effects (Table 71–2).

ACUTE OVERDOSE

Many drugs (most commonly alcohol, amphetamines, opiates, and cocaine) can result in a toxicologic emergency. This situation most often occurs the first time an adolescent uses a substance, sometimes being unaware of its nature. Such an initial reaction makes identification of the offending agent difficult (see Table 71–2). Initial management should be directed at appropriate supportive medical treatment, with follow-up counseling after the toxic effects have diminished.

ACUTE ILLNESS

Heavy alcohol use can cause acute gastritis and acute pancreatitis. IV drug use can result in hepatitis B, bacterial endocarditis, osteomyelitis, septic pulmonary embolism, infection, or AIDS. Chronic marijuana or tobacco use is associated with bronchoconstriction and bronchitis.

CHRONIC USE

Compulsive drug or alcohol use results in an adolescent being unable to help himself or herself out of drug dependency and the psychosocial sequelae that attend such habituation (e.g., stealing, prostitution, drug dealing, unemployment, school failure, social isolation).

TABLE 71–1. CRAFFT: A Screening Tool for Adolescent Substance Abuse

C	Car	Driving under the influence of drugs
R	Relax	Using drugs to relax, fit in, feel better
A	Alone	Drugs/alcohol consumption while alone
F	Forgetting	Forgetting things as a result of drugs/alcohol
F	Family/Friends	Family and friends tell teen to stop/cut down
T	Trouble	Getting into trouble because of drugs/alcohol

TABLE 71–2.   Substances Abused by Adolescents: Effects and Facts, Route of Administration, Detection

Substance (Street/Alternative Name)	Effects and Facts	Route of Administration (Time of Action)	Detection
Alcohol (Meths)	Disinhibition, ataxia, slurred speech, respiratory and CNS depression	Ingested (depends on amount and tolerance)	Urine and Blood
Nicotine Snuff, dipping, chewed	Relaxation, CNS dependence, ↑ BP, ↑ HR, ↓ temperature	Inhaled (minutes)	
Marijauna (Cannabis) (Hashish, joints)	Euphoria, relaxation, ↑ appetite, ↓ reaction time	Inhaled (minutes) Tablets (30 min +)	Urine up to 1 mo
Stimulants Cocaine (crack) Amphetamines (ice)	Alertness, euphoria Insomia, ↓ appetite	Inhaled and snorted (Quick high) Tablets (longer effect)	Urine up to 48 h
Hallucinogens Mescaline Psilocybin (magic mushrooms) LSD PCP Phencyclidine (angel dust)	Hallucination, anxiety Psychosis, dilated pupils Dysphoria "Artistic high" "Lucy in the sky with diamonds" Microdots in many colors Can induce suicide attempts	Orally Injected, sniffed, ingested 2-12 hr "trip"	E.M.I.T. E.M.I.T. for PCP
EDMA **Ecstasy** (Club drugs: combinations, i.e., of hallucinogens and amphetamines)			Ecstasy *not* detected by urine screen
Opiates Heroin Opium and Heroin (freebase) Oxycontin (cotton, hillbilly) — new	Euphoria, ataxia, miosis, slurred speech A common adolescent mix	Orally, IV, smoked, snorted, and sniffed	
Tranquilizers Flunitrazepam (Rohypnol "roofies" ("date rape" drugs) Sedatives — Barbituates "downers"		Small white pills; dissolve easily, odorless, colorless, tasteless (often mixed in alcohol)	Urine 1-24 h
Inhalants (Solvents, gasoline)	Like alcohol	Inhaled	
Anabolic steroids	To enhance athletic performance	Tablets	Urine

Common side effects (treatment) of substance abuse drugs are:
Paranoia (haloperidol), Seizures (diazepam), Hyperthermia (slow cooling), Hypertension (β-blockers), Opiate overdose (naloxone)

Smoking information for Professions: www.surgeongeneral.gov
click on: Publications
click on: Reports of the Surgeon General
click on: Reducing Tobacco Use: A Report of the Surgeon General

TREATMENT

Specific management of substance use by adolescents depends on many individual patient factors. Because of the highly addictive (physical and psychological) nature of most substances, residential drug treatment facilities are being used, especially for younger adolescents.

SUGGESTED READING

American Academy of Child and Adolescent Psychiatry. http://www.aacap.org.

Behrman RE, Kliegman RM, Jenson HB (eds): Nelson Textbook of Pediatrics, 17th ed. Philadelphia, WB Saunders, 2003.

Braverman PK: Sexually transmitted diseases in adolescents. Med Clin North Am 84:869-889, 2000.

Brill SR, Rosenfeld WD: Contraception. Med Clin North Am 84:907-925, 2000.

Bryant-Waugh R, Lask B: Annotation: Eating disorders in children. J Child Psychol Psychiatry 36:191-202, 1995.

Centers for Disease Control and Prevention: 1998 STD treatment guidelines. MMWR Morb Mortal Wkly Rep 47(RR-1):1-11, 1998.

Centers for Disease Control and Prevention: CDC surveillance summaries: Youth risk behavior surveillance—United States, 1999. MMWR Morb Mortal Wkly Rep 49(SS-5):1-96, 2000.

Coupey SM: Interviewing adolescents. Pediatr Clin North Am 47:1349-1364, 1997.

Ehrman W, Matson S: Approach to assessing adolescents on serious or sensitive issues. Pediatr Clin North Am 45:189-204, 1998.

Gusella J: Thin and heavy children and adolescents. Can J CME 9:21-27, 1997.

Hogan MJ: Diagnosis and treatment of teen drug use. Med Clin North Am 84:927-966, 2000.

Kreijpe RE, Birndorf SA: Eating disorders in adolescents and young adults. Med Clin North Am 84:1027-1049.

Minjarez DA, Bradshaw KD: Abnormal uterine bleeding in adolescents. Obstet Gynecol Clin North Am 27:63-78, 2000.

Mitan LA, Slap GB: Adolescent menstrual disorders: Update. Med Clin North Am 84: 851-868, 2000.

National Institute on Drug Abuse (NIDA). http://www.drugabuse.gov/.

National Youth Anti-Drug Media Campaign: Tools for Parents and Adult Caregivers. www.theantidrug.com.

Office of National Drug Control Policy: National Youth Anti-Drug Media Campaign. www.mediacampaign.org/mg/print.html.

Sacks D, Westwood M: An approach to interviewing adolescents. Paediatr Child Health 8:554-556, 2003.

Schwartz RH: Marijuana: A decade and a half later, still a crude drug with underappreciated toxicity. Pediatrics 109:284-289, 2002.

Strasburger VC: Sex, drugs, rock 'n' roll revisited. Clin Pediatr 39:657-658, 2000.

The Emergency Contraception Website, Office of Population Research, Princeton, NJ. http://ec.princeton.edu/.

SECTION **XIII**

IMMUNOLOGY

Ramsay Fuleihan

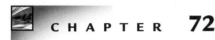

CHAPTER **72**

Assessment

Primary immunodeficiency diseases result from gene defects that affect one or more components of the immune system, leading to an increased susceptibility to infection. When functioning effectively, host defenses rapidly eliminate pathogens and toxins. Frequent, chronic, or unusually severe infections, the hallmarks of immunodeficiency, occur when the immune system is ineffective or deficient. The major components of host defense include an anatomic barrier, innate immunity, and adaptive immunity. Integrity of the **anatomic-mucociliary barrier** at the interface between the body and its environment (skin and mucous membranes) is essential for protection against infection (Table 72–1). Anatomic defects must not be overlooked as a potential source of recurrent infection in children. The innate immune system, which includes cellular components and soluble factors, initiates antigen-nonspecific mechanisms as a first line of defense against pathogens, before the development of more versatile adaptive immune responses, which involve antigen-specific T lymphocytes and B lymphocytes.

The **innate immune system** consists of serum proteins and cellular components that respond rapidly to pathogens early after infection. Soluble factors of the innate immune response include complement proteins that are activated in a cascade-like, sequential pattern, killing pathogens by facilitating their uptake by phagocytic cells or by antibody-independent lysis of pathogens. Other important soluble factors in innate immunity are acute-phase proteins, cytokines, and chemokines (Table 72–2). Proinflammatory acute-phase proteins include C-reactive protein and mannose-binding lectin, which are involved in recog-

nition of damaged cells and pathogens. In addition, they can activate complement and induce production of inflammatory cytokines. Chemokines have a broad range of activities, including the recruitment and activation of inflammatory cells. The pattern of chemokines produced determines the type and location of inflammatory infiltrate. Cytokines are involved in the regulation of the immune response and may have a direct role in defense.

The **cellular arm** of innate immunity includes phagocytic cells that engulf and digest foreign antigens and microorganisms. Phagocytic cells include polymorphonuclear neutrophils, which ingest pyogenic bacteria and some fungi, *Aspergillus* in particular, and macrophages, which develop from circulating monocytes and are effective in killing facultative intracellular organisms, such as *Mycobacterium, Toxoplasma,* and *Legionella*. In addition, natural killer (NK) lymphocytes play a major role in innate immunity by mediating cytotoxic activity against virally infected cells and cancer cells. Recognition of pathogens by the innate immune system is facilitated by receptors on macrophages, NK cells, and neutrophils, which recognize conserved pathogen motifs called **pathogen-associated molecular patterns**, which include lipopolysaccharide in gram-negative bacteria, lipoteichoic acid in gram-positive bacteria, mannans in yeast, and specific nucleotide sequences (cytosine adjacent to guanine) in bacterial and viral DNA. The innate immune system responds rapidly to pathogens early during immune responses and is required for activation of the adaptive immune response.

The key features of the **adaptive immune system** are antigen specificity and the development of immunologic memory, produced by the expansion and maturation of antigen-specific T cells and B cells. Antibodies (immunoglobulin), produced by B cells, protect against infection by neutralizing toxins released by pathogens, facilitating opsonization of the pathogen

---

TABLE 72–1.   Anatomic and Mucociliary Defects That Result in Recurrent or Opportunistic Infections

Anatomic Defects in Upper Airways

Aspiration syndromes (gastroesophageal reflux, ineffective cough, foreign body)
Cleft palate, eustachian tube dysfunction
Adenoidal hypertrophy
Nasal polyps
Obstruction of paranasal sinus drainage (osteomeatal complex disease), encephaloceles
Post-traumatic or congenital sinus tracts (CSF rhinorrhea)

Anatomic Defects in the Tracheobronchial Tree

Tracheal esophageal fistula, bronchobiliary fistula
Pulmonary sequestration, bronchogenic cysts, vascular ring
Tumor, foreign body, or enlarged nodes

Physiologic Defects in Upper and Lower Airways

Primary ciliary dyskinesia syndromes, Young syndrome
Cystic fibrosis, bronchopulmonary dysplasia, bronchiectasis
Allergic disease (allergic rhinitis, asthma)
Chronic cigarette smoke exposure

Other Defects

Burns
Chronic atopic dermatitis
Ureteral obstruction, vesicoureteral reflux
IV drug use
Central venous line, artificial heart value, CSF shunt, peritoneal dialysis catheter, urinary catheter

---

by phagocytic cells, activating complement causing cytolysis of the pathogen, or directing NK cells to kill infected cells by antibody-mediated cytotoxicity. **T cells** play a central role in the adaptive immune response by killing virus-infected or cancer cells, by delivering the necessary signals for B cell antibody synthesis and memory B cell formation, and by activating macrophages to kill intracellular pathogens. T cells are necessary for immunity to intracellular organisms, such as viruses; *Mycobacterium, Toxoplasma, Legionella,* and *Brucella;* fungi, such as *Histoplasma* and *Candida;* and protozoa.

Immunodeficiency can result from defects in any one or more components of innate or adaptive immunity, leading to recurrent, opportunistic, or life-threatening infections. Primary immunodeficiency diseases are relatively rare diseases individually, but together amount to a significant cause of chronic disease, morbidity, and mortality. Affected children are susceptible to frequent, severe infections. The pediatrician must be able to distinguish the rare child with true immunodeficiency from an immunologically normal child who has recurrent infections. The evaluation of children with recurrent infections must be based on a comprehensive understanding of the immune system, the patient's age, the site, and the pathogens involved (Table 72–3).

HISTORY

The history is probably the most important element in determining the need for evaluation for immunodeficiency disease. Early diagnosis of a primary immunodeficiency disease and initiation of therapy before serious and chronic infections result in a better outcome. The difficulty lies in identifying the individual child with immunodeficiency disease from among numerous pediatric patients with common infections. A **family history** of primary immunodeficiency disease or of infants dying from infection warrants an immunologic evaluation, especially in the presence of recurrent infections.

The frequency, severity, and location of the infection and the pathogens involved can help differentiate infections in a normal host from infections in an immunodeficient patient (see Table 72–3). Patients with primary immunodeficiency acquire infection with opportunistic organisms that do not ordinarily cause disease; however, antibody deficiency diseases initially manifest with common infections, such as otitis media and sinusitis, but at a higher frequency than in immunocompetent children. A total of eight or more episodes of otitis media, two or more serious sinus infections, or two or more episodes of pneumonia in 1 year suggests an antibody deficiency, especially if the infections are difficult to treat. Protection against sinopulmonary infections with encapsulated bacteria requires antibody-mediated immunity because these pathogens evade phagocytosis by cells of the innate immune system. Failure to thrive, diarrhea, malabsorption, and fungal infections suggest T cell immunodeficiency. Recurrent viral infections can result from T cell or NK cell deficiency. Opportunistic infections with organisms such as *Pneumocystis jirovecii (carinii)* suggest a T cell disorder, such as severe combined immunodeficiency (SCID), or T cell dysfunction, as in X-linked hyper-IgM. Deep-seated abscesses and infections with *Staphylococcus aureus, Serratia marcescens,* and *Aspergillus* suggest a disorder of neutrophil function, such as chronic granulomatous disease. Delayed separation of the umbilical cord, especially in the presence of omphalitis, and periodontal disease in addition to abscesses indicate leukocyte adhesion deficiency, whereas hyper-IgE syndrome is associated with cold abscesses, eczema, and frequent fractures. Deep-seated infections can help differentiate hyper-IgE syndrome from atopic dermatitis, which can be associated with extremely elevated levels of IgE. Onset of symptoms in

TABLE 72–2. Cytokines and Chemokines and Their Functions

Factor	Source	Function
IL-1	Macrophages	Costimulatory effect on T cells enhances antigen presentation
IL-2	T cells	Primary T cell growth factor; B and NK cell growth factor
IL-3	T cells	Mast cell growth factor; multicolony-stimulating factor
IL-4	T cells	T cell growth factor; enhances IgE synthesis; enhances B cell differentiation; mast cell growth
IL-5	T cells	Enhances immunoglobulin synthesis; enhances IgA synthesis; enhances eosinophil differentiation
IL-6	T cells, macrophages, fibroblasts, endothelium	Enhances immunoglobulin synthesis, antiviral activity, and hepatocyte-stimulating factor
IL-7	Stromal cells	Enhances growth of pre-B cells and pre-T cells
IL-8	T cells, macrophages, epithelium	Neutrophil-activating protein; T lymphocyte, neutrophil chemotactic factor
IL-9	T cells	Acts in synergy with IL-4 to induce IgE production, mast cell growth
IL-10	T cells, macrophages	Cytokine synthesis inhibitory factor; suppresses macrophage function; enhances B-cell growth; inhibits IL-12 production
IL-12	Macrophages, neutrophils	NK cell stimulatory factor; cytotoxic lymphocyte maturation factor; enhances IFN-γ synthesis; inhibits IL-4 synthesis
IL-13	T cells	Enhances IgE synthesis; enhances B cell growth; inhibits macrophage activation; causes airway hyperreactivity
IL-18	Macrophages	Enhances IFN-γ synthesis
IFN-γ	T cells	Macrophage activation; inhibits IgE synthesis; antiviral activity
TGF-β	T cells, many cells	Inhibits T cell and B cell proliferation and activation
RANTES	T cells, endothelium	Chemoattractant (chemokine) for monocytes, T cells, eosinophils
MIP-1α	Mononuclear cells, endothelium	Chemoattractant for T cells; enhances differentiation of CD4$^+$ T cells
Eotaxin 1, 2, and 3	Epithelium, endothelium, eosinophils, fibroblasts, macrophages	Chemoattractant for eosinophils, basophils, and Th2 cells
IP-10	Monocytes, macrophages, endothelium	Chemoattractant for activated T cells, monocytes, and NK cells; T cells activate NK cells

IFN, interferon; NK, natural killer; RANTES, regulated on activation, normal T expressed and secreted; Th2, T helper 2.

the teens or 20s suggests common variable immuno-deficiency (CVID) rather than agammaglobulinemia, although milder phenotypes of primary immunodeficiency disease may not present until later in life. The presence of associated problems such as congenital heart disease and tetany from hypocalcemia suggests DiGeorge syndrome. Ataxia-telangiectasia is associated with history of abnormal gait and telangiectasia on the skin. Atopic dermatitis is present in patients with hyper-IgE syndrome and is associated with easy bruising or a bleeding disorder in patients with Wiskott-Aldrich syndrome.

PHYSICAL EXAMINATION

Recurrent infection in immunologically deficient children is associated with incomplete recovery at sites of infection; this leads to scarring of the skin or of the tympanic membrane, abnormal hearing, persistent perforation of the tympanic membrane, persistent ear drainage, chronic lung disease, persistent cough and sputum production, failure to thrive, digital clubbing, or anemia of chronic disease. The accrual of substantial morbidity from repeated infections (including minor infections) suggests the presence of significant immunologic disease. Height and weight percentiles, nutritional status, and presence of subcutaneous fat should be assessed. Oral thrush, purulent nasal or otic discharge, chronic rales, and scarring of the tympanic membranes or of the skin may be evidence of persistent infection. Lymphoid tissue, such as the tonsils, and lymph nodes should be examined. Absence of tonsils suggests X-linked agammaglobulinemia or SCID, whereas increased size of lymphoid tissue suggests CVID, chronic granulomatous disease, or HIV infection. Cerebellar ataxia and telangiectasia indicate

---

TABLE 72–3. Clinical Characteristics of Primary Immunodeficiencies

B Cell Defects

Recurrent pyogenic infections with extracellular encapsulated organisms, such as pneumococci, *Haemophilus influenzae,* and streptococci

Otitis, sinusitis, recurrent pneumonia, bronchiectasis, and conjunctivitis

Few problems with fungal or viral infections (except enterovirus encephalitis and poliomyelitis)

Decreased levels of immunoglobulins in serum and secretions

Diarrhea common, especially secondary to infection with *Giardia lamblia*

Growth retardation not striking

Compatible with survival to adulthood or for several years after onset unless complications occur

Complement Defects

Recurrent bacterial infections with extracellular encapsulated organisms, such as pneumococcus and *H. influenzae*

Unusual susceptibility to recurrent gonococcal and meningococcal infections

Increased incidence of autoimmune disease (SLE)

Severe or recurrent skin and respiratory tract infection

T Cell Defects

Recurrent infections with less virulent or opportunistic organisms, such as fungi, mycobacteria, viruses, and protozoa

Growth retardation, malabsorption, diarrhea, and failure to thrive common

Anergy

Susceptible to graft-versus-host reactions if given unirradiated blood

Fatal reactions may occur from live virus or BCG vaccination

High incidence of malignancy

Poor survival beyond infancy or childhood

Neutrophil Defects

Recurrent dermatologic infections with bacteria and fungi, such as *Staphylococcus, Pseudomonas, Escherichia coli,* and *Aspergillus*

Subcutaneous, lymph node, lung, and liver abscesses

Pulmonary infections common, including abscess and pneumatocele formation, contributing to chronic disease

Bone and joint infection common

BCG, bacille Calmette-Guérin; SLE, systemic lupus erythematosus.

ataxia-telangiectasia. Eczema and petechiae or bruises suggest Wiskott-Aldrich syndrome.

DIFFERENTIAL DIAGNOSIS

Separate episodes must be differentiated from a relapse or recurrence of a single episode, which often occurs when episodes of otitis media or sinusitis are treated inadequately. Recurrent episodes of severe infection, such as meningitis or sepsis, are much more worrisome than recurrent otitis media, but antibody deficiency states initially manifest with common infections, such as otitis media and sinusitis. In patients with antibody deficiency states, ciliary dyskinesia, T cell deficiencies, or neutrophil disorders, infections develop at multiple sites (ears, sinuses, lungs, skin), whereas in individuals with anatomic problems (sequestered pulmonary lobe, ureteral reflux), infections are confined to a single anatomic site, such as a single pulmonary lobe or the urinary tract. Asplenia is associated with recurrent and severe infections even in the presence of protective antibody titers. Infection with HIV should be ruled out in any patient presenting with a history suggesting a T cell immunodeficiency. There are many causes of secondary immunodeficiency (Table 72–4).

DIAGNOSTIC EVALUATION

The diagnosis and effective treatment of patients with primary immunodeficiency diseases depend on early recognition of signs and symptoms suggesting immunodeficiency and the use of laboratory tests to evaluate immune function. The pediatrician or primary care physician needs to recognize the patient who might have an immunodeficiency disease and initiate an evaluation or a referral to an immunologist (Fig. 72–1).

Laboratory Tests

A diagnosis of primary immunodeficiency disease cannot be established without the use of laboratory tests. The choice of test and the extent of testing depend on the clinical history. Several tests are used in the diagnosis of primary immunodeficiency disease (Table 72–5).

A **complete blood count with differential** always should be obtained. A complete blood count can identify patients with low numbers of neutrophils (neutropenia) or lymphocytes (SCID) and the presence of eosinophils (allergic disease) and anemia (chronic disease).

Serum immunoglobulin levels vary with age, with normal adult values of IgG at full-term birth from transplacental transfer of maternal IgG, a physiologic nadir occurring at 6 to 8 months of age, and a gradual increase to adult values over several years. IgA can be absent at birth, and IgA and IgM levels increase gradually over several years with IgA taking the longest to

response to the immunization. Inadequate responses to bacterial polysaccharide antigens normally occur before age 2 years, but they also are associated with IgG subclass deficiency in older children. The development of protein-conjugate polysaccharide vaccines, especially to *H. influenzae* type b, has prevented infections with these organisms in early childhood. This situation has made it difficult, however, to assess antibody responses to polysaccharide vaccines in children older than 2 years. Antibody responses to the *Streptococcus pneumoniae* serotypes found in the 23-valent polysaccharide vaccine, but not in the conjugate vaccine, can be used to test antibody responses to polysaccharide antigens. Low or absent specific antibody responses confirm the diagnosis of antibody deficiency even if B cells are

reach normal adult values. Low albumin levels with low immunoglobulin levels suggest low synthetic rates for all proteins or increased loss of proteins, as in protein-losing enteropathy. High immunoglobulin levels suggest intact B cell immunity and can be found in diseases with recurrent infections, such as chronic granulomatous disease, immotile cilia syndrome, cystic fibrosis, or HIV infection. Elevated IgE levels can be found in hyper-IgE syndrome or in atopic dermatitis.

Specific antibody titers after childhood vaccination (tetanus, diphtheria, *Haemophilus influenzae,* or pneumococcal vaccine) determine the capacity of the immune system to synthesize antibodies and to develop memory B cells (see Table 72–5). If titers are low, the patient can be immunized with the particular vaccine and titers obtained 4 to 6 weeks later to check for

TABLE 72–4. Causes of Secondary Immunodeficiency

Viral Infections

Measles (inhibits interleukin-12 production in macrophages)
Roseola (human herpesvirus-6)
Epstein-Barr virus (X-linked lymphoproliferative disease or Duncan syndrome)
Cytomegalovirus
HIV (destroys CD4$^+$ T cells)

Metabolic Disorders

Diabetes mellitus
Malnutrition
Uremia
Sickle cell disease
Zinc deficiency
Multiple carboxylase deficiency
Burns

Protein-Losing States

Nephrotic syndrome
Protein-losing enteropathy

Other Causes

Prematurity
Immunosuppressive agents (e.g., corticosteroids, radiation, and antimetabolites)
Malignancy (leukemia, Hodgkin disease, nonlymphoid cancer)
Acquired asplenia
Periodontitis
Chronic (acute) blood transfusions
Acquired neutropenia (autoimmune, viral, or drug induced)
Bone marrow transplantation/graft-versus-host disease
Systemic lupus erythematosus
Sarcoidosis

TABLE 72–5. Tests for Suspected Immune Deficiency

General

Complete blood count, including hemoglobin, differential white blood cell count and morphology, and platelet count
Radiographs to document infection in chest, sinus, mastoids, and long bones, if indicated by clinical history
Cultures, if appropriate
Erythrocyte sedimentation rate

Antibody-Mediated Immunity

Quantitative immunoglobulin levels: IgG, IgA, IgM, IgE
Isohemagglutinin titers (anti-A, anti-B): measures IgM function
Specific antibody levels: diphtheria, tetanus, polio, rubella, *Haemophilus influenzae, Streptococcus pneumoniae*
B cell numbers and subsets by flow cytometry

Cell-Mediated Immunity

Lymphocyte count and morphology
Delayed hypersensitivity skin tests (*Candida,* tetanus toxoid, tuberculin, mumps): measures T cell and macrophage function
T and B cell numbers and subsets by flow cytometry
T lymphocyte function analyses

Phagocytosis

Neutrophil cell count and morphology
Nitroblue tetrazolium dye test
Staphylococcal killing, chemotaxis assay
Myeloperoxidase stain

Complement

Total hemolytic complement CH$_{50}$: measures complement activity
AP$_{50}$: measures alternative pathway complement activity
Levels of individual complement components
C1-inhibitor level and function

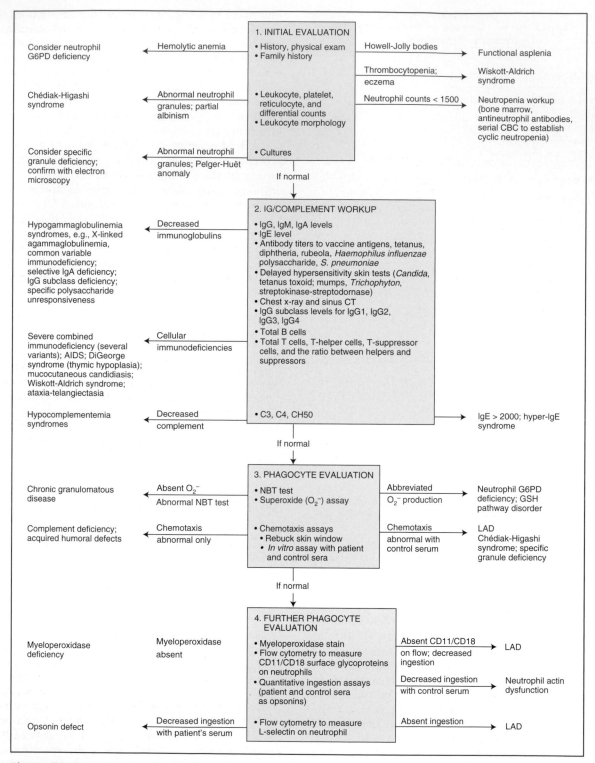

Figure 72–1

Algorithm for workup of a patient with recurrent infections. CBC, complete blood count; G6PD, glucose-6-phosphate dehydrogenase; GSH, reduced glutathione; NBT, nitroblue tetrazolium; LAD, leukocyte adhesion deficiency syndrome. (Modified from Curnutte JT, Boxer LA: Clinically significant phagocyte cell defects. In Remington JS, Swartz MN [eds]: Current Clinical Topics in Infectious Diseases, 6th ed. New York, McGraw-Hill, 1985, p 144.)

present, and serum immunoglobulin levels are in the normal range.

Lymphocyte phenotyping by flow cytometry enumerates the percentage and absolute numbers of T cell, B cell, and NK cell subsets and the presence of surface proteins that are necessary for normal immunity, such as MHC molecules or adhesion molecules. Absent T cells in the presence or absence of B cells indicates SCID, whereas isolated deficiency of B cells characterizes agammaglobulinemia.

Delayed-type hypersensitivity (DTH) skin tests to antigens, such as tetanus, diphtheria, *Candida*, or mumps, show the presence of antigen-specific memory T cells and functioning antigen presenting cells. T cells recognize peptide fragments derived from antigens and presented by MHC molecules on the surface of antigen presenting cells. If delayed-type hypersensitivity skin test results are negative, patients should receive a booster vaccination and be retested 4 weeks later. If the results remain negative, in vitro T cell proliferation assays should be performed to confirm or rule out the lack of T cell responsiveness.

T cell proliferation assays to mitogens (phytohemagglutinin, concanavalin A, or pokeweed mitogen) or antigens (tetanus toxoid or *Candida*) are in vitro assays that determine the capacity of T cells to proliferate in response to a nonspecific stimulus (mitogens, which are plant lectins) or the presence of antigen-specific memory T cells (antigens).

Tests for cytokine synthesis or expression of activation markers by T cells may be performed in specialized research laboratories and can help identify defects in T cell function when T cells are present by flow cytometry, but the clinical history suggests a T cell disorder.

Complement assays include the total hemolytic activity of serum (CH_{50}), which is a widely available test depending on the presence of normal levels of the major components of complement. Activation of the alternative pathway of complement is performed by the AP_{50} test, which is available in some, but not all, clinical laboratories. If the CH_{50} or AP_{50} level is abnormal, tests for individual complement components must be analyzed in specialized laboratories. Tests for C1-inhibitor antigen and function are used to diagnose hereditary or acquired angioneurotic edema. The commercially available test for C1-inhibitor function that is used by most clinical laboratories can miss some patients with abnormal C1-inhibitor function, and testing by specialized laboratories should be performed if the diagnosis of angioneurotic edema is suspected.

Tests for neutrophil function include the nitroblue tetrazolium test for chronic granulomatous disease (CGD), in which a soluble yellow dye turns into an insoluble blue dye inside activated neutrophils that have generated oxygen radicals to kill bacteria. Patients with CGD have no blue-staining neutrophils, whereas carriers of the disease have, on average, half of their neutrophils turn blue in the nitroblue tetrazolium test. In vitro tests for evaluation of neutrophil phagocytosis, chemotaxis, and bacterial killing and for the presence of myeloperoxidase activity are available in some laboratories, and tests for the expression of adhesion molecules such as CD18 (leukocyte function–associated antigen type 1 [LFA-1]) can be performed by flow cytometry.

Genetic testing to confirm the diagnosis of a primary immunodeficiency disease can be performed in specialized laboratories and may be helpful for deciding on a course of treatment and determining the natural history and prognosis of the disease, genetic counseling, and prenatal diagnosis. In patients suspected to have DiGeorge syndrome, fluorescent in situ hybridization studies for deletions of chromosome 22 can be helpful. In patients suspected of having ataxia-telangiectasia, chromosomal studies for breakage in chromosomes 7 and 14 are useful.

Diagnostic Imaging

The absence of a thymus on chest x-ray suggests DiGeorge syndrome. Abnormalities in the cerebellum are found in patients with ataxia-telangiectasia. Otherwise, the use of diagnostic imaging in the evaluation of immunodeficiency diseases is essentially limited to the diagnosis of infectious diseases, such as pneumonia and sinusitis, and complications of recurrent infections, such as bronchiectasis.

CHAPTER **73**

Lymphocyte Disorders

Disorders that affect lymphocyte development or function result in significant immunodeficiency because lymphocytes play a major role in the adaptive immune response by providing antigen specificity and memory responses. Lymphocytes develop from hematopoietic stem cells through a series of stages that culminate in a common lymphoid progenitor, which gives rise to T lymphocytes, B lymphocytes, and NK lymphocytes. B cells complete their development in the bone marrow, whereas T cells develop in the thymus from bone marrow–derived precursors (Fig. 73–1). Isolated B cell disorders result in **antibody deficiency diseases**, whereas T cell disorders usually cause **combined immunodeficiency** because they are necessary for cell-mediated immunity, immunity to intracellular pathogens, and antibody synthesis by B cells (Fig. 73–2). NK cells are an important component of the **innate**

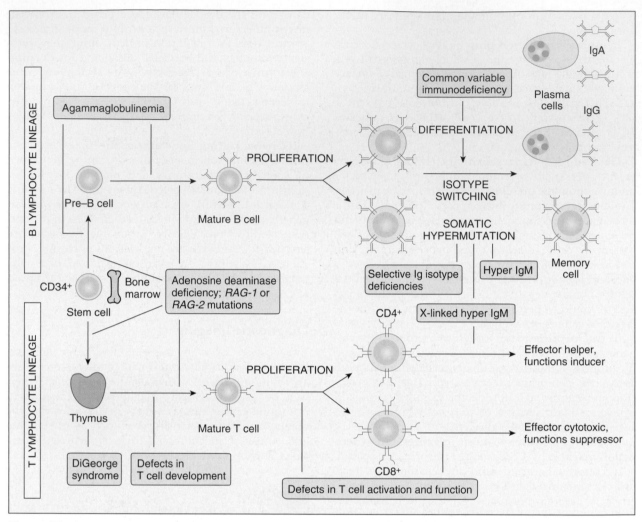

Figure 73–1

Sites of cellular abnormalities in congenital immunodeficiencies. In different congenital (primary) immunodeficiencies, the maturation or activation of B or T lymphocytes may be blocked at different stages. (Adapted from Abbas AK, Lichtman AH, Pober JS: Cellular and Molecular Immunology, 3rd ed. Philadelphia, WB Saunders, 1997.)

immune response. NK cells can kill virus-infected cells and tumor cells, and antibodies can enhance their function by antibody-mediated cellular cytotoxicity.

ETIOLOGY AND CLINICAL MANIFESTATIONS

Antibody Deficiency Diseases

B cells synthesize antibodies that can kill pathogens in conjunction with complement proteins, facilitate uptake of pathogens by phagocytic cells, and neutralize toxins secreted by pathogens. Disorders of B cells result in an increased susceptibility to infections by encapsulated bacteria because these pathogens resist uptake by phagocytic cells, and antibodies are necessary for their clearance. A variety of defects can affect the development or function of B cells leading to the inability to synthesize specific antibodies, the common underlying problem in all B cell disorders.

Agammaglobulinemia results from the absence of B cells with subsequent absence or severe decrease in immunoglobulin levels and a total absence of specific antibody. **X-linked agammaglobulinemia** is a congenital immunodeficiency that affects males and is characterized by a profound deficiency of B cells, resulting in severe hypogammaglobulinemia and absence of lymphoid tissue (Table 73–1; see Fig. 73–1). The defect

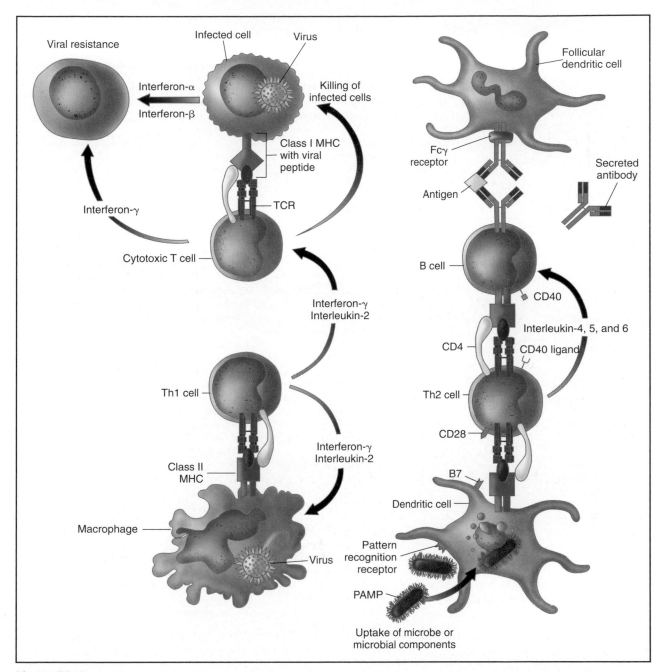

Figure 73–2

Overview of lymphocyte responses. *Left,* T cells characteristically possess T cell receptors (TCRs) that recognize processed antigen presented by MHC molecules. Most cytotoxic T cells are positive for CD8, recognize processed antigen presented by MHC class I molecules, and kill infected cells, preventing viral replication. Activated cytotoxic T cells secrete interferon-γ, which, together with interferon-α and interferon-β produced by the infected cells themselves, sets up a state of cellular resistance to viral infection. *Right,* Helper T cells are generally positive for CD4, recognize processed antigen presented by MHC class II molecules, and can be divided into two major populations. Type 1 (Th1) helper T cells secrete interferon-γ and interleukin (IL)-2, which activate macrophages and cytoxic T cells to kill intracellular organisms; type 2 (Th2) helper T cells secrete IL-4, IL-5, and IL-6, which help B cells secrete protective antibodies. B cells recognize antigen either directly or in the form of immune complexes on follicular dendritic cells in germinal centers. (Modified from Delves PJ, Roitt IM: The immune system. Second of two parts. N Engl J Med 343:108-117, 2000.)

TABLE 73–1. Disorders of Lymphocyte Function

Disorder	Genetics	Onset	Manifestations	Pathogenesis	Associated Features
Bruton agammaglobulinemia	X-linked (Xq22)	Infancy (6-9 mo)	Recurrent high-grade infections, sinusitis, pneumonia, meningitis	Arrest in B cell differentiation (pre-B level); mutation in the *Btk* gene	Lymphoid hypoplasia
Common variable immunodeficiency	AR; AD	Second to third decade	Sinusitis, bronchitis, pneumonia, chronic diarrhea	Arrest in B cell-to-plasma cell differentiation	Autoimmune disease, RA, SLE, Graves disease, ITP, malignancy
Transient hypogammaglobulinemia of infancy		Infancy (3-7 mo)	Recurrent viral and pyogenic infections	Delayed development of plasma cell maturation	Frequently in families with immuno-deficiencies
IgA deficiency	X-linked, AR, ?6p21.3	Variable	Sinopulmonary infections	Failure of IgA expressing B cell differentiation	IgG subclass deficiency, common variable immunodeficiency, autoimmune diseases
IgG subclass deficiency	AR 2p11; 14q32.3	Variable	Gastrointestinal infections; may be normal	Defect in isotype IgG production	IgA deficiency, ataxia-telangiectasia
IgM deficiency	AR	First year	Variable (normal to recurrent sinopulmonary infections and gastrointestinal infections)	Defective helper T cell–B cell interaction	Whipple disease, regional enteritis, lymphoid hyperplasia
Immunodeficiency with increased IgM	X-linked, AR, (Xq26)	First year	Sinopulmonary infections, opportunistic infections, *Pneumocystis carinii*	Defect in CD40 ligand/CD40 signaling	Neutropenia
DiGeorge anomaly	?22q11.2	Early infancy	Recurrent pyogenic infections (e.g., otitis media, sinusitis, tonsillitis, pneumonia)	Hypoplasia of third and fourth pharyngeal pouch	Hypoparathyroidism, aortic arch anomalies, micrognathia, hypertelorism
Wiskott-Aldrich syndrome	X-linked, (Xp11.22)	Early infancy	Variable	53-kD protein (WASP) defect	Recurrent infections, atopic dermatitis, platelet dysfunction, thrombocytopenia
Ataxia-telangiectasia	AR (11q22.3)	2-5 yr	Recurrent otitis media, pneumonia, meningitis with encapsulated organisms	AT gene mutation (PI3 kinase)	Neurologic and endocrine dysfunction, malignancy, telangiectasis; sensitive to radiation
Nijmegen breakage syndrome	AR (8q21)	Infancy	Sinopulmonary infections, bronchiectasis, urinary tract infections	Defect in chromosomal repair mechanisms	Sensitivity to ionizing radiation; microcephaly with mild neurologic impairment; malignancy
Cartilage-hair hypoplasia (short-limbed dwarf)	AR (9p13-21)	Birth	Variable	Unknown	Metaphyseal dysplasia, short extremities
Severe combined immunodeficiency (common gamma chain)	X-linked (Xq13.1), AR	1-3 mo	Candidiasis, all types of infections (bacterial, viral, fungal, protozoal)	IL-2R common gamma chain mutation (severe T cell depletion) ZAP-70 (2q12), Jak-3 kinase (19p13.1), or IL-7R alpha chain deficiency (15p13 deficiency)	Severe graft-versus-host disease from maternal fetal transfusions

TABLE 73–1.   Disorders of Lymphocyte Function—cont'd

Disorder	Genetics	Onset	Manifestations	Pathogenesis	Associated Features
Severe combined immunodeficiency (ADA deficiency)	AR (20q13.11)	1-3 mo	Candidiasis, all types of infections (bacterial, viral, fungal, protozoal)	Adenosine deaminase deficiency resulting in dATP-induced lymphocyte toxicity	Multiple skeletal abnormalities, chondro-osseous dysplasia
Severe combined immunodeficiency (PNP deficiency)	AR (14q13.1)	1-3 mo	Candidiasis, all types of infections (bacterial, viral, fungal, protozoal)	Purine nucleosidase deficiency resulting in dGTP-induced T cell toxicity	Neurologic disorders, severe graft-versus-host disease from transfusions
Severe combined immunodeficiency (reticular dysgenesis)	AR	1-3 mo	Candidiasis, all types of infections (bacterial, viral, fungal, protozoal)	Defective maturation of common stem cell affecting myeloid and lymphoid cells	Agammaglobulinemia, alymphocytosis, agranulocytosis
Omenn syndrome	AR (11p13)	1-3 mo	Candidiasis, all types of infections (bacterial, viral, fungal, protozoal)	Mutations of recombinase-activating genes (RAG-1 and RAG-2)	Exfoliative erythroderma, eosinophilia, elevated IgE, lymphadenopathy, hepatosplenomegaly
Bare lymphocyte syndrome (MHC class I)	AR (6p21.3)	First decade	Sinopulmonary infections	TAP1 (transporter associated with antigen processing) and TAP2 mutations	Chronic lung inflammation
Bare lymphocyte syndrome (MHC class II)	AR	Early infancy	Respiratory tract infections, chronic diarrhea, CNS viral infections	Mutations in RFX5, RFXAP, CIITA, and RFX-B (DNA binding factors)	Autoimmune disease
Chronic mucocutaneous candidiasis	AR	3-5 yr	Candidal infections of mucous membranes, skin, and nails	Unknown	Autoimmune endocrinopathies
Lymphoproliferative syndrome	X-linked (Xq25)	Variable	Variable decrease in T, B, and NK cell function and hypogammaglobulinemia following EBV infection	SAP (SLA-associated protein) defect	Life-threatening EBV infection, lymphoma or Hodgkin disease, aplastic anemia, lymphohistiocytic disorder
Lymphoproliferative syndrome	AR (10p14-15)	Variable	IL-2 receptor alpha-chain gene defect	CD25 deficiency, with autoimmunity	
Hyper-IgE syndrome	AD?	Variable	Skin and pulmonary abscesses, fungal infections, skin rash, elevated IgE	Unknown	Coarse facial features, failure to shed primary teeth, frequent fractures

AD, autosomal dominant; AR, autosomal recessive; dATP, deoxyadenosine triphosphate; dGTP, deoxyguanosine triphosphate; IL, interleukin; IL-2R γ, interleukin-2 receptor gamma chain; ITP, idiopathic thrombocytopenic purpura; PNP, purine nucleoside phosphorylase; RA, rheumatoid arthritis.
Modified from Boxer L, Blackwood K: Recurrent infection. In Kliegman RM, Nieder ML, Super DM (eds): Practical Strategies in Pediatric Diagnostics and Therapy. Philadelphia, WB Saunders, 1996, p 866.

is caused by mutations in a gene encoding for the tyrosine kinase *Btk* on chromosome Xq22 that is involved in signaling via the pre–B cell receptor and the B cell antigen receptor. The major consequence is the arrest of B cell development at the pre–B cell state. During development from a common lymphoid progenitor, B cell precursors progress through a variety of stages that are characterized by recombination of the variable region of the heavy and light chains of an immunoglobulin molecule, which serves as the antigen receptor on the surface of mature B cells. The B cell antigen receptor consists of an immunoglobulin molecule in association with several transmembrane and cytoplasmic molecules that function in signal transduction, including B cell linker protein and *Btk*. At the pre–B cell stage, a rearranged heavy chain associates with surrogate light chain genes λ5 and VpreB and the other component of the B cell antigen receptor to generate a pre–B cell receptor. Signaling via the pre–B cell receptor is necessary for rearrangement of a light chain molecule that associates with a heavy chain molecule to form the B cell antigen receptor. Defects in any of the genes that encode for structural or signaling molecules associated with the pre–B cell and B cell receptors can lead to agammaglobulinemia. These gene defects are inherited in an autosomal recessive manner and include mutations in the μ heavy chain gene on chromosome 14, the λ5 and VpreB surrogate light chains, Igα, Igβ, and B cell linker. X-linked agammaglobulinemia is more common than the autosomal recessive forms of agammaglobulinemia because only one copy of the gene needs to be defective to express the disease. Some patients with agammaglobulinemia do not have any defects in the above-described genes.

Patients with agammaglobulinemia usually present during the first 6 to 12 months of life, as maternal antibodies are waning. Some patients do not present with symptoms until 12 months or 3 to 5 years of age. These patients develop infections with *S. pneumoniae, H. influenzae, S. aureus,* and *Pseudomonas,* organisms for which antibody is an important opsonin. Gastrointestinal problems except for enteroviral infection and giardiasis are relatively rare, in contrast to the frequency of gastrointestinal symptoms seen in CVID. Patients with agammaglobulinemia also are susceptible to viral infections, such as chronic enteroviral meningoencephalitis and attenuated live virus vaccine–associated poliomyelitis.

CVID is a heterogeneous disorder characterized by hypogammaglobulinemia developing after an initial period of normal immune function, most commonly in the teens and 20s (see Table 73–1). Serum IgG levels are less than 500 mg/dL (usually <300 mg/dL) with IgA levels less than 10 mg/dL and low IgM levels. Antibody titers to protein antigens, such as tetanus and diphtheria, and to polysaccharide antigens, such as pneumococcus, are absent. T cell function is variable; patients may have decreased numbers of CD4 T cells, may have decreased lymphocyte proliferation to mitogens and antigens, or may be normal. B cells may be present at low or normal numbers, and affected patients exhibit normal-sized or enlarged tonsils and lymph nodes and may have splenomegaly. CVID patients have a susceptibility to frequent respiratory tract infections; bronchiectasis; autoimmune diseases, such as hemolytic anemia, thrombocytopenia, and neutropenia; gastrointestinal disease (malabsorption, chronic diarrhea, liver dysfunction, and *Helicobacter pylori* infection); granulomatous disease; and cancer, especially lymphoma. CVID is observed frequently in families with IgA deficiency. The gene defects leading to CVID are unknown. Some patients have a defect in the gene encoding for ICOS, the "inducible costimulator" on activated T cells. These patients had normal T cell numbers and function, but had a decrease in naive and memory B cells. Some patients who were thought to have CVID were found by genetic studies to have X-linked agammaglobulinemia, X-linked lymphoproliferative disease, or hyper-IgM syndrome. It is important to exclude these disorders and other causes of hypogammaglobulinemia, such as hypogammaglobulinemia associated with thymoma or secondary to immunoglobulin loss (intestinal loss), before making the diagnosis of CVID.

Selective **IgA deficiency** is defined as serum IgA levels less than 5 to 10 mg/dL accompanied by normal or increased levels of other immunoglobulins. It occurs in approximately 1 in 500 individuals. Many patients with selective IgA deficiency are asymptomatic. In others, it is associated with recurrent sinopulmonary infections, IgG₂ subclass deficiency, antibody deficiency, food allergy, autoimmune disease, or celiac disease. IgA deficiency occurs in families, suggesting an autosomal inheritance. It also is seen in families with CVID. The genes for IgA deficiency (and for some forms of CVID) may reside in the MHC class III (complement) region on chromosome 6.

IgG subclass deficiency occurs when the level of antibodies in one or more of the four IgG subclasses is selectively decreased, while total IgG levels are normal or only slightly decreased. The IgG_1 subclass is the most prevalent of the IgG subclasses, and deficiency in IgG_1 usually is reflected as hypogammaglobulinemia. IgG_2 subclass deficiency is the most common of these deficiencies and often is associated with IgA deficiency, ataxia-telangiectasia, and reduced capacity to produce antibody against polysaccharide antigens. IgG_3 subclass deficiency also has been associated with recurrent infections. The significance of IgG_4 deficiency is unknown; absent IgG_4 levels are not considered to be clinically significant. An inability to synthesize specific antibody titers to protein or polysaccharide antigens provides the best association of IgG subclass deficiency with recurrent infections and need for therapy.

Transient hypogammaglobulinemia of infancy is a temporary condition characterized by delayed immunoglobulin production. The pathogenesis of this disorder is unknown, but it is thought to result from a prolongation of the physiologic hypogammaglobulinemia of infancy. The normal immunoglobulin nadir at 6 months of age is accentuated, with immunoglobulin levels less than 200 mg/dL. B and T cells are present, and antibodies can be synthesized to protein antigens, such as diphtheria and tetanus toxoid. Immunoglobulin levels remain diminished throughout the first year of life, but increase to normal, age-appropriate levels usually by 2 to 4 years of age; however, the low levels may persist longer. The incidence of sinopulmonary infection is increased in some patients. This diagnosis can be suspected especially if hypogammaglobulinemia is associated with normal antibody titers to protein antigens. The transient nature of this disorder cannot be confirmed, however, until immunoglobulin levels return to the normal range.

Antibody deficiency syndrome is characterized by recurrent infections with normal immunoglobulin levels and normal lymphocyte numbers and subsets, but an inability to synthesize specific antibody to polysaccharide antigens, such as to the 23-valent pneumococcal vaccine. The pathogenesis of this disorder is unknown, but the lack of specific antibody titers explains the recurrent infections and justifies appropriate therapy.

Combined Immunodeficiency Diseases

Disorders that affect T cell development or function usually result in combined immunodeficiency because T cells provide necessary signals for B cell differentiation. **Hyper-IgM syndrome** usually is classified under antibody deficiency diseases or B cell disorders. The most common form of hyper-IgM, X-linked hyper-IgM, is a combined immunodeficiency disease, however, with deficient T cell function. Hyper-IgM syndrome is characterized by a failure of immunoglobulin isotype switching from IgM and IgD to IgG, IgA, or IgE and a lack of memory responses. Affected patients have normal or elevated serum levels of IgM with low or absent IgG, IgA, and IgE. Immunoglobulin isotype switching allows a B cell to maintain antigen specificity while altering immunoglobulin function, which resides in the constant region of the immunoglobulin heavy chain. Immunoglobulin isotype switching is directed by cytokines and requires direct interaction between CD40 ligand on a CD4 T cell and CD40 on a B cell (Fig. 73-3). Subsequent signal transduction via CD40 leads to activation of several signaling molecules and transcription factors, including nuclear factor κB (NF-κB) and two enzymes necessary for immunoglobulin isotype switching and somatic hypermutation, activation-induced cytidine deaminase (AID) and uracil DNA-glycosylase (UNG). Somatic hypermutation is a process by which the variable region of immunoglobulin is mutated to generate antibody molecules with a higher affinity to antigen. In addition, signaling via CD40 on B cells and other antigen presenting cells is important for T cell priming by up-regulation of costimulatory molecules that signal back to the T cell via CD28 and secretion of cytokines, such as interleukin (IL)-12.

X-linked hyper-IgM results from defects in the CD40 ligand gene that inhibit its capacity to bind to CD40, and no signal reaches the B cell for immunoglobulin isotype switching or antigen presenting cells for costimulation for T cell priming. Defects in CD40, inherited in an autosomal recessive manner, lead to a similar immunodeficiency as X-linked hyper-IgM because there is no signaling via CD40. Other forms of autosomal recessive hyper-IgM involve defects in AID or UNG, however, which are restricted to B cells and present with a failure of immunoglobulin isotype switching without abnormality in T cell priming. These forms of hyper-IgM are an antibody disorder and not a combined immunodeficiency. Patients with defects in CD40 ligand or CD40 have small lymph nodes with no germinal centers, whereas patients with defects in AID or UNG have large germinal centers and lymphadenopathy.

All patients have a susceptibility to sinopulmonary infections; however, patients with defects in CD40 ligand or CD40 also are susceptible to opportunistic infections, such as *P. jirovecii* (*carinii*) and *Cryptosporidium parvum*. The hyper-IgM phenotype also is found in an X-linked disorder associated with ectodermal dysplasia resulting from the defects in the gene encoding the NF-κB essential modulator that is necessary for signaling via NF-κB and results in low IgG, IgA, and IgE with normal or elevated IgM. NF-κB signaling also is important for several functions of the innate immune system, and these patients present with a different susceptibility to infection, such as meningitis and infection with atypical mycobacteria.

SCID is characterized by a profound lack of T cell function and B cell dysfunction resulting from the gene defect itself or secondary to lack of T cell function (see Fig. 73-1). T cells develop from bone marrow–derived precursors in the thymus (see Fig. 73-3), where they undergo several stages of development characterized by recombination of the variable region of T cell antigen receptor chains α and β (or γ and δ) in an analogous manner to the variable region of immunoglobulin in the B cell antigen receptor. In addition, thymocytes differentiate into CD4 or CD8 T cells if they interact with MHC class II or class I molecules, respectively. The T cell antigen receptor can recognize only peptide fragments from antigens that are presented via MHC molecules, CD4 T cells by MHC class II, and CD8 T cells by MHC class I. Because the variable region of the T cell antigen receptor rearranges randomly to provide as much variability as possible, not all T cell antigen receptors can interact with the MHC molecules present in the individual. A process of positive selection occurs in the thymus that selects thymocytes with antigen receptors that can interact with the expressed MHC molecules in the individual (Fig. 73-4). All other thymocytes die in the thymus. Some of the positively selected thymocytes have antigen receptors, however, that recognize self-antigens presented by

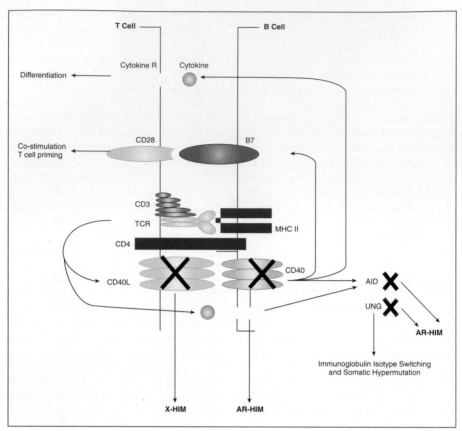

Figure 73–3

Schematic representation of the interaction between a CD4 T cell and a B cell. T cell activation follows T cell receptor (TCR) recognition of peptide antigen presented via MHC class II molecules resulting in CD40 ligand (CD40L) expression and cytokine synthesis. CD40L stimulates the B cell via CD40, resulting in expression of costimulatory molecules (B7) that are important in T cell priming and cytokine synthesis that drives T cell differentiation. CD40 signaling and signaling by cytokines in B cells activate activation-induced cytidine deaminase (AID) and uracil DNA-glycosylase (UNG) to promote immunoglobulin isotype switching and somatic hypermutation. Defects in CD40L cause X-linked hyper-IgM (X-HIM), and defects in CD40, AID, or UNG cause autosomal recessive hyper-IgM (AR-HIM). Defects in either CD40L or CD40 affect T cell costimulation and priming, leading to T cell defects, whereas defects in AID and UNG maintain normal T cell costimulation and function.

MHC molecules in the thymus. These cells are deleted in the thymus by a process of negative selection. Positive selection and negative selection in the thymus ensure that the mature T cells that leave the thymus for the peripheral lymphoid tissues can function with the individual's MHC molecules and do not mount autoimmune responses. SCID can result from any specific genetic mutation that interferes with T cell development in the thymus or T cell function in the periphery.

X-linked SCID, the most common form of SCID, is caused by mutations in the gene on chromosome Xq13.1 coding for the common gamma chain of the IL-2, IL-4, IL-7, IL-9, IL-15, and IL-21 receptors. Affected patients have no T cells or NK cells in the peripheral blood, but have normal numbers of B cells. Immunoglobulin levels are low or undetectable, however, and lymph nodes and tonsils are absent. The defect in T cell and NK cell development results from a failure of signaling via the IL-7 and IL-15 receptors because defects in the IL-7 receptor alpha chain also result in absent T cells, but normal numbers of B cells and NK cells, whereas IL-15 is necessary for NK cell

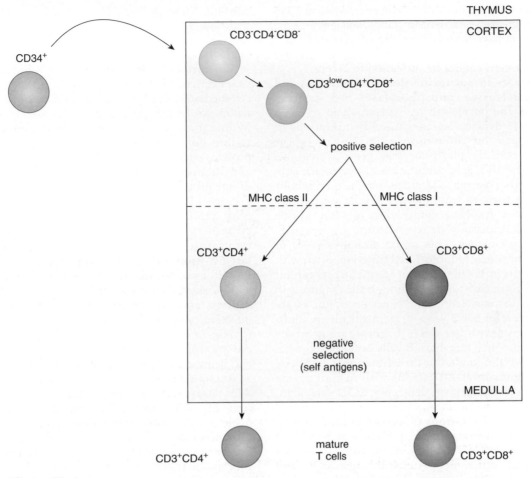

Figure 73-4

Schematic representation of T cell development in the thymus. CD34⁺ T cell precursors leave the bone marrow and go to the thymus, where they develop from CD3⁻CD4⁻CD8⁻ into mature CD4 or CD8 T cells via a CD4⁺CD8⁺ immature thymocyte stage. Positive selection selects thymocytes that can interact with MHC class I and II molecules to survive, and negative selection deletes autoreactive CD4 or CD8 thymocytes before their release into the periphery.

development. **Autosomal recessive SCID** results from defects in signaling molecules, such as Janus tyrosine kinase 3 (Jak3), which signals downstream of the common gamma chain, or ZAP-70 kinase, which is important in signaling via the T cell antigen receptor. In Jak3 deficiency, T cells and NK cells are absent, whereas B cells are present in normal numbers but are not functional. In ZAP-70 deficiency, there is a marked decrease in CD8 T cells with normal numbers of CD4 T cells that are not functional because ZAP-70 is necessary for CD4 T cell signaling.

Recombination of the variable regions of the T cell receptor and immunoglobulin molecules requires two genes called *recombinase activating gene (RAG) 1 and 2*. Defects in either gene that abolish its function result

in autosomal recessive SCID with no T cells or B cells present. Mutations in *RAG1* or *RAG2* that preserve limited function result in **Omenn syndrome**, a variant form of SCID that is characterized by exfoliative erythroderma, lymphadenopathy, hepatosplenomegaly, marked eosinophilia, elevated serum IgE, and impaired T cell function. Patients with Omenn syndrome have T cells in the periphery, but these T cells have a limited repertoire.

Bare lymphocyte syndrome results from defects in transcription factors that regulate expression of class II molecules or genes that affect transport of antigen peptides, which leads to absence of either MHC class I or MHC class II molecules. Lymphoid tissue and B cells may be present in normal amounts, but CD4 T cells are decreased or absent in class II deficiency, whereas CD8 cells are decreased or absent in class I deficiency. Some patients may have normal numbers of CD4 or CD8 T cells, but none of the T cells are functional because peptide antigens cannot be presented to T cells.

Deficiencies in **adenosine deaminase (ADA)** and **purine nucleoside phosphorylase**, two enzymes involved in the purine salvage pathway, also result in SCID. These deficiencies are caused by mutations in the ADA gene on chromosome 20q12-q13.1 or the purine nucleoside phosphorylase gene located on chromosome 14q13. Accumulation of nucleoside substrates in the plasma and urine or their metabolic products is toxic to lymphocytes. T cells are particularly sensitive to the accumulation of toxic purine metabolites, especially deoxyadenosine triphosphate and deoxyadenosine. This accumulation results in absent or markedly reduced T cell function, often with absent B cells or B cell function. Most patients exhibit severe infection early in life, although the diagnosis in patients with partial immune function is not established until after age 5 years or occasionally in adulthood. Patients with late-onset diagnosis are generally lymphopenic; they may have B cells and normal total immunoglobulin levels, but little functional anti-body (**Nezelof syndrome**). All patients with ADA or purine nucleoside phosphorylase deficiency SCID have lymphopenia and loss of immune function over time.

Clinical manifestations of SCID include failure to thrive, severe bacterial infection in the first month of life, chronic candidiasis, infection with *P. jirovecii* (*carinii*) and other opportunistic organisms, and intractable diarrhea. Patients often have skin disease similar to eczema, possibly related to graft-versus-host disease (GVHD) from engraftment of maternal lymphocytes, which is not usually fatal. Patients with SCID are extremely susceptible to fatal GVHD, however, from lymphocytes in blood transfusions. Patients with T cell disorders always should receive irradiated blood products.

DiGeorge syndrome is the classic example of T cell deficiency that is the result of dysmorphogenesis of the third and fourth pharyngeal pouches, resulting in hypoplasia of the thymus through which T cells must mature. Most, but not all, patients with DiGeorge syndrome represent a subset of patients with a field defect on chromosome 22q11.2, including the **velocardiofacial syndrome** and **CATCH 22 syndrome** (**c**ardiac anomalies, **a**bnormal facies, **t**hymic hypoplasia, **c**left palate, and **h**ypocalcemia). DiGeorge syndrome is classically characterized by hypocalcemic tetany, conotruncal and aortic arch anomalies (e.g., interrupted aortic arch type B, tetralogy of Fallot, and truncus arteriosus), and increased infections. The diagnosis of CATCH 22 is established by fluorescent in situ hybridization with a DNA probe to detect deletions in chromosome 22q11.2. Most patients have partial immune defects with low T cell numbers and function that improve with age. Severe T cell deficiency is rare, but results in SCID (lack of T cell and B cell function).

Wiskott-Aldrich syndrome is an X-linked disorder characterized by thrombocytopenia, eczema, defects in cell-mediated and humoral immunity, and a predisposition to lymphoproliferative disease. It is caused by mutations of the gene on chromosome Xp11.22 coding for the 53-kD Wiskott-Aldrich syndrome protein, which is expressed in lymphocytes, platelets, and monocytes. Deficiency of Wiskott-Aldrich syndrome protein results in elevated levels of IgE and IgA, decreased IgM, poor responses to polysaccharide antigens, waning T cell function, and profound thrombocytopenia. Opportunistic infections and autoimmune cytopenias become problematic in older children. **Isolated X-linked thrombocytopenia** also results from mutations of the identical gene. One third of patients with Wiskott-Aldrich syndrome die as a result of hemorrhage, and two thirds die as a result of recurrent infection caused by bacteria, cytomegalovirus, *P. jirovecii* (*carinii*), or herpes simplex virus. Bone marrow or stem cell transplantation has corrected the immunologic and hematologic problems in some patients.

Ataxia-telangiectasia is a syndrome caused by the *ATM* (ataxia-telangiectasia, mutated) gene on chromosome 11q22.3, which codes for a phosphatidylinositol-3 kinase. Patients have cutaneous and conjunctival telangiectasias and progressive cerebellar ataxia with degeneration of Purkinje cells. IgA deficiency, IgG$_2$ subclass deficiency of variable severity, low IgE levels, and variably depressed T cell function also may be seen. The normal function of the *ATM* gene is not clear, but it seems to be involved in detecting DNA damage, blocking cell growth division until the damage is repaired, or both. Ataxia-telangiectasia cells are exquisitely sensitive to irradiation. Leukemias, lymphomas, and diabetes also may be present, and sexual maturation is delayed. There is no uniformly effective therapy for this disease, but antimicrobial therapy and IV immunoglobulin (IVIG) replacement therapy may be helpful.

Chronic mucocutaneous candidiasis is characterized by chronic or recurrent candidal infections of the mucous membranes, skin, and nails. There is normal antibody production, but significantly decreased or absent lymphocyte proliferation and delayed skin reactivity to *Candida*. Patients usually do not respond to topical antifungal therapy and must be treated with oral antifungal agents. In most patients, an autoimmune endocrine disorder, such as hypoparathyroidism and Addison disease, develops by early adulthood. Other autoimmune disorders, such as autoimmune hemolytic anemia, also have been reported. Because the onset of these endocrine disorders can be insidious, patients must be evaluated frequently for autoimmune endocrine diseases. This disease has been found to result from a defect in the gene for the transcription factor autoimmune regulator *(AIRE)*, which seems to be necessary for expression of peripheral tissue antigens in the thymus, resulting in tolerance to these tissues.

Patients with **X-linked lymphoproliferative** disease have a defect in immune responsiveness to Epstein-Barr virus (EBV). Boys with this disease are essentially normal, until they become infected with EBV (infectious mononucleosis), which is fatal in 80% of patients. The disease is caused by a mutation in the gene called *SH2D1A* at chromosome Xq25, which codes for an adapter protein that normally inhibits signal transduction in proliferating T cells. In EBV infection, the mutation results in extensive expansion of CD8 T cells, hepatic necrosis, and death. Boys who survive the EBV infection have significant hypogammaglobulinemia associated with aplastic anemia and lymphoma. Treatment of the acute EBV infection with prednisone and acyclovir may be helpful; also, VP-16 and anti-CD20 monoclonal antibody may be helpful. IVIG for hypogammaglobulinemia also is indicated. Bone marrow transplantation has been attempted in some patients and has prevented disease progression.

Hyper-IgE syndrome is characterized by markedly elevated serum IgE levels, a rash that resembles atopic dermatitis, eosinophilia, and staphylococcal abscesses of the skin, lungs, joints, and viscera. Infections with *H. influenzae, Candida,* and *Aspergillus* also may occur. These patients have coarse facial features, develop osteopenia, and may have giant pneumatoceles in the lungs after staphylococcal pneumonias. Although serum IgG, IgA, and IgM concentrations are near-normal, humoral immune responses to specific antigens are reduced, as is cell-mediated immunity. Long-term treatment with antistaphylococcal medications is indicated, and IVIG therapy may be helpful.

TREATMENT

The approach to therapy of lymphocyte disorders depends on the diagnosis, clinical findings, and laboratory findings (Table 73-2). When immunodeficiency is suspected, and while the workup is in process, all blood products to be transfused need to be irradiated and ascertained to be cytomegalovirus negative because lymphocytes present in blood products can cause fatal **graft-versus-host disease (GVHD)** in patients with SCID. Cytomegalovirus infection can be fatal in an immunodeficiency patient undergoing bone marrow transplantation. Live viral vaccines need to be withheld from patients and household members until a diagnosis is established because patients with T cell

---

TABLE 73–2. General Management of Patients with Immunodeficiency

Avoid transfusions with blood products unless they are irradiated and cytomegalovirus negative

Avoid live virus vaccines, especially in patients with severe T cell deficiencies or severe agammaglobulinemia, and in household members

Follow pulmonary function in patients with recurrent pneumonia

Use chest physiotherapy, postural drainage in patients with recurrent pneumonia

Use prophylactic antibiotics because minor infections can quickly disseminate

Examine diarrheal stools for *Giardia* and *Clostridium difficile*

Avoid unnecessary exposure to individuals with infection

Use IV immunoglobulin for severe antibody deficiency states at a dose of 400-500 mg/kg q3-4 wk IV

---

deficiency or agammaglobulinemia are susceptible to infection from attenuated live viral vaccines.

Acute and chronic infections should be treated with appropriate antibiotics. Prevention of recurrent infections provides a better quality of life, however, and decreases the consequences of recurrent infections. Patients with milder forms of antibody deficiency diseases may benefit from **vaccination** with protein-conjugated polysaccharide vaccines to *H. influenzae* type b and *S. pneumoniae* (seven-valent), with postvaccination titers assayed at least 1 month later. These vaccines are administered routinely to young children; however, older children and adults with antibody deficiency syndrome also should receive these vaccines because they may generate protective antibody levels to *H. influenzae* type b and to some of the more common *S. pneumoniae* serotypes. Other microorganisms, including nonvaccine *S. pneumoniae* serotypes, can cause infections in susceptible patients. In addition to immunization, antibiotic prophylaxis or IVIG can be used to prevent recurrent infections.

Antibiotic prophylaxis can be attempted with once-daily administration of trimethoprim-sulfamethoxazole or amoxicillin at one half of the therapeutic dose, especially if the patient does not have a severe antibody deficiency and does not have a complicated infection. Therapy with antibiotics may be complicated by the development of immediate, autoimmune, immune complex, and delayed-type hypersensitivity drug reactions. Alternating prophylactic antibiotics on a monthly basis may help reduce the incidence of drug-resistant microorganisms.

Immunoglobulin replacement therapy with IVIG is a lifesaving therapy for patients with severe antibody deficiency diseases. It provides passive immunity against common infectious microorganisms and reduces the frequency and severity of infection in most patients with antibody deficiency diseases. IVIG is indicated in patients with agammaglobulinemia, hyper-IgM syndrome, other antibody deficiency diseases and combined immunodeficiency diseases; patients with infections requiring hospitalization, especially in ICUs, or infections that affect growth, development, or hearing and speech development; and patients who have failed antibiotic prophylaxis. IVIG usually is administered at a dose of 400 to 500 mg/kg of body weight every 3 to 4 weeks. IVIG therapy should be monitored by regularly measuring trough IgG levels, antibody titers to *H. influenzae* type b, and, most importantly, the clinical course. Patients who continue to have recurrent infections, especially in the last week before the administration of IVIG, may require higher doses or more frequent administration. A combination of prophylactic antibiotics and IVIG therapy may be indicated in some patients who continue to have recurrent infections. Other causes of recurrent infections should be reconsidered, however. **Complications of IVIG** therapy include transfusion reactions with chills, fever, and myalgia, which usually can be prevented in subsequent infusions by pretreatment with an antihistamine and an antipyretic and by a slower rate of infusion. Headache from aseptic meningitis can develop after IVIG therapy, usually in the first 24 hours, and it most often responds to treatment with ibuprofen. Allergic reactions to IVIG can occur in patients with absent IgA if the patient develops IgE antibodies to the IgA present in IVIG. Allergic reactions are rare and should not be a problem in patients who have detectable serum IgA levels or patients who cannot synthesize any antibodies. IVIG is a blood product that is prepared from pooled plasma from large numbers of selected donors through numerous steps that include testing for infectious organisms and inactivation of the viruses that can be transmitted via blood products. The risk for transmission of infectious agents is low, but the potential remains.

Therapy for severe T cell disorders is stem cell transplantation, preferably from an HLA-matched sibling (see Chapter 76). IVIG also is useful to provide passive antibody-mediated immunity. Some patients continue to have poor B cell function after bone marrow transplantation and require IVIG. **GVHD**, in which the transplanted cells initiate an immune response against the host tissues, is the main complication of bone marrow transplantation. Patients with the ADA deficiency form of SCID who lack histocompatible sibling donors can receive repeated intramuscular replacement doses of ADA, stabilized by coupling to polyethylene glycol. Gene therapy has been performed in several patients with the common gamma chain deficiency form and ADA deficiency form of SCID by transfer of a normal gene into bone marrow stem cells, which are infused into the patient. Gene therapy for ADA deficiency has not been successful yet, whereas gene therapy for common gamma chain deficiency was successful in most of the treated patients; however, it was complicated by the development of leukemia in some of the patients.

PREVENTION

Prenatal diagnosis is possible for all immunodeficiency diseases with an identified gene defect. Testing can be performed in specialized laboratories by gene sequencing, especially when the mutation in the index case has been identified.

CHAPTER **74**
Neutrophil Disorders

Neutrophils play important roles in immunity and wound healing. The major function of neutrophils is to ingest and kill pathogens. Neutrophil disorders can result from deficient cell numbers, defective chemotaxis, or defective function (Table 74–1). Patients with neutrophil disorders are susceptible to infections with *S. aureus,* certain fungi, and gram-negative bacteria. They may present with mucous membrane infections (gingivitis), abscesses in the skin and viscera, lymphadenitis, poor wound healing, delayed umbilical cord separation, or absence of pus. Neutrophils develop in the bone marrow from hematopoietic stem cells by the action of several colony-stimulating factors, including stem cell factor, granulocyte-monocyte colony-stimulating factor (GM-CSF), granulocyte colony-stimulating factor (G-CSF), and IL-3. Mature neutrophils leave the bone marrow for the periphery, where they are found in the circulation or reside in the marginating pool. Chemotactic factors, including the complement fragment C5a, IL-8, and bacterial formylated peptides, mobilize neutrophils to enter tissues and sites of infections. Adhesion molecules are necessary for neutrophils to roll and adhere to vascular endothelium and extravasate from the blood into sites of infection, where they encounter, phagocytose, and kill pathogens, especially if the pathogens are coated by complement or antibodies. Neutrophils kill ingested pathogens by enzymes found in granules or by activation of oxygen radicals. Immunodeficiency can result from defects in neutrophil production, survival, chemotaxis, or function.

Name	Defect	Comment
Chronic granulomatous disease	Bactericidal	X-linked recessive (66%), autosomal recessive (33%); eczema, osteomyelitis, granulomas, abscesses caused by *Staphylococcus aureus, Burkholderia cepacia, Aspergillus fumigatus;* X-linked defect in cytochrome b produces negative result on nitroblue tetrazolium test
Chédiak-Higashi syndrome (1q42I-44)	Bactericidal plus chemotaxis; poor natural killer function	Autosomal recessive; oculocutaneous albinism, neuropathy, giant neutrophilic cytoplasmic inclusions; malignancy, neutropenia
Hyperimmunoglobulin E (Job syndrome)	Chemotaxis, opsonization	Eczema, staphylococcal abscesses, granulocyte and monocyte chemotaxis affected; antistaphylococcal IgE
Myeloperoxidase deficiency	Bactericidal, fungicidal	Reduced chemiluminescence; autosomal recessive (1:4000); persistent candidiasis in diabetics
Glucose-6-phosphate dehydrogenase deficiency	Bactericidal	Phenotypically similar to chronic granulomatous disease
Burns, malnutrition	Bactericidal plus chemotaxis	Reversible defects
Lazy leukocyte syndrome	Chemotaxis	Normal bone marrow cells but poor migration; granulocytopenia
Leukocyte adhesion deficiency; CD18 deficiency (21q22.3)	Adherence, chemotaxis, phagocytosis; reduced lymphocyte cytotoxicity	Delayed separation or infection of umbilical cord; lethal bacterial infections without pus; autosomal recessive; neutrophilia; deficiency of LFA-1, Mac-1, CR3
Shwachman-Diamond syndrome	Chemotaxis, neutropenia	Pancreatic insufficiency, metaphyseal chondrodysplasia; autosomal recessive

TABLE 74–1. Phagocytic Disorders

ETIOLOGY AND CLINICAL MANIFESTATIONS

Disorders of Neutrophil Numbers

The normal neutrophil count varies with age. Neutropenia may be caused by decreased marrow production or peripheral neutrophil destruction. **Neutropenia** is defined as an absolute neutrophil count (ANC) less than 1500/mm³ for white children 1 year old or older. African-American children normally have lower total white blood cell and neutrophil counts. The effect of neutropenia depends on its severity. The increased susceptibility to infection is minimally increased until the ANC is less than 1000/mm³, and most patients do well with an ANC greater than 500/mm³. At these levels of circulating neutrophils, localized infections are more common than generalized bacteremia. Serious bacterial infections are common with an ANC less than 200/mm³. In the absence of an adequate neutrophil count, migration of neutrophils to areas of damage in the skin and mucous membrane is delayed. Neutropenia may be congenital or acquired (Table 74–2). Neutropenia may be associated with specific diseases, especially infections (Table 74–3), or may result from drug reactions (Table 74–4). The major types of infection associated

with neutropenia are cellulitis, pharyngitis, gingivitis, lymphadenitis, abscesses (cutaneous or perianal), enteritis (typhlitis), and pneumonia. The sites of the infection usually are colonized heavily with normal bacterial flora that becomes invasive in the presence of neutropenia.

There are several forms of **congenital neutropenia**, which is caused by an inadequate production of cells. **Severe congenital neutropenia (Kostmann syndrome)** is inherited as an autosomal recessive disorder and may present in infancy. In severe congenital neutropenia, myeloid cells within the marrow fail to mature beyond the early stages of the promyelocyte. The peripheral blood may show an impressive monocytosis. Endogenous G-CSF levels are increased; nevertheless, exogenous G-CSF produces a rise in the neutrophil count. Treatment with G-CSF has improved the care of these children. Acute myeloid leukemia has developed in a few patients who have survived into adolescence. Bone marrow transplantation may be curative.

Severe congenital neutropenia that may be either persistent or cyclic also is a component of **Shwachman-Diamond syndrome**, an autosomal recessive syndrome of pancreatic insufficiency accompanying bone marrow dysfunction. This is a panmyeloid

TABLE 74–2.   Mechanisms of Neutropenia

Abnormal Bone Marrow

Marrow Injury

Drugs: idiosyncratic, cytotoxic (myelosuppressive)
Radiation
Chemicals: DDT, benzene
Hereditary
Immune-mediated: T and B cell and immunoglobulin
Infection: HIV, hepatitis B
Infiltrative processes: tumor, storage disease

Maturation Defects

Folic acid deficiency
Vitamin B_{12}
Glycogen storage disease type Ib
Shwachman-Diamond syndrome
Organic acidemias
Clonal disorders: congenital
Cyclic neutropenia

Peripheral Circulation

Pseudoneutropenia: Shift to Bone Marrow

Hereditary
Severe infection

Intravascular

Destruction: neonatal isoimmune, autoimmune,
   hypersplenism
Leukoagglutination: lung, after cardiac bypass surgery

Extravascular Mechanisms

Increased use: severe infection, anaphylaxis
Destruction: antibody-mediated, hypersplenism

Adapted from Moore JO, Oritel TL, Rosse WF: Disorders of granulocytes
and monocytes: In Andreoli TE, Bennett JC, Carpenter CC, Plum F (eds):
Cecil Essentials of Medicine, 4th ed. Philadelphia, WB Saunders, 1997.

TABLE 74–3.   Infections Associated with Neutropenia

Bacterial

Typhoid-paratyphoid
Brucellosis
Neonatal sepsis
Meningococcemia
Overwhelming sepsis
Congenital syphilis
Tuberculosis

Viral

Measles
Hepatitis B
HIV
Rubella
Cytomegalovirus
Influenza
Epstein-Barr virus

Rickettsial

Rocky Mountain spotted fever
Typhus
Ehrlichiosis
Rickettsialpox

and in some instances are transmitted as an autosomal dominant disorder. Severe congenital neutropenia also may be associated with SCID in **reticular dysgenesis**, a disorder of hematopoietic stem cells affecting all lineages.

TABLE 74–4.   Drugs Associated with Neutropenia

Cytotoxic

Myelosuppressive, chemotherapeutic agents
Immunosuppressive agents

Idiosyncratic

Chloramphenicol
Sulfonamides
Propylthiouracil
Penicillins
Trimethoprim-sulfamethoxazole
Carbamazepine
Phenytoin
Cimetidine
Methyldopa
Indomethacin
Chlorpromazine
Penicillamine
Gold salts

disorder in which neutropenia is the most prominent manifestation. Patients may have all the common complications of neutropenia, including gingivitis, which may be severe and lead to serious oral infections and alveolar bone destruction. Patients may become edentulous at an early age. Metaphyseal dysostosis and dwarfism also may occur. Patients usually respond to G-CSF.

Other congenital neutropenias caused by deficient production of neutrophils vary in severity and are poorly characterized. **Benign congenital neutropenia** is a functional diagnosis for patients with significant neutropenia in whom major infectious complications do not develop. Many patients whose ANC ranges from 100 to 500/mm^3 have an increased frequency of infections, particularly respiratory infections, but the major problem is the slow resolution of the infections that develop. These disorders may be sporadic or familial

Cyclic neutropenia is a stem cell disorder in which all marrow elements cycle; it may be transmitted as an autosomal dominant, recessive, or sporadic disorder. The only clinically significant abnormality is neutropenia, however, because of the short half-life of neutrophils in the blood (6 to 7 hours) compared with platelets (10 days) and red blood cells (120 days). The usual cycle is 21 days, with neutropenia lasting 4 to 6 days, accompanied by monocytosis and often by eosinophilia. Clinical manifestations of stomatitis or oral ulcers, pharyngitis, lymphadenopathy, fever, and cellulitis are present at the time of neutropenia. Severe, debilitating bone pain is common in these patients when the neutrophil count is low. Cyclic neutropenia responds to G-CSF with a reduced number of days of neutropenia and an overall increase in neutrophil numbers.

Isoimmune neutropenia occurs in neonates and is the result of transplacental transfer of maternal antibodies to fetal neutrophil antigens. The mother is sensitized to specific neutrophil antigens on fetal leukocytes that are inherited from the father and are not present on maternal cells. Isoimmune neonatal neutropenia, similar to isoimmune anemia and thrombocytopenia, is a transient process (see Chapters 62 and 151). Cutaneous infections are common, whereas sepsis is rare. Early treatment of infection while the infant is neutropenic is the major goal of therapy. Administration of IVIG may decrease the duration of neutropenia.

Autoimmune neutropenia usually develops early in childhood (5 to 24 months old) and often persists for prolonged periods. Neutrophil autoantibodies may be IgG, IgM, IgA, or a combination of these. Usually the condition resolves in 6 months to 4 years. Clinical symptoms may dictate treatment. Although IVIG and corticosteroids have been used in the past, most patients respond to G-CSF. Most patients do not progress to more generalized autoimmune disorders; autoimmune neutropenia rarely may be an early manifestation of systemic lupus erythematosus or rheumatoid arthritis. The marrow in autoimmune neutropenia and systemic lupus erythematosus shows myeloid hyperplasia except that if antibody is directed against myeloid precursors, it reveals hypoplasia.

Neutropenia is common in stressed neonates. Virtually any major illness, including asphyxia, may precipitate transient neonatal neutropenia. Maternal conditions, such as hypertension and eclampsia, can induce neonatal neutropenia. Significant neutropenia may develop in infected neonates partly secondary to depletion of bone marrow stores. The bone marrow stores, which are seven times as great as the circulating pool of neutrophils in adults, are far less extensive in neonates. Infectious processes readily deplete their marrow reserve.

Disorders of Neutrophil Migration

Neutrophils normally adhere to endothelium and migrate to areas of inflammation by the interaction of membrane proteins called *integrins* and *selectins* with endothelial cell adhesion molecules. A hallmark of defects in neutrophil migration is the absence of pus at sites of infection. The presence of neutrophils in abscesses or other sites of infections rules out a chemotactic defect. In **leukocyte adhesion deficiency type I (LAD-I)**, infants lacking the β_2 integrin CD18 exhibit the condition early in infancy with failure of separation of the umbilical cord (often 2 months after birth) with attendant omphalitis and sepsis (see Table 74–1). The neutrophil count usually is greater than 20,000/mm³ because of failure of the neutrophils to adhere normally to vascular endothelium and to migrate out of blood to the tissues (Fig. 74–1). Cutaneous, respiratory, and mucosal infections occur, and children with this condition usually have severe gingivitis. Sepsis usually leads to death in early childhood. This disorder is transmitted as an autosomal recessive trait. Bone marrow transplantation may be lifesaving.

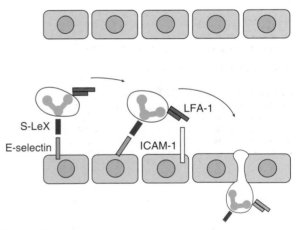

Figure 74–1

Schematic representation of neutrophil migration from the vascular space across the vascular endothelium into tissues. Neutrophils bind to selectin molecules on the surface of vascular endothelium via sialylated and fucosylated tetrasaccharides related to the sialylated Lewis X blood group (S-LeX) found on the surface of neutrophils. The bound neutrophils roll along the endothelium and become tightly bound by the interaction of the adhesion molecule leukocyte function–associated antigen type 1 (LFA-1) on the neutrophil and intercellular adhesion molecule type 1 (ICAM-1) on vascular endothelium, allowing neutrophils to move through the endothelium and into the tissue spaces. (Adapted from Janeway CA, Travers P, Walport M, Capra JD: Immunobiology: The Immune System in Health and Disease, 4th ed. New York, Elsevier, 1999.)

LAD-II results from impairment of neutrophil rolling along the vascular wall, which is the first step in neutrophil migration into tissues and sites of infection. Rolling is mediated by sialylated and fucosylated tetrasaccharides related to the sialylated Lewis X blood group found on the surface of neutrophils, monocytes, and activated lymphocytes binding to selectin molecules on vascular endothelium (see Fig. 74–1). LAD-II results from a general defect in fucose metabolism leading to the absence of sialylated Lewis X blood group on the surface of neutrophils and other leukocytes.

A variety of conditions are associated with chemotactic defects in neutrophils. **Hyper-IgE syndrome** is characterized by eczema, hyperimmunoglobulinemia E, an extrinsic chemotactic defect, absent T cell and B cell responses to antigens, and recurrent cold boils (characteristically caused by *S. aureus*) that do not become markedly red or drain (see Table 74–1).

Disorders of Neutrophil Function

Defects in neutrophil function are relatively rare inherited disorders and tend to be associated with a marked susceptibility to bacterial and fungal infection. **CGD** is a rare disorder of white blood cells that results from defective intracellular killing of bacteria and intracellular pathogens by neutrophils and macrophages because of an inability to activate the "respiratory burst," the catalytic conversion of molecular oxygen to superoxide (O_2^-). Reduced nicotinamide adenine dinucleotide phosphate oxidase, the enzyme that catalyzes the respiratory burst, consists of four subunits, two subunits of cytochrome b558, gp91^{phox} and p22^{phox}, and two cytosolic oxidase components, p47^{phox} and p67^{phox}. Defects in any of these enzymes lead to an inability to kill catalase-positive pathogens, such as *S. aureus*, enteric gram-negative bacteria (*Salmonella, Proteus, Klebsiella, Escherichia coli, Serratia marcescens, Burkholderia cepacia*), and fungi (*Aspergillus fumigatus, Candida albicans, Torulopsis glabrata*). The gp91^{phox} gene is located on chromosome Xp21.1 and is the more common form of the disease because only one copy of the gene needs to be defective for the disease to be expressed in males. The other gene defects are inherited in an autosomal recessive manner because the chromosome locations for these genes are 16q24 for p22^{phox}, 7q11.23 for p47^{phox}, and 1q25 for p67^{phox}. Glucose-6-phosphate dehydrogenase also is involved in the production of superoxide, and severe forms of glucose-6-phosphate dehydrogenase deficiency also result in CGD. Patients characteristically have lymphadenopathy, hypergammaglobulinemia, hepatosplenomegaly, dermatitis, failure to thrive, anemia, chronic diarrhea, and abscesses. Infections occur in the lungs, resulting in chronic bronchitis, and in the middle ear, gastrointestinal tract, skin, urinary tract, lymph nodes, liver, and bones. Granulomas may obstruct the pylorus or ureters.

Chédiak-Higashi syndrome, an abnormality of secondary granules, is an autosomal recessive disorder caused by a mutation in a cytoplasmic protein (CHS1) of unknown function, thought to be involved in organellar protein trafficking, resulting in fusion of the primary and secondary granules in neutrophils. Giant granules are present in many cells, including lymphocytes, platelets, and melanocytes. Patients usually have partial oculocutaneous albinism. The defect in Chédiak-Higashi syndrome results in defective neutrophil and NK cell function, leading to recurrent and sometimes fatal infections with streptococci and staphylococci. Most patients progress to an accelerated phase associated with EBV infection and characterized by a **lymphoproliferative syndrome** with generalized lymphohistiocytic infiltrates, fever, jaundice, hepatomegaly, adenopathy, and pancytopenia. The condition resembles familial erythrophagocytic lymphohistiocytosis and virus-associated hemophagocytic syndrome more than a malignant lymphoma.

LABORATORY DIAGNOSIS

The evaluation of a neutropenic child depends on associated clinical abnormalities, such as signs of infection, family and medication history, age of the patient, cyclic or persistent nature of the condition, signs of bone marrow infiltration (malignancy or storage disease), and evidence of involvement of other cell lines (Fig. 74–2). Neutropenia is confirmed by a complete blood count and differential. A bone marrow aspirate and biopsy may be necessary to determine if the neutropenia is due to a failure of production in the bone marrow, infiltration of the bone marrow, or loss of neutrophils in the periphery. Antineutrophil antibodies are helpful to diagnose autoimmune neutropenia.

Neutrophil chemotactic defects can be excluded by the presence of neutrophils at the site of infection. Chemotactic assays are performed in specialized laboratories. The **Rebuck skin window** is a 4-hour in vivo test for neutrophil chemotaxis that is not performed routinely by most laboratories. Flow cytometry for the presence of adhesion molecules, such as CD18, can help diagnose leukocyte adhesion defects. Point mutations that affect the function of the adhesion molecule but do not alter antibody binding are missed using flow cytometry, however.

CGD can be diagnosed by flow cytometry tests or the **nitroblue tetrazolium** test. In this test, a soluble yellow dye is normally reduced to an insoluble blue compound in activated neutrophils that have generated oxygen radicals.

Light microscopy of neutrophils for the presence of giant granules can help diagnose Chédiak-Higashi

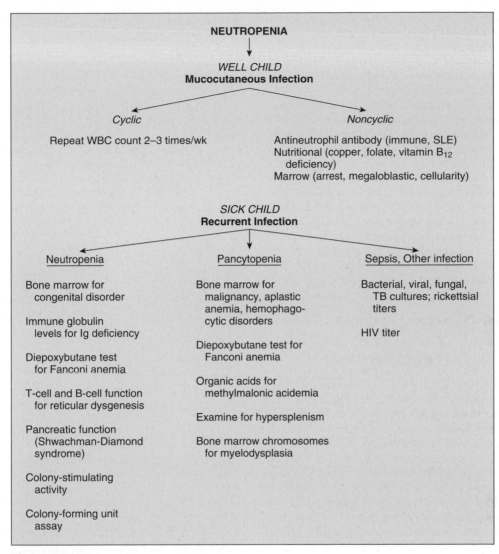

Figure 74-2

Algorithm for evaluation of neutropenia. SLE, systemic lupus erythematosus; TB, tuberculosis; WBC, white blood cell.

syndrome. The presence of an elevated IgE level, especially in association with poor antibody and T cell responses to antigens, suggests hyper-IgE syndrome.

DIFFERENTIAL DIAGNOSIS

Episodes of bacteremia are associated with the presence of indwelling catheters or other foreign bodies, mucosal injury secondary to cytotoxic agents, and immunosuppressive agents. The presence of an underlying malignancy, treatment with chemotherapy, or immunodeficiency disorder also increases the risk for serious bacterial or fungal infection.

Neutropenia can result from bone marrow infiltration from malignancy or from a storage disease. The differential diagnosis of autoimmune neutropenia includes systemic lupus erythematosus, rheumatoid arthritis (Felty syndrome), immunodeficiency, or drug-induced neutropenia. Atopic dermatitis can be associated with elevated IgE levels and superficial skin infections, but not with deep-seated infections and abscesses.

TREATMENT

Therapy for neutropenia depends on the underlying cause. Patients with severe bacterial infections require broad-spectrum antibiotics; the resolution of neutropenia during an infection is a good prognostic sign. Most patients with severe congenital neutropenia or autoimmune neutropenia respond to therapy with G-CSF. Granulocyte transfusion should be reserved for life-threatening infection; even with transfusion, the results of such treatment have been disappointing. Chronic mild neutropenia not associated with immunosuppression can be managed expectantly with prompt antimicrobial treatment of soft tissue infections, which usually are caused by *S. aureus* or group A streptococci.

Frequent courses of antibiotics, including trimethoprim-sulfamethoxazole prophylaxis, and surgical débridement of infections are required in **CGD**. Because *A. fumigatus* can cause serious infection in patients with CGD, moldy hay, decomposing compost, and other nests of fungi must be avoided. The frequency of infection in CGD also is lessened by treatment with **recombinant interferon-γ** administered subcutaneously three times a week. Stem cell transplantation (see Chapter 76) may be lifesaving in CGD, LAD-1, and Chédiak-Higashi syndrome.

PROGNOSIS AND PREVENTION

The prognosis depends on the particular defect. Milder and transient defects in neutrophil numbers have a better prognosis. Prolonged absence of neutrophils or their function has a poor prognosis, especially with the risk of bacterial and fungal sepsis. Treatment with interferon-γ has improved the prognosis of patients with CGD; however, successful bone marrow transplantation is the only currently available mode of therapy that can reverse the poor prognosis of severe neutrophil defects. As in other genetic defects, prenatal diagnosis and genetic counseling are possible for all known gene mutations.

TABLE 75–1.   Deficiency of Complement and Associated Disease

Deficient Protein	Associated Disease
C1q, C1r	SLE, glomerulonephritis; occasional pneumococcal infection
C2	SLE, arthritis, JRA, recurrent infections in some patients, rare glomerulonephritis
C3	Recurrent infections, rare glomerulonephritis, or SLE
C4	SLE-like disease, pyogenic infection
C5	Recurrent meningococcal or gonococcal infections, rare glomerulonephritis, or SLE
C6	Recurrent meningococcal or gonococcal infections, rare glomerulonephritis, or SLE
C7	Recurrent meningococcal or gonococcal infections, Raynaud phenomenon
C8	Recurrent meningococcal or gonococcal infections
C9	Occasional meningococcal infection, autoimmune disease in some patients
Properdin	Recurrent infections, meningococcal infection (often fatal)
Factor H	Glomerulonephritis, meningococcal infection
Factor I	Recurrent infections
C4-binding protein	Collagen vascular disease
C5a inhibitor	Familial Mediterranean fever
C3b receptor	SLE
C1 inhibitor	Hereditary angioedema

JRA, juvenile rheumatoid arthritis; SLE, systemic lupus erythematosus.

CHAPTER 75

Complement

The **complement system** consists of several plasma and membrane proteins that function in the innate immune response and in adaptive immunity by complementing antibody-mediated immunity. **Complement proteins** can kill pathogens with or without antibody, opsonize pathogens to facilitate their uptake by phagocytes, or mediate inflammation. The complement system can be activated through three pathways—the classic, alternative, or lectin pathways—that involve a cascade-like, sequential activation of complement factors resulting in an amplified response (Fig. 75–1). Disorders of the complement system predispose to recurrent infection, autoimmunity, or angioedema (Table 75–1).

ETIOLOGY

The three pathways for complement activation are initiated by different mechanisms. The **classic pathway** is activated by antigen-antibody complexes or by C-reactive protein and trypsin-like enzymes. The **alternative pathway** may be activated by C3b generated through classic complement activation or by endotoxin or fungal antigens (zymogen). The **lectin**

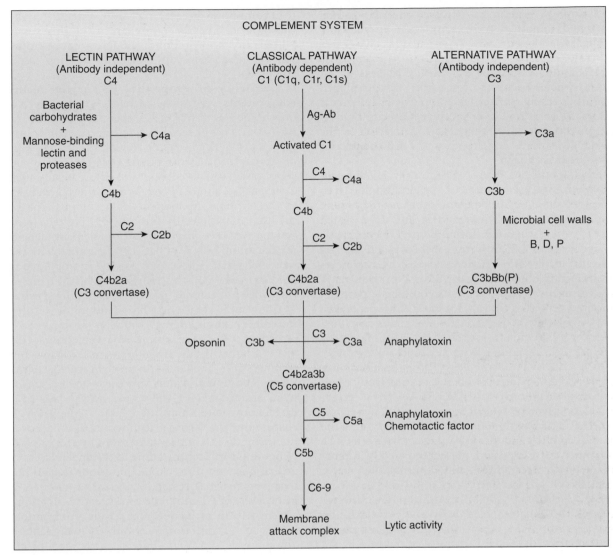

Figure 75-1

Complement component cascade involving the classic, alternate, and lectin pathways. The initiating events for the pathways differ, but result in production of C3 cleaving enzyme activity, which is the pivotal step as the three pathways converge to the terminal activation sequences. Ag-Ab, antigen-antibody complex; B, factor B; D, factor D (factor B clearing enzyme); P, properdin.

pathway is initiated by the interaction of mannose-binding lectin (MBL) with microbial carbohydrate. The three pathways lead to the generation of a C3 convertase, which activates the complement protein C3 and initiates a cascade common to the three pathways and culminates in the formation of a **membrane attack complex (MAC)**, which can lyse pathogens and other target cells (see Fig. 75-1). C3 convertase cleaves C3 into C3a, an anaphylatoxin, and C3b, which can act as an opsonin or can combine with (either

classic pathway or alternative pathway) C3 convertase to form a C5 convertase. C5 is cleaved into C5a, an anaphylatoxin, and C5b, which combines with C6 to initiate the formation of the MAC, a complex of C5b, C6, C7, C8, and several C9 molecules. The MAC generates pores in the cell membrane, leading to lysis of the cells. The MAC without C9 can form small pores; however, the addition of C9 leads to a large trans-membrane pore that enhances lysis of the target cell. C3a and C5a can release histamine from mast cells and basophils, leading to increased vascular permeability and smooth muscle contraction. In addition, C5a has chemotactic activity, attracting phagocytes to the site of complement activation, and can cause degranulation of phagocytic cells. C3b acts as an opsonin when attached to the surface of a pathogen by binding to phagocytes via complement receptor 1 (CR1), and its degradation product iC3b can bind to CR3 on the surface of phagocytes. Activation of the phagocyte leads to ingestion of the C3b-coated or iC3b-coated pathogen.

Activation of the classic pathway by an antigen-antibody complex is initiated by the binding of C1q to the Fc portion of an antibody molecule in the immune complex. C1r autoactivates and cleaves C1s, which cleaves C4 and then C2, forming the C3 convertase C4b2a. The same C3 convertase, C4b2a, is activated by the lectin pathway when lectins such as mannose-binding protein bind to sugar residues on the surface of pathogens, and mannose-binding protein–associated proteases cleave C4 and C2. The alternative pathway is always active at a low level and is amplified when active C3 binds to a surface that lacks regulatory proteins. C3b generated from C3 binds to factor B, which is cleaved by factor D to form the alternative pathway C3 convertase C3bBb. Properdin binds to and stabilizes the C3 convertase (see Fig. 75–1).

The complement system is under tight regulation because it has potent inflammatory activity and the potential to cause significant damage to host cells. The complement cascade is inherently regulated by a short half-life of the sites on C4b and C3b that allow them to bind to cell surfaces and by instability of the C3 convertases, C4b2a and C3bBb. In addition, C1-inhibitor regulates the cascade at an early stage by blocking active sites on C1r, C1s, and the proteases associated with the lectin pathway. Factor I destabilizes the C3 convertase complexes and degrades the active fragments. Other inhibitors include membrane proteins, such as decay accelerating factor, CR1, membrane cofactor protein, and plasma proteins such as C4b-binding protein and factor H. Formation of the MAC can be blocked by cell surface CD59, protein S, and other plasma proteins. Deficiency of any of these regulatory proteins can result in an inflammatory response, tissue damage, or excessive complement consumption.

Disorders of complement proteins can result from inherited deficiency or can be secondary to increased consumption. The consequences of decreased complement depend on the affected factor (see Table 75–1). **Deficiencies of early components** of the classic pathway, C1, C2, or C4, are not usually associated with severe infections, although patients with C2 deficiency may present with milder recurrent infections. Patients with C1, C2, or C4 deficiency are susceptible to autoimmune diseases, especially systemic lupus erythematosus. The exact mechanism of this susceptibility is not known, but is thought to arise from the role of these early components in clearing immune complexes.

Deficiency of properdin, C3, or the terminal components predisposes patients to severe recurrent infections. Deficiency of C3, the major opsonin, from a genetic defect or secondary to excessive consumption from a deficiency in factor H, factor I, or the presence of C3 nephritic factor predisposes patients to infections, especially with encapsulated organisms such as *S. pneumoniae* and *H. influenzae* type b. Deficiency of one of the terminal components that compose the MAC predisposes patients to infection with *Neisseria meningitidis* or *Neisseria gonorrhoeae*. Complement deficiency may be found in 40% of patients presenting with recurrent neisserial infections. Deficiency of mannose-binding lectin (MBL) also is associated with an increased frequency of bacterial infections, including sepsis.

Congenital deficiency of C1-inhibitor results in **hereditary angioedema**, which is characterized by recurrent episodes of nonpruritic angioedema lasting 48 to 72 hours, occurring spontaneously or after minor trauma, stress, or anxiety. Angioedema can occur in any tissue. Abdominal edema can cause acute abdominal pain, and edema of the upper airway can be life-threatening and may necessitate emergency tracheostomy. The disorder is inherited as an autosomal dominant disease and results from a heterozygous deficiency of C1-inhibitor leading to serum levels less than 30% of normal values. Some mutations (type II hereditary angioedema) result in normal or elevated antigenic levels of C1-inhibitor but defective function. An acquired form of angioedema results from autoantibodies to C1-inhibitor in lymphoid malignancies or autoimmune disorders, but is uncommon in childhood. The mechanism by which angioedema occurs in C1-inhibitor deficiency is not known. C1-inhibitor is a regulator of Hageman factor, clotting factor XI, plasma kallikrein, and plasmin in addition to C1r and C1s, and angioedema may be the result of loss of regulation of one of these pathways.

LABORATORY STUDIES

The **CH$_{50}$ test** is a widely available test of classic complement pathway function based on an antibody-dependent hemolytic assay of sheep red blood cells, which measures the serum dilution that results in lysis of 50% of sheep red blood cells. The CH$_{50}$ test depends on the function of all nine complement proteins, C1 through C9, and is the best screen for complement function. The **AP$_{50}$ test**, which measures complement activation via the alternative pathway using red blood cells from different species (e.g., rabbit) that can activate the alternative pathway, is less widely available than the CH_{50} test. Abnormal results in both tests indicate a deficiency in a terminal component common to both pathways, whereas abnormal results in one or the other pathway indicates a deficiency of an early component of the respective pathway. If the CH_{50} or AP_{50} levels are abnormal, individual components can be analyzed in specialized laboratories.

Determination of C1-inhibitor levels and function is needed to diagnose hereditary angioedema. Some functional tests can miss rare mutations that allow C1-inhibitor to bind C1s, but not one or more of the other enzymes with which it interacts. Low C1-inhibitor levels or function results in chronically decreased C4 levels and decreased C2 levels during acute attacks. Low C1q levels are found in acquired C1-inhibitor deficiency, which distinguishes it from hereditary angioedema. Tests for autoantibodies to C1-inhibitor and C1q can be performed by enzyme-linked immunosorbent assay.

TREATMENT

Specific treatment of complement deficiencies with component replacement is not available; long, frequent courses of antibiotics constitute the therapy. Immunization of patients and close contacts with pneumococcal and meningococcal vaccines may be useful, but may provide a false sense of security because infections still can occur in immunized complement-deficient patients. Replacement of complement proteins by plasma transfusion has been used in some patients with C2 deficiency or factor H deficiency.

Patients with C1-inhibitor deficiency and frequent episodes of angioedema respond to prophylactic use of an oral attenuated androgen (**stanozolol** or **danazol**), which increases serum concentrations of C1-inhibitor. The use of androgens should be limited, however, because of adverse effects, which include masculinization in females, growth arrest, and hepatitis. Care must be taken in using plasma transfusions for angioedema. Prophylactic administration of fresh frozen plasma before surgery can prevent angioedema, but administration during an acute episode may exacerbate the episode. Angioedema of the airway can present as an acute emergency, necessitating tracheostomy because administration of epinephrine, antihistamines, or corticosteroids is ineffective in reversing this type of angioedema. Purified C1-inhibitor can be used prophylactically (before surgery) and during acute episodes of angioedema. Angiotensin-converting enzyme inhibitors, such as captopril, should be avoided in patients with C1-inhibitor deficiency because they can precipitate episodes of angioedema by inhibiting degradation of kinins that mediate edema formation.

CHAPTER 76
Hematopoietic Stem Cell Transplantation

Hematopoietic stem cell transplantation is the only therapy available that can cure patients with primary immunodeficiency disease (Table 76–1). It is not available to all patients, however. Use of hematopoietic stem cell transplantation is limited to immunodeficiency diseases with T cell defects, some metabolic storage diseases (see Chapters 55 and 56), malignancies (see Chapter 154), aplastic anemia (see Chapter 150), and a few other disorders. The principle of hematopoietic stem cell transplantation is to replace a patient's defective bone marrow stem cells with normal stem cells.

Hematopoietic stem cells reside in the bone marrow, but also can be obtained from peripheral blood or cord blood. Peripheral blood does not contain a significant proportion of stem cells, unless the donor's bone marrow is actively stimulated to generate stem cells, and is not always used as a source of stem cells. Cord blood is a good source of stem cells and is used for sibling and unrelated hematopoietic stem cell transplantation.

TABLE 76–1. Immunodeficiency Diseases Curable by Stem Cell Transplantation

Severe combined immunodeficiency (SCID)
  X-linked SCID (γ_c deficiency)
  Jak 3 kinase deficiency
  ZAP 70 deficiency and other T cell activation defects
  RAG1/RAG2 deficiency and other T^-B^- SCID
  Omenn syndrome
  Adenosine deaminase deficiency
  Purine nucleoside phosphorylase deficiency
  Reticular dysgenesis
  Bare lymphocyte syndrome
Wiskott-Aldrich syndrome
X-linked hyper-IgM
X-linked lymphoproliferative syndrome
Cartilage hair hypoplasia
Autoimmune lymphoproliferative syndrome (Fas defect)
Severe congenital neutropenia
Shwachman-Diamond syndrome
Cyclic neutropenia
Chédiak-Higashi syndrome
Leukocyte adhesion deficiency type I
Familial hemophagocytic lymphohistiocytosis

MHC compatibility is important in the choice of stem cell donor to avoid rejection of the donor cells by the host immune system and to prevent GVHD from contaminating mature T cells. The donor stem cells give rise to T cells that develop in the host thymus and need to interact with donor and host antigen presenting cells. Stem cells from a partially mismatched donor, such as a parent, can give rise to a functioning immune system because the patient shares at least half of the MHC molecules with the donor stem cells. Mature T cells need to be removed from the bone marrow, however, before transplantation. The reduction in risk of **GVHD** outweighs the disadvantage of a prolonged time of 90 to 120 days before T cells develop in patients with SCID. Patients with other immunodeficiency diseases are at risk for developing **lymphoproliferative disease**, especially from EBV, with T cell–depleted stem cell transplantation probably because of the delay in T cell engraftment. Hematopoietic stem cells can be obtained from MHC-identical siblings (25% chance of a matched sibling), matched unrelated cord blood or bone marrow or, for patients with SCID, haploidentical bone marrow from a parent (preferred) or a sibling.

MHC molecules are highly polymorphic; typing is performed at the DNA level rather than by serology. Bone marrow and cord blood registries are available worldwide. Searching and identifying a donor can be a lengthy process, especially for some underrepresented ethnic backgrounds. Finding a suitable cord blood donor is faster because the cord blood already has been obtained and stored, whereas bone marrow donors have to be identified, located, and tested. A matched sibling, if available, is the preferred source of hematopoietic stem cells.

Patients with SCID are ideal candidates for hematopoietic stem cell transplantation. Stem cell transplantation is the only option for treatment of SCID at this time. Patients are unlikely to survive beyond 1 to 2 years old without transplantation, and they have no T cell function to reject donor cells. Patients with SCID may not need to undergo preconditioning with chemotherapy or irradiation before transplantation. The development of transplantation using T cell–depleted, haploidentical bone marrow from a parent for SCID has provided almost every patient with SCID a potential donor. The mother is the preferred source for haploidentical bone marrow, if she in able to donate bone marrow, because some transfer of maternal T cells can occur during pregnancy, and these maternal T cells can reject cells obtained from the father. The survival rate after hematopoietic stem cell transplantation for SCID is 84% with MHC-identical and 61% with haploidentical bone marrow transplantation. The earlier the patient is transplanted, the better the outcome. Because the outcome of stem cell transplantation as soon after birth as possible is excellent, the risks of in utero transplantation and the inability to observe the fetus for signs of GVHD in utero make it difficult to justify this type of transplantation.

The decision to treat other patients with primary immunodeficiency diseases is more difficult because hematopoietic stem cell transplantation is not always successful. Patients with some, albeit decreased, T cell function require preconditioning, with the risks that it entails. It is difficult to predict the prognosis of a particular patient because of the variability in clinical course of most primary immunodeficiency diseases, although there is only a small chance of reaching adulthood. The availability of a matched related sibling favors the decision to perform hematopoietic stem cell transplantation. Disorders of B cells have not been treated with hematopoietic stem cell transplantation because in many cases donor B cells do not engraft and because patients with antibody diseases usually do well with IVIG. If hematopoietic stem cell transplantation techniques improve to allow for better B cell engraftment and reduce the risks of GVHD and preconditioning, however, treatment of agammaglobulinemia and other immune system diseases with hematopoietic stem cell transplantation may be possible.

COMPLICATIONS

Rejection of the grafted cells is the first potential complication of hematopoietic stem cell transplantation; this depends on the immunocompetence of the patient, the degree of MHC incompatibility, and the number of cells administered. Preconditioning the patient with myeloablative drugs, such as busulfan and cyclophosphamide, can prevent graft rejection. Preconditioning can be complicated, however, by pulmonary toxicity requiring prolonged oxygen therapy and by veno-occlusive disease of the liver, which results from damage to the hepatic vascular endothelium and can be fatal. Myeloablation results in anemia, leukopenia, and thrombocytopenia, making patients susceptible to infection and bleeding disorders. Neutropenic precautions should be maintained and patients supported with red blood cell and platelet transfusions until the red blood cell, platelet, and neutrophil lineages engraft. **Lymphoproliferative** disease can develop after T cell–depleted bone marrow transplantation.

Hematopoietic stem cell transplantation, in contrast to solid organ transplantation, can be complicated by rejection of the host by mature T cells from the donor. **GVHD** can arise from an MHC-mismatched transplantation or from mismatch in minor histocompatibility antigens that are not tested for before transplantation. T cell depletion of haploidentical bone marrow reduces the risk of GVHD, and patients with

SCID transplanted with T cell–depleted haploidentical bone marrow do not usually develop severe GVHD. Acute GVHD begins 6 or more days after transplantation and can result from transfusion of nonirradiated blood products in patients with no T cell function. **Acute GVHD** presents with fever, skin rash, and severe diarrhea. Patients develop a high, unrelenting fever; a morbilliform maculopapular erythematous rash that is painful and pruritic; hepatosplenomegaly and abnormal liver function tests; and nausea, vomiting, abdominal pain, and watery diarrhea. Acute GVHD is staged from grade 1 to 4 depending on the degree of skin, fever, gastrointestinal, and liver involvement. **Chronic GVHD** can result from acute GVHD lasting longer than 100 days, can develop separately without acute GVHD, or can develop after acute GVHD has resolved. Chronic GVHD is characterized by skin lesions (hyperkeratosis, reticular hyperpigmentation, fibrosis, and atrophy with ulceration), limitation of joint movement, interstitial pneumonitis, and immune dysregulation with autoantibody and immune complex formation.

Hematopoietic stem cell transplantation can be used for any disorder of hematopoiesis, such as aplastic anemia, sickle cell disease, and other hemoglobinopathies. It is also used in treatment of malignancy, such as leukemia, lymphoma, and solid tumors. In some cases of solid tumor therapy, autologous bone marrow is harvested before high-dose chemotherapy, then reinfused into the patient to rescue the hematopoietic system.

SUGGESTED READING

Behrman RE, Kliegman RM, Jenson HB (eds): Nelson Textbook of Pediatrics, 17th ed. Philadelphia, WB Saunders, 2004.

Bonilla FA, Geha RS: Primary immunodeficiency diseases. J Allergy Clin Immunol 111(Suppl):S571-S581, 2003.

Buckley RH: A historical review of bone marrow transplantation for immunodeficiencies. J Allergy Clin Immunol 113:793-800, 2004.

Buckley RH: Primary cellular immunodeficiencies. J Allergy Clin Immunol 109:747-757, 2002.

Fischer A: Human primary immunodeficiency diseases: A perspective. Nat Immunol 5:23-30, 2004.

Rosenzweig SD, Holland SM: Phagocyte immunodeficiencies and their infections. J Allergy Clin Immunol 113:620-626, 2004.

Tangsinmankong N, Bahna SL, Good RA: The immunologic workup of the child suspected of immunodeficiency. Ann Allergy Asthma Immunol 87:362-370, 2001.

Walport MJ: Advances in immunology: Complement—first of two parts. N Engl J Med 344:1058-1066, 2001.

Walport MJ: Advances in immunology: Complement—second of two parts. N Engl J Med 344:1140-1144, 2001.

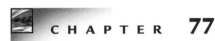

CHAPTER **77**

Assessment

Atopy is a result of a complex interaction between multiple genes and environmental factors. Atopy implies specific IgE-mediated diseases, including allergic rhinitis, asthma, and atopic dermatitis. An **allergen** is an antigen that triggers an IgE response in genetically predisposed individuals.

Hypersensitivity disorders of the immune system are classified into four groups based on the mechanism that leads to tissue inflammation (Table 77–1). **Type I reactions** are triggered by the binding of antigen to high-affinity IgE receptors on the surface of tissue mast cells or circulating basophils or both. This binding and cross-linking of IgE causes the release of preformed chemical mediators, such as histamine and tryptase, and newly generated mediators, such as leukotrienes, prostaglandins, and platelet-activating factor, which contribute to the clinical development of allergic symptoms, with anaphylaxis as the most profound symptom. Several hours after the initial response, a **late-phase reaction** may develop, in which there is an influx of other inflammatory cells, such as basophils, eosinophils, monocytes, lymphocytes, and neutrophils, and their inflammatory mediators. Recruitment of these cells leads to more persistent and chronic symptoms.

Type II (antibody cytotoxicity) reactions involve IgM, IgG, or IgA antibodies binding to the cell surface. This binding can activate the entire complement pathway, resulting in lysis of the cell or release of anaphylatoxins, such as C3a, C4a, and C5a (see Chapter 75). These anaphylatoxins trigger mast cell degranulation, resulting in inflammatory mediator release. The target antigens can be cell surface membrane antigens, such as red blood cells (hemolytic anemia); platelet cell surface molecules (thrombocytopenia); basement membrane molecules in the kidney (Goodpasture syndrome); the alpha chain of the acetylcholine receptor at the neuromuscular junction (myasthenia gravis); and thyroid-stimulating hormone receptor on thyroid cells (Graves disease). A classic example of a type II reaction is hemolytic disease of the newborn resulting from Rh incompatibility (see Chapter 62).

Type III (immune complex) reactions involve the formation of antigen-antibody or immune complexes, which enter into the circulation and are deposited in tissue, such as blood vessels and filtering organs (liver, spleen, kidney). These complexes initiate tissue injury by activating the complement cascade and by recruiting neutrophils that release their toxic mediators. Local reactions caused by the injection of antigen into tissue are called **Arthus reactions**. Administration of large amounts of antigen leads to serum sickness, a classic example of a type III reaction. Other type III–mediated reactions include hypersensitivity pneumonitis and some vasculitic syndromes (Henoch-Schönlein purpura).

Type IV (cellular immune–mediated or delayed-hypersensitivity) reactions involve recognition of antigen by sensitized T cells. Antigen presenting cells form peptides that are expressed on the cell surface in association with MHC class II molecules. Memory T cells recognize the antigen peptide/MHC class II complexes. Cytokines, such as interferon-γ, tumor necrosis factor-α, and granulocyte-macrophage colony-stimulating factor, are secreted from this interaction, which activates and attracts tissue macrophages. Contact allergies (nickel, poison ivy, topical medications) and immunity to tuberculosis are type IV reactions.

HISTORY

A family history of allergic disease is often present in affected patients. Multiple genes predispose to atopy, including the linkage of atopy with chromosome 5.

TABLE 77–1. Gell and Coombs Classification of Hypersensitivity Disorders

Type	Interval Between Exposure and Reaction	Effector Cell or Antibody	Target or Antigen	Examples of Mediators	Examples
I—Anaphylactic Immediate Late phase	<30 min 2-12 hr	IgE	Pollens, food, venom, drugs	Histamine, tryptase, leukotrienes, prostaglandins, platelet-activating factor	Anaphylaxis, urticaria (penicillin), allergic rhinitis, allergic asthma
II—Cytotoxic antibody	Variable (minutes to hours)	IgG, IgM, IgA	Red blood cells, platelets	Complement	Rh hemolytic anemia, thrombocytopenia, hemolysis (quinidine), Goodpasture syndrome
III—Immune complex reactions	4-8 hr	Antigen with antibody	Blood vessels, liver, spleen, kidney, lung	Complement, anaphylatoxin	Serum sickness (cefaclor), hypersensitivity pneumonitis
IV—Delayed type	24-48 hr	Lymphocytes	*Mycobacterium tuberculosis,* chemicals	Cytokines (IFN-γ, TNF-α, GM-CSF)	TB skin test reactions, contact dermatitis (neomycin), graft-versus-host disease

GM-CSF, granulocyte-macrophage colony-stimulating factor; IFN-γ, interferon-γ; TNF-α, tumor necrosis factor-α.

Allergic parents often ask whether their child will have the same disease. If one parent has allergies, the risk is 25% that a child will develop allergic disease. If both parents have allergies, the risk increases to 50% to 70%. Similar allergic diseases tend to occur in families; if both parents have allergic rhinitis, their offspring also will have allergic rhinitis.

PHYSICAL EXAMINATION

Children with allergic rhinitis exhibit frequent nasal itching and rubbing of the nose with the palm of the hand, the **allergic salute**, which can lead to a transverse nasal crease found across the lower bridge of the nose. **Allergic shiners**, blue-gray to purple discoloration below the lower eyelids that is attributed to venous congestion, are often present in children along with swollen eyelids or conjunctival injection. Cutaneous findings of atopy include hyperlinearity of the palms and soles, white dermatographism, pityriasis alba, and **Dennie-Morgan folds** or **Dennie lines** (prominent creases under the lower eyelids).

COMMON MANIFESTATIONS

Cutaneous manifestations are most common, ranging from generalized **xerosis** (dry skin) to urticaria to the pruritic, erythematous papules and vesicles of atopic dermatitis. There may be involvement of the upper res-piratory tract with allergic rhinitis and the lower respiratory tract with asthma.

DISTINGUISHING FEATURES

Allergic disease may involve only the skin or the nose, eyes, lungs, and gastrointestinal tract alone or in combination. Allergic disease is distinguished by environmental exposure to an inciting trigger and usually a history of previous similar disease or development of symptoms after a suspected trigger. Many patients have more than one allergic symptom.

INITIAL DIAGNOSTIC EVALUATION

Diagnosis begins with a thorough history with description of all symptoms, exposure to common allergens, and responses to previous therapies. In vivo skin testing and in vitro serum testing are crucial to accurate diagnosis.

SCREENING TESTS

Atopy is characterized by elevated levels of IgE (Table 77–2) and eosinophilia (3% to 10% of white blood cells or an absolute eosinophil count of >250 eosinophils/mm^3) with a predominance of Th2 cytokines, including interleukin (IL)-4, IL-5, and IL-13. Extreme eosinophilia suggests a nonallergic disorder,

TABLE 77-2. Disorders Associated with Elevated Serum Immunoglobulin E

Allergic disease
Atopic dermatitis (eczema)
Helminthic infections
Hyperimmunoglobulin-E syndrome
Allergic bronchopulmonary aspergillosis
Wiskott-Aldrich syndrome
Bone marrow transplantation
Hodgkin disease
Bullous pemphigoid
Idiopathic nephrotic syndrome
Mononucleosis

TABLE 77-4. Comparison of In Vivo Skin Tests and In Vitro Serum IgE Antibody Immunoassay in Allergic Diagnosis

In Vivo—Skin Test	In Vitro—Serum Immunoassay
Less expensive	No patient risk
Greater sensitivity	Patient/physician convenience
Wide allergen selection	Not suppressed by antihistamines
Results available immediately	Preferable to skin testing for Dermatographism Widespread dermatitis Uncooperative children

From Skoner DP: Allergic rhinitis: Definition, epidemiology, pathophysiology, detection, and diagnosis. J Allergy Clin Immunol 108:S2-S8, 2001.

such as infections with tissue-invasive parasites, drug reactions, or malignancies (Table 77-3). A classic example of a type IV reaction is the tuberculin skin test. A small amount of purified protein derivative from *Mycobacterium tuberculosis* is injected intradermally. In a previously sensitized individual, a type IV inflammatory reaction develops over the next 24 to 72 hours.

There are two methods for identifying allergen-specific IgE: in vivo skin testing and in vitro serum testing (Table 77-4). **In vivo skin testing** is a method by which allergen is introduced into the skin via a

TABLE 77-3. Disorders Associated with Eosinophilia

Allergic disease
    Allergic rhinitis
    Atopic dermatitis
    Asthma
Gastrointestinal
    Eosinophilic gastroenteritis
    Allergic colitis
    Inflammatory bowel disease
Infectious
    Tissue-invasive parasitic infections
Neoplastic
    Eosinophilic leukemia
    Hodgkin disease
Respiratory
    Eosinophilic pneumonia
    Allergic bronchopulmonary aspergillosis
Systemic
    Idiopathic hypereosinophilic syndrome
    Mastocytosis
Iatrogenic
    Drug induced

prick/puncture or intradermal injection. The allergen diffuses through the skin to interact with IgE that is bound to mast cells. Cross-linking of IgE causes mast cell degranulation, which results in histamine release. Histamine release prompts the development of a **central wheal and erythematous flare**. The wheal and flare are measured 15 to 20 minutes after the allergen has been placed. Properly performed skin tests are the best available method for detecting the presence of allergen-specific IgE.

In vitro serum testing is indicated for patients who have abnormal cutaneous conditions, such as dermatographism or extensive dermatitis; who cannot discontinue medications, such as antihistamines, that interfere with test results; who are very allergic by history, and anaphylaxis is a possible risk; or who are noncompliant for skin testing. The presence of specific IgE antibodies alone is not sufficient for the diagnosis of allergic diseases. Diagnosis must be based on the physician's assessment of the entire clinical picture, including the history and physical examination, the presence of specific IgE antibodies, and the correlation of symptoms to IgE-mediated inflammation.

DIAGNOSTIC IMAGING

Diagnostic imaging has a limited role in the management of allergic disease. Chest radiography is helpful with the differential diagnosis of asthma. Sinus radiography and CT may be used to evaluate sinus disease, but when these images are abnormal, they do not distinguish allergic disease from nonallergic disease.

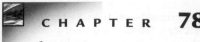

CHAPTER 78

Asthma

ETIOLOGY

Inflammatory cells (mast cells, eosinophils, T lymphocytes, neutrophils), chemical mediators (histamine, leukotrienes, platelet-activating factor, bradykinin), and chemotactic factors (cytokines, eotaxin) result in the underlying inflammation found in asthmatic airways. Inflammation contributes to airway **hyperresponsiveness**, which is the tendency for the airways to constrict in response to allergens, irritants, viral infections, and exercise. It also results in edema, increased mucus production in the lungs, influx of inflammatory cells into the airway, and epithelial cell denudation. Chronic inflammation can lead to **airway remodeling**, which results from a proliferation of extracellular matrix proteins and vascular hyperplasia and may lead to irreversible structural changes and a progressive loss of pulmonary function.

EPIDEMIOLOGY

Asthma is the most common chronic disease of childhood, affecting nearly 5 million children younger than age 18 in the U.S. Asthma affects 1 in 13 school-age children and is a leading cause of office and emergency department visits, hospitalizations, and school absenteeism. Asthma mortality nearly doubled between 1980 and 1993, with more than 5500 fatalities annually.

CLINICAL MANIFESTATIONS

Children with asthma have symptoms of coughing, wheezing, shortness of breath or rapid breathing, and chest tightness. The history should elicit the frequency and severity and factors that may worsen the child's symptoms. Exacerbating factors include viral infections, exposure to allergens and irritants (smoke, strong odors, fumes), exercise, emotions, and change in weather/humidity. Nighttime symptoms are common. Rhinosinusitis, gastroesophageal reflux, and sensitivity to nonsteroidal anti-inflammatory drugs (especially aspirin) can aggravate asthma. Treatment of these conditions may lessen the frequency and severity of the asthma. Obtaining a family history of allergy and asthma is useful because allergic diseases occur in families.

During acute episodes, the **physical examination** may reveal tachypnea, tachycardia, cough, wheezing, and a prolonged expiratory phase. Physical findings may be subtle, and classic wheezing may not be prominent if there is minimal air movement. As the attack progresses, cyanosis, diminished air movement (tight chest), retractions, agitation, inability to speak, tripod sitting position, diaphoresis, and pulsus paradoxus (decrease in blood pressure with inspiration of >15 mm Hg) may be observed. Physical examination may show evidence of other atopic diseases, such as eczema or allergic rhinitis.

LABORATORY AND IMAGING STUDIES

Objective measurements of pulmonary function (spirometry) help to establish the diagnosis and treatment of asthma. Spirometry can help monitor the patient's response to the treatment plan, assess degree of reversibility with therapeutic intervention, and measure the severity of an asthma exacerbation. Generally, children older than 5 years of age can perform spirometry maneuvers.

Allergy skin testing should be a part of the evaluation of all children with persistent asthma. Testing should not be done during an exacerbation of wheezing. An allergist offers the special skill of administering and interpreting skin tests to determine immediate hypersensitivity to aeroallergens. Studies have shown that positive skin test results correlate strongly with bronchial allergen provocative challenges. In vitro serum tests, such as radioallergosorbent test (RAST) and enzyme-linked immunosorbent assay, are another option to measure levels of antigen-specific IgE. Compared with in vivo skin testing, in vitro serum testing is generally less sensitive in defining clinically pertinent allergens, it is more expensive, and results take several days compared with several minutes (see Table 77-4).

A **chest radiograph** should be performed with the first episode of asthma or with recurrent episodes of undiagnosed cough or wheeze or both to exclude anatomic abnormalities. Children with a history of asthma do not need repeat chest radiograph with each episode, unless there is fever that suggests pneumonia, or if there are localized findings on physical examination.

DIFFERENTIAL DIAGNOSIS

Many childhood conditions cause the wheeze and cough of asthma (Table 78-1). Not all cough and wheeze is asthma, and misdiagnosis can delay correcting the underlying cause and expose children to inappropriate prolonged asthma therapy. Wheezing and cough, especially in young infants, suggest other conditions that should be excluded before the diagnosis of asthma is made (Table 78-2).

Allergic bronchopulmonary aspergillosis occurs in a few patients who have a hypersensitivity type of reaction to antigens of the mold *Aspergillus fumigatus*.

TABLE 78–1. Differential Diagnosis of Cough and Wheeze in Infants and Children

Upper Respiratory Tract	Middle Respiratory Tract	Lower Respiratory Tract
Allergic rhinitis	Bronchial stenosis	Asthma
Adenoid/tonsillar hypertrophy	Enlarged lymph nodes	Bronchiectasis
Foreign body	Epiglottitis	Bronchopulmonary dysplasia
Infectious rhinitis	Foreign body	*Chlamydia trachomatis*
Sinusitis	Laryngeal webs	Chronic aspiration
	Laryngomalacia	Congestive heart failure
	Laryngotracheobronchitis	Cystic fibrosis
	Mediastinal lymphadenopathy	Foreign body
	Pertussis	Gastroesophageal reflux
	Toxic inhalation	Hyperventilation syndrome
	Tracheoesophageal fistula	Obliterative bronchiolitis
	Tracheal stenosis	Pulmonary hemosiderosis
	Tracheomalacia	Toxic inhalation, including smoke
	Tumor	Tumor
	Vascular rings	Viral bronchiolitis
	Vocal cord dysfunction	

From Lemanske RF Jr, Green CG: Asthma in infancy and childhood. In Middleton E Jr, Reed CE, Ellis EF, et al (eds): Allergy: Principles and Practice, 5th ed. St Louis, Mosby–Year Book, 1998, p 878.

This condition is observed in patients with steroid-dependent asthma and children with cystic fibrosis.

TREATMENT

Optimal medical treatment of asthma includes the following key components: environmental control, pharmacologic therapy, and patient education including attainment of self-management skills. Because many children with asthma have coexisting allergies, steps to minimize allergen exposure should be taken (Table 78–3). For all children with asthma, exposures to tobacco and wood smoke and exposure to viral infections should be minimized. Asthma medications can be divided into long-term control medications and quick-relief medications.

Long-Term Control Medications

Inhaled Corticosteroids

Inhaled corticosteroids are the most effective anti-inflammatory medications for the treatment of chronic, persistent asthma. Regular use reduces airway hyperreactivity, the need for rescue bronchodilator therapy, the risk of hospitalization, and the risk of death from asthma. Inhaled corticosteroids are available as a metered-dose inhaler (MDI), dry powder inhaler (DPI), and nebulizer solution. Inhaled corticosteroids available in the U.S. include beclomethasone, budesonide, flunisolide, fluticasone, and triamcinolone, with mometasone forthcoming.

There is little risk of systemic effects if inhaled corticosteroids are used in doses of less than 400 µg/day (beclomethasone equivalent). In short-term studies, inhaled corticosteroids reduce rates of linear growth. This finding is offset by the fact that long-term studies show apparent similarity of heights of asthmatic children prescribed inhaled corticosteroids compared with normal peers. Results from the Childhood Asthma Management Program (CAMP), the largest and longest prospective clinical trial of inhaled corticosteroids in children with mild to moderate asthma, showed a decrease in growth velocity within the first year of inhaled corticosteroid therapy without additional effect as treatment continued. The measured difference

TABLE 78–2. Mnemonic of Causes of Cough in the First Months of Life

C—Cystic fibrosis
R—Respiratory tract infections
A—Aspiration (swallowing dysfunction, gastroesophageal reflux, tracheoesophageal fistula, foreign body)
D—Dyskinetic cilia
L—Lung and airway malformations (laryngeal webs, laryngotracheomalacia, tracheal stenosis, vascular rings and slings)
E—Edema (heart failure, congenital heart disease)

From Schidlow DV: Cough. In Schidlow DV, Smith DS (eds): A Practical Guide to Pediatric Disease. Philadelphia, Hanley & Belfus, 1994.

TABLE 78–3.　Controlling Factors Contributing to Asthma Severity

Major Indoor Triggers for Asthma	Suggestions for Reducing Exposure
Viral upper respiratory tract infections (RSV, influenza virus)	Limit exposure to viral infections (daycare with fewer children) Annual influenza immunization for children with persistent asthma
Tobacco smoke, wood smoke	No smoking around the child or in child's home Help parents and caregivers quit smoking Eliminate use of wood stoves and fireplaces
Dust mites	Essential actions 　Encase pillow, mattress, and box spring in allergen-impermeable encasement 　Wash bedding in hot water weekly Desirable actions 　Avoid sleeping or lying on upholstered furniture 　Minimize number of stuffed toys in child's bedroom 　Reduce indoor humidity to <50% 　If possible, remove carpets from bedroom and play areas; if not possible, vacuum frequently
Animal dander	Remove the pet from the home or keep outdoors; if removal is not acceptable 　Keep pet out of bedroom 　Use a filter on air ducts in child's room 　Wash pet weekly (the evidence to support this has not been firmly established)
Cockroach allergens	Do not leave food or garbage exposed Use boric acid traps Reduce indoor humidity to <50% Fix leaky faucets, pipes
Indoor mold	Fix leaky faucets, pipes Avoid vaporizers Reduce indoor humidity to <50%

RSV, respiratory syncytial virus.
From American Academy of Allergy, Asthma and Immunology: Pediatric Asthma: Promoting Best Practice. Milwaukee, Wis, American Academy of Allergy, Asthma, and Immunology, 1999, p 50.

in growth between children on inhaled corticosteroids and children assigned to placebo was 1.1 cm. The practitioner should monitor potential growth suppression by regularly scheduled height measurements preferably with a stadiometer. Rinsing the mouth after inhalation and using spacers help to lessen local adverse effects of dysphonia and candidiasis and to decrease systemic absorption from the gastrointestinal tract. The goal is to use the lowest effective dose that controls the child's asthma. For children with severe asthma, high-dose inhaled corticosteroids may be needed to minimize the oral steroid dose.

Leukotriene Modifiers

Leukotriene modifiers are oral, daily-use, asthma medications. Leukotrienes, synthesized via the arachidonic acid metabolism cascade, are potent mediators of inflammation and smooth muscle bronchoconstriction. Leukotriene modifiers have been designed to inhibit these biologic effects in the airway. Two classes of leukotriene modifiers include cysteinyl leukotriene receptor antagonists (zafirlukast and montelukast) and leukotriene synthesis inhibitors (zileuton). The leukotriene receptor antagonists have much wider appeal than zileuton. Zafirlukast has been approved for children older than age 5 years and is given twice daily. Montelukast is dosed once daily at night as 4-mg granules or chewable tablets for children age 12 months to 5 years and 5-mg chewable tablets for children age 6 to 14 years. For adolescents older than 15 years, 10-mg tablets are available. Pediatric studies show the usefulness of leukotriene modifiers in mild asthma and the attenuation of exercise-induced bronchoconstriction. These agents may be helpful as steroid-sparing agents in patients with asthma that is more difficult to control.

Long-Acting β_2-Agonists

Long-acting β_2-agonists, formoterol and salmeterol, have twice-daily dosing and relax airway smooth muscle for 12 hours, but they do not have any significant anti-inflammatory effects. Adding a long-acting bronchodilator to inhaled corticosteroid therapy is more beneficial than doubling the dose of inhaled corticosteroids. Formoterol, available in the DPI form, is approved for use in children 5 years and older for maintenance asthma therapy and for prevention of exercise-induced asthma. Formoterol has a rapid onset of action similar to albuterol (15 minutes), whereas salmeterol begins bronchodilating within 30 minutes. Salmeterol is available in the DPI form and is approved for children 4 years old and older.

A fluticasone/salmeterol combination product (Advair) is available as a DPI in three doses, varying by the amount of corticosteroid available (100 µg, 250 µg, or 500 µg). Each of these strengths contains 50 µg of salmeterol. Patients 4 years to 11 years old use Advair 100 and those 12 years and older use Advair 100, 250, or 500. This agent has advantages in terms of compliance because it is administered 1 puff twice daily, and it combines two potent asthma medications.

Theophylline

Theophylline was more widely used previously, but with current management aimed at inflammatory control, its popularity has declined. It is considered as an alternative add-on treatment to low-dose and medium-dose inhaled corticosteroids. Theophylline is available in syrup, tablet, and capsule formulation. It is mildly to moderately effective as a bronchodilator. Serum levels must be monitored routinely and maintained generally between 5 and 15 µg/mL. Levels can be affected by febrile illnesses, diet, and medications, such as macrolide antibiotics, cimetidine, and oral antifungal agents. Adverse effects associated with elevated theophylline levels include nausea, insomnia, headaches, hyperreactivity, and seizures.

Novel Therapies

Subcutaneous therapy with omalizumab (Xolair), a humanized anti-IgE monoclonal antibody, is approved for moderate to severe allergic asthma in children 12 years old and older.

Quick-Relief Medications

Short-Acting β₂-Agonists

Short-acting β₂-agonists, such as albuterol, levalbuterol, and pirbuterol, are the most effective bronchodilators. They exert their effect by relaxing bronchial smooth muscle within 5 to 10 minutes of administration and last for 4 to 6 hours. Generally, patients are prescribed a short-acting β₂-agonist for acute symptoms and as prophylaxis before allergen exposure and exercise. The inhaled route is preferred because there are fewer adverse effects of tremor, prolonged tachycardia, and irritability. **Overuse** of β₂-agonists implies that asthma may not be in adequate control and that a change in medications may be warranted. The definition of "overuse" depends on the severity of the child's asthma; use of more than one MDI canister per month or more than 8 puffs per day suggests poor control.

Anticholinergic Agent

Ipratropium bromide is an anticholinergic bronchodilator that relieves bronchoconstriction, decreases mucus hypersecretion, and counteracts cough-receptor irritability by binding acetylcholine at the muscarinic receptors found in bronchial smooth muscle. It seems to have an additive effect with β₂-agonists when used for acute asthma exacerbations. Long-term use of anticholinergic medications is not supported by the literature.

Oral Corticosteroids

Short bursts of oral corticosteroids (3 to 10 days) are administered to children with acute asthma exacerbations. The initial starting dose is 1 to 2 mg/kg/day of prednisone followed by 1 mg/kg/day over the next 2 to 5 days. Oral corticosteroids are available in various liquid or tablet formulations. Prolonged use of oral corticosteroids can result in systemic adverse effects, such as hypothalamic-pituitary-adrenal suppression, cushingoid features, weight gain, hypertension, diabetes, cataracts, glaucoma, osteoporosis, and growth suppression. For children with severe asthma, oral corticosteroids may be needed for extended periods. When possible, the dose should be tapered to the minimum effective dose, preferably administered on alternate days.

Approach to Therapy

Current therapy is based on the concept that chronic inflammation is a fundamental feature of asthma. A stepwise approach is used for management of infants and young children (Fig. 78–1) and children 5 years old and older (Fig. 78–2). A short-acting bronchodilator should be available for all children with asthma. A child with intermittent asthma has asthma symptoms fewer than two times per week. To determine if a child is having more persistent asthma, the **rule of twos** is helpful. Daytime symptoms occurring two or more times per week or nighttime awakening two or more times per month implies a need for daily anti-inflammatory medication. In infants and young children

STEPWISE APPROACH FOR MANAGING ACUTE OR CHRONIC ASTHMA IN INFANTS AND YOUNG CHILDREN (≤AGE 5)

Classify Severity: Clinical Features Before Treatment or Adequate Control		Medications Required To Maintain Long-Term Control
	Symptoms/Day	
	Symptoms/Night	Daily Medications
Step 4 *Severe Persistent*	Continual Frequent	**Preferred treatment:** **High-dose inhaled corticosteroids AND long-acting inhaled beta$_2$-agonists** **AND,** if needed, Corticosteroid tablets or syrup long term (2 mg/kg/day, generally do not exceed 60 mg per day). (Make repeat attempts to reduce systemic corticosteroids and maintain control with high-dose inhaled corticosteroids.)
Step 3 *Moderate Persistent*	Daily >1 night/week	**Preferred treatments:** **Low-dose inhaled corticosteroids and long-acting inhaled beta$_2$-agonists** **OR** **Medium-dose inhaled corticosteroids.** *Alternative treatment:* Low-dose inhaled corticosteroids and either leukotriene receptor antagonist or theophylline. . . . . If needed (particularly in patients with recurring severe exacerbations): **Preferred treatment:** **Medium-dose inhaled corticosteroids and long-acting beta$_2$-agonists.** *Alternative treatment:* Medium-dose inhaled corticosteroids and either leukotriene receptor antagonist or theophylline.
Step 2 *Mild Persistent*	>2/week but <1x/day >2 nights/month	**Preferred treatment:** **Low-dose inhaled corticosteroids (with nebulizer or MDI with holding chamber with or without face mask or DPI).** *Alternative treatment (listed alphabetically):* Cromolyn (nebulizer is preferred or MDI with holding chamber) *OR* leukotriene receptor antagonist.
Step 1 *Mild Intermittent*	2 days/week 2 nights/month	**No daily medication needed.**

Quick Relief *All Patients*	•Bronchodilator as needed for symptoms. Intensity of treatment will depend upon severity of exacerbation. 　*Preferred treatment:* **Short-acting inhaled beta$_2$-agonists** by nebulizer or face mask and space/holding chamber 　*Alternative treatment:* Oral beta$_2$-agonists •With viral respiratory infection 　Bronchodilator, q 4–6 hours up to 24 hours (longer with physician consent); in general, repeat no more than once every 6 weeks 　Consider systemic corticosteroid if exacerbation is severe or patient has a history of previous severe exacerbations •Use of short-acting beta$_2$-agonists >2 times a week in intermittent asthma (daily, or increasing use in persistent asthma) may indicate the need to initiate (increase) long-term-control therapy.

 Step down
Review treatment every 1 to 6 months:
a gradual stepwise reduction in treatment
may be possible.

 Step up
If control is not maintained, consider step up.
First, review patient medication technique,
adherence, and environmental control.

Goals of Therapy: Asthma Control

Minimal or no chronic symptoms day or night

Minimal or no exacerbations

No limitations on activities; no school/parent's work missed

Minimal use of short-acting inhaled beta$_2$-agonist

Minimal or no adverse effects from medications

Notes
The stepwise approach is intended to assist, not replace, the clinical decision-making required to meet individual patient needs.
Classify severity: assign patient to most severe step in which any feature occurs. There are very few studies on asthma therapy for infants.
Gain control as quickly as possible (a course of short systemic corticosteroids may be required); then step down to the least medication necessary to maintain control.
Minimize use of short-acting inhaled beta$_2$-agonists. Overreliance on short-acting inhaled beta$_2$-agonists (e.g., use of short-acting inhaled beta$_2$-agonist every day, increasing use or lack of expected effect, or use of approximately one canister a month even if not using it every day) indicates inadequate control of asthma and the need to initiate or intensify long-term control therapy.
Provide parent education on asthma management and controlling environmental factors that make asthma worse (e.g., allergens and irritants).
Consultation with an asthma specialist is recommended for patients with moderate or severe persistent asthma. Consider consultation for patients with mild persistent asthma.

Figure 78–1

Approach for managing acute or chronic asthma in infants and young children. MDI, metered-dose inhaler; DPI, dry powder inhaler. (From NHLBI, National Asthma Education and Prevention Program: Expert Panel Report: Guidelines for the Diagnosis and Management of Asthma—Update on Selected Topics. NIH Publication No. 02-5075. Bethesda, MD, U.S. Department of Health and Human Services, 2002, p 115. http://www.nhlbi.nih.gov/guidelines/asthma/asthupdt.htm.)

STEPWISE APPROACH FOR MANAGING ASTHMA IN ADULTS AND CHILDREN (>AGE 5)

Classify Severity: Clinical Features Before Treatment or Adequate Control			Medications Required To Maintain Long-Term Control
	Symptoms/Day Symptoms/Night	PEF or FEV$_1$ PEF Variability	Daily Medications
Step 4 *Severe Persistent*	Continual Frequent	≤60% >30%	***Preferred treatment:*** **High-dose inhaled corticosteroids AND long-acting inhaled beta$_2$-agonists** ***AND,*** if needed, Corticosteroid tablets or syrup long term (2 mg/kg/day, generally do not exceed 60 mg per day). (Make repeat attempts to reduce systemic corticosteroids and maintain control with high-dose inhaled corticosteroids.)
Step 3 *Moderate Persistent*	Daily >1 night/week	>60%–<80% >30%	***Preferred treatment:*** **Low- to medium-dose inhaled corticosteroids and long-acting inhaled beta$_2$-agonists.** *Alternative treatment (listed alphabetically):* Increase inhaled corticosteroids with medium-dose range ***OR*** Low- to medium-dose inhaled corticosteroids and either leukotriene modifier or theophylline. ⋯⋯⋯⋯⋯⋯⋯⋯⋯⋯⋯⋯⋯⋯⋯ If needed (particularly in patients with recurring severe exacerbations): ***Preferred treatment:*** **Increase inhaled corticosteroids with medium-dose range and add long-acting inhaled beta$_2$-agonists.** *Alternative treatment:* Increase inhaled corticosteroids with medium-dose range and add either leukotriene modifier or theophylline.
Step 2 *Mild Persistent*	>2/week but <1x/day >2 nights/month	≥80% 20–30%	***Preferred treatment:*** **Low-dose inhaled corticosteroids.** *Alternative treatment (listed alphabetically):* Cromolyn, leukotriene modifier, nedocromil, *OR* sustained-release theophylline to serum concentration of 5–15 mcg/mL.
Step 1 *Mild Intermittent*	≤2 days/week ≤2 nights/month	≥80% <20%	**No daily medication needed.** Severe exacerbations may occur, separated by long periods of normal lung function and no symptoms. A course of systemic corticosteroids is recommended.

Quick Relief

All Patients

- Short-acting bronchodilator: 2–4 puffs **short-acting inhaled beta$_2$-agonists** as needed for symptoms.
- Intensity of treatment will depend upon severity of exacerbation; up to 3 treatments at 20-minute intervals or a single nebulizer treatment as needed. Course of systemic corticosteroids may be needed.
- Use of short-acting beta$_2$-agonists >2 times a week in intermittent asthma (daily, or increasing use in persistent asthma) may indicate the need to initiate (increase) long-term-control therapy.

Step down
Review treatment every 1 to 6 months: a gradual stepwise reduction in treatment may be possible.

Step up
If control is not maintained, consider step up. First, review patient medication technique, adherence, and environmental control.

Goals of Therapy: Asthma Control

Minimal or no chronic symptoms day or night
Minimal or no exacerbations
No limitations on activities; no school/work missed
Maintain (near) normal pulmonary function
Minimal use of short-acting inhaled beta$_2$-agonist
Minimal or no adverse effects from medications

Notes
The stepwise approach is intended to assist, not replace, the clinical decision-making required to meet individual patient needs.
Classify severity: assign patient to most severe step in which any feature occurs. (PEF is % of personal best; FEV$_1$ is % predicted).
Gain control as quickly as possible (consider a short course of systemic corticosteroids); then step down to the least medication necessary to maintain control.
Minimize use of short-acting inhaled beta$_2$-agonists. Overreliance on short-acting inhaled beta$_2$-agonists (e.g., use of short-acting inhaled beta$_2$-agonist every day, increasing use or lack of expected effect, or use of approximately one canister a month even if not using it every day) indicates inadequate control of asthma and the need to initiate or intensify long-term control therapy.
Provide education on self-management and controlling environmental factors that make asthma worse (e.g., allergens and irritants).
Refer to an asthma specialist if there are difficulties controlling asthma or if step 4 care is required. Referral may be considered if step 3 care is required.

Figure 78–2

Approach for managing acute or chronic asthma in adults and children older than age 5. PEF, peak expiratory flow; FEV$_1$, forced expiratory volume in 1 second. (From NHLBI, National Asthma Education and Prevention Program: Expert Panel Report: Guidelines for the Diagnosis and Management of Asthma—Update on Selected Topics. NIH Publication No. 02-5075. Bethesda, MD, U.S. Department of Health and Human Services, 2002, p 116. http://www.nhlbi.nih.gov/guidelines/asthma/asthupdt.htm.)

who have had three episodes of wheezing in the previous year along with risk factors for the development of asthma or have had severe exacerbations less than 6 weeks apart, controller medications are desirable.

The preferred first-line controller medication for children of all ages with persistent asthma is inhaled corticosteroids. For children with mild persistent asthma, low-dose inhaled corticosteroids are recommended. For children older than 5 years with moderate persistent asthma, combining long-acting bronchodilators with low to medium doses of inhaled corticosteroids improves lung function and reduces rescue medication usage. For children younger than 5 years with moderate persistent asthma, medication combinations have not been as well studied. The preferred therapy is either low doses of inhaled corticosteroid with long-acting bronchodilator or medium doses of inhaled corticosteroid. For children with severe persistent asthma, high-dose inhaled corticosteroid and long-acting bronchodilator are the preferred therapy. The guidelines also recommend that patients be seen every 1 to 6 months so that medications can be reduced (step-down) or increased (step-up) depending on the child's control.

COMPLICATIONS

Most asthma exacerbations can be managed at home successfully. **Status asthmaticus** is an acute exacerbation of asthma that does not respond adequately to therapeutic measures and may require hospitalization. Exacerbations may progress over several days or occur suddenly and can range in severity from mild to life-threatening. Significant respiratory distress, dyspnea, wheezing, cough, and a decrease in peak expiratory flow rates characterize deterioration in asthma control. During severe episodes of wheezing, pulse oximetry is helpful in monitoring oxygenation. In status asthmaticus, arterial blood gases may be necessary for measurement of ventilation. As airway obstruction worsens and chest compliance decreases, carbon dioxide retention can occur. In the face of tachypnea, a "normal" PCO_2 (40 mm Hg) indicates impending respiratory arrest.

First-line management of asthma exacerbations includes supplemental oxygen, repetitive or continuous administration of short-acting bronchodilators, and oral or IV corticosteroids (Fig. 78-3). Coadministration of anticholinergic agents (ipratropium) with bronchodilators has been shown to decrease rates of hospitalization and duration of time in the emergency department. Early administration of oral corticosteroids is important in treating the underlying inflammation. IM epinephrine or SC terbutaline is rarely used with the exception of severe asthma associated with anaphylaxis or unresponsive to continuous administration of short-acting bronchodilators.

PROGNOSIS

For some children, symptoms of wheezing with respiratory infections subside in the preschool years, whereas other children have more persistent asthma symptoms. Prognostic indicators have been identified for children younger than 3 years old who are at risk for asthma (Table 78-4). The strongest predictor for wheezing continuing into persistent asthma is atopy (Table 78-5).

PREVENTION

Education plays an important role in helping patients and their families adhere to the prescribed therapy and needs to begin at the time of diagnosis. Successful education involves teaching basic asthma facts, explaining the role of medications, teaching environmental control measures, and improving patient skills in the use of spacer devices for MDIs and peak flow monitoring. Families should have an asthma management plan (Fig. 78-4) for daily care and for exacerbations.

Peak flow monitoring is a self-assessment tool that is helpful for children older than age 5. It is advisable for children who are "poor perceivers" of airway obstruction, have moderate to severe asthma, or have a history of severe exacerbations. Peak flow monitoring also can be useful in children recently diagnosed with asthma who are still learning to recognize asthma symptoms.

To use a peak flow meter, a child should be standing with the indicator placed at the bottom of the scale. The child must inhale deeply, place the device in the mouth, bite down on the mouthpiece, seal the lips around the mouthpiece, and blow out forcefully and rapidly. The indicator moves up the numeric scale. The **peak expiratory flow rate (PEFR)** is the highest number achieved. The test is repeated three times to obtain the best possible effort. Peak flow meters are available as low range (measurement ≤300 L/sec) and high range (measurement ≤700 L/sec). For children, it

---

TABLE 78–4. Predictive Measures of Increased Risk for Asthma for Wheezing Children Younger than 3 Years Old

1 Major Criterion *and*	2 Minor Criteria
Parental asthma	Allergic rhinitis
Eczema	Wheezing apart from colds
	Eosinophilia ≥4%

From Castro-Rodriguez JA, Holberg CJU, Wright AL, Martinez FD: A clinical index to define risk of asthma in young children with recurrent wheezing. Am J Respir Crit Care Med 162: 1403-1406, 2000.

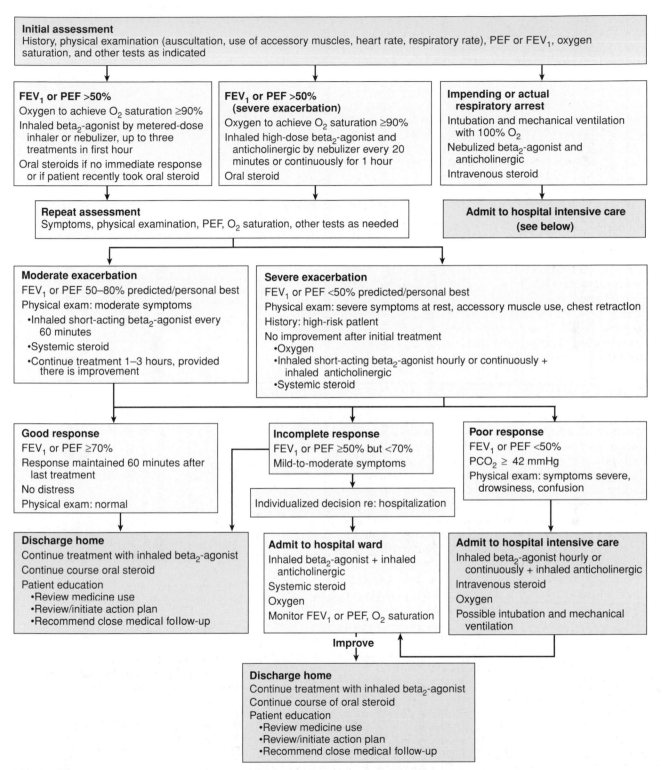

Figure 78–3

Management of asthma exacerbations. Emergency department and hospital-based care. PEF, peak expiratory flow; FEV_1, forced expiratory volume in 1 second. (From NHLBI, National Asthma Education and Prevention Program: Expert Report 2: Practical Guide for the Diagnosis and Management of Asthma. NIH Publication No. 97-4053. Bethesda, MD, U.S. Department of Health and Human Services, 1997, p 29. http://www.nhlbi.nih.gov/health/prof/lung/asthma/practgde.htm.)

Asthma Action Plan for _____ Doctor's name _____ Date _____

Doctor's phone number _____ Hospital/emergency room phone number _____

Take These Long-Term-Control Medicines Each Day (include an anti-inflammatory)

GREEN ZONE: Doing well

Medicine	How much to take	When to take it

- No cough, wheeze, chest tightness, or shortness of breath during the day or night
- Can do usual activities

And, if a peak flow meter is used,

Peak flow: more than _____ (80% or more of my best peak flow)

My best peak flow is: _____

Before exercise ☐ _____ ☐ 2 or ☐ 4 puffs   5 to 60 minutes before exercise

---

FIRST **Add: Quick-relief medicine—and keep taking your GREEN ZONE medicine**

☐ _____ ☐ 2 or ☐ 4 puffs, every 20 minutes for up to 1 hour
(short-acting beta₂-agonist) ☐ Nebulizer, once

SECOND **If your symptoms (and peak flow, if used) return to GREEN ZONE after 1 hour of above treatment:**

☐ Take the quick-relief medicine every 4 hours for 1 to 2 days.
☐ Double the dose of your inhaled steroid for _____ (7–10) days.

OR

If your symptoms (and peak flow, if used) do not return to GREEN ZONE after 1 hour of above treatment:

☐ Take: _____ ☐ 2 or ☐ 4 puffs or ☐ Nebulizer
(short-acting beta₂-agonist)
☐ Add: _____ _____ mg per day For _____ (3–10) days
(oral steroid)
☐ Call the doctor ☐ before/ ☐ within _____ hours after taking the oral steroid.

YELLOW ZONE: Asthma is getting worse

- Cough, wheeze, chest tightness, or shortness of breath, or
- Waking at night due to asthma, or
- Can do some, but not all, usual activities

OR

Peak flow: _____ to _____ (50%–80% of my best peak flow)

Take this medicine:

☐ _____ ☐ 4 or ☐ 6 puffs or ☐ Nebulizer
(short-acting beta₂-agonist)
☐ _____ _____ mg.
(oral steroid)

Then call your doctor NOW. Go to the hospital or call for an ambulance if:
- You are still in the red zone after 15 minutes AND
- You have not reached your doctor

RED ZONE: Medical alert!

- Very short of breath, or
- Quick-relief medicines have not helped, or
- Cannot do usual activities, or
- Symptoms are same or get worse after 24 hours in Yellow Zone

OR

Peak flow: less than _____ (50% of my best peak flow)

DANGER SIGNS

- Trouble walking and talking due to shortness of breath
- Lips or fingernails are blue

■ Take ☐ 4 or ☐ 6 puffs of your quick-relief medicine AND
■ Go to the hospital or call for an ambulance (_____) NOW!

Figure 78–4

Asthma self-management guideline. (From NHLBI, National Asthma Education and Prevention Program: Expert Report 2: Practical Guide for the Diagnosis and Management of Asthma. NIH Publication No. 97-4053. Bethesda, MD, U.S. Department of Health and Human Services, 1997, p 46. http://www.nhlbi.nih.gov/health/prof/lung/asthma/practgde.htm.)

TABLE 78–5. Risk Factors for Persistent Asthma

Allergy
  Atopic dermatitis
  Allergic rhinitis
  Elevated total serum IgE levels (first year of life)
  Peripheral blood eosinophilia >4% (2-3 yr old)
  Food and inhalant allergen sensitization
Gender
  Boys
    Transient wheezing
    Persistent allergy-associated asthma
  Girls
    Asthma associated with obesity and early-onset puberty
    Triad asthma (adulthood)
Parental asthma
Lower respiratory tract infection
  Respiratory syncytial virus, parainfluenza
  Severe bronchiolitis (e.g., requiring hospitalization)
  Pneumonia
Environmental tobacco smoke exposure (including
    prenatal)

From Liu A, Martinez FD, Taussig LM: Natural history of allergic diseases and asthma. In Leung DYM, Sampson HA, Geha RS, Szefler SJ (eds): Pediatric Allergy: Principles and Practice. St Louis, Mosby, 2003, p 15.

is important to provide the appropriate range meter so that accurate measurements can be obtained, and children do not become discouraged because their blows barely move the indicator.

A child's personal best is the highest PEFR achieved over a 2-week period when stable. Based on the child's personal best, a written action plan can be established. The **written action plan** is divided into three zones similar to a stoplight. The green zone indicates a PEFR 80% to 100% of the child's personal best value. In this zone, the child is likely asymptomatic and should continue with medications as usual. The yellow zone indicates a PEFR 50% to 80% of the child's personal best value, which generally coincides with the child having more asthma symptoms. Rescue medications, such as albuterol, are added, and a telephone call to the physician may be warranted if the peak flows do not return to the green zone within the next 24 to 48 hours or if asthma symptoms are deteriorating. The red zone indicates a PEFR less than 50% and is a medical emergency. The rescue medication should be taken immediately. If the PEFR remains in the red zone or the child is having significant airway compromise, a phone call to the physician or emergency care is needed.

A key message for families is that children with asthma should be seen not only when they are ill, but also when they are healthy. Regular office visits allow the healthcare team to review adherence to medication and control measures and to determine if doses of medications need adjustment.

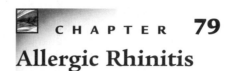

CHAPTER 79
Allergic Rhinitis

ETIOLOGY

Rhinitis describes diseases that involve inflammation of the nasal epithelium and is characterized by sneezing, itching, rhinorrhea, and congestion. There are many different causes of rhinitis in children, but approximately half of all cases of rhinitis are caused by allergies.

Allergic rhinitis is caused by a type I, IgE-mediated allergic response. During the early allergic phase, mast cells degranulate and release preformed chemical mediators, such as histamine and tryptase, and newly generated mediators, such as leukotrienes, prostaglandins, and platelet-activating factor. After a quiescent phase in which other cells are recruited, a late phase occurs approximately 4 to 8 hours later. Eosinophils, basophils, CD4 T cells, monocytes, and neutrophils release their chemical mediators, which leads to the development of chronic nasal inflammation.

Allergic rhinitis can be seasonal, perennial, or episodic depending on the particular allergen and the child's exposure. Some children experience perennial symptoms with seasonal exacerbations. **Seasonal allergic rhinitis** is caused by airborne pollen with a seasonal pattern. Insect-pollinated plants (flowers, flowering trees) are not a cause of allergic rhinitis. Typically, trees pollinate in the spring, grasses in late spring to summer, and weeds in the summer and fall. The pollen, microscopic in size, can travel airborne hundreds of miles and be inhaled easily into the respiratory tract. **Perennial allergic rhinitis** is primarily caused by indoor allergens, such as house dust mites, animal dander, mold, and cockroaches. **Episodic rhinitis** occurs with intermittent exposure to allergens, such as visiting a friend's home where a pet dwells.

Genetic predisposition and repeated exposure to allergens are important factors that contribute to the development of allergic rhinitis. It often takes weeks, months, or years to sensitize the immune system to produce sufficient allergen-specific IgE. When an atopic child inhales airborne allergens, these proteins penetrate the nasal mucosal epithelium and interact with allergen-specific IgE on tissue mast cells. Allergic rhinitis is relatively rare in children younger than 6 months old, and if it is present in infancy, it is due to foods or household inhalants rather than seasonal pollens. Typically, seasonal allergic rhinitis presents in children older than 3 years.

EPIDEMIOLOGY

Chronic rhinitis is one of the most common disorders encountered in infants and children. Overall, allergic rhinitis is observed in 10% to 25% of the population, with children and adolescents more commonly affected than adults. The prevalence of physician-diagnosed allergic rhinitis may be 40%.

CLINICAL MANIFESTATIONS

Clear, thin rhinorrhea; nasal congestion; paroxysms of sneezing; and pruritus of the eyes, nose, ears, and palate are hallmarks of the disease. Postnasal drip may result in frequent attempts to clear the throat, nocturnal cough, and hoarseness. It is important to correlate the onset, duration, and severity of symptoms with seasonal or perennial exposures, changes in the home or school environment, and exposure to nonspecific irritants, such as tobacco smoke. Children with allergic rhinitis may experience sleep disturbances, limitations of activity, irritability, and mood and cognitive disorders that adversely affect their performance at school and their sense of well-being.

The physical examination includes a thorough nasal examination and an evaluation of the eyes, ears, throat, chest, and skin. Physical findings may be subtle. Classic physical findings include pale pink or bluish gray, swollen, boggy nasal turbinates with clear, watery secretions. Frequent nasal itching and rubbing of the nose with the palm of the hand, the **allergic salute**, can lead to a transverse nasal crease found across the lower bridge of the nose. Children may produce clucking sounds by rubbing the soft palate with their tongue. Oropharyngeal examination may reveal lymphoid hyperplasia of the soft palate and posterior pharynx or visible mucus or both. Orthodontic abnormalities may be seen in children with chronic mouth breathing. **Allergic shiners**, dark periorbital swollen areas caused by venous congestion, are often present in children along with swollen eyelids or conjunctival injection. Retracted tympanic membranes from eustachian tube dysfunction or serous otitis media also may be present. Other atopic diseases, such as asthma or eczema, may be present, which helps lead the clinician to the correct diagnosis.

LABORATORY AND IMAGING STUDIES

Allergy testing can be performed by in vivo skin tests or by in vitro serum tests (RAST) to pertinent allergens found in the patient's environment (see Table 77–4).

Skin tests (prick/puncture) provide immediate and accurate results because positive tests correlate strongly with nasal and bronchial allergen provocative challenges. In vitro serum tests are useful for patients with abnormal skin conditions, patients with a tendency for anaphylaxis, and patients taking medications that interfere with skin testing. Disadvantages of serum tests include increased cost, inability to obtain immediate results, and reduced sensitivity compared with skin tests. Widespread screening with serum testing without regard to a patient's symptoms is not recommended. Measurement of total serum IgE or blood eosinophils generally is not helpful in the differential diagnosis of rhinitis. The presence of eosinophils on the nasal smear suggests a diagnosis of allergy, but eosinophils also can be found in patients with nonallergic rhinitis with eosinophilia. Nasal smear eosinophilia is often predictive of a good clinical response to nasal corticosteroid sprays.

DIFFERENTIAL DIAGNOSIS

Rhinitis can be divided into allergic and nonallergic rhinitis (Table 79–1). Nonallergic rhinitis describes a group of nasal diseases in which there is no evidence of allergic etiology and can be divided further into nonanatomic and anatomic etiologies. The most common form of nonallergic rhinitis in children is infectious rhinitis, which may be acute or chronic. Acute infectious rhinitis, or the common cold, is caused by viruses, including rhinoviruses and coronaviruses, and typically resolves within 7 to 10 days. An average child has three to six common colds per year, with younger children and children attending

TABLE 79–1. Classification of the Etiology of Rhinitis in Children

	Nonallergic	
Allergic	*Nonanatomic*	*Anatomic*
Seasonal	Nonallergic,	Adenoidal
Perennial	noninfectious	hypertrophy
Episodic	(vasomotor) rhinitis	CSF rhinorrhea
	Infectious	Choanal atresia
	rhinosinusitis	Congenital
	Nonallergic rhinitis	anomalies
	with eosinophilia	Foreign body
	Physical rhinitis	Nasal polyps
	Rhinitis	Septal deviation
	medicamentosa	Tumors
		Turbinate
		hypertrophy

daycare the most affected. Infection is suggested by the presence of sore throat, fever, and poor appetite, especially with a history of exposure to other children with colds. Chronic infectious rhinosinusitis, or sinusitis, should be suspected if there is mucopurulent nasal discharge with symptoms that persist beyond 10 days. Classic signs of acute sinusitis among older children and adults include facial tenderness, tooth pain, headache, and fever. In young children, these classic signs usually are not present. Younger children may present with symptoms of postnasal drainage with cough, throat clearing, halitosis, and rhinorrhea. The character of the nasal secretions with infectious rhinitis varies from purulent to minimal or absent. Coexistence of middle ear disease, such as otitis media or eustachian tube dysfunction, may be additional clues of infection.

Nonallergic, noninfectious rhinitis, formerly known as *vasomotor rhinitis,* can manifest as rhinorrhea and sneezing in children with profuse clear nasal discharge. Exposure to irritants, such as cigarette smoke and dust, and strong fumes and odors, such as perfumes and chlorine in swimming pools, can trigger these nasal symptoms. Nonallergic rhinitis with eosinophilia syndrome is associated with clear nasal discharge and eosinophils on nasal smear and is seen infrequently in children. Cold air (**skier's nose**), hot/spicy food ingestion (**gustatory rhinitis**), and exposure to bright light (**reflex rhinitis**) are examples of physical rhinitis. Treatment with topical ipratropium before exposure may be helpful.

Rhinitis medicamentosa, which is due primarily to overuse of topical nasal decongestants such as oxymetazoline, phenylephrine, or cocaine, is not a common condition of younger children. Adolescents or young adults may become dependent on these over-the-counter medications. Treatment requires discontinuation of the offending decongestant spray, the addition of topical corticosteroids, and frequently a short course of oral corticosteroids.

The most common anatomic problem seen in young children is obstruction secondary to adenoidal hypertrophy, which can be suspected from symptoms such as mouth breathing, snoring, hyponasal speech, and persistent rhinitis with or without chronic otitis media. Infection of the nasopharynx may be secondary to infected hypertrophied adenoid tissue.

Choanal atresia is the most common congenital anomaly of the nose and consists of a bony or membranous septum between the nose and pharynx, either unilateral or bilateral. Bilateral choanal atresia classically presents in neonates as cyclic cyanosis because neonates are preferential nose breathers. Airway obstruction and cyanosis are relieved when the mouth is opened to cry and recurs when the calming infant reattempts to breathe through the nose. Some newborns show respiratory difficulty only while feeding. Nearly half of infants with choanal atresia have other congenital anomalies as a part of the **CHARGE association** (**c**oloboma, congenital **h**eart disease, choanal **a**tresia, **r**etardation, **g**enitourinary defects, **e**ar anomalies). Unilateral choanal atresia may go undiagnosed until later in life and presents with symptoms of unilateral nasal obstruction and discharge.

Nasal polyps typically appear as bilateral, gray, glistening sacs originating from the ethmoid sinuses and may be associated with clear or purulent nasal discharge. Nasal polyps are rare in children younger than 10 years old, but if present warrant evaluation for an underlying disease process, such as cystic fibrosis or primary ciliary dyskinesia. **Triad asthma** is asthma, aspirin sensitivity, and nasal polyps with chronic or recurrent sinusitis.

Foreign bodies are seen more commonly in young children who hide food, small toys, stones, or erasers in their nose. The index of suspicion should be raised by a history of unilateral, purulent nasal discharge, or foul odor. The foreign body can often be seen on examination with a nasal speculum.

Nasal septal deviation in infants can be congenital or the result of birth trauma. In older children, facial trauma from contact sports, automobile or bicycle accidents, or play activities can result in septal deformity. Hypertrophy of the turbinates causing nasal symptoms also can be seen in children. Severe anatomic abnormalities of the septum or turbinates may benefit from surgical intervention.

A rare cause of rhinitis is CSF rhinorrhea. This condition should be suspected in the presence of unilateral, clear nasal discharge and may occur even in the absence of trauma or recent surgery.

Tumors are extremely rare causes of anatomic obstruction in children and include hemangioma, rhabdomyosarcoma, lymphoma, and olfactory neuroblastoma. Other unusual congenital nasal lesions include dermoid cysts, teratomas, gliomas, and encephaloceles that present as insidious nasal obstruction in children. In adolescent boys, nasal obstruction and severe, recurring nosebleeds may be a sign of **angiofibroma**, a benign tumor.

TREATMENT

Management of allergic rhinitis is based on disease severity, impact of the disease on the patient, and the ability of the patient to comply with recommendations. Treatment modalities include allergen avoidance, pharmacologic therapy, and immunotherapy. Environmental control and steps to minimize allergen exposure, similar to preventive steps for asthma, should be implemented whenever possible (see Table 78-3).

Pharmacotherapy

Intranasal corticosteroids are the most potent pharmacologic therapy for treatment of allergic and nonallergic rhinitis. These include beclomethasone (Beconase, Vancenase), fluticasone (Flonase), triamcinolone (Nasacort), mometasone (Nasonex), flunisolide (Nasarel), and budesonide (Rhinocort). These agents work topically to reduce inflammation, edema, and mucus production and are effective for symptoms of nasal congestion, rhinorrhea, itching, and sneezing. They are less effective for ocular symptoms. Nasal corticosteroid sprays have been used safely in long-term therapy. Deleterious effects on adrenal function or nasal membranes have not been reported when used appropriately. The most common adverse effects include local irritation, burning, and, sneezing, which occur in 10% of patients. Nasal bleeding from improper technique also can occur, which is related to spraying the nasal septum. Rare cases of nasal septal perforation have been reported.

Antihistamines are the medications used most frequently to treat allergic rhinitis. They are useful in treating the symptoms of rhinorrhea, sneezing, nasal itching, and ocular itching but are less helpful in treating nasal congestion. First-generation antihistamines, such as diphenhydramine (Benadryl) and hydroxyzine (Atarax), easily cross the blood-brain barrier, with sedation as the most common reported adverse effect. Use of first-generation antihistamines in children has shown a negative effect on cognitive and academic function. In very young children, a paradoxical stimulatory CNS effect resulting in irritability and restlessness has been noted. Other adverse effects of first-generation antihistamines include anticholinergic effects, such as blurred vision, urinary retention, dry mouth, tachycardia, and constipation. Second-generation antihistamines, such as cetirizine (Zyrtec), fexofenadine (Allegra), desloratadine (Clarinex), and loratadine (Claritin), are less likely to cross the blood-brain barrier and are less sedating. Cetirizine, desloratadine, and loratadine are available in a syrup formulation; cetirizine and desloratadine are approved for children older than 6 months of age, and loratadine is approved for children older than 2 years. Loratadine has been approved for nonprescription use. Azelastine (Astelin), a topical nasal antihistamine spray, also is available and approved for children older than age 5. Drawbacks to its use include its bitter taste and that it may cause sedation.

Decongestants may be used to relieve nasal congestion and can be taken orally or intranasally. Oral medications, such as pseudoephedrine and phenylephrine, are available either alone or in combination with antihistamines. Adverse effects of oral decongestants include insomnia, nervousness, irritability, tachycardia, tremors, and palpitations. For older children participating in sports, oral decongestant use may be restricted. Topical nasal decongestant sprays are effective for immediate relief of nasal obstruction but should be used for fewer than 5 to 7 days to prevent occurrence of rebound nasal congestion (rhinitis medicamentosa).

Topical ipratropium bromide (Atrovent), an anticholinergic nasal spray, is used primarily for nonallergic rhinitis and rhinitis associated with viral upper respiratory infection. Leukotriene modifiers have been studied in the treatment of allergic rhinitis. Montelukast (Singulair) is approved for use in seasonal allergic rhinitis.

Immunotherapy

If environmental control measures and medication intervention are only partially effective or produce unacceptable adverse effects, immunotherapy may be recommended. The mechanism of action for allergen immunotherapy is complex but includes increased production of an IgG-blocking antibody, decreased production of specific IgE, and alteration of cytokine expression produced in response to an allergen challenge. Immunotherapy is effective for desensitization to pollens, dust mites, and cat and dog protein. In young children, its use may be limited by the need for frequent injections. Immunotherapy must be administered in a physician's office, where the patient is observed for 20 to 30 minutes after the allergen injection. Anaphylaxis may occur, and the physician must be experienced in the treatment of these severe adverse allergic reactions.

COMPLICATIONS

Approximately 60% of children with allergic rhinitis have symptoms of reactive airways disease/asthma (see Chapter 78). Chronic allergic inflammation leads to chronic cough from postnasal drip; eustachian tube dysfunction and otitis media; tonsillar and adenoid hypertrophy, which may lead to obstructive sleep apnea; marked sinus mucosal thickening and sinus opacification on radiography; and development of nasal polyposis. Children with allergic rhinitis may experience sleep disturbances, limitations of activity, irritability, and mood and cognitive disorders that adversely affect their performance at school and their sense of well-being.

PROGNOSIS

Seasonal allergic rhinitis is a common and prominent condition that may not improve as children grow older, although they become more adept at self-management of symptoms. Perennial allergic rhinitis improves with allergen control of indoor allergens.

PREVENTION

Removal or avoidance of the offending allergen is advised. The only effective measure for minimizing animal allergens from pets is removal of the pet from the home. Avoidance of pollen and outdoor molds can be accomplished by staying indoors in a controlled environment. Air conditioning and keeping windows and doors closed lower exposure to pollen. HEPA filters reduce the counts of airborne mold spores. Sealing the mattress, pillow, and covers in allergen-proof encasings is the most effective strategy for reduction of mite allergen. Bed linens and blankets should be washed in hot water (>130°F) every week.

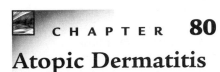

CHAPTER 80
Atopic Dermatitis

ETIOLOGY

The precise mechanism producing atopic dermatitis, a form of eczema, is unclear; genetics, environmental factors, and cutaneous immunologic factors play a role. Children with primary T cell immunodeficiency disorders, such as Wiskott-Aldrich and Omenn syndromes, frequently have atopic dermatitis. When these children undergo stem cell transplantation, the procedure corrects the immunologic defect and the dermatitis.

Several immunoregulatory abnormalities have been described in patients with atopic dermatitis (Fig. 80–1). There is an exaggerated cutaneous inflammatory response to environmental triggers, including irritants and allergens. Activated Langerhans cells in the dermis expressing surface-bound IgE stimulate T cells. In acute lesions, activated Th2 lymphocytes infiltrate the dermis. They initiate and maintain local tissue inflammation primarily through IL-4 and IL-13, which promotes IgE production; and IL-5, which promotes eosinophil differentiation. As the disease progresses from an acute to a chronic phase, there is a switch from Th2 to Th1 cellular response. Chronic lesions are characterized by increased IL-12 and IFN-γ.

Patients with atopic dermatitis have hyperirritable skin; many factors can cause the disease to worsen or relapse. Known triggers include anxiety and stress, climate factors (extremes of temperature and humidity), irritants, allergens, and infections. Approximately 35% to 40% of children with moderate to severe atopic dermatitis have coexistent food allergies. The more severe the atopic dermatitis and the younger the patient, the more likely food allergy is a contributing factor. Egg allergy is the most common cause of food-induced eczematous reactions. Eggs, milk, peanuts, soy, wheat, fish, shellfish, and tree nuts account for 90% of food allergy in children.

EPIDEMIOLOGY

Atopic dermatitis commonly affects infants and children. Atopic dermatitis is the first clinical manifestation of a child prone to atopic diseases. Approximately 50% of all children develop atopic dermatitis in the first year of life, with 80% of these children experiencing disease onset before age 5 years. Approximately 80% of children with atopic dermatitis develop asthma or allergic rhinitis, with many losing symptoms of dermatitis at the onset of respiratory allergy.

CLINICAL MANIFESTATIONS

During infancy, atopic dermatitis involves the face, scalp, cheeks, and extensor surfaces of the extremities with the diaper area being spared. In older children, the rash localizes to the antecubital and popliteal flexural surfaces. **Acute atopic dermatitis** is characterized by intensely pruritic, ill-defined plaques of erythema and scale with excoriations and serous exudates. **Chronic atopic dermatitis** is characterized by generalized xerosis (dry skin), lichenification, and fibrotic papules. Physical examination may show hyperlinearity of the palms and soles, white dermatographism, pityriasis alba, creases under the lower eyelids (**Dennie-Morgan folds**), and **keratosis pilaris** (asymptomatic horny follicular papules on the extensor surfaces of the arms).

LABORATORY AND IMAGING STUDIES

The diagnosis is based on the clinical diagnostic criteria rather than laboratory tests. Skin biopsy may be needed in some situations to exclude other diseases that imitate atopic dermatitis. Allergy skin testing or, alternatively, CAP-RAST may be helpful if specific allergies are suspected.

DIFFERENTIAL DIAGNOSIS

Diagnostic criteria have been established for the diagnosis of atopic dermatitis (Table 80–1). According to the criteria, three of the four major features along with at least three of the minor features must be present for a diagnosis of atopic dermatitis. Pruritus is the hallmark of the disease. No diagnostic test is available, but skin biopsy shows hyperkeratosis of the epidermis with perivascular inflammation in the dermis.

Many conditions share signs and symptoms of atopic dermatitis (Table 80–2). Infants presenting in the first year of life with failure to thrive, recurrent

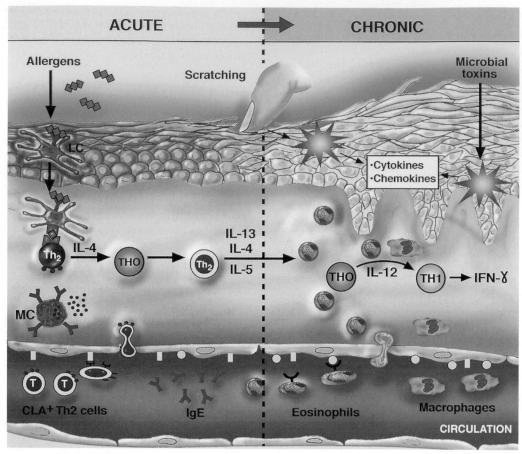

ACUTE → CHRONIC

Allergens

Scratching

Microbial toxins

LC

·Cytokines
·Chemokines

Th2 — IL-4 → THO → Th2 — IL-13 IL-4 IL-5 → THO — IL-12 → TH1 → IFN-γ

MC

CLA⁺ Th2 cells   IgE   Eosinophils   Macrophages

CIRCULATION

Figure 80–1

The immunologic pathways involved in the progression of atopic dermatitis. Patients with atopic dermatitis have a systemic Th2 response with elevated IgE and eosinophilia. The acute skin lesion is associated with infiltration of Th2 cells. Chronic atopic dermatitis is associated with the infiltration of eosinophils and macrophages, and there is a switch to Th1 cellular responses. This biphasic Th2/Th1 switch in immune responses is paralleled clinically and histologically by acute population and spongiosus followed by the development of lichenification, hyperkeratosis, and dermal fibrosis. CLA, cutaneous lymphoid antigen; IFN, interferon; LC, Langerhans cells; MC, mast cells; Th, T helper cell type; THO, naïve T cell. (From J Allergy Clin Immunol, cover, May 2000; with permission from the American Academy of Allergy, Asthma, and Immunology.)

skin or systemic infections, and scaling, erythematous rash should be evaluated for immunodeficiency disorders. Wiskott-Aldrich syndrome is an X-linked recessive syndrome characterized by atopic dermatitis, thrombocytopenia, small-sized platelets, and recurrent infections. Histiocytosis X (Letterer-Siwe disease) is characterized by hemorrhagic or petechial lesions. Scabies is an intensely pruritic skin condition caused by the human scabies mite. The presence of a burrow found in the web spaces of the fingers, the flexor surfaces of the wrists, elbows, axilla, or genitals is pathognomonic. Burrows may be few in number or absent, however.

TREATMENT

Successful management involves skin hydration, pharmacologic therapy to reduce pruritus, and identification and avoidance of triggers. Patients with atopic dermatitis have a decrease in skin barrier function and enhanced transepidermal water loss. Daily, lukewarm baths for 15 to 20 minutes followed immediately by the application of fragrance-free emollients to retain moisture are a major component of therapy. Prevention of xerosis is important for control of pruritus and for maintaining the integrity of the epithelial barrier. Emollients should be ointments or creams, such as

TABLE 80–1. Criteria for the Diagnosis of Atopic Dermatitis in Children

Major Features (Must Have Three)

1. Pruritus
2. Typical morphology and distribution
   a. Facial and extensor involvement during infancy and early childhood
   b. Flexural lichenification by adolescence
3. Chronic or chronically relapsing dermatitis
4. Personal or family history of atopy

Minor or Less Specific Features

1. Xerosis
2. Periauricular fissures
3. Ichthyosis, hyperlinear palms, or keratosis pilaris
4. IgE reactivity (increased serum IgE, RAST, or prick test positivity)
5. Hand or foot dermatitis
6. Cheilitis
7. Scalp dermatitis (cradle cap)
8. Susceptibility to cutaneous infections (especially *Staphylococcus aureus* and herpes simplex)
9. Perifollicular accentuation (especially in pigmented races)

Modified from Hanifin JM: Atopic dermatitis in infants and children. Pediatr Clin North Am 38:763-789, 1991.

petrolatum, Aquaphor, Eucerin, or Cetaphil. Lotions are not as effective because they contain water or alcohol and may have a drying effect owing to evaporation. A mild nonsoap cleanser also is recommended.

Topical anti-inflammatory agents, including corticosteroids and immunomodulators, are the cornerstone of therapy for acute flares and prevention of relapses. Topical corticosteroids are used for reducing inflammation and pruritus and are effective for the acute and chronic phases of the disease. Ointments generally are preferred over creams because of enhanced potency and skin penetration and work best when applied after bathing. Corticosteroids are ranked by potency into seven classes. Low-potency, nonfluorinated corticosteroids should be used on the face, groin area, and intertriginous areas. Higher potency corticosteroids may be necessary to diminish the dermatitis flare but should be used for limited periods. Adverse effects, such as skin atrophy, striae, and hypothalamic-pituitary-adrenal axis and growth suppression, are related to the potency, length of use, and extent of medication application. In infants and younger children, the possibility for corticosteroid adverse effects may be greater. When control of inflammatory lesions is achieved, most patients can be managed with emollients and low-potency topical corticosteroids.

The use of oral corticosteroids is rarely indicated in the treatment of chronic atopic dermatitis. The dramatic improvement frequently is associated with a severe rebound flare of atopic dermatitis after the oral corticosteroid has been discontinued.

Other effective therapies for atopic dermatitis include the topical immunomodulating drugs tacrolimus (Protopic) and pimecrolimus (Elidel). Their mechanism of action is to reduce the generation of inflammatory cytokines through inhibition of calcineurin and blocking of calcineurin-dependent transcription of early cytokine genes necessary for T cell activation. These agents may be used on all body locations without the adverse effect of cutaneous atrophy seen with topical corticosteroids. Adverse effects include local burning and the need for sun protection. Both agents have been approved for children 2 years old and older. Patients should apply a thin layer of ointment twice

TABLE 80–2. Differential Diagnosis of Atopic Dermatitis

Congenital disorders
  Netherton syndrome
  Familial keratosis pilaris
Chronic dermatoses
  Seborrheic dermatitis
  Contact dermatitis (allergic or irritant)
  Nummular eczema
  Psoriasis
  Ichthyoses
Infections and infestations
  Scabies
  HIV-associated dermatitis
  Dermatophytosis
Malignancies
  Cutaneous T cell lymphoma (mycosis fungoides/Sézary syndrome)
  Histiocytosis X (Letterer-Siwe disease)
Autoimmune disorders
  Dermatitis herpetiformis
  Pemphigus foliaceus
  Graft-versus-host disease
  Dermatomyositis
Immunodeficiencies
  Wiskott-Aldrich syndrome
  Severe combined immunodeficiency
  Hyper-IgE syndrome
Metabolic disorders
  Zinc deficiency
  Pyridoxine (vitamin B_6) and niacin deficiency
  Multiple carboxylase deficiency
  PKU

From Leung DYM: Atopic dermatitis. In Leung DYM, Sampson HA, Geha RS, Szefler SJ (eds): Pediatric Allergy: Principles and Practice. St Louis, Mosby, 2003, p 562.

daily and continue to use for approximately 1 week after lesions have cleared. Long-term studies with these agents showed that using emollients regularly with immunomodulating drugs at the earliest sign or symptom of atopic dermatitis, with mid-potency topical corticosteroids reserved for breakthrough flares, resulted in fewer flares and less use of topical steroids.

Antihistamines are used at bedtime to help control the nighttime itching. The older antihistamines, diphenhydramine and hydroxyzine, are preferred because they also cause sedation. Although the non-sedating antihistamines are less effective in treating pruritus, cetirizine may be helpful in younger atopic children in delaying asthma onset.

COMPLICATIONS

Staphylococcal and streptococcal infections can complicate atopic dermatitis, and treating these infections can improve recurrent dermatitis. Secondarily infected atopic dermatitis often presents as impetiginous pustular lesions with crusting and honey-colored exudate. Mupirocin, a topical antibiotic, can be used to treat local areas of infection, or oral antibiotics, such as cephalexin and dicloxacillin, can be used for multifocal disease or for infection around the eyes and mouth that is difficult to treat topically. Bacterial cultures may be helpful in patients who do not respond to oral antibiotics or who have infection after multiple antibiotic courses.

Herpes simplex superinfection of affected skin, or **Kaposi varicelliform eruption** or **eczema herpeticum**, results in vesiculopustular lesions that appear in crops and can become hemorrhagic. Herpes simplex virus infection can be misdiagnosed as bacterial infection and should be considered if skin lesions fail to respond to antibiotics.

In individuals with atopic dermatitis, smallpox vaccination or exposure to a vaccinated individual may lead to **eczema vaccinatum**, a localized vaccinial superinfection of affected skin. Eczema vaccinatum may progress to generalized vaccinia with vaccinial lesions appearing at sites distant from the inoculation and in patients with underlying immunodeficiencies may be life-threatening.

PROGNOSIS

Atopic dermatitis is a chronic skin disorder that tends to be more severe and prominent in young children. Symptoms become less severe in two thirds of children, with complete remission into at least 20%. Risk factors for persistent atopic dermatitis into adulthood include widespread dermatitis in childhood, concomitant allergic rhinitis or asthma, family history of atopic dermatitis, early age of onset, and high serum IgE levels.

PREVENTION

An important step in the management of atopic dermatitis is to help patients and families identify and avoid allergens and irritants. Common irritants include soaps, detergents, fragrances, chemicals, smoke, and extremes of temperature and humidity. Wool and synthetic fabrics can be irritating to the skin; 100% cotton fabric is preferred. Sweating also is a recognized trigger. Fingernails should be trimmed frequently to minimize scratching.

In infants and younger children who do not respond to the usual therapies, identifying and removing a food allergen from the diet may lead to clinical improvement of the skin. Food allergy is not a common trigger for older patients with atopic dermatitis. Other environmental allergies, such as dust mites, pet dander, or pollens, also can play a role in atopic dermatitis. It is also important to inform the family that flares do occur and that there is not a "cure," but that atopic dermatitis can be controlled.

CHAPTER 81
Urticaria, Angioedema, and Anaphylaxis

ETIOLOGY

Urticaria and angioedema are caused by an allergic, IgE-mediated reaction to an allergen that activates mast cells in the skin. **Anaphylactic reactions**, which are mediated by IgE, and **anaphylactoid reactions**, which result from mechanisms that are not IgE mediated, are acute, severe, life-threatening reactions caused by a massive release of inflammatory mediators. Urticaria, angioedema, and anaphylaxis are best considered as symptoms because they have a variety of causes.

Urticaria and angioedema occur in response to the release of inflammatory mediators, including histamine, leukotrienes, platelet-activating factor, prostaglandins, and cytokines from mast cells present in the skin. A variety of stimuli can trigger mast cells and basophils to release their chemical mediators. Typically, mast cell degranulation results when cross-linking of the membrane-bound IgE occurs. Release of these mediators results in vasodilation, increased vascular leakage, and pruritus. Basophils from the circulatory system also can localize in tissue and release mediators similar to mast cells. Patients with urticaria have elevated histamine content in the skin that is more readily released.

TABLE 81–1.   Etiology of Acute Urticaria

Foods	Egg, milk, wheat, peanuts, tree nuts, soy, shellfish, fish, strawberries (direct mast cell degranulation)
Medications	Suspect all medications, even over-the-counter or homeopathic
Insect stings	Hymenoptera (honeybee, yellow jacket, hornets, wasp, fire ants), biting insects (papular urticaria)
Infections	Bacterial (streptococcal pharyngitis, *Mycoplasma*, sinusitis); viral (hepatitis, mononucleosis [EBV], coxsackievirus A and B); parasitic (*Ascaris, Ancylostoma, Echinococcus, Fasciola, Filaria, Schistosoma, Strongyloides, Toxocara, Trichinella*); fungal (dermatophytes, *Candida*)
Contact allergy	Latex, pollen, animal saliva, nettle plants, caterpillars
Transfusion reactions	Blood, blood products, or IV immunoglobulin administration
Idiopathic	

EBV, Epstein-Barr virus.
From Lasley MV, Kennedy MS, Altman LC: Urticaria and angioedema. In Altman LC, Becker JW, Williams PV (eds): Allergy in Primary Care. Philadelphia, WB Saunders, 2000, p 232.

Not all mast cell activation is IgE mediated. Immunologic, nonimmunologic, physical, and chemical stimuli can produce degranulation of mast cells and basophils. **Anaphylatoxins**, C3a and C5a, can cause histamine release in a non–IgE-mediated reaction. Anaphylatoxins are generated in serum sickness, which occurs in reactions to blood transfusions and with infectious, neoplastic, and rheumatic diseases. In addition, mast cell degranulation can occur from a direct pharmacologic effect or physical or mechanical activation, such as urticaria after exposure to opiate medications and dermatographism.

By definition, **acute urticaria and angioedema** are hives and diffuse swelling that last less than 6 weeks. Often the patient's history is quite helpful in eliciting the cause of this acute reaction (Table 81–1). An IgE mechanism is more common in acute urticaria than in chronic urticaria. **Chronic urticaria and angioedema** are characterized by persistence of symptoms beyond 6 weeks (Table 81–2). Some have daily symptoms of hives and swelling, whereas others have intermittent or recurrent episodes. Most cases of chronic urticaria do not have a determinable cause and are labeled **chronic idiopathic urticaria**, which is a diagnosis of exclusion.

Physical urticaria and angioedema are characterized by environmental factors triggering these reactions. The most common physical urticaria is dermatographism, affecting 2% to 5% of the general population. **Dermatographism** means "writing on the skin" and is easy to diagnose by firmly scratching the skin with a blunt point, such as the wooden tip of a cotton swab or tongue depressor. It is characterized by an urticarial reaction localized to the site of skin trauma. It has been suggested that trauma induces an IgE-mediated reaction causing histamine to be released from the mast cells.

Cholinergic urticaria, characterized by the appearance of 1- to 3-mm wheals surrounded by large erythematous flares after an increase in core body temperature, occurs commonly in young adults. Lesions may develop during strenuous exercise after a hot bath or emotional stress. It may be confused with exercise-induced anaphylaxis, although there are no airway symptoms with cholinergic urticaria.

Cold urticaria occurs with exposure to cold and may develop within minutes on areas directly exposed to cold or on rewarming of the affected parts. Ingestion of cold drinks may result in lip swelling. Cold urticaria syndromes can be categorized into acquired and familial disorders. Severe reactions resulting in death can occur with swimming or diving into cold water. It is imperative

TABLE 81–2.   Etiology of Chronic Urticaria

Idiopathic	75%-90% of cases
	25%-50% of adult patients have IgG, anti-IgE, and anti-FcεRI (high-affinity IgE receptor alpha chain) autoantibodies
Physical	Dermatographism
	Cholinergic urticaria
	Cold urticaria
	Delayed pressure urticaria
	Solar urticaria
	Vibratory urticaria
	Aquagenic urticaria
Rheumatologic	Systemic lupus erythematosus
	Juvenile rheumatoid arthritis
Endocrine	Hyperthyroidism
	Hypothyroidism
Neoplastic	Lymphoma
	Mastocytosis
	Leukemia
Angioedema	Hereditary angioedema (autosomal dominant inherited deficiency of C1-esterase inhibitor)
	Acquired angioedema
	Angiotensin-converting enzyme inhibitors

From Lasley MV, Kennedy MS, Altman LC: Urticaria and angioedema. In Altman LC, Becker JW, Williams PV (eds): Allergy in Primary Care. Philadelphia, WB Saunders, 2000, p 234.

that patients never swim alone, avoid total body exposure to cold, and have injectable epinephrine available.

Autoimmune diseases have been associated with urticaria and angioedema and are more commonly found in adults than children. Connective tissue diseases that have been associated with chronic urticaria and angioedema include systemic lupus erythematosus, Sjögren syndrome, polymyositis, and various forms of leukocytoclastic vasculitis. A specific autoimmune disorder causing urticaria has been identified in patients who seem to have IgG anti-IgE receptor antibody directed against IgE and the IgE receptor. These antibodies trigger the mast cell and basophils to degranulate. Skin testing with autologous serum elicits an immediate wheal and flare response and cellular degranulation.

Hereditary angioedema is an uncommon but treatable type of angioedema that involves an autosomal dominant inherited deficiency of C1-esterase inhibitor (see Chapter 75). Deficiency of this regulatory protein results in complement activation. Most patients have type I hereditary angioedema with low levels of C1-esterase inhibitor; approximately 15% have type II hereditary angioedema with normal levels but dysfunctional C1-esterase inhibitor protein. Patients with hereditary angioedema have recurrent, circumscribed edema typically affecting the extremities and face brought about by minor tissue trauma. One fourth of affected patients die as a result of laryngeal edema. These patients rarely have urticaria associated with angioedema. A low C4 level serves as a good initial screening test. During acute attacks, patients also may have reduced levels of C2. Patients with reduced C4 should have quantitative and functional levels of C1-esterase inhibitor measured. Angiotensin-converting enzyme inhibitors also account for an increasing proportion of angioedema, especially in elderly patients.

Anaphylactic reactions are type I, IgE-mediated reactions and result from many causes (Table 81–3). Cross-linking of the IgE molecule with the allergen leads to IgE receptor activation on the mast cell and basophil. The activated cells release their mediators, including histamine, tryptase, tumor necrosis factor, platelet-activating factor, leukotrienes, prostaglandins, and cytokines. Other cell types involved in the reactions include monocytes, macrophages, eosinophils, neutrophils, and platelets. The mediator release results in the clinical picture of anaphylaxis.

Anaphylactoid reactions are due to nonimmunologic mechanisms. Mast cells and basophils can be activated by direct, nonspecific stimulation, although the exact underlying mechanism is unknown. Reactions to agents such as opiates and radiocontrast material are classic examples. Complement system activation also can result in mast cell and basophil activation. **Anaphylatoxins**, C3a and C5a, are named because of

TABLE 81–3. Common Causes of Anaphylaxis in Children*	
Foods	Peanuts, tree nuts, milk, eggs, fish, shellfish, seeds, fruits, grains
Drugs	Penicillins, cephalosporins, sulfonamides, nonsteroidal anti-inflammatory drugs, opiates, muscle relaxants, vancomycin, dextran, thiamine, vitamin B_{12}, insulin, thiopental, local anesthetics
Hymenoptera venom	Honeybee, yellow jacket, wasp, hornet, fire ant
Latex	
Allergen immunotherapy	
Exercise	Food-specific exercise, postprandial (non–food-specific) exercise
Vaccinations	Tetanus, measles, mumps, influenza
Miscellaneous	Radiocontrast media, immunoglobulin, cold temperature, chemotherapeutic agents, blood products, inhalants
Idiopathic	

*In order of frequency.
From Young MC: General treatment of anaphylaxis. In Leung DYM, Sampson HA, Geha RS, Szefler SJ (eds): Pediatric Allergy: Principles and Practice. St Louis, Mosby, 2003, p 644.

their ability to trigger mediator release and are generated in serum sickness. The most common cause of this type of reaction is transfusion with blood products. There are other causes of anaphylactoid reactions for which the mechanism has not been clarified.

EPIDEMIOLOGY

Urticaria and angioedema are common conditions affecting children and adults. Acute urticaria and angioedema are more common in children and young adults, whereas chronic urticaria and angioedema are more common in adults. The incidence of anaphylaxis in children is unknown.

CLINICAL MANIFESTATIONS

Raised, erythematous lesions with pale centers that are intensely pruritic characterize **urticaria**, commonly called **hives**. The lesions vary in size and can occur anywhere on the body. Typically, urticaria arises suddenly and may resolve within 1 to 2 hours or may persist for 24 hours. **Angioedema** is a similar process that involves the deeper dermis or subcutaneous tissue, with swelling as the principal symptom. Generally, angioedema is not pruritic, may be mildly painful, and persists longer than 24 hours. In rare cases, it may become life-threatening when swelling affects the upper airway.

The clinical manifestations of **anaphylaxis** and **anaphylactoid** reactions are the same for children and adults. The signs and symptoms vary and can range from mild dermatologic symptoms to a fatal reaction, with 90% of patients presenting with cutaneous symptoms, including urticaria, angioedema, flushing, and warmth. The absence of cutaneous symptoms does not exclude the diagnosis of anaphylaxis. Other affected organ systems include the respiratory tract (with rhinorrhea, oropharyngeal edema, laryngeal edema, hoarseness, stridor, wheezing, dyspnea, and asphyxiation), cardiovascular system (with tachycardia, hypotension, shock, syncope, and arrhythmias), gastrointestinal tract (with nausea, abdominal pain, crampy diarrhea, and vomiting) and neurologic system (with syncope, seizure, dizziness, and a sense of impending doom). The severity of an anaphylactic reaction is often proportional to the speed of symptom onset.

LABORATORY AND IMAGING STUDIES

The laboratory evaluation of patients with urticaria and angioedema must be tailored to the clinical situation. Acute urticaria and angioedema do not require specific laboratory evaluation except to document the suspected cause. For patients with chronic urticaria and angioedema, laboratory evaluation should be performed to exclude important underlying diseases (Table 81–4). Patients with recurrent angioedema without urticaria should be evaluated for hereditary angioedema (Table 81–5).

Measurement of the mast cell mediators histamine and tryptase may be helpful when the diagnosis of anaphylaxis is in question. A tryptase level is a more useful test because histamine is released quickly, has a short half-life, and is often difficult to detect in the serum. Serum tryptase levels peak 1 to 1.5 hours after anaphylaxis, and elevated levels may be helpful in establishing the diagnosis of anaphylaxis. Normal tryptase levels do not rule out this diagnosis, however. It is best to measure a serum tryptase level 1 to 2 hours after the onset of symptoms. It also can be ordered retrospectively on stored serum that is 1 to 2 days old.

DIFFERENTIAL DIAGNOSIS

The diagnosis of urticaria and angioedema is straightforward; finding the etiology may be more difficult. Other dermatologic conditions can mimic urticaria. **Erythema multiforme** has target-shaped, erythematous, macular or papular lesions that may look similar to the lesions seen in urticaria. A differentiating feature

TABLE 81–4. Suggested Testing for Chronic Urticaria/Angioedema of Unknown Etiology

Basic Tests	Discretionary Tests Based on
Complete blood count with differential	If vasculitis is suspected
Erythrocyte sedimentation rate	Antinuclear antibody
	Skin biopsy
	CH50
Urinalysis	If liver function tests abnormal
Liver function tests	Serology for viral hepatitis
Thyroid function and autoantibodies	
Anti-FcεR autoantibody (if available)	

From Zuraw B: Urticaria and angioedema. In Leung DYM, Sampson HA, Geha RS, Szefler SJ (eds): Pediatric Allergy: Principles and Practice. St Louis, Mosby, 2003, p 580.

TABLE 81–5. Complement Evaluation of Patients with Recurrent Angioedema

Assay	Idiopathic Angioedema	Type I Hereditary Angioedema	Type II Hereditary Angioedema	Acquired C1-Esterase Inhibitor Deficiency	Vasculitis
C4	Normal	Low	Low	Low	Low or normal
C4d/C4 ratio	Normal	High	High	High	High or normal
C1-esterase inhibitor level	Normal	Low	Normal	Low	Normal
C1-esterase inhibitor function	Normal	Low	Low	Low	Normal
C1q	Normal	Normal	Normal	Low	Low or normal
C3	Normal	Normal	Normal	Normal	Low or normal

From Zuraw B: Urticaria and angioedema. In Leung DYM, Sampson HA, Geha RS, Szefler SJ (eds): Pediatric Allergy: Principles and Practice. St Louis, Mosby, 2003, p 580.

of erythema multiforme is that the lesions are fixed, last for several days, and do not respond to subcutaneous epinephrine. Other dermatologic diseases include dermatitis herpetiformis and bullous pemphigoid, which are quite pruritic, and early on, the lesions may resemble urticaria. Mastocytosis is characterized by mast cell infiltration of various organs, including the skin. Some patients have skin lesions similar in appearance to urticaria rather than the classic urticaria pigmentosa. Urticaria pigmentosa appears as hyperpigmented, red-brown macules, which may coalesce. When these lesions are stroked, they urticate, which is called *Darier sign*. A rare disorder that should be included in the differential diagnosis of urticaria is **Muckle-Wells syndrome**. It is an autosomal dominant disorder characterized by episodic urticaria presenting in infancy, with sensorineural deafness, amyloidosis, arthralgias, and skeletal abnormalities. Another rare syndrome is **Schnitzler syndrome**, which is characterized by chronic urticaria and macroglobulinemia. These patients also have bone pain, anemia, fever, fatigue, and weight loss. **Urticarial vasculitis** represents a small vessel vasculitis with histologic features of a leukocytoclastic response. The main distinguishing feature of urticarial vasculitis is that the lesions last longer than 24 hours, may be tender, and leave behind skin pigmentation. Skin biopsy is required for definitive diagnosis.

The diagnosis of anaphylaxis is usually apparent from the acute and often dramatic onset of multisystem involvement of the skin, respiratory tract, and cardiovascular system. Sudden cardiovascular collapse in the absence of cutaneous symptoms suggests vasovagal collapse, seizure disorder, aspiration, pulmonary embolism, or myocardial infarction. Laryngeal edema, especially with abdominal pain, suggests hereditary angioedema. Many patients with anaphylaxis are initially thought to have septic shock (see Chapter 40).

TREATMENT

Avoidance of triggering agents is important in management of urticaria and angioedema. The mainstay of pharmacologic treatment is H_1 antihistamines. Second-generation H_1 antihistamines, such as cetirizine, fexofenadine, loratadine, and desloratadine, are preferred because they have fewer adverse effects. If a second-generation H_1 antihistamine by itself does not provide adequate relief, the next step is to add a sedating H_1 antihistamine given at bedtime or H_2 antihistamines, such as cimetidine or ranitidine. Tricyclic antidepressants, such as doxepin and amitriptyline, block H_1 and H_2 histamine receptors. Corticosteroids are effective in treating urticaria and angioedema, although adverse effects from long-term use mandate that they be used at the lowest dose for the shortest time. When urticaria is resistant to treatment, other immunomodulating agents have been used, including cyclosporine, hydroxychloroquine, and IV immunoglobulin. These modalities require more intensive monitoring and cost.

Anaphylaxis is a medical emergency; prompt recognition and immediate treatment are crucial (Table 81–6). Early administration of IM epinephrine is the mainstay of therapy and should be given at the same time basic measures of cardiopulmonary resuscitation are being performed. If the child is not in a medical setting, emergency medical services should be called.

TABLE 81–6. Management of Acute Anaphylaxis

Immediate

Rapid assessment of airway, breathing, circulation; dermatologic examination; mental status assessment
Epinephrine, 0.01 mg/kg (1 : 1000) IM; repeat every 20 min as needed*
Oxygen 100%, secure and maintain airway
Start large-bore IV line for venous access and fluids
IV isotonic fluids, 20 mL/kg, repeat as necessary
Frequent vital signs, cardiac monitor, pulse oximetry
Rapid history for acute triggering event, known allergy and anaphylaxis history, current medications, history of asthma symptoms, concomitant medical conditions

Subacute

H_1 antagonist, diphenhydramine, 1-2 mg/kg PO, IM, IV
Corticosteroids, administered PO, prednisone, 1 mg/kg, or IV, methylprednisolone, 1-2 mg/kg
Nebulized albuterol, 1.25-2.5 mg every 20 minutes or continuously

Secondary

H_2 antagonist, ranitidine, 1.5 mg/kg administered PO or IV
Glucagon, 0.1 mg/kg IV, if refractory to initial treatment above and if patient is receiving β-blockers
Observe at least 4 hr for biphasic anaphylaxis

Disposition

If still symptomatic, admit for further treatment
If unstable vital signs, angioedema of upper airway, or refractory bronchospasm, admit patient to ICU
If symptoms have resolved without biphasic response, discharge patient on 72 hr of antihistamine, prednisone, and, if bronchospasm occurred with episode, albuterol metered-dose inhaler
Discuss allergen trigger and avoidance and EpiPen instructions and prescriptions
Follow-up with allergist

*May require continuous IV epinephrine infusion.
From Young MC: General treatment of anaphylaxis. In Leung DYM, Sampson HA, Geha RS, Szefler SJ (eds): Pediatric Allergy: Principles and Practice. St Louis, Mosby, 2003, p 646.

Supplemental 100% oxygen and IV fluid should be administered. Intubation or tracheotomy may be required. Additional pharmacologic therapies, such as corticosteroids, antihistamines, H₂-receptor antagonists, and bronchodilators, may be given to improve symptoms and lessen the biphasic response. A **biphasic reaction** can occur in 5% to 20% of patients with anaphylaxis with recurrence of symptoms 4 to 6 hours after the initial event.

PREVENTION

Prevention of urticaria, angioedema, and anaphylaxis focuses on avoidance of known triggers. A referral to an allergy specialist for a thorough history, diagnostic testing, and recommendations for avoidance is suggested for patients with severe reactions or anaphylaxis. Skin testing and serum IgE-specific testing are available for foods, inhalants, insect venoms, drugs (penicillin), vaccines, and latex. Educating the patient and family members about the signs and symptoms of anaphylaxis and using self-administered epinephrine early result in better outcomes. Fatal anaphylaxis has occurred, however, despite timely and appropriate treatment. A **MedicAlert bracelet** with appropriate information should be worn. Medications such as β-blockers, angiotensin-converting enzyme inhibitors, and monoamine oxidase inhibitors should be discontinued because they may exacerbate anaphylaxis or interfere with treatment.

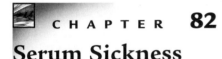

CHAPTER 82
Serum Sickness

ETIOLOGY

Serum sickness is a type III hypersensitivity reaction (see Table 77-1). Antigen-antibody or immune complexes form and enter into the circulation, where they are deposited in blood vessels and in filtering organs. These complexes cause tissue injury by activating the complement cascade and by recruiting neutrophils, resulting in increased capillary permeability, toxic mediator release, and tissue damage.

EPIDEMIOLOGY

Immune complexes were first described after administration of heterologous serum, such as horse serum for diphtheria. The availability of biologicals of human origin, bioengineered antibodies, and alternative pharmacotherapies has reduced greatly the incidence of serum sickness. Common inciting agents include blood products and foreign proteins, such as anti-thymocyte globulin and antivenoms. Medications frequently implicated include penicillin, sulfonamides, minocycline, cefaclor, hydantoins, and thiazides.

CLINICAL MANIFESTATIONS

The symptoms of serum sickness typically occur 7 to 12 days (up to 3 weeks) after the administration of drugs, foreign proteins, or infections. The illness can occur in 12 to 36 hours in previously sensitized individuals. Serum sickness is manifested by fever, malaise, lymphadenopathy, polyarticular arthralgias and arthritis, nephritis, hepatitis, and vasculitis. Cutaneous lesions vary and include urticaria, angioedema, morbilliform rashes, palpable purpura, and a characteristic serpiginous rash at the interface of the dorsal and palmar or plantar aspects of the hands and feet.

LABORATORY AND IMAGING STUDIES

Laboratory tests may show an elevated erythrocyte sedimentation rate, presence of circulating immune complexes measured by ^{125}I-C1q binding assay, and depressed complement (C3 and C4) levels. Skin biopsy specimens show immune deposits of IgM, IgA, IgE, or C3. Hematuria or proteinuria or both may be present.

DIFFERENTIAL DIAGNOSIS

The diagnosis is established by history of exposure to an inciting cause, characteristic clinical manifestations, and laboratory testing showing circulating immune complexes and depressed complement levels.

TREATMENT

Because serum sickness is self-limited and resolves within 1 to 2 weeks, treatment is symptomatic relief. Antihistamines may be administered to relieve pruritus. Aspirin and other nonsteroidal anti-inflammatory drugs are given for fever and joint pain, and if necessary, prednisone (1 to 2 mg/kg orally daily) is administered with a tapering dose. Allergy skin testing does not predict the likelihood of serum sickness development.

COMPLICATIONS

Carditis, glomerulonephritis, Guillain-Barré syndrome, and peripheral neuritis are rare complications.

PREVENTION

The primary means of prevention is to avoid use of the implicated agents.

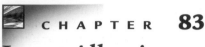

CHAPTER 83

Insect Allergies

ETIOLOGY

Systemic allergic reactions usually result from stinging insects of the order **Hymenoptera**, which include **apids** (honeybee and bumblebee), **vespids** (yellow jacket, wasp, yellow-face and white-face hornets), and **formicids** (fire and harvester ants). Honeybees have a barbed stinger that remains embedded after a sting. Yellow jackets are responsible for most allergic reactions in most parts of the U.S., whereas wasps are the most frequent cause of sting reactions in Texas. Fire ants are a wingless Hymenoptera found in the southeastern and south central U.S.

Biting insects rarely cause anaphylaxis. Anaphylaxis has been described, however, after the bites of kissing bug (*Triatoma*), bed bug, blackfly, and deerfly. Large local reactions from biting insects, such as mosquitoes, fleas, and flies, are a more common occurrence. The reaction appears urticarial and is caused by the salivary secretions deposited by the biting insect and does represent an allergic response.

EPIDEMIOLOGY

Allergic reactions to insect stings are a relatively common medical problem, estimated to affect at least 0.3% to 3% of the population. Reactions in adults are generally more severe than in children and can result in death.

CLINICAL MANIFESTATIONS

Symptoms may occur several days to weeks after the sting (Table 83–1). **Normal reactions** to insect stings, which are observed in 90% of children, include localized pain, swelling, and erythema at the sting site that usually subsides within 24 hours. **Large local reactions** occur in approximately 10% of patients and resemble IgE-mediated, late-phase reactions with prolonged swelling over a large area. **Systemic reactions** are IgE mediated and occur in 1% of children. They can be mild and non–life-threatening with cutaneous symptoms only or life-threatening with respiratory and cardiovascular symptoms of anaphylaxis (see Chapter 81). **Toxic reactions** may result if a person receives a large number of stings (50 to 100), such as occurs when a nest is disturbed. Symptoms include malaise, nausea, and emesis resulting from the toxic effects of the venom. **Unusual reactions**, such as vasculitis,

TABLE 83–1.	**Classification of Insect Sting Reactions**
Reaction Type	**Characteristics**
Normal	<2 inches in diameter
	Transient pain and erythema
	Duration <24 hr
Large local reaction	>2 inches in diameter
	Swelling contiguous to the site
	Duration 2-7 days
Systemic	
Non–life-threatening	Immediate generalized reaction confined to the skin (erythema, urticaria, angioedema)
Life-threatening	Immediate generalized reaction not confined to the skin with respiratory (laryngeal edema, bronchospasm) or cardiovascular (hypotension, shock) symptoms
Toxic	Follows multiple stings, produced by exogenous vasoactive amines in venom
Unusual	Serum sickness, vasculitis, nephrosis, neuritis, encephalitis
	Symptoms start several days to weeks after the insect sting

nephrosis, neuritis, serum sickness, and encephalitis, rarely are associated with insect stings.

LABORATORY AND IMAGING STUDIES

Skin testing with insect venom is the most sensitive method to determine the insect responsible. A positive skin test result shows only the presence of venom-specific IgE. The strength of the reaction does not correlate with the severity of the prior reaction or the likelihood or severity of possible future reactions. Future reactions correlate more with past individual patterns than with the strength of the skin test response. Venom-specific IgE antibodies also may be measured by in vitro serum tests (RAST); this technique has a 15% to 20% false-negative rate compared with skin tests. RAST may be positive in 5% to 10% of patients with negative skin test results; patients with a clinical history of a systemic reaction with negative skin tests also should undergo RAST.

DIFFERENTIAL DIAGNOSIS

A history of an immediate systemic reaction is necessary before venom testing and immunotherapy should be considered. Identification of the offending insect is often unreliable. Honeybee stings may be identified by the stinger that remains in place. Vespid stings are usually unprovoked and occur at summer's end when the insects are more aggressive.

TREATMENT

Local reactions should be treated by cleaning the site, applying cold compresses, and administering oral antihistamines and analgesics. In cases of large local reactions, a short course of prednisone may be advisable. Secondary infection, if present, should be treated with antibiotics.

Treatment of systemic reactions is guided by the severity of the reaction, but epinephrine is the cornerstone of therapy and should be administered without delay. Antihistamines may be administered concurrently with epinephrine. Corticosteroids should be given to prevent recurrent or prolonged symptoms. For severe reactions, IV fluids and epinephrine, oxygen, and respiratory support in an ICU may be needed.

COMPLICATIONS

Anaphylaxis may follow an insect sting and requires appropriate treatment (see Chapter 81). Secondary infection, usually with *Staphylococcus aureus* or *Streptococcus pyogenes,* may complicate insect stings.

PROGNOSIS

Successfully avoiding the stinging insect is the most important prognostic factor. Greater than 85% of adults who complete 5 years of immunotherapy tolerate challenge stings without systemic reactions for 5 to 10 years after completion.

PREVENTION

Commonsense measures to reduce the chance of accidental sting include exterminating infested areas, not eating or drinking outdoors, wearing long pants and shoes, and avoiding brightly colored clothing, fragrances, or hairspray when outdoors. Common insect repellents are not effective against Hymenoptera.

Current recommendations are to administer **venom immunotherapy** to children who have had a systemic life-threatening reaction from an insect sting and have positive venom skin tests or elevated levels of venom-specific IgE. In children younger than 16 years with a cutaneous reaction only, the risk of subsequent severe systemic reaction is the same as that of the general population. Because these reactions have a benign prognosis, they do not require immunotherapy and can be managed with the availability of epinephrine.

Children with a history of systemic reactions to insects should be instructed in the use of an epinephrine autoinjector, such as EpiPen (0.3 mg) or EpiPen Jr. (0.15 mg). A **MedicAlert bracelet** with appropriate information should be worn.

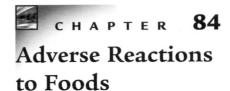

CHAPTER 84

Adverse Reactions to Foods

ETIOLOGY

An **adverse reaction to food** is a generic description of any untoward reaction after food ingestion. Adverse food reactions include toxic reactions, such as food poisoning, and nontoxic reactions, which can be subdivided further into nonimmune and immune reactions. An example of a nonimmune reaction is lactose intolerance. Food allergy or hypersensitivity reactions encompass immune reactions to food and can be divided further into IgE-mediated reactions, which are typically rapid in onset, and non–IgE-mediated reactions.

Food allergy or hypersensitivity reactions are the result of reactions to glycoproteins and develop in genetically predisposed individuals. In children, cow's milk, eggs, peanuts, soybean, wheat, tree nuts, fish, and shellfish cause 90% of IgE-mediated reactions. In older children and adults, peanuts, tree nuts, fish, and shellfish account for most reactions. Exposure to the allergenic food protein results in cross-linking of the IgE receptor found on the mast cells and basophils, which become activated and degranulate, releasing numerous potent mediators and cytokines. Non–IgE-mediated reactions typically occur hours to days after the allergen ingestion and typically involve the gastrointestinal tract. A cell-mediated immune mechanism may be responsible.

EPIDEMIOLOGY

Approximately 6% to 8% of children are affected with food allergy, which declines to a 1% to 2% prevalence in adulthood.

CLINICAL MANIFESTATIONS

Symptoms of hypersensitivity reactions vary from involvement of the skin, gastrointestinal tract, and respiratory tract to anaphylaxis. Non–IgE-mediated food allergy typically presents during infancy as proctitis/proctocolitis, enteropathy, or enterocolitis (Table 84–1).

TABLE 84–1. Non–IgE-Mediated Gastrointestinal Food Allergy or Hypersensitivity in Children

Feature	Proctitis/Proctocolitis	Enteropathy	Enterocolitis
Age of onset	Usually first 2-8 wk of life	Infancy to 24 mo	First 6 mo of life
Proteins involved	Usually cow's milk or egg or soy via maternal breast milk	Cow's milk, soy, cereals, egg, fish	Usually cow's milk, soy (both in 50%); also grains, poultry
IgE-mediated	No	No	No
Failure to thrive	No	Yes, with malabsorption, edema	Yes
Diarrhea	No	Yes	Yes
Vomiting	No	Mild	Yes
Hypotension	No	No	Possible
Blood in stool	Yes	No	Yes
Natural history	Tolerant by age 1 yr	Resolves by 2-3 yr of age	Usually resolves by 3 yr of age. Re-exposure before tolerance can result in delayed-onset (2 hr) vomiting and shock in 20%

From Sampson HA, Anderson JA: Summary and recommendations: Classification of gastrointestinal manifestations due to immunologic reactions to foods in infants and young children. J Pediatr Gastroenterol Nutr 30:S87-S94, 2000.

LABORATORY AND IMAGING STUDIES

In acute IgE reactions, skin prick allergy testing and serum testing to foods may help confirm the suspect food.

DIAGNOSIS

A careful history focuses on the symptoms, the time interval from ingestion to onset of symptoms, the quantity of food necessary to evoke the reaction, the most recent reaction and patterns of reactivity, and any associated factors, such as exercise and medication use. Skin prick testing can be performed to confirm IgE-mediated food allergies. A negative skin test virtually excludes an IgE-mediated reaction (unless the clinical history suggests a severe reaction after an isolated ingestion of the food). A positive skin test indicates sensitization, but does not prove clinical reactivity and must be interpreted based on the history.

In vitro RAST can be obtained for specific allergens. The CAP-RAST is a quantitative measurement of food-specific IgE antibodies and offers improved specificity and reproducibility compared with other RAST methods. These tests provide supplementary information to skin tests. Researchers have tried to determine concentrations of food-specific IgE at which clinical reactions are highly likely to occur (Table 84-2). Patients with CAP-RAST levels greater than the 95% predictive value may be considered allergic, and there is no need for an oral food challenge. Monitoring the CAP-RAST level may be helpful in predicting whether a child has "outgrown" the food allergy. Oral food challenges remain the "gold standard" and can be performed to determine if a child can eat the food safely.

TREATMENT

Injectable epinephrine, such as EpiPen (0.3 mg) or EpiPen Jr. (0.15 mg), is the initial treatment for severe allergic reactions to foods. Candidates include individuals with previous severe reactions, with allergy to foods that commonly cause severe reactions, and with food allergy and underlying asthma. Diphenhydramine can be used to treat mild reactions. Promising future therapies include injections with humanized monoclonal anti-IgE.

TABLE 84–2. Interpretation of Serum IgE Antibody Concentrations

Food	Food-Specific IgE Antibody Concentrations at or Above Which Clinical Reactions Are Highly Likely (IU/L)	Positive Predictive Value (%)
Egg	7	98
≤2 yr old	2	95
Milk	15	95
<2 yr old	5	95
Peanut	14	95-100
Fish	20	100
Soybean	30	73
Wheat	26	74
Tree nuts	~15	~95

From Sampson HA: Food Allergy. J Allergy Clin Immunol 111:S544, 2003.

COMPLICATIONS

Anaphylaxis is the most serious complication of allergic food reactions and can result in death (see Chapter 81).

PROGNOSIS

Approximately 85% of children have resolution of their hypersensitivity to egg, milk, wheat, and soy within the first 3 to 5 years of life. Sensitivity to certain foods, such as peanuts, tree nuts, fish, and shellfish, tends to be life-long. Twenty percent of children who first manifested peanut allergy at younger than 2 years old may outgrow it, however.

PREVENTION

Avoidance of the suspect food is paramount. Careful reading of food labels is a priority. A **MedicAlert bracelet** with appropriate information should be worn. The Food Allergy Network (www.foodallergy.org) is a useful educational resource for families and physicians.

Food allergy prevention is aimed at the "high-risk" newborn. Avoidance diets during pregnancy seem to have little benefit; however, avoiding peanuts may be prudent. Exclusive breastfeeding for the first 6 months is recommended and seems to be generally protective of food allergy. A lactating mother should avoid peanuts and tree nuts and, depending on the clinical history, possibly eggs, milk, and fish. An extensively hydrolyzed protein formula (e.g., Nutramigen or Alimentum) is recommended if the infant is to be bottle-fed or a supplement to breast milk is needed. The AAP recommends that solid food not be introduced until 6 months of age, dairy products deferred until 1 year of age, eggs until 2 years, and peanuts, nuts, and fish until 3 years.

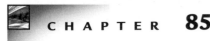

C H A P T E R 85
Adverse Reactions to Drugs

ETIOLOGY

Adverse drug reactions are commonly seen in the pediatric population and usually are caused by antibiotics. Drug reactions can be **predictable**, which are dose dependent and related to the pharmacologic actions of the drug, or **unpredictable**, which are independent of dose and often not related to the pharmacologic actions of the drug (Table 85–1). The Gell and Coombs classification can be used to describe some drug-induced allergic reactions (see Table 77–1). Many other

TABLE 85–1. Classification of Adverse Drug Reactions

Reactions	Example (Drug: Reaction)
Predictable	
Overdosage	Acetaminophen: hepatic necrosis
Adverse effect	Albuterol: tremor
Secondary effect	Clindamycin (and other antibiotics): *Clostridium difficile*–associated colitis (pseudomembranous colitis)
Drug-drug interaction	Terfenadine/erythromycin: torsades de pointes arrhythmia
Unpredictable	
Intolerance	Aspirin, at usual dose: tinnitus
Idiosyncratic	Chloroquine: hemolytic anemia in G6PD-deficient persons
Allergic	Penicillin: anaphylaxis
Pseudoallergic	Radiocontrast media: anaphylactoid

G6PD, glucose-6-phosphate dehydrogenase.
From Solensky R, Mendelson LM: Drug allergy. In Leung DYM, Sampson HA, Geha RS, Szefler SJ (eds): Pediatric Allergy: Principles and Practice. St Louis, Mosby, 2003, p 612.

drug reactions cannot be classified, however, because the exact immune mechanism has not been defined. Most drugs cannot elicit an immune response because of their small size; rather the drug or a metabolite acts as a hapten and binds to larger molecules, such as tissue or serum proteins, a process called **haptenation**. The multivalent hapten-protein complex forms a new immunogenic epitope that elicits T and B lymphocyte responses. Drug reactions to penicillins and cephalosporins are the most common allergic drug reactions encountered in the pediatric population.

EPIDEMIOLOGY

Approximately 6% to 10% of children are labeled as being "penicillin allergic." Risk factors for drug reactions include previous drug exposure, increasing age (>20 years old), parenteral or topical administration, higher dose, intermittent repeated exposure, and a genetic predisposition of slow drug metabolism. An atopic background does not predispose an individual to the development of drug reactions, but may indicate a greater risk of serious reaction.

CLINICAL MANIFESTATIONS

Allergic reactions can be classified into **immediate (anaphylactic) reactions**, which occur within 60 minutes of drug administration; **accelerated reac-**

tions, which begin 1 to 72 hours after drug administration; and **late reactions**, which occur after 72 hours. The most common form of adverse drug reaction is cutaneous. Accelerated reactions are usually dermatologic or serum sickness reactions. Late reactions include desquamating dermatitis, Stevens-Johnson syndrome, toxic epidermal necrolysis, and serum sickness.

LABORATORY AND IMAGING STUDIES

Skin testing is recommended as part of the diagnosis, but other laboratory testing and imaging studies are unnecessary.

DIFFERENTIAL DIAGNOSIS

The broadest experience with managing adverse drug reactions is with penicillin. Penicillin allergy should be evaluated when the individual is well and not in acute need of treatment. Penicillin skin testing is helpful for IgE-mediated reactions because of its negative predictive value; only 1% to 3% of patients with negative skin tests have a reaction, which is mild, when re-exposed to penicillin. Skin testing for penicillin should be performed using the **major determinant, penicilloyl-polylysine** (available as Pre-Pen), and **minor determinants**, which include penicillin G, penicilloate, and penilloate. The minor determinants are not commercially produced but are available at some medical centers. Skin testing to penicillin does not predict non–IgE-mediated reactions. In patients with a history consistent with serum sickness or desquamative-type reactions, skin testing should not be performed, and penicillin should be avoided indefinitely.

TREATMENT

If penicillin skin testing is positive, penicillin should be avoided, and an alternative antibiotic should be used. If there is a definite need for penicillin, **desensitization** can be accomplished by administration of increasing amounts of drug over a short time in a hospital setting. The exact mechanism of desensitization is unclear; however, it is thought to render mast cells unresponsive to the drug. To maintain desensitization, the drug must be given at least twice daily. If the drug is stopped for more than 48 hours, the patient is no longer considered "desensitized," and future courses of the antibiotic must be administered using the same protocol.

For other antibiotics, the relevant allergenic determinants that are produced by metabolism or degradation are not well defined. In these cases, skin testing to the native antibiotic in nonirritating concentrations can be performed. A negative response does not exclude allergy; however, a positive response suggests the presence of IgE-mediated allergy. In the case of a negative skin test response, a graded challenge or test dose may be administered, depending on the clinical history of the reaction. Patients who have experienced Stevens-Johnson syndrome, toxic epidermal necrolysis, or serum sickness should not be challenged.

COMPLICATIONS

Anaphylaxis is the most serious complication of allergic drug reactions and can result in death (see Chapter 81).

PROGNOSIS

Most drug reactions do not seem to be allergic in nature. Repeated, intermittent exposure during childhood or early adulthood contributes to an increased incidence of adverse drug reactions in adults.

PREVENTION

Avoidance of the suspect drug is paramount. A **MedicAlert bracelet** with appropriate information should be worn. One of the most common concerns in regards to allergic drug reactions is cross-reactivity between penicillin and cephalosporins because they both have a β-lactam ring in their structure. In children with a history of penicillin allergy, it is important to determine if they are truly allergic by skin testing to penicillin using the major determinant and minor determinants. If the penicillin skin test is negative, there is not an increased risk for an allergic reaction to cephalosporins. If there is a positive penicillin skin test, the patient can receive an alternate non–cross-reacting antibiotic, a graded challenge to the required cephalosporin under appropriate monitoring, or desensitization to the required cephalosporin.

For children with a history of a cephalosporin allergy who require another cephalosporin, two approaches may be considered. A graded challenge with a cephalosporin that does not share the same side chain determinant can be performed, or skin testing with the same or a different cephalosporin can be performed. A positive response suggests the presence of IgE-mediated allergy; the value of a negative test is unknown. Skin testing with cephalosporins has not been standardized or validated.

SUGGESTED READING

American Academy of Allergy, Asthma and Immunology: Pediatric Asthma: Promoting Best Practice. Milwaukee, Wis, American Academy of Allergy, Asthma, and Immunology, 1999.

Behrman RE, Kliegman RM, Jenson HB (eds): Nelson Texbook of Pediatrics, 17th ed. Philadelphia, WB Saunders, 2004.

Leung DYM, Sampson HA, Geha RS, Szefler SJ (eds): Pediatric Allergy: Principles and Practice. St Louis, Mosby, 2003.

NHLBI, National Asthma Education and Prevention Program: Expert Panel Report: Guidelines for the Diagnosis and Management of Asthma—Update on Selected Topics. NIH Publication No. 02-5075. Bethesda, MD, U.S. Department of Health and Human Services, 2002. http://www.nhlbi.nih.gov/guidelines/asthma/index.htm.

NHLBI, National Asthma Education and Prevention Program: Expert Panel Report II: Guidelines for the Diagnosis and Management of Asthma. NIH Publication No. 97-4051. Bethesda, MD, U.S. Department of Health and Human Services, 1997.

The Childhood Asthma Management Program Research Group: Long-term effects of budesonide or nedocromil in children with asthma. N Engl J Med 343:1054-1063, 2000.

RHEUMATIC DISEASES
OF CHILDHOOD

Hilary M. Haftel

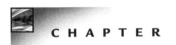

CHAPTER **86**

Assessment

The **rheumatic diseases (collagen vascular or connective tissue diseases)** of childhood are characterized by autoimmunity and inflammation, which may be localized or generalized. Vasculitis is a component of many rheumatic diseases and is the prominent element of Henoch-Schönlein purpura (HSP) and Kawasaki disease (KD). The classic rheumatic diseases of children include juvenile rheumatoid arthritis (JRA), systemic lupus erythematosus (SLE), and juvenile dermatomyositis (JDM). The musculoskeletal pain syndromes are a set of overlapping conditions characterized by poorly localized pain involving the extremities. Scleroderma, Behçet disease, and Sjögren syndrome are rare in childhood. The differential diagnosis of rheumatologic disorders includes postinfectious diseases, active infectious diseases, and malignancies (Table 86-1).

HISTORY

The history is important in identifying a possible rheumatologic condition. Symptoms reflect the source of the inflammation, including whether it is localized or systemic. Symptoms of systemic inflammation tend to be nonspecific. **Fever,** caused by cytokine release, can take many forms. A hectic fever, or fever without periodicity or pattern, is commonly found in vasculitides such as KD, but also occurs in children with underlying infection. Certain illnesses, such as systemic-onset JRA, produce a patterned fever with regular temperature spikes once or twice a day. Many other rheumatic illnesses cause low-grade fevers. Having family members chart the child's fever pattern, particularly in the absence of antipyretics, is useful. Rashes can occur in many forms (see Table 86–1). Other systemic symptoms include malaise, anorexia, weight loss, and fatigue, which can vary from mild to debilitating.

Symptoms of localized inflammation vary depending on the involved site. **Arthritis,** or inflammation of the synovium (**synovitis**), leads to joint pain, swelling, and impaired ability to use the affected joint. Morning stiffness or gelling is described. Parents may notice that the child is slow to arise in the morning and may have a limp. Children may elect to refrain from previous activities, such as athletics. **Enthesitis** is inflammation at the insertion of a ligament to a bone. **Serositis,** or inflammation of serosal linings, such as pleuritis, pericarditis, or peritonitis, gives rise to chest pain, shortness of breath, or abdominal pain. **Myositis,** or inflammation of the muscle, may lead to symptoms of muscle pain, weakness, or difficulty performing tasks of daily living. **Vasculitis,** or inflammation of the blood vessels, of small vessels deep in the papillary dermis leads to nonspecific symptoms of rash (petechiae, purpura) and edema; involvement of medium-sized vessels results in a circumscribed tender nodule.

PHYSICAL EXAMINATION

The combination of a thorough history and physical examination is frequently sufficient to narrow the differential diagnosis and elicit the appropriate diagnosis. An assessment of the child's overall appearance, evidence of growth failure, or evidence of failure to thrive may point to a significant underlying inflammatory disorder. The head and neck examination may show evidence of mucosal ulceration seen in diseases such as SLE. The eye examination may show pupillary

TABLE 86–1. Differential Diagnosis of Pediatric Arthritis Syndromes

Characteristic	Systemic Lupus Erythematosus	Juvenile Rheumatoid Arthritis	Rheumatic Fever
Sex	F > M	Type-dependent	M = F
Age	10-20 yr	1-16 yr	5-15 yr
Arthralgia	Yes	Yes	Yes
Morning stiffness	Yes	Yes	No
Rash	Butterfly; discoid	Salmon-pink macules (systemic onset)	Erythema marginatum
Monarticular, pauciarticular	Yes	50%	No
Polyarticular	Yes	Yes	Yes
Small joints	Yes	Yes	No
Temporomandibular joint	No	Rare	No
Eye disease	Uveitis/retinitis	Iridocyclitis (rare in systemic)	No
Total WBC count	Decreased	Increased (decreased in macrophage activation syndrome)	Normal to increased
ANA	Positive	Positive (50%)	Negative
Rheumatoid factor	Positive	Positive (10%) (polyarticular)	Negative
Other laboratory results	↓Complement ↑Antibodies to double-stranded DNA		↑ASO anti-DNase B
Erosive arthritis	Rare	Yes	Rare
Other clinical manifestations	Proteinuria, serositis	Fever, serositis (systemic onset)	Carditis, nodules, chorea
Pathogenesis	Autoimmune	Autoimmune	Group A streptococcus
Treatment	NSAIDs, steroids, hydroxychloroquine, immunosuppressive agents	NSAIDs, etanercept, methotrexate for resistant disease	Penicillin prophylaxis, aspirin, steroids

ANA, antinuclear antibody; ASO, antistreptolysin-O titer; GC, gonococcus; NSAID, nonsteroidal anti-inflammatory drug; WBC, white blood cell.

irregularity and synechiae from uveitis or the conjunctivitis of KD. Diffuse lymphadenopathy may be found and is nonspecific. The respiratory and cardiac examinations may show pericardial or pleural friction rubs, indicating serositis. Splenomegaly or hepatomegaly may be found on abdominal examination, raising suspicion of activation of the reticuloendothelial system that occurs in systemic-onset JRA or SLE.

The joint examination is crucial for the diagnosis of arthritis and may identify evidence of joint swelling, effusion, tenderness, and erythema from increased blood flow. Joint contractures may be seen. The joint lining, or synovium, may be thickened from chronic inflammation. Activation of epiphyseal growth plates in an area of arthritis can lead to localized, bony proliferation and limb length discrepancies (see Chapter 199). Conversely, inflammation at sites of immature growth centers may lead to maldevelopment of bones, such as the carpals or tarsals, resulting in crowding, or

the temporomandibular joints, resulting in micrognathia. The skin examination may show rash or may show evidence of underlying skin disorders, such as skin thickening from scleroderma or sclerodactyly. Chronic Raynaud phenomenon may result in nail-fold capillary changes, ulceration, or digital tuft wasting.

COMMON MANIFESTATIONS

The rheumatic diseases of childhood encompass a heterogeneous group of diseases with a shared underlying pathogenesis: disordered functioning of the immune system leading to inflammation directed against native proteins, with secondary increases in numbers of activated lymphocytes, inflammatory cytokines, and circulating antibodies. This antibody production can be nonspecific, but in certain diseases, antibodies can be targeted against specific native proteins, leading to subsequent disease manifestations (Table 86–2).

TABLE 86–1. Differential Diagnosis of Pediatric Arthritis Syndromes—cont'd

Lyme Disease	Leukemia	Gonococcemia	Kawasaki Disease
M = F	M = F	F > M	M = F
≥5-20 yr	2-10 yr	>12 yr	<5 yr
Yes	Yes	Yes	Yes
No	No	No	No
Erythema migrans	No	Palms/soles papulopustules	Diffuse maculopapular (nonspecific), desquamation
Yes	Yes	Yes	—
No	Yes	No	Yes
Rare	Yes	No	Yes
Rare	No	No	No
Conjunctivitis, keratitis	No	No	Conjunctivitis, uveitis
Normal	Increased or neutropenia ± blasts	Increased	Increased
Negative	Negative	Negative	Negative
Negative	Negative	Negative	Negative
↑Cryoglobulin, ↑Immune complexes	+ Bone marrow	+ Culture for GC	Thrombocytosis, ↑immune complexes
Rare	No	Yes	No
Carditis, neuropathy, meningitis	Thrombocytopenia	Sexual activity, menses	Fever, lymphadenopathy, swollen hands/feet, mouth lesions
Borrelia burgdorferi	Acute lymphoblastic leukemia	*Neisseria gonorrhoeae*	Unknown
Penicillin, doxycycline, ceftriaxone	Steroids, chemotherapy	Ceftriaxone	Aspirin, intravenous immunoglobulin

Although immune system hyperactivity can be self-limited, the hallmark of most rheumatic diseases of childhood is chronicity, or the perpetuation of the inflammatory process. This chronic inflammation can lead to long-term disability. Rheumatologic diseases often require the long-term use of immunosuppressive medications to control symptoms and prevent complications.

INITIAL DIAGNOSTIC EVALUATION

Although the rheumatic diseases sometimes can present with nonspecific symptoms, especially early in the course, each disease over time develops a characteristic set of symptoms and physical findings that can be elicited by careful history and physical examination. These data, in conjunction with carefully chosen confirmatory laboratory tests, help develop the appropriate differential diagnosis and eventually determine the correct diagnosis and treatment plan. The correct diagnosis is imperative to prevent any long-term disability associated with untreated chronic inflammation.

Most rheumatologic diagnoses are established by clinical findings or fulfillment of classification criteria. Use of laboratory testing should be judicious and based on a differential diagnosis rather than random screening in search of a diagnosis. Laboratory tests are used to confirm clinical diagnoses rather than develop them.

SCREENING TESTS

Evidence of an underlying systemic inflammation may be indicated by elevated acute phase reactants, especially the erythrocyte sedimentation rate (ESR), but also the white blood cell (WBC) count, platelet count, and C-reactive protein (CRP). The complete blood count may show evidence of a normochromic, normo-

TABLE 86–2. Manifestations of Autoantibodies

Coombs-positive hemolytic anemia
Immune neutropenia
Immune thrombocytopenia
Thrombosis (anticardiolipin, antiphospholipid, lupus anticoagulant)
Immune lymphopenia
Antimitochondrial (primary biliary cirrhosis, SLE)
Antimicrosomal (chronic active hepatitis, SLE)
Antithyroid (thyroiditis, SLE)
Antineutrophil cytoplasmic antibody (ANCA-cytoplasmic) (Wegener granulomatosis)
ANCA-perinuclear (microscopic polyangiitis)

Antinuclear Antibodies to Specific Nuclear Antigens and Associated Manifestations

Single-stranded DNA* (nonspecific, indicates inflammation)
Double-stranded DNA* (SLE, renal disease)
DNA-histone (drug-induced SLE)
Sm (Smith) (SLE, renal, CNS)
RNP (ribonucleoprotein) (SLE, Sjögren syndrome, scleroderma, polymyositis, MCTD)
Ro (Robert: SSA) (SLE, neonatal lupus–congenital heart block, Sjögren syndrome)
La (Lane: SSB) (SLE, Sjögren syndrome)
Jo-1 (polymyositis, dermatomyositis)
Scl-70 (scleroderma)
Centromere (CREST syndrome variant of scleroderma)
PM-Scl (scleroderma, UCTD)

*Because antibodies to single-stranded DNA (ssDNA) are a nonspecific response to inflammatory diseases and because ssDNA may contaminate double-stranded DNA (dsDNA) preparations, the purer, circular dsDNA of *Crithidia luciliae* (crithidia test) is preferred.
CREST syndrome, calcinosis, Raynaud phenomenon, esophageal dysfunction, sclerodactyly, telangiectasia; MCTD, mixed connective tissue disease; SLE, systemic lupus erythematosus; SSA, Sjögren syndrome antigen A; SSB, Sjögren syndrome antigen B; UCTD, undifferentiated connective tissue disease.
Adapted from Condemi J: The autoimmune diseases. JAMA 268:2882-2892, 1992.

cytic anemia of chronic disease. All of these laboratory findings are nonspecific for any particular rheumatologic diagnosis. Certain laboratory tests may help confirm a diagnosis, such as autoantibody production in SLE or muscle enzyme elevation in JDM.

DIAGNOSTIC IMAGING

Radiologic studies should focus on areas of concern identified by history or physical examination. Radiography of joints in patients with arthritis on examination may be beneficial, but radiographic abnormalities may lag far behind the clinical examination. More sen-

sitive tests, such as bone scan, CT scan, and MRI, may be useful when trying to differentiate between frank synovitis from traumatic soft tissue injury. MRI also can be useful to identify evidence of CNS involvement with SLE or for evidence of myositis with JDM.

CHAPTER 87

Henoch-Schönlein Purpura

ETIOLOGY

HSP is a vasculitis of unknown etiology characterized by inflammation of small blood vessels with associated leukocytic infiltration of tissue, hemorrhage, and ischemia. The immune complexes associated with HSP are predominantly composed of IgA, raising the suggestion that this illness may be allergy mediated, although this has not been proved. It also has been postulated that HSP is associated with group A streptococcal infection, but no causal association has been proved.

EPIDEMIOLOGY

HSP is the most common systemic vasculitis of childhood and of nonthrombocytopenic purpura, with an incidence of 13 per 100,000 children. It occurs primarily in children age 3 to 15 years, although it has been described in adults. HSP is slightly more common in boys than girls and occurs more frequently in the winter than the summer months.

CLINICAL MANIFESTATIONS

HSP is characterized by rash, arthritis, and, less frequently, gastrointestinal or renal vasculitis. The hallmark of HSP is the rash of **palpable purpura**, which is caused by small vessel inflammation in the skin leading to extravasation of blood into the surrounding tissues. IgA often is deposited in the lesions. Although the rash can occur anywhere on the body, it is classically found in dependent areas, below the waist on the buttocks and lower extremities. The rash can begin as small macules or urticarial lesions, but rapidly progresses to purpura with areas of ecchymosis. The rash also can be accompanied by edema, particularly of the calves and dorsum of the feet and the scalp and scrotum or labia. HSP occasionally is associated with encephalopathy, pancreatitis, and orchitis.

Arthritis occurs in 80% of patients with HSP and can occur in any joint, but tends to affect the lower extremities, most commonly the ankles and knees. Joint swelling can be confused with the peripheral edema that can be seen with the rash of HSP. The arthritis is acute and can be painful with refusal to bear weight.

Gastrointestinal involvement occurs in about half of affected children and most typically presents as mild to moderate crampy abdominal pain, which is thought to be due to small vessel involvement of the gastrointestinal tract leading to ischemia. Less commonly, significant abdominal distention, bloody diarrhea, intussusception, or abdominal perforation occurs and requires emergent intervention. Gastrointestinal involvement is typically during the acute phase of the illness and sometimes can precede the onset of rash.

One third of children with HSP develop renal involvement, which can occur as an acute or chronic event. Acute glomerulonephritis manifested by hematuria, hypertension, or acute renal failure can occur, although in most cases renal involvement is mild. Most cases of glomerulonephritis occur within the first few months of presentation, but rarely patients develop late renal disease, which ultimately can lead to decreased renal function and chronic renal failure.

LABORATORY AND IMAGING STUDIES

Patients with HSP show evidence of systemic inflammation with elevated ESR, CRP, and WBC count. The platelet count is the most important test because HSP is characterized by nonthrombocytopenic purpura with a normal, or even high, platelet count. The presence of normal platelet numbers differentiates HSP from other causes of purpura that are associated with thrombocytopenia, such as autoimmune thrombocytopenia, SLE, or leukemia. The urine should be screened by urinalysis for evidence of hematuria, and serum BUN and creatinine should be obtained to evaluate renal function. Testing the stool for blood may identify evidence of gut ischemia. Any question of gut perforation requires radiologic investigation.

DIFFERENTIAL DIAGNOSIS

The diagnosis of HSP is based on the presence of two of four criteria (Table 87–1), which provides 87.1% sensitivity and 87.7% specificity for the disease. The differential diagnosis includes other systemic vasculitides (Table 87–2) and diseases associated with thrombocytopenic purpura, such as idiopathic thrombocytopenic purpura and leukemia.

TREATMENT

Therapy for HSP is supportive. A short-term course of nonsteroidal anti-inflammatory drugs (NSAIDs) can be administered for the acute arthritis. Use of systemic

TABLE 87–1. Criteria for Diagnosis of Henoch-Schönlein Purpura*

Criteria	Definition
Palpable purpura	Raised, palpable hemorrhagic skin lesions in the absence of thrombocytopenia
Bowel angina	Diffuse abdominal pain or the diagnosis of bowel ischemia
Diagnostic biopsy	Histologic changes showing granulocytes in the walls of arterioles or venules
Pediatric age group	Age ≤20 years at onset of symptoms

*The diagnosis of Henoch-Schönlein purpura is based on the presence of two of four criteria.

corticosteroids usually is reserved for children with gastrointestinal disease and provides significant relief of abdominal pain. A typical dosing regimen is prednisone, 1 mg/kg/day for 1 to 2 weeks followed by a taper schedule. It is possible, however, for the abdominal pain to return as corticosteroids are being weaned, necessitating a longer course of treatment. Acute nephritis

TABLE 87–2. Classification of Vasculitides

Antineutrophil Cytoplasmic Antibody–Associated Vasculitis
Wegener granulomatosis Polyarteritis nodosa Churg-Strauss syndrome
Hypersensitivity Syndromes
Henoch-Schönlein purpura Serum sickness (e.g., drug-related) Vasculitis associated with infections
Connective Tissue Diseases
Systemic lupus erythematosus Dermatomyositis Juvenile rheumatoid arthritis
Giant Cell Arteritis
Temporal arteritis Takayasu arteritis
Others
Behçet syndrome Kawasaki disease Hypocomplementemic urticarial vasculitis

typically is treated with corticosteroids, but may require more aggressive immunosuppressive therapy.

COMPLICATIONS

Most cases of HSP are uniphasic in nature, lasting 3 to 4 weeks, then resolving completely. The rash can wax and wane, however, for 1 year after HSP, and parents should be warned regarding possible recurrences. The arthritis of HSP does not leave any permanent joint damage, and it does not typically recur. Gastrointestinal involvement can lead to temporary abnormal peristalsis that poses a risk for intussusception, which may be followed by complete obstruction or infarction with bowel perforation. Any child with a recent history of HSP who presents with acute abdominal pain, obstipation, or diarrhea should be evaluated for intussusception. Renal involvement rarely may lead to acute renal failure.

PROGNOSIS

The prognosis of HSP is excellent because most children have complete resolution of the illness without any significant sequelae. Patients with HSP renal disease (elevated BUN, persistent high-grade proteinuria) are at highest risk for long-term complications, such as hypertension or renal insufficiency, particularly if the initial course was marked by significant nephritis. There is a long-term risk of progression to end-stage renal disease in less than 1% of children with HSP. The rare patients who develop end-stage renal disease may require renal transplantation. HSP may recur in the transplanted kidney.

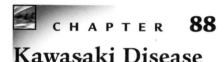

C H A P T E R **88**

Kawasaki Disease

ETIOLOGY

KD is a vasculitis of unknown etiology that is characterized by multisystem involvement and inflammation of small to medium-sized arteries with resulting aneurysm formation. Although many causes of KD have been hypothesized, no single underlying etiology has been ascertained.

EPIDEMIOLOGY

KD is a common vasculitis of childhood that has been described in variable frequency in all parts of the world, the highest of which is in Japan. The incidence in the U.S. is approximately 6 per 100,000 children younger than age 5 years. Although KD can affect children of all races, it is more common among children of Asian descent. KD most commonly occurs in children younger than age 5, with a peak between ages 2 and 3 years, and is rare in children older than age 7. A seasonal variability has been described with a peak between February and May, but the disease occurs throughout the year.

CLINICAL MANIFESTATIONS

The clinical course of KD can be divided into three phases, each with its own unique manifestations. Aneurysmal involvement of the coronary arteries is the most important manifestation of KD.

Acute Phase

The acute phase of KD, which lasts 1 to 2 weeks, is marked by sudden onset of a high, hectic fever (≥40°C) without an apparent source. The onset of fever is followed by conjunctival erythema; mucosal changes, including dry, cracked lips and a strawberry tongue; cervical lymphadenopathy; and swelling of the hands and feet. The conjunctivitis is bilateral and nonsuppurative. Cervical lymphadenopathy is found in 70% of children and should be greater than 1.5 cm in diameter for the purposes of diagnosis. A rash, which can vary in appearance, occurs in 80% of children with KD and may be particularly accentuated in the inguinal area and on the chest. Extreme irritability is prominent, especially in infants. Abdominal pain and hydrops of the gallbladder, CSF pleocytosis, and arthritis, particularly of medium-sized to large joints, can arise. Carditis in the acute phase may be manifested by tachycardia, shortness of breath, or overt congestive heart failure. **Giant coronary artery aneurysms**, which are rare but occur most commonly in very young children, can appear during this phase.

Subacute Phase

The subacute phase, which lasts until about the fourth week, is characterized by gradual resolution of fever (if untreated) and other symptoms. **Desquamation** of the skin, particularly of the fingers and toes, appears at this point. The platelet count, previously normal or slightly elevated, increases to a significant degree (often >1 million/mm^3). This phase heralds the onset of **coronary artery aneurysms**, which usually appear in the subacute and convalescent phases, and pose the highest risk of sudden death. Risk factors for development of coronary artery aneurysms include prolonged fever, prolonged elevation of inflammatory parameters such as the ESR, age younger than 1 year, and male gender.

Convalescent Phase

The convalescent phase begins with the disappearance of clinical symptoms and continues until the ESR returns to normal, usually 6 to 8 weeks after the onset of illness. Beau lines of the fingernails may appear during this phase.

LABORATORY AND IMAGING STUDIES

It is particularly important to exclude other causes of fever, notably infection. It is appropriate to obtain blood and urine cultures and to perform a chest x-ray. In the acute phase, inflammatory parameters are elevated, including WBC count, platelet count, and the ESR, which can be profoundly elevated (often >80 mm/hr). A lumbar puncture, if performed to exclude infection, may show pleocytosis. Tests of hepatobiliary function may be abnormal. Greatly elevated platelet counts develop during the subacute phase. The development of coronary artery aneurysms is identified by performing two-dimensional echocardiograms, usually during the acute phase, at 2 to 3 weeks, and at 6 to 8 weeks. More frequent echocardiograms and, potentially, coronary angiography are indicated for patients who develop coronary artery abnormalities.

DIFFERENTIAL DIAGNOSIS

The diagnosis of KD is based on the presence of fever for more than 5 days without an identifiable source and the presence of four of five other clinical criteria (Table 88–1). It is possible to establish a diagnosis of **atypical KD** if only three clinical criteria are present if the coronary artery aneurysms can be identified. Because many of the manifestations of KD are found in other illnesses, many diagnoses must be considered and excluded before the diagnosis of KD can be established (Table 88–2).

TREATMENT

IV immunoglobulin (IVIG) is the mainstay of therapy for KD, although the mechanism of action is unknown. A single dose of IVIG (2 g/kg over 12 hours) results in rapid defervescence and resolution of clinical illness in most patients and more importantly reduces the incidence of coronary artery aneurysms in patients with KD. Aspirin is initially given in **anti-inflammatory doses** (80 to 100 mg/kg/day divided every 6 hours) in the acute phase. When the fever has resolved for at least 48 hours, the dose of aspirin is decreased to **antithrombotic doses** (3 to 5 mg/kg/day as a single dose). This dose is continued through the subacute and convalescent phases, usually for 6 to 8 weeks, until follow-up echocardiography fails to show the presence of coronary artery aneurysms.

TABLE 88–1. Criteria for Diagnosis of Kawasaki Disease

Fever of ≥5 days' duration associated with at least 4* of the following 5 changes
  Bilateral nonsuppurative conjunctivitis
  One of more changes of the mucous membranes of the upper respiratory tract, including pharyngeal injection, dry fissured lips, injected lips, and "strawberry" tongue
  One or more changes of the extremities, including peripheral erythema, peripheral edema, periungual desquamation, and generalized desquamation
  Polymorphous rash, primarily truncal
  Cervical lymphadenopathy >1.5 cm in diameter
Disease cannot be explained by some other known disease process

*A diagnosis of Kawasaki disease can be made if fever and only 3 changes are present in conjunction with coronary artery disease documented by two-dimensional echocardiography or coronary angiography.

Approximately 3% to 5% of children with KD initially fail to respond satisfactorily to IVIG therapy. Most of these patients respond to retreatment with IVIG (2 g/kg over 12 hours). Corticosteroids are rarely used in KD, as opposed to other vasculitides, but may have a role during the acute phase if active carditis is apparent and for children with persistent fever after two doses of IVIG.

TABLE 88–2. Differential Diagnosis of Kawasaki Disease

Infectious

Scarlet fever
Epstein-Barr virus
Adenovirus
Meningococcemia
Measles
Rubella
Roseola infantum
Staphylococcal toxic shock syndrome
Scalded skin syndrome
Toxoplasmosis
Leptospirosis
Rocky Mountain spotted fever

Inflammatory

Juvenile rheumatoid arthritis (systemic onset)
Polyarteritis nodosa
Behçet syndrome

Hypersensitivity

Drug reaction
Stevens-Johnson syndrome (erythema multiforme)

TABLE 88–3.   Complications of Kawasaki Disease
Coronary artery thrombosis
Peripheral artery aneurysm
Coronary artery aneurysms
Myocardial infarction
Myopericarditis
Congestive heart failure
Hydrops of gallbladder
Aseptic meningitis
Irritability
Arthritis
Sterile pyuria (urethritis)
Thombocytosis (late)
Diarrhea
Pancreatitis
Peripheral gangrene

COMPLICATIONS

There are few long-term complications of KD because most cases resolve without sequelae. There have been reports of sudden cardiac death in older children who have been shown on autopsy to have coronary artery aneurysms, which may have been due to past KD. Myocardial infarction also has been documented, most likely caused by stenosis of a coronary artery at the site of an aneurysm. Other complications are listed in Table 88-3.

PROGNOSIS

IVIG reduces the prevalence of coronary artery disease from 20% to 25% in children treated with aspirin alone to 2% to 4% in children treated with IVIG and aspirin. Other than the risk for persistent coronary artery aneurysms, KD has an excellent prognosis.

C H A P T E R **89**

Juvenile Rheumatoid Arthritis

ETIOLOGY

The chronic arthritides of childhood include several types of childhood arthritis, the most common of which is JRA, also known as **juvenile chronic arthritis**. The etiology of this autoimmune disease is unknown. The common underlying manifestation of this group of ill-nesses is the presence of chronic **synovitis**, or inflam-mation of the joint synovium. The synovium becomes

thickened and hypervascular with infiltration by lym-phocytes, which also can be found in the synovial fluid along with inflammatory cytokines. The inflammation leads to the production and release of tissue proteases and collagenases, which if left untreated can lead to tissue destruction, particularly of the articular cartilage and eventually the underlying bony structures.

EPIDEMIOLOGY

JRA is the most common chronic rheumatologic disease of childhood, with a prevalence of 1 : 1000. The disease has two peaks, one at ages of 1 to 3 years and another, broader, peak at ages 8 to 12 years, but JRA can occur in any age group. Girls are affected more commonly than boys, particularly with respect to the pauciarticular form of the illness.

CLINICAL PRESENTATION

JRA can be divided into three subtypes—pauciarticular, polyarticular, and systemic onset—each with particular disease characteristics (Table 89-1). Chronic arthritis typically presents with swelling of the joint with accom-panying effusion. Although the onset of the arthritis is slow, the actual joint swelling is often noticed by the child or parent acutely, such as after an accident or fall, and can be confused with trauma (although traumatic effusions are rare in children). The child may develop pain and stiffness in the joint and limit the use of the affected joint. The child rarely refuses to use the joint at all, although this does occur occasionally. Morning stiffness and gelling also can occur in the joint and, if present, can be followed in response to therapy.

On physical examination, signs of inflammation are present, including joint tenderness, erythema, and effusion (Fig. 89-1). Joint range of motion may be

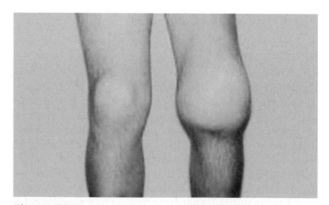

Figure 89–1

An affected knee in a patient with pauciarticular juvenile rheumatoid arthritis. Note sizeable effusion, bony proliferation, and flexion contracture.

TABLE 89–1. Features of Juvenile Rheumatoid Arthritis Subgroups

Feature	Pauciarticular	Polyarticular	Systemic Onset
No. joints	<5	≥5	Varies, usually ≥5
Types of joints	Medium to large	Small to medium	Small to medium
Gender predominance	F > M (especially in younger children)	F > M	F = M
Systemic features	None	Some constitutional	Prominent
Uveitis	+++	+	+
ANA positivity	++	+	–
RF positivity	–	+ (in older children with early onset RA)	–
Outcomes	Excellent, >90% complete remission	Good, >50% complete remission, some risk for disability	Variable, depends on extent of arthritis

ANA, antinuclear antibody; RA, rheumatoid arthritis; RF, rheumatoid factor.

limited because of pain, swelling, or contractures from lack of use. In children, owing to the presence of an active growth plate, it may be possible to find bony abnormalities of the surrounding bone, causing bony proliferation and localized growth disturbance. In a lower extremity joint, a leg length discrepancy may be appreciable if the arthritis is asymmetric.

All children with chronic arthritis are at risk for chronic **iridocyclitis** or **uveitis**. There is an association with the presence of HLA-DR5, HLA-DR6, and HLA-DR8 and uveitis. The presence of a positive **antinuclear antibody (ANA)** identifies children with arthritis who are at higher risk for chronic uveitis. Although all children with JRA are at increased risk, the subgroup of children, particularly young girls, with pauciarticular JRA and a positive ANA are at highest risk, with an incidence of uveitis of 80%. The uveitis associated with JRA can be asymptomatic until the point of visual loss, making it the primary treatable cause of blindness in children. It is crucial for children with JRA to undergo regular ophthalmologic screening with a slit-lamp examination to identify anterior chamber inflammation and to initiate prompt treatment of any active disease.

Pauciarticular Juvenile Rheumatoid Arthritis

Pauciarticular JRA is defined as the presence of arthritis in fewer than five joints within the first 6 months from diagnosis. This is the most common form of JRA, accounting for approximately 50% of cases. Pauciarticular JRA presents in young children, with a peak at ages 1 to 3 years and another broader peak at ages 8 to 12 years. The arthritis is found in medium-sized to large joints, with the knee being the most common joint involved followed by the ankle and the wrist. It is unusual for small joints, such as the fingers or toes, to be involved, although this may occur. Neck involvement and hip involvement also are uncommon. Children with pauciarticular JRA may be otherwise well and not show any evidence of systemic inflammation (fever, weight loss, or failure to thrive) or have any laboratory evidence of systemic inflammation (elevated WBC count or ESR).

Polyarticular Juvenile Rheumatoid Arthritis

Polyarticular JRA describes children with arthritis in five or more joints within the first 6 months of diagnosis and accounts for about 40% of cases. Children with polyarticular JRA tend to have symmetric arthritis, which can affect any joint, but typically involves the small joints of the hands, feet, ankles, wrists, and knees. The cervical spine can be involved, leading to fusion of the spine over time. In contrast to pauciarticular JRA, children with polyarticular disease can present with evidence of systemic inflammation, including malaise, low-grade fever, growth retardation, anemia of chronic disease, and elevated markers of inflammation. Polyarticular JRA can present at any age, although there is a peak in early childhood. There is a second peak in adolescence, but these children differ from the other group by the presence of a positive **rheumatoid factor**. Children with rheumatoid factor–positive polyarticular JRA most likely represent a subgroup with true adult rheumatoid arthritis, with a clinical course and prognosis that are similar to the adult entity.

Systemic-Onset Juvenile Rheumatoid Arthritis

A small subgroup of patients (approximately 10%) with juvenile arthritis do not present with onset of arthritis, but rather with preceding **systemic inflammation**.

This form of JRA is manifested by the presence of a typical recurring spiking fever, usually once or twice a day, which can occur for several weeks to months. This inflammation is accompanied by a rash, typically **morbilliform** and **salmon colored**. The rash may be evanescent and occur only at times of high fever. Rarely the rash can be urticarial in nature. Internal organ involvement also occurs. Serositis, such as pleuritis and pericarditis, occurs in half of children. Pericardial tamponade rarely may occur. Hepatosplenomegaly also is common, occurring in 70% of children. Children with systemic-onset JRA appear sick; they have significant constitutional symptoms, including malaise and failure to thrive. Laboratory findings also show the inflammation, with elevated ESR, CRP, WBC count, and platelet counts and anemia. The arthritis of JRA follows the systemic inflammation by 6 weeks to 6 months. The arthritis is typically polyarticular in nature and can be extensive and resistant to treatment, placing these children at highest risk for long-term disability.

LABORATORY AND IMAGING STUDIES

Most children with pauciarticular JRA may have no laboratory abnormalities. Children with polyarticular and systemic-onset disease commonly show elevated acute phase reactants and anemia of chronic disease, however. In all pediatric patients with joint or bone pain, a complete blood count should be performed to exclude leukemia, which also can present with limb pain (see Chapters 155 and 185). Other indicators for leukemia include a low WBC count or platelet count, instead of elevated values, or significantly lower hemoglobin than would be expected with anemia of chronic disease alone. All patients with pauciarticular JRA should have an ANA to help identify patients at higher risk for uveitis. Older children and adolescents with polyarticular disease should have a rheumatoid factor performed to identify children with early onset adult rheumatoid arthritis.

Diagnostic arthrocentesis may be necessary to exclude suppurative arthritis in children who present with acute onset of monarticular symptoms. The synovial fluid WBC count is typically less than 50,000 to 100,000/mm^3 and should be predominantly lymphocytes, rather than neutrophils seen with suppurative arthritis and should have a negative Gram stain and culture (see Chapter 118).

The most common radiologic finding in the early stages of JRA is a normal bone x-ray. Over time, periarticular osteopenia resulting from decreased mineralization is most commonly found. Growth centers may be slow to develop, whereas there may be accelerated maturation of growth plates or evidence of bony proliferation. Erosions of bony articular surfaces may be a late finding. If the cervical spine is involved, fusion of C1-4 may occur, and atlantoaxial subluxation may be demonstrable.

DIFFERENTIAL DIAGNOSIS

The diagnosis of JRA is established by the presence of arthritis, the duration of the disease for at least 6 weeks, and the exclusion of other possible diagnoses. Although a presumptive diagnosis of systemic-onset JRA can be established for a child during the systemic phase, a definitive diagnosis is not possible until arthritis develops. Children must be younger than 16 years old at time of onset of disease; the diagnosis of JRA does not change when the child becomes an adult. Because there are so many other causes of arthritis, these disorders need to be excluded before providing a definitive diagnosis of JRA (Table 89–2). The acute arthritides can affect the same joints as JRA, but have a shorter time course. In particular, JRA can be confused with the spondyloarthropathies, which are associated with spinal involvement, and enthesitis, which is inflammation of tendinous insertions. All of the pediatric spondyloarthropathies can present with peripheral arthritis before other manifestations and initially may be diagnosed as JRA (Table 89–3).

TREATMENT

The treatment of JRA focuses on suppressing inflammation, preserving and maximizing function, preventing deformity, and preventing blindness. NSAIDs are the first choice in the treatment of JRA. Naproxen, sulindac, ibuprofen, indomethacin, and others all have been used successfully. Aspirin products, the mainstay of arthritis treatment in the past, have been replaced in large part by NSAIDs, not only because of concerns about Reye syndrome, but also because of the convenience of twice daily rather than four times daily dosing. Systemic corticosteroid medications, such as prednisone and prednisolone, should be avoided in all but the most extreme circumstances, such as for severe systemic-onset JRA with internal organ involvement or for significant active arthritis leading to inability to ambulate. In this circumstance, it is used as **bridging therapy** until other medications take effect. For patients with a few isolated inflamed joints, intra-articular corticosteroids may be helpful.

Second-line medications, such as hydroxychloroquine and sulfasalazine, have been used in patients whose arthritis does not come under complete control with NSAIDs alone. **Methotrexate**, given either orally or subcutaneously, has become the drug of choice for polyarticular and systemic-onset JRA, which may not respond to baseline agents alone. Methotrexate can cause bone marrow suppression and hepatotoxicity; regular monitoring can minimize these risks. For

TABLE 89–2. Differential Diagnosis of Juvenile Arthritis

Connective Tissue Diseases

Juvenile rheumatoid arthritis
Systemic lupus erythematosus
Juvenile dermatomyositis
Scleroderma with arthritis

Seronegative Spondyloarthropathies

Seronegative enthesopathy/arthropathy
  syndrome
Juvenile ankylosing spondylitis
Psoriatic arthritis
Reiter syndrome
Arthritis associated with inflammatory bowel
  disease

Infectious Arthritis

Bacterial arthritis
Viral arthritis
Fungal arthritis
Lyme disease

Reactive Arthritis

Poststreptococcal arthritis
Rheumatic fever
Toxic synovitis
Henoch-Schönlein purpura

Orthopedic Disorders

Traumatic arthritis
Legg-Calvé-Perthes disease
Slipped capital femoral epiphysis
Osteochondritis dissecans
Chondromalacia patellae

Musculoskeletal Pain Syndromes

Growing pains
Hypermobility syndromes
Myofascial pain syndromes/fibromyalgia
Reflex sympathetic dystrophy

Hematologic/Oncologic Disorders

Leukemia
Lymphoma
Sickle cell disease
Thalassemia
Malignant and benign tumors of bone, cartilage, or
  synovium
Metastatic bone disease

Miscellaneous

Rickets/metabolic bone disease
Lysosomal storage diseases
Heritable disorders of collagen

patients who do not respond to NSAIDs, second-line medications, or methotrexate, there are now agents available to control arthritis by blocking the cytokine tumor necrosis factor-α. These medications, including **etanercept** and **infliximab**, have been shown to be effective in the treatment of JRA by blocking the inflammatory cascade.

COMPLICATIONS

Complications with JRA result primarily from the loss of function of an involved joint secondary to joint contractures or bony fusion or loss of joint space. Physical and occupational therapy, professionally and through home programs, are crucial to the treatment of the

TABLE 89–3. Comparison of Juvenile Rheumatoid Arthritis and Spondyloarthropathies

Clinical Manifestations	JRA	JAS	PsA	IBD
Gender predominance	F	M	Equal	Equal
Peripheral arthritis	+++	+	++	+
Back symptoms	–	+++	+	++
Family history	–	++	++	+
ANA positivity	++	–	–	–
HLA-B27 positivity	–	++	–	+
RF positivity	+ (in early-onset JRA)	–	–	–
Extra-articular manifestations	Systemic symptoms (systemic-onset JRA)	Enthesopathy	Psoriasis, nail changes	Bowel symptoms
Eye disease	Anterior uveitis	Iritis	Posterior uveitis	Anterior uveitis

ANA, antinuclear antibody; IBD, inflammatory bowel disease; JAS, juvenile ankylosing spondylitis; JRA, juvenile rheumatoid arthritis; PsA, poststreptococcal arthritis; RF, rheumatoid factor.

disease to preserve and maximize function. More serious complications stem from the associated uveitis, which if left untreated can lead to serious visual loss or blindness.

PROGNOSIS

The prognosis of JRA is excellent, with an overall 85% complete remission rate. Children with pauciarticular JRA uniformly tend to do well, whereas children with polyarticular disease and systemic-onset disease constitute most children with functional disability. Systemic-onset disease, a positive rheumatoid factor, poor response to therapy, and the presence of erosions on x-ray all connote a poorer prognosis. The importance of physical and occupational therapy cannot be overstated because when the disease remits, the physical limitations remain with the patient into adulthood.

CHAPTER 90
Systemic Lupus Erythematosus

ETIOLOGY

SLE is a multisystem disorder of unknown etiology characterized by the production of large amounts of **circulating autoantibodies**. This antibody production may be due to loss of T lymphocyte control on B lymphocyte activity, leading to hyperactivity of B lymphocytes, which leads to nonspecific and specific antibody and autoantibody production. These antibodies form immune complexes, which can get trapped in the microvasculature, leading to inflammation and ischemia.

EPIDEMIOLOGY

Although SLE is thought to affect women of childbearing age, approximately 5% of SLE presents in childhood, mostly around puberty. SLE is rare in children younger than 9 years old. Although there is a female predominance of this disease in adulthood and in the teenage years, there is an equal gender distribution in children. The overall prevalence of SLE in the pediatric population is 10 to 25 per 100,000.

CLINICAL MANIFESTATIONS

Patients with SLE can present in an abrupt fashion with fulminant disease, or in an indolent manner (Tables 90–1 and 90–2). Nonspecific symptoms are common

TABLE 90–1.　Criteria for Diagnosis of Systemic Lupus Erythematosus*

Physical Signs

Malar (butterfly) rash
Discoid lupus
Photosensitivity
Oral and nasopharyngeal ulcers
Nonerosive arthritis (≥2 joints with effusion and tenderness)
Pleuritis *or* pericarditis (serositis)
Seizures *or* psychosis in absence of metabolic toxins or drugs

Laboratory Data

Renal Disease (Nephritis)
　Proteinuria (>500 mg/24 hr) *or*
　Cellular casts (RBC, granular, or tubular)

Hematologic Disease
　Hemolytic anemia with reticulocytosis *or*
　Leukopenia (<4000 on 2 occasions) *or*
　Lymphopenia (<1500 on 2 occasions) *or*
　Thrombocytopenia (<100,000/mm³)

Serologic Data

Positive anti-dsDNA *or*
Positive anti-Sm *or*
Evidence of presence of antiphospholipid antibodies
　IgG or IgM anticardiolipin antibodies *or*
　Lupus anticoagulant *or*
　False-positive VDRL for >6 mo
Positive ANA in absence of drugs known to induce lupus

*These are the 1997 revised criteria for diagnosing systemic lupus erythematosus (SLE). A patient must have 4 of the 11 criteria to establish the diagnosis of SLE. These criteria may be present at the same or at different times during the patient's illness. Additional, less diagnostic manifestations are noted in Table 90–2.
ANA, antinuclear antibody; RBC, red blood cell; VDRL, Venereal Disease Research Laboratory.

but can be quite profound and may include significant fatigue and malaise, low-grade fever, and weight loss.

　Skin disease can be a prominent finding. A raised, erythematous rash on the cheeks, called a **malar "butterfly" rash**, is common. This rash also can occur across the bridge of the nose, on the forehead, and chin. **Photosensitivity** also can be problematic, particularly during the summer months. Both of these rashes are improved with appropriate therapy. The rash of **discoid lupus**, by contrast, is an inflammatory process that leads to disruption of the dermal-epidermal junction, resulting in permanent scarring and loss of pigmentation in the affected area. If discoid lupus occurs in the scalp, alopecia ensues because of loss of hair follicles. **Raynaud phenomenon**, although not specific

TABLE 90–2. Additional Manifestations of Systemic Lupus Erythematosus

Systemic

Fever
Malaise
Weight loss
Fatigue

Musculoskeletal

Myositis, myalgia
Arthralgia

Cutaneous

Raynaud phenomenon
Alopecia
Urticaria-angioedema
Panniculitis
Livedo reticularis

Neuropsychiatric

Personality disorders
Stroke
Peripheral neuropathy
Chorea
Transverse myelitis
Migraine headaches
Depression

Cardiopulmonary

Endocarditis
Myocarditis
Pneumonitis

Ocular

Episcleritis
Sicca syndrome
Retinal cytoid bodies

Gastrointestinal

Pancreatitis
Mesenteric arteritis
Serositis
Hepatomegaly
Hepatitis (chronic lupoid)
Splenomegaly

Renal

Nephritis
Nephrosis
Uremia
Hypertension

Reproduction

Repeat spontaneous abortions
Neonatal lupus erythematosus
Congenital heart block

for SLE, also can occur in these patients, as can livedo reticularis.

Mouth and **nasal sores** resulting from mucosal ulceration are a common complaint in patients with SLE. This condition can lead to ulceration and perforation of the nasal septum, a finding that can be seen on physical examination. Because of reticuloendothelial system stimulation, lymphadenopathy and splenomegaly are common findings in SLE. In particular, axillary lymphadenopathy can be a sensitive indicator of disease activity. Serositis can be seen, with chest pain and pleural or pericardial friction rubs or frank effusion.

Renal involvement is one of the most serious manifestations of SLE and is common in pediatric SLE, occurring in 50% to 70% of children. Renal disease may range from microscopic proteinuria or hematuria to gross hematuria, nephrotic syndrome, and renal failure. Hypertension or the presence of edema should clue the clinician to the risk of lupus renal disease.

Arthralgias and arthritis also are common. The arthritis is rarely deforming and typically involves the small joints of the hands, although any joint may be involved. Patients with SLE also can develop myalgias or frank myositis, with muscle weakness and muscle fatigability. SLE can affect the CNS, leading to a myriad of symptoms ranging from subtle symptoms, such as poor school performance and difficulty concentrating, to seizures, psychosis, and stroke.

LABORATORY AND IMAGING STUDIES

Testing for SLE is performed for several reasons: to make the diagnosis, to determine prognosis, and to monitor response to therapy. Although a nonspecific test, a positive **ANA** is found in more than 97% of patients with SLE, usually at high titers. Because of its high sensitivity, a negative ANA has a high negative predictive value for SLE so that it is unlikely for a patient with a negative ANA to have SLE. The presence of **antibodies to double-stranded DNA** should raise suspicion for SLE because these antibodies are present in most patients with SLE and are found almost exclusively in the disease, as are antibodies directed against Sm (Smith). Antibodies to Sm are found in only approximately 30% of persons with SLE, limiting its clinical utility. Antibodies to Ro (SSA) and La (SSB) also can be found in patients with SLE, but were originally described in patients with Sjögren syndrome and are not specific to SLE. Likewise, patients with SLE can have antibodies directed against phospholipids, which also can be seen in other rheumatologic diseases and in primary antiphospholipid syndrome. These antibodies lead to an increased risk of arterial and venous thrombosis and can be detected by the presence of anticardiolipin antibodies, a false-positive Venereal Disease

Research Laboratory (VDRL) test, or a prolonged activated partial thromboplastin time.

Hematologic abnormalities also are prevalent in patients with SLE. Leukopenia, primarily manifested as lymphopenia, is common. Thrombocytopenia and anemia of chronic disease may be found. Rarely, patients with SLE develop Coombs-positive autoimmune hemolytic anemia, which is manifested by the presence of schistocytes and fragmented cells on peripheral blood smear. Excessive antibody production can lead to polyclonal hypergammopathy, with an elevated globulin fraction in the serum. Excessive circulating antibodies and immune complexes also lead to the consumption of complement proteins, with low levels of C3 and C4 and decreased complement function as measured by CH50. Effective therapy returns the low complement levels to normal. This is one way to monitor therapy except in some patients with familial deficiency in complement components, which itself predisposes to SLE.

Urinalysis shows hematuria and proteinuria, which is crucial in identifying patients with lupus nephritis. Serum BUN and creatinine should be obtained to evaluate renal function. Hypoalbuminemia and hypoproteinemia may be present. Elevation of muscle enzymes may be a clue for the presence of myositis. Elevated CSF protein and an elevated IgG-to-albumin ratio when comparing CSF with serum (IgG index) can indicate antibody production in the CSF and help diagnose SLE affecting the CNS.

DIFFERENTIAL DIAGNOSIS

Because SLE is a multisystem disease, it can be difficult to diagnosis early in the disease course. Suspicion for SLE must be high in patients who present with diffuse symptoms, particularly in adolescent girls. Many of the clinical manifestations of SLE are found in other inflammatory illnesses and during acute or chronic infection. Criteria have been developed for the diagnosis of SLE (see Table 90-1). The presence of 4 of 11 of these criteria has 98% sensitivity and 97% specificity for SLE.

TREATMENT

Corticosteroids have been the mainstay of treatment for SLE for decades. Initial use of pulse methylprednisolone and high-dose oral prednisone (up to 2 mg/kg) frequently are required to treat SLE, followed by cautious tapering to minimize recurrence of symptoms. NSAIDs have been used to treat the arthralgias and arthritis associated with SLE. Hydroxychloroquine is used not only for the treatment of lupus skin disease, such as discoid lupus, but also has been found to be helpful as maintenance therapy in the disease. Patients with SLE who take hydroxychloroquine have been

shown to have longer periods of wellness between flares of disease and decreased numbers of flares.

For lupus nephritis or cerebritis, corticosteroids and hydroxychloroquine frequently are not sufficient therapies. Cyclophosphamide is effective for the worst forms of lupus nephritis, with significant improvements in outcome and decreased rates of progression to renal failure. Similarly, CNS lupus has been shown to respond to cyclophosphamide. For patients who are not able to tolerate the tapering of their corticosteroids, the use of steroid-sparing agents, such as azathioprine, methotrexate, or mycophenolate mofetil, may be indicated.

Patients with SLE should be counseled to wear sun block and stay out of the sun because the sun has been shown to lead to flares of the disease. Because of this prohibition, patients benefit from supplementation with calcium and vitamin D to reduce the risk of osteoporosis that may result from prolonged corticosteroid use.

COMPLICATIONS

Long-term complications include avascular necrosis owing to corticosteroid use, infections, and myocardial infarction. Adult patients with SLE develop accelerated atherosclerosis, based not only on prolonged corticosteroid use, but also on the disease. All patients with SLE should be counseled regarding their weight and to maintain an active lifestyle to reduce other cardiac risk factors.

PROGNOSIS

Outcomes for SLE have improved significantly over the last several decades and depend largely on the organ systems that are involved. Worse prognoses are seen in patients with severe lupus nephritis or cerebritis, with risk of chronic disability or progression to renal failure. With current therapy for the disease and the success of renal transplantation, however, most patients live well into adulthood.

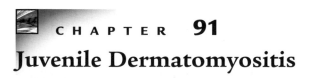

CHAPTER **91**

Juvenile Dermatomyositis

ETIOLOGY

The etiology of JDM is unknown, but it is characterized by activation of T and B lymphocytes, leading to vasculitis affecting small vessels of skeletal muscle, with immune complex deposition and subsequent inflammation of blood vessels and muscle. JDM has been documented to follow infections, allergic reactions, or sun exposure, but no causal relationship has been shown.

EPIDEMIOLOGY

JDM is a rare disease, with an incidence of less than 0.1 : 100,000. JDM can occur in all age groups, but has a peak incidence between ages 4 and 10 years. The disease is slightly more common in girls than boys.

CLINICAL MANIFESTATIONS

Dermatomyositis tends to present in a slow, progressive fashion with insidious onset of fatigue, malaise, and progressive muscle weakness, accompanied by low-grade fevers and rash. Some children can present in an acute fashion, however, with rapid onset of severe disease.

The muscle disease of JDM primarily affects the proximal muscles, particularly the hip and shoulder girdles, and the abdominal and neck muscles. Children have difficulty climbing steps, getting out of chairs, and getting off the floor. The patient may have a positive **Gower sign** (needing to lean on legs while getting up from the ground). In severe cases, the patient is not able to sit up from a supine position or even lift the head off the examination table (see Chapter 182). If muscles of the upper airway and pharynx are involved, the patient's voice will sound nasal and the patient may have difficulty swallowing.

Several cutaneous findings are associated with JDM. The classic **JDM rash** occurs on the face and across the cheeks, but also can be found on the shoulders and back (shawl sign). Patients may have **heliotrope discoloration** of the eyelids. Scaly, red plaques, called **Gottron papules**, classically are found across the knuckles, but can be found on the extensor surfaces of any joint. Patients may have periungual erythema and **dilated nail-fold capillaries**. Less commonly, patients develop cutaneous vasculitis, with inflammation, erythema, and skin breakdown.

At some point in their illness, 15% of patients with JDM develop arthritis. The arthritis commonly affects small joints, but can occur in any joint. Raynaud phenomenon, hepatomegaly, and splenomegaly also have been known to occur.

LABORATORY AND IMAGING STUDIES

Many patients with JDM have no evidence of systemic inflammation, with a normal blood count and ESR, indicating inflammation isolated to the muscle and skin. Evidence of myositis can be identified in 98% of children with active JDM by elevated serum muscle enzymes, including aspartate aminotransferase, alanine aminotransferase, creatine phosphokinase, aldolase, and lactate dehydrogenase. Electromyography and muscle biopsy can be used to document the myositis; MRI is a noninvasive means of showing muscle inflammation.

DIFFERENTIAL DIAGNOSIS

Diagnosis of JDM is based on the presence of documented muscle inflammation in the setting of classic rash (Table 91–1). A small percentage of children have muscle disease without skin manifestations, but polymyositis is sufficiently rare in children that they should have a muscle biopsy to exclude other causes of muscle weakness, such as muscular dystrophy, particularly boys. The differential diagnosis also includes postinfectious myositis and other myopathies (see Chapter 182).

TREATMENT

Systemic corticosteroids are the cornerstone of therapy for JDM. Initial treatment is high-dose oral prednisone (2 mg/kg/day in divided doses), which may be preceded by pulse IV methylprednisolone. Because of the toxicity associated with long-term corticosteroid therapy, it is common practice to add a steroid-sparing agent early, such as methotrexate. In severe or refractory cases, it may be necessary to use cyclosporine or cyclophosphamide. IVIG also has been shown to be useful as adjunctive therapy. Hydroxychloroquine or dapsone has been used for the skin manifestations; they do not significantly affect the muscle disease. Exposure to the sun worsens the cutaneous manifestations, but also exacerbates the muscle disease; sunlight may lead to flare. Patients should be advised

---

TABLE 91–1. Criteria for Diagnosis of Juvenile Dermatomyositis*

Rash typical of dermatomyositis
Symmetric proximal muscle weakness
Elevated muscle enzymes (SGOT, SGPT, LDH, CPK, and aldolase)
EMG abnormalities typical of dermatomyositis (fasciculations, needle insertion irritability, and high-frequency discharges)
Positive muscle biopsy specimen with chronic inflammation

*To make definitive diagnosis of dermatomyositis, 4 of 5 criteria are required.
ALT, alanine aminotransferase; AST, aspartate aminotransferase; CPK, creatine phosphokinase; EMG, electromyography; LDH, lactate dehydrogenase.

to wear sun block and refrain from prolonged sun exposure.

COMPLICATIONS

The most serious complication of JDM is the development of **calcinosis**. Dystrophic calcification can occur in the skin and soft tissues in any area of the body and can range from mild to extensive (**calcinosis universalis**). Although it is difficult to predict which patients will develop calcinosis, it seems to occur more commonly in children who have had cutaneous vasculitis, prolonged disease activity, or delays in onset of therapy. JDM patients who develop vasculitis also are at risk for gastrointestinal perforation and gastrointestinal bleeding. JDM also has been associated with lipoatrophy and insulin resistance, which can progress to frank type 2 diabetes. In these patients, control of insulin resistance frequently leads to improvement in muscle disease.

PROGNOSIS

The outcomes in patients with JDM depend greatly on the extent of muscle disease and the time between disease onset and initiation of therapy. JDM follows one of three clinical courses: a uniphasic course, in which patients are treated and improve without significant sequelae; a chronic recurrent course; and a chronic progressive course, marked by poor response to therapy and resulting loss of function. Patients who ultimately develop calcinosis also are at risk for chronic loss of mobility depending on the extent of calcium deposition. The association of polymyositis with malignancy is seen in adults and not in children.

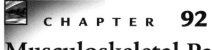

CHAPTER 92
Musculoskeletal Pain Syndromes

GROWING PAINS

Growing pains, or benign musculoskeletal pain syndrome, occur in 10% to 20% of school-age children. The peak age range is 3 to 7 years, and the syndrome seems to be more common in boys than girls. There is no known etiology, although there seems to be a familial predisposition.

Children with growing pains complain of deep, crampy pain in the calves and thighs. It most typically occurs in the evening or as nocturnal pain that occa-

sionally can awake the child from sleep. Growing pains tend to be more common in children who are extremely active; bouts are exacerbated by increased physical activity. The physical examination is unremarkable; there is no evidence of arthritis or muscular tenderness or weakness. Laboratory studies or x-rays, if performed, are normal.

The **diagnosis** of growing pains is based on a typical history and a normal physical examination. The presence of **hypermobility** excludes the diagnosis of growing pains. It is important to consider leukemia as a cause of nocturnal leg pain in children of this age group, so it is prudent to document a normal complete blood count. If the symptoms have persisted for some time, however, it is unlikely that an underlying malignancy is present.

The **treatment** of growing pains consists of reassurance and a regular bedtime ritual of stretching and relaxation. The pain can be relieved by massage. Some patients may benefit from a nighttime dose of acetaminophen or an analgesic dose of an NSAID. Occasionally, nocturnal awakening has been of long duration, leading to disruptive behavior patterns. In these cases, intervention must be aimed at decreasing the secondary gain associated with nighttime parental attention and should focus on sleep hygiene. Other than the negative behavioral patterns that can occur in the context of growing pains, there are no significant complications. Growing pains are not associated with other illnesses and resolve over time.

BENIGN HYPERMOBILITY

Hypermobility syndromes are disorders of unknown etiology that cause musculoskeletal pain secondary to excessive mobility of joints. These disorders most commonly present in children 3 to 10 years old. Girls are more commonly affected than boys. There is a familial predisposition to hypermobility syndromes.

Hypermobility can be isolated to a specific joint group or can present as a generalized disorder. Symptoms vary depending on the joints involved. The most consistent symptom is pain, occurring either during the day or at night. The discomfort can be increased after exertion, but rarely interferes with regular physical activity. Children with hypermobility of the ankles or feet may complain of chronic leg or back pain.

Joint hypermobility may be quite marked (Fig. 92–1). Range of motion may be exaggerated with excessive flexion or extension at the metacarpophalangeal joints, wrists, elbows, or knees (genu recurvatum). There may be excessive pronation of the ankles. Hypermobility of the foot (flat foot; pes planus) is shown by the presence of a longitudinal arch of the foot that disappears with weight bearing and may be associated with a shortened Achilles tendon (see Chapter 200).

These physical findings are rarely associated with tenderness on examination. No laboratory test abnormalities are associated with these disorders. Radiographs of affected joints are normal.

Excessive skin elasticity or mitral valve prolapse suggests **Ehlers-Danlos syndrome** or **Marfan syndrome** rather than benign hypermobility. The diagnosis of isolated hypermobility is made on the basis of physical examination with demonstration of exaggerated mobility of a joint. Generalized hypermobility is diagnosed by the presence of sufficient criteria (Table 92–1) and the absence of evidence of other underlying disorders.

The treatment of hypermobility consists of reassurance and regular stretching, similar to treatment for other benign musculoskeletal disorders. NSAIDs can be administered as needed, but do not need to be prescribed on a regular basis. Arch supports can be helpful in children with symptomatic pes planus, but are not indicated in the absence of symptoms. Benign hypermobility tends to improve with increasing age and is not associated with long-term complications.

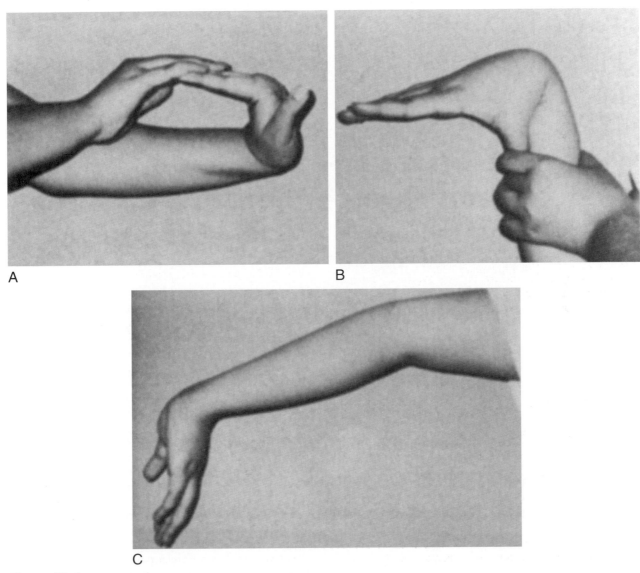

A

B

C

Figure 92–1

Features of hypermobility in children. **A,** Hyperextension of fingers. **B,** Apposition of thumbs. **C,** Hyperextension of elbows.

Continued

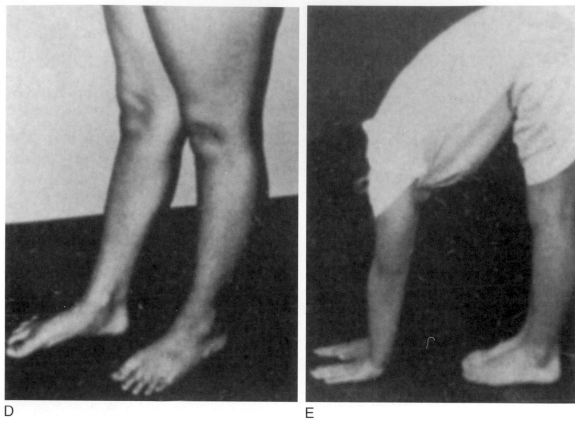

D

E

Figure 92–1, cont'd

D, Hyperextension of knees. **E,** Flexion of trunk. (From Gedalia A, Brewer EJ: Joint hypermobility in pediatric practice—a review. J Rheumatol 20:371-374, 1993.)

TABLE 92–1. Criteria for Diagnosis of Benign Hypermobility*

Touch thumb to flexor aspect of the forearm	1 point each for right and left
Extend fifth metacarpophalangeal joint to 90 degrees	1 point each for right and left
>10 degrees hyperextension of elbow	1 point each for right and left
>10 degrees hyperextension of knee	1 point each for right and left
Touch palms to floor with knees straight	1 point

*≥6 points defines hypermobility.

MYOFASCIAL PAIN SYNDROMES AND FIBROMYALGIA

The myofascial pain syndromes are a group of non-inflammatory disorders characterized by the presence of multiple **trigger points**, which are discrete painful sites, and fatigue, malaise, and poor sleep patterns. The etiology of these disorders is unknown, although there seems to be a familial predisposition. Although these disorders sometimes follow viral infection or trauma, no causal relationship has been shown. The myofascial pain syndromes are most common in adults but can occur in children (particularly >12 years old). The syndromes are more common in girls than boys. The prevalence of fibromyalgia in children has been reported to be 6%.

Patients with myofascial pain syndromes complain of long-standing diffuse pain in muscles and in the soft tissues around joints that can occur at any time of day, awaken the patient from sleep, and interfere with regular activities. Patients with these disorders frequently have high degrees of school absenteeism, despite maintaining adequate school performance. Patients with myofascial pain syndromes complain of malaise and fatigue and have a history of poor sleep hygiene and nonrestorative sleep. A significant percentage of patients with myofascial pain syndromes exhibit symptoms consistent with depression.

Physical examination is typically unremarkable, with the exception of the presence of trigger points that are painful—not just tender—to digital palpation. Trigger points often are located on the neck, back, lateral epicondyles, greater trochanter, and knees. There is no evidence of arthritis or muscular weakness on examination.

Patients with myofascial pain syndromes frequently undergo extensive medical testing because of the concern for underlying inflammatory disease associated with significant disability. These tests are invariably normal in the setting of myofascial pain syndromes. Children may have a false-positive ANA, which is found in 20% of the normal pediatric population.

The **diagnosis** of myofascial pain syndrome is based on the presence of multiple trigger points in the absence of other underlying illness. To fulfill strict criteria for a diagnosis of fibromyalgia, the patient must have a history of diffuse pain for at least 3 months and the presence of 11 of 18 specific tender points on examination. It is important to exclude underlying inflammatory diseases, such as SLE, or the postinfectious fatigue that characteristically follows Epstein-Barr virus and influenza virus infection. Mood and conversion disorders also should be considered.

Treatment consists of pain control, usually using NSAIDs, physical therapy, relaxation techniques, and education regarding sleep hygiene. Patients may require low doses of medications such as amitriptyline to regulate sleep. Education and reassurance are crucial in the treatment of these disorders: Because of the disability associated with myofascial pain syndromes, patients and parents frequently believe that the child has a serious underlying condition and may be resistant to reassurance. It should be emphasized to patients and parents that there is no simple cure for these illnesses, and time and perseverance are required.

The long-term outcomes in the myofascial pain syndromes vary. Patients and families who focus on therapy and are positive in their approach tend to have better outcomes. Patients who demand prolonged evaluations, especially from multiple healthcare providers, in search of a more defined diagnosis may do more poorly. Overall, children with fibromyalgia and myofascial pain syndromes have better prognoses than their adult counterparts.

SUGGESTED READING

Ballinger S: Henoch-Schönlein purpura. Curr Opin Rheumatol 15:591-594, 2003.

Barron KS: Kawasaki disease: Etiology, pathogenesis, and treatment. Cleve Clin J Med 69(Suppl 2):SII69-SII78, 2002.

Behrman RM, Kliegman RM, Jenson HB (eds): Nelson Textbook of Pediatrics, 17th ed. Philadelphia, WB Saunders, 2004.

Boon SJ, McCurdy D: Childhood systemic lupus erythematosus. Pediatr Ann 31:407-417, 2002.

Ilowite NT: Current treatment of juvenile rheumatoid arthritis. Pediatrics 109:109-115, 2002.

Klein-Gitelman M, Reiff A, Silverman ED: Systemic lupus erythematosus in childhood. Rheum Dis Clin North Am 28:561-577, 2002.

Nocton J: Arthritis. In Kliegman RM, Greenbaum LA, Lye PS (eds): Practical Strategies in Pediatric Diagnosis and Therapy, 2nd ed. Philadelphia, WB Saunders, 2004.

Rennebohm R: Juvenile dermatomyositis. Pediatr Ann 31:426-433, 2002.

Schneider R, Passo MH: Juvenile rheumatoid arthritis. Rheum Dis Clin North Am 28:503-530, 2002.

Sherry DD: Pain syndromes in children. Curr Rheumatol Rep 2:337-342, 2000.

Yalcindag A, Sundel R: Vasculitis in childhood. Curr Opin Rheumatol 13:422-427, 2001.

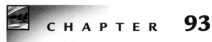

CHAPTER 93

Assessment

Infectious diseases range from minor upper respiratory tract infection to lethal sepsis. Occasionally, presumed noninfectious signs or symptoms are due to an infectious disease. Many nonspecific disease manifestations are presumed to be infectious. The foremost reason is the fear that an untreated minor infection may progress to a life-threatening illness if antibiotic treatment is not given. Many infections can be treated relatively easily with antimicrobial agents; a good clinical response while receiving antibiotic treatment is taken as evidence that it is not necessary to pursue noninfectious diagnoses. Nonetheless, many illnesses are short-lived and would resolve without antibiotics. The consequence is that many individuals are treated unnecessarily with antimicrobial agents. This unnecessary treatment has resulted in the serious problem of the development of antibiotic-resistant bacteria. Appropriate diagnosis of infectious and noninfectious diseases and providing specific treatment only as indicated would help reduce the unnecessary use of antibiotics.

HISTORY

A complete medical history is essential for assessment of infectious risk. The principal symptom can suggest a primary infectious disease or infection that is secondary to another disease, such as immunodeficiency or cystic fibrosis. The history may provide many potential clues for diagnosis of infection (Table 93-1). Family history, especially of unexpected deaths of male infants, may suggest familial immunodeficiency (see Chapters 73 through 76). Localization of the site of infection also is helpful (Table 93-2).

PHYSICAL EXAMINATION

A complete physical examination is essential to identify the signs of infection, which may be systemic, such as fever, or focal, such as localized signs of inflammation, including swelling, erythema, tenderness, and limitation of function. Many infectious diseases have associated cutaneous signs, which require firsthand examination of the patient to characterize the lesions accurately (see Table 97-1). Accurate otolaryngologic examination is key to diagnosing upper respiratory tract infections and otitis media, the most common childhood infectious diseases in the U.S.

COMMON MANIFESTATIONS

Attention to the common manifestations of infectious diseases usually leads to an appropriate diagnosis (see Table 93-2). Infections often have signs and symptoms recognizable at respiratory and gastrointestinal mucosal surfaces, where microbes first interface with the host. Viral infections of the respiratory tract rarely are limited to one target site. Pharyngitis with coryza and conjunctivitis suggests a viral (adenovirus) upper respiratory infection; if there is also cough, the diagnosis may be viral bronchitis. If there are signs of respiratory distress and crackles, viral or bacterial pneumonia is likely. Alternatively, if the only manifestation is severe conjunctivitis, the diagnosis is more likely to be a bacterial conjunctivitis (see Chapter 119). Table 93-3 presents variables that may help in differentiating viral and bacterial infections.

The host immune response varies with age, and neonates are at risk for different types of infections and have different clinical manifestations than school-age children or adolescents (see Chapters 65 and 66). The clinical manifestations and consequences of the inflammatory response may be more deleterious than the injury directly attributed to the pathogen.

TABLE 93–1. Clues from the History for Risk of Infection

Season of year
Age
General health
Weight change
Fever—presence, duration, and pattern
Previous similar symptoms
Previous infections and other illnesses
Previous surgeries
Preceding trauma
Presence of outbreaks or epidemics in the community
Similar illness in close contacts
Exposures to infected individuals
Exposures to farm or feral animals and pets
Exposures to ticks and mosquitoes
Sexual history, including possibility of sexual abuse
Illicit drug use
Place of residence
Travel history
Daycare or school attendance
Sources of water
Food and ingestion history, especially of undercooked meat or unpasteurized dairy products
Home sanitary facilities and hygiene
Presence of foreign bodies (e.g., indwelling catheters, shunt, grafts)
Immunization history
Current medications

Certain presentations of infections are medical emergencies. Severe gastroenteritis with extreme dehydration or sepsis with hypotension can lead to multiorgan damage and requires immediate fluid resuscitation and appropriate antibiotics (see Chapter 40). Infections of the airway, such as croup, epiglottitis, retropharyngeal abscess, peritonsillar abscess, or tonsillitis with obstruction from severe Epstein-Barr infection, can result in airway obstruction that may require emergent intubation or rarely tracheostomy (see Chapter 135). Fever, headache, vomiting, changes in sensorium, and signs of nuchal rigidity suggest bacterial meningitis and necessitate emergent lumbar puncture and examination of the CSF and a CT scan if indicated (see Chapter 100).

DIFFERENTIAL DIAGNOSIS

Fever does not always represent infection; children with overwhelming infection may be afebrile or hypothermic. Rheumatologic disease, inflammatory bowel disease, Kawasaki disease, poisoning, and malignancy also may present with fever. The varied manifestations of infectious diseases frequently mimic rheumatoid arthritis, lupus erythematosus, inflammatory bowel disease, leukemia, and lymphoma.

Many manifestations of infectious diseases mimic noninfectious diseases. Symptoms such as bone pain or lymphadenopathy that suggest infection also are symptoms that could be due to leukemia, lymphoma, juvenile rheumatoid arthritis, or Kawasaki disease (see Chapters 88, 89, and 153). Acute mental status changes or focal neurologic impairment could be due to infections, such as encephalitis, meningitis, or brain abscess; manifestations of brain or spinal tumors; inflammatory conditions, such as multiple sclerosis; postinfectious sequelae, such as acute demyelinating encephalomyelitis; or impairment owing to toxic ingestions or inhalants. If the underlying cause is an infection, the presenting manifestation may be CNS infection of bacterial, viral, fungal, or parasitic origin.

Certain infections are more common in specific geographic areas; parasitic infections are more common in tropical climates. Diarrhea may be bacterial, viral, or parasitic in the tropics, but in temperate climates parasitic causes of diarrhea other than giardiasis are much less likely. Certain fungal infections are common in specific geographic areas, such as coccidioidomycosis in the southwestern U.S., blastomycosis in the upper Midwest, and histoplasmosis in the central part of the U.S., especially in the states bordering the Mississippi and Ohio Rivers. In other areas, fungal pneumonias are rare except in immunocompromised persons.

Some infections are prone to recurrence, especially if the treatment is suboptimal or for a shorter duration than is recommended. Recurrent, severe, or unusual (opportunistic) infections suggest the possibility of immunodeficiency (see Chapters 72 and 125). Many manifestations of mucosal allergy (rhinitis, diarrhea) may mimic an infectious disease (see Chapter 77).

DISTINGUISHING FEATURES

Signs of inflammation, including fever, are routinely associated with infection, but inflammation is not specific and may reflect rheumatologic diseases, inflammatory bowel diseases, and cancer. The absence of fever may suggest an allergic etiology, unless secondary infection (sinusitis) occurs.

Initial complaints of infection may be nonspecific, especially in infants who present with fever, lethargy, irritability, excessive sleeping, or poor feeding. Certain individual physical findings, such as unique rashes, may be diagnostic (see Chapter 97). Because of the varied presentations of infectious diseases, it is important to investigate thoroughly every objective finding from the history and physical examination.

TABLE 93–2.   Localizing Manifestations of Infection

Site	Localizing Symptoms	Localizing Signs*
Upper respiratory tract	Rhinorrhea, sore throat, cough, drooling, stridor, trismus, sinus pain, tooth pain, hoarse voice	Nasal congestion, pharyngeal erythema, enlarged tonsils with exudate, swollen red epiglottis, regional lymphadenopathy
Ear	Ear pain or drainage	Red bulging tympanic membrane, drainage from ear canal
Lower respiratory tract	Cough, chest pain, dyspnea, sputum production, cyanosis	Tachypnea, crackles, wheezing, localized diminished breath sounds, intercostal retractions
Gastrointestinal tract	Nausea, vomiting, diarrhea, abdominal pain, anorexia	Hypoactive or hyperactive bowel sounds, abdominal tenderness (generalized or focal), hematochezia
Liver	Anorexia, vomiting, dark urine, light stools	Jaundice, hepatomegaly, hepatic tenderness, bleeding diatheses, coma
Genitourinary tract	Dysuria, frequency, urgency, flank or suprapubic pain, vaginal discharge	Costovertebral angle or suprapubic tenderness, cervical motion and adnexal tenderness
CNS	Lethargy, irritability, headache, neck stiffness, seizures	Nuchal rigidity, Kernig sign, Brudzinski sign, bulging fontanel, altered mental status, focal neurologic deficits, coma
Cardiovascular	Dyspnea, palpitations, fatigue, exercise intolerance, chest pain	Tachycardia, hypotension, cardiomegaly, hepatomegaly, splenomegaly, crackles, petechiae, Osler nodes, Janeway lesions, Roth spots, new or change in murmur, distended neck veins, pericardial friction rub, muffled heart sounds
Skeletal	Limp, bone pain, limited function (pseudoparalysis)	Local swelling, erythema, warmth, limited range of motion, point bone tenderness, joint line tenderness

*Fever usually accompanies infection as a systemic manifestation.

INITIAL DIAGNOSTIC EVALUATION

The ability to diagnose specific infection accurately in pediatric patients begins with an understanding of the epidemiology and risk factors associated with each infectious agent and the age-related susceptibility, which reflects the maturity of the immune system. Initial diagnostic evaluation requires accurately recognizing the site of the infection (see Table 93–2), recognizing all of the manifestations that are present, knowing all of the risk factors, recognizing exposure to potential infectious agents, and knowing the most likely organisms causing each infection and the usual host immune response to the infection. Obtaining a thorough history identifies most of these risk factors (see Table 93–1).

Antibiotics often are begun before a definitive diagnosis is established, which complicates the ability to rely on cultures for microbiologic diagnosis (see Chapter 95). Although persistent or progressive symptoms despite antibiotic treatment may indicate the need to change the regimen, they more frequently indicate the need to stop all antibiotics to facilitate definitive diagnosis by obtaining appropriate cultures. Antibiotics should not be given before obtaining appropriate cultures, unless there is a life-threatening situation (e.g., septic shock).

SCREENING TESTS

Laboratory diagnosis of infection includes examination of bacterial morphology using Gram stain, various culture techniques, molecular microbiologic methods such as polymerase chain reaction (PCR), and assessment of the immune response with antibody titers or skin testing (e.g., tuberculosis). The **acute phase response** is the nonspecific metabolic and inflammatory response to infection, trauma, autoimmune disease, and some malignancies. **Acute phase reactants,** such as erythrocyte sedimentation rate (ESR) and C-reactive protein (CRP), are commonly elevated during an infection, but are not specific for infection and do not identify any specific infection. These tests

TABLE 93–3. Differentiating Viral from Bacterial Infections

Variable	Viral	Bacterial
Petechiae	Present	Present
Purpura	Rare	If severe
Leukocytosis	Uncommon*	Common
Shift to left (↑ bands)	Uncommon	Common
Neutropenia	Possible	Suggests overwhelming infection
↑ESR	Unusual*	Common
↑CRP	Unusual	Common
↑TNF, IL-1, PAF	Uncommon	Common
Meningitis (pleocytosis)	Lymphocytic†	Neutrophilic
Meningeal signs positive‡	Present	Present

*Adenovirus and herpes simplex may cause leukocytosis and increased ESR; Epstein-Barr virus may cause petechiae and increased ESR.
†Early viral (enterovirus, arbovirus) meningitis initially may have a neutrophilic pleocytosis.
‡Nuchal rigidity, bulging fontanel, Kernig or Brudzinski sign.
CRP, C-reactive protein; ESR, erythrocyte sedimentation rate; IL, interleukin; PAF, platelet-activating factor; TNF, tumor necrosis factor.

are often useful to show response to therapy (e.g., osteomyelitis).

The **complete blood count** frequently is obtained to identify evidence of bone marrow response to infection. The initial response to infection, especially in children, is usually a **leukocytosis**, which is an increase in the number of circulating leukocytes, with a neutrophilic response to bacterial and viral infections. With most viral infections, the initial neutrophilic response is transient and is followed quickly by the characteristic mononuclear response. In general, bacterial infections are associated with greater neutrophilia than are viral infections. A **shift to the left** is an increase in the numbers of circulating immature cells of the neutrophil series, including band forms, metamyelocytes, and myelocytes. A shift to the left indicates the rapid release of cells from the bone marrow and characteristically is seen in the early stages of infection and with bacterial infections. Transient lymphopenia at the beginning of illness and lasting 24 to 48 hours has been described with many viral infections. **Atypical lymphocytes** are mature T lymphocytes with larger, eccentrically placed, and indented nuclei that classically are seen with infectious mononucleosis caused by Epstein-Barr virus (EBV). Other infections associated with atypical lymphocytosis include cytomegalovirus (CMV) infection, toxoplasmosis, viral hepatitis, rubella, roseola, mumps, and some drug reactions. **Eosinophilia** is characteristic of tissue-invasive multicellular parasites, such as the migration of the larval stages of the parasite through skin, connective tissue, and viscera. High-grade eosinophilia (>30% eosinophils, or a total eosinophil count >3000/μL) frequently occurs during the muscle invasion phase of **trichinellosis**, the pulmonary phases of **ascariasis** and **hookworm** infection (eosinophilic pneumonia), and the hepatic and CNS phases of **visceral larva migrans**.

Other common screening tests include **urinalysis** for urinary tract infections (UTIs), transaminases for liver function, and **lumbar puncture** for evaluation of the CSF if there is concern for meningitis or encephalitis (see Chapters 100 and 101). A grouping of various tests may help distinguish viral versus bacterial infection, but definitive diagnosis requires culture or PCR.

Cultures are the mainstay of diagnosis. Blood cultures are sensitive and specific for bacteremia that may be primary or secondary to a focus (osteomyelitis, gastroenteritis, urinary tract, endocarditis). Urine cultures confirm UTI, which may be occult in young infants. CSF cultures should be obtained with any lumbar puncture. Other cultures are determined by the presence of fluid collections or masses that are suspected to be infectious. Tissue culture techniques help identify viruses and intracellular pathogens. Rapid tests are useful for preliminary diagnosis and are included in numerous bacterial, viral, fungal, and parasitic antigen detection tests. Serologic tests, using enzyme-linked immunosorbent assay (ELISA) or Western blotting, showing an IgM response, high IgG, or seroconversion between acute and convalescent sera can be used for diagnosis. Molecular detection methods, such as **PCR** for DNA or RNA, offer the specificity of culture, high sensitivity, and rapid results. When an unusual infection is suspected, the laboratory must be notified before the sample is obtained.

DIAGNOSTIC IMAGING

The choice of diagnostic imaging mode should be based on the location of the findings. In the absence of localizing signs and an acute infection, imaging of the entire body is rarely productive. There is often more than one suitable approach to diagnostic imaging of suspected infections. Plain x-rays are useful for the middle and lower respiratory tract, but they have been superseded by cross-sectional imaging techniques. **Ultrasonography** is a noninvasive, nonirradiating technique well suited to infants and children for solid organs, such as the kidneys, liver, pancreas, and spleen. It also is useful to identify soft tissue abscesses with lymphadenitis and to diagnose suppurative arthritis of the hip. **CT** (with contrast enhancement) and **MRI** (with gadolinium enhancement) allow characterization of lesions and precise anatomic localization and are the modalities of choice for the brain. CT shows greater bone detail, and MRI shows greater tissue detail. High-resolution CT is useful for complicated chest infections. Contrast studies (upper gastrointestinal series, barium enema) are used to identify mucosal lesions of the gastrointestinal tract, with CT or MRI for evaluation of appendicitis and intra-abdominal masses. A voiding cystourethrogram (VCUG) is used to evaluate for ureteral reflux, which is a predisposing factor for upper UTIs. MRI is especially useful for diagnosis of osteomyelitis, myositis, and necrotizing fasciitis. Radionuclide scans, such as technetium-99m for osteomyelitis and dimercaptosuccinic acid (DMSA) for acute pyelonephritis or chronic renal scarring, are often informative.

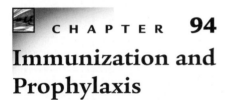

CHAPTER 94

Immunization and Prophylaxis

IMMUNIZATION

Childhood immunization has reduced the impact of major infectious diseases markedly. **Active immunization** is the process of inducing immunity by vaccination with a **vaccine** or **toxoid** (inactivated toxin). **Passive immunization** includes transplacental transfer of maternal antibodies and the administration of antibody, either as immunoglobulin or monoclonal antibody.

Vaccinations may be with live attenuated viruses (measles, mumps, rubella, varicella), inactivated or killed viruses (polio, hepatitis A [HAV], influenza), recombinant products (hepatitis B [HBV]), or immunogenic components of bacteria (pertussis, *Haemophilus influenzae* type b [Hib], and *Streptococcus pneumoniae*), including toxoids (diphtheria, tetanus). Many purified polysaccharides are T-independent antigens that initiate B cell proliferation without involvement of CD4 T lymphocytes and are poor immunogens in children younger than 2 years old. Conjugation of a polysaccharide to a **protein carrier** induces a T-dependent response in infants and creates immunogenic vaccines for Hib, *S. pneumoniae*, and *Neisseria meningitidis*.

Childhood immunization standards and recommendations in the U.S. are formulated by the Advisory Committee on Immunization Practices of the Centers for Disease Control and Prevention, the AAP, and the American Academy of Family Physicians. In the U.S., rates of 95% composite immunization in school-age children were achieved in the 1980s and 1990s, in part because of state laws requiring immunization for school entry. Children in the U.S. routinely receive vaccines against 12 diseases: diphtheria, tetanus, pertussis, poliomyelitis, measles, mumps, rubella, Hib infection, *S. pneumoniae* infection, HBV, influenza, and varicella (Fig. 94–1). This schedule of 12 vaccines requires up to 21 injections in four to five visits by 18 months of age. Children and adolescents who are at increased risk should receive additional immunizations as recommended for hepatitis A, pneumococcus (polysaccharide vaccine), and meningococcus. Children who are behind in immunization should receive catch-up immunizations as rapidly as feasible (Table 94–1). Infants born prematurely, regardless of birth weight, should be vaccinated at the same chronologic age and according to the same schedule and precautions as full-term infants and children (with the exception of HBV vaccine for infants weighing <2000 g if the mother is hepatitis B virus surface antigen (HB$_s$Ag)–negative, which should begin a 1 month instead of at birth). For adolescents, vaccines should be given at 11 to 12 years of age. Many colleges and universities require or recommend meningococcal vaccine before matriculation because of the increased risk of meningococcal disease, especially for freshmen living in dormitories.

Vaccines should be administered after obtaining informed consent. The National Childhood Vaccine Injury Act requires that all healthcare providers provide parents or patients with copies of **Vaccine Information Statements**, prepared by the Centers for Disease Control and Prevention (http://www.cdc.gov/nip/publications/vis) before administering each vaccine dose.

Most vaccines are administered by IM or SC injection. The preferred sites for administration are the anterolateral aspect of the thigh in infants and the deltoid region in children and adults. Multiple vaccines can be administered simultaneously at anatomically separate sites without diminishing the immune response. Measles, mumps, and rubella (MMR) and varicella vaccines should be administered simultaneously or at least 30 days apart. Administration of blood products and immunoglobulin can diminish the response to live virus vaccines if administered before the recommended interval.

General **contraindications** to vaccination include serious allergic reaction (anaphylaxis) after a previous vaccine dose or to a vaccine component, immunocompromised states or pregnancy for live virus vaccines, and moderate or severe acute illness with or without fever. History of anaphylactic-like reactions to eggs is a contraindication to influenza and yellow fever vaccines, which are produced in embryonated chicken eggs. Current preparations of measles and mumps vaccines,

TABLE 94–1

Catch-up Immunization Schedule for Children and Adolescents Who Start Late or Who Are >1 Month Behind, by Age Group, Vaccine, and Dosage Interval — United States, 2005

Catch-up Schedule for Children Age 4 Months Through 6 Years

Vaccine	Minimum Age for Dose 1	Minimum Interval Between Doses			
		Dose 1 to Dose 2	*Dose 2 to Dose 3*	*Dose 3 to Dose 4*	*Dose 4 to Dose 5*
DTAP[1]	6 wk	4 wk	4 wk	6 mo	6 mo[1]
IPV[2]	6 wk	4 wk	4 wk	4 wk[2]	
HepB[3]	Birth	4 wk	8 wk (and 16 wk after first dose)		
MMR[4]	12 mo	4 wk[4]			
Varicella	12 mo				
Hib[5]	6 wk	**4 wk:** if first dose given at age <12 mo **8 wk (as final dose):** if first dose given at age 12-14 mo **No further doses needed:** if first dose given at age ≥15 mo	**4 wk[6]:** if current age <12 mo **8 wk (as final dose)[6]:** if current age ≥12 mo and second dose given at age <15 mo **No further doses needed:** if previous dose given at age ≥15 mo	**8 wk (as final dose):** this dose only necessary for children age 12 mo-5 yr who received 3 doses before age 12 mo	
PCV[7]	6 wk	**4 wk:** if first dose given at age <12 mo and current age ≤24 mo **8 wk (as final dose):** if first dose given at age ≥12 mo or current age 24-59 mo **No further doses needed:** for healthy children if first dose given at age ≥24 mo	**4 wk:** if current age <12 mo **8 wk (as final dose):** if current age ≥12 mo **No further doses needed:** for healthy children if previous dose given at age ≥24 mo	**8 wk (as final dose):** this dose only necessary for children age 12 mo-5 yr who received 3 doses before age 12 mo	

Catch-up Schedule for Children Age 7 Through 18 Years

Vaccine	Minimum Interval Between Doses		
	Dose 1 to Dose 2	*Dose 2 to Dose 3*	*Dose 3 to Booster Dose*
Td[8]	4 wk	6 mo	**6 mo[8]:** if first dose administered at age <12 mo and current age <11 yr **5 y[8]:** if first dose administered at age <12 mo and third dose administered at age <7 yr and current age ≥11 yr **10 yr[8]:** if third dose administered at age ≥7 yr
IPV[9]	4 wk	4 wk	
HepB	4 wk	8 wk (and 16 wk after first dose)	
MMR	4 wk[4]		
Varicella[10]	4 wk		

Note: A vaccine series does not require restarting, regardless of the time that has elapsed between doses.

1. Diphtheria and tetanus toxolds and acellular pertussis (DTaP) vaccine. The fifth dose is not necessary if the fourth dose was administered after the fourth birthday.

2. Inactivated poliovirus (IPV) vaccine. For children who received an all-IPV or all-oral poliovirus (OPV) series, a fourth dose is not necessary if the third dose was administered at age ≥4 years. If both OPV and IPV were administered as part of a series, a total of 4 doses should be administered, regardless of the child's current age.

3. Hepatitis B (HepB) vaccine. All children and adolescents who have not been immunized against hepatitis B should begin the HepB immunization series during any visit. Providers should make special efforts to immunize children who were born in, or whose parents were born in, areas of the world where hepatitis B virus infection is moderately or highly endemic.

4. Measles, mumps, and rubella (MMR) vaccine. The second dose of MMR is recommended routinely at age 4–6 years but may be administered earlier if desired.

5. *Haemophilus influenzae* type b (Hib) Vaccine. Vaccine is not generally recommended for children aged ≥5 years.

6. Hib vaccine. If current age is <12 months and the first 2 doses were PRP-OMP (PedvaxHIB® or ComVax® [Merck]), the third (and final) dose should be administered at age 12–15 months and at least 8 weeks after the second dose.

7. Pneumococcal conjugate vaccine (PCV). Vaccine is not generally recommended for children aged ≥5 years.

8. Tetanus and diphtheria toxoids (Td). For children aged 7–10 years, the interval between the third and booster dose is determined by the age when the first dose was administered. For adolescents aged 11–18 years, the interval is determined by the age when the third dose was administered.

9. IPV. Vaccine is not generally recommended for persons aged ≥18 years.

10. Varicella vaccine. Administer the 2-dose series to all susceptible adolescents aged ≥13 years.

which are produced in chick embryo fibroblast tissue culture, do not contain significant amounts of egg proteins and may be administered without testing children with history of egg allergy. Mild acute illness with or without fever, convalescent phase of illness, recent exposure to infectious diseases, current antimicrobial therapy, breastfeeding, mild to moderate local reaction or low-grade to moderate fever after previous vaccination, and history of penicillin or other nonvaccine allergy or receiving allergen extract immunotherapy are **not contraindications** to immunization.

Severe immunosuppression resulting from congenital immunodeficiency, HIV infection, leukemia, lymphoma, cancer therapy, or a prolonged course of high-dose corticosteroids (≥ 2 mg/kg/day for >2 weeks) predisposes to complications and is a contraindication for live virus vaccines. MMR vaccination is recommended at 12 months of age, with a second dose 1 month later rather than waiting until 4 to 6 years, for all HIV-infected children who do not have evidence of severe immunosuppression. Varicella vaccine is contraindicated for persons with cellular immunodeficiency, but is recommended for persons with impaired humoral immunity (hypogammaglobulinemia or dysgammaglobulinemia) and at 12 months of age for HIV-infected children who do not have evidence of severe immunosuppression, given as two doses 3 months apart.

The National Childhood Vaccine Injury Act also requires that clinically significant adverse events after vaccination be reported to the **Vaccine Adverse Event Reporting System (VAERS)** (http://www.vaers.org or

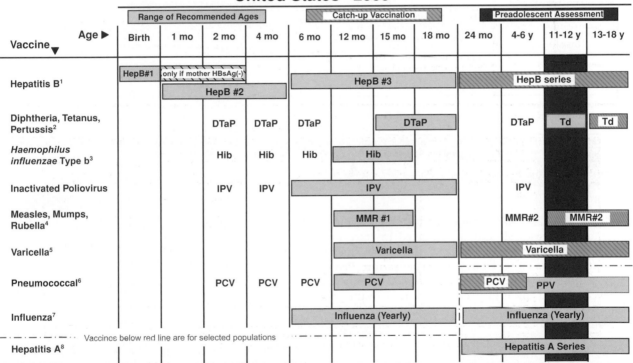

Recommended Childhood and Adolescent Immunization Schedule
United States · 2005

This schedule indicates the recommended ages for routine administration of currently licensed childhood vaccines, as of December 1, 2004, for children through age 18 years. Any dose not given at the recommended age should be given at any subsequent visit when indicated and feasible. ▓▓▓ Indicates age groups that warrant special effort to administer those vaccines not previously given. Additional vaccines may be licensed and recommended during the year. Licensed combination vaccines may be used whenever any components of the combination are indicated and the vaccine's other components are not contraindicated. Providers should consult the manufacturers' package inserts for detailed recommendations. Clinically significant adverse events that follow immunization should be reported to the Vaccine Adverse Event Reporting System (VAERS). Guidance about how to obtain and complete a VAERS form can be found on the Internet: www.vaers.org or by calling 800-822-7967.

Figure 94–1

Recommended childhood and adolescent immunization schedule for U.S. (2005). Approved by the Advisory Committee on Immunization Practices (http://www.cdc.gov/nip/acip), the AAP (http://www.aap.org), and the American Academy of Family Physicians (http://www.aafp.org). (From Centers for Disease Control and Prevention: Recommended childhood and adolescent immunization schedule—United States, 2005. MMWR 53:Q1-Q3, 2005.)   *Continued*

1. Hepatitis B (HepB) vaccine. All infants should receive the first dose of hepatitis B vaccine soon after birth and before hospital discharge; the first dose may also be given by age 2 months if the infant's mother is hepatitis B surface antigen (HBsAg) negative. Only monovalent HepB can be used for the birth dose. Monovalent or combination vaccine containing HepB may be used to complete the series. Four doses of vaccine may be administered when a birth dose is given. The second dose should be given at least 4 weeks after the first dose, except for combination vaccines which cannot be administered before age 6 weeks. The third dose should be given at least 16 weeks after the first dose and at least 8 weeks after the second dose. The last dose in the vaccination series (third or fourth dose) should not be administered before age 24 weeks.

Infants born to HBsAg-positive mothers should receive Hep B and 0.5 mL of Hepatitis B Immune Globulin (HBIG) within 12 hours of birth at separate sites. The second dose is recommended at age 1–2 months. The last dose in the immunization series should not be administered before age 24 weeks. These infants should be tested for HBsAg and antibody to HBsAg (anti-HBs) at age 9–15 months.

Infants born to mothers whose HBsAg status is unknown should receive the first dose of the HepB series within 12 hours of birth. Maternal blood should be drawn as soon as possible to determine the mother's HBsAg status; if the HBsAg test is positive, the infant should receive HBIG as soon as possible (no later than age 1 week). The second dose is recommended at age 1–2 months. The last dose in the immunization series should not be administered before age 24 weeks.

2. Diphtheria and tetanus toxoids and acellular pertussis (DTaP) vaccine. The fourth dose of DTaP may be administered as early as age 12 months, provided 6 months have elapsed since the third dose and the child is unlikely to return at age 15–18 months. The final dose in the series should be given at age ≥4 years. **Tetanus and diphtheria toxoids (Td)** is recommended at age 11–12 years if at least 5 years have elapsed since the last dose of tetanus and diphtheria toxoid-containing vaccine. Subsequent routine Td boosters are recommended every 10 years.

3. Haemophilus influenzae **type b (Hib) conjugate vaccine.** Three Hib conjugate vaccines are licensed for infant use. If PRP-OMP (PedvaxHIB or ComVax [Merck]) is administered at ages 2 and 4 months, a dose at age 6 months is not required. DTaP/Hib combination products should not be used for primary immunization in infants at ages 2, 4 or 6 months but can be used as boosters following any Hib vaccine. The final dose in the series should be given at age ≥12 months.

4. Measles, mumps, and rubella vaccine (MMR). The second dose of MMR is recommended routinely at age 4–6 years but may be administered during any visit, provided at least 4 weeks have elapsed since the first dose and both doses are administered beginning at or after age 12 months. Those who have not previously received the second dose should complete the schedule by the visit at age 11–12 years.

5. Varicella vaccine. Varicella vaccine is recommended at any visit at or after age 12 months for susceptible children (i.e., those who lack a reliable history of chickenpox). Susceptible persons age ≥13 years should receive 2 doses, given at least 4 weeks apart.

6. Pneumococcal vaccine. The heptavalent **pneumococcal conjugate vaccine (PCV)** is recommended for all children age 2–23 months. It is also recommended for certain children age 24–59 months. The final dose in the series should be given at age >12 months. **Pneumococcal polysaccharide vaccine (PPV)** is recommended in addition to PCV for certain high-risk groups. See MMWR 2000;49(RR-9):1-35.

7. Influenza vaccine. Influenza vaccine is recommended annually for children aged ≥6 months with certain risk factors (including but not limited to asthma, cardiac disease, sickle cell disease, HIV, and diabetes), healthcare workers, and other persons (including household members) in close contact with persons in groups at high risk (see MMWR 2004;53[RR-6]:1-40) and can be administered to all others wishing to obtain immunity. In addition, healthy children aged 6–23 months and close contacts of healthy children aged 0–23 months are recommended to receive influenza vaccine, because children in this age group are at substantially increased risk for influenza-related hospitalizations. For healthy persons aged 5–49 years, the intranasally administered live, attenuated influenza vaccine (LAIV) is an acceptable alternative to the intramuscular trivalent inactivated influenza vaccine (TIV). See MMWR 2004;53[RR-6]:1-40. Children receiving TIV should be administered a dosage appropriate for their age (0.25 mL if 6–35 months or 0.5 mL if ≥3 years). Children aged ≤8 years who are receiving influenza vaccine for the first time should receive 2 doses (separated by at least 4 weeks for TIV and at least 6 weeks for LAIV).

8. Hepatitis A vaccine. Hepatitis A vaccine is recommended for children and adolescents in selected states and regions and for certain high-risk groups; consult your local public health authority. Children and adolescents in these states, regions, and high-risk groups who have not been immunized against hepatitis A can begin the hepatitis A immunization series during any visit. The 2 doses in the series should be administered at least 6 months apart. See MMWR 1999;48(RR-12):1-37.

For additional information about vaccines, including precautions and contraindications for immunization and vaccine shortages, please visit the National Immunization Program Web site at (**www.cdc.gov/nip/acip/**) or call the National Immunization Information Hotline at 800-232-2522 (English) or 800-232-0233 (Spanish).

Approved by the Advisory Committee on Immunization Practices (www.cdc.gov/nip/acip), the American Academy of Pediatrics (www.aap.org), and the American Academy of Family Physicians (www.aafp.org).

Figure 94–1, cont'd

---

telephone 800-822-7967). Suspected cases of vaccine-preventable diseases should be reported to state or local health departments. The Act also established the **National Vaccine Injury Compensation Program**, a no-fault system in which persons thought to have suffered an injury or death as a result of administration of a covered vaccine can seek compensation.

PROPHYLAXIS

Prophylaxis is used in many situations, such as post-exposure, perinatal exposure, and pre-exposure for persons at increased risk of infection. **Primary prophylaxis** is used to prevent infection before a first occurrence. **Secondary prophylaxis** is used to prevent recurrence of infection after a first episode. Prophylaxis may include antibiotics, immunoglobulin or monoclonal antibody, vaccine, or a combination (Table 94–2).

Meningococcus

Prophylaxis to all contacts of index cases of *N. meningitidis* infection should be administered as soon as possible (see Chapter 100). Prophylaxis is recommended for all household contacts, especially young children; childcare or nursery school contacts in the previous 7 days; direct exposure to the index patient's secretions through kissing or sharing of toothbrushes or eating utensils; mouth-to-mouth resuscitation or unprotected contact during endotracheal intubation within 7 days before onset of illness; and for contacts who frequently sleep or eat in the same dwelling as the index patient. Chemoprophylaxis is not recommended for casual contacts with no history of direct exposure to the index patient's oral secretions (school or work mate), indirect contact with no direct contact with the index patient, or medical personnel without direct exposure to the patient's oral secretions. Rifampin twice daily for 2 days, ceftriaxone once, and ciprofloxacin once (≥18 years old) are the recommended regimens.

TABLE 94–2.   Summary of Pre-exposure and Postexposure Prophylaxis for Children

Disease	Prophylactic Agents
Animal bites (postexposure)	Amoxicillin-clavulanate
Asplenia (anatomic or functional, includes sickle cell disease)	Penicillin, amoxicillin
Streptococcus pneumoniae	
Haemophilus influenzae type b	
Chlamydia trachomatis, urogenital or neonatal exposure	Tetracycline, erythromycin, azithromycin
Diphtheria (*Corynebacterium diphtheriae*)	Penicillin, erythromycin, vaccination
Endocarditis, for individuals with structural heart defects undergoing procedures	Amoxicillin, others
Fever and neutropenia (with malignancy or transplantation)	
Bacterial infections	Broad-spectrum antibiotics
Fungal infections	Antifungal agents
Group B streptococcus (neonatal sepsis)	Penicillin or ampicillin administered to the mother peripartum
Hepatitis A	Immunoglobulin, vaccine
Hepatitis B	Hepatitis B immunoglobulin (HBIG), vaccine
H. influenzae type b	Rifampin (to all close contacts if there are ≥1 children <48 months old who are not fully immunized or are immunocompromised)
HIV-1	Antiretroviral agents for perinatal exposure and postexposure after needle-stick injury
Influenza	
Influenza A viruses	Amantadine, rimantadine, oseltamivir
Influenza B viruses	Oseltamivir
Lyme disease	Doxycycline
Malaria (*Plasmodium*)	Chloroquine, others
Measles	Immunoglobulin, vaccine
Mycobacterium avium-complex (MAC) in patients with AIDS	Clarithromycin, azithromycin, rifabutin
Mycobacterium tuberculosis (primary and secondary prevention of tuberculosis)	Isoniazid (BCG vaccine rarely used in U.S.)
Neonatal omphalitis (*Staphylococcus aureus*)	Triple dye to umbilical stump
Neisseria meningitidis (meningococcus)	Rifampin, ceftriaxone, sulfadiazine (if susceptible), ciprofloxacin (≥18 years old)
Ophthalmia neonatorum (*Neisseria gonorrhoeae*)	Topical silver nitrate, erythromycin, tetracycline
Otitis media (recurrent)	Amoxicillin, sulfisoxazole
Pertussis (*Bordetella pertussis*)	Erythromycin, vaccine
Plague (*Yersinia pestis*)	Tetracycline, sulfonamide
Pneumocystis jirovecii (*carinii*) pneumonia (primary and secondary prevention in immunocompromised persons)	TMP-SMZ, aerosolized pentamidine, others
Rabies	Rabies immune globulin, vaccine
Respiratory syncytial virus (bronchiolitis)	Palivizumab
Rheumatic fever (group A streptococcal pharyngitis, secondary prevention)	Penicillin, sulfadiazine
Syphilis (*Treponema pallidum*)	Penicillin
Tetanus (*Clostridium tetani*)	Tetanus immune globulin (TIG), vaccine
Transplant recipients	
Bacterial infections	IV immunoglobulin
Cytomegalovirus	Cytomegalovirus immunoglobulin
Fungal infections	Fluconazole
Herpes simplex virus infection	Acyclovir, famciclovir, valacyclovir
Urinary tract infections (recurrent)	TMP-SMZ, nitrofurantoin, amoxicillin
Varicella-zoster virus (chickenpox)	Acyclovir, vaccine, varicella-zoster immunoglobulin (VZIG)

BCG, bacille Calmette-Guérin; TMP-SMZ, trimethoprim-sulfamethoxazole.

TABLE 94–3. Guide to Tetanus Prophylaxis in Wound Management

Previous Tetanus Immunization (Doses)	Clean Minor Wounds		All Other Wounds*	
	Td	TIG†	Td	TIG†
Uncertain or <3 doses	Yes	No	Yes	Yes
≥3 doses	Yes, if only 3 doses have been given or >10 yr since the last dose	No	Yes, if >5 yr since the last dose	No

*Including but not limited to wounds contaminated with dirt, soil, feces, or saliva; puncture wounds; avulsions; and wounds resulting from missiles, crushing, burns, and frostbite.
†Equine tetanus antitoxin should be used if TIG is not available.
Td, tetanus-diphtheria toxoid; TIG, tetanus immunoglobulin.

Tetanus

All postexposure wound treatment begins with immediate thorough cleansing using soap and water, removal of foreign bodies, and débridement of devitalized tissue. Tetanus prophylaxis after wounds and injuries includes vaccination of persons with incomplete immunization and tetanus immunoglobulin for contaminated wounds (soil, feces, saliva), puncture wounds, avulsions, and wounds resulting from missiles, crushing, burns, and frostbite (Table 94–3).

Rabies

Rabies immunoglobulin (RIG) and vaccine are extremely effective for prophylaxis after exposure to rabies, but are of no known benefit after symptoms have appeared. Because rabies is one of the deadliest infections, recognition of potential exposure and prophylaxis are crucial. Any healthy-appearing domestic dog, cat, or ferret responsible for an apparently unprovoked bite should be captured and observed for 10 days by a veterinarian for signs of rabies, without immediate treatment of the victim. Prophylaxis should be administered if the animal is rabid or suspected to be rabid, or if the animal develops signs of rabies while under observation. Captured wild animals should be killed (by animal control officials) without a period of observation. If the biting animal is not captured, particularly if it is a wild animal of a species known to harbor the virus in the region, rabies should be assumed to be present, and the victim should be given prophylaxis. Skunks, raccoons, foxes, most other carnivores, and bats are regarded as rabid unless proved negative by testing. Holding these animals for observation is not recommended. Prophylaxis also should be provided for persons exposed to a bat who might be unaware of the bat or unable to relate that a bite or direct contact with a bat has occurred, such as a mentally disabled or intoxicated person, a sleeping child, or an unattended young infant.

All rabies postexposure management begins with immediate thorough cleansing of the bite using soap and water and, if available, irrigation with a virucidal agent such as povidone-iodine. RIG in a dosage of 20 IU/kg should be administered with the full dose of RIG infiltrated subcutaneously into the area around the wound, if possible. Any remaining RIG that cannot be infiltrated into the wound should be administered as an IM injection. Inactivated rabies vaccine should be administered simultaneously as soon as possible with additional vaccine doses on days 3, 7, 14, and 28.

CHAPTER 95
Anti-infective Therapy

Empirical or presumptive anti-infective therapy is based on a **clinical diagnosis** combined with evidence from the literature and from experience of the probable pathogens causing the infection. **Definitive therapy** depends on **microbiologic diagnosis** by isolation or other direct evidence of the pathogen. Microbiologic diagnosis permits characterization of the pathogen's anti-infective drug susceptibility and delivery of the appropriate anti-infective agent to the site of infection in sufficient quantities to kill the pathogen or alter it to facilitate the immune response to kill it eventually. Antiviral therapy must take into consideration the intracellular nature of viral replication and, to avoid toxicity to the host's cells, must be directed at viral-specific proteins, such as the thymidine kinase of herpesviruses or reverse transcriptase of HIV. The choice of antimicrobial therapy depends on the site of infection, probable causative agents, host immunity, and pathogens susceptible to the antimicrobial agent (Table 95–1).

Text continued on p. 459

TABLE 95–1. Anti-infective Agents Commonly Used in Pediatrics

Agent	Mechanism of Action/ Activity and Spectrum	Major Susceptible Bacteria and Indications	Comments
Antibiotics			
Penicillins	Bind to penicillin-binding proteins; inhibit transpeptidation reaction of cell wall, causing eventual cell lysis		No activity for coagulase-negative staphylococci, *Mycoplasma, Chlamydia*
Penicillin G (IV or IM), penicillin V (PO)		Group A streptococci, *Streptococcus pneumoniae, Neisseria meningitidis, Neisseria gonorrhoeae,* anaerobic bacteria (Prevotella melaninogenica) *Pasteurella multocida, Actinomyces*	Penicillinase-producing *N. gonorrhoeae,* some *S. pneumoniae,* and many anaerobes are resistant
Ampicillin (IV), amoxicillin (PO)	β-lactamase susceptible	*Haemophilus influenzae, Listeria monocytogenes, Escherichia coli, Salmonella, Shigella, Proteus mirabilis, Enterococcus*	Many strains of these organisms produce β-lactamases and are resistant
Amoxicillin-clavulanic acid (PO)	Extended spectrum	As for ampicillin, plus *Staphylococcus aureus, Enterococcus, Bacteroides fragilis, Moraxella catarrhalis*	Clavulanic acid inhibits β-lactamases
Ampicillin-sulbactam (IV)	Extended spectrum	As for amoxicillin-clavulanic acid, plus anaerobes	Sulbactam inhibits β-lactamases; IV drug
Ticarcillin-clavulanic acid (IV)	Extended spectrum	As above, plus broader gram-negative coverage; not *Enterococcus*	
Piperacillin-tazobactam (IV)	Extended spectrum, including *Pseudomonas*	*Pseudomonas aeruginosa, Klebsiella, Citrobacter, Acinetobacter, S. aureus, Enterococcus,* anaerobes	Tazobactam inhibits β-*lactamases*
Oxacillin or nafcillin (IV)	Gram-positive only	*S. aureus, Streptococcus;* not *Enterococcus* or anaerobes	Penicillinase-resistant penicillins; most coagulase-negative staphylococci usually are resistant
Cephalosporins	Bind to penicillin-binding proteins; inhibit cell wall cross-linking; produce cell lysis		No activity against *Listeria* or *Enterococcus*
First-Generation			
Cefazolin (IV), cephalothin (IV), cephalexin (PO)		*S. aureus, E. coli, Klebsiella*	Good for *S. aureus,* other gram-positive organisms; *H. influenzae* type b is resistant
Second-Generation Cefuroxime (IV), cefuroxime axetil (PO)	β-lactamase stable	*H. influenzae, S. aureus,* many strains of *Klebsiella, E. coli*	Poor CSF drug levels
Cephamycins	Excellent anaerobic coverage		
Cefoxitin (IV), cefotetan (IV)		*P. melaninogenica, B. fragilis, E. coli,* gonococcus	Abdominal and genital tract infections

Continued

TABLE 95–1. Anti-infective Agents Commonly Used in Pediatrics—cont'd

Agent	Mechanism of Action/ Activity and Spectrum	Major Susceptible Bacteria and Indications	Comments
Third-Generation Cefotaxime (IV), ceftriaxone (IV), ceftibuten (PO), cefpodoxime proxetil (PO), ceftizoxime (PO)	Broad spectrum	*N. gonorrhoeae, H. influenzae, S. pneumoniae, N. meningitidis, E. coli, Klebsiella, S. aureus* (but not as good as first-generation cephalosporins for *S. aureus*)	Better gram-negative enteric coverage, good penetration of CNS; ceftriaxone has longer half-life; oral agents useful for treating *Shigella*
Ceftazidime (IV), cefoperazone (IV)		Same as above, gram-negative plus *Pseudomonas*; not uniformly active against *Burkholderia cepacia*	Resistance may be induced during therapy
Carbapenems	Thienamycin drug: binds to penicillin-binding proteins; very broad spectrum		
Imipenem/cilastatin (IV), meropenem (IV)		Most gram-positive and gram-negative bacteria, *Listeria monocytogenes, Bacillus, Pseudomonas, Acinetobacter,* most anaerobes	*Stenotrophomonas maltophilia,* methicillin-resistant *S. aureus,* and *Enterococcus* are resistant; requires cilastatin to inhibit renal degradation
Monobactam Aztreonam (IV)	Monobactam drug: binds to penicillin-binding proteins of Enterobacteriaceae only; narrow spectrum	Most gram-negative bacteria	No action against anaerobic or gram-positive bacteria; *B. cepacia* is resistant; does not induce β-lactamase production
Aminoglycosides (all IV or IM)	Inhibition of bacterial protein synthesis at ribosomes		Ototoxicity and nephrotoxicity, must monitor peak and trough serum concentrations
Gentamicin, tobramycin, netilmicin		Gram-negative Enterobacteriaceae including *Pseudomonas,* plague, tularemia, brucellosis (plus tetracycline)	Broad spectrum, synergy with β-lactams; *Enterococcus* resistant
Amikacin		Same as above	Less susceptible to aminoglycoside-inactivating enzymes
Streptomycin		Tuberculosis	
Macrolides Erythromycin (PO)	Inhibit protein synthesis	Pneumococcus, streptococci, *Corynebacterium diphtheriae, Mycoplasma, Chlamydia, Bordetella pertussis, Haemophilus ducreyi, Legionella, Campylobacter*	Often used as an alternative to penicillin G; nausea, hepatotoxicity (estolate ester); increases theophylline and carbamazepine blood levels; associated with pyloric stenosis in infants
Azithromycin (PO)		Less active than erythromycin against *S. aureus,* pneumococcus, streptococci, more active against *H. influenzae, Mycoplasma, Chlamydia,* gram-negative bacilli; active against *M. catarrhalis, Chlamydia pneumoniae, Legionella pneumophila, Borrelia burgdorferi, N. gonorrhoeae*	Possible efficacy for *Mycobacterium avium, Toxoplasma* encephalitis, cryptosporidiosis; long half-life: single-dose treatment for uncomplicated *Chlamydia* urethritis or cervicitis; prolonged use may cause hearing loss

TABLE 95–1. Anti-infective Agents Commonly Used in Pediatrics—cont'd

Agent	Mechanism of Action/ Activity and Spectrum	Major Susceptible Bacteria and Indications	Comments
Clarithromycin (PO)		More active than erythromycin for *S. aureus, Streptococcus*	Similar to azithromycin
Other Antibiotics			
Trimethoprim-sulfamethoxazole (IV or PO)	Inhibition of bacterial folate synthesis at 2 separate sites of the folate pathway	*E. coli, Proteus mirabilis, Salmonella, Shigella, H. influenzae, Yersinia, Streptococcus, S. aureus, Pneumocystis jirovecii (carinii), M. catarrhalis, Nocardia*	*P. aeruginosa* and *Enterococcus* are resistant; group A streptococci may be resistant; associated with Stevens-Johnson syndrome, anemia, neutropenia, glucose-6-phosphate dehydrogenase hemolysis
Metronidazole (IV or PO)	Damage of DNA by free radicals	*Bacteroides, Clostridium difficile,* anaerobic bacteria, *Gardnerella vaginalis, Capnocytophaga, Giardia lamblia, Entamoeba histolytica*	Seizures, encephalopathy, disulfiram reaction, metallic taste
Tetracyclines (IV or PO), doxycycline	Inhibition of protein synthesis	*Chlamydia, Mycoplasma, N. gonorrhoeae, Actinomyces,* Lyme disease, pelvic inflammatory disease, Rocky Mountain spotted fever, urethritis, *Brucella,* tularemia, plague	Stains teeth; contraindicated in children <8 yr old
Rifampin (PO)	Inhibition of DNA-dependent RNA polymerase	*S. aureus, Mycobacterium tuberculosis, H. influenzae, N. meningitidis*	Red discoloration of secretions; increases metabolism of drugs (e.g., oral contraceptives); resistance develops rapidly, if used alone
Clindamycin (IV or PO)	Inhibits protein synthesis	*S. aureus, Streptococcus,* most anaerobic bacteria, *Actinomyces* (penicillin-allergic patients)	Pseudomembranous colitis, toxicity
Vancomycin (IV)	Inhibits cell wall synthesis	Methicillin-resistant *S. aureus,* coagulase-negative staphylococci, JK diphtheroids, *C. difficile, Enterococcus*	Red man syndrome if injected too fast; nephrotoxic; resistance in enterococci a major problem
Linezolid (IV or PO)	Inhibits protein synthesis	Gram-positive bacteria, including vancomycin-resistant *Enterococcus faecium* and *Enterococcus faecalis, S. aureus,* coagulase-negative staphylococci	Reserved for antibiotic-resistant isolates; kinetics not fully known in children
Daptomycin (IV)	Binds to the bacterial cell membrane causing rapid depolarization of membrane potential, inhibiting protein and nucleic acid synthesis	Gram-positive bacteria, including vancomycin-resistant *E. faecium* and *E. faecalis, S. aureus,* coagulase-negative staphylococci	Reserved for antibiotic-resistant isolates; kinetics not fully known in children
Quinupristin-dalfopristin (IV)	Dalfopristin inhibits the early phase of protein synthesis, while quinupristin inhibits the late phase of protein synthesis	Gram-positive bacteria, including vancomycin-resistant *E. faecium* and *E. faecalis, S. aureus,* coagulase-negative staphylococci	Reserved for antibiotic-resistant isolates; kinetics not fully known in children

Continued

TABLE 95–1. Anti-infective Agents Commonly Used in Pediatrics—cont'd

Agent	Mechanism of Action/ Activity and Spectrum	Major Susceptible Bacteria and Indications	Comments
Ciprofloxacin (IV or PO) (many other fluoroquinolones are available, but they have limited use in pediatrics)	Inhibition of bacterial DNA gyrase (similar to nalidixic acid); broad spectrum	*P. aeruginosa, Shigella, Salmonella, E. coli, Klebsiella, Proteus, S. aureus, H. influenzae, N. gonorrhoeae, Chlamydia, L. monocytogenes*	May be given by mouth; arthritis; neurotoxicity; not approved for children <18 years old except for complicated urinary tract infection and prevention of anthrax; widely used among adults
Antifungals			
Amphotericin B, liposomal amphotericin B, amphotericin B lipid complex, amphotericin B cholesteryl complex (all IV)	Binds to sterols in the fungal cell membrane of susceptible fungi with a resultant change in membrane permeability and leakage of cellular contents	*Candida, Aspergillus, Coccidioides, Cryptococcus, Blastomyces, Histoplasma,* Zygomycetes	Most broadly active of the antifungals, but causes fever, hypotension, hypokalemia, and renal failure. Lipid formulations have less nephrotoxicity
Azoles	Inhibit cytochrome P-450-dependent 14-α-sterol demethylase, a crucial step in the synthesis of ergosterol		
Fluconazole (IV or PO)		*Candida, Coccidioides, Cryptococcus,* dermatophytes	
Itraconazole (IV or PO)		*Candida, Aspergillus, Coccidioides, Cryptococcus, Blastomyces, Histoplasma, Sporothrix,* dermatophytes	
Voriconazole (IV or PO)		*Candida, Aspergillus, Coccidioides, Cryptococcus,* dermatophytes	Preferred azole for *Aspergillus*
Flucytosine (PO)	Incorporated into fungal RNA inhibiting cell growth	*Candida, Cryptococcus*	Used in combination with amphotericin B
Caspofungin (IV)	Inhibits β-1,3-D glucan synthase, a crucial component in fungal cell walls	Mainly for *Aspergillus;* also *Candida, Coccidioides, Cryptococcus, Blastomyces, Histoplasma*	Causes fever and hepatotoxicity; limited data in children
Antivirals			
Acyclovir (IV or PO), valacyclovir (PO), famciclovir (PO, with increased absorption of prodrug)	Require viral thymidine kinase to produce acyclovir monophosphate, which inhibits DNA polymerase	HSV 1 and 2, VZV	VZV requires higher drug levels; toxic encephalopathy, renal dysfunction
Ganciclovir (PO, IV, ocular implant)	Same as acyclovir	CMV, HSV 1 and 2	Neutropenia, recurrence when discontinued
Foscarnet (IV)	Inhibits viral DNA polymerase	CMV retinitis, ganciclovir-resistant CMV; acyclovir-resistant HSV and VZV	Not myelosuppressive; nephrotoxic
Amantadine (PO), rimantadine (PO)	Inhibits viral replication	Influenza A only	Prophylaxis and therapy; neurotoxicity with poor concentration, confusion
Oseltamivir (PO)	Neuraminidase inhibitor	Influenza A and B	Therapy or prevention
Zanamivir (inhalation)	Neuraminidase inhibitor	Influenza A and B	Therapy only
Ribavirin (IV or inhalation)	Inhibits RNA synthesis and reverse transcriptase	Parenteral use for influenza, Lassa virus; use for RSV is controversial	Aerosol has few adverse effects; avoid exposure in pregnancy

CMV, cytomegalovirus; HSV, herpes simplex virus; RSV, respiratory syncytial virus; VZV, varicella-zoster virus.

Empirical therapy usually is initiated after obtaining appropriate laboratory tests, including cultures of appropriate fluids or tissues. In high-risk circumstances, such as neonatal sepsis or bacteremia in immunocompromised persons, empirical therapy includes broad-spectrum antibiotics (see Chapters 96 and 120). Empirical antibiotic therapy may be tailored to specific pathogens based on the clinical diagnosis (e.g., streptococcal pharyngitis) or for persons at defined risks (e.g., close exposure to tuberculosis or meningococcal disease). Definitive therapy is based on culture and susceptibility results, choosing therapy that minimizes drug toxicity, development of resistant microorganisms, superinfection by fungi, and cost.

Antibiotic effectiveness may be influenced by host factors. Antimicrobial agents are an adjunct to the normal host immune response. Infections associated with a foreign body, such as an intravascular catheter or a prosthetic device, are difficult to eradicate because polymorphonuclear leukocytes and macrophages may not effectively engulf organisms on artificial surfaces. Similarly, it is difficult for phagocytic cells to eradicate bacteria amid vegetations of fibrin and platelets on infected heart valves. For these types of infections to be sterilized, prolonged therapy with bactericidal antibiotics is required and does not always result in a satisfactory outcome. Foreign body devices may have to be removed if sterilization does not occur promptly. Chronic osteomyelitis, with organisms sequestered from the circulation in abscesses or poorly perfused bone, is similarly difficult to cure without surgical drainage and débridement of the infected tissue and re-establishment of a good vascular supply. Antimicrobial therapy alone may not cure infections in closed spaces with limited perfusion, such as abscesses.

Optimal antimicrobial therapy requires an understanding of the **pharmacokinetic properties** of the drugs being administered to specific patient populations. Drug dosage in a premature neonate must account for the immaturity of renal function by increasing dosing intervals to allow time for drug excretion. In patients with cystic fibrosis, who often have larger volume of distribution of hydrophilic antibiotics and increased renal clearance, larger doses are required to achieve therapeutic levels. Obese children may receive significant antibiotic overdoses if they are given dosage regimens on a per-kilogram basis that exceed the maximum recommended adult doses. These patients may have a significantly smaller volume of distribution for hydrophilic drugs and do not require the large doses required by a leaner child of equivalent weight. Determining peak and trough drug levels for antibiotics with lower safety margins (e.g., aminoglycosides and vancomycin) prevents adverse effects of treatment.

Oral absorption may affect the choice of antimicrobial therapy. The bioavailability of orally administered antibiotics varies depending on the acid stability of the drug, the amount of gastric acidity, and whether it is taken with food, antacids, H_2 blockers, or other medications. Patients with ileus may have an abnormal transit time and unpredictable absorption.

The **site and nature** of the infection may affect the choice of antimicrobial therapy. Aminoglycosides, which are active only against aerobic organisms, have significantly reduced activity in abscesses with low pH and oxygen tension. Infections of the CNS or the eye necessitate treatment with antimicrobial agents that penetrate and achieve therapeutic levels in these sites.

Drug interactions must be considered when multiple antimicrobial agents are used to treat infection. For the empirical treatment of life-threatening infection, the use of two or more antimicrobial agents may be justified when broad-spectrum activity is indicated, before the identification of the organism. Such indications include the continuation of two drugs to treat infection, such as the use of a cell wall–active agent (β-lactam or vancomycin) plus an aminoglycoside to treat effectively infections caused by the highly resistant enterococci. Two drugs with different mechanisms of action are often used against serious *Pseudomonas aeruginosa* infections. Several drugs are administered in combination (trimethoprim-sulfamethoxazole [TMP-SMZ], amoxicillin-clavulanate, ampicillin-sulbactam, and ticarcillin-clavulanate) because of their **synergism**, or significantly greater bacterial killing than when either is used alone. The addition of clavulanic acid (a β-lactamase inhibitor with modest antibacterial activity) to amoxicillin broadens the spectrum of the penicillin, allowing it to be used against gram-negative β-lactamase–producing bacteria such as *H. influenzae*, gram-positive organisms such as *Staphylococcus aureus*, and anaerobes. The use of a bacteriostatic drug, such as a tetracycline, along with a β-lactam agent, which is effective only against growing organisms, may result in antibiotic **antagonism**, or less bacterial killing in the presence of both drugs than if either were used alone.

CHAPTER **96**
Fever without a Focus

Core body temperature is normally maintained within 1°C to 1.5°C in a range of 37°C to 38°C. Normal body temperature is often considered to be 37°C (98.6°F; range 97°F to 99.6°F). Rectal temperatures greater than 38°C (>100.4°F) generally are considered abnormal.

There is normal diurnal variation, with maximum temperature in the late afternoon.

The normal body temperature is maintained by a complex regulatory system in the anterior hypothalamus. Development of fever begins with the release of endogenous pyrogens into the circulation as the result of infection, inflammatory processes (rheumatic disease), or malignancy. Microbes and microbial toxins act as **exogenous pyrogens** by stimulating release of **endogenous pyrogens**, which include cytokines such as interleukin-1, interleukin-6, tumor necrosis factor, and interferons that are released by monocytes, macrophages, mesangial cells, glial cells, epithelial cells, and B lymphocytes. Endogenous pyrogens reach the anterior hypothalamus via the arterial blood supply, liberating arachidonic acid, which is metabolized to prostaglandin E_2, resulting in an elevation of the hypothalamic thermostat. Endotoxin stimulates endogenous pyrogen release and directly affects thermoregulation in the hypothalamus.

Antipyretics (acetaminophen, ibuprofen, and aspirin) inhibit hypothalamic cyclooxygenase, inhibiting production of prostaglandin E_2. Aspirin is associated with Reye syndrome in children and is not recommended as an antipyretic. The response to antipyretics does not distinguish bacterial from viral infections.

Malignant hyperthermia can follow intense muscle contraction (cocaine overdose) or muscle metabolism altered by drugs (neuroleptic agents) or anesthetics. **Heatstroke**, a potentially fatal febrile illness, is caused by excessively high environmental temperatures and failure of physiologic body heat–losing mechanisms.

The **pattern of fever** in children may vary depending on the age of the child and the nature of the illness. Neonates may not have a febrile response and may be hypothermic despite significant infection, whereas older infants and children younger than 5 years old may have an exaggerated febrile response with temperatures of up to 105°F (40.6°C) in response to either a serious bacterial infection or an otherwise benign viral infection. Fever to this degree is unusual in older children and adolescents and suggests a serious process. The fever pattern does not distinguish fever caused by bacterial, viral, fungal, or parasitic organisms from that resulting from malignancy, autoimmune diseases, or drugs.

Children with fever without a focus present a diagnostic challenge that includes identifying bacteremia and sepsis. **Bacteremia** is defined as a positive blood culture and may be primary or secondary to a focal infection. **Sepsis** is the systemic response to infection that is manifested by hyperthermia or hypothermia, tachycardia, tachypnea, and shock (see Chapter 40). Children with septicemia and signs of CNS dysfunction (irritability, lethargy), cardiovascular impairment (cyanosis, poor perfusion), and disseminated intravascular coagulation (petechiae, ecchymosis) are readily recognized as **toxic appearing** or **septic**. Most febrile illness in children may be categorized as follows:

- **Fever of short duration** accompanied by localizing signs and symptoms, in which a diagnosis can be established by clinical history and physical examination
- **Fever without localizing signs** (without a focus), frequently occurring in a child younger than 3 years old, in which a history and physical examination fail to establish a cause, although a diagnosis of occult bacteremia may be suggested by laboratory studies
- **Fever of unknown origin (FUO)**, which defines fever for more than 14 days without an identified etiology despite history, physical examination, and routine laboratory tests or after 1 week of hospitalization and evaluation

FEVER IN INFANTS YOUNGER THAN 3 MONTHS OLD

Fever or **temperature instability** in infants younger than 3 months old is associated with a higher risk of **serious bacterial infections** than in older infants. These younger infants usually exhibit only fever and poor feeding, without localizing signs. Most febrile illnesses in this age group are caused by common viral pathogens, but serious bacterial infections that are seen frequently include **bacteremia** (caused by *S. pneumoniae*, Hib, nontyphoidal *Salmonella*, group B streptococcus, or *N. meningitidis*), **UTI** (*Escherichia coli*), **pneumonia** (*S. aureus*, *S. pneumoniae*, or group B streptococcus), **meningitis** (*S. pneumoniae*, Hib, group B streptococcus, meningococcus, herpes simplex virus [HSV], enteroviruses), **bacterial diarrhea** (*Salmonella*, *Shigella*, *E. coli*), and **osteomyelitis** or **septic arthritis** (*S. aureus* or group B streptococcus).

Differentiation between viral and bacterial infections in young infants is difficult. Febrile infants younger than 3 months old who appear ill and all febrile infants younger than 4 weeks old usually are admitted to the hospital for empirical antibiotics pending culture results, especially if there is uncertainty of follow-up. After blood, urine, and CSF specimens are obtained for culture, broad-spectrum parenteral antibiotics (cefotaxime and ampicillin) are administered. The choice of antibiotics depends on the pathogens suggested by localizing findings, which may indicate possible pneumonia, infectious arthritis, osteomyelitis, or meningitis. Well-appearing febrile infants 4 weeks of age or older without an identifiable focus, with good follow-up, with no history of prematurity or prior antimicrobial therapy, with a white blood cell (WBC) count of 5000 to 15,000/μL, with urine with less than 10 WBCs/high-power field, with stool with less than 5 WBCs/high-power field (for infants with diarrhea), and with normal chest x-ray (for infants with respiratory signs) may be followed as outpatients without empirical antibiotic treatment or sometimes are treated with the long-acting antibiotic ceftriaxone given intramuscularly. Regardless of antibiotic treatment, close follow-up for at least 72 hours, including re-evaluation in 24 hours or immediately with any clinical change, is essential.

FEVER IN CHILDREN YOUNGER THAN 3 YEARS OLD

A common clinical pediatric problem is the evaluation of a febrile but well-appearing child younger than 3 years old with no localizing signs of infection. Although most of these children have self-limited viral infections, some have **occult bacteremia** (bacteremia without an identifiable focus), and a few have severe and potentially life-threatening illnesses, such as bacterial meningitis. Particularly in the early stages of such illness, it is difficult even for experienced clinicians to differentiate patients with bacteremia from patients with benign illnesses.

Children between 2 months and 3 years of age are at increased risk for infection with organisms with polysaccharide capsules, including *S. pneumoniae*, Hib, *N. meningitidis*, and nontyphoidal *Salmonella*. Effective phagocytosis of these organisms requires opsonic antibody. Transplacental maternal IgG initially provides immunity to these organisms, but as the IgG gradually dissipates over the first several months of life, the infant is at increased risk for infection. In the U.S., use of conjugate Hib and *S. pneumoniae* vaccines has reduced the incidence of these infections dramatically. In this age group, the most common identified serious bacterial infection is a urinary tract infection.

The **observational assessment** is a key part of the assessment. Descriptions of normal appearance and behavior of **alertness** include "child looking at the observer" and "looking around the room," with eyes that are "shiny" or "bright," whereas descriptions that indicate severe impairment include "glassy" and "stares vacantly into space." Observations such as "sitting," "moving arms and legs on table or lap," and "sits without support" reflect normal motor ability, whereas "no movement in mother's arms" and "lays limply on table" indicate severe impairment. Normal behaviors such as "vocalizing spontaneously," "playing with objects," "reaching for objects," "smiling," and "crying with noxious stimuli" reflect **playfulness**; abnormal behaviors reflect **irritability**. Another common observation is the response of a crying child to being held by the parent. A normal response is "stops crying when held by the parent," whereas severe impairment is indicated by "continual cry despite being held and comforted." These observations represent a more precise description of what is called **consolability**.

Most episodes of fever in children younger than 3 years old have a demonstrable source of infection that is elicited by history or physical examination or a simple laboratory test; usually a common cold, otitis media, pneumonia, or UTI. Among well-appearing febrile children 3 to 36 months old without localizing signs, approximately 1.5% have occult bacteremia. Risk factors for occult bacteremia include temperature 102.2°F (39°C) or greater, WBC count 15,000/mm³ or greater, and elevated absolute neutrophil count, band count, ESR, or CRP. No combination of clinical parameters or laboratory tests reliably predicts occult bacteremia, however. Socioeconomic status, race, gender, and age (within the range of 3 to 36 months) do not affect the risk for occult bacteremia.

Occult bacteremia in otherwise healthy children is usually transient and self-limited, but may progress to serious localizing infections, such as pneumonia, meningitis, infectious arthritis, and pericarditis. All children with fever without localizing signs should have blood culture and urinalysis and urine culture to evaluate for a UTI. Patients with diarrhea should have a stool evaluation for leukocytes. Ill-appearing children should be admitted to the hospital and treated with antibiotics. Well-appearing children usually are followed as outpatients without empirical antibiotic treatment or sometimes treated with IM ceftriaxone. Regardless of antibiotic treatment, close follow-up for at least 72 hours, including re-evaluation in 24 hours or immediately with any clinical change, is essential. Children with a positive blood culture require immediate re-evaluation, repeat blood culture, consideration for lumbar puncture, and empirical antibiotic treatment.

Children with sickle cell disease have impaired splenic function and properdin-dependent opsonization that places them at increased risk for bacteremia, especially during the first 5 years of life. Children with sickle cell disease and fever who appear seriously ill, have a temperature 104°F (40°C) or greater, or have a WBC count less than 5000/mm³ or greater than 30,000/mm³ should be hospitalized and treated empirically with antibiotics. Other children with sickle cell disease and fever should have blood culture, empirical treatment with ceftriaxone, and close outpatient follow-up. Osteomyelitis resulting from *Salmonella* or *S. aureus* is also more common in children with sickle cell disease; the blood culture is not always positive in the presence of osteomyelitis.

FEVER OF UNKNOWN ORIGIN

FUO is defined as temperature greater than 100.4°F (38°C) lasting for more than 14 days with no obvious cause despite a complete history, physical examination, and routine screening laboratory evaluation. Imaging and special diagnostic techniques, including imaging-guided biopsy, have decreased greatly the number of patients with FUO. It is important to distinguish persistent fever from recurrent fever, which usually represents serial acute illnesses.

The initial evaluation of FUO requires a thorough history and physical examination supplemented with a few screening laboratory tests (Fig. 96–1). Additional laboratory and imaging tests are determined by abnormalities on initial evaluation. Important elements of the history include the impact the fever has had on the child's health and activity; weight loss; the use of drugs, medications, or immunosuppressive therapy; history of unusual, severe, or chronic infection suggesting immunodeficiency (see Chapter 72); immunizations; exposure to unprocessed or raw foods; history of pica and exposure to soil-borne or waterborne organisms;

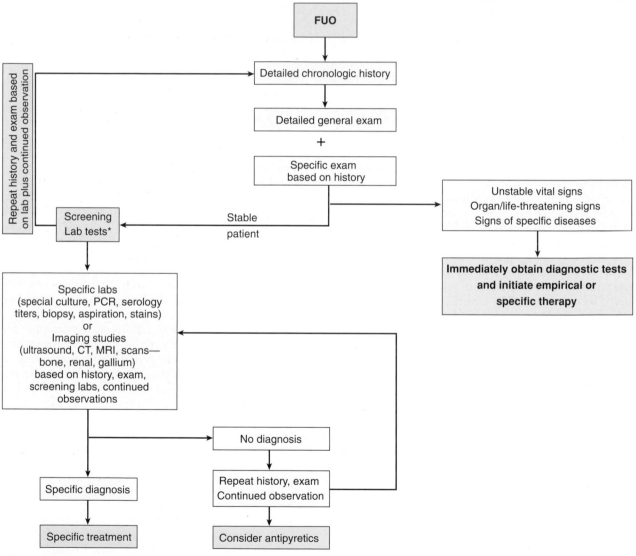

Figure 96–1

Approach to the evaluation of fever of unknown origin (FUO) in children. *Screening laboratory tests (labs) include a complete blood cell count, measurement of erythrocyte sedimentation rate, urinalysis, blood and urine cultures, and a chest radiograph. PCR, polymerase chain reaction. (From McCoy ACS, Aronoff SC: Fever of unknown origin. In Kliegman RM, Greenbaum LA, Lye PS [eds]: Practical Strategies in Pediatric Diagnosis and Therapy, 2nd ed. Philadelphia, WB Saunders, 2004, p 990.)

exposure to industrial or hobby-related chemicals; blood transfusions; domestic or foreign travel; exposure to animals; exposure to ticks or mosquitoes; genetic background; recent surgical procedures or dental work; tattooing and body piercing; and sexual activity. The etiology of most occult infections causing FUO is an unusual presentation of a common disease.

Localizing symptoms and signs, such as heart murmur, abdominal pain, or abnormal liver function, should be investigated fully. Entities such as sinusitis, endocarditis, intra-abdominal abscesses (perinephric,

intrahepatic, or subdiaphragmatic), and CNS lesions (tuberculoma, cysticercosis, abscess, or toxoplasmosis) may be relatively asymptomatic. FUO also may be the presentation of an immunodeficiency disease.

The most common categories of FUO in children are infectious diseases, inflammatory or rheumatologic diseases, and malignancies (Table 96–1). Systemic infections commonly presenting as FUO include cat-scratch disease (*Bartonella henselae*), ehrlichiosis, *Salmonella*, mycobacteria, brucellosis, tularemia, leptospirosis, Lyme disease, rat-bite fever, syphilis, HIV, CMV, hepati-

TABLE 96–1. Causes of Fever of Unknown Origin in Children

Infections

Bacterial Diseases

Brucellosis
Campylobacter
Cat-scratch disease (*Bartonella henselae*)
Gonococcemia (chronic)
Meningococcemia (chronic)
Salmonellosis
Streptobacillus moniliformis
Tuberculosis
Tularemia
Localized infections
  Abscesses: abdominal, dental, hepatic, pelvic, perinephric, rectal, subphrenic, splenic, periappendiceal, psoas
  Cholangitis
  Endocarditis
  Mastoiditis
  Osteomyelitis
  Pneumonia
  Pyelonephritis
  Sinusitis

Spirochetal Diseases

Leptospirosis
Lyme disease (*Borrelia burgdorferi*)
Relapsing fever (*Borrelia recurrentis*, other *Borrelia*)
Spirillum minus
Syphilis

Viral Diseases

Cytomegalovirus
Hepatitis
HIV (and associated opportunistic infections)
Infectious mononucleosis (Epstein-Barr virus)

Chlamydial Diseases

Lymphogranuloma venereum
Psittacosis

Rickettsial Diseases

Ehrlichiosis
Q fever
Rocky Mountain spotted fever

Fungal Diseases

Blastomycosis (extrapulmonary)
Coccidioidomycosis (disseminated)
Histoplasmosis (disseminated)

Parasitic Diseases

Extraintestinal amebiasis
Babesiosis
Giardiasis
Malaria
Toxoplasmosis
Trypanosomiasis
Visceral larva migrans

Autoimmune Hypersensitivity Diseases

Drug fever
Hypersensitivity pneumonitis
Juvenile rheumatoid arthritis (systemic onset, Still disease)
Polyarteritis nodosa
Rheumatic fever
Serum sickness
Systemic lupus erythematosus

Malignancies

Atrial myxoma
Ewing sarcoma
Hepatoma
Hodgkin disease
Leukemia

Lymphoma
Neuroblastoma

Granulomatous Diseases

Granulomatous hepatitis
Sarcoidosis
Crohn disease

Familial-Hereditary Diseases

Anhidrotic ectodermal dysplasia
Cyclic neutropenia
Deafness, urticaria, amyloidosis syndrome
Fabry disease
Familial dysautonomia
Familial Mediterranean fever
Hypertriglyceridemia
Ichthyosis

Miscellaneous

Behçet syndrome
Chronic active hepatitis
Diabetes insipidus (central and nephrogenic)
Factitious fever
Hemophagocytic syndromes
Histiocytosis syndromes
Hypothalamic-central fever
Infantile cortical hyperostosis
Inflammatory bowel disease
Kawasaki disease
Pancreatitis
Periodic fever
Postoperative (pericardiotomy, craniectomy)
Pulmonary embolism
Spinal cord injury—crisis
Thyrotoxicosis
Central fever

Modified from Powell KR: Fever without a focus. In Behrman RE, Kliegman RM, Jenson HB (eds): Nelson Textbook of Pediatrics, 17th ed. Philadelphia, WB Saunders, 2004, p 844.

tis, and EBV. Localized bacterial infections commonly include endocarditis, intra-abdominal or liver abscess, sinusitis, mastoiditis, osteomyelitis, pneumonia, and pyelonephritis or perinephric abscess.

A history of unusual, severe, or chronic infection suggests immunodeficiency (see Chapter 72). Immunocompromised children require an aggressive evaluation to identify the occult infection. Common infections causing FUO in these patients include viral hepatitis, EBV, CMV, *B. henselae*, ehrlichiosis, *Salmonella*, and tuberculosis. **Inflammatory diseases** commonly presenting as FUO include juvenile rheumatoid arthritis, systemic lupus erythematosus, polyarteritis nodosa, rheumatic fever, Kawasaki disease, and inflammatory bowel disease. **Malignancies** are a less common cause of FUO in children than in adults, accounting for only about 10% of all episodes. Malignancies that may present as FUO in children include Hodgkin and non-Hodgkin lymphoma, leukemia, Ewing sarcoma, and neuroblastoma.

Factitious fever, or fever produced or feigned intentionally by the patient (**Munchausen syndrome**) or the parent of a child (**Munchausen syndrome by proxy**), is an important consideration, particularly if family members are familiar with health care (see Chapter 22). Fever should be recorded in the hospital by a reliable individual who remains with the patient when the temperature is taken. Psychiatric disorders frequently are masked by family members' denial and desire to find an organic cause for the child's problems. Continuously observing the patient over a long period and repetitive evaluation are essential.

Screening tests for FUO include complete blood count with WBC and differential count, platelet count, ESR, hepatic transaminase levels, urinalysis, bacterial cultures of urine and blood, chest radiograph, and evaluation for rheumatic disease with antinuclear antibody, rheumatoid factor, and serum complement (C3, C4, CH$_{50}$). Additional tests for FUO that may be indicated include throat culture, stool culture, tuberculin skin test (TST) with controls, HIV antibody, EBV antibody profile, and *B. henselae* antibody. Consultation with infectious disease, immunology, rheumatic disease, or oncology specialists should be considered. Further tests may include lumbar puncture for CSF analysis and culture; CT or MRI of the chest, abdomen, and head; and bone marrow biopsy for cytology and culture.

Compared with adults, children with FUO have a better prognosis, although the outcome depends on the underlying disease. An etiology is not identified in 25% of cases, even after thorough evaluation. Fever eventually resolves in many of these cases, usually without sequelae, although some of these patients may develop definable signs of rheumatic disease over time.

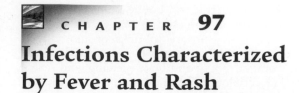

CHAPTER **97**

Infections Characterized by Fever and Rash

Rashes are a common manifestation of many infections. Skin lesions evolve over time, but the characteristic distribution and appearance provide important clues to the diagnosis (Table 97–1). Several classic pediatric illnesses are characterized primarily by fever and generalized rash: measles, rubella, roseola infantum (exanthem subitum), erythema infectiosum (fifth disease), and chickenpox.

MEASLES (RUBEOLA)

Etiology

Measles (rubeola) is caused by a single-stranded RNA paramyxovirus with one antigenic type. Humans are the only natural host. Measles virus infects the upper respiratory tract and regional lymph nodes and is spread systemically during a brief, low-titer primary viremia. A secondary viremia occurs within 5 to 7 days when virus-infected monocytes spread the virus to the respiratory tract, skin, and other organs. The characteristic histologic finding is the presence of large, multinucleated giant cells (**Warthin-Finkeldey cells**) and syncytium formation in respiratory epithelia and reticuloendothelial cells.

Virus is present in respiratory secretions, blood, and urine of infected individuals. Measles virus is transmitted by large droplets from the upper respiratory tract and requires close contact. The virus is stable at room temperature for 1 to 2 days. Infected persons are contagious from 1 to 2 days before symptoms (about 5 days before onset of rash) to 4 days after the appearance of the rash.

Epidemiology

Measles is endemic in regions where measles vaccination is not available; worldwide it is responsible for about 1 million deaths per year. There are less than 100 cases reported annually in the U.S., although outbreaks may occur as a result of low immunization rates among susceptible children in crowded urban areas or from internationally imported cases. Most young infants are protected from measles by transplacental antibody, but infants become susceptible toward the end of the first year of life. Passive immunity may interfere with effective vaccination until 12 to 15 months of age.

TABLE 97–1. Differential Diagnosis of Fever and Rash

Lesion	Pathogen or Disease
Macular or Maculopapular Rash	
Viruses	Measles
	Rubella
	Roseola (HHV-6 or HHV-7)
	Erythema infectiosum (fifth disease, parvovirus B19)
	Epstein-Barr virus
	Echoviruses
	HBV (papular acrodermatitis or Gianotti-Crosti syndrome)
	HIV
Bacteria	Erythema marginatum (rheumatic fever)
	Scarlet fever (group A streptococcus)
	Erysipelas (group A streptococcus)
	Arcanobacterium haemolyticum
	Secondary syphilis
	Leptospirosis
	Pseudomonas
	Meningococcal infection (early)
	Salmonella typhi (typhoid fever)
	Lyme disease (erythema migrans)
	Mycoplasma pneumoniae
Rickettsiae	Rocky Mountain spotted fever (early)
	Typhus (scrub, endemic)
	Ehrlichiosis
Other	Kawasaki disease
	Rheumatoid arthritis
	Drug reaction
Diffuse Erythroderma	
Bacteria	Scarlet fever (group A streptococcus)
	Staphylococcal scalded skin syndrome
	Toxic shock syndrome (*Staphylococcus aureus*)
Fungi	*Candida albicans*
Other	Kawasaki syndrome
Urticarial Rash	
Viruses	Epstein-Barr virus
	HBV
	HIV
Bacteria	*M. pneumoniae*
	Group A streptococcus
Other	Drug reaction

Lesion	Pathogen or Disease
Vesicular, Bullous, Pustular	
Viruses	Herpes simplex viruses
	Varicella-zoster virus
	Coxsackievirus
Bacteria	Staphylococcal scalded skin syndrome
	Staphylococcal bullous impetigo
	Group A streptococcal crusted impetigo
Rickettsiae	Rickettsialpox
Other	Toxic epidermal necrolysis
	Erythema multiforme (Stevens-Johnson syndrome)
Petechial-Purpuric	
Viruses	Atypical measles
	Congenital rubella
	Congenital cytomegalovirus
	Enterovirus
	Papular-purpuric gloves and socks (parvovirus B19)
	HIV
	Hemorrhagic fever viruses
Bacteria	Sepsis (meningococcal, gonococcal, pneumococcal, *Haemophilus influenzae* type b)
	Infective endocarditis
	Ecthyma gangrenosum (*Pseudomonas aeruginosa*)
Rickettsiae	Rocky Mountain spotted fever
	Epidemic typhus
	Ehrlichiosis
Fungi	Necrotic eschar (*Aspergillus, Mucor*)
Other	Vasculitis
	Thrombocytopenia
	Henoch-Schönlein purpura
	Malaria
Erythema Nodosum	
Viruses	Epstein-Barr virus
	HBV
Bacteria	Group A streptococcus
	Mycobacterium tuberculosis
	Yersinia
	Cat-scratch disease (*Bartonella henselae*)
Fungi	Coccidioidomycosis
	Histoplasmosis
Other	Sarcoidosis
	Inflammatory bowel disease
	Estrogen-containing oral contraceptives
	Systemic lupus erythematosus
	Behçet disease

HBV, hepatitis B virus; HHV, human herpesvirus.

Clinical Manifestations

Measles infection is divided into four phases: incubation, prodromal (catarrhal), exanthematous (rash), and recovery. The incubation period is 8 to 12 days from exposure to the onset of symptoms and 14 days from exposure to the onset of rash. The classic symptoms of cough, coryza, and conjunctivitis occur during the secondary viremia of the exanthematous phase.

The manifestations of the 3-day prodromal period are cough, coryza, conjunctivitis, and the pathognomonic **Koplik spots** (gray-white, sand grain–sized dots on the buccal mucosa opposite the lower molars) that last 12 to 24 hours. The conjunctiva may reveal a characteristic transverse line of inflammation along the eyelid margin (**Stimson line**). The rash phase often is accompanied by high fever (40°C to 40.5°C [104°F to 105°F]). The macular rash begins on the head (often above the hairline) and spreads over most of the body in 24 hours in a descending fashion. It is often confluent. The rash fades in the same manner. The severity of the illness is related to the extent of the rash. It may be petechial or hemorrhagic (**black measles**). As the rash fades, it undergoes brownish discoloration and desquamation.

Cervical lymphadenitis, splenomegaly, and mesenteric lymphadenopathy with abdominal pain may be noted. Otitis media, pneumonia, and diarrhea are more common in infants. Liver involvement is more common in adults.

The term **modified measles** is used to describe mild cases of measles occurring in persons with partial protection against measles. Modified measles occurs in persons vaccinated before 12 months of age or with coadministration of immune serum globulin, in infants with disease modified by transplacental antibody, or in persons receiving immunoglobulin.

Laboratory and Imaging Studies

Routine laboratory findings are nonspecific and do not aid in diagnosis. Leukopenia is characteristic. In patients with acute encephalitis, the CSF reveals an increased protein, a lymphocytic pleocytosis, and normal glucose levels. Measles virus can be cultivated in human or monkey cells, but culture is not generally available. Serologic testing for IgM antibodies, which appear within 1 to 2 days of the rash and persist for 1 to 2 months, is used to confirm the clinical diagnosis. Chest x-rays may show interstitial or perihilar infiltrates, but do not distinguish measles pneumonia and bacterial superinfection.

Differential Diagnosis

The clinical presentation is characteristic. Confirmation is by identification of multinucleated giant cells in nasal mucosal smears, virus isolation in culture, and diagnostic antibody increases in acute and convalescent serum. The rash must be differentiated from rubella, roseola, enteroviral or adenoviral infection, infectious mononucleosis, toxoplasmosis, meningococcemia, scarlet fever, rickettsial disease, Kawasaki syndrome, serum sickness, and drug rash. The constellation of fever, rash, cough, and conjunctivitis is diagnostic for measles. Koplik spots are pathognomonic, but are not always present at the time the rash is most pronounced.

Treatment

There is no specific therapy for measles. Routine supportive care includes maintaining adequate hydration and antipyretics. Photophobia is intensified by strong light, which should be avoided. IV ribavirin may be beneficial in severe infections.

High-dose vitamin A supplementation improves the outcome in infected malnourished infants and should be considered for populations at risk for severe complications, including infants 6 months to 2 years old requiring hospitalization, HIV-infected infants, and infants from endemic areas in developing countries.

Complications

Measles is often complicated by otitis media. Measles virus may cause interstitial pneumonia or, more commonly, pneumonia may result from secondary bacterial infection. Persons with impaired cell-mediated immunity may develop **giant cell (Hecht) pneumonia**, which is usually fatal. Anergy associated with measles may activate latent tuberculosis. Myocarditis and mesenteric lymphadenitis are infrequent complications. Encephalomyelitis occurs in 1 to 2 per 1000 cases and usually occurs 2 to 5 days after the onset of the rash. Early encephalitis probably is caused by direct viral infection of brain tissue, whereas later onset encephalitis is a demyelinating and probably an immunopathologic phenomenon. **Subacute sclerosing panencephalitis** is a late neurologic complication of slow measles infection that occurs in approximately 1 in every 1 million cases of measles, developing an average of 8 to 10 years after measles.

Prognosis

Deaths most frequently result from bronchopneumonia or encephalitis, with much higher risk among persons with underlying malignancy or HIV infection. Deaths among adolescents and adults usually result from subacute sclerosing panencephalitis, which leads to death in all cases. Other forms of measles encephalitis in immunocompetent persons are associated with a mortality rate of approximately 15%, with 20% to 30% of survivors having serious neurologic sequelae.

Prevention

Live measles vaccine prevents infection and is recommended as MMR for children at age 12 to 15 months and 4 to 6 years (see Fig. 94–1). The second dose is not a booster dose, but significantly reduces the primary vaccine failure rate, which is 5% or less. Severe immunosuppression predisposes to complications and is a contraindication for live virus vaccines. Contraindications to measles vaccine include immunocompromised states resulting from congenital immunodeficiency, severe HIV infection, leukemia, lymphoma, cancer therapy, or an immunosuppressive course of corticosteroids (≥2 mg/kg/day for ≥14 days); pregnancy; or recent administration of immunoglobulin (3 to 11 months depending on dose). MMR vaccination is recommended for all HIV-infected persons who do not have evidence of severe immunosuppression (low age-specific total CD4 T lymphocyte count or a low CD4 T lymphocyte count as a percentage of total lymphocytes), children with cancer in remission who have not received chemotherapy in the previous 3 months, and children who previously have received immunosuppressive doses of corticosteroids but who have not received corticosteroids in the previous month. Susceptible household contacts with a chronic disease or who are immunocompromised who are exposed to measles should receive **postexposure prophylaxis** with measles vaccine, within 72 hours of exposure, or immunoglobulin within 6 days of exposure.

RUBELLA (GERMAN OR 3-DAY MEASLES)

Etiology

Rubella, also known as **German measles** and **3-day measles**, is caused by a single-stranded, positive-sense RNA virus with a glycolipid envelope, which is a member of the togavirus family. Humans are the only natural host. Rubella virus invades the respiratory epithelium and disseminates via a primary viremia. After replication in the reticuloendothelial system, a secondary viremia ensues, and virus can be isolated from peripheral blood monocytes, CSF, and urine.

Infection **in utero** results in significant morbidity from **congenital rubella syndrome** (see Chapter 66). Maternal infection during the first trimester results in fetal infection in more than 90% of cases with a generalized vasculitis. Rubella virus is most contagious from 2 days before until 5 to 7 days after onset of the rash. Infants with congenital rubella may shed virus in nasopharyngeal secretions and urine for longer than 1 year after birth and may transmit the virus to susceptible contacts.

Epidemiology

In unvaccinated populations, rubella usually occurs in the spring, with epidemics occurring in cycles of every 6 to 9 years. Subclinical cases outnumber clinically apparent cases by a ratio of 2 : 1. Fewer than 20 cases of rubella occur annually in the U.S. Outbreaks of rubella in nonvaccinated groups occasionally occur in adults in workplaces, prisons, colleges, and healthcare centers from internationally imported cases. Transplacental antibody is protective during the first 6 months of life.

Clinical Manifestations

The incubation period for postnatal rubella is 14 to 21 days. The mild catarrhal symptoms of the prodromal phase of rubella may go unnoticed. The characteristic signs of rubella are retroauricular, posterior cervical, and posterior occipital lymphadenopathy accompanied by an erythematous, maculopapular, discrete rash. The rash begins on the face and spreads to the body and lasts for 3 days. The rash is less extensive than in measles. An enanthem consisting of rose-colored spots on the soft palate, known as **Forschheimer spots**, develops in 20% of patients and may appear before the rash. Other manifestations of rubella include mild pharyngitis, conjunctivitis, anorexia, headache, malaise, and low-grade fever. Polyarthritis, usually of the hands, may occur, especially among older women, but usually resolves without sequelae. Paresthesias and tendinitis may occur.

Laboratory and Imaging Studies

Routine laboratory findings in cases of rubella are nonspecific and generally do not aid in diagnosis. The WBC count usually is normal or low, and thrombocytopenia rarely occurs.

Differential Diagnosis

The rash must be differentiated from measles, roseola, enteroviral or adenoviral infection, infectious mononucleosis, toxoplasmosis, scarlet fever, rickettsial disease, Kawasaki syndrome, serum sickness, and drug rash. Diagnosis is confirmed by serologic testing for IgM antibodies or by a fourfold or greater increase in specific IgG antibodies in paired acute and convalescent sera.

Treatment

There is no specific therapy for rubella. The efficacy of corticosteroids for rubella encephalitis is unproved. Routine supportive care includes maintaining adequate hydration and antipyretics.

Complications

Complications of rubella are rare. Rubella infection during pregnancy may result in **congenital rubella syndrome** with intrauterine growth retardation, cataracts, deafness, and a patent ductus arteriosus (see Chapter 66).

Prognosis

The prognosis for rubella is excellent. Deaths rarely occur with rubella encephalitis.

Prevention

Live rubella vaccine prevents infection and is recommended as MMR for children at age 12 to 15 months and at 4 to 6 years (see Fig. 94–1). After vaccination, rubella virus is shed from the nasopharynx for several weeks, but it is not communicable. Pregnant women who are susceptible to rubella should be immunized after delivery. Rubella vaccine rarely is associated with adverse effects in children, but in postpubertal females causes arthralgias in 25% of vaccinees and acute arthritis-like symptoms in 10% of vaccinees. These symptoms typically develop 1 to 3 weeks after vaccination and last 1 to 3 days.

Contraindications to rubella vaccine include immunocompromised states resulting from congenital immunodeficiency, HIV infection, leukemia, lymphoma, cancer therapy, or an immunosuppressive course of corticosteroids (≥2 mg/kg/day for ≥14 days); pregnancy; or recent administration of immunoglobulin (3 to 11 months depending on dose). Vaccine virus has been recovered from fetal tissues, although no cases of congenital rubella syndrome have been identified among infants born to women who were vaccinated inadvertently against rubella in pregnancy. Nevertheless, women are cautioned to avoid pregnancy after receipt of rubella-containing vaccine for 28 days. Inadvertent vaccination of pregnant women with rubella vaccine is not an indication for abortion. All pregnant women should have prenatal serologic testing to determine their immune status to rubella, and susceptible mothers should be vaccinated after delivery and before hospital discharge.

Susceptible, nonpregnant persons exposed to rubella should receive rubella vaccination. Immunoglobulin should be administered to susceptible, pregnant women exposed to rubella if elective abortion is not an option.

ROSEOLA INFANTUM (EXANTHEM SUBITUM)

Etiology

Roseola infantum (exanthem subitum, sixth disease) is caused by human herpesvirus (HHV) type 6 (HHV-6) and in 10% to 30% of cases by HHV-7. HHV-6 and HHV-7 are large, enveloped double-stranded DNA viruses, which are members of the herpesvirus family. They infect mature mononuclear cells and cause a relatively prolonged (3 to 5 days) viremia during primary infection. They can be detected in the saliva of healthy adults, which suggests, as with other herpesviruses, the development of lifelong latent infection and intermittent shedding of virus.

Epidemiology

Transplacental antibody protects most infants until 6 months of age. The incidence of infection increases as maternally derived antibody levels decline. By 12 months of age, approximately 60% to 90% of children have antibodies to HHV-6, and essentially all children are seropositive by 2 to 3 years of age. HHV-6 is a major cause of acute febrile illnesses in infants and may be responsible for 20% of visits to the emergency department for children 6 to 18 months old. The virus is likely acquired from asymptomatic adults who periodically shed these viruses. HHV-6 and HHV-7 can cause encephalitis in immunocompromised persons.

Clinical Manifestations

Roseola is characterized by high fever (often ≥40°C) with an abrupt onset and lasting 3 to 5 days with a maculopapular, rose-colored rash that erupts coincident with defervescence, although it also may be present earlier. The rash usually lasts 1 to 3 days but may fade rapidly. Not all infants with HHV-6 infection have a rash. Upper respiratory symptoms, nasal congestion, erythematous tympanic membranes, and cough may occur. Gastrointestinal symptoms are described. Most children with roseola are irritable and appear toxic. Roseola is associated with approximately one third of febrile seizures. Roseola caused by HHV-6 and HHV-7 is clinically indistinguishable, although HHV-6–associated roseola typically occurs in younger infants. Reactivation of HHV-6 may cause bone marrow suppression after bone marrow transplantation.

Laboratory and Imaging Studies

Routine laboratory findings are nonspecific and do not aid in diagnosis. Encephalitis with roseola is characterized by mild pleocytosis (30 to 200 cells/mm^3) with mononuclear cell predominance, elevated protein concentration, and normal glucose concentration. The diagnosis can be confirmed by serologic testing showing a fourfold rise in acute and convalescent sera.

Differential Diagnosis

Children with roseola may present during the febrile period, before the rash appears, or after the rash has appeared. Many febrile illnesses may be easily confused with roseola during the pre-eruptive stage. The pattern of high fever for 3 to 5 days without significant physical findings followed by onset of rash with defervescence of fever is characteristic. Serious infections as the cause of high fever must be excluded, although, in marked contrast to the high fever, most children are alert, behave normally, and continue with their usual play and daily activities.

Treatment

There is no specific therapy for roseola. Routine supportive care includes maintaining adequate hydration and antipyretics.

Complications and Prognosis

The prognosis for roseola is excellent. A few deaths have been attributed to HHV-6, usually in cases complicated by encephalitis or virus-associated hemophagocytosis syndrome.

Prevention

There are no guidelines for prevention of roseola.

ERYTHEMA INFECTIOSUM (FIFTH DISEASE)

Etiology

Erythema infectiosum (fifth disease) is caused by the human parvovirus B19, a single-stranded DNA virus. This is a benign viral exanthem in healthy children. The affinity of this virus to red blood cell progenitor cells makes it an important cause of aplastic crisis in patients with hemolytic anemias, including sickle cell disease, spherocytosis, and thalassemia. Parvovirus B19 also causes fetal anemia and hydrops fetalis after primary infection during pregnancy. The cell receptor for parvovirus B19 is the **erythrocyte P antigen**, a glycolipid present on erythroid cells. The virus replicates in actively dividing erythroid stem cells, leading to cell death that results in erythroid aplasia and anemia.

Epidemiology

Erythema infectiosum is common. Parvovirus B19 seroprevalence is only 2% to 9% in children younger than 5 years old, but increases to 15% to 35% in older children (5 to 18 years old) and 30% to 60% in adults. Community epidemics usually occur in the spring. The virus is transmitted by respiratory secretions and by blood product transfusions.

Clinical Manifestations

The incubation period is typically 4 to 14 days and rarely may last 21 days. Parvovirus B19 infections usually begin with a mild, nonspecific illness characterized by fever, malaise, myalgias, and headache. In some cases, this illness is followed by the characteristic rash 7 to 10 days later. Erythema infectiosum is manifested by rash, low-grade or no fever, and occasionally pharyngitis and mild conjunctivitis. The rash appears in three stages. The initial stage typically is apparent by erythematous cheeks, appearing as a **"slapped cheek" rash** with circumoral pallor. An erythematous symmetric, maculopapular, truncal rash appears 1 to 4 days later, but later fades as central clearing takes place, giving a distinctive **lacy, reticulated rash** that lasts 2 to 40 days (mean 11 days). This rash may be pruritic, does not desquamate, and may recur with exercise, bathing, rubbing, or stress. Adolescents and adults may experience myalgia, significant arthralgia or arthritis, headache, pharyngitis, coryza, and gastrointestinal upset.

Children with an increased erythroid production requirement because of shortened erythrocyte life span (e.g., sickle cell disease) may develop a **transient aplastic crisis** that is characterized by ineffective erythroid production (see Chapter 150). Most children with parvovirus B19–induced transient aplastic crisis have multiple symptoms, including fever, lethargy, malaise, pallor, headache, gastrointestinal symptoms, and respiratory symptoms. The reticulocyte count is extremely low or zero, and the hemoglobin level is lower than usual for the patient. Transient neutropenia and thrombocytopenia also commonly occur.

Persistent parvovirus B19 infection may develop in children with immunodeficiency, causing severe anemia resulting from pure red blood cell aplasia. These children do not display the typical manifestations of erythema infectiosum.

Laboratory and Imaging Studies

Many abnormalities occur with parvovirus infection, including reticulocytopenia lasting 7 to 10 days, mild anemia, thrombocytopenia, lymphopenia, and neutropenia. Parvovirus B19 can be detected by PCR and by electron microscopy of erythroid precursors in the bone marrow. Serologic tests showing antibody response to parvovirus, especially the presence of specific IgM antibody to parvovirus, are diagnostic.

Differential Diagnosis

The diagnosis of erythema infectiosum in children is established on the basis of the clinical findings of typical facial rash with absent or mild prodromal symptoms, followed by a reticulated rash over the body that waxes and wanes. The differential diagnosis includes measles, rubella, scarlet fever, enteroviral or adenoviral infection, infectious mononucleosis, scarlet fever, Kawasaki disease, systemic lupus erythematosus, serum sickness, and drug rash.

Treatment

There is no specific therapy. Routine supportive care includes maintaining adequate hydration and antipyretics. Transfusions may be required for transient aplastic crisis. Intrauterine transfusion has been performed for hydrops fetalis associated with fetal parvovirus B19 infection. IV immunoglobulin may be used for immunocompromised persons with severe anemia.

Complications and Prognosis

The prognosis for erythema infectiosum is excellent. Fatalities associated with transient aplastic crisis are rare. Parvovirus B19 is not teratogenic, but in utero infection of fetal erythroid cells may result in fetal heart failure, hydrops fetalis, and fetal death. Of the approximately 50% of women of childbearing age susceptible to parvovirus B19 infection, 30% of exposed women develop infection, with 25% of exposed fetuses becoming infected and 10% of these culminating in fetal death.

Prevention

The greatest risk is to pregnant women from infected children 5 to 7 years old, in the household, at daycare, and in schools. Effective control measures are limited. Exclusion of affected children from school is not recommended because children generally are not infectious by the time the rash is present. Good hand washing and hygiene are practical measures that should help reduce transmission.

VARICELLA-ZOSTER VIRUS INFECTION (CHICKENPOX AND ZOSTER)

Etiology

Chickenpox and zoster are caused by varicella-zoster virus (VZV), an enveloped, icosahedral, double-stranded DNA virus that is a member of the herpesvirus family. Humans are the only natural host. **Chickenpox (varicella)** is the manifestation of primary infection. VZV infects susceptible individuals via the conjunctivae or respiratory tract and replicates in the nasopharynx and upper respiratory tract. It disseminates by a primary viremia and infects regional lymph nodes, the liver, the spleen, and other organs. A secondary viremia follows, resulting in a cutaneous infection with the typical vesicular rash. After resolution of chickenpox, the virus persists in latent infection in the dorsal root ganglia cells. **Zoster (shingles)** is the manifestation of reactivated latent infection of endogenous VZV. VZV (chickenpox) is highly communicable among susceptible individuals, with a secondary attack rate of more than 90%. The period of communicability ranges from 2 days before to 7 days after the onset of the rash, when all lesions are crusted.

Epidemiology

In the prevaccine era, the peak age of occurrence was 5 to 10 years, with peak seasonal infection in late winter and spring. Transmission is by direct contact, droplet, and air. **Zoster** is a recurrence of latent VZV. Only 5% of cases of zoster occur in children younger than 15 years old. The overall incidence of zoster (215 cases per 100,000 person-years) results in a cumulative lifetime incidence of approximately 10% to 20%, with 75% of cases occurring after 45 years of age. The incidence of zoster is increased among immunocompromised persons.

Clinical Manifestations

The incubation period of varicella is generally 14 to 16 days, with a range of 11 to 20 days after contact. Primary infection with VZV results in chickenpox. Prodromal symptoms of fever, malaise, and anorexia may precede the rash by 1 day. The characteristic rash appears initially as small red papules that rapidly progress to nonumbilicated, oval, "teardrop" vesicles on an erythematous base. The fluid progresses from clear to cloudy, and the vesicles ulcerate, crust, and heal. New crops appear for 3 to 4 days, usually beginning on the trunk followed by the head, the face, and, less commonly, the extremities. There may be a total of 100 to 500 lesions, with all forms of lesions being present at the same time. Pruritus is universal and marked. Lesions also may be present on mucous membranes. Lymphadenopathy may be generalized. The severity of the rash varies, as do systemic signs and fever, which generally abate after 3 to 4 days.

The pre-eruption phase of **zoster** includes intense localized pain and tenderness along a dermatome, accompanied by malaise and fever. In adults, the pain of **acute neuritis** in the affected dermatomes is characteristically intense and constant. In several days, the eruption of papules, which quickly vesiculate, occurs in the dermatome or in two adjacent dermatomes. Groups of lesions occur for 1 to 7 days, then progress to crusts and healing. The typical areas involved are dorsal and lumbar, although cephalic and sacral lesions may develop. Lesions generally are unilateral and are accompanied by regional lymphadenopathy. In one third of patients, a few vesicles occur outside the primary dermatome. Any branch of cranial nerve V may be involved, which also may cause corneal and intraoral lesions. Involvement of cranial nerve VII may result in facial paralysis and ear canal vesicles (**Ramsay Hunt syndrome**). Ophthalmic zoster may be associated with ipsilateral cerebral angiitis and stroke. Immunocompromised persons may have unusually severe, painful herpes zoster that involves cutaneous and, rarely, visceral dissemination (to liver, lungs, and CNS). **Postherpetic neuralgia** is pain persisting longer than 1 month and is uncommon in children.

Laboratory and Imaging Studies

Laboratory testing confirmation for diagnosis is usually unnecessary. Vesicles exhibit polymorphonuclear leukocytes. Cytology and electron microscopy of vesicular fluid or scrapings may reveal intranuclear inclusions, giant cells, and virus particles. VZV is fastidious and difficult to culture, in contrast to HSV. A cytology that is consistent with either HSV or VZV in the presence of a negative culture suggests VZV. Infection can be confirmed by detection of varicella-specific antigen in vesicular fluid by immunofluorescence using monoclonal antibodies, or by demonstration of a fourfold antibody increase of acute and convalescent sera.

Differential Diagnosis

The diagnosis of varicella and zoster is based on the distinctive characteristics of the rash. **Eczema herpeticum**, or **Kaposi varicelliform eruption**, is a localized, vesicular eruption caused by HSV that develops on skin that is affected by underlying eczema or trauma. The differentiation between zoster and HSV infection may be difficult because HSV may cause eruption that appears to be in a dermatomal distribution. A previously healthy patient with more than one recurrence probably has HSV infection, which can be confirmed by viral culture.

Treatment

Symptomatic therapy of varicella includes nonaspirin antipyretics, cool baths, and careful hygiene. In immunocompromised persons, early therapy with antivirals is effective in preventing severe complications, including pneumonia, encephalitis, and death from varicella. Early administration of acyclovir, famciclovir, or valacyclovir for chickenpox may decrease the incidence of varicella pneumonia and is recommended for nonpregnant persons 13 years old and older and children 12 months old and older with chronic cutaneous or pulmonary disease; receiving short-course, intermittent, or aerosolized corticosteroids; or receiving long-term salicylate therapy. The dose of acyclovir for VZV infections is much higher than for HSV. The routine oral administration of acyclovir is not recommended in **otherwise healthy children** because of the marginal therapeutic benefit, the lack of difference in complications, and the cost of acyclovir treatment.

Antiviral treatment of zoster accelerates cutaneous healing, hastens the resolution of acute neuritis, and reduces the risk of postherpetic neuralgia. Oral famciclovir and valacyclovir have much greater oral bioavailability than acyclovir and are recommended for treatment of zoster in adults. Acyclovir is recommended for children and is an alternative therapy for adults. The necessity of concomitant oral corticosteroids for zoster is controversial, but oral corticosteroids are recommended for relatively healthy persons older than 50 years of age with moderate or severe pain at presentation.

Complications

Although VZV infection is generally a mild disease, complications are common. Varicella is a more severe disease for neonates, adults, and immunocompromised persons. HIV-infected children frequently have a prolonged course and may have recurrent episodes.

Secondary infection of skin lesions by streptococci or staphylococci is the most common complication. These infections may be mild, resembling impetigo, or life-threatening with toxic shock syndrome or necrotizing fasciitis. Thrombocytopenia and hemorrhagic lesions or bleeding also may occur, known as **varicella gangrenosa**. Pneumonia is uncommon in healthy children, but occurs in 15% to 20% of healthy adults and immunocompromised persons. Myocarditis, pericarditis, orchitis, hepatitis, ulcerative gastritis, glomerulonephritis, and arthritis may complicate varicella. Reye syndrome may follow varicella; aspirin use is **contraindicated** during varicella infection.

Neurologic complications frequently include postinfectious encephalitis, cerebellar ataxia, nystagmus, and tremor. Less common neurologic complications include Guillain-Barré syndrome, transverse myelitis, cranial nerve palsies, optic neuritis, and hypothalamic syndrome.

Primary varicella can be a fatal disease in immunocompromised persons as a result of visceral dissemination, encephalitis, and pneumonitis. The mortality rate approaches 10% in children with leukemia who do not receive prophylaxis or therapy for varicella (see Chapter 66).

Primary varicella in a pregnant woman may result in fetal varicella infection, characterized by low birth weight, cortical atrophy, seizures, mental retardation, chorioretinitis, cataracts, microcephaly, intracranial calcifications, and diagnostic cicatricial scarring of the body or extremities. Children exposed in utero to VZV may develop zoster early in life without ever exhibiting varicella.

A severe form of neonatal varicella may develop in newborns of mothers with varicella (but not shingles) occurring 5 days before or 2 days after delivery. The fetus is exposed to a large inoculum of virus, but is born before the maternal antibody response develops. These infants should be treated as soon as possible with varicella-zoster immunoglobulin (VZIG) to attempt to prevent or ameliorate the infection.

Prognosis

Primary varicella usually resolves spontaneously. The mortality rate is much higher for persons older than age 20 years and for immunocompromised persons. Zoster usually is self-limited, especially in children. Advanced age and severity of pain at presentation and at 1 month are predictors of prolonged pain. Scarring is more common with zoster because of involvement of the deeper layers of the skin.

Prevention

Children with chickenpox should not return to school until all vesicles have crusted. A hospitalized child with chickenpox should be isolated in a negative-pressure room to prevent transmission.

A live attenuated varicella vaccine is recommended as a single dose for all children at age 12 to 18 months and for children age 19 months to the 13th birthday without a history of chickenpox (see Fig. 94–1). Susceptible persons 13 years old or older at high risk of exposure also should be immunized with two doses 4 weeks apart. Varicella vaccine is 85% effective in preventing any disease and is 97% effective in preventing moderately severe and severe disease. Transmission of the vaccine virus from a healthy vaccinee is possible.

Passive immunity can be provided by VZIG, which is indicated within 96 hours of exposure for susceptible individuals at increased risk for severe illness, including immunocompromised persons, neonates of infected mothers who had onset of chickenpox within 5 days before delivery or 48 hours after delivery, premature infants younger than 28 weeks or born to mothers without a history of chickenpox, and possibly children older than 15 years or adults with a close exposure to varicella. Administration of VZIG does not eliminate the possibility of disease in recipients and prolongs the incubation period to 28 days.

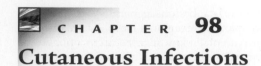

CHAPTER 98

Cutaneous Infections

SUPERFICIAL BACTERIAL INFECTIONS

Impetigo

Nonbullous or crusted impetigo is caused most often by *S. aureus,* occasionally with group A streptococcus, and begins as a single erythematous papulovesicule that progress to one or many honey-colored, crusted lesions weeping serous drainage. **Bullous impetigo** is an uncommon variant with thin-walled (0.5 to 3 cm) bullae, with erythematous margins resembling second-degree burns, and is associated with *S. aureus* phage type 71. Impetigo most frequently occurs on the face, around the nares and mouth, and on the extremities. Fever is uncommon. The **diagnosis** usually is established by the clinical appearance alone, without the need for culture.

Recommended **treatment** is topical 2% mupirocin or oral antibiotics. Extensive or disseminated lesions or lesions around the eyes or that otherwise are not amenable to topical therapy are treated with oral antibiotics with good activity against *S. aureus,* such as cephalexin. Streptococcal impetigo is associated with increased risk for poststreptococcal glomerulonephritis but not acute rheumatic fever (see Chapter 163). Antibiotic treatment for streptococcal impetigo may not decrease the risk for poststreptococcal glomerulonephritis, but treatment is recommended to decrease possible spread of nephritogenic strains to close contacts. Children with impetigo should remain out of school or daycare until 24 hours of antibiotic therapy has been completed.

Cellulitis

Cellulitis is infection involving the subcutaneous tissues and the dermis. It usually is caused by *S. aureus,* group A streptococcus, *S. pneumoniae.* Hib cellulitis, especially of the face, was common before routine vaccination for Hib. Cellulitis typically presents with indurated, warm, and erythematous macules with indistinct borders that expand rapidly. Additional manifestations commonly include fever, lymphangitis, regional lymphadenitis, and less often bacteremia, which may lead to secondary foci and sepsis. **Erysipelas** is a superficial variant of cellulitis usually caused by group A streptococcus that involves only the dermis. The rapidly advancing lesions are tender, are bright red in appearance, have sharp margins, and have an "orange peel" quality. Aspiration of the leading edge of the cellulitis reveals positive Gram stain and culture in a few cases. Blood cultures are recommended. Empirical antibiotic treatment is recommended with a first-generation cephalosporin (cefazolin, cephalexin). Hospitalization and initial IV antibiotic treatment is recommended for cellulitis of the face, hands, feet, or perineum or with lymphangitis. Many patients may be managed with oral antibiotics with close outpatient follow-up.

Ecthyma usually is caused by group A streptococcus and frequently complicates impetigo. Initially, ecthyma is characterized by a lesion with a rim of erythematous induration surrounding an eschar, which, if removed, reveals a shallow ulcer. **Ecthyma gangrenosum** is a serious skin infection that occurs in immunocompromised persons that results from hematogenous spread of septic emboli to the skin. It classically is caused by *P. aeruginosa* or other gram-negative organisms or occasionally *Aspergillus*. The lesions begin as purple macules that undergo central necrosis to become exquisitely tender, deep, punched-out ulcers 2 to 3 cm in diameter with a dark necrotic base, raised red edges, and sometimes a yellowish green exudate. Fever usually is present.

Necrotizing fasciitis is the most extensive form of cellulitis and involves the deeper subcutaneous tissues and fascial planes and may progress to **myonecrosis**, with involvement of the underlying muscle. It usually is caused by *S. aureus* and group A streptococcus alone or in combination with anaerobic organisms, such as *Clostridium perfringens*. Risk factors include underlying immunodeficiency, recent surgery or trauma, and varicella infection. The lesions progress rapidly with raised or sharply demarcated margins. Subcutaneous gas formation confirms anaerobic infection. MRI delineates the extent of deep tissue involvement. Necrotizing fasciitis is a medical emergency that is associated with systemic toxicity and shock. Treatment includes surgical débridement of all necrotic tissues and IV antibiotics, such as clindamycin plus cefotaxime or ceftriaxone, with or without an aminoglycoside.

Folliculitis

Folliculitis refers to small, dome-shaped pustules or erythematous papules located in the hair follicle predominantly caused by *S. aureus,* with superficial, limited inflammatory reaction in the surrounding tissue. A **furuncle (boil)** represents deeper infections of the hair follicle that manifest as nodules with more intense surrounding inflammatory reaction. These occur most frequently on the neck, trunk, axillae, and buttocks. A **carbuncle** represents the deepest and most complicated of hair follicle infections and is characterized by multiseptate, loculated abscesses that frequently require incisional drainage. Superficial folliculitis can be treated with topical therapy, such as an antibacterial chlorhexidine wash or an antibacterial lotion or solution such as clindamycin 1%, applied twice a day for 7 to 10 days. Oral antibiotics are necessary for unresponsive or persistent cases, cases with widespread involvement, or furuncles or carbuncles. Furuncles and carbuncles may need incision and drainage.

P. aeruginosa **folliculitis (hot tub folliculitis)** is associated with hot tubs. It presents as pruritic papules, pustules, or deeper, purple-red nodules that are predominantly on areas of skin that were covered by a swimsuit. The folliculitis develops 8 to 48 hours after exposure, usually without associated systemic symptoms. It usually is self-limited and resolves in 1 to 2 weeks without treatment.

Perianal Dermatitis

Perianal dermatitis (perianal streptococcal disease) is caused by group A streptococcus and is characterized by well-demarcated, tender perianal erythema extending 2 cm from the anus. Manifestations include anal pruritus and painful defecation, sometimes with blood-streaked stools. The differential diagnosis includes diaper dermatitis, candidiasis, pinworm infection, and simple anal fissures. Treatment is oral penicillin V or erythromycin.

Anthrax

Cutaneous anthrax is caused by *Bacillus anthracis,* a gram-positive bacillus that forms spores that remain viable for decades. Cutaneous anthrax is transmitted via spores from the soil or animal hides that contaminate abraded or traumatized skin. After a 2- to 5-day incubation period, a small, painless, erythematous papule develops at the site of inoculation that rapidly enlarges and becomes edematous and hemorrhagic. The center of the lesion becomes necrotic, and a black eschar develops. Despite destructive local involvement, the lesion is characteristically painless. There may be regional lymphadenopathy and fever. Dissemination and systemic manifestations are uncommon. The recommended treatment of cutaneous anthrax is high-dose penicillin G.

Cutaneous Nontuberculous Mycobacterial Infections

Cutaneous mycobacterial infections are usually the result of inoculation with *Mycobacterium marinum* (**swimming pool granuloma** or **fish tank granuloma**) or *Mycobacterium fortuitum* complex. *M. marinum* frequently is isolated from freshwater, salt water, swimming pool walls, tropical fish aquaria, and marine animals. The initial papule or nodule usually is located on the extremities, elbows, or knees where abrasions and trauma may have occurred and slowly enlarges and ulcerates. Skin biopsy and acid-fast stain may be necessary to confirm the diagnosis. Infection in healthy children is often self-limited, but resolution without treatment may require several years. Prolonged therapy with antimycobacterial drugs may be necessary.

SUPERFICIAL FUNGAL INFECTIONS

Cutaneous Dermatophyte Infections

Dermatophytoses (tinea) of glabrous, or non–hair-bearing, skin are classified according to their anatomic location and are caused by three genera: *Microsporum, Trichophyton,* and *Epidermophyton.* Tinea corporis and tinea capitis are more common among young children, whereas tinea versicolor, tinea pedis, and tinea cruris are more common after puberty among adolescents and young adults. These are common infections; estimated lifetime risk of developing a dermatophytosis is 10% to 20%. Dermatophytes are spread by person-to-person transmission or via fomites, such as combs, brushes, or bedding. Some also can be transmitted by contact with infected animals (Table 98–1).

Tinea corporis (ringworm) is caused by *Trichophyton rubrum, Trichophyton mentagrophytes,* and *Microsporum canis.* It presents as a pruritic annular papule or plaque that expands outward with a raised ring of erythema and scale surrounding a central area of clearing. Multiple secondary lesions may merge to form one large area that may be several centimeters in diameter. Autoinoculation facilitates spread to other parts of the body. The diagnosis usually is established by visual inspection. The primary lesion must be differentiated from psoriasis; nummular eczema; granuloma annulare, the herald patch of pityriasis rosea; and erythema migrans, the primary lesion of Lyme disease.

Tinea pedis (athlete's foot) commonly affects adolescents and young adults. Tinea pedis is acquired through direct contact with contaminated surfaces, especially the warm, moist environments of showers and locker room floors. It presents with fissuring, scaling, and cracking of the skin between the toes and over the dorsum of the foot. Symptoms include intense burning sensation, pruritus, and foul odor. It also may present as a chronic, diffuse plantar hyperkeratosis with mild erythema. The differential diagnosis for tinea pedis includes simple maceration and peeling of the interdigital spaces, contact dermatitis, dyshidrotic eczema, and juvenile plantar dermatosis (a friction-induced disorder characterized by plantar erythema, maceration, and fissuring that spares the web spaces).

Tinea cruris (jock itch) commonly affects adolescents and young adults. Risk factors for tinea cruris include hyperhidrosis, obesity, and wearing tight-fitting or occlusive garments. It begins as a scaly erythematous patch on the inner aspect of the thigh that spreads peripherally. Vesiculation is frequent at the margins of the spreading lesion. Eventually the lesion evolves into an irregular, well-demarcated patch with a hyperpigmented, scaling center. The penis and scrotum usually are not involved. The differential diagnosis for tinea cruris includes intertrigo, contact dermatitis, and candidal dermatitis.

The **diagnosis of a cutaneous dermatophytosis** usually is established by visual inspection and may be confirmed by potassium hydroxide (KOH) examination and fungal culture of skin scrapings from the margins of the lesion. **Recommended treatment** of tinea corporis, tinea pedis, and tinea cruris is with topical antifungal cream (e.g., miconazole, clotrimazole, terbinafine, econazole, ketoconazole, tolnaftate) for about 2 weeks or for 1 week after resolution.

Onychomycosis, or dermatophyte infection of the nail, is uncommon in children but occurs with increasing frequency after puberty. Subungual onychomycosis is characterized by thickening and yellowing of the distal fingernail or toenail. *T. rubrum* is isolated most frequently. The **diagnosis** of onychomycosis always should be confirmed by KOH examination and fungal culture. Recommended **treatment** is terbinafine or itraconazole for at least 12 weeks.

Tinea Versicolor

Tinea versicolor (pityriasis versicolor) is a dermatophytosis mainly affecting adolescents and young adults that is caused by *Malassezia furfur,* a saprophytic yeast that infects the stratum corneum. *M. furfur* is part of the normal cutaneous flora in adults but not infants. The lesions of tinea versicolor are scaly, oval, hyperpigmented or hypopigmented macules usually 1 to 2 cm in diameter located on the upper chest, back, or arms. They tend to coalesce and form irregularly shaped patches involving most of the trunk. The lesions have a fine scale and are usually asymptomatic or may be mildly pruritic.

The characteristic clinical presentation usually permits the diagnosis by visual inspection. Wood lamp examination usually shows copper-orange fluorescence. The diagnosis is confirmed by KOH examination of scrapings from the lesion that show the characteristic short "cigar-butt" hyphae and round spores, referred to as a "spaghetti and meatballs" appearance. *M. furfur* requires specialized medium with lipids for culture.

Isolated lesions are **treated** with twice-daily application of an antifungal cream, such as miconazole 2%, clotrimazole 1%, econazole nitrate 1%, or ketoconazole 2%. Widespread involvement is treated with selenium sulfide 2.5% lotion applied twice daily for 30 minutes

TABLE 98-1. Superficial Fungal Infections

Name	Etiology	Manifestations	Diagnosis	Therapy
Tinea capitis (ringworm)	*Microsporum audouinii, Trichophyton tonsurans, Microsporum canis*	Prepubertal infection of scalp, hair-shafts; "black dot" alopecia; *T. tonsurans* common in blacks	*M. audouinii* fluorescence: blue-green with Wood lamp*; +KOH, culture	Griseofulvin; terbinafine, itraconazole
Kerion	Inflammatory reaction to tinea capitis	Swollen, boggy, crusted, purulent, tender mass with lymphadenopathy; secondary distal "id" reaction common	As above	As above, plus steroids for "id" reactions
Tinea corporis (ringworm)	*M. canis, Trichophyton rubrum,* others	Slightly pruritic ringlike, erythematous papules, plaques with scaling and slow outward expansion of the border; check cat or dog for *M. canis*	+KOH, culture; *M. canis* fluorescence: blue-green with Wood lamp; differential diagnosis: granuloma annulare, pityriasis rosea, nummular eczema, psoriasis	Topical miconazole, clotrimazole, terbinafine, econazole, ketoconazole, or tolnaftate
Tinea cruris (jock itch)	*Epidermophyton floccosum, Trichophyton mentagrophytes, T. rubrum*	Symmetric, pruritic, scrotal sparing, scaling plaques	+KOH, culture; differential diagnosis: erythrasma (*Corynebacterium minutissimum*)	See "Tinea Corporis"; wear loose cotton underwear
Tinea pedis (athlete's foot)	*T. rubrum, T. mentagrophytes*	Moccasin or interdigital distribution, dry scales, interdigital maceration with secondary bacterial infection	+KOH, culture; differential diagnosis: *C. minutissimum* erythrasma	Medications as above; wear cotton socks
Tinea unguium (onychomycosis)	*T. mentagrophytes, T. rubrum, Candida albicans*	Uncommon before puberty; peeling of distal nail plate; thickening, splitting of nails	+KOH, culture	Oral terbinafine or itraconazole
Tinea versicolor	*Malassezia furfur*	Tropical climates, steroids or immunosuppressive drugs; uncommon before puberty; chest, back, arms; oval hypopigmented or hyperpigmented in blacks, red-brown in whites; scaling patches	+KOH; orange-gold fluorescence with Wood lamp; differential diagnosis: pityriasis alba	Topical selenium sulfide, oral ketoconazole
Candidiasis	*C. albicans*	Diaper area, intense erythematous plaques or pustules, isolated or confluent	+KOH, culture	Topical nystatin; oral nystatin treats concomitant oral thrush

*Wood lamp examination uses an UV source in a completely darkened room. *Trichophyton* usually has no fluorescence. KOH, potassium hydroxide.

or oral ketoconazole for 7 to 10 days. Hypopigmentation may persist for weeks to months after successful therapy. Recurrences are common.

Tinea Capitis

Tinea capitis is infection of the scalp and hair shafts. *Microsporum audouinii* previously was responsible for most cases, but *Trichophyton tonsurans* now causes more than 90% of cases. Most cases occur in children, with higher incidence among African American and Hispanic children. **Black dot tinea** presents with discrete scaly areas of patchy alopecia with short, broken hairs at the scalp surface, resulting from brittle hairs from intrapilar sporulation. Other *T. tonsurans* infections present with only mild scalp erythema and fine scaling that may be itchy or asymptomatic and is easily confused with seborrheic dermatitis (dandruff) and atopic dermatitis. Diffuse hair loss may complicate long-standing infection. *T. tonsurans* does not fluoresce on Wood light. A **kerion** is the result of an intense inflammatory response with perifollicular pustules on a boggy, nontender scalp mass. Tinea capitis may be accompanied by a pruritic, papular eruption on the face, neck, and trunk known as an **id reaction**, which represents a hypersensitivity reaction to fungal allergens and may be mistaken for an allergic reaction to drug therapy.

The **diagnosis** is established by clinical appearance and may be confirmed by KOH examination of a hair plucked from the scalp or by fungal culture. Tinea capitis is treated with oral griseofulvin (microsize or ultramicrosize) for 6 to 8 weeks or terbinafine or itraconazole for 2 to 4 weeks. Topical therapy alone is not effective. Adjunctive use of selenium sulfide or ketoconazole shampoo may decrease spore shedding and reduce transmission. A short course of oral prednisone may hasten resolution and reduce the risk of scarring from a kerion.

SUPERFICIAL VIRAL INFECTIONS

Herpes Simplex Virus

Primary herpetic infections can occur after inoculation of the virus at any mucocutaneous site. HSV type 1 is common in children and classically infects skin and mucous membranes above the waist. HSV type 2 is rare in childhood and classically infects the genitalia as a sexually transmitted infection (STI) (see Chapter 116).

Herpes gingivostomatitis is a primary HSV infection that involves the gingivae and the vermilion border of the lips. **Herpes labialis** is limited to the vermilion border involving skin and mucous membrane. Clinical manifestations of primary HSV gingivostomatitis include the typical oropharyngeal vesicular lesions with high fever, malaise, stinging mouth pain, drooling, fetor oris (fetid breath), and cervical lymphadenopathy.

Herpetic skin lesions characteristically begin as erythematous papules that quickly progress to the characteristically grouped, 2- to 4-mm, fluid-filled vesicles on an erythematous base. Removal of the vesicle roof reveals a small, sharply demarcated ulcer with a "punched-out" appearance. Herpetic lesions are quite painful. The characteristic grouped vesicles distinguish HSV from chickenpox (see Chapter 97). Within several days, the vesicles become pustular, rupture, become crusted and may appear as impetigo, and gradually heal. Scarring is uncommon, but there may be residual hyperpigmentation. After primary infection, the virus remains latent in the dorsal root ganglia. Recurrences occur in roughly the same location and may be preceded by prodromal symptoms of tingling or burning, but without fever and lymphadenopathy.

Viral paronychia (herpetic whitlow) is painful, localized infection of a digit with erythematous and occasionally vesiculopustular eruption. It occurs among children who suck their thumbs and bite their nails and especially among older children with herpetic gingivostomatitis. **Herpes gladiatorum** occurs among wrestlers and rugby players who acquire cutaneous herpes from close body contact with the cutaneous infections of other players. Cutaneous HSV infection in persons with an underlying skin disorder, often atopic dermatitis, can result in **eczema herpeticum (Kaposi varicelliform eruption)**, which is a disseminated cutaneous infection. There may be hundreds of herpetic vesicles over the body, usually concentrated in the areas of skin affected by the underlying disorder.

Erythema multiforme is associated with HSV infection (see Chapter 194). After primary HSV gingivostomatitis, HSV establishes latency in the trigeminal ganglion. About 20% to 40% of adults experience recurrent oral episodes of HSV labialis (cold sores or fever blisters) that occur intermittently throughout life.

Treatment with oral valacyclovir or famciclovir may shorten duration of disease for primary and recurrent infection. Topical antiviral therapy, with penciclovir cream, is effective only for recurrent gingivostomatitis and must be started with the first symptoms. Infants, persons with eczema, and persons with immunodeficiency are at increased risk for disseminated and severe HSV disease and should receive IV acyclovir therapy.

Human Papillomaviruses (Warts)

Warts are caused by the human papillomaviruses (HPV), which infect keratinocytes of the skin and mucous membranes but do not cause systemic disease. More than 70 serotypes of HPV have been identified, with different serotypes accounting for the variation in location and clinical presentation of warts. **Common warts (verruca vulgaris)** are associated with HPV types 2 and 4; **flat warts (verruca plana)** are associated with HPV types 2, 3, and 5; and **genital warts (condylomata acuminata)** are associated with HPV types 6 and 11 (see Chapter 116). Regardless of the infecting serotype, all warts are associated with the basic pathologic finding of hyperplasia of the epidermal cells.

Warts can occur at any age. They are transmitted by direct contact or by fomites and have an incubation period of approximately 1 month before clinical presentation. The most typical lesion is the common wart, a painless, well-circumscribed, small (2 to 5 mm) papule with a papillated or verrucous surface. Common warts are classically distributed on the fingers, toes, elbows, and knees. They also may be found on the nose, ears, and lips. **Filiform warts** are verrucous, exophytic, 2-mm papules that have a narrow or pedunculated base. **Flat warts** are multiple, flat-topped 2- to 4-mm papules clustered on the dorsal surface of the hands, on the soles of the feet (**plantar warts**), or on the face. Plantar warts may be painful because of the effect of pressure and friction on the lesions. Genital warts are flesh-colored, hyperpigmented, or erythematous lesions that are filiform, fungating, or plaquelike in appearance and involve multiple sites on the vulva, vagina, penis, or perineum.

Warts typically are self-limited and resolve spontaneously over years without specific treatment. Genital warts carry the risk of malignant transformation, which is low with HPV types 6 and 11, but is high among patients with infection resulting from HPV types 16 and 18. Genital warts are more common and associated with higher risk of recurrence and malignant transformation among patients with immunodeficiencies.

Treatment options are available for common and flat warts and for condylomata acuminata. For common and flat warts, destructive modalities, such as cryotherapy with liquid nitrogen, electrodesiccation, and vesicant therapy with cantharidin, are available. These treatments are painful and are not always effective. Topical 5-fluorouracil ointment (5%) may be applied to treat refractory lesions. Plantar warts may be treated with topical application of 10% to 17% salicylic and lactic acids in collodion or topical 40% salicylic acid alone. Newer treatment methods include laser ablation and immunotherapy with intralesional interferon; immunotherapy may be associated with significant toxicities.

Molluscum Contagiosum

Molluscum contagiosum virus is a poxvirus that replicates in host epithelial cells. The lesions of molluscum contagiosum are discrete, small (2 to 4 mm), pearly flesh-colored or pink, nontender, dome-shaped papules with central umbilication. Papules occur most commonly in intertriginous regions, such as the axillae, groin, and neck. They rarely occur on the face, in the periocular region. The infection typically affects toddlers and young children and is acquired through direct contact with an infected individual, with additional spread by autoinoculation. Infection with molluscum contagiosum may be complicated by a surrounding dermatitis. Severely immunocompromised persons or persons with extensive atopic dermatitis often have widespread lesions.

Lesions are self-limited, resolving over months to years, and usually no specific treatment is recommended. Available treatment options are limited to destructive modalities, such as cryotherapy with topical liquid nitrogen, vesicant therapy with topical 0.9% cantharidin, or removal by curettage.

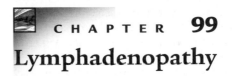

CHAPTER **99**

Lymphadenopathy

ETIOLOGY

Lymphoid tissue steadily enlarges until puberty, when it undergoes progressive atrophy throughout life. Lymph nodes are most prominent among children 4 to 8 years old. Normal lymph node size is 10 mm in diameter, with the exceptions of 15 mm for inguinal nodes, 5 mm for epitrochlear nodes, and 2 mm for supraclavicular nodes, which are usually undetectable. **Lymphadenopathy** is disease or enlargement of lymph nodes and occurs in response to a wide variety of infectious, inflammatory, and malignant processes. **Generalized lymphadenopathy** is enlargement of two or more noncontiguous lymph node groups, whereas **regional lymphadenopathy** involves only one lymph node group.

Lymphadenitis is acute or chronic inflammation of lymph nodes and indicates acute inflammation and enlargement. Acute lymphadenitis usually results as bacteria and toxins from a site of acute inflammation are carried via lymph to regional nodes. There are numerous infectious causes of generalized lymphadenopathy, regional lymphadenopathy, and lymphadenitis (Tables 99–1 and 99–2). Causes of inguinal regional lymphadenopathy also include STIs (see Chapter 116). **Lymphocutaneous syndromes** are characterized by regional lymphadenitis associated with a characteristic skin lesion at the site of inoculation. **Lymphangitis** is an inflammation of subcuta-

TABLE 99–1. Infectious Causes of Generalized Lymphadenopathy

Viral

Epstein-Barr virus (infectious mononucleosis)
Cytomegalovirus (infectious mononucleosis–like syndrome)
HIV (acute retroviral syndrome)
Hepatitis B virus
Hepatitis C virus
Varicella
Adenoviruses
Rubeola (measles)
Rubella

Bacterial

Endocarditis
Brucella (brucellosis)
Leptospira interrogans (leptospirosis)
Streptobacillus moniliformis (bacillary rat-bite fever)
Mycobacterium tuberculosis (tuberculosis)
Treponema pallidum (secondary syphilis)

Fungal

Coccidioides immitis (coccidioidomycosis)
Histoplasma capsulatum (histoplasmosis)

Protozoal

Toxoplasma gondii (toxoplasmosis)

neous lymphatic channels that usually presents as an acute bacterial infection, usually caused by *S. aureus* and group A streptococcus.

Cervical lymphadenitis is the most common regional lymphadenitis among children and is associated most commonly with pharyngitis caused by group A streptococcus (see Chapter 103) and EBV. Other common infectious causes of cervical lymphadenitis include *B. henselae* (cat-scratch disease) and atypical mycobacteria, or nontuberculous mycobacteria.

EBV is the primary cause of **infectious mononucleosis**, a clinical syndrome that is characterized by fever, fatigue and malaise, cervical or generalized lymphadenopathy, tonsillitis, and pharyngitis. EBV, a member of the herpesvirus family, infects B lymphocytes and is spread by salivary secretions. After primary infection, EBV is maintained latently in multiple episomes in the cell nucleus of resting B lymphocytes and establishes lifelong infection that remains clinically inapparent. Most persons shed EBV intermittently, with approximately 20% of healthy individuals shedding EBV at any given time. CMV, *Toxoplasma gondii*, adenoviruses, HBV, hepatitis C (HCV), and the initial HIV infection, known as **acute retroviral syndrome**,

can cause an infectious mononucleosis–like syndrome with lymphadenopathy. CMV is commonly transmitted in daycare environments and by transfusion of blood products.

The cause of **cat-scratch disease** is *B. henselae,* which is a small, pleomorphic, gram-negative bacillus that stains with Warthin-Starry silver stain. *B. henselae* does not seem to cause disease in cats, which may be bacteremic, especially kittens. The cat flea, *Ctenocephalides felis,* can harbor *B. henselae* and may be the major vector for transmission among cats. *B. henselae* is transmitted to humans by bites and scratches, which may appear minor. *B. henselae* also causes bacillary angiomatosis and peliosis hepatis in persons with HIV infection (see Chapter 125).

Atypical mycobacteria are ubiquitous in soil, vegetation, dust, and water. Atypical *Mycobacterium* species commonly causing lymphadenitis in children include

TABLE 99–2. Infectious Causes of Regional Lymphadenopathy and Lymphadenitis

Nonvenereal Origin

Staphylococcus aureus
Group A streptococci
Group B streptococci (in infants)
Bartonella henselae (cat-scratch disease)
Yersinia pestis (plague)
Francisella tularensis (glandular tularemia)
Mycobacterium tuberculosis
Atypical mycobacteria
Sporothrix schenckii (sporotrichosis)
Epstein-Barr virus
Toxoplasma gondii

Sexually Transmitted Infections (Primarily Inguinal Lymphadenopathy)

Neisseria gonorrhoeae (gonorrhea)
Treponema pallidum (syphilis)
Herpes simplex virus
Haemophilus ducreyi (chancroid)
Chlamydia trachomatis serovars L$_{1-3}$ (lymphogranuloma venereum)

Lymphocutaneous Syndromes

Bacillus anthracis (anthrax)
F. tularensis (ulceroglandular tularemia)
B. henselae (cat-scratch disease)
Pasteurella multocida (dog or cat bite)
Spirillum minus (spirillary rat-bite fever)
Y. pestis (plague)
Nocardia (nocardiosis)
Cutaneous diphtheria (*Corynebacterium diphtheriae*)
Cutaneous coccidioidomycosis (*Coccidioides immitis*)
Cutaneous histoplasmosis (*Histoplasma capsulatum*)
Cutaneous sporotrichosis (*S. schenckii*)

M. avium complex, *M. scrofulaceum,* and *M. kansasii. M. tuberculosis* is an important but uncommon cause of cervical lymphadenitis.

EPIDEMIOLOGY

Cervical lymphadenitis as a complication of group A streptococcal infection parallels the incidence of streptococcal pharyngitis (see Chapter 103). Many cases also are caused by *S. aureus.* EBV and CMV are ubiquitous, with most infections occurring in young children, who are likely to be asymptomatic or only mildly symptomatic. Approximately one third of adolescents and young adults with primary EBV infection develop symptomatic disease. EBV disease is most commonly observed among adolescents and young adults dispite the higher incidence of EBV infection among young children. Risk factors for specific causes of lymphadenopathy may be indicated by past medical and surgical history; preceding trauma; exposure to animals; contact with persons infected with tuberculosis; sexual history; travel history; food and ingestion history, especially of undercooked meat or unpasteurized dairy products; and current medications.

CLINICAL MANIFESTATIONS

Cervical lymphadenopathy associated with pharyngitis is characterized by small and rubbery lymph nodes in the anterior cervical chain with minimal to moderate tenderness. Suppurative cervical lymphadenitis, frequently caused by *S. aureus,* group A streptococcus, *B. henselae,* or atypical mycobacteria, shows erythema and warmth of the overlying skin with moderate to exquisite tenderness.

The characteristic triad of EBV infectious mononucleosis is fever, pharyngitis, and lymphadenopathy. The pharynx shows enlarged tonsils and exudate and sometimes an enanthem with pharyngeal petechiae. Lymphadenopathy is most prominent in the anterior and posterior cervical and submandibular lymph nodes and less commonly involves axillary and inguinal lymph nodes. Other findings include splenomegaly in 50% of cases, hepatomegaly in 10% to 20%, and maculopapular or urticarial rash in 5% to 15%. A diffuse, erythematous rash developed in approximately 80% of patients treated with oral ampicillin, known as **ampicillin rash**. Compared with EBV infection, infectious mononucleosis–like illness caused by CMV has minimal pharyngitis and often more prominent splenomegaly; it often presents only with fever. The most common manifestation of toxoplasmosis is asymptomatic cervical lymphadenopathy, but approximately 10% of cases of acquired toxoplasmosis develop chronic posterior cervical lymphadenopathy and fatigue, usually without significant fever.

Cat-scratch disease typically presents with a cutaneous papule or conjunctival granuloma followed by lymphadenopathy localized to the draining regional nodes. The nodes are tender, with suppuration in approximately 10% of cases. Lymphadenopathy may persist 1 to 4 months. Less common features of cat-scratch disease include erythema nodosum, osteolytic lesions, encephalitis, oculoglandular (Parinaud) syndrome, hepatic or splenic granulomas, endocarditis, polyneuritis, and transverse myelitis.

Lymphadenitis caused by atypical mycobacteria usually is unilateral in the cervical, submandibular, or preauricular nodes. The nodes usually are relatively painless and firm initially, but over time they gradually soften, then rupture and drain. The local reaction is circumscribed, and although the skin overlying the node may develop a pinkish discoloration, it is not warm to the touch. Fever and systemic symptoms are minimal or absent.

LABORATORY AND IMAGING STUDIES

Initial laboratory tests of regional lymphadenopathy include a complete blood count and ESR. Infectious mononucleosis is characterized by a lymphocytosis with atypical lymphocytes, which are T lymphocytes in response to EBV-infected B lymphocytes. Thrombocytopenia and elevated hepatic enzymes are common.

Cultures of infected skin lesions and tonsillar exudates should be obtained. Isolation of group A streptococci from the nasopharynx suggests but does not confirm streptococcal cervical lymphadenitis. A blood culture should be obtained from children with systemic signs and symptoms of bacteremia.

Serologic testing for EBV should be obtained and for *B. henselae* (cat-scratch disease) if there is a history of exposure to cats. The most reliable test for diagnosis of acute EBV infection is the IgM anti–viral capsid antigen (Fig. 99–1). Heterophil antibody also is diagnostic, but this test is not reliably positive in children younger than 4 years old with infectious mononucleosis.

Extended diagnostic workup is guided by the history and physical examination and may include chest radiograph, throat culture, antistreptolysin O titer, and serologic tests for CMV, toxoplasmosis, syphilis, tularemia, *Brucella,* histoplasmosis, and coccidioidomycosis. Genital tract evaluation and specimens should be obtained with regional inguinal lymphadenopathy (see Chapter 116). Intradermal skin testing for tuberculosis can be performed using the standard (5 TU) Mantoux test, which also may be positive with atypical mycobacterial infection.

Aspiration is indicated for acutely inflamed, fluctuant cervical lymph nodes, especially if greater than 3 cm in diameter. Ultrasound or CT may be extremely useful in establishing the extent of lymphadenopathy and defining whether the mass is solid, cystic, or suppura-

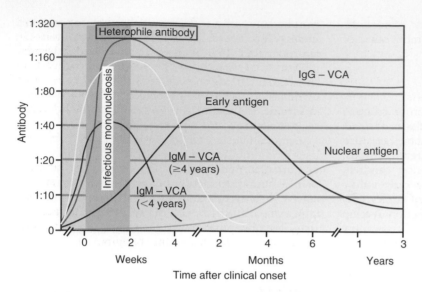

Figure 99-1

The development of antibodies to various Epstein-Barr virus antigens in patients with infectious mononucleosis. The titers are geometric mean values expressed as reciprocals of the serum dilution. The IgM response to viral capsid antigen (VCA) is divided because of the significant differences noted according to age of the patient. (From Jenson HB, Ench Y: Epstein-Barr virus. In Rose NR, Hamilton RG, Detrick B [eds]: Manual of Clinical Laboratory Immunology, 6th ed. Washington, DC, American Society for Microbiology, 2002, p 617.)

tive with formation of an abscess. Pus from fluctuant should be examined by Gram stain and acid-fast stain and cultured for aerobic and anaerobic bacteria and mycobacteria. Biopsy should be performed if lymphoma is suspected because of firm, matted, nontender nodes and other findings (see Chapter 156).

If the diagnosis remains uncertain, and the lymphadenopathy persists and fails to respond to empirical antibiotic therapy for presumed *S. aureus* and group A streptococcus, excisional biopsy should be performed. The entire node should be excised if possible, which is curative for atypical mycobacterial lymphadenitis. Biopsy material should be submitted for histopathology, Gram, acid-fast, Giemsa, periodic acid–Schiff, Warthin-Starry silver (*B. henselae*), and methenamine silver stains. Cultures for aerobic and anaerobic bacteria, mycobacteria, and fungi should be performed.

DIFFERENTIAL DIAGNOSIS

Physical examination should include noting exact location and detailed measurement of the size and number of involved nodes and assessment of the shape and character of the nodes, including consistency, mobility, tenderness, warmth, fluctuant nature, firmness, and adherence to adjacent tissues. The physical examination should include assessment of presence or absence of dental disease, oropharyngeal or skin lesions, ocular disease, other nodal enlargement, and any other signs of systemic illness, including hepatosplenomegaly and skin lesions.

Noninfectious causes of cervical lymphadenopathy include congenital and acquired cysts, juvenile rheumatoid arthritis, systemic lupus erythematosus, Kawasaki disease, sarcoidosis, benign neoplasms,

malignancies, and serum sickness and other adverse drug reactions, especially with phenytoin and other antiepileptic medications, allopurinol, isoniazid, antithyroid medications, and pyrimethamine. Lymphadenopathy is a diagnostic criterion of Kawasaki disease, but is not consistently present (see Chapter 88). Leukemia, lymphoma, and occasionally neuroblastoma may have lymph nodes that are usually painless, not inflamed, matted, and firm in consistency (see Chapters 155 and 156). A syndrome of **periodic fever, aphthous stomatitis, pharyngitis, and adenitis** is an occasional cause of recurrent fever and cervical lymphadenitis (see Chapter 103).

TREATMENT

Management of lymphadenopathy and lymphadenitis depends on the age of the patient, associated findings, size and location of the nodes, and severity of the acute systemic symptoms. In children, most cases of cervical lymphadenopathy, without other signs of acute inflammation, require no specific therapy and usually regress within 2 to 3 weeks. Progression to lymphadenitis or development of generalized lymphadenopathy requires further evaluation.

The specific treatment of cervical lymphadenitis depends on the underlying etiology. The most common causes of acute suppurative cervical lymphadenitis are *S. aureus* and group A streptococcus. Empirical treatment should include an antibiotic, such as a penicillinase-resistant penicillin or first-generation cephalosporin. For patients with hypersensitivity to β-lactam antibiotics, or if community-acquired methicillin-resistant *S. aureus* is suspected, clindamycin is appropriate. Children with isolated suppurative cervical lymphadenitis often respond to empirical antibiotic therapy, obviating the need for further evaluation. Absence of a clinical response within 48 to 72 hours is an indication for further laboratory evaluation and possible excisional biopsy and culture.

There is no specific treatment for infectious mononucleosis. Definitive therapy of persistent lymphadenitis should be guided initially by Gram stain and acid-fast stain and ultimately by serologic tests and culture, if obtained. Cat-scratch disease usually does not require treatment because the lymphadenopathy resolves in 2 to 4 months with sequelae. Aspiration is indicated for suppurative nodes. Azithromycin may hasten resolution and reduces node size at 30 days, but there is no benefit of treatment at 90 days. The recommended treatment of cervical lymphadenitis caused by nontuberculous mycobacteria is complete surgical excision. Antimycobacterial drugs are necessary only if there is recurrence or inability to excise the infected nodes completely, or if *M. tuberculosis* is identified, which requires 6 months of antituberculous chemotherapy (see Chapter 124). Localized cutaneous or lymphocutaneous sporotrichosis is treated with oral itraconazole.

COMPLICATIONS AND PROGNOSIS

Most acute infections caused by *S. aureus* and group A streptococcus respond to treatment and have an excellent prognosis. Complications such as abscess formation, cellulitis, and bacteremia may occur. Abscess formation is treated with incision and drainage in conjunction with appropriate antibiotic therapy.

Infectious mononucleosis usually resolves in 2 to 4 weeks, but fatigue and malaise may wax and wane for several weeks to months. EBV also is associated with numerous complications during the acute illness. Splenic rupture is rare but may be life-threatening. Neurologic complications include seizures, aseptic meningitis syndrome, Bell palsy, transverse myelitis, encephalitis, and Guillain-Barré syndrome. Other complications include Coombs-positive hemolytic anemia, antibody-mediated thrombocytopenia, hemophagocytic syndrome, and, rarely, aplastic anemia. Corticosteroids have been used for respiratory difficulty resulting from tonsillar hypertrophy, which responds rapidly, and for thrombocytopenia, hemolytic anemia, and neurologic complications. **X-linked lymphoproliferative disease** is manifested as fulminant infectious mononucleosis with primary EBV infection, malignant lymphoproliferative disease, or dysgammaglobulinemia that results from a mutation of the *SH2D1A* gene located in the Xq25 region.

EBV infection, as with other herpesviruses, persists for life, but no symptoms are attributed to intermittent reactivation. EBV is causally associated with nasopharyngeal carcinoma, Burkitt lymphoma, Hodgkin

disease, and EBV lymphoproliferative disease and leiomyosarcoma in immunocompromised persons, especially post-transplant patients and AIDS patients.

Lymphadenitis caused by nontuberculous mycobacteria has an excellent prognosis. Surgical excision of cervical lymphadenitis caused by nontuberculous mycobacteria is curative in greater than 97% of cases.

PREVENTION

The incidence of suppurative regional lymphadenitis reflects the incidence of predisposing conditions, such as dental disease, streptococcal pharyngitis, otitis media, impetigo, and other infections involving the face and scalp. There are no guidelines to prevent lymphadenitis caused by nontuberculous mycobacteria.

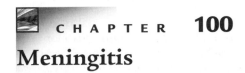

CHAPTER **100**
Meningitis

ETIOLOGY

Meningitis, inflammation of the leptomeninges, can be caused by bacteria, viruses, or, rarely, fungi. The term **aseptic meningitis** refers principally to viral meningitis, but a similar picture may be seen with other infectious organisms (Lyme disease, syphilis, tuberculosis), parameningeal infections (brain abscess, epidural abscess, venous sinus empyema), chemical exposure (nonsteroidal anti-inflammatory drug, IV immunoglobulin), autoimmune disorders, and many other diseases.

The organisms commonly causing bacterial meningitis (Table 100–1) before the availability of current conjugate vaccines were Hib, *S. pneumoniae*, and *N. meningitidis*. In the U.S., the rate of Hib has declined to less than 5% of its previous rate, the rate of *S. pneumoniae* meningitis is declining, and a conjugate meningococcal vaccine is being introduced. The bacteria causing neonatal meningitis are the same as the bacteria that cause neonatal sepsis (see Chapter 65). Staphylococcal meningitis occurs in patients who have had neurosurgery or penetrating head trauma.

Viral meningitis is caused principally by enteroviruses, including coxsackieviruses, echoviruses, and, in unvaccinated individuals, polioviruses. Fecal excretion and transmission are continuous and persist for several weeks. Enteroviruses and arboviruses (St. Louis, LaCrosse, California encephalitis viruses) are the principal causes of meningoencephalitis (see Chapter 101). Other viruses that cause meningitis include HSV, EBV, CMV, lymphocytic choriomeningitis virus, and HIV.

TABLE 100–1.   Bacterial Causes of Meningitis

Age	Most Common	Less Common
Neonatal	Group B streptococci *Escherichia coli* *Klebsiella* *Enterobacter*	*Staphylococcus aureus* Coagulase-negative staphylococci *Enterococcus faecalis* *Citrobacter diversus* *Salmonella* *Listeria monocytogenes* *Pseudomonas aeruginosa* *Haemophilus influenzae* types a, b, c, d, e, f, and nontypable
>1 mo	*Streptococcus pneumoniae* *Neisseria meningitidis*	*H. influenzae* type b Group A streptococci Gram-negative bacilli *L. monocytogenes*

Mumps virus is a common cause of viral meningitis in unvaccinated children. Uncommon causes of meningitis include *Borrelia burgdorferi* (Lyme disease), *B. henselae* (cat-scratch disease), *M. tuberculosis, Toxoplasma,* fungi (*Cryptococcus, Histoplasma,* and *Coccidioides*), and parasites (*Angiostrongylus cantonensis, Naegleria fowleri, Acanthamoeba*).

EPIDEMIOLOGY

The incidence of bacterial meningitis is highest among children younger than 1 year of age. Extremely high rates are found among Native Americans, Alaskan Natives, and Australian aboriginals, suggesting that genetic factors play a role in susceptibility. Other risk factors include acquired or congenital immunodeficiencies, hemoglobinopathies such as sickle cell disease, functional or anatomic asplenia, and crowding such as occurs in some households, daycare centers, or college and military dormitories. A CSF leak resulting from congenital anomaly or after a basilar skull fracture increases the risk for meningitis, especially caused by *S. pneumoniae.*

Enteroviruses cause meningitis with peaks during the summer and fall. These infections are more prevalent in people from low socioeconomic groups, young children, and immunocompromised persons. The prevalence of arboviral meningitis is determined by the geographic distribution and seasonal activity of the arthropod vectors (mosquito). In the U.S., most arboviral infections occur during the summer and fall.

CLINICAL MANIFESTATIONS

Preceding upper respiratory tract symptoms are common. Rapid onset is typical of *S. pneumoniae* and *N. meningitidis.* Indications of meningeal inflammation include headache, irritability, nausea, nuchal rigidity, lethargy, photophobia, and vomiting. Fever usually is present. Kernig and Brudzinski signs of meningeal irritation usually are positive in children older than 12 months of age. In young infants, signs of meningeal inflammation may be minimal with only irritability, restlessness, depressed mental status, and poor feeding. Focal neurologic signs, seizures, arthralgia, myalgia, petechial or purpuric lesions, sepsis, shock, and coma may occur.

Increased intracranial pressure is reflected in complaints of headache, diplopia, and vomiting. A bulging fontanel may be present in infants. Ptosis, sixth nerve palsy, anisocoria, bradycardia with hypertension, and apnea are signs of increased intracranial pressure with brain herniation. Papilledema is uncommon, unless there is occlusion of the venous sinuses, subdural empyema, or brain abscess.

LABORATORY AND IMAGING STUDIES

If bacterial meningitis is suspected, a lumbar puncture should be performed. A lumbar puncture should be avoided in the presence of cardiovascular instability or signs of increased intracranial pressure, other than a bulging fontanel, because of the risk of herniation. Routine CSF examination includes WBC count, differential, protein and glucose levels, and Gram stain (Table 100–2). Bacterial meningitis is characterized by neutrophilic pleocytosis, moderately to markedly elevated protein, and low glucose. Viral meningitis is characterized by mild to moderate lymphocytic pleocytosis, normal or slightly elevated protein, and normal glucose. CSF should be cultured for bacteria and, when appropriate, fungi, viruses, and mycobacteria. PCR is used to diagnose enteroviruses and HSV; it is more sensitive and more rapid than viral culture. Leukocytosis is common. Blood cultures are positive in 90% of

TABLE 100–2.   Cerebrospinal Fluid Findings in Various Central Nervous System Disorders

Condition	Pressure	Leukocytes (/μL)	Protein (mg/dL)	Glucose (mg/dL)	Comments
Normal	50-180 mm H₂O	<4; 60-70% lymphocytes, 30-40% monocytes, 1-3% neutrophils	20-45	>50 or 75% blood glucose	
Acute bacterial meningitis	Usually elevated	100-60,000+; usually a few thousand; PMNs predominate	100-500	Depressed compared with blood glucose; usually <40	Organism may be seen on Gram stain and recovered by culture
Partially treated bacterial meningitis	Normal or elevated	1-10,000; PMNs usual but mononuclear cells may predominate if pretreated for extended period	>100	Depressed or normal	Organisms may be seen; pretreatment may render CSF sterile in pneumococcal and meningococcal disease, but antigen may be detected
Tuberculous meningitis	Usually elevated; may be low because of CSF block in advanced stages	10-500; PMNs early but lymphocytes and monocytes predominate later	100-500; may be higher in presence of CSF block	<50 usual; decreases with time if treatment not provided	Acid-fast organisms may be seen on smear; organism can be recovered in culture or by PCR; PPD, chest x-ray positive
Fungal	Usually elevated	25-500; PMNs early; mononuclear cells predominate later	20-500	<50; decreases with time if treatment not provided	Budding yeast may be seen; organism may be recovered in culture; India ink preparation or antigen may be positive in cryptococcal disease
Viral meningitis or meningoencephalitis	Normal or slightly elevated	PMNs early; mononuclear cells predominate later; rarely more than 1000 cells except in eastern equine	20-100	Generally normal; may be depressed to 40 in some viral diseases (15-20% of mumps)	Enteroviruses may be recovered from CSF by appropriate viral cultures or PCR; HSV by PCR
Abscess (parameningeal infection)	Normal or elevated	0-100 PMNs unless rupture into CSF	20-200	Normal	Profile may be completely normal

HSV, herpes simplex virus; PCR, polymerase chain reaction; PMNs, polymorphonuclear leukocytes; PPD, purified protein derivative of tuberculin.

cases. An electroencephalogram (EEG) may confirm an encephalitis component (see Chapter 101).

DIFFERENTIAL DIAGNOSIS

Many disorders may show signs of meningeal irritation and increased intracranial pressure, including the many infectious causes of meningitis, encephalitis, hemorrhage, rheumatic diseases, and malignancies.

Seizures are associated with meningitis, encephalitis, and intracranial abscess or can be the sequelae of brain edema, cerebral infarction or hemorrhage, or vasculitis.

TREATMENT

Treatment of bacterial meningitis focuses on sterilization of the CSF by antibiotics (Table 100–3) and maintenance of adequate cerebral and systemic perfusion.

TABLE 100–3.   Initial Antimicrobial Therapy by Age for Presumed Bacterial Meningitis

Age	Recommended Treatment	Alternative Treatments
Newborns (0-28 days)	Cefotaxime or ceftriaxone plus ampicillin with or without gentamicin	Gentamicin plus ampicillin Ceftazidime plus ampicillin
Infants and toddlers (1 mo-4 yr)	Ceftriaxone or cefotaxime plus vancomycin	Cefotaxime or ceftriaxone plus rifampin
Children and adolescents (5-13 yr) and adults	Ceftriaxone or cefotaxime plus vancomycin	Ampicillin plus chloramphenicol

Because of increasing resistance of *S. pneumoniae,* many of which are relatively resistant to penicillin or cephalosporins, cefotaxime (or ceftriaxone) *plus* vancomycin should be administered until antibiotic susceptibility testing is available. Cefotaxime or ceftriaxone also is adequate to cover *N. meningitidis* and *H. influenzae* types *a* through *f.* For infants younger than 2 months of age, ampicillin is added to cover the possibility of *Listeria monocytogenes.* Duration of treatment is 10 to 14 days for *S. pneumoniae,* 5 to 7 days for *N. meningitidis,* and 7 to 10 days for *H. influenzae.*

Supportive therapy involves treatment of dehydration with replacement fluids and treatment of shock, disseminated intravascular coagulation, inappropriate antidiuretic hormone secretion, seizures, increased intracranial pressure, apnea, arrhythmias, and coma. Supportive therapy also involves the maintenance of adequate cerebral perfusion in the presence of cerebral edema.

COMPLICATIONS

Syndrome of inappropriate antidiuretic hormone may complicate meningitis and necessitates monitoring of urine output and judicious fluid administration, balancing the need for fluid administration for hypotension and hypoperfusion. CT or MRI commonly detects subdural effusions with *S. pneumoniae* and Hib meningitis. Most effusions are asymptomatic and do not necessitate drainage unless associated with increased intracranial pressure or focal neurologic signs. Persistent fever is common during treatment of meningitis, but also may be related to infective or immune complex–mediated pericardial or joint effusions, thrombophlebitis, drug fever, or nosocomial infection. A repeat lumbar puncture is not indicated for fever in the absence of other signs of persistent CNS infection.

PROGNOSIS

Even with appropriate antibiotic therapy, the mortality rate for bacterial meningitis in children is significant: 25% for *S. pneumoniae,* 15% for *N. meningitidis,* and 8% for Hib. Of survivors, 35% have some sequelae, particularly after pneumococcal infection, including deafness, seizures, learning disabilities, blindness, paresis, ataxia, or hydrocephalus. All patients with meningitis should have hearing evaluation before discharge and at follow-up. Poor prognosis is associated with young age, long duration of illness before effective antibiotic therapy, seizures, coma at presentation, shock, low or absent CSF WBC count in the presence of visible bacteria on Gram stain of the CSF, and immunocompromised status.

Rarely, **relapse** may occur 3 to 14 days after treatment, possibly from parameningeal foci or resistant organisms. **Recurrence** may indicate an underlying immunologic or anatomic defect that predisposes the patient to meningitis.

PREVENTION

Routine **immunizations** against Hib and *S. pneumoniae* are recommended for children beginning at 2 months of age. Vaccines against *N. meningitidis* are recommended for young adolescents and college freshmen as well as military personnel and travelers to highly endemic areas. **Chemoprophylaxis** is recommended for close contacts of *N. meningitidis* infections and the index case and for close contacts of Hib and the index case; rifampin, ciprofloxacin, or ceftriaxone is recommended (see Chapter 94).

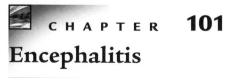

CHAPTER   101
Encephalitis

ETIOLOGY

Encephalitis is an inflammatory process of the brain parenchyma that usually is an acute process, but may be a postinfectious encephalomyelitis, a chronic degenerative disease, or a slow viral infection. Encephalitis results from inflammation of the brain parenchyma, leading to cerebral dysfunction. Encephalitis may be diffuse or localized. Organisms cause encephalitis by one of two mechanisms: (1) direct infection of the brain parenchyma or (2) an apparent immune-mediated response in the CNS that usually begins several days after the appearance of extraneural manifestations of the infection.

Viruses are the principal causes of acute infectious encephalitis (Table 101–1). Encephalitis also may result from other types of infection and metabolic, toxic, and neoplastic disorders. The most common viral causes of encephalitis in the U.S. are the arboviruses (St. Louis, LaCrosse, California, West Nile encephalitis viruses), enteroviruses, and herpesviruses. HIV is an important cause of encephalitis in children and adolescents and may present as an acute febrile illness, but more commonly is insidious in onset (see Chapter 125).

Acute disseminated encephalomyelitis (ADEM) is the abrupt development of multiple neurologic signs related to an inflammatory, demyelinating disorder of the brain and spinal cord. Acute disseminated encephalomyelitis follows childhood viral infections, such as measles and chickenpox or vaccinations. Acute disseminated encephalomyelitis resembles multiple sclerosis.

EPIDEMIOLOGY

Arboviral and enteroviral encephalitides characteristically appear in clusters or epidemics that occur from midsummer to early fall, although sporadic cases of enteroviral encephalitis occur throughout the year. Herpesviruses and other infectious agents account for additional sporadic cases throughout the year.

Arboviruses tend to be limited to certain geographic areas. St. Louis encephalitis virus, which is spread from the bird reservoir, is present throughout the U.S. California encephalitis virus, common in the Midwest, is carried by rodents and spread by mosquitoes. Eastern equine encephalitis virus is limited to the East Coast, in mosquitoes and birds. Western equine encephalitis virus is present throughout the Midwest and West in mosquitoes and birds. West Nile virus is endemic throughout Africa and Asia. In North America, it causes outbreaks of summer encephalitis. The principal vector for West Nile virus is the *Culex pipiens* mosquito, but the organism can be isolated in nature from a wide variety of *Culex* and *Aedes* species. A broad range of birds serves as the major reservoir for West Nile virus.

CLINICAL MANIFESTATIONS

Acute infectious encephalitis usually is preceded by a prodrome of several days of nonspecific symptoms, such as cough, sore throat, fever, headache, and abdominal complaints, which are followed by the characteristic symptoms of progressive lethargy, behavioral changes, and neurologic deficits. Seizures are common at presentation. Children with encephalitis also may have a maculopapular rash and severe complications, such as fulminant coma, transverse myelitis, anterior horn cell disease (polio-like illness), or peripheral neuropathy.

West Nile encephalitis produces a broad spectrum of illness, from asymptomatic infection to death. Symptoms usually include mild, nonspecific extraneurologic illness characterized by fever, rash, arthralgias, lymphadenopathy, gastrointestinal complaints, and conjunctivitis. Occasional cases are complicated by hepatitis or pancreatitis.

TABLE 101–1.   Viral Causes of Encephalitis

Acute

Adenoviruses
Arboviruses
 In North America
  Eastern equine encephalitis
  Western equine encephalitis
  St. Louis encephalitis
  California encephalitis
  West Nile encephalitis
  Colorado tick fever
 Outside North America
  Venezuelan equine encephalitis
  Japanese encephalitis
  Tick-borne encephalitis
  Murray Valley encephalitis
Enteroviruses
Herpesviruses
 Herpes simplex viruses
 Epstein-Barr virus
 Varicella-zoster virus
 Human herpesvirus-6
 Human herpesvirus-7
HIV
Influenza viruses
Lymphocytic choriomeningitis virus
Measles virus (native or vaccine)
Mumps virus (native or vaccine)
Rabies virus
Rubella virus

Subacute

HIV
JC virus
Prion-associated encephalopathies (Creutzfeldt-Jakob
  disease, kuru)

LABORATORY AND IMAGING STUDIES

The diagnosis of viral encephalitis is supported by examination of the CSF, which typically shows a lymphocytic pleocytosis, slight elevation in protein content, and normal glucose level. Increased erythrocytes and CSF protein may occur with HSV. Extreme elevations of protein and reductions of glucose suggest tuberculosis, cryptococcal infection, or meningeal carcinomatosis. The CSF occasionally may be normal. The EEG is the definitive test and shows diffuse, slow wave activity, although focal changes may be present. Neuroimaging studies may be normal or may show diffuse cerebral swelling of the parenchyma or focal abnormalities. A temporal lobe focus on EEG or brain imaging characterizes HSV infection.

Serologic studies should be obtained for arboviruses, EBV, *Mycoplasma pneumoniae,* cat-scratch disease, and Lyme disease. An IgM assay of serum or CSF for West Nile viral infection is available, but cross-reactivity with other flaviviruses (St. Louis encephalitis) may occur. Additional serologic testing for the less common pathogens should be performed as indicated by the travel, social, or medical history. In addition to serologic testing, a sample of CSF and stool and a nasopharyngeal swab should be obtained for viral culture. In most cases of viral encephalitis, the virus is difficult to isolate from the CSF. PCR tests for HSV, enteroviruses, and other viruses are available. Even with extensive testing and the use of PCR assays, the cause of encephalitis remains undetermined in one third of cases.

Brain biopsy may be necessary for definitive diagnosis of the cause of encephalitis, especially in patients with focal neurologic findings. Brain biopsy may be appropriate for patients with severe encephalopathy who show no clinical improvement if the diagnosis remains obscure. HSV, rabies encephalitis, prion-related diseases (Creutzfeldt-Jakob disease and kuru) may be routinely diagnosed by culture or pathologic examination of brain biopsy tissue. Brain biopsy may be important to identify arbovirus and enterovirus infections, tuberculosis, fungal infections, and non-infectious illnesses, particularly primary CNS vasculopathies or malignancies.

DIFFERENTIAL DIAGNOSIS

The diagnosis is established presumptively in the presence of characteristic neurologic signs, epidemiology, and evidence of infection by CSF analysis, EEG, and brain imaging techniques. Brain biopsy may be diagnostic but is seldom performed. Encephalitis may result from infections with bacteria, *Mycoplasma, Rickettsia,* fungi, and parasites and from many non-infectious diseases, including metabolic diseases (encephalopathy) such as Reye syndrome, hypoglycemia, collagen vascular disorders, drugs, hypertension, and malignancies.

TREATMENT

With the exception of HSV and HIV, there is no specific therapy for viral encephalitis. Management is supportive and frequently requires ICU admission, which allows aggressive therapy for seizures, timely detection of electrolyte abnormalities, and, when necessary, airway monitoring and protection and reduction of increased intracranial pressure.

IV acyclovir is the treatment of choice for HSV infections. HIV infections may be treated with a combination of antiretroviral agents. *M. pneumoniae* infections may be treated with doxycycline, erythromycin, azithromycin, or clarithromycin, although the value of treating CNS mycoplasmal disease with these agents is disputed. Supportive care is crucial to decrease elevated intracranial pressure and to maintain adequate cerebral perfusion pressure and oxygenation.

ADEM has been treated with high-dose IV corticosteroids. It is unclear whether the improved outcome with corticosteroids reflects milder cases recognized by MRI, fewer cases of ADEM caused by measles (which causes severe ADEM), or improved supportive care.

COMPLICATIONS AND PROGNOSIS

Among survivors, symptoms usually resolve over several days to 2 to 3 weeks. Although most patients with epidemic forms of infectious encephalitis (St. Louis, California, and enterovirus infections) in the U.S. recover without sequelae, severe cases leading to death or substantial neurologic sequelae can occur with virtually any of these neurotropic viruses. The overall mortality for infectious encephalitis is approximately 5%. About two thirds of patients recover fully before being discharged from the hospital. The remainder show clinically significant residua, including paresis or spasticity, cognitive impairment, weakness, ataxia, and recurrent seizures. Most patients with neurologic sequelae of infectious encephalitis at the time of hospital discharge gradually recover some or all of their function.

Disease caused by HSV, eastern equine encephalitis, or *M. pneumoniae* is associated with a poorer prognosis. The prognosis may be poorer for encephalitis in children younger than 1 year old or with coma. Rabies is universally fatal.

Relapses of ADEM have occurred in 14%, usually within 1 year with the same or new clinical signs. Recurrences of ADEM may represent childhood multiple sclerosis.

PREVENTION

The best prevention for arboviral encephalitis is to avoid mosquito-borne or tick-borne infections and to remove ticks carefully (see Chapter 122). There are no vaccines in use in the U.S. for prevention of arboviral infection or for enteroviruses except for poliomyelitis. There are no specific preventive measures for HSV encephalitis except for cesarean section for mothers with active genital lesions (see Chapter 65). Rabies can be prevented by pre-exposure or postexposure vaccination. Influenza encephalitis can be prevented by use of influenza vaccination. Reye syndrome can be prevented by avoiding use of aspirin or aspirin-containing compounds for children with fever, and use of varicella and influenza vaccines.

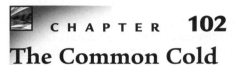

CHAPTER 102
The Common Cold

ETIOLOGY

The common cold is a viral infection with prominent symptoms of rhinorrhea and nasal obstruction, absent or mild fever, and lacking systemic manifestations. It is often referred to as rhinitis, but usually also involves the sinus mucosa and is more correctly termed **rhinosinusitis**.

The viruses primarily associated with colds are rhinoviruses and, less commonly, coronaviruses. Other viruses that cause common cold symptoms as part of broader clinical syndromes include respiratory syncytial virus (RSV) and, less commonly, influenza viruses, parainfluenza viruses, and adenoviruses. Viral infection of the nasal epithelium causes an acute inflammatory response with mucosal infiltration by inflammatory cells and release of inflammatory cytokines. The inflammatory response is partly responsible for many of the symptoms.

EPIDEMIOLOGY

Colds occur throughout the year, but have peak incidence from early fall through late spring, reflecting the seasonal prevalence of the viral pathogens. Young children have an average of 6 to 7 colds each year, and 10% to 15% of children have at least 12 colds each year. The annual number of colds decreases with age, to 2 to 3 colds each year by adulthood. Children in out-of-home daycare during the first year of life have 50% more colds than children cared for only at home. This difference diminishes during subsequent years in daycare.

CLINICAL MANIFESTATIONS

Common cold symptoms typically develop 1 to 3 days after viral infection and include nasal obstruction, rhinorrhea, sore or "scratchy" throat, and occasional nonproductive cough. Colds usually persist about 1 week, although 10% last 2 weeks. There is often a change in the color or consistency of nasal secretions, which is not indicative of sinusitis or bacterial superinfection. Examination of the nasal mucosa may reveal swollen, erythematous nasal turbinates.

LABORATORY AND IMAGING STUDIES

Laboratory studies often are not helpful. A nasal smear for eosinophils may be useful in the evaluation for allergic rhinitis (see Chapter 79).

DIFFERENTIAL DIAGNOSIS

Rhinorrhea is a frequent manifestation of infection and allergic disease. The differential diagnosis of the common cold includes allergic rhinitis, foreign body (especially with unilateral nasal discharge), sinusitis, pertussis, and streptococcal nasopharyngitis. Allergic rhinitis is characterized by absence of fever, eosinophils in the nasal discharge, and other allergic manifestations, such as allergic shiners, nasal polyps, a transverse crease on the nasal bridge, and pale, edematous, nasal turbinate mucosa. Rare causes of rhinorrhea are choanal atresia or stenosis, CSF fistula, diphtheria, tumor, congenital syphilis (with "snuffles"), nasopharyngeal malignancy, and Wegener granulomatosis.

TREATMENT

There is no specific therapy for the common cold. Antibacterial therapy is not beneficial for the common cold. Management consists of symptomatic therapies. Use of symptomatic therapies in children is based on effectiveness that has been shown in adults; few studies have shown a significant benefit in children. It is prudent to target therapy to the most bothersome symptoms. Fever infrequently is associated with an uncomplicated common cold and antipyretic treatment is usually unnecessary, although acetaminophen may reduce symptoms of sore throat. Cough suppressants and expectorants are usually unnecessary and have not been shown to be beneficial.

Either topical or oral adrenergic agents may be used as nasal decongestants. Reduced strength formulations of effective topical adrenergic agents, such as xylometazoline, oxymetazoline, or phenylephrine, are available as intranasal drops or nasal sprays, but are not approved for use in children younger than 2 years old. Prolonged use may lead to **rhinitis medicamentosa**, a rebound effect that causes the sensation of nasal obstruction when the drug is discontinued. Oral adrenergic agents are less effective than the topical preparations and are associated with systemic effects, such as CNS stimulation, hypertension, and arrhythmias.

First-generation antihistamines reduce rhinorrhea by 25% to 30%, which seems to be related to the anticholinergic effect rather than the antihistaminic properties. Second-generation or "nonsedating" antihistamines have no effect on common cold symptoms. The major adverse effect associated with the use of antihistamines is sedation, which may be less bothersome in children than in adults. Rhinorrhea also may be treated with ipratropium bromide, a topical anticholinergic agent that produces an effect comparable to antihistamines but is not associated with sedation. The most common adverse effects of ipratropium are nasal irritation and bleeding. Vitamin C, guaifenesin, and inhalation of warm, humidified air are no more effective than placebo. The benefit of zinc lozenges or sprays has been inconsistent.

COMPLICATIONS AND PROGNOSIS

Otitis media is the most common complication and occurs in 5% to 20% of children with a cold (see Chapter 105). Other complications include bacterial sinusitis, which should be considered if rhinorrhea or daytime cough persists without improvement for at least 10 to 14 days or if severe signs of sinus involvement develop, such as fever, facial pain, or facial swelling (see Chapter 104). Colds may lead to exacerbation of asthma and may result in inappropriate antibiotic treatment.

PREVENTION

There are no proven methods for prevention of colds other than good hand washing and avoiding contact with infected persons. No significant effect of vitamin C or echinacea for prevention of the common cold has been confirmed.

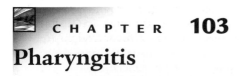

CHAPTER 103
Pharyngitis

ETIOLOGY

Many infectious agents can cause pharyngitis (Table 103–1). Group A streptococci (*Streptococcus pyogenes*) are gram-positive, nonmotile cocci that are facultative anaerobes. On sheep blood agar, the colonies are small (1 to 2 mm in diameter) and have a surrounding zone of beta (clear) hemolysis. Other bacterial organisms less often associated with pharyngitis include group C beta-hemolytic streptococcus; *Arcanobacterium haemolyticum,* which is a hemolytic, gram-positive rod; and *Francisella tularensis,* the gram-negative coccobacillus that is the cause of tularemia. *Chlamydophila pneumoniae,* strain TWAR, is associated with lower respiratory disease, but also causes sore throat. *M. pneumoniae* is associated with atypical pneumonia, but also can cause mild pharyngitis without distinguishing clinical manifestations. Other bacteria, including *S. aureus,* Hib, and *S. pneumoniae* are cultured frequently from the throats of children with pharyngitis, but their role in causing pharyngitis is unclear.

Many viruses cause acute pharyngitis. Some viruses, such as adenoviruses, are more likely than others to cause pharyngitis as a prominent symptom, whereas other viruses, such as rhinoviruses, are more likely to cause pharyngitis as a minor part of an illness that primarily features other symptoms, such as rhinorrhea or cough. EBV (mononucleosis), enteroviruses (herpangina), and primary HIV infection also produce pharyngitis.

EPIDEMIOLOGY

Infections of the upper respiratory tract account for a substantial proportion of illnesses in children. Sore throat is the primary symptom in approximately one third of such illnesses. Streptococcal pharyngitis is relatively uncommon before 2 to 3 years of age, but the incidence increases in young school-age children, then declines in late adolescence and adulthood. Streptococcal pharyngitis occurs throughout the year in temperate climates, with a peak during the winter and spring. The illness often spreads to siblings and classmates. Viral infections generally spread via close contact with an infected person and peak during winter and spring.

CLINICAL MANIFESTATIONS

The inflammation of pharyngitis causes cough, sore throat, dysphagia, and fever. If involvement of the tonsils is prominent, the term **tonsillitis** or **tonsillopharyngitis** is often used.

The onset of streptococcal pharyngitis is often rapid and associated with prominent sore throat and moderate to high fever. Headache, nausea, vomiting, and abdominal pain are frequent. In a typical, florid case, the pharynx is distinctly red, and the tonsils are enlarged and covered with a yellow, blood-tinged exudate. There may be petechiae or "doughnut-shaped" lesions on the soft palate and posterior pharynx, and the uvula may be red, stippled, and swollen. The anterior cervical lymph nodes are enlarged and tender to touch. The clinical spectrum of disease is broad, however, and many children present with only mild

TABLE 103–1. Major Microbial Causes of Acute Pharyngitis

Agent	Syndrome or Disease	Estimated Occurrence (%)
Bacterial		
Group A streptococcus (*Streptococcus pyogenes*)	Pharyngitis, tonsillitis	15-30
Group C streptococcus	Pharyngitis, tonsillitis	1-5
Other (e.g., *Corynebacterium diphtheriae*)	Pharyngitis, laryngitis	<5
Viral		
Rhinoviruses (>100 types)	Common cold	20
Coronaviruses (≥4 types)	Common cold	≥5
Adenoviruses (types 3, 4, 7, 14, 21)	Pharyngoconjunctival fever, acute respiratory disease	5
Herpes simplex viruses (types 1 and 2)	Gingivitis, stomatitis, pharyngitis	4
Parainfluenza viruses (types 1-4)	Common cold, croup	2
Influenza viruses (types A and B)	Influenza	2
Epstein-Barr virus	Mononucleosis	Unknown
Unknown		40

Adapted from Hayden GF, Hendley JO, Gwaltney JM Jr: Management of the ambulatory patient with a sore throat. Curr Clin Top Infect Dis 1988;9:63.

pharyngeal erythema without tonsillar exudate or cervical lymphadenitis.

In addition to sore throat and fever, some patients exhibit the stigmata of **scarlet fever**: circumoral pallor, strawberry tongue, and a fine diffuse erythematous macular-papular rash that has the feeling of goose flesh. The tongue initially has a white coating, but red and edematous lingual papillae later project through this coating, producing a **white strawberry tongue**. When the white coating peels off, the resulting **red strawberry tongue** is a beefy red tongue with prominent papillae.

Compared with classic streptococcal pharyngitis, the onset of viral pharyngitis is typically more gradual, and symptoms more often include rhinorrhea, cough, and diarrhea. Many illnesses fall in the general category of upper respiratory tract infection, in which the symptoms of rhinorrhea and nasal obstruction are prominent, and systemic symptoms and signs, such as myalgia and fever, are absent or mild.

Gingivostomatitis is characteristic of HSV-1 and usually occurs in children 1 to 5 years old, with the highest incidence from 9 to 36 months of age. It is transmitted primarily by direct contact with draining mucosal lesions or from asymptomatic shedding. The incubation period of oral HSV illness is 7 days (range 2 to 25 days). Primary HSV infection is more severe than recurrent illness. Clinical features of primary HSV gingivostomatitis include high fever, poor intake of liquid and solid food, dehydration, malaise, stinging mouth pain, drooling, fetid breath, oropharyngeal vesicular lesions, and lymphadenopathy. Grouped lesions on an erythematous base are present around the stomal opening and on the tongue, gums, lips, and oral mucosa and on the soft and hard palate. The lesions usually become crusted and heal within 5 to 10 days, but occasionally they may last 3 weeks. Primary infection usually is accompanied by fever and tender lymphadenopathy, which are often absent with recurrent disease. The lesions persist for 12 days (range 9 to 15 days) and heal without scarring. Limited involvement to only a portion of the vermilion is more characteristic of recurrent illness than primary HSV infection; this presentation is often called **herpes labialis**.

Herpangina is an enteroviral infection with major symptoms of sudden onset of high fever, vomiting, headache, malaise, myalgia, backache, conjunctivitis, poor intake, drooling, sore throat, and dysphagia. The oral lesions of herpangina may be nonspecific, but classically there are one or more small, tender, papular, or pinpoint vesicular lesions on an erythematous base scattered over the soft palate, uvula, fauces, and tongue. These vesicles enlarge from 1 to 2 mm to 3 to 4 mm over 3 to 4 days, rupture, and produce small, punched-out ulcers that persist for several days.

Mononucleosis

▶ SEE CHAPTER 99.

LABORATORY EVALUATION

The principal challenge is to distinguish pharyngitis caused by group A streptococci from pharyngitis caused by nonstreptococcal (usually viral) organisms.

A rapid streptococcal antigen test or a throat culture or both are often performed to improve diagnostic precision and to help identify children who are most likely to benefit from antibiotic therapy of streptococcal disease.

The predictive values of WBC count, ESR, and CRP are not sufficient to distinguish streptococcal from nonstreptococcal pharyngitis, and these tests are not routinely recommended. The complete blood count in patients with infectious mononucleosis may show a predominance of atypical lymphocytes.

Many rapid diagnostic techniques for streptococcal pharyngitis are available, with excellent specificity of 95% to 99%. The sensitivity of these rapid tests varies, however, and a negative rapid test ideally should be confirmed with a negative culture, especially when the clinical suspicion of streptococcal illness is great.

Throat culture is the diagnostic "gold standard" for establishing the presence of streptococcal pharyngitis. False-positive cultures can occur if other organisms are incorrectly identified as group A streptococcus. A proportion of positive cultures reflects streptococcal carriage, but not the etiology of the acute pharyngitis.

DIFFERENTIAL DIAGNOSIS

The differential diagnosis of infectious pharyngitis includes other local infections of the oral cavity, retropharyngeal abscesses (*S. aureus,* streptococci, anaerobes), diphtheria (if unimmunized), peritonsillar abscesses (with quinsy sore throat or unilateral tonsil swelling caused by streptococci, anaerobes, or, rarely, *S. aureus*), and epiglottitis. In addition, neutropenic mucositis (leukemia, aplastic anemia), thrush (candidiasis secondary to T cell immune deficiency), autoimmune ulceration (systemic lupus erythematosus, Behçet disease), and Kawasaki disease may cause pharyngitis. Pharyngitis is often a prominent feature of EBV-associated mononucleosis (see Chapter 99).

Vincent infection or **trench mouth** is a fulminant form of **acute necrotizing ulcerative gingivitis** with synergistic infection with certain spirochetal organisms, notably *Treponema vincentii,* with anaerobic *Selenomonas* and *Fusobacterium*. **Vincent angina** refers to a virulent form of anaerobic pharyngitis wherein gray pseudomembranes are found on the tonsils, accounting for the synonym **false diphtheria**.

Noma, also known as **cancrum oris** or **gangrenous stomatitis**, may be related in pathophysiology to Vincent infection, but typically begins as a focal gingival lesion and rapidly progresses to gangrene and consequent destruction of bone, teeth, and soft tissues. Mortality rates of 70% to 90% occur in the absence of prompt surgical intervention. Noma has been associated with infection by *Borrelia vincentii* and *Fusobac-*

terium nucleatum. Noma seems to be related to severe malnutrition or to immunodeficiency states.

Ludwig angina is a mixed anaerobic bacterial cellulitis of the submandibular and sublingual regions. Although often applied to any infection of the sublingual or submandibular region, the term *Ludwig angina* originally was reserved for a rapidly spreading bilateral cellulitis of the sublingual and submandibular spaces. It is often odontogenic in origin, typically spreading from a periapical abscess of the second or third mandibular molar. It also has been associated with tongue piercing. A propensity for rapid spread, glottic and lingual swelling, and consequent airway obstruction makes prompt intervention imperative.

A syndrome of **periodic fever, aphthous stomatitis, pharyngitis, and cervical adenitis (PFAPA)** is a rare cause of recurrent fever in children. This syndrome is characterized by recurring nonspecific pharyngitis accompanied by fever and aphthae, which are painful solitary vesicular lesions in the mouth. The fevers begin at a young age (usually <5 years old). Episodes last approximately 5 days; duration is shorter with treatment with oral prednisone. There is a mean of 28 days between episodes. Episodes are unresponsive to nonsteroidal anti-inflammatory drugs or antibiotics. The syndrome resolves in some children, whereas symptoms persist in other children. Long-term sequelae do not develop.

TREATMENT

Even if untreated, most episodes of streptococcal pharyngitis resolve uneventfully over a few days. If instituted early in the course of illness, however, antimicrobial therapy accelerates clinical recovery by 12 to 24 hours. The major benefit of antimicrobial therapy is the prevention of acute rheumatic fever (see Chapter 146). Because the latent (incubation) period of acute rheumatic fever is relatively long (1 to 3 weeks), treatment instituted within 9 days of illness is virtually 100% successful in preventing rheumatic fever. Treatment begun more than 9 days after the onset of illness is less than 100% successful, but may have some preventive value. Antibiotic therapy should be started immediately in children with a positive rapid test for group A streptococcus, scarlet fever, symptomatic pharyngitis whose siblings are ill with documented streptococcal pharyngitis, symptomatic pharyngitis and a past history of rheumatic fever or a recent history of rheumatic fever in a family member, or symptomatic pharyngitis who are living in an area experiencing an epidemic of acute rheumatic fever or poststreptococcal glomerulonephritis.

A variety of antimicrobial agents can be used to treat streptococcal pharyngitis (Table 103-2). Penicillin has a narrow spectrum, is inexpensive, and has relatively

TABLE 103–2. Antimicrobial Treatment of Group A Streptococcal Pharyngitis

Penicillin
  Intramuscular benzathine penicillin G (single dose)
    For children <60 lb: 600,000 U
    For larger children and adults: 1.2 million U
  or
  Oral penicillin V (3 or 4 times daily for 10 days)
    For children <60 lb: 125 mg/dose
    For larger children and adults: 250 mg/dose
For persons allergic to β-lactams
Erythromycin
  For larger children and adults:
    1 g/day in 2-4 divided doses for 10 days
  For smaller children:
    Erythromycin ethyl succinate: 40-50 mg/kg/day in
      3-4 doses for 10 days
    Erythromycin estolate: 20-40 mg/kg/day in 2-4 doses
      for 10 days

few adverse effects. It usually is given orally three or four times daily for a full 10 days. The taste of oral amoxicillin is preferred over oral penicillin by many children. A single IM dose of benzathine penicillin (or a benzathine-procaine combination) is painful, but it ensures adherence and provides adequate blood levels for more than 10 days. For patients allergic to penicillins, erythromycin is the drug of choice.

Some drugs (oral first-generation cephalosporins) seem to be as good as, or better than, penicillin in eradicating the streptococci. One proposed explanation is that staphylococci or anaerobes in the pharynx produce β-lactamase, which inactivates penicillin and reduces its efficacy. Another possible explanation is that these other drugs are more effective than penicillin in eradicating streptococcal carriage. Some drugs also may offer convenience, such as once-daily administration or shorter length of therapy, which may translate into improved compliance. These drugs are more expensive than penicillin and usually have more adverse effects.

Children with recurrent episodes of pharyngitis with throat cultures positive for group A streptococcus pose a particular problem. An alternative antibiotic may be chosen to treat pharyngeal flora producing β-lactamase, which may be responsible for the recurrences. Either amoxicillin-clavulanate or clindamycin is an effective regimen for eliminating streptococcal carriage.

Specific antiviral therapy is unavailable for most cases of viral pharyngitis. Patients with primary herpetic gingivostomatitis benefit from early treatment with oral acyclovir.

COMPLICATIONS AND PROGNOSIS

Pharyngitis caused by streptococci or respiratory viruses usually resolves completely. The complications of group A streptococcal pharyngitis include local suppurative complications, such as parapharyngeal abscess and other infections of the deep fascial spaces of the neck, and nonsuppurative complications, such as acute rheumatic fever and acute postinfectious glomerulonephritis. Viral respiratory tract infections, including infections caused by influenza A, adenoviruses, parainfluenza type 3, and rhinoviruses, may predispose to bacterial middle ear infections.

PREVENTION

Antimicrobial prophylaxis with daily oral penicillin prevents recurrent streptococcal infections and is recommended only to prevent recurrences of rheumatic fever.

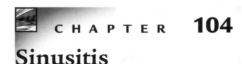

CHAPTER 104

Sinusitis

ETIOLOGY

Sinusitis is a suppurative infection of the paranasal sinuses and often complicates the common cold and allergic rhinitis. The maxillary and ethmoid sinuses are present at birth, but only the ethmoidal sinuses are pneumatized. The maxillary sinuses become pneumatized at 4 years of age. The frontal sinuses begin to develop at 7 years of age and are not completely developed until adolescence. The sphenoid sinuses are present by 5 years of age. The ostia draining the sinuses are narrow (1 to 3 mm) and drain into the middle meatus in the **ostiomeatal complex**. The mucociliary system maintains the sinuses as normally sterile.

Obstruction to mucociliary flow, such as mucosal edema resulting from a viral rhinosinusitis (common cold), impedes sinus drainage and predisposes to bacterial proliferation. Bacteria causing sinusitis include *S. pneumoniae,* nontypable *H. influenzae, Moraxella catarrhalis,* and less commonly *S. aureus,* other streptococci, and anaerobes. Indwelling nasogastric and nasotracheal tubes predispose to nosocomial sinusitis, which is often caused by gram-negative bacteria (*Klebsiella* and *Pseudomonas*). Antibiotic therapy predisposes to infection with antibiotic-resistant organisms. Sinusitis in neutropenic and immunocompromised persons may be caused by *Aspergillus* and the Zygomycetes (e.g., *Mucor, Rhizopus*).

EPIDEMIOLOGY

The common cold is the major predisposing factor for developing sinusitis at all ages. Other risk factors include cystic fibrosis, immunodeficiency, HIV infection, nasogastric or nasotracheal intubation, immotile cilia syndrome, nasal polyps, and nasal foreign body. Sinusitis also is a frequent problem in immunocompromised children after organ transplantation.

CLINICAL MANIFESTATIONS

Clinical manifestations most commonly include persistent, mucopurulent, unilateral or bilateral rhinorrhea, nasal stuffiness, and cough, especially at night. Less common symptoms include a nasal quality to the voice, halitosis, facial swelling, facial tenderness and pain, and headache. Sinusitis may exacerbate asthma.

LABORATORY AND IMAGING STUDIES

Culture of the nasal mucosa is not useful. Sinus aspirate culture is the most accurate diagnostic method but is not practical or necessary. Transillumination may show evidence of fluid, but this is difficult to perform in children and is not reliable.

Plain film and CT may reveal sinus clouding, mucosal thickening, or an air-fluid level. Abnormal radiographic findings are not consistently diagnostic of sinusitis; CT and MRI frequently show abnormalities, including air-fluid levels, in the sinuses of asymptomatic persons. Abnormal radiographic findings do not differentiate infection from allergic disease. Conversely, normal radiographs have high negative predictive value for bacterial sinusitis.

DIFFERENTIAL DIAGNOSIS

The diagnosis usually is based on history and physical findings for longer than 10 to 14 days without improvement or increased severity of symptoms compared with the common cold.

TREATMENT

Amoxicillin continued for 7 days after resolution of symptoms is recommended for treatment of uncomplicated sinusitis. Alternative antibiotics for penicillin-allergic patients include cefuroxime axetil, cefpodoxime, clarithromycin, and azithromycin. For children at increased risk for resistant bacteria (antibiotic treatment in the preceding 1 to 3 months, daycare attendance, age <2 years), and for children who fail to respond to initial therapy with amoxicillin within 72 hours, treatment with high-dose amoxicillin-clavulanate (80 to 90 mg/kg/day of amoxicillin and 6.4 mg/kg/day of clavulanate) is recommended. Failure to respond to this regimen necessitates referral to an otolaryngologist.

COMPLICATIONS

Complications include orbital cellulitis, epidural or subdural empyema, brain abscess, dural sinus thrombosis, osteomyelitis of the outer or inner table of the frontal sinus (**Pott puffy tumor**), and meningitis. These complications should be managed with sinus drainage and broad-spectrum parenteral antibiotics. Sinusitis also may exacerbate bronchoconstriction in asthmatic patients.

Orbital cellulitis is a serious complication of sinusitis in adolescents that follows spread of bacteria into the orbit through the wall of the infected sinus. It typically begins as ethmoid sinusitis and spreads through the lamina papyracea, which is a thin, bony plate that separates the medial orbit and the ethmoid sinus. Orbital involvement can lead to subperiosteal abscess, proptosis, ophthalmoplegia, cavernous sinus thrombosis, and vision loss. Manifestations of orbital cellulitis include orbital pain, proptosis, chemosis, ophthalmoplegia and limited extraocular muscle motion, diplopia, and reduced visual acuity. Infection of the orbit must be differentiated from that of the preseptal (anterior to the palpebral fascia) or periorbital space. **Preseptal cellulitis (periorbital cellulitis)** usually occurs in children younger than 3 years old; these children do not have proptosis or ophthalmoplegia. Periorbital cellulitis usually is associated with a skin lesion or trauma and usually is caused by *S. aureus* or group A streptococcus.

The diagnosis of orbital cellulitis is confirmed by a CT scan of the orbit, which determines the extent of orbital infection and the need for surgical drainage. Disorders to be considered in the differential diagnosis are zygomycosis (mucormycosis), aspergillosis, rhabdomyosarcoma, neuroblastoma, Wegener granulomatosis, inflammatory pseudotumor of the orbit, and trichinosis. Therapy for orbital cellulitis involves broad-spectrum parenteral antibiotics, such as oxacillin and ceftriaxone.

PROGNOSIS

More than half of children with acute bacterial sinusitis recover without any antimicrobial therapy. Fever and nasal discharge should improve dramatically within 48 hours of initiating treatment for sinusitis. Persistent symptoms suggest another etiology.

PREVENTION

The best means of prevention are good hand washing to minimize acquisition of colds and management of allergic rhinitis, both of which are risk factors for sinusitis.

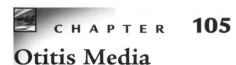

CHAPTER 105

Otitis Media

ETIOLOGY

Otitis media is suppurative infection of the middle ear cavity. Bacteria gain access to the middle ear when the normal patency of the eustachian tube is blocked by infection, pharyngitis, or hypertrophied adenoids. Air trapped in the middle ear is resorbed, creating negative pressure in this cavity and facilitating reflux of nasopharyngeal bacteria. Obstructed flow of secretions from the middle ear to the pharynx combined with bacterial reflux leads to infected middle ear effusion.

The common bacterial pathogens are *S. pneumoniae,* nontypable *H. influenzae, M. catarrhalis,* and, less frequently, group A streptococcus. *S. pneumoniae* that is **relatively resistant** to penicillin (minimal inhibitory concentration 0.1 to 1 µg/mL) or **highly resistant** to penicillin (minimal inhibitory concentration >2 µg/mL) is isolated with increasing frequency from young children, particularly from children who attend daycare or who have received antibiotics recently. Viruses, including rhinoviruses and RSV, are recovered alone or as copathogens in 20% to 25% of patients.

EPIDEMIOLOGY

Diseases of the middle ear account for approximately one third of office visits to pediatricians. The peak incidence of acute otitis media is in the second 6 months of life. By the first birthday, 62% of children experience at least one episode. Few first episodes occur after 18 months of age. Otitis media is more common in boys and in patients of lower socioeconomic status. There is increased incidence of otitis media among Native Americans and Alaskan Natives and in certain high-risk populations, such as children with HIV, cleft palate, and trisomy 21. In most of the U.S., otitis media is a seasonal disease with a distinct peak in January and February, which corresponds to the rhinovirus, RSV, and influenza seasons. It is less common from July to September. The major risk factors for acute otitis media are young age, bottle-feeding as opposed to breastfeeding, drinking a bottle in bed, parental history of ear infection, the presence of a sibling in the home (especially a sibling with a history of ear infection), sharing a room with a sibling, passive exposure to tobacco smoke from parental smoking, and increased exposure to infectious agents (daycare).

As defined by the presence of six or more acute otitis media episodes in the first 6 years of life, at least 12% of children in the general population have **recurrent otitis media** and would be considered **otitis-prone**. Craniofacial anomalies and immunodeficiencies often are associated with recurrent otitis media; most children with recurrent acute otitis media are otherwise healthy.

CLINICAL MANIFESTATIONS

In infants, the most frequent symptoms of acute otitis media are nonspecific and include fever, irritability, and poor feeding. In older children and adolescents, acute otitis media usually is associated with fever and **otalgia** (acute ear pain). Acute otitis media also may present with **otorrhea**, or ear drainage, after spontaneous rupture of the tympanic membrane. Signs of a common cold, which predisposes to acute otitis media, are often present (see Chapter 102).

LABORATORY AND IMAGING STUDIES

Routine laboratory studies, including complete blood count and ESR, are not useful in the evaluation of otitis media. Tympanometry provides objective acoustic measurements of the tympanic membrane–middle ear system by reflection or absorption of sound energy from the external ear duct as pressure in the duct is varied (just as in pneumatic otoscopy). Measurements of the resulting **tympanogram** correlate well with the presence or absence of middle ear effusion.

Instruments using acoustic reflectometry are available for office and home use. Use of reflectometry as a screening test for acute otitis media should be followed by examination with pneumatic otoscopy when abnormal reflectometry is identified.

Bacteria recovered from the nasopharynx do not correlate with bacteria isolated by tympanocentesis. Tympanocentesis and culture of the middle ear exudate is not always necessary, but is required for accurate identification of bacterial pathogens present in the middle ear and may be useful in neonates, immunocompromised patients, and patients not responding to therapy.

DIFFERENTIAL DIAGNOSIS

Examination of the ears is essential for diagnosis and should be part of the physical examination of any child with fever. The hallmark of otitis media is the presence of effusion in the middle ear cavity (Table 105–1). The presence of an effusion does not define its nature or potentially infectious etiology, but does define the need for appropriate diagnosis and therapy.

Pneumatic otoscopy, using a pneumatic attachment to a hermetically sealed otoscope, allows evaluation of ventilation of the middle ear and is a standard

TABLE 105–1. Definition of Acute Otitis Media

A diagnosis of AOM requires
  History of acute onset of signs and symptoms
  Presence of middle ear effusion
  Signs and symptoms of middle ear inflammation
The definition of AOM includes all of the following:
  Recent, usually abrupt, onset of signs and symptoms of
    middle ear inflammation and middle ear effusion
  The presence of middle ear effusion that is indicated by
    any of the following:
    Bulging of the tympanic membrane
    Limited or absent mobility of the tympanic membrane
    Air-fluid level behind the tympanic membrane
    Otorrhea
  Signs or symptoms of middle ear inflammation as
    indicated by either
    Distinct erythema of the tympanic membrane *or*
    Distinct otalgia (discomfort clearly referable to the ear
      that results in interference with or precludes normal
      activity or sleep)

AOM, acute otitis media.

TABLE 105–2. Criteria for Initial Antibiotic Treatment or Observation in Children with Acute Otitis Media*		
Age	**Certain Diagnosis**	**Uncertain Diagnosis**
<6 mo	Antibiotic therapy	Antibiotic therapy
6 mo-2 yr	Antibiotic therapy	Antibiotic therapy for severe illness
		Observation option† for severe illness
≥2 yr	Antibiotic therapy for nonsevere illness	Observation option†
	Observation option† for nonsevere illness	

*A certain diagnosis of acute otitis media meets all 3 criteria: (1) rapid onset, (2) signs of middle ear effusion, and (3) signs and symptoms of middle ear inflammation.
†Observation is appropriate only when follow-up can be ensured and antibiotic treatment can be started if symptoms persist or worsen. Nonsevere illness is mild otalgia and fever <39°C in the preceding 24 hr. Severe illness is moderate to severe otalgia or fever ≥39°C.
Data from the New York Region Otitis Project: Observation Option tool kit for acute otitis media. Publication 4894. New York, State of New York Department of Health, 2002.

for clinical diagnosis. The tympanic membrane of the normal, air-filled middle ear has much greater compliance than if the middle ear is fluid-filled. With acute otitis media, the tympanic membrane is characterized by hyperemia, or red color rather than the normal pearly gray color, but it can be pink, white, or yellow with a full to bulging position and with poor mobility to negative and positive pressure. The light reflex is lost, and the middle ear structures are obscured and difficult to distinguish. A hole in the tympanic membrane or purulent drainage confirms perforation. Occasionally, bullae are present on the lateral aspect of the tympanic membrane, which characteristically are associated with severe ear pain.

The major difficulty is differentiation of acute otitis media from **otitis media with effusion**, which also is referred to as **chronic otitis media**. Acute otitis media is accompanied by signs of acute illness, such as fever, pain, and upper respiratory tract inflammation. Otitis media with effusion is the presence of effusion without any of the other signs and symptoms.

TREATMENT

Recommendations for treatment are based on certainty of diagnosis and severity of illness (Table 105–2). The recommended first-line therapy for most children with acute otitis media is amoxicillin (80 to 90 mg/kg/day in two divided doses). Failure of initial therapy with amoxicillin at 3 days suggests infection with β-lactamase–producing *H. influenzae* or *M. catarrhalis* or relatively or highly resistant *S. pneumoniae*. Recommended next-step treatments include high-dose amoxicillin-clavulanate (amoxicillin 80 to 90 mg/kg/day), cefuroxime axetil, cefdinir, or ceftriaxone (50 mg/kg intramuscularly in one to three daily doses). IM ceftriaxone is especially appropriate for children younger than 3 years old with vomiting that precludes oral treatment. Tympanocentesis may be required for patients who are difficult to treat or who do not respond to therapy, but this is not a routine procedure in most pediatric offices.

Acetaminophen and ibuprofen are recommended for fever. Decongestants or antihistamines are not effective alone or when combined with antibiotics.

COMPLICATIONS

The complications of otitis media are chronic effusion, hearing loss, cholesteatoma (masslike keratinized epithelial growth), petrositis, intracranial extension (brain abscess, subdural empyema, or venous thrombosis), and mastoiditis. **Acute mastoiditis** is a suppurative complication of otitis media with inflammation and potential destruction of the mastoid airspaces. The disease progresses from a periostitis to an osteitis with mastoid abscess formation. Posterior auricular tenderness and swelling and erythema, in addition to the signs of otitis media, are present. The pinna is displaced downward and outward. Radiographs or CT scan of the mastoid reveals clouding of the air cells, demineralization, or bone destruction. The bacteria that cause acute otitis media also are those responsible for acute mastoiditis. Treatment includes systemic antibiotics and drainage if the disease has progressed to abscess formation.

PROGNOSIS

Otitis media with effusion is the most frequent sequela of acute otitis media and occurs most frequently in the first 2 years of life. **Persistent middle ear effusion** may last for many weeks or months in some children. The condition should be sought at all well-child examinations of young children.

Conductive hearing loss should be assumed to be present with persistent middle ear effusion; the loss is mild to moderate and often is transient or fluctuating. **Glue ear** is used to describe the presence of a viscous, gluelike effusion that is produced when the chronically inflamed middle ear mucosa produces an excess of mucus that, because of absence of the normal clearance of the middle ear cavity, is retained for prolonged periods.

Normal tympanograms after 1 month of treatment obviate the need for further follow-up. In children at developmental risk or with frequent episodes of recurrent acute otitis media, 3 months of persistent effusion with significant bilateral hearing loss is a reasonable indicator of need for intervention with insertion of pressure equalization tubes.

PREVENTION

Parents should be encouraged to continue exclusive breastfeeding as long as possible and should be cautioned about the risks of "bottle-propping" and of children taking a bottle to bed. The home should be a smoke-free environment.

Children identified at high-risk for recurrent acute otitis media are candidates for prolonged courses of antimicrobial prophylaxis, which can reduce recurrences significantly. Amoxicillin (20 to 30 mg/kg/day) or sulfisoxazole (50 mg/kg/day) given once daily at bedtime for 3 to 6 months or longer is used for prophylaxis.

Pneumococcal vaccine and influenza vaccine may reduce marginally the incidence of otitis media. The conjugate *S. pneumoniae* vaccine seems to reduce pneumococcal otitis media caused by vaccine serotypes by half, all pneumococcal otitis media by one third, and all otitis media by 6%. Annual immunization against influenza virus may be helpful in high-risk children.

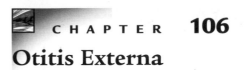

CHAPTER 106
Otitis Externa

ETIOLOGY

Otitis externa, also known as **swimmer's ear**, is defined by inflammation and exudation in the external auditory canal in the absence of other disorders, such as otitis media or mastoiditis. It results from the interaction of host, environmental, and microbial factors.

The most common bacterial pathogen is *P. aeruginosa,* especially in association with swimming in pools or lakes. Other common pathogens may be associated with **tympanostomy tubes**. Otitis externa develops in approximately 20% of children with tympanostomy tubes, associated with *S. aureus, S. pneumoniae, M. catarrhalis, Proteus, Klebsiella,* and occasionally anaerobes. Coagulase-negative staphylococci and *Corynebacterium* are isolated frequently from cultures of the external canal but represent normal flora. **Malignant otitis externa** is caused by *P. aeruginosa* in immunocompromised persons and adults with diabetes.

EPIDEMIOLOGY

Otitis externa is a frequent complaint in summer, in contrast to otitis media, which occurs primarily in colder seasons in association with viral upper respiratory tract infections. Disruption of the integrity of the cutaneous lining of the ear canal and local defenses, as occurs with cleaning of the auditory canal, swimming, and, in particular, diving, predisposes to otitis externa.

CLINICAL MANIFESTATIONS

Pain, tenderness, and aural discharge are the characteristic clinical findings of otitis externa. Fever is notably absent, and hearing is unaffected. Tenderness with movement of the pinnae, especially the tragus, and with chewing is particularly typical. This is not present in otitis media, and is a valuable diagnostic criterion. The most common symptoms of malignant otitis externa are severe ear pain, tenderness on movement of the pinna, drainage from the canal, and occasionally facial nerve palsy. Inspection usually reveals that the lining of the auditory canal is inflamed with mild to severe erythema and edema. There may be a scant to copious discharge from the auditory canal, often obscuring the tympanic membrane. In **malignant otitis externa**, the most common physical findings are swelling and granulation tissue in the canal, usually with a discharge from the external auditory canal.

LABORATORY AND IMAGING STUDIES

The diagnosis of uncomplicated otitis externa usually is established solely on the basis of the clinical symptoms and physical examination findings without the need for additional laboratory or microbiologic evaluation. In malignant otitis externa, an elevated ESR is a constant finding. The diagnosis requires documentation of the extent of involvement with diagnostic imaging studies, such as CT or MRI. Cultures are required to identify the etiologic agent, which is usually *P. aeruginosa*, and the antimicrobial susceptibility.

DIFFERENTIAL DIAGNOSIS

Otitis media with tympanic perforation and discharge into the auditory canal may be confused with otitis externa, particularly in infants in whom it may be difficult to clear the discharge. Pain on movement of the pinnae or the tragus, which is typical of otitis externa, is not present. Local and systemic signs of mastoiditis, of swelling and tenderness over the mastoid, indicate a process more extensive than otitis externa. **Tuberculous otitis media** is marked by a chronic, painless aural discharge, further suggested by skin testing and chest x-ray. **Malignancies** presenting in the auditory canal are rare in children, but may occur with discharge, unusual pain, or hearing loss.

TREATMENT

The most widely used topical otic preparations contain a combination of an aminoglycoside, such as neomycin and polymyxin B, with a topical corticosteroid. Topical **quinolone** antibiotic drops (ciprofloxacin, ofloxacin) are more popular despite the cost. They are active against *S. aureus* and most gram-negative bacteria, including *P. aeruginosa*. None of these antibiotics has any antifungal activity.

Local therapy with acetic acid preparations (2%) designed to restore the acid pH of the auditory canal is usually effective. It may be necessary to remove the aural exudate with a swab or with suction to permit instillation of the solution. The predisposing activity, such as swimming or diving, that produced the condition should be avoided until the inflammation has resolved. Topical acetic acid preparations have indirect antibacterial and antifungal effects by acidification.

Otic solutions containing corticosteroids are used frequently and reduce local inflammation when there is no infection. Solutions that combine antibiotics and corticosteroids are a reasonable choice in severe cases and when therapy with acetic acid preparations has not been effective. Treatment with topical otic analgesics and ceruminolytics is usually unnecessary.

Fungi such as *Aspergillus*, *Candida*, and dermatophytes occasionally are isolated from the external ear. It may be difficult to determine whether they represent normal flora or are the cause of inflammation. In most cases, local therapy and restoration of normal pH as recommended for bacterial otitis externa are sufficient.

Tympanostomy tube otorrhea is best treated with quinolone otic drugs because they are considered less likely to be ototoxic. There are theoretical risks of ototoxicity with neomycin and polymyxin B, which should be avoided in the presence of tympanic perforation.

Malignant otitis externa is treated by parenteral antimicrobials with activity against *P. aeruginosa*, such as an expanded-spectrum penicillin (mezlocillin, piperacillin-tazobactam) or a cephalosporin with activity against *P. aeruginosa* (ceftazidime, cefepime) plus an aminoglycoside.

COMPLICATIONS AND PROGNOSIS

Acute otitis externa usually resolves promptly without complications within 1 to 2 days of initiating treatment. Persistent pain, especially if severe or if accompanied by other symptoms, such as fever, should prompt re-evaluation for other conditions.

Malignant otitis externa frequently is accompanied by complications. Invasion of the bones of the base of the skull may cause cranial nerve palsies, such as facial nerve palsy. A mortality of 15% to 20% occurs in adults with malignant otitis media. Relapses within the first year after treatment are common.

PREVENTION

Overly vigorous cleaning of an asymptomatic auditory canal should be avoided. Drying the auditory canals with acetic acid (2%), Burow solution, or diluted isopropyl alcohol (rubbing alcohol) after swimming may be used prophylactically to help prevent the maceration that may facilitate bacterial invasion. Often underwater gear, such as earplugs or diving equipment, must be avoided to prevent recurrent disease. There is no role for prophylactic otic antibiotics.

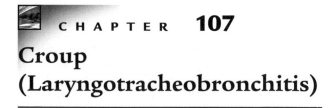

CHAPTER 107

Croup (Laryngotracheobronchitis)

ETIOLOGY

Croup, or laryngotracheobronchitis, is the most common infection of the middle respiratory tract (Table 107–1). The most common causes of croup are parainfluenza viruses (types 1, 2, and 3) and RSV. Laryngotracheal

TABLE 107–1.   Clinical Features of Laryngotracheal Respiratory Tract Infections

Feature	Viral Laryngotracheobronchitis	Epiglottitis	Bacterial Tracheitis	Spasmodic Croup
Viral prodromal illness	++	–	+	–
Mean age	6-36 mo (60% <24 mo)	3-4 yr (25% <2 yr)	4-5 yr	6-36 mo (60% <24 mo)
Onset of illness	Gradual (2-3 days)	Acute (6-24 hr)	Acute (1-2 days)	Sudden (at night)
Fever	±	+	+	–
Toxicity	–	+	++	–
Inspiratory stridor	Harsh	Mild	Harsh	Harsh
Drooling, neck hyperextension	–	++	+	–
Cough	++	–	++	++
Sore throat	±	++	±	–
Positive blood culture	–	+	±	–
Leukocytosis	–	+	+	–
Recurrence	+	–	–	++
Hospitalization and endotracheal intubation	Rare	Frequent	Frequent	Rare

+ = frequently present; – = absent; ± = may or may not be present; ++ = present and usually pronounced.
From Bell LM: Middle respiratory tract infections. In Jenson HB, Baltimore RS (eds): Pediatric Infectious Diseases: Principles and Practice, 2nd ed. Philadelphia, WB Saunders, 2002, p 772.

airway inflammation disproportionately affects children because a small decrease in diameter secondary to mucosal edema and inflammation exponentially increases airway resistance and significantly increases the work of breathing. During inspiration, the walls of the subglottic space are drawn together, aggravating the obstruction and producing the stridor characteristic of croup.

EPIDEMIOLOGY

Croup is most common in children 6 months to 3 years old, with a peak in fall and early winter. Episodes typically follow a common cold. Symptomatic reinfection is common; reinfections are usually mild.

CLINICAL MANIFESTATIONS

The manifestations of croup are cough, hoarseness, inspiratory stridor, low-grade fever, and respiratory distress that may develop slowly or quickly. **Stridor** is a harsh, high-pitched respiratory sound produced by turbulent airflow that is usually inspiratory, but may be biphasic; it is a sign of upper airway obstruction (Table 107–2). Croup is characterized by a harsh cough that is described as **barking** or **brassy** in quality. Signs of upper airway obstruction, such as labored breathing and marked suprasternal, intercostal, and subcostal retractions, may be evident on examination (see Chapter 135). Wheezing may be present if there is associated lower airway involvement.

TABLE 107–2.   Differential Diagnosis of Stridor

Infections	Noninfectious Conditions
Acute laryngotracheobronchitis	Foreign body aspiration
Epiglottitis	Angioneurotic edema
Pharyngitis	Spasmodic croup
Parapharyngeal abscess	Ingestion of caustic or hot fluid
Bacterial tracheitis	Trauma, smoke inhalation
Laryngopharyngeal diphtheria	Laryngomalacia
Laryngeal papillomatosis	Congenital subglottic stenosis
Extrinsic inflammatory mass compressing the trachea (e.g., tuberculosis)	Extrinsic mass compressing the trachea (cystic hygroma, hemangioma, vascular malformation)
	Hypocalcemia
	Vocal cord paralysis

From Bell LM: Middle respiratory tract infections. In Jenson HB, Baltimore RS (eds): Pediatric Infectious Diseases: Principles and Practice, 2nd ed. Philadelphia, WB Saunders, 2002, p 771.

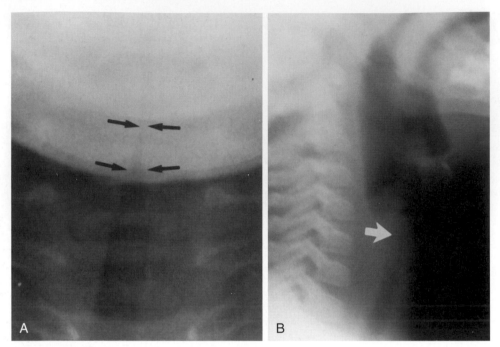

Figure 107–1

Croup, or laryngotracheobronchitis. A, Posteroanterior view of the upper airway shows the so-called steeple sign, the tapered narrowing of the immediate subglottic airway *(arrows)*. **B,** Lateral view of the upper airway shows good delineation of the supraglottic anatomy. The subglottic trachea is hazy and poorly defined *(arrow)* because of the inflammatory edema that has obliterated the sharp undersurface of the vocal cords and extends down the trachea in a diminishing manner. (From Bell LM: Middle respiratory tract infections. In Jenson HB, Baltimore RS [eds]: Pediatric Infectious Diseases: Principles and Practice, 2nd ed. Philadelphia, WB Saunders, 2002, p 774.)

LABORATORY AND IMAGING STUDIES

Anteroposterior radiographs of the neck often, but not always, show the diagnostic subglottic narrowing of croup, known as the **steeple sign** (Fig. 107–1). Routine laboratory studies are not useful in establishing the diagnosis. Leukocytosis is uncommon and suggests epiglottitis or bacterial tracheitis. Many rapid tests (PCR or antigen) are available for parainfluenza viruses and RSV and other less common viral causes of croup, such as influenza and adenoviruses. The sensitivity of the RSV indirect immunofluorescence tests is 75% to 97%; the sensitivity and positive predictive values for parainfluenza viruses appear to be less than those for RSV.

DIFFERENTIAL DIAGNOSIS

The diagnosis of croup usually is established by clinical manifestations. Stridor in infants younger than 4 months old or persistence of symptoms for more than

1 week indicates an increased probability of another lesion (subglottic stenosis or hemangioma) and the need for direct laryngoscopy (see Chapter 135).

Epiglottitis typically occurs in children 1 to 5 years old and is a medical emergency because of the risk of sudden airway obstruction. Hib is historically the principal causative agent, but immunization has reduced Hib infections markedly. Stridor is common, but is distinguished from croup by sudden onset and rapid progression, high fever, muffled rather than hoarse voice, dysphagia and drooling of secretions, refusal to eat or drink, refusal to sleep, and preference for sitting, often with the head held forward, the mouth open, and the jaw thrust forward (**sniffing position**). Lateral radiograph reveals thickened and bulging epiglottis (**thumb sign**) and swelling of the aryepiglottic folds. The diagnosis is confirmed by direct observation of the inflamed and swollen supraglottic structures and swollen, cherry-red epiglottitis, which should be performed only in the operating room with a competent surgeon and anesthesiologist prepared to place an endotracheal tube or less often to perform a tracheostomy. Epiglottitis requires endotracheal intubation to maintain the airway and antibiotic therapy. Clinical recovery is rapid, and most children can be extubated safely within 48 to 72 hours.

Bacterial tracheitis is a rare but serious superinfection of the trachea that may follow viral croup and is most commonly caused by *S. aureus*. Symptoms include high fever with cough and stridor. The diagnosis requires visualization of the middle airway, with culture of the thick, mucopurulent subglottic debris. Treatment includes endotracheal intubation and antibiotic therapy.

Spasmodic croup describes sudden onset of croup symptoms, usually at night, but without an upper respiratory tract prodrome. These episodes may be recurrent and severe but usually are of short duration. Spasmodic croup has a milder course than viral croup and responds to relatively simple therapies, such as exposure to cool or humidified air. The etiology is not well understood but may be allergic.

TREATMENT

Administration of aerosolized racemic (D- and L-) or L-epinephrine reduces subglottic edema by α-adrenergic vasoconstriction, temporarily producing marked clinical improvement. The peak effect is within 10 to 30 minutes, but fades within 2 hours. A rebound effect may occur, with worsening of symptoms as the effect of the drug dissipates. Aerosol treatment may need to be repeated every 20 minutes (for no more than 1 to 2 hours) in severe cases. Oral or IM dexamethasone for children with mild or moderate croup reduces the need for hospitalization and shortens hospital stays.

Children should be kept as calm as possible to minimize forceful inspiration. One useful calming method is for a child with croup to sit in the parent's lap. Sedatives should be used cautiously and only in the ICU. Cool mist administered by tent or facemask may help prevent drying of the secretions around the larynx.

Hospitalization often is required for children with stridor at rest. Children receiving aerosol treatment should be hospitalized or observed for at least 2 to 3 hours because of the risk of rebound. Subsidence of symptoms may indicate improvement or fatigue and impending respiratory failure.

COMPLICATIONS

The most common complication of croup is viral pneumonia, which occurs in 1% to 2% of children with croup. Parainfluenza pneumonia and secondary bacterial pneumonia are more common among immunocompromised persons.

PROGNOSIS

The prognosis for croup is excellent. Illness usually lasts approximately 5 days. As children grow, they become less susceptible to the airway effects of viral infections of the middle respiratory tract.

PREVENTION

There is no vaccine for parainfluenza or RSV.

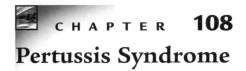

CHAPTER 108
Pertussis Syndrome

ETIOLOGY

The pertussis syndrome includes disease caused by *Bordetella pertussis* and certain other infectious agents. Classic pertussis, the **whooping cough syndrome**, usually is caused by *B. pertussis,* a gram-negative pleomorphic bacillus with fastidious growth requirements. Some cases of pertussis syndrome are caused by other organisms, including *Bordetella parapertussis,* which causes a similar but milder illness that is not affected by *B. pertussis* vaccination. *B. pertussis* and *B. parapertussis* infect only humans and are transmitted person to person by coughing. Asymptomatic carriage is rare. Adenoviruses have been associated with the pertussis syndrome. Dual infection with *B. pertussis* and adenovirus occurs more frequently than expected.

EPIDEMIOLOGY

The mean incubation period is 6 days. Patients are most contagious during the earliest stage. The annual rate of pertussis was approximately 100 to 200 cases per 100,000 population in the prevaccination era, and presently it may be higher in developing countries. In the U.S., the incidence of pertussis has increased steadily since the 1980s, with 5000 to 10,000 cases reported each year. The peak age incidence of pertussis in the U.S. is younger than 4 months of age—among infants too young to be completely immunized and most likely to have the complications of pneumonia and severe infection that are associated with a high mortality.

If vaccination rates are not high, pertussis rates increase. In the United Kingdom, there was a steady decline in the incidence of pertussis until the late 1970s, when the incidence increased dramatically as the rate of vaccination declined. These data, a similar episode in Japan at about the same time, and the decline in the incidence of cases when vaccines were first tested are major events indicating the efficacy of vaccination.

CLINICAL MANIFESTATIONS

Classic pertussis is the syndrome seen in most infants beyond the neonatal period through school age. The progression of the disease is divided into catarrhal, paroxysmal, and convalescent stages. The **catarrhal stage** is marked by nonspecific signs (injection, increased nasal secretions, and low-grade fever) that last 1 to 2 weeks. The **paroxysmal stage** is the most distinctive stage of pertussis. Coughing occurs in **paroxysms** during expiration, causing young children to lose their breath. This pattern of coughing is due to the need to dislodge plugs of necrotic bronchial epithelial tissues and thick mucus. It lasts approximately 2 to 4 weeks. The forceful inhalation against a narrowed glottis that follows this paroxysm of cough produces the characteristic **whoop**. Post-tussive emesis is common. The **convalescent stage** is marked by gradual resolution of symptoms over 1 to 2 weeks. Coughing becomes less severe, and the paroxysms and whoops slowly disappear. Although the disease typically lasts 6 to 8 weeks, residual cough may persist for months, especially with physical stress or respiratory irritants.

Young infants may not display the classic pertussis syndrome; the first signs may be episodes of apnea. Young infants are unlikely to have the classic whoop, are more likely to have CNS damage as a result of hypoxia, and are more likely to have secondary bacterial pneumonia. Adolescents and adults with pertussis usually present with a prolonged bronchitic illness that often begins as a nonspecific upper respiratory tract infection. This illness is not much different from pertussis in children, but generally adolescents and adults do not have a whoop with the cough, although they may have severe paroxysms. The cough may persist many weeks to months.

LABORATORY AND IMAGING STUDIES

The diagnosis depends on isolation of *B. pertussis*, which is usually accomplished during the early phases of illness by culture of nasopharyngeal swabs on Regan-Lowe medium or classically on glycerin-potato-blood agar medium (Bordet-Gengou) to which penicillin has been added to inhibit growth of other organisms. Direct fluorescent antibody staining to detect the organism is technically difficult, dependent on the skills of the technologist, and has low specificity. PCR is useful. Available serologic tests are not useful for diagnosis of acute infection.

A characteristic feature of pertussis in patients beyond the neonatal age is an abnormally high absolute number and relative percentage of lymphocytes in the peripheral blood. In classic *B. pertussis*–associated pertussis, **lymphocytosis** is found in 75% to 85% of patients, although in young infants the rate is much less. The WBC count may increase from 20,000 cells/mm^3 to more than 50,000 cells/mm^3, consisting mostly of mature lymphocytes.

It is not unusual for physical and radiographic signs of segmental lung atelectasis to develop during pertussis, especially during the paroxysmal stage. Perihilar infiltrates are common and are similar to what is seen in viral pneumonia.

DIFFERENTIAL DIAGNOSIS

For a young child with classic pertussis syndrome, the diagnosis based on recognition of the pattern of illness is quite accurate. The paroxysmal stage is the most distinctive part of the syndrome. Respiratory viruses such as RSV, parainfluenza virus, and *C. pneumoniae* can produce bronchitic illnesses among infants. In older children and young adults, *M. pneumoniae* may produce a prolonged bronchitic illness that is not distinguished easily from pertussis in this age group.

TREATMENT

Erythromycin, given early in the course of illness, eradicates nasopharyngeal carriage of organisms within 3 to 4 days and ameliorates the effects of the infection. Treatment is not effective in the paroxysmal stage. When given to neonates younger than 4 weeks old, erythromycin has been associated rarely with pyloric stenosis, but treatment is still recommended because of the seriousness of pertussis at this age. Azithromycin and clarithromycin can be given for a shorter duration and are associated with fewer gastrointestinal adverse effects. TMP-SMZ may be beneficial as an alternative, but this remains unproven. Pertussis-specific immunoglobulin may be effective in reducing the symptoms of the paroxysmal stage.

COMPLICATIONS

Major complications are most common among infants and young children and include hypoxia, apnea, pneumonia, seizures, encephalopathy, and malnutrition. The most frequent complication is pneumonia caused by *B. pertussis* itself or resulting from secondary bacterial infection from *S. pneumoniae*, Hib, and *S. aureus*. Atelectasis may develop secondary to mucous plugs. The force of the paroxysm may rupture alveoli and produce pneumomediastinum, pneumothorax, or interstitial or subcutaneous emphysema; epistaxis; hernias; and retinal and subconjunctival hemorrhages. Otitis media and sinusitis may occur.

PROGNOSIS

Most children do well with complete healing of the respiratory epithelium and have normal pulmonary function after recovery. Young children can die from pertussis; 13 children died in the U.S. from pertussis in 2003. Most deaths occurred in unvaccinated children or infants too young to be vaccinated. Most permanent disability is a result of encephalopathy.

PREVENTION

Active immunity can be induced with acellular pertussis vaccine, given in combination with the toxoids of tetanus and diphtheria (DTaP). Pertussis vaccine has an efficacy of 70% to 90%; efficacy declines with fewer vaccinations. The acellular vaccines contain one or more antigens isolated from *B. pertussis,* such as pertussis toxin, pertactin, or filamentous hemagglutinins. Each preparation currently licensed seems to provide equivalent protection. DTaP vaccine is available for adolescents. Compared with older, whole cell pertussis vaccines, acellular vaccines have fewer adverse effects and local reactions.

Erythromycin and other macrolides are effective in preventing disease in contacts exposed to pertussis. Close contacts younger than 7 years old who have received four doses of vaccine should receive a booster dose of DTaP, unless a booster dose has been given within the preceding 3 years. They also should be given a macrolide antibiotic. Close contacts older than age 7 should receive prophylactic macrolide antibiotic for 10 to 14 days, but not the vaccine.

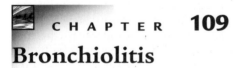

CHAPTER 109
Bronchiolitis

ETIOLOGY

Bronchiolitis is the term used for first-time wheezing with a viral respiratory infection. The distinctive element of acute bronchiolitis is respiratory tract inflammation with airway obstruction resulting from swelling of small bronchioles, which leads to inadequate expiratory airflow. Most severe cases of bronchiolitis occur among infants, probably as a consequence of narrow-sized airways and an immature immune system. Bronchiolitis is potentially life-threatening.

RSV is the primary cause, followed in frequency by human metapneumovirus, parainfluenza viruses, influenza viruses, adenoviruses, rhinoviruses, and, infrequently, *M. pneumoniae.* Viral bronchiolitis is extremely contagious and is spread by contact with infected respiratory secretions. Although coughing does produce aerosols, hand carriage of contaminated secretions is the most frequent mode of transmission.

EPIDEMIOLOGY

Bronchiolitis is the leading cause of hospitalization of infants. Approximately 50% of children experience bronchiolitis during the first 2 years of life, with a peak age at 2 to 6 months. The incidence falls rapidly between the ages of 1 and 5 years, after which bronchiolitis is uncommon. It is estimated that only 10% of healthy children with bronchiolitis and wheezing require hospitalization.

Children acquire infection after exposure to infected family members, who typically have symptoms of an upper respiratory tract infection, or from infected children in daycare. In the U.S., annual peaks are usually in the late winter months from December through March. Boys are affected more commonly than girls in a ratio of 1.5:1.

CLINICAL MANIFESTATIONS

Bronchiolitis caused by RSV has an incubation period of 4 to 6 days. Bronchiolitis classically presents as a progressive respiratory illness that is similar to the common cold in its early phase with cough, coryza, and rhinorrhea. It progresses over 3 to 7 days to noisy, raspy breathing and audible wheezing. There is usually a low-grade fever accompanied in young children by irritability, which may reflect the increased work of breathing and may increase itself with increased respiratory effort. In contrast to the classic progression of disease, young infants infected with RSV may not have a prodrome and may have apnea as the first sign of infection.

Physical signs of bronchiolar obstruction include prolongation of the expiratory phase of breathing, intercostal retractions with inward drawing of the lower ribs, suprasternal retractions, and air trapping with hyperexpansion of the lungs. During the wheezing phase of the illness, percussion of the chest usually reveals only hyperresonance, but auscultation usually reveals diffuse wheezes and crackles throughout the breathing cycle. With more severe disease, grunting and cyanosis may be present.

LABORATORY AND IMAGING STUDIES

Routine laboratory tests lack specificity for diagnosing bronchiolitis and are not required to confirm the diagnosis. A mild leukocytosis of 12,000 to 16,000/μL is encountered frequently but is not specific. In severe cases of bronchiolitis, it is important to assess gas exchange. Visual assessment of oxygenation correlates poorly with actual blood gas values. Pulse oximetry is generally adequate for monitoring oxygen saturation. Frequent, regular visual assessments and cardiorespiratory monitoring of infants are necessary because respiratory failure may develop precipitously in very tired infants even though blood gas values taken before rapid decompensation are not alarming.

Antigen tests (usually by immunofluorescence or ELISA) of nasopharyngeal secretions for RSV, parainfluenza viruses, influenza viruses, and adenoviruses are the most sensitive tests to confirm the infection. Rapid viral diagnosis also is performed by PCR and is helpful for cohorting children with the same infection.

The chest radiograph frequently shows the signs of hyperexpansion of the lungs, including increased lung radiolucency and flattened or depressed diaphragms. The lung fields may appear normal or may show areas of increased density, which may represent either viral pneumonia or localized atelectasis.

DIFFERENTIAL DIAGNOSIS

The major difficulty in the diagnosis of bronchiolitis is to differentiate other diseases associated with wheezing. It may be impossible to differentiate asthma from bronchiolitis by physical examination, but age of presentation, presence of fever, and no history (personal or family) of asthma are the major differential factors. Bronchiolitis occurs primarily in the first year of life and is accompanied by a fever, whereas asthma usually presents in older children with wheezing episodes that usually are not accompanied by fever unless a respiratory tract infection is the trigger for the asthma attack.

Wheezing also may be due to other causes, such as a foreign body in the airway, congenital airway obstructive lesion, cystic fibrosis, exacerbation of bronchopulmonary dysplasia, viral or bacterial pneumonia, and other lower respiratory tract diseases (see Chapter 78). **Cardiogenic asthma**, which can be confused with bronchiolitis in infants, is wheezing associated with pulmonary congestion secondary to left-sided heart failure.

Wheezing associated with gastroesophageal reflux is likely to be chronic or recurrent, and the patient may have a history of frequent emesis. Cystic fibrosis is associated with poor growth, chronic diarrhea, and a positive family history. A focal area on radiography that does not inflate or deflate suggests a **foreign body**.

TREATMENT

Treatment of bronchiolitis consists of supportive therapy, including monitoring, control of fever, good hydration, upper airway suctioning, and oxygen administration. Supplemental oxygen by nasal cannula is often necessary, with intubation and ventilatory assistance for respiratory failure or apnea.

Indications for hospitalization include young age (<6 months old), moderate to marked respiratory distress (sleeping respiratory rate of >50 to 60 breaths/min), hypoxemia (PO_2 <60 mm Hg or oxygen saturation <92% on room air), apnea, inability to tolerate oral feeding, and lack of appropriate care available at home. Children with chronic lung disease such as bronchopulmonary dysplasia, hemodynamically significant cyanotic and acyanotic congenital heart disease, neuromuscular weakness, or immunodeficiency are at increased risk of severe, potentially fatal disease. Hospitalization of high-risk children with bronchiolitis should be considered.

Temporary use of bronchodilators possibly may improve wheezing and respiratory distress in infants and young children being treated as outpatients. Nonetheless, the benefits are inconsequential in that they are modest, are short-lived, and do not seem to reduce hospitalization.

COMPLICATIONS

Most hospitalized children show marked improvement in 2 to 5 days with supportive treatment alone. The course of the wheezing phase varies, however. There may be tachypnea and hypoxia after admission, progressing to respiratory failure requiring assisted ventilation. Apnea is a major concern for very young infants with bronchiolitis.

PROGNOSIS

Most cases of bronchiolitis resolve completely, although minor abnormalities of pulmonary function and bronchial hyperreactivity may persist for years. Recurrence is common, but tends to be mild, and should be assessed and treated similarly to the first episode. The incidence of asthma seems to be higher for children hospitalized for bronchiolitis as infants, but it is unclear whether this is causal or if children prone to having asthma are more likely to be hospitalized when they develop bronchiolitis. There is a 1% to 2% mortality rate, which is highest among infants with preexisting cardiopulmonary or immunologic impairment.

PREVENTION

Monthly injections of **palivizumab**, an RSV-specific monoclonal antibody, initiated just before the onset of the RSV season confers some protection from severe RSV disease. Palivizumab is indicated for some infants younger than 2 years old with chronic lung disease (bronchopulmonary dysplasia), very low birth weight infants, and infants with hemodynamically significant cyanotic and acyanotic congenital heart disease.

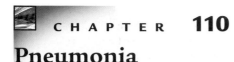

CHAPTER 110

Pneumonia

ETIOLOGY

Pneumonia is an infection of the lower respiratory tract that involves the airways and parenchyma with consolidation of the alveolar spaces. The term **lower respiratory tract infection** is often used to encompass bronchitis (see Chapter 108), bronchiolitis (see Chapter 109), or pneumonia or any combination of the three, which may be difficult to distinguish clinically. **Pneumonitis** is a general term for lung inflammation that may or may not be associated with consolidation. **Lobar pneumonia** describes "typical" pneumonia localized to one or more lobes of the lung in which the affected lobe or lobes are completely consolidated. **Atypical pneumonia** describes patterns other than lobar pneumonia. **Bronchopneumonia** refers to inflammation of the lung that is centered in the bronchioles and leads to the production of a mucopurulent exudate that obstructs some of these small airways and causes patchy consolidation of the adjacent lobules. **Interstitial pneumonitis** refers to inflammation of the interstitium, which is composed of the walls of the alveoli, the alveolar sacs and ducts, and the bronchioles. Interstitial pneumonitis is characteristic of acute viral infections, but also may be a chronic process.

Defects in host defenses increase the risk of pneumonia. Lower airways and secretions are sterile as a result of a multicomponent cleansing system. Airway contaminants are caught in the mucus secreted by the goblet cells. Cilia on epithelial surfaces, composing the **ciliary elevator system**, beat synchronously to move particles upward toward the central airways and into the throat, where they are swallowed or expectorated. Polymorphonuclear neutrophils from the blood and tissue macrophages ingest and kill microorganisms. IgA secreted into the upper airway fluid protects against invasive infections and facilitates viral neutralization.

The infectious agents that commonly cause community-acquired pneumonia vary by age (Table 110–1). The most common causes are RSV in infants (see Chapter 109), respiratory viruses (RSV, parainfluenza viruses, influenza viruses, adenoviruses) in children younger than 5 years old, and *M. pneumoniae* and *S. pneumoniae* in children older than age 5. *M. pneumoniae* and *C. pneumoniae* are the principal causes of **atypical pneumonia**. Additional agents occasionally or rarely cause pneumonia as hospital-acquired pneumonia, as zoonotic infections, in endemic areas, or among immunocompromised persons. Severe acute respiratory syndrome (SARS) describes an outbreak of SARS-associated coronavirus (SARS-CoV) in 2002 in Southern China that spread worldwide during 2003. The epidemic (with >8000 cases and >700 deaths) has since been contained. Avian influenza, also known as bird flu, is a highly contagious viral disease of poultry and other birds that is caused by influenza A (H5N1). There were outbreaks among humans in South East Asia in 1997 and 2003-2004, with high mortality rates. Hantavirus cardiopulmonary syndrome is caused by Sin Nombre virus, which is carried by *Peromyscus maniculatus* (the deer mouse) and transmitted to humans by aerosolized rodent excreta. *Legionella pneumophila* (legionnaires' disease) is a rare cause of pneumonia in children.

Chlamydia trachomatis and less commonly *Mycoplasma hominis*, *Ureaplasma urealyticum*, and CMV cause a similar respiratory syndrome in infants 1 to 3 months of age with subacute onset of an **afebrile pneumonia** with cough and hyperinflation as the predominant signs. These infections are difficult to diagnose and to distinguish from each other. In adults, these organisms are spread by sexual transmission and are carried primarily as part of the genital mucosal flora. Women who harbor these agents may transmit them perinatally to newborns, and the epidemiology of much infant pneumonia is linked to sexually transmitted agents in adults.

Causes of pneumonia in immunocompromised persons include gram-negative enteric bacteria, mycobacteria (*M. avium* complex), fungi (aspergillosis, histoplasmosis), viruses (CMV), and *Pneumocystis jirovecii* (*carinii*). Pneumonia in patients with cystic fibrosis usually is caused by *S. aureus* in infancy and *P. aeruginosa* or *Burkholderia cepacia* in older patients.

EPIDEMIOLOGY

Immunizations have had a great impact on the incidence of pneumonia caused by pertussis, diphtheria, measles, Hib, and *S. pneumoniae*. Where used, bacille Calmette-Guérin (BCG) for tuberculosis also has had a significant impact. More than 4 million deaths each year in developing countries are due to acute respiratory tract infections. Risk factors for lower respiratory tract infections include gastroesophageal reflux, neurologic impairment (aspiration), immunocompromised states, anatomic abnormalities of the respiratory tract, residence in residential care facilities for handicapped children, and hospitalization, especially in an ICU or requiring invasive procedures.

CLINICAL MANIFESTATIONS

Age is a determinant in the clinical manifestations of pneumonia. Neonates may have fever only with subtle or no physical findings of pneumonia (see Chapter 65).

TABLE 110–1.   Etiologic Agents and Empirical Antimicrobial Therapy for Pneumonia without Recent Antibiotic Therapy

Age Group	Frequent Pathogens* (in order of frequency)	Outpatients[†] (7-10 days total duration of treatment)	Patients Requiring Hospitalization[‡] (10-14 days total duration of treatment)	Patients Requiring Intensive Care*[‡] (10-14 days total duration of treatment)
Neonates (<1 mo)	Group B streptococcus, *Escherichia coli*, other gram-negative bacilli, *Streptococcus pneumoniae, Haemophilus influenzae* (type b,[§] nontypable)	Outpatient management not recommended	Ampicillin *plus* cefotaxime or an aminoglycoside *plus* an antistaphylococcal agent if *Staphylococcus aureus* is suspected	Ampicillin *plus* cefotaxime or an aminoglycoside *plus* an antistaphylococcal agent if *S. aureus* is suspected
1-3 mo Febrile pneumonia	Respiratory syncytial virus, other respiratory viruses (parainfluenza viruses, influenza viruses, adenoviruses), *S. pneumoniae, H. influenzae* (type b,[§] nontypable)	Initial outpatient management not recommended	Cefuroxime *or* cefotaxime or ceftriaxone *plus* nafcillin or oxacillin	Cefotaxime or ceftriaxone *plus* nafcillin or oxacillin
Afebrile pneumonia	*Chlamydia trachomatis, Mycoplasma hominis, Ureaplasma urealyticum,* cytomegalovirus	Erythromycin, azithromycin, or clarithromycin with close follow-up	Erythromycin, azithromycin, or clarithromycin	Erythromycin, azithromycin, or clarithromycin *plus* cefotaxime or ceftriaxone *plus* nafcillin or oxacillin
3-12 mo	Respiratory syncytial virus, other respiratory viruses (parainfluenza viruses, influenza viruses, adenoviruses), *S. pneumoniae, H. influenzae* (type b,[§] nontypable), *C. trachomatis, Mycoplasma pneumoniae,* group A streptococcus	Amoxicillin, erythromycin, azithromycin, or clarithromycin	Ampicillin or cefuroxime	Cefuroxime or ceftriaxone *plus* erythromycin or clarithromycin
2-5 yr	Respiratory viruses (parainfluenza viruses, influenza viruses, adenoviruses), *S. pneumoniae, H. influenzae* (type b,[§] nontypable), *M. pneumoniae, Chlamydophila pneumoniae, S. aureus,* group A streptococcus	Amoxicillin, erythromycin, azithromycin, or clarithromycin	Ampicillin or cefuroxime	Cefuroxime or ceftriaxone *plus* erythromycin, azithromycin, or clarithromycin
5-18 yr	*M. pneumoniae, S. pneumoniae, C. pneumoniae, H. influenzae* (type b,[§] nontypable), influenza viruses, adenoviruses, other respiratory viruses	Erythromycin, azithromycin, or clarithromycin	Erythromycin, azithromycin, or clarithromycin with or without cefuroxime or ampicillin	Cefuroxime or ceftriaxone *plus* erythromycin or clarithromycin
≥18 yr[¶]	*M. pneumoniae, S. pneumoniae, C. pneumoniae, H. influenzae* (type b,[§] nontypable), influenza viruses, adenoviruses, *Legionella pneumophila*	Erythromycin, azithromycin or clarithromycin, doxycycline, moxifloxacin, gatifloxacin, levofloxacin, or gemifloxacin	Moxifloxacin, gatifloxacin, levofloxacin, or gemifloxacin *or* azithromycin or clarithromycin *plus* cefotaxime, ceftriaxone, or ampicillin-sulbactam	Cefotaxime, ceftriaxone, or ampicillin-sulbactam *plus either* azithromycin or clarithromycin *or* moxifloxacin, gatifloxacin, levofloxacin, or gemifloxacin

*Severe pneumonia requiring admission to an ICU from *S. pneumoniae, S. aureus,* group A streptococcus, *H. influenzae* type b, or *M. pneumoniae.* Antipseudomonal agents should be added if *Pseudomonas* is suspected.

[†]Oral administration.

[‡]IV administration for inpatients except for the macrolides (erythromycin, azithromycin, and clarithromycin), which are given orally.

[§]*H. influenzae* type b is uncommon with universal *H. influenza* type b immunization.

[¶]Fluoroquinolones are contraindicated for children, adolescents <18 years old, and pregnant and lactating women. Tetracyclines are not recommended for children <9 years old.

The typical clinical patterns of viral and bacterial pneumonias usually differ between older infants and children, although the distinction is not always clear for a particular patient. Fever, chills, tachypnea, cough, malaise, pleuritic chest pain, retractions, and apprehension, because of difficulty breathing or shortness of breath, are common to older infants and children.

Viral pneumonias are associated more often with cough, wheezing, or stridor; fever is less prominent than with bacterial pneumonia. The chest radiograph in viral pneumonia shows diffuse, streaky infiltrates of bronchopneumonia, and the WBC count often is normal or mildly elevated, with a predominance of lymphocytes. Bacterial pneumonias typically are associated with higher fever, chills, cough, dyspnea, and auscultatory findings of lung consolidation. The chest radiograph often shows lobar consolidation (or a round pneumonia) and pleural effusion (10% to 30%). The WBC count is elevated (>20,000/mm^3) with a predominance of neutrophils.

Afebrile pneumonia in young infants is characterized by tachypnea, cough, crackles on auscultation, and often concomitant chlamydial conjunctivitis. The WBC count typically shows mild eosinophilia, and there is hyperinflation on chest radiograph. All significant pneumonias have localized crackles and decreased breath sounds; a pleural effusion also has dullness to percussion.

LABORATORY AND IMAGING STUDIES

The diagnosis of lower respiratory tract infections in children is hampered by difficulty in obtaining material for culture that truly represents the infected tissue. The upper respiratory tract bacterial flora is not an accurate reflection of the causes of lower respiratory tract infection, and good quality sputum is rarely obtainable from children. In otherwise healthy children without life-threatening disease, invasive procedures to obtain lower respiratory tissue or secretions usually are not indicated. Serologic tests are not useful for the most common causes of bacterial pneumonia.

The WBC count with viral pneumonias is often normal or mildly elevated, with a predominance of lymphocytes, whereas with bacterial pneumonias the WBC count is elevated (>20,000/mm^3) with a predominance of neutrophils. Mild eosinophilia is characteristic of infant *C. trachomatis* pneumonia. Blood cultures should be performed to attempt to diagnose a bacterial cause of pneumonia. Blood cultures are positive in 10% to 20% of bacterial pneumonia and are considered to be confirmatory of the cause of pneumonia if positive for a recognized respiratory pathogen. Urinary antigen tests are useful for *L. pneumophila* (legionnaires' disease).

Cultures of upper respiratory secretions or serologic tests with paired sera are relatively accurate for the diagnosis of viral and mycoplasmal lower respiratory disease. A pneumolysin-based PCR test for pneumococcus is available at some centers and may aid in the diagnosis of pneumococcal pneumonia. CMV and enterovirus can be cultured from the nasopharynx, urine, or bronchoalveolar lavage fluid. *M. pneumoniae* should be suspected if cold agglutinins are present in peripheral blood samples; this may be confirmed by *Mycoplasma* IgM or more specifically PCR. The diagnosis of *M. tuberculosis* is established by TSTs and analysis of sputum or gastric aspirates by culture, antigen detection, or PCR.

The need to establish an etiologic diagnosis of pneumonia is greater for patients who are ill enough to require hospitalization, immunocompromised patients (persons with HIV infection, cancer or transplant therapies, congenital immunodeficiencies), patients with recurrent pneumonia, or patients with pneumonia unresponsive to empirical therapy. For these patients, bronchoscopy with bronchoalveolar lavage and brush mucosal biopsy, needle aspiration of the lung, and open lung biopsy are methods of obtaining material for microbiologic diagnosis.

When there is effusion or empyema, performing a thoracentesis to obtain pleural fluid can be diagnostic and therapeutic. Evaluation differentiates between empyema and a sterile parapneumonic effusion caused by irritation of the pleura contiguous with the pneumonia. Gram stain and culture may lead to microbiologic diagnosis. The pleural fluid should be cultured for bacteria, mycobacteria, fungi, and viruses. If the fluid is grossly purulent, removal reduces the patient's toxicity and associated discomfort and may facilitate more rapid recovery. If the accumulation is large and impairs the ability of the lung to expand, removal of the fluid improves pulmonary mechanics and gas exchange.

Frontal and lateral radiographs are required to localize the diseased segments and to visualize adequately infiltrates behind the heart or the diaphragmatic leaflets. There are characteristic radiographic findings of pneumonia, although there is much overlap that precludes definitive diagnosis by radiography alone. Bacterial pneumonia characteristically shows lobar consolidation, or a round pneumonia, with pleural effusion in 10% to 30% of cases (Fig. 110–1). Viral pneumonia characteristically shows diffuse, streaky infiltrates of bronchopneumonia (Fig. 110–2). Atypical pneumonia, such as with *M. pneumoniae* and *C. pneumoniae*, shows increased interstitial markings or bronchopneumonia (Fig. 110–3). The chest radiograph may be normal in early pneumonia, with appearance of an infiltrate during the treatment phase of the disease when edema fluid is greater. Hilar lymphadenopathy is

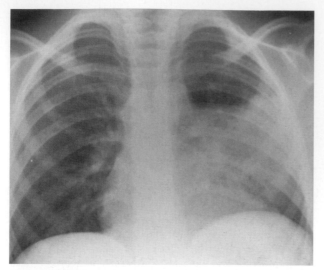

Figure 110–1

Acute lobar pneumonia of the lingula in a 6-year-old child with high fever, cough, and chest pain. Frontal chest radiograph shows airspace consolidation, which obliterates the silhouette of the heart border on the left. The left hemidiaphragm is mildly elevated as a result of splinting. (From Markowitz RI: Diagnostic imaging. In Jenson HB, Baltimore RS [eds]: Pediatric Infectious Diseases: Principles and Practice, 2nd ed. Philadelphia, WB Saunders, 2002, p 133.)

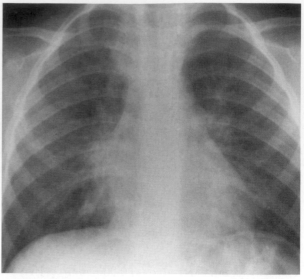

Figure 110–2

Diffuse viral bronchopneumonia in a 12-year-old boy with cough, fever, and wheezing. Frontal chest radiograph shows bilateral, perihilar, peribronchial thickening and shaggy infiltrate. Focal airspace disease representing consolidation or atelectasis is present in the medial portion of the right upper lobe. The findings are typical of bronchopneumonia. (From Markowitz RI: Diagnostic imaging. In Jenson HB, Baltimore RS [eds]: Pediatric Infectious Diseases: Principles and Practice, 2nd ed. Philadelphia, WB Saunders, 2002, p 132.)

uncommon with bacterial pneumonia, but may be a sign of tuberculosis, histoplasmosis, or an underlying malignant neoplasm. Unusual etiologies or recurrent pneumonias require special considerations (Table 110–2). Lung abscesses, pneumatoceles, and empyema all require special management. Decubitus views or ultrasound should be used to assess size of pleural effusions and whether they are freely mobile. CT is used to evaluate serious disease, pleural abscesses, bronchiectasis, and delineating effusions.

DIFFERENTIAL DIAGNOSIS

Complete examination is important to identify other foci of disease or associated findings that may suggest the etiology. Mucosal congestion and inflammation of the upper airway suggest a viral infection. Breathing should be observed for rate and pattern. Tachypnea can be caused by airway inflammation resulting in obstruction or by pneumonia resulting in inadequate gas exchange and hypoxia. Other signs of respiratory distress include flaring of the alae of the nose, intercostal and subcostal retractions, and grunting. Generalized or peripheral cyanosis indicates hypoxia with severe diffuse or multilobular pneumonia or a large pleural

effusion. With a young infant, apneic spells may be the first sign of pneumonia.

Asymmetry or shallow breathing may be due to splinting from pain. Low diaphragms by percussion indicate air trapping, which is common in asthma, but also frequently accompanies viral lower respiratory infections. Poor diaphragmatic excursion may indicate hyperexpanded lungs or an inability for expansion because a large consolidation is causing poor lung compliance. Hyperexpansion may push the diaphragm and liver downward. Dullness to percussion may be due to lobar or segmental infiltrates or pleural fluid. Auscultation may be normal in early or very focal pneumonia, but the presence of localized crackles, rhonchi, and wheezes may help one to detect and locate pneumonia. Distant breath sounds may indicate a large, poorly ventilated area of consolidation or pleural fluid.

The various types of pneumonia—lobar pneumonia, bronchopneumonia, interstitial and alveolar pneumonias—need to be differentiated on the basis of radiologic or pathologic diagnosis. Pneumonia must be differentiated from other acute lung diseases, including lung edema caused by heart failure, allergic pneumonitis, and aspiration, and autoimmune diseases, such as rheumatoid disease and systemic lupus

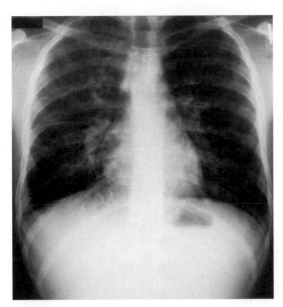

Figure 110–3

Mycoplasma pneumoniae **infection (atypical pneumonia) in a 14-year-old boy with malaise, dry cough, and mild shortness of breath for 1 week.** Frontal chest radiograph shows a diffuse pattern of increased interstitial markings, including Kerley lines. The heart is normal, and there are no focal infiltrates. Cold agglutinins were markedly elevated, and the patient responded to erythromycin. This radiographic pattern of reticulonodular interstitial disease is observed in 25% to 30% of patients with pneumonia caused by *M. pneumoniae*. (From Baltimore RS: Pneumonia. In Jenson HB, Baltimore RS [eds]: Pediatric Infectious Diseases: Principles and Practice, 2nd ed. Philadelphia, WB Saunders, 2002, p 808.)

erythematosus. Radiographically, pneumonia must be differentiated from lung trauma and contusion, hemorrhage, foreign body obstruction, and irritation from subdiaphragmatic inflammation.

TREATMENT

Therapy for pneumonia includes supportive and specific treatment. The appropriate treatment plan depends on the degree of illness, complications, and knowledge of the infectious agent or of the agent that is likely causing the pneumonia. Age, severity of the illness, complications noted on the chest radiograph, degree of respiratory distress, and ability of the family to care for the child and to assess the progression of the symptoms all must be taken into consideration in the choice of ambulatory treatment over hospitalization (Table 110-3). Most cases of pneumonia in healthy children can be managed on an outpatient basis.

Although viruses cause most community-acquired pneumonias in young children, in most situations experts recommend empirical treatment for the most probable treatable causes. Treatment recommendations are based on the age of the child, severity of the pneumonia, and antimicrobial activity of agents against the expected pathogens that cause pneumonia

TABLE 110–2. Differential Diagnosis of Recurrent Pneumonia
Hereditary Disorders
Cystic fibrosis Sickle cell disease
Disorders of Immunity
AIDS Bruton agammaglobulinemia Selective IgG subclass deficiencies Common variable immunodeficiency syndrome Severe combined immunodeficiency syndrome
Disorders of Leukocytes
Chronic granulomatous disease Hyperimmunoglobulin E syndrome (Job syndrome) Leukocyte adhesion defect
Disorders of Cilia
Immotile cilia syndrome Kartagener syndrome
Anatomic Disorders
Sequestration Lobar emphysema Esophageal reflux Foreign body Tracheoesophageal fistula (H type) Gastroesophageal reflux Bronchiectasis Aspiration (oropharyngeal incoordination)

TABLE 110–3. Factors Suggesting Need for Hospitalization of Children with Pneumonia
Age <6 mo Immunocompromised state Toxic appearance Severe respiratory distress Requirement for supplemental oxygen Dehydration Vomiting No response to appropriate oral antibiotic therapy Noncompliant parents
Adapted from Baltimore RS: Pneumonia. In Jenson HB, Baltimore RS (eds): Pediatric Infectious Diseases: Principles and Practice. Philadelphia, WB Saunders, 2002, p 801.

TABLE 110–4. Antimicrobial Therapy for Pneumonia Caused by Specific Pathogens*

Pathogen	Recommended Treatment	Alternative Treatment
Streptococcus pneumoniae[†]	Ceftriaxone, cefotaxime, penicillin G, or penicillin V	Cefuroxime axetil, erythromycin, or vancomycin
Group A streptococcus	Penicillin G	Cefuroxime, cefuroxime axetil, or erythromycin
Group B streptococcus	Penicillin G	
Haemophilus influenzae type b	Ceftriaxone, cefotaxime, amoxicillin, or ampicillin	Cefuroxime or cefuroxime axetil
Mycoplasma pneumoniae	Erythromycin, azithromycin, or clarithromycin	Doxycycline (if >9 years old) or a respiratory fluoroquinolone (if ≥18 years old)[‡]
Gram-negative aerobic bacilli (except *Pseudomonas aeruginosa*)	Cefotaxime (or ceftriaxone) with or without an aminoglycoside[§]	Piperacillin-tazobactam plus an aminoglycoside[§]
P. aeruginosa	Ceftazidime with or without an aminoglycoside[§]	Piperacillin-tazobactam plus an aminoglycoside[§]
Staphylococcus aureus	Nafcillin or oxacillin	Vancomycin
Chlamydophila pneumoniae	Erythromycin, azithromycin, or clarithromycin	Doxycycline (if >9 years old) or a respiratory fluoroquinolone (if ≥18 years old)[‡]
Chlamydia trachomatis (afebrile pneumonia in infants)	Erythromycin, azithromycin, or clarithromycin	TMP-SMZ
Herpes simplex virus	Acyclovir	

*Oral outpatient therapy may be used for mild illness. IV inpatient therapy should be used for moderate to severe illness.
[†]Antibiotic should be chosen on the basis of antibiotic susceptibility of the isolate or susceptibility of the prevalent isolates in the community.
[‡]Respiratory fluoroquinolones include moxifloxacin, gatifloxacin, levofloxacin, and gemifloxacin. Fluoroquinolones are contraindicated for children, adolescents <18 years old, and pregnant and lactating women. Tetracyclines are not recommended for children <9 years old.
[§]Aminoglycoside dosing should be guided by serum antibiotic concentrations after a steady state has been reached.
TMP-SMZ, trimethoprim-sulfamethoxazole.

at different ages (Table 110–4). Pneumonia caused by *S. pneumoniae* presents a problem because of increasing antibiotic resistance. In contrast to pneumococcal meningitis, presumed pneumococcal pneumonia can be treated with high-dose penicillin or cephalosporin therapy, even with high-level penicillin resistance. Vancomycin can be used if the isolate shows high-level resistance and the patient is severely ill.

Empirical antibiotic treatment is sufficient for management of pneumonia in children, unless there is an exceptional need to know the pathogen to guide management. Such exceptional situations include lack of response to empirical therapy, unusually severe presentations, nosocomial pneumonia, and immunocompromised children susceptible to infections with opportunistic pathogens. Infants 4 to 18 weeks old with afebrile pneumonia most likely have infection with *C. trachomatis,* and erythromycin is the recommended treatment.

COMPLICATIONS

Bacterial pneumonias frequently cause inflammatory fluid to collect in the adjacent pleural space, causing a **parapneumonic effusion** or, if grossly purulent, an **empyema**. Small effusions may not require any special therapy. Large effusions usually restrict breathing and require drainage. Air dissection within lung tissue may result in a **pneumatocele**, or air pocket. Scarring of the airways and lung tissue may leave dilated bronchi, resulting in **bronchiectasis** and increased risk for recurrent infection.

Pneumonia that causes necrosis of lung tissue may evolve into a **lung abscess**. Lung abscess is an uncommon problem in children and usually is caused by aspiration or infection behind an obstructed bronchus. The most commonly involved sites are the posterior segments of the upper lobes and the superior segments of the lower lobes, where aspirated material drains when the child is recumbent. Anaerobic bacteria usually predominate, along with various streptococci, *E. coli, Klebsiella pneumoniae, P. aeruginosa,* and *S. aureus.* Chest radiograph or CT scan reveals a cavitary lesion, often with an air-fluid level, surrounded by parenchymal inflammation. If the cavity communicates with the bronchi, organisms may be isolated from sputum. Diagnostic bronchoscopy may be indicated to exclude a foreign body and obtain microbiologic specimens. Lung abscesses usually respond to appropriate antimicrobial therapy, usually with clindamycin, penicillin G, or ampicillin-sulbactam.

PROGNOSIS

Most children recover from pneumonia rapidly and completely. The radiographic abnormalities may take 6 to 8 weeks to return to normal. In a few children, pneumonia may persist longer than 1 month or may be recurrent. In such cases, the possibility of underlying disease must be investigated further, such as with TST, sweat chloride determination for cystic fibrosis, serum immunoglobulin and IgG subclass determinations, bronchoscopy to identify anatomic abnormalities or foreign body, and barium swallow for gastroesophageal reflux (see Table 110–2).

Severe adenovirus pneumonia may result in **bronchiolitis obliterans**, a subacute inflammatory process in which the small airways are replaced by scar tissue, resulting in a reduction in lung volume and lung compliance. The syndrome of **unilateral hyperlucent lung**, or **Swyer-James syndrome**, seems to be a focal sequela of severe necrotizing pneumonia in which all or part of a lung has increased translucency radiographically and has been linked to adenovirus type 21.

PREVENTION

Immunizations have had a great impact on reducing the incidence of vaccine-preventable causes of pneumonia. RSV infections can be reduced in severity by use of palivizumab (see Chapter 109). Reducing the length of mechanical ventilation and using antibiotic treatment only when necessary can reduce ventilator-associated pneumonias. The head of the bed should be raised to 30 to 45 degrees to prevent aspiration, and all suctioning equipment and saline should be sterile. Hand washing before and after every patient contact and use of gloves for invasive procedures are important measures to prevent nosocomial transmission of infections. Hospital staff with respiratory illnesses or who are carriers of certain organisms, such as methicillin-resistant *S. aureus,* should use masks or be reassigned to non–patient care duties. Treating sources of aerosols, such as air coolers, can prevent *Legionella* pneumonia.

CHAPTER 111
Infective Endocarditis

ETIOLOGY

Infective endocarditis is an infection on the endothelial surface of the heart, including the heart valves. Infections on the endothelial surface of blood vessels may act as an "endocarditis equivalent." The infectious endothelial lesions, called **vegetations**, usually occur on the valve leaflets. These lesions are composed of microorganisms trapped in a fibrin mesh that extends into the bloodstream. Because antibiotics must reach the organisms by passive diffusion through the fibrin, high doses of antibiotics are required for an extended period of treatment.

Although many microorganisms have been reported to cause endocarditis, there are only a few principal causes in children (Table 111–1). Viridans streptococci are the principal causes in children with congenital heart diseases without previous surgery. *S. aureus* and coagulase-negative staphylococci are important causes of endocarditis that assume greater prominence after cardiac surgical procedures and with prosthetic cardiac and endovascular material. Nonetheless, *S. aureus* can cause endocarditis on previously healthy native valves.

EPIDEMIOLOGY

Infective endocarditis among children is primarily a complication of congenital heart disease. High-risk cardiac lesions include tetralogy of Fallot, ventricular septal defect, aortic stenosis, aortic regurgitation, patent ductus arteriosus, and transposition of the great vessels. The risk is increased after dental and oral procedures or instrumentation or surgical procedures

---

TABLE 111–1.   Causes of Infective Endocarditis in Children

Bacteria

Viridans streptococci (the most common at all ages)*
*Enterococcus**
*Staphylococcus aureus**
Coagulase-negative staphylococci*
Hemolytic streptococci: groups A, B (in neonates and elderly), C, G, D
Streptococcus pneumoniae
Gram-negative enteric bacilli
HACEK organisms (*Haemophilus aphrophilus, Actinobacillus actinomycetemcomitans, Cardiobacterium hominis, Eikenella corrodens,* and *Kingella kingae*)

Fungi

Candida albicans
Non-*albicans Candida*
Aspergillus
Cryptococcus neoformans

Others

Coxiella burnetii (Q fever)
Chlamydia
Culture-negative endocarditis

*Most common causes of endocarditis in children.

of the respiratory tract, genitourinary tract, or gastrointestinal tract. Rheumatic heart disease is a rare risk factor. Neonatal endocarditis is associated with the use of central vascular catheters and surgery in neonates. Endocarditis is a sporadic disease with no geographic predisposition and little gender or socioeconomic predisposition in children. In adults, there is a male preponderance and association with social and behavioral factors, such as IV drug abuse and atherosclerotic heart disease.

CLINICAL MANIFESTATIONS

The most common early symptoms of infective endocarditis are nonspecific and include fever, malaise, and weight loss (Table 111–2). The subtle and nonspecific findings underscore the need to obtain blood cultures if endocarditis is suspected, especially for children with congenital heart disease and for unexplained illness after dental or surgical procedures. Endocarditis is usually a subacute, slowly progressive disorder, but acute endocarditis is often due to *S. aureus* and may resemble sepsis.

LABORATORY STUDIES AND IMAGING

The key to diagnosis is showing continuous bacteremia or less often fungemia by culturing the blood. Multiple blood cultures are performed before initiating antibiotic therapy. Three separate venipunctures for blood culture represent near-maximal sensitivity (about 95%) among patients who have not been treated recently with antibiotics. Patients who have been treated with antibiotics recently or who are currently receiving antibiotics should have additional cultures performed. Despite adequate blood culture techniques, 10% to 15% of cases of endocarditis are culture-negative.

Echocardiography visualizes endocardial and valvular vegetations measuring greater than or equal to 2 mm. Transesophageal echocardiography is more sensitive than transthoracic echocardiography for adolescents and adults and for patients with prosthetic valves, but is often unnecessary in children.

DIFFERENTIAL DIAGNOSIS

Infective endocarditis must be differentiated from other causes of bacteremia or other cardiac conditions using the **Duke criteria** for categorizing the strength of the endocarditis diagnosis (Table 111–3). Noninfectious causes of endocardial vegetations must be excluded, such as sterile clots and vegetations associated with rheumatoid disease and lupus erythematosus. Prolonged bacteremia can be caused by infectious endothelial foci outside of the heart, often associated with congenital malformations, vascular trauma, an infected venous thrombosis, and post-vascular surgery.

TABLE 111–2. Symptoms, Signs, and Laboratory Findings Associated with Infective Endocarditis in Children

Symptoms	Signs	Laboratory Findings
Common	**Common**	**Common**
Fever	Fever	Positive blood culture
Malaise	Tachycardia	Elevated ESR, CRP
Anorexia or weight loss	New or changed murmur	Leukocytosis
	Heart failure	Anemia
Uncommon	Splenomegaly	Positive rheumatoid factor
	Petechiae	Hematuria
Chills	Embolic phenomena	Echocardiographic evidence of vegetation
Chest pain		
Dyspnea	**Uncommon**	**Uncommon**
Arthralgia		
Myalgia	Dysrhythmia	Hypergammaglobulinemia
Focal neurologic deficit	Embolic phenomena (Osler nodes,	
(aseptic meningitis)	Roth spots, Janeway lesions, splinter	
	hemorrhages, conjunctival	
	hemorrhages)	
	Clubbing	

CRP, C-reactive protein; ESR, erythrocyte sedimentation rate.

TABLE 111–3. Duke Clinical Criteria for Diagnosis of Infective Endocarditis

Definite Infective Endocarditis

Pathologic Criteria

Microorganisms shown by culture or histologic findings in a vegetation, or in a vegetation that has embolized, or in an intracardiac abscess *or*

Pathologic lesion—vegetation or intracardiac abscess present, confirmed by histologic findings showing active endocarditis

Clinical Criteria (2 Major Criteria or 1 Major and 3 Minor Criteria or 5 Minor Criteria)

Major Criteria

Blood culture positive for infective endocarditis
  Typical microorganisms for infective endocarditis from two separate blood cultures
  Viridans streptococci,* *Streptococcus bovis,* HACEK (*Haemophilus aphrophilus, Actinobacillus actinomycetemcomitans, Cardiobacterium hominis, Eikenella corrodens,* and *Kingella kingae*) group, *or*
  Community-acquired *Staphylococcus aureus* or *Enterococcus* in the absence of a primary focus, *or*
  Persistently positive blood culture result, defined as recovery of a microorganism consistent with endocarditis from blood culture specimens drawn >12 hr apart *or*
    All of 3 or a majority of ≥4 separate blood culture specimens, with first and last drawn at least 1 hr apart
Evidence of endocardial involvement
  Echocardiogram positive for infective endocarditis
  Oscillating intracardiac mass on valve or supporting structures *or* in path of regurgitant jets *or* on implanted material in the absence of an alternative anatomic explanation, *or*
  Abscess *or*
  New partial dehiscence of prosthetic valve *or*
  New valvular regurgitation (increase or change in preexisting murmur not sufficient)

Minor Criteria

Predisposition—predisposing heart condition *or* IV drug use
Fever ≥38°C (≥100.4°F)
Vascular phenomena—major arterial emboli, septic pulmonary infarcts, mycotic aneurysm, intracranial hemorrhage, conjunctival hemorrhages, Janeway lesions
Immunologic phenomena—glomerulonephritis, Osler nodes, Roth spots, rheumatoid factor
Microbiologic evidence—positive blood culture result, but not meeting major criteria as noted previously[†] *or* serologic evidence of active infection with organism consistent with infective endocarditis
Echocardiogram—consistent with infective endocarditis, but not meeting major criteria as noted previously

Possible Infective Endocarditis

Findings consistent with infective endocarditis that fall short of "definite" but not "rejected"

Rejected

Firm alternate diagnosis for manifestations of endocarditis *or*
Resolution of manifestations of endocarditis with antibiotic therapy for ≤4 days *or*
No pathologic evidence of endocarditis at surgery or autopsy after antibiotic therapy of ≤4 days

*Including nutritionally variant strains.
[†]Excluding single cultures positive for coagulase-negative staphylococci and organisms that do not cause endocarditis.
From Durack DT, Lukas AS, Bright DK, et al: New criteria for diagnosis of infective endocarditis: Utilization of specific echocardiographic findings. Duke Endocarditis Services. Am J Med 96:200-209, 1994.

TREATMENT

Severely ill patients must be stabilized with supportive therapies for cardiac failure, pulmonary edema, and low cardiac output (see Chapter 145). Multiple blood cultures should be obtained before initiating antibiotic therapy. Empirical antibiotic therapy may be started for acutely ill persons. With subacute disease, it is recommended to await results of blood cultures to confirm the diagnosis and to treat according to the susceptibility of the isolate. Treatment of a culture-positive case is directed against the particular bacterium using bactericidal antibiotics continued for 4 to 8 weeks. Infective carditis from viridans streptococci can be treated with traditional monotherapy with penicillin G for 4 weeks. A 2-week regimen of penicillin G plus an aminoglycoside is effective in adults. Surgery is indicated if medical treatment is unsuccessful or if there is persistent bacteremia, an unusual pathogen (fungal endocarditis), abscess of the valve annulus or of the myocardium, rupture of a valve leaflet, valvular insufficiency with refractory heart failure, recurrent serious embolic complications, or refractory prosthetic valve disease.

COMPLICATIONS

The major complications of infective endocarditis are direct damage to the heart and heart valves and distant complications secondary to sterile and septic emboli from vegetations. Damage to the heart and heart valves may include regurgitation with vegetations or actual defects in the leaflets resulting from embolization of the leaflet tissue, abscess of the valve ring, or myocardial abscess. These complications can be monitored by physical examination and echocardiography. Cerebral abscesses or aneurysms can cause a strokelike picture. Splenic abscesses can cause fatal bleeding.

PROGNOSIS

The outcome of infective endocarditis caused by the most common organisms is good. In uncomplicated endocarditis caused by viridans streptococci on a natural valve, the cure rate is greater than 90%. The cure rate for *Enterococcus* endocarditis treated by a synergistic combination of antibiotics is 75% to 90%. The presentation and course of *S. aureus* endocarditis may be acute and severe, and the cure rate is 60% to 75%. The prognosis for endocarditis caused by gram-negative bacilli and rarer organisms is poor. Fungal endocarditis has the poorest prognosis, with a cure rate of about 50%, even with valve replacement.

PREVENTION

Surgical repair of congenital heart disease reduces the risk for endocarditis. In patients with preexisting endothelial or endocardial lesions, prophylactic antibiotics before and during procedures in which bacteremia is common may prevent endocarditis. Such procedures include invasive dental procedures in which the gingivae are cut, colonoscopy, and urinary tract instrumentation in patients who have bacteriuria. The antibiotic regimen to prevent endocarditis during dental or respiratory procedures is oral amoxicillin taken 1 hour before the procedure. Preventive treatment for gastrointestinal or genitourinary manipulation includes oral amoxicillin or parenteral ampicillin and gentamicin. The latter recommendation is for high-risk patients, such as patients with prosthetic heart valves, systemic-to-pulmonary shunts, or previous endocarditis. Clindamycin is indicated for most patients allergic to penicillin. Prolonged or continuous antibiotic prophylaxis is not recommended.

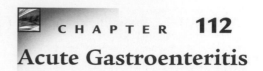

CHAPTER 112
Acute Gastroenteritis

ETIOLOGY AND EPIDEMIOLOGY

Acute enteritis or acute gastroenteritis refers to **diarrhea**, which is abnormal frequency and liquidity of fecal discharges. Diarrhea is caused by many different infectious or inflammatory processes in the intestine (Table 112–1). These processes directly affect enterocyte secretory and absorptive functions. Some of these processes act by increasing cyclic AMP levels (*Vibrio cholerae*, *E. coli* heat-labile toxin, vasoactive intestinal peptide–producing tumors). Other processes (*Shigella* toxin, congenital chloridorrhea) cause secretory diarrhea by affecting ion channels or by unknown mechanisms. Enteritis has many viral, bacterial, and parasitic causes (Table 112–2).

Diarrhea is the leading cause of morbidity and the second most common disease in children in the U.S. In the developing world, it is a major cause of childhood mortality. The epidemiology of gastroenteritis depends on the specific organisms. Some organisms are spread person to person, others are spread via contaminated food or water, and some are spread from animal to human. Many organisms spread by multiple routes. The ability of an organism to infect relates to its mode of spread, its ability to colonize the gastrointestinal tract, and the number of organisms required to cause disease.

Viral causes of gastroenteritis in children include rotaviruses, caliciviruses (including the noroviruses), astroviruses, and enteric adenoviruses (serotypes 40 and 41). Rotavirus invades the epithelium and damages villi of the upper small intestine and in severe cases involves the entire small bowel and colon. Rotavirus is the most frequent cause of diarrhea during the winter months. Vomiting may last 3 to 4 days, and diarrhea may last 7 to 10 days. Dehydration is common in younger children. Primary infection with rotavirus in infancy may cause moderate to severe disease but is less severe later in life.

Typhoid fever is caused by *Salmonella typhi* and occasionally *Salmonella paratyphi*. These infections are distinguished by their potential for prolonged fever, inconsistent presence of diarrhea, and extraintestinal manifestations. In the U.S., approximately 400 cases of typhoid fever occur each year. The incubation period of typhoid fever is usually 7 to 14 days (range 3 to 60 days). Most cases are imported from other countries. Worldwide there are an estimated 16 million cases of typhoid fever annually, resulting in 600,000 deaths. The typhoid bacillus infects humans only, and chronic carriers are responsible for new cases.

TABLE 112–1. Mechanisms of Diarrhea

Primary Mechanism	Defect	Stool Examination	Examples	Comment
Secretory	Decreased absorption, increased secretion: electrolyte transport	Watery, normal osmolality; osmols $= 2 \times (Na^+ + K^+)$	Cholera, toxigenic *Escherichia coli;* carcinoid, VIP, neuroblastoma, congenital chloride diarrhea, *Clostridium difficile,* cryptosporidiosis (AIDS)	Persists during fasting; bile salt malabsorption also may increase intestinal water secretion; no stool leukocytes
Osmotic	Maldigestion, transport defects, ingestion of unabsorbable solute	Watery, acidic, + reducing substances; increased osmolality; osmosis $>2 \times (Na^+ + K^+)$	Lactase deficiency, glucose-galactose malabsorption, lactulose, laxative abuse	Stops with fasting, increased breath hydrogen with carbohydrate malabsorption, no stool leukocytes
Motility Increased motility	Decreased transit time	Loose to normal-appearing stool, stimulated by gastrocolic reflex	Irritable bowel syndrome, thyrotoxicosis, postvagotomy dumping syndrome	Infection also may contribute to increased motility
Decreased motility	Defect in neuromuscular unit(s) Stasis (bacterial overgrowth)	Loose to normal-appearing stool	Pseudo-obstruction, blind loop	Possible bacterial overgrowth
Mucosal inflammation	Inflammation, decreased mucosal surface area and/or colonic reabsorption, increased motility	Blood and increased WBCs in stool	Celiac disease, *Salmonella, Shigella,* amebiasis, *Yersinia, Campylobacter,* rotavirus enteritis	Dysentery = blood, mucus, and WBCs

VIP, vasoactive intestinal peptide; WBCs, white blood cells.
From Wyllie R: Major symptoms and signs of digestive tract disorders. In Behrman RE, Kliegman RM, Jenson HB (eds): Nelson Textbook of Pediatrics, 17th ed. Philadelphia, WB Saunders, 2004, p 1200.

Nontyphoidal *Salmonella* produce diarrhea by invading the intestinal mucosa. The organisms are transmitted through contact with infected animals (chickens, pet iguanas, other reptiles, turtles) or from contaminated food products, such as dairy products, eggs, and poultry. Infected persons without symptoms, or **chronic carriers**, serve as reservoirs and sources of continuous spread. Carriers often have cholelithiasis. A large inoculum, of 1000 to 10 billion organisms, is required because *Salmonella* are killed by gastric acidity. The incubation period for gastroenteritis ranges from 6 to 72 hours, but usually is less than 24 hours.

Shigella dysenteriae may cause disease by producing **Shiga toxin**, either alone or combined with tissue invasion. The incubation period is 1 to 7 days, and infected adults may shed organisms for 1 month. Infection is spread by person-to-person contact or by the ingestion of contaminated food with 10 to 100 organisms. The colon is selectively affected. High fever and seizures may occur, in addition to diarrhea.

Only certain strains of *E. coli* produce diarrhea. *E. coli* strains associated with enteritis are classified by the mechanism of diarrhea: enteropathogenic (EPEC), enterotoxigenic (ETEC), enteroinvasive (EIEC), enterohemorrhagic (EHEC), or enteroaggregative (EAEC). EPEC is responsible for many of the epidemics of diarrhea in newborn nurseries and in daycare centers. ETEC produce **heat-labile (cholera-like) enterotoxin**, **heat-stable enterotoxin**, or both. ETEC causes 40% to 60% of cases of **traveler's diarrhea**. EPEC and ETEC adhere to the epithelial cells in the upper small intestine and produce disease by liberating toxins that induce intestinal secretion and limit absorption. EIEC invades the colonic mucosa, producing widespread mucosal damage with acute inflammation, similar to *Shigella.* EHEC, especially the *E. coli* O157:H7 strain, produce a

TABLE 112–2. Common Infectious Causes of Diarrhea and Their Virulence Mechanisms

Organisms	Virulence Properties
Viruses	
Rotaviruses	Damage to microvilli
Caliciviruses	Mucosal lesion
Astroviruses	Mucosal lesion
Enteric adenoviruses (serotypes 40 and 41)	Mucosal lesion
Bacteria	
Campylobacter jejuni	Invasion, enterotoxin
Clostridium difficile	Cytotoxin, enterotoxin
Escherichia coli	
Enteropathogenic (EPEC)	Adherence, effacement
Enterotoxigenic (ETEC) (traveler's diarrhea)	Enterotoxins (heat-stable or heat-labile)
Enteroinvasive (EIEC)	Invasion of mucosa
Enterohemorrhagic (EHEC) (includes O157:H7 causing HUS)	Adherence, effacement, cytotoxin
Enteroaggregative (EAEC)	Adherence, mucosal damage
Salmonella	Invasion, enterotoxin
Shigella	Invasion, enterotoxin, cytotoxin
Vibrio cholerae	Enterotoxin
Vibrio parahaemolyticus	Invasion, cytotoxin
Yersinia enterocolitica	Invasion, enterotoxin
Parasites	
Entamoeba histolytica	Invasion, enzyme and cytotoxin production; cyst resistant to physical destruction
Giardia lamblia	Adheres to mucosa; cyst resistant to physical destruction
Spore-forming intestinal protozoa	Adherence, inflammation
Cryptosporidium parvum	
Isospora belli	
Cyclospora cayetanensis	
Microsporida (*Enterocytozoon bieneusi, Encephalitozoon intestinalis*)	

HUS, hemolytic uremic syndrome.

Shiga-like toxin that is responsible for a hemorrhagic colitis and most cases of **hemolytic uremic syndrome (HUS)**, which is a syndrome of microangiopathic hemolytic anemia, thrombocytopenia, and renal failure (see Chapter 164). EHEC is associated with contaminated food, including unpasteurized fruit juices and especially undercooked beef. EHEC is associated with a self-limited form of gastroenteritis, usually with bloody diarrhea, but production of this toxin blocks host cell protein synthesis and affects vascular endothelial cells and the glomeruli, resulting in the clinical manifestations of HUS.

Campylobacter jejuni accounts for 15% of bacterial diarrhea. The infection is spread by person-to-person contact and by contaminated water and food, especially poultry, raw milk, and cheese. The organism invades the mucosa of the jejunum, ileum, and colon, producing enterocolitis.

Yersinia enterocolitica is transmitted by pets and contaminated food, especially chitterlings. Infants and young children characteristically have a diarrheal disease, whereas older children usually have acute lesions of the terminal ileum or acute mesenteric lymphadenitis mimicking appendicitis or Crohn disease. Arthritis, rash, and spondylopathy may develop.

Clostridium difficile causes **C. difficile–associated diarrhea**, or antibiotic-associated diarrhea secondary to its toxin. The organism produces spores that spread from person to person. *C. difficile*–associated diarrhea may follow exposure to any antibiotics, but is classically associated with clindamycin.

Entamoeba histolytica (amebiasis), *Giardia lamblia,* and *Cryptosporidium parvum* are important enteric parasites found in North America. Amebiasis occurs in warmer climates, whereas giardiasis is endemic throughout the U.S. and is common among infants in daycare centers. *E. histolytica* infects the colon; amebae may pass through the bowel wall and invade the liver, lung, and brain. Diarrhea is of acute onset, is bloody, and contains WBCs. *G. lamblia* is transmitted through ingestion of cysts, either from contact with an infected individual or from food or freshwater or well water contaminated with infected feces. The organism adheres to the microvilli of the duodenal and jejunal epithelium. *Cryptosporidium* causes mild, watery diarrhea in immunocompetent persons that resolves without treatment. It produces severe, prolonged diarrhea in persons with AIDS (see Chapter 125).

CLINICAL MANIFESTATIONS

Gastroenteritis may be accompanied by systemic findings, such as fever, lethargy, and abdominal pain. Patients with diarrhea and possible dehydration should be evaluated to assess the degree of dehydration as evident from clinical signs and symptoms, ongoing losses, and daily requirements (see Chapter 33).

Viral diarrhea is characterized by watery stools, with no blood or mucus. Vomiting may be present, and dehydration may be prominent. Fever, when present, is low grade. **Typhoid fever**, caused by *S. typhi* and *S. paratyphi*, is characterized by bacteremia and fever that usually precede the final enteric phase. There is fever, headache, and abdominal pain that worsen over 48 to 72 hours with nausea, decreased appetite, and constipation over the first week. If untreated, the disease persists for 2 to 3 weeks marked by significant weight loss and occasionally hematochezia or melena. Bowel perforation is a common complication in adults, but is rare in children. **Dysentery** is diarrhea involving the colon and rectum, with blood and mucus, possibly foul smelling, and fever. *Shigella* is the prototype, which must be differentiated from infection with EIEC, EHEC, *E. histolytica* (**amebic dysentery**), *C. jejuni, Y. enterocolitica*, and nontyphoidal *Salmonella*. Gastrointestinal bleeding and blood loss may be significant. **Enterotoxigenic disease** is caused by agents that produce enterotoxins, such as *V. cholerae* and ETEC, the organism associated with 40% to 60% of cases of traveler's diarrhea. Fever is absent or only low grade. Diarrhea usually involves the ileum with watery stools without blood or mucus and usually lasts 3 to 4 days with four to five loose stools per day. Insidious onset of progressive anorexia, nausea, gaseousness, abdominal distention, watery diarrhea, secondary lactose intolerance, and weight loss is characteristic of giardiasis.

A chief consideration in management of a child with diarrhea is to assess the degree of dehydration. The degree of dehydration dictates the urgency of the situation and the volume of fluid needed for rehydration. **Mild dehydration (3% to 5%)** is characterized by normal pulse rate or minimal tachycardia, decreased urine output, thirst, and normal physical examination. **Moderate dehydration (5% to 10%)** is characterized by tachycardia, little or no urine output, irritability or lethargy, sunken eyes and fontanel, decreased tears, dry mucous membranes, mild tenting of the skin, and delayed capillary refill ($\leq$2 seconds) with cool and pale skin. **Severe dehydration (10% to 15%)** is characterized by tachycardia with a weak pulse, hypotension and widened pulse pressure, no urine output, extremely sunken eyes and fontanel, no tears, parched mucous membranes, tenting of the skin, and extremely delayed capillary refill ($\geq$3 seconds) with cold and mottled skin. As the degree of dehydration increases, the requirement to provide immediate medical intervention also increases. Mild to moderate dehydration usually can be treated with oral rehydration, whereas severe dehydration usually requires IV rehydration. Severe dehydration may require ICU admission.

LABORATORY AND IMAGING STUDIES

Initial laboratory evaluation of moderate to severe diarrhea includes a complete blood count, electrolytes, BUN, creatinine, and urinalysis for specific gravity as an indicator of hydration. Stool specimens should be examined for mucus, blood, and leukocytes, which indicate colitis. Fecal leukocytes are present in response to bacteria that diffusely invade the colonic mucosa. A positive fecal leukocyte examination indicates the presence of an invasive or cytotoxin-producing organism, such as *Shigella, Salmonella, C. jejuni*, and invasive *E. coli*. Patients infected with Shiga toxin–producing *E. coli* and *E. histolytica* generally have minimal fecal leukocytes.

A rapid diagnostic test for rotavirus in stool should be performed, especially during the winter. Stool cultures are recommended for patients with fever, profuse diarrhea, and dehydration or if HUS is suspected. If the stool test result is negative for blood and WBCs, and there is no history to suggest contaminated food ingestion, a viral etiology is most likely. Stool evaluation for parasitic agents should be considered for acute dysenteric illness or in protracted cases of diarrhea in which no bacterial agent is identified.

Positive blood cultures are uncommon with bacterial enteritis except for *S. typhi* (typhoid fever) and for nontyphoidal *Salmonella* and *E. coli* enteritis in very young infants. In typhoid fever, blood cultures are positive early in the disease, whereas stool cultures become positive only after the secondary bacteremia.

The diagnosis of *E. histolytica* is based on identification of the organism in the stool. Serologic tests are useful for diagnosis of extraintestinal amebiasis, including amebic hepatic abscess.

Giardiasis can be diagnosed by identifying trophozoites or cysts in stool; less often a duodenal aspirate or biopsy of the duodenum or upper jejunum is needed. *Giardia* is excreted intermittently; three specimens are required. The Entero-Test is a nylon string affixed to a gelatin capsule, which is swallowed. After several hours, the string is withdrawn and duodenal contents are examined for *G. lamblia* trophozoites.

DIFFERENTIAL DIAGNOSIS

Diarrhea can be caused by infection, toxins, gastrointestinal allergy including allergy to milk or its components, malabsorption defects, inflammatory bowel disease, celiac disease, or any injury to enterocytes. Specific infections are differentiated from each other by the use of stool cultures and ELISA or PCR tests, when necessary. Acute enteritis may mimic other acute diseases, such as intussusception and acute appendicitis, which are best identified by diagnostic imaging. Many noninfectious causes of diarrhea produce chronic diarrhea, with persistence for more than 14 days. Persistent or chronic diarrhea may require tests for malabsorption or invasive studies, including endoscopy and small bowel biopsy (see Chapter 129).

Common-source diarrhea usually is associated with ingestion of contaminated food. In the U.S., the most common bacterial food-borne causes (in order of frequency) are nontyphoidal *Salmonella, Campylobacter, Shigella, E. coli* O157:H7, *Yersinia, L. monocytogenes,* and *V. cholerae.* The most common parasitic food-borne causes are *C. parvum* and *Cyclospora cayetanensis.* Common-source diarrhea also includes ingestion of preformed enterotoxins produced by bacteria, such as *S. aureus* and *Bacillus cereus,* which multiply in contaminated foods, and nonbacterial toxins, such as from fish, shellfish, and mushrooms. After a short incubation period, vomiting and cramps are prominent symptoms, and diarrhea may or may not be present. Heavy metals that leach into canned food or drinks causing gastric irritation and emetic syndromes may mimic symptoms of acute infectious enteritis.

TREATMENT

Most infectious causes of diarrhea in children are self-limited. Management of viral and most bacterial causes of diarrhea is primarily supportive and consists of correcting dehydration and ongoing fluid and electrolyte deficits and managing secondary complications resulting from mucosal injury. Antibiotic treatment is recommended for only some bacterial and parasitic causes of diarrhea (Table 112–3).

Treatment of fluid deficits requires an estimation of the degree of dehydration and the determination of any electrolyte imbalance. Hyponatremia is common, and hypernatremia is less common. Metabolic acidosis results from losses of bicarbonate in stool, lactic acidosis resulting from malabsorption or shock, and phosphate retention resulting from transient prerenalrenal insufficiency. Traditionally, therapy for 24 hours with oral rehydration solutions alone is effective for viral diarrhea. Therapy for severe fluid and electrolyte losses involves IV hydration, whereas less severe degrees of dehydration (<10%) in children without excessive vomiting or shock may be managed with oral rehydration solutions containing glucose and electrolytes. The World Health Organization oral rehydration solution contains 90 mEq/L of sodium, 20 mEq/L of potassium chloride, and 111 mEq/L of glucose.

Antibiotic treatment of mild illness with *Salmonella* does not shorten the clinical course, but does prolong bacterial excretion. Antibiotic therapy is necessary only for patients with *S. typhi* (typhoid fever) and sepsis or bacteremia with signs of systemic toxicity, metastatic foci, or age younger than 3 months with nontyphoidal salmonella.

Antibiotic treatment of *Shigella* produces a bacteriologic cure in 80% of patients after 48 hours, reducing the spread of the disease. Many *Shigella sonnei* isolates, the predominant strain affecting children, are resistant to amoxicillin and TMP-SMZ. Recommended treatment for children is an oral third-generation cephalosporin (ceftriaxone, cefixime, cefpodoxime) or a fluoroquinolone for persons 18 years old or older.

Antibiotic treatment of *E. coli* enteritis is indicated for infants younger than 3 months old with EPEC and patients who remain symptomatic (see Table 112–3). Antibiotic treatment is not recommended for patients with *E. coli* O157:H7 or HUS because release of toxin may precipitate or worsen the course of HUS.

Most patients with *Campylobacter* recover spontaneously before the diagnosis is established. Treatment with erythromycin, azithromycin, or ciprofloxacin (for persons >18 years old) initiated within 5 days of the onset of illness speeds recovery and reduces the duration of the carrier state.

The course of *Y. enterocolitica* usually is self-limited, lasting 3 days to 3 weeks. The efficacy of antibiotic treatment is questionable, but children with septicemia or focal infection, such as mesenteric lymphadenopathy, should be treated with cefotaxime. Treatment of *C. difficile* includes discontinuation of the antibiotic and, if diarrhea is severe, oral metronidazole or vancomycin. *E. histolytica* dysentery is treated with metronidazole followed by a luminal agent, such as iodoquinol. The treatment of *G. lamblia* is with albendazole, metronidazole, furazolidone, or quinacrine. No specific treatment is recommended for *Cryptosporidium* in otherwise healthy persons. Drugs such as loperamide, paregoric, and diphenoxylate are potentially dangerous and have no place in the management of acute infectious diarrhea in children

TABLE 112–3.   Antibiotic Therapy for Infectious Diarrhea*

Organism	Treatment	Comment
Salmonella typhi, Salmonella paratyphi	Ampicillin,[†] chloramphenicol,[†] TMP-SMZ, cefotaxime, ciprofloxacin[‡]	Invasive, bacteremic disease (typhoid fever or enteric fever)
Nontyphoidal *Salmonella*	Usually none (if ≥3 months old); ampicillin, cefotaxime, ciprofloxacin[‡]	Treatment indicated if <3 months old, malignancy, sickle cell disease, HIV/AIDS, or evidence of nongastrointestinal foci of infection is present
Shigella	Children: Third-generation cephalosporin, TMP-SMZ[†] Adults: fluoroquinolones[‡]	High prevalence of resistance to amoxicillin Increasing prevalence of resistance to TMP-SMZ Treatment reduces infectivity and improves outcome
Escherichia coli		
Enterotoxigenic	Usually none if endemic; TMP-SMZ or ciprofloxacin for traveler's diarrhea	Prevention of traveler's diarrhea with bismuth subsalicylate, doxycycline, or ciprofloxacin[‡]
Enteroinvasive	TMP-SMZ, ampicillin if susceptible	
Enteropathogenic	TMP-SMZ or an aminoglycoside	
Enterohemorrhagic	Usually none	No treatment if HUS is suspected
Enteroaggregative	TMP-SMZ or an aminoglycoside	
Campylobacter jejuni	Mild disease needs no treatment; erythromycin or azithromycin for diarrhea; aminoglycoside, ciprofloxacin,[‡] meropenem, or imipenem for systemic illness	If started early (days 1-3), treatment reduces symptoms and fecal organisms
Yersinia enterocolitica	None for uncomplicated diarrhea; TMP-SMZ; gentamicin or cefotaxime for extraintestinal disease	Value of treatment of mesenteric lymphadenitis with antibiotics is not established
Vibrio cholerae	Tetracycline, doxycycline, TMP-SMZ	Fluid maintenance crucial
Clostridium difficile	Oral metronidazole,[§] oral vancomycin	*C. difficile* is agent of antibiotic-associated diarrhea (pseudomembranous colitis)
Entamoeba histolytica	Metronidazole[§] followed by iodoquinol to treat luminal infection	Treatment determined by degree of tissue invasion
Giardia lamblia	Metronidazole,[§] quinacrine, furazolidone, others	Furazolidone is only preparation available in liquid form
Cryptosporidium parvum	None; azithromycin or paromomycin and octreotide in persons with HIV/AIDS	A serious infection in immunocompromised persons

*All treatment is predicated on knowledge of antimicrobial sensitivities.
[†]Commonly resistant.
[‡]Fluoroquinolone antibiotics are contraindicated in children, adolescents <18 years old, or pregnant or lactating women.
[§]The safety of metronidazole in children is unproven.
HUS, hemolytic uremic syndrome; TMP-SMZ, trimethoprim-sulfamethoxazole.

COMPLICATIONS

The major complication of gastroenteritis is dehydration and the cardiovascular compromise that can occur with severe hypovolemia. In disease caused by *Shigella,* high fever and seizures may occur. Intestinal abscesses can form with *Shigella* and *Salmonella* infections, especially typhoid fever, leading to intestinal perforation, which is a life-threatening complication. Severe vomiting associated with gastroenteritis can cause esophageal tears or aspiration.

PROGNOSIS

Deaths resulting from diarrhea reflect the principal problem of disruption of fluid and electrolyte homeostasis, which leads to dehydration, electrolyte imbalance, vascular instability, and shock. In the U.S., approximately 75 to 150 deaths occur annually from diarrheal disease, primarily in children younger than 1 year old. These deaths occur in a seasonal pattern between October and February, concurrent with the rotavirus season.

At least 10% of patients who have typhoid fever shed *S. typhi* for about 3 months, and 4% become chronic carriers. The risk of becoming a chronic carrier is low in children. Ciprofloxacin is recommended for adult carriers with persistent *Salmonella* excretion.

PREVENTION

The most important means of preventing childhood diarrhea is the provision of clean, uncontaminated water and proper hygiene in growing, collecting, and preparing foods. Although these are expectations in the developed world, for a large proportion of the world, these basic goals have not been achieved.

Only two vaccines for the prevention of diarrheal diseases are available. Three different types of typhoid vaccines have been licensed in the U.S.: (1) an oral live attenuated vaccine (Ty 21a); (2) a parenteral heat-phenol inactivated, killed whole cell vaccine; and (3) a parenteral capsular polysaccharide vaccine (Vi CPS). These are not routinely recommended except for international travelers to endemic areas. A rotavirus vaccine was removed from the market because of the association with intussusception.

Good hygienic measures, especially good hand washing with soap and water, are the best means of controlling person-to-person spread of most organisms causing gastroenteritis. Similarly, poultry products, such as eggs, should be considered potentially contaminated with *Salmonella* and should be handled and cooked appropriately.

Families should be aware of the risk of acquiring salmonellosis from household reptile pets. Transmission of *Salmonella* from reptiles can be prevented by thorough hand washing with soap and water after handling reptiles or reptile cages. Children younger than 5 years old and immunocompromised persons should avoid contact with reptiles. Pet reptiles should not be allowed to roam freely in the home or living areas and should be kept out of kitchens and food preparation areas to prevent contamination.

Traveler's diarrhea, caused primarily by ETEC, may be prevented by avoiding uncooked food and untreated drinking water. Prophylaxis with bismuth subsalicylate (Pepto-Bismol) is effective but unnecessary and is not recommended for children. Recommendations for travelers are for **presumptive self-treatment** for 3 days with TMP-SMZ for children, and ciprofloxacin, norfloxacin, or ofloxacin for adults, which are initiated at the first signs of diarrhea, nausea, bloating, or urgency.

Lactobacillus acidophilus has been recommended as a probiotic to prevent antibiotic-associated diarrhea. Studies have shown the value of *Lactobacillus* in reducing the incidence of community-acquired and antibiotic-associated diarrhea in children treated with oral antibiotics for other infectious diseases.

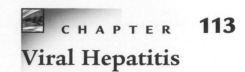

CHAPTER 113
Viral Hepatitis

ETIOLOGY

There are five primary hepatotropic viruses, which differ in their virologic characteristics, transmission, severity, likelihood of persistence, and subsequent risk of hepatocellular carcinoma (Table 113–1). HAV and hepatitis E virus (HEV) are transmitted by the fecal-oral route. HBV, HCV, and hepatitis D virus (HDV) are transmitted parenterally by IV drug use and sexual and perinatal modes. HDV, also known as the **delta agent**, is a defective virus that requires HBV for spread and causes either coinfection with HBV or superinfection in chronic HB$_s$Ag carriers. HBV, HCV, and HDV infections can result in chronic hepatitis, or a chronic carrier state, which facilitates spread. Other hepatitis viruses include hepatitis G virus (HGV), also known as hepatitis GB virus type C (HGBV-C), and members of the Circoviridae family of viruses, including TT virus (TTV) and SEN virus (SEN-V). The causes of 10% to 15% of cases of acute hepatitis are unknown.

EPIDEMIOLOGY

HAV causes approximately half of viral hepatitis in the U.S. Among children in the U.S., approximately 70% to 80% of all new cases of viral hepatitis are related to HAV, 5% to 30% are related to HBV, and 5% to 15% are related to HCV. The major risk factors for HBV and HCV are injection drug use, frequent exposure to blood products (hemophilia, organ transplants, chronic renal failure), and maternal infection. HEV follows travel to endemic areas outside the U.S. HGV is prevalent in HIV-infected persons. HBV and HCV cause chronic infection, which may lead to cirrhosis and is a significant risk factor for hepatocellular carcinoma and represents a persistent risk of transmission.

CLINICAL MANIFESTATIONS

There is considerable overlap in the characteristic clinical courses for HAV, HBV, and HCV (Fig. 113–1). The **preicteric phase**, which lasts approximately 1 week, is characterized by headache, anorexia, malaise, abdominal discomfort, nausea, and vomiting and usually precedes the onset of clinically detectable disease. Infants with perinatal HBV may have immune complexes accompanied by urticaria and arthritis before the onset of icterus. Jaundice and tender hepatomegaly are the most common physical findings and are characteristic of the **icteric phase**. Prodromal symptoms, particularly

TABLE 113–1. Characteristics of Agents Causing Acute Viral Hepatitis

Hepatitis	Hepatitis A Virus (enterovirus 72)	Hepatitis B Virus	Hepatitis C Virus (formerly post-transfusion non-A, non-B virus)	Hepatitis D Virus	Hepatitis E Virus (formerly enteral, non-A, non-B virus)	Hepatitis G Virus	TTV, SEN-V
Virus	27 nm ssRNA virus	42 nm dsDNA virus	30-60 nm ssRNA virus	36 nm circular ssRNA hybrid particle with HB$_s$Ag coat	27-34 nm ssRNA virus	50-100 nm ssRNA virus	30-50 nm ssDNA virus
Family	Picornavirus	Hepadnavirus	Flavivirus	Satellite	Flavivirus	Flavivirus	Circovirus
Transmission	Fecal-oral, rarely parenteral	Transfusion, sexual, inoculation, perinatal	Parenteral, transfusion, perinatal	Similar to HBV	Fecal-oral (endemic and epidemic)	Parenteral, transfusion	Parenteral, perinatal
Incubation period	15-30 days	60-180 days	30-60 days	Coinfection with HBV	35-60 days	Unknown	Unknown
Serum markers	Anti-HAV	Surface-antigen HB$_s$Ag, a core antigen HB$_c$Ag, an e-antigen HB$_e$Ag, anti-HB$_s$, anti-HB$_c$	Anti-HCV (IgG, IgM), RIBA, PCR for HCV RNA	Anti-HDV, RNA	Anti-HEV	RNA by RT-PCR	
Fulminant liver failure	Rare	<1% unless coinfection with HDV	Uncommon	2-20%	20%	Probably no	
Persistent infection	No	5-10% (90% with perinatal infection)	85%	2-70%	No	Persistent infection common; chronic disease rare	
Increased risk of hepatocellular carcinoma	No	Yes	Yes	No	No	Unknown	
Prophylaxis	Vaccine: immune serum globulin Good hygiene	Vaccine: Hepatitis B immunoglobulin					
Prevention	Good hygiene	Screen donated blood for elevated hepatic transaminases and HB$_s$Ag	Screen donated blood for elevated hepatic transaminases and anti-HCV (appears 4 mo postinfection, 6 mo post-transfusion)	Screen donated blood for elevated hepatic transaminases and HB$_s$Ag	Good hygiene	Screen donated blood for elevated hepatic transaminases	

PCR, polymerase chain reaction; RIBA, recombinant immunoblot assay; RT-PCR, reverse transcriptase polymerase chain reaction.

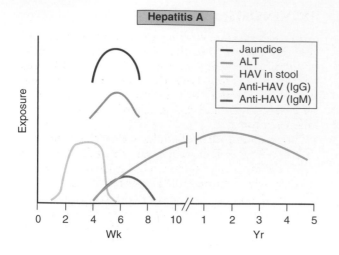

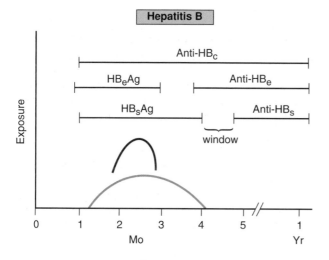

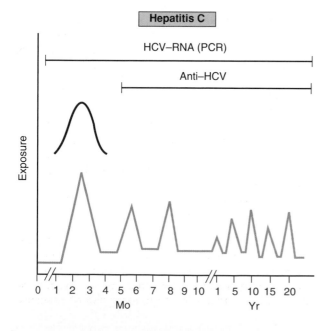

in children, may abate during the icteric phase. Asymptomatic or mild, nonspecific illness without icterus is common with HAV, HBV, and HCV, especially in young children. Hepatitic enzymes may increase 15-fold to 20-fold. Resolution of the hyperbilirubinemia and normalization of the transaminases may take 6 to 8 weeks.

LABORATORY AND IMAGING STUDIES

Alanine aminotransferase and aspartate aminotransferase levels are elevated and generally reflect the degree of parenchymal inflammation. Alkaline phosphatase, 5′-nucleotidase, and total and direct (conjugated) bilirubin levels indicate the degree of cholestasis, which results from hepatocellular and bile duct damage. The prothrombin time is a good predictor of severe hepatocellular injury and progression to fulminant hepatic failure (see Chapter 130).

The diagnosis of viral hepatitis is confirmed by characteristic serologic testing (see Table 113–1 and Fig. 113–1). The presence of IgM-specific antibody to HAV with low or absent IgG antibody to HAV is presumptive evidence of HAV. There is no chronic carrier state of HAV. The presence of HB$_s$Ag signifies acute or chronic infection with HBV. Antigenemia appears early in the illness and is usually transient, but also is diagnostic of the carrier state. Maternal HB$_s$Ag status always should be determined when HBV infection is diagnosed in infants younger than 1 year old because of the likelihood of vertical transmission. Hepatitis B e antigen (HB$_e$Ag) appears in the serum with acute HBV. The continued presence of HB$_s$Ag and HB$_e$Ag in the absence of antibody to e antigen (anti-HB$_e$) indicates high risk of transmissibility that is associated with ongoing viral replication. Clearance of HB$_s$Ag from the serum precedes a variable **window period** followed by the emergence of the antibody to surface antigen (anti-HB$_s$), which indicates development of lifelong immunity. Antibody to core antigen (anti-HB$_c$) a useful marker for recognizing HBV infection during the window phase (when HB$_s$Ag has disappeared, but before the appearance of anti-HB$_s$). Anti-HB$_e$ is useful in predicting a low degree of infectivity during the carrier state. Seroconversion after HCV infection may occur 6 months after

Figure 113–1

Clinical course and laboratory findings associated with hepatitis A, hepatitis B, and hepatitis C. ALT, alanine aminotransferase; HAV, hepatitis A virus; anti-HB$_c$, antibody to hepatitis B core antigen; HB$_e$Ag, hepatitis B early antigen; anti-HB$_e$, antibody to hepatitis B early antigen; HB$_s$Ag, hepatitis B surface antigen; anti-HB$_s$, antibody to hepatitis B surface antigen; HCV, hepatitis C virus; PCR, polymerase chain reaction.

infection. A positive result of HCV ELISA should be confirmed with the more specific recombinant immunoblot assay, which detects antibodies to multiple HCV antigens. Detection of HCV RNA by PCR is a sensitive marker for active infection, and results of this test may be positive 3 days after inoculation.

DIFFERENTIAL DIAGNOSIS

Many other viral infections may cause hepatitis as part of systemic infection, including EBV, CMV, VZV (chickenpox), herpes simplex, and adenoviruses. Bacterial infections include *E. coli* sepsis and leptospirosis. Patients with cholecystitis, cholangitis, and choledocholithiasis may present with acute symptoms and jaundice. Other causes of acute liver disease in childhood include drugs (isoniazid, phenytoin, valproic acid, carbamazepine, oral contraceptives, acetaminophen), toxins (ethanol, mushroom poisoning), Wilson disease, metabolic disease (galactosemia, tyrosinemia), α_1-antitrypsin deficiency, tumor, shock, anoxia, and graft-versus-host disease (see Chapter 130).

TREATMENT

The treatment of acute hepatitis is largely supportive and involves rest, hydration, and adequate dietary intake. Hospitalization is indicated for persons with severe vomiting and dehydration, a prolonged prothrombin time, or signs of hepatic encephalopathy. When the diagnosis of viral hepatitis is established, attention should be directed toward preventing its spread to close contacts. For HAV, hygienic measures include hand washing and careful disposal of excreta, contaminated diapers or clothing, needles, and other blood-contaminated items.

Chronic HBV infection may be treated with interferon alfa-2b or lamivudine, and HCV may be treated with interferon alfa alone or more often in combination with oral ribavirin. Most experience with these treatment regimens is in adults. The decision to treat is based on the patient's current age, age at HBV acquisition, development of viral mutations during therapy, and stage of viral infection. Transmission of HBV by vertical transmission or infection early in life often results in chronic HBV infection in an immune tolerant phase, in which interferon usually is not effective.

COMPLICATIONS

A protracted or relapsing course may develop in 10% to 15% of cases of HAV in adults, lasting for 6 months with an undulating course before eventual clinical resolution. **Fulminant hepatitis** with hepatic encephalopathy, gastrointestinal bleeding from esophageal varices or coagulopathy, and profound jaundice is uncommon, but is associated with a high mortality rate.

PROGNOSIS

Most cases of acute viral hepatitis resolve without specific therapy, with less than 0.1% of cases progressing to fulminant hepatic necrosis. HAV and HEV cause only acute infection. HBV, HCV, and HDV may persist as chronic infection with chronic inflammation, fibrosis, and cirrhosis and the associated risk of hepatocellular carcinoma.

Five percent to 10% of adults with HBV develop persistent infection, defined by persistence of HB_sAg in the blood for more than 6 months compared with 90% of children who acquire HBV by perinatal transmission. Chronic HB_sAg carriers are usually HB_eAg-negative and have no clinical, biochemical, or serologic evidence of active hepatitis, unless there is superinfection with HDV. Approximately 10% to 15% of HB_sAg carriers eventually clear HB_sAg.

Approximately 85% of persons infected with HCV remain chronically infected, which is characterized by fluctuating transaminase levels (see Fig. 113-1). There is poor correlation of symptoms with ongoing liver damage. Approximately 20% of persons with chronic infection develop cirrhosis, and approximately 25% of those develop hepatocellular carcinoma. HIV infection and ethanol use increase the risk of HCV progression.

PREVENTION

Good hygienic practices significantly reduce the risk of fecal-oral transmission of HAV. Screening blood donors for evidence of hepatitis significantly reduces the risk of blood-borne transmission. Vaccines are available for HAV and HBV, which have reduced the incidence of both infections. Specific postexposure measures are recommended to prevent secondary cases in susceptible persons.

HAV vaccination is recommended for all children living in 11 Western states with historically high levels of HAV: Arizona, Alaska, Oregon, New Mexico, Utah, Washington, Oklahoma, South Dakota, Idaho, Nevada, and California (see Fig. 94-1). Vaccination should be considered for all children in six additional states (Missouri, Texas, Colorado, Arkansas, Montana, Wyoming) or living in communities with high rates of HAV (Native American reservations, Alaskan Native villages), travelers to countries with intermediate or high endemicity of HAV, men who have sex with men, injection drug users, laboratory workers who work with HAV, persons who use clotting factor concentrates, and persons with chronic liver disease.

HBV vaccine is recommended for routine immunization of all infants beginning at birth and for all children and adolescents through 18 years of age who have not been immunized previously (see Fig. 94-1). It also is recommended as a pre-exposure vaccination for older children and adults at increased risk of exposure to HBV, including persons undergoing hemodialysis, persons with hemophilia or other recipients of clotting factor concentrates, residents and staff of institutions for developmentally disabled persons, men who have sex with men, injection drug users, inmates of juvenile detention and other correctional facilities, and healthcare workers. HBV vaccine already has shown effectiveness in reducing the incidence of hepatocellular carcinoma in high-risk populations.

Unvaccinated household and sexual contacts of persons with HAV should receive immunoglobulin (0.02 mL/kg) intramuscularly as soon as possible, but not more than 2 weeks after the last exposure. Immunoglobulin also is used for prophylaxis among unvaccinated staff and children in daycare facilities. If HAV is diagnosed in a food handler, immunoglobulin should be administered to other unvaccinated food handlers at the same establishment and can be considered for patrons if they can receive prophylaxis within 2 weeks after the last exposure.

Postexposure prophylaxis using hepatitis B immunoglobulin (HBIG) and vaccine, is recommended for household members with intimate contact including sex partners. Prophylaxis is given to unvaccinated persons following needle stick injuries with blood from an HB$_s$Ag-positive patient.

Routine prenatal screening for HB$_s$Ag is recommended for all pregnant women in the U.S. Infants born to HB$_s$Ag-positive mothers should receive HBV vaccine and HBIG (0.5 mL) within 12 hours of birth, with subsequent vaccine doses at 1 to 2 months of age and 6 months of age. Infants born to mothers whose HB$_s$Ag status is unknown should receive vaccine within 12 hours of birth. If maternal testing is positive for HB$_s$Ag, the infant should receive HBIG as soon as possible (no later than 1 week of age). The combination of HBIG and vaccination is 98% to 99% effective in preventing vertical transmission of HBV. Vaccination alone without HBIG may prevent 75% of cases of perinatal HBV transmission and approximately 95% of cases of symptomatic childhood HBV infection.

CHAPTER 114
Urinary Tract Infection

ETIOLOGY

UTIs include **cystitis** (infection localized to the bladder), **pyelonephritis** (infection of the renal parenchyma, calyces, and renal pelvis), and **renal abscess**, which may be intrarenal or perinephric. The urinary tract and urine are normally sterile. *E. coli,* ascending from bowel flora, accounts for 90% of first infections and 75% of recurrent infections. Ninety percent of nephritogenic *E. coli* possess P-fimbriae, which facilitates adherence to uroepithelial cells via cell surface receptors, such as the disaccharide **α-Gal(1 → 4)β-Gal** (gal-gal) receptor, which is genetically determined and related to the P blood group. Other bacteria commonly causing infection include *Klebsiella, Proteus, Enterococcus,* and *Pseudomonas. Staphylococcus saprophyticus* is associated with UTI in some children and in sexually active adolescent girls. *S. saprophyticus, C. trachomatis,* and *E. coli* are the chief causes of the **acute urethral syndrome**, or **postcoital urethritis**, which typically occurs 12 to 72 hours after sexual intercourse.

EPIDEMIOLOGY

Approximately 5% of girls and 1% of boys have a UTI by 11 years of age. The lifetime incidence of UTI in females is about 30% and only 1% in males. Approximately 75% of infants younger than 3 months old with bacteriuria are male compared with only 10% between the ages of 3 and 8 months. After 12 months of age, UTI in healthy children usually is seen in girls.

A short urethra predisposes girls to UTI. Uncircumcised male infants (<1 year old) are at 5-fold to 12-fold increased risk for UTI. Obstruction to urine flow and urinary stasis is the major risk factor and may result from anatomic abnormalities, nephrolithiasis, renal tumor, indwelling urinary catheter, ureteropelvic junction obstruction, megaureter, extrinsic compression, and pregnancy. Vesicoureteral reflux, whether primary (70% of cases) or secondary to urinary tract obstruction, predisposes to chronic infection and renal scarring. Scarring also may develop in the absence of reflux.

CLINICAL MANIFESTATIONS

The symptoms and signs of UTI vary markedly with age (Table 114–1). In neonates, failure to thrive and feeding problems are the most consistent symptoms. Direct hyperbilirubinemia may occur. Infants 1 month to 2 years old present with feeding problems, failure to thrive, diarrhea, vomiting, or unexplained fever. The symptoms may masquerade as gastrointestinal illness with "colic," irritability, and screaming periods. At 2 years of age, children begin to show the classic signs of UTI, such as urgency, dysuria, frequency, and abdominal pain. The presence of UTI should be suspected in all infants and young children with unexplained fever and in patients of all ages with fever and congenital anomalies of the urinary tract.

LABORATORY AND IMAGING STUDIES

The diagnosis of UTI requires a culture of the urine. Urine samples for urinalysis should be examined promptly (within 20 minutes) or refrigerated until

TABLE 114–1. Symptoms and Signs of Urinary Tract Infection in Children by Age Group

Symptom or Sign	Frequency of Occurrence (%) by Age			
	0-1 mo	1-24 mo	2-5 yr	5-12 yr
Failure to thrive	53	36	7	0
Jaundice	44	0	0	0
Vomiting	24	29	16	3
Diarrhea	18	16	0	3
Fever	11	38	57	50
Convulsions	2	7	9	5
Irritability	0	13	7	0
Changes in urine	0	9	13	0
Hematuria	0	7	16	8
Frequency, dysuria	0	4	34	41
Enuresis	0	0	27	29
Abdominal pain	0	0	23	0
Flank pain	0	0	0	0

Adapted from Smellie JM, Hodson CJ, Edwards D, et al: Clinical and radiological features of urinary tract infection in childhood. BMJ 2:1222-1226, 1964.

cultured. A voided urine sample with greater than 10^5 cfu/mL of a single organism has a 95% positive correlation with positive culture by suprapubic aspiration. Urine obtained by midstream, clean-catch technique (for older children and adolescents) is considered significant with bacterial growth of greater than 100,000 cfu/mL; urine obtained by catheterization is considered significant with bacterial growth of greater than 10,000 cfu/mL; and urine obtained by suprapubic aspiration is considered significant with bacterial growth of greater than 1000 cfu/mL. Suprapubic percutaneous aspiration of the bladder may be performed in young infants who have not voided for 1 to 3 hours. Perineal bags for urine collection are prone to contamination and are not recommended for urine collection for culture.

For infants and young children with unexplained fever who require immediate antibiotic therapy, a urine specimen should be obtained by catheterization or suprapubic percutaneous aspiration. For infants and young children with unexplained fever who do not require antibiotic treatment, a urine specimen should be obtained by catheterization or suprapubic aspiration or alternatively by the most convenient method with a repeat urine collection by catheterization or suprapubic aspiration if the urinalysis suggests a UTI.

Urinalysis showing **pyuria** (leukocyturia of >10 WBC/mm^3) suggests infection, but also is consistent with urethritis, vaginitis, nephrolithiasis, glomerulonephritis, and interstitial nephritis. The leukocyte esterase dipstick test has poor sensitivity (50%) for pyuria, and the urinary nitrate dipstick test has poor sensitivity (30%) for bacterial counts greater than 10^5 cfu/mL. The presence of numerous motile bacteria in freshly voided, uncentrifuged urine from symptomatic infants and children has a 94% correlation with a positive culture by suprapubic aspiration. The presence of even scant bacteria has an 82% correlation with a positive culture by suprapubic aspiration.

Ultrasonography, VCUG, radionuclide cystography, renal nucleotide scans, and CT or MRI can be used for anatomic and functional assessment of the urinary tract. Ultrasound provides limited information about renal scarring and is performed to exclude an anatomic abnormality. VCUG is the best imaging study for determining the presence or absence of vesicoureteral reflux, which is ranked from grade I (ureter only) to grade V (complete gross dilation of the ureter and obliteration of caliceal and pelvic anatomy) (see Chapter 167). A technetium-99m DMSA scan can identify acute pyelonephritis, but is most useful to define renal scarring as a late effect of UTI.

DIFFERENTIAL DIAGNOSIS

The diagnosis of a UTI is confirmed by a positive culture of bacteria in the urine, although this does not distinguish between upper tract and lower tract infection. Localization of a UTI is important because upper UTI is associated more frequently with bacteremia and with anatomic abnormalities than is uncomplicated cystitis. The clinical manifestations of UTI do not reliably distinguish the site of infection in neonates, infants, and toddlers. Fever and abdominal pain may occur with either lower or upper UTI, although high fever, costovertebral tenderness, high ESR, leukocytosis, and bacteremia each suggest upper tract involvement. Indirect findings, such as WBC casts, inability to concentrate urine maximally, presence of antibody-coated bacteria detected by immunofluorescence, and β_2-microglobulin excretion or ratios are of limited value in localizing the site of the UTI to the upper tract. DMSA scan is sensitive for detecting acute pyelonephritis.

The manifestations of UTI overlap with signs of sepsis seen in young children and with enteritis, appendicitis, mesenteric lymphadenitis, and pneumonia in older children. Dysuria may indicate pinworm infection, hypersensitivity to soaps or detergents, vaginitis, or sexual abuse and infection.

TREATMENT

Empirical therapy should be initiated for symptomatic children and for all children with a urine culture confirming UTI. For a child who does not appear ill but with a positive urine culture, antibiotic therapy should be initiated either parenterally or orally. For a child with suspected UTI who appears toxic, appears dehydrated, or is unable to retain oral fluids, initial antibiotic therapy should be administered parenterally, and hospitalization should be considered.

Neonates with UTI are treated for 10 to 14 days with parenteral antibiotics because of the higher rate of bacteremia. Older children with acute cystitis are treated for 7 to 14 days with an oral antibiotic. Increasing bacterial resistance has limited the usefulness of some antibiotics, such as amoxicillin. TMP-SMZ is used frequently, although resistance to this drug also is increasing. Oral third-generation cephalosporins (cefixime, cefpodoxime) are effective but expensive. Children with high fever or other manifestations of acute pyelonephritis often are hospitalized for initial treatment with parenteral antibiotics, such as cefotaxime. Patients with systemic toxicity (chills and high fever) should be hospitalized and treated with IV cefotaxime and gentamicin (or another aminoglycoside). When the patient has improved and is afebrile, oral therapy with an agent to which the cultured organism is sensitive is administered to complete 7 to 14 days of total therapy.

The degree of toxicity, dehydration, and ability to retain oral intake of fluids should be assessed carefully. Restoring or maintaining adequate hydration, including correction of electrolyte abnormalities that are often associated with vomiting or poor oral intake, is important.

Infants and children who do not show the expected clinical response within 2 days of starting antimicrobial therapy should be re-evaluated, have another urine specimen obtained for culture, and undergo ultrasound promptly and either VCUG or radionuclide cystography, which should be performed at the earliest convenient time.

COMPLICATIONS

Bacteremia occurs in 2% to 5% of episodes of pyelonephritis and is more likely in infants than in older children. Focal renal abscesses are an uncommon complication.

PROGNOSIS

The relapse rate of UTI is approximately 25% to 40%, with most relapses occurring within 2 to 3 weeks of treatment. Follow-up urine cultures should be obtained 1 to 2 weeks after completing therapy to document sterility of the urine. Prophylactic antibiotics should be administered until the VCUG has been completed, and the presence of reflux is known. TMP-SMZ (2 mg/kg TMP, 10 mg/kg SMZ) and nitrofurantoin (1 to 2 mg/kg) given once daily at bedtime are recommended as prophylactic agents, which, in contrast to amoxicillin and cephalosporins, are associated with low rates of developing antibiotic resistance. Clinical

follow-up for at least 2 to 3 years, with repeat urine culture as indicated, is prudent. Some experts recommend that follow-up urine cultures should be obtained after recurrent cystitis or pyelonephritis, monthly for 3 months, at 3-month intervals for 6 months, then yearly for 2 to 3 years.

Grade 1 to 3 reflux resolves at a rate of about 13% per year for the first 5 years, then at a rate of 3.5% per year. Grade 4 to 5 reflux resolves at a rate of about 5% per year. Bilateral reflux resolves more slowly than unilateral reflux (see Chapter 167).

PREVENTION

Primary prevention is achieved by promoting good perineal hygiene and managing underlying risk factors for UTI, such as chronic constipation, encopresis, and daytime and nighttime urinary incontinence. Secondary prevention of UTI with antibiotic prophylaxis given once daily is directed toward preventing recurrent infections, although the impact of secondary prophylaxis to prevent renal scarring is unknown. Acidification of the urine with cranberry juice is not recommended as the sole means of preventing UTI in children at high risk.

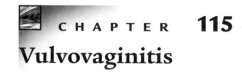

CHAPTER 115

Vulvovaginitis

ETIOLOGY

Vulvovaginitis, which is inflammation of the vulva or the vagina or both, is the most common gynecologic problem in children. The low prepubertal levels of estrogen result in thin, atrophic vaginal epithelium that is susceptible to bacterial invasion. At puberty, estrogen increases, and the pH of the vagina becomes more acidic. There are several specific causes of vulvovaginitis (Table 115–1), including STIs such as *Trichomonas vaginalis* and HSV (see Chapter 116). **Nonspecific vaginitis** results from overgrowth of normal aerobic vaginal flora that is associated with poor hygiene. **Bacterial vaginosis** is caused by *Gardnerella vaginalis,* which interacts synergistically with vaginal anaerobes, including *Bacteroides, Mobiluncus,* and *Peptostreptococcus.*

EPIDEMIOLOGY

Nonspecific vaginitis is the most common cause of vulvovaginitis in young girls. *G. vaginalis* is often present as part of the normal vaginal flora in preadolescent

TABLE 115–1.   Characteristics of Vulvovaginitis

Etiology	Presentation	Diagnosis	Treatment
Physiologic vaginal discharge (physiologic leukorrhea)	Minimal, clear, thin discharge without pruritus or inflammation; occurs soon after birth and again at 6-12 mo before menarche	No pathogenic organisms on culture	Reassurance
Nonspecific vaginitis	Vaginal discharge, dysuria, itching; fecal soiling of underwear	Evidence of poor hygiene; no pathogenic organisms on culture	Improved hygiene, sitz baths
Bacterial vaginosis (*Gardnerella vaginalis* and anaerobes)	Often asymptomatic; possible thin vaginal discharge with a "fishy" odor	At least 3 of the following 4 criteria: (1) thin, homogeneous vaginal discharge; (2) vaginal pH ≥4.5; (3) a fishy odor of volatile amines on the addition of a drop of 10% potassium hydroxide to a drop of vaginal discharge (the whiff test); and (4) the presence of clue cells on a saline wet mount of vaginal discharge	Metronidazole, clindamycin
Candida	Itching, dysuria, white "cottage cheese" vaginal discharge	*Candida* on saline wet mount of vaginal discharge	Topical antifungal (e.g., butoconazole, clotrimazole, miconazole, nystatin, tioconazole, terconazole, fluconazole)
Enterobiasis (pinworms)	Perineal pruritus (nocturnal); gastrointestinal symptoms; variable vulvovaginal contamination from feces	Adult worms in stool or eggs on perianal skin	Mebendazole or albendazole
Giardiasis	Asymptomatic fecal contaminant, vaginal discharge, diarrhea, malabsorption syndrome	Protozoal flagellate (cyst or trophozoites) in feces	Metronidazole or albendazole
Molluscum contagiosum	Vulvar lesions, nodules with umbilicated area; white core of curdlike material	Isolation of poxvirus	Dermal curettage of papule
Phthirus pubis (pediculosis pubis)	Pruritus, excoriation, sky blue macules; inner thigh or lower abdomen	Nits on hair shafts, lice on skin or clothing	Lindane lotion
Sarcoptes scabiei (scabies)	Nocturnal pruritus, pruritic vesicles, pustules in runs	Mites; ova black, dots of feces (microscopic)	1% lindane
Shigella	Bloody vaginal discharge; fever, malaise, fecal contamination, diarrhea; blood and mucus, cramps, pus in stool	Stools: white blood cells and red blood cells, positive for *Shigella*	Oral third-generation cephalosporin
Staphylococcus, Streptococcus	Vaginal discharge, possibly bloody; spread from primary lesion	Bacterial culture	First-generation cephalosporin or dicloxacillin
Foreign body	Foul-smelling vaginal discharge, sometimes bloody	Foreign body on physical examination	Removal of foreign body

girls, but is more common in girls who are sexually active. *Candida* is much less common in preadolescent girls than in women.

CLINICAL MANIFESTATIONS

The primary symptoms of vulvovaginitis are vaginal discharge, erythema, and pruritus. A thin, gray, homogeneous discharge with a "fishy" odor suggests bacterial vaginosis. A white "cottage cheese" discharge suggests *Candida*. Bloody discharge suggests group A streptococcus or *Shigella*. Foul-smelling discharge suggests a foreign body.

LABORATORY AND IMAGING STUDIES

Wet mount microscopic examination, prepared by mixing vaginal secretions with normal saline solution, and culture may be used to confirm a specific diagnosis (see Table 115–1). The diagnosis of bacterial vaginosis is established by the presence of at least three of the following four criteria: (1) thin, homogeneous vaginal discharge, (2) vaginal pH 4.5 or greater, (3) a characteristic **fishy odor** after release of volatile amines on the addition of a drop of 10% KOH to a drop of vaginal discharge (the **whiff test**), and (4) the presence of clue cells on a saline wet mount of vaginal discharge. **Clue cells** are vaginal epithelial cells that are covered with *G. vaginalis* and have a granular appearance. Vaginal cultures for *G. vaginalis* are not useful. *Candida* may be shown by saline wet mount or by culture.

DIFFERENTIAL DIAGNOSIS

Noninfectious causes of vulvovaginitis include physical agents (foreign body, sand), chemical agents (bubble bath, soap, detergent), and vulvar skin disease (atopic dermatitis, seborrhea, psoriasis). **Physiologic vaginal discharge** or **physiologic leukorrhea** of desquamated vaginal cells and mucus occurs normally in girls soon after birth, with discharge lasting for about 1 week, and again at 6 to 12 months before menarche. There is minimal, clear, thin discharge without pruritus or inflammation. No treatment is necessary.

TREATMENT

The treatment of vulvovaginitis depends on the etiology (see Table 115–1). Treatment of nonspecific vaginitis includes improving perineal hygiene and sitz baths two to three times a day as needed. The recommended treatment for bacterial vaginosis is oral metronidazole. Imidazole creams and vaginal tablets and suppositories all are effective for the treatment of acute vulvovaginal candidiasis. Douching or vaginal irrigation is not beneficial and is not recommended.

COMPLICATIONS AND PROGNOSIS

Complications are rare. The prognosis is excellent.

PREVENTION

There are no recognized prophylactic measures for bacterial vaginosis or nonspecific vaginitis. Douching reduces normal vaginal flora, which are protective against pathogenic organisms, and is not protective.

CHAPTER **116**

Sexually Transmitted Infections

Adolescents have the highest rates of STIs. Biologic factors may predispose adolescents to certain STIs, such as *C. trachomatis*. Compared with adults, sexually active adolescents are more likely to believe that they will not contract an STI, more likely to come into contact with an infected sexual partner, less likely to receive health care when an STI develops, and less likely to be compliant with treatment for an STI.

Although numerous organisms cause STIs, the diseases can be grouped by the characteristic clinical presentation. **Urethritis** and **cervicitis**, or, more correctly, **endocervicitis** (Table 116–1), are characteristic of *Neisseria gonorrhoeae* and *C. trachomatis,* which are the most common STIs. More than 70% of genital chlamydial infections in women are asymptomatic. **Genital ulcers** (Table 116–2) are characteristic of syphilis (*Treponema pallidum*), genital HSV, chancroid *(Haemophilus ducreyi),* and granuloma inguinale, also known as donovanosis (*Calymmatobacterium granulomatis*). **Vaginal discharge** (Table 116–3) is a symptom of trichomoniasis (*T. vaginalis*) and is part of the spectrum of vulvovaginitis (see Chapter 115), which is not always associated with sexual activity. HPV cause **condylomata acuminata,** or **genital warts** (Table 116–4).

STIs are associated with significant physiologic and psychological morbidity. Early diagnosis and treatment are important for preventing medical complications and infertility. All STIs are preventable; primary prevention of STIs should be a goal for all healthcare providers for adolescents. Diagnosis of an STI necessitates evaluation or treatment for concomitant STIs and notification and treatment of sexual partners.

Many infections that are not traditionally considered STIs are sexually transmissible, including HIV, human T cell leukemia viruses types I and II, CMV, EBV, HHV-6, HHV-7, HBV, molluscum contagiosum

TABLE 116–1. Features of Sexually Transmitted Infections Characterized by Mucopurulent Cervicitis, Urethritis, and Pelvic Inflammatory Disease

	Gonorrhea	Chlamydial Infection
Agent	*Neisseria gonorrhoeae*	*Chlamydia trachomatis*
Incubation period	3-14 days	5-12 days
Possible presentations	**The following possible presentations apply to both infections:**	
	Female	*Male*
	Asymptomatic	Asymptomatic
	Urethritis	Urethritis
	Skenitis/bartholinitis	Epididymo-orchitis
	PID	Neonatal conjunctivitis (inclusion conjunctivitis)
	Proctitis	
	Pharyngitis	
	Conjunctivitis (including neonatal conjunctivitis)	
	Disseminated gonorrhea infection (arthritis, dermatitis, endocarditis, meningitis)	
Typical findings of mucopurulent cervicitis or urethritis	**The following possible presentations apply to both infections:**	
	Female	*Male*
	Cervical erythema, friability, with thick, creamy discharge	Penile discharge
	>10 PMNs/hpf	>10 PMNs/hpf
	Mild cervical tenderness	
	Gram-negative intracellular diplococci on Gram stain	Often coexists with gonorrhea
PID (females)	**The following possible presentations apply to both infections:**	
	Onset day 3-10 of menstrual period	
	Lower abdominal pain (95%)	
	Adnexal tenderness, mass (95%)	
	Pain on cervical motion (95%)	
	Fever (35%)	
	Mucopurulent cervical discharge (variable)	
	Menstrual irregularities (variable)	
	Nausea, vomiting (variable)	
	Weakness, syncope, dizziness (variable)	
	Perihepatitis (5%)	
Diagnosis	Gram stain (in cervicitis: 60% sensitivity, 95% specificity; diagnostic in males)	Antigen detection by PCR amplification (LCR, TMA, EIA)
	Culture (Thayer-Martin selective medium)	Culture
	Antigen detection by PCR amplification (LCR)	
Treatment		
Uncomplicated cervicitis, urethritis, pharyngitis, proctitis	Ceftriaxone *or* cefixime *plus* doxycycline (for *Chlamydia*)	Doxycycline *or* azithromycin
PID (females)		
Outpatient	Ofloxacin *or* levofloxacin *with or without* metronidazole (all for 14 days) *or* ceftriaxone (1 dose) *plus* doxycycline for 14 days *with or without* metronidazole for 14 days	
Inpatient	Cefotetan *or* cefoxitin (until improved for 24 hr) *plus* doxycycline to complete 14 days	
Disseminated gonococcal infection	Ceftriaxone	

EIA, enzyme immunoassay; LCR, ligase chain reaction; PCR, polymerase chain reaction; PID, pelvic inflammatory disease; PMNs, polymorphonuclear cells; TMA, transcription-mediated amplification.

TABLE 116–2.   Features of Sexually Transmitted Infections Characterized by Genital Ulcers

	Syphilis	Genital Herpes	Chancroid	Granuloma Inguinale (Donovanosis)
Agent	*Treponema pallidum*	HSV-1, HSV-2	*Haemophilus ducreyi*	*Calymmatobacterium granulomatis*
Incubation	10-90 days	4-14 days	3-10 days	8-80 days
Systemic findings	Fever, rash, malaise, anorexia, arthralgia, lymphadenopathy	Headache, fever, malaise, myalgia in one third of cases	None	Local spread only
Inguinal lymphadenopathy	Late, bilateral, nontender, no suppuration	Early, bilateral, tender, no suppuration	Early, rapid, tender, and unilateral; suppuration likely	Lymphatic obstruction
Primary lesion	Papule	Vesicle	Papule to pustule	Papule
Ulcer characteristics				
Number	≥1	Multiple	<3	≥1, may coalesce
Edges	Distinct	Reddened, ragged	Ragged, undermined	Rolled, distinct
Depth	Shallow	Shallow	Deep	Raised
Base	Red, smooth	Red, smooth	Necrotic	Beefy red, clean
Secretion	Serous	Serous	Pus, blood	None
Induration	Firm	None	None	Firm
Pain	None	Usual	Often	None
Diagnosis				
Serology	VDRL *or* RPR MHA-TP *or* FTA-ABS	Seroconversion (primary infection only)	None	None
Isolation	No in vitro test; rabbit inoculation	Culture	Aspirate of node, swab of ulcer on selective medium	None
Microscopic	Dark-field examination	Pap smear; Tzanck smear; direct FA staining	Gram-negative pleomorphic rods	Staining of ulcer biopsy material for Donovan bodies
Treatment	*Early:* Benzathine penicillin G (2.4 million U IM) once *Late (>1 yr duration):* Benzathine penicillin G (2.4 million U IM) weekly × 3 doses	Acyclovir *or* famciclovir *or* valacyclovir	Aspirate fluctuant nodes Incision and drainage of buboes >5 cm Azithromycin *or* ciprofloxacin *or* erythromycin	Doxycycline *or* TMP-SMZ

FTA-ABS, fluorescent treponemal antibody–absorption; HSV, herpes simplex virus; MHA-TP, microhemagglutination assay–*Treponema pallidum*; RPR, rapid plasma reagin; TMP-SMZ, trimethoprim-sulfamethoxazole; VDRL, Venereal Disease Research Laboratory.

virus, and *Sarcoptes scabiei*. The presence of any STI suggests behavior that increases risk for HIV (see Chapter 125), and HIV counseling and testing should be provided to all adolescents with STIs. Acquisition of gonorrhea, syphilis, HSV-2, and trichomoniasis in prepubertal children beyond the neonatal period indicates sexual contact and signifies the need to investigate for possible sexual abuse (see Chapter 22). The association of vulvovaginitis and genital HPV infec-

tion, which may result from skin or genital HPV types, with sexual abuse is less certain.

GONORRHEA (*NEISSERIA GONORRHOEAE*)

N. gonorrhoeae, a gram-negative coccus, is often seen as diplococci. Gonorrhea is a common STI among adolescents. The greatest increase in incidence is in the

TABLE 116–3.   Features of Sexually Transmitted Infections Characterized by Vaginal Discharge

	Physiologic Leukorrhea (Normal)	Trichomoniasis	Bacterial Vaginosis (Gardnerella vaginalis–Associated Vaginitis)
Agent	Normal flora	*Trichomonas vaginalis*	*G. vaginalis* and anaerobes
Incubation	—	3-28 days	Not necessarily sexually transmitted
Predominant symptoms			
Pruritus	None	Mild to moderate	None to mild
Discharge	Minimal	Moderate to severe	Mild to moderate
Pain	None	Mild	Uncommon
Vulvar inflammation	None	Common	Uncommon
Characteristics of discharge			
Amount	Small	Profuse	Moderate
Color	Clear, milky	Yellow-green or gray	Gray
Consistency	Flocculent	Frothy	Homogeneous
Viscosity	Thin	Thin	Thin
Foul odor	None	None	Yes
Odor with KOH	None	Possible	Characteristic fishy odor (amine)
pH	<4.5	>5.0	>4.5
Diagnosis			
Saline drop	Squamous and few WBCs	Motile flagellates, slightly larger than WBCs, and WBCs	Squamous cells studded with bacteria ("clue cells") and WBCs
Gram stain	Gram-positive and gram-negative rods and cocci	*Trichomonas* killed	Predominance of gram-negative rods
Culture	Mixed flora with *Lactobacillus* predominant	Culture generally not indicated; antigen detection and antibody tests available	Culture not useful
Treatment	Reassurance	Metronidazole	Metronidazole or clindamycin

KOH, potassium hydroxide; WBCs, white blood cells.

15- to 19-year-old age group, especially among girls. The organism causes infection at the site of acquisition, which commonly results in mucopurulent cervicitis and urethritis (see Table 116–1). Cervicitis is often asymptomatic. Infection may include the periurethral Skene glands, labial Bartholin glands, rectum (proctitis), pharynx, and conjunctiva. In males, the urethra, epididymis, and prostate can be infected. **Dissemination** to the joints, skin, meninges, and endocardium can occur via the hematogenous route. Perinatal transmission of maternal infection can lead to neonatal sepsis and meningitis (see Chapter 65) and ophthalmia neonatorum (see Chapter 119).

Treatment regimens should be effective against *N. gonorrhoeae* and *C. trachomatis* because of the high frequency of concomitant infection. A single dose of IM ceftriaxone (125 mg) or oral cefixime (400 mg) is recommended for uncomplicated gonococcal infection of the cervix, urethra, and rectum. Ciprofloxacin or ofloxacin may be used in persons 18 years old or

older. Disseminated gonococcal infection results in petechial or pustular acral skin lesions, asymmetric arthralgia, tenosynovitis or septic arthritis, and occasionally endocarditis or meningitis. Hospitalization and treatment with ceftriaxone are recommended. For all gonococcal infections, azithromycin or doxycycline also is administered, unless chlamydial infection is excluded. Sexual partners should be notified and treated.

Pelvic Inflammatory Disease

Direct extension of *N. gonorrhoeae,* often in combination with *C. trachomatis,* to the endometrium, fallopian tubes, and peritoneum causes **pelvic inflammatory disease**. Complications of pelvic inflammatory disease include tubo-ovarian abscess and **Fitz-Hugh–Curtis syndrome**, which is inflammation of the capsule of the liver. A major sequela of pelvic inflammatory disease is infertility. The differential diagnosis of pelvic

TABLE 116–4. Features of Sexually Transmitted Infections Characterized by Nonulcerative External Genital Symptoms

	Genital Warts	Vulvovaginal Candidiasis	Pediculosis Pubis (Crabs)
Agent	Human papillomavirus	*Candida albicans*	*Phthirus pubis*
Incubation	30-90 days	Uncommon sexual transmission	5-10 days
Presenting complaints	Genital warts are seen or felt	Vulvar itching or discharge	Pubic itching, live organisms may be seen; sexual partner has "crabs"
Signs	Firm, gray-to-pink, single or multiple, fimbriated, painless excrescences on vulva, introitus, vagina cervix, perineum, anus	Inflammation of vulva, with thick, white, "cottage cheese" discharge, pH < 5; friable mucosa that easily bleeds	Eggs (nits) at base of pubic hairs, lice may be visible; excoriated, red skin secondary to infestation
Clinical associations	Cervical neoplasia, dysplasia	Oral contraceptives, diabetes, antibiotics	
Diagnosis	Clinical appearance; most infections asymptomatic; acetowhite changes on colposcopy; enlarged cells with perinuclear halo and hyperchromatic nuclei	KOH (10%): pseudohyphae; Gram stain: gram-positive pseudohyphae; Nickerson or Sabouraud medium for culture	History and clinical appearance
Treatment	*Patient-applied therapies:* Podofilox solution or gel *or* Imiquimod cream *Provider-applied therapies:* cryotherapy with liquid nitrogen or cryoprobe *or* topical podophyllin resin *or* trichloroacetic acid or dichloroacetic acid *or* surgical removal	*Intravaginal agents:* butoconazole *or* clotrimazole *or* miconazole *or* nystatin *or* tioconazole *or* terconazole *Oral agent:* fluconazole	Permethrin 1% cream *or* lindane 1% shampoo *or* pyrethrin with piperonyl butoxide

KOH, potassium hydroxide.

inflammatory disease includes ectopic pregnancy, septic abortion, ovarian cyst torsion or rupture, UTI, appendicitis, mesenteric lymphadenitis, and inflammatory bowel disease. Pelvic ultrasound may detect thickened adnexal structures and is the imaging study of choice for other possible diagnoses. Clinical criteria for diagnosis of pelvic inflammatory disease are lower abdominal tenderness, uterine/adnexal tenderness, and cervical motion tenderness. Additional criteria that support the diagnosis are fever, mucopurulent vaginal discharge, elevated WBCs (in 45%), elevated ESR (in 65%) or CRP, and documented infection with *N. gonorrhoeae* or *C. trachomatis*. Adolescents should be hospitalized for treatment if the diagnosis is uncertain and other etiologies (appendicitis) cannot be excluded, the patient is pregnant, there has not been clinical response to oral therapy with 72 hours, the patient is unable to adhere to or tolerate oral therapy, there is a tubo-ovarian abscess, or there is severe illness with high fever, nausea, and vomiting. The recommended parenteral **treatment** is cefotetan or cefoxitin plus doxycycline orally. The recommended oral treatment of

pelvic inflammatory disease for women 18 years old or older is ofloxacin or levofloxacin, with or without metronidazole, for 14 days. The recommended oral treatment of pelvic inflammatory disease for younger persons is ceftriaxone in a single dose, plus doxycycline orally for 14 days, with or without metronidazole for 14 days. Follow-up examination should be performed within 72 hours, with hospitalization for parenteral therapy if there has not been clinical improvement.

CHLAMYDIA TRACHOMATIS

Chlamydiae are obligate intracellular bacteria with a biphasic life cycle, existing as relatively inert elementary bodies in their extracellular form and as **reticulate bodies** when phagocytosed and replicating within a phagosome. Reticulate bodies divide by binary fission and after 48 to 72 hours reorganize into elementary bodies that are released from the cell. *Chlamydia* infects nonciliated squamocolumnar cells and the transitional epithelial cells that line the mucosa of the urethra, cervix, rectum, and conjunctiva.

C. trachomatis serovars D-K cause urethritis, cervicitis, pelvic inflammatory disease, inclusion conjunctivitis in the newborn, and infant pneumonia. *C. trachomatis* serovars L₁,₃ cause lymphogranuloma venereum, an uncommon STI that is characterized by unilateral, painful inguinal lymphadenitis. *C. trachomatis* serovars A, B, Ba, and C produce trachoma (hyperendemic blinding), which eventually leads to blindness from extensive local scarring.

Chlamydia is the most frequently diagnosed bacterial STI in adolescents and accounts for most cases of **nongonococcal urethritis and cervicitis** (see Table 116-1). There is a 5:1 female-to-male ratio. Males often have dysuria and a mucopurulent discharge, although approximately 25% may be asymptomatic. Women are more often asymptomatic (approximately 70%) or may have minimal symptoms, including dysuria, mild abdominal pain, or a vaginal discharge. Prepubertal girls may have vaginitis. At least 30% of persons with gonococcal cervicitis, urethritis, proctitis, or epididymitis have a concomitant *C. trachomatis* infection.

Chlamydia infection usually is diagnosed by PCR tests, using ligase chain reaction and transcription-mediated amplification, of cervical, urethral, and early morning first-voided urine specimens. Amplification tests have supplanted less sensitive culture and ELISA tests. Because of false-positive results, only culture should be used for legal purposes to confirm *C. trachomatis* infection in cases of suspected sexual abuse.

Treatment regimens should be effective against *C. trachomatis* and *N. gonorrhoeae* because of the high frequency of concomitant infection. A single oral dose of azithromycin (1 g) or doxycycline for 7 days is recommended, which can be combined with a single oral dose of cefixime (400 mg) to treat concomitant gonorrhea infection. Alternative regimens include erythromycin and, in persons 18 years old and older, ofloxacin and levofloxacin for 7 days. Sexual partners should be notified and treated.

SYPHILIS (*TREPONEMA PALLIDUM*)

Syphilis is caused by *T. pallidum,* a long, slender, coiled spirochete. It cannot be cultivated routinely in vitro, but can be observed by dark-field microscopy. Untreated infection progresses through several clinical stages (see Table 116-2). **Primary syphilis** is manifested as a single, painless genital ulcer, or **chancre**, usually on the genitalia that appears 3 to 6 weeks after inoculation. **Secondary syphilis** follows 6 to 8 weeks later and is manifested as fever, generalized lymphadenopathy, and a disseminated maculopapular rash that also is present on the palms and soles. Plaque-like skin lesions, **condylomata lata**, and mucous membrane lesions also occur and are infectious. **Tertiary** syphilis is a slowly progressive disease that involves the cardiovascular, neurologic, and musculoskeletal systems and is not seen in children. **Latent syphilis** is asymptomatic infection that is detected by serologic testing. **Early latent syphilis** indicates acquisition within the preceding year; all other cases of latent syphilis are either **late latent syphilis** or designated **latent syphilis of unknown duration**.

The diagnosis of syphilis is based on serologic testing. **Nontreponemal antibody tests**, the **Venereal Disease Research Laboratory (VDRL) test**, and the **rapid plasma reagin test** are screening tests and can be quantified as titers increase with increasing duration of infection and decrease in response to therapy. A nonquantitative VDRL test can be performed on CSF, but is insensitive. Rheumatic disease and other infectious diseases may cause biologic false-positive results. Confirmatory, specific **treponemal antibody tests**, the **microhemagglutination assay–*T. pallidum*** and **fluorescent treponemal antibody-absorption**, are more specific and are used to confirm the diagnosis of syphilis. These tests usually remain positive for life even if the infection is treated and cured. Dark-field examination of chancres, mucous membranes, or cutaneous lesions may reveal motile organisms.

The **treatment** of choice for all stages of syphilis is penicillin G. Primary syphilis, secondary syphilis, and early latent syphilis is treated with a single IM dose of benzathine penicillin G. Tertiary syphilis, late latent syphilis, and latent syphilis of unknown duration is treated with three doses at 1-week intervals. Neurosyphilis is treated with IV aqueous crystalline penicillin G for 10 to 14 days. A systemic, febrile **Jarisch-Herxheimer reaction** occurs in 15% to 20% of syphilitic patients treated with penicillin.

HERPES SIMPLEX VIRUS INFECTION

HSV-1 and HSV-2 are large, double-stranded DNA viruses of the herpesvirus family that have a linear genome contained within an icosahedral capsid. There is significant DNA homology between types 1 and 2. The virus initially infects mucosal surfaces and enters cutaneous neurons, where it migrates along the axons to the sensory ganglia. As viral replication occurs in the ganglia, infectious virus moves down the axon to infect and destroy the epithelial cells. Infection may disseminate to other organs in immunocompromised patients. Virus latency is maintained in the ganglia, where it undergoes periodic reactivation and replication triggered by undefined events. Although either virus can be found in any site, nongenital type 1 (HSV-1) more commonly occurs above the waist (CNS, eyes, mouth), and genital type 2 (HSV-2) more commonly involves the genitalia and skin below the waist. Reinfection can occur with exposure to the other type or even a second strain of the same type.

Genital herpes is characterized by painful, multiple, grouped vesicles or ulcerative and crusted external genital lesions on an erythematous base (see Table 116–2). In females, the cervix also is involved. Primary illness lasts 10 to 20 days. Primary genital herpes also may include regional lymphadenopathy, discharge, and dysuria. Recurrences occur in 50% to 80% of patients with symptomatic primary infection. Some primary and many secondary lesions are asymptomatic. Secondary, recurrent, or reactivation eruptions are not as dramatic and are not associated with systemic symptoms. In primary herpes simplex infection, viral shedding lasts 10 to 14 days, and vesicles and ulcers resolve in 16 to 20 days. In recurrent disease, often with several episodes annually, virus shedding lasts for less than 7 days, and vesicles resolve in 8 to 10 days. Many persons experience five to eight recurrences per year.

Viral cultures show cytopathic effect in 2 to 5 days. The diagnosis is suggested by a Tzanck smear or Papanicolaou smear showing characteristic multinucleated giant cells with intranuclear inclusions. Latency develops as the virus becomes dormant in the sacral nerve ganglion. Serologic testing is useful only for primary infection, to show seroconversion between acute and convalescent sera. There is much overlap between types 1 and 2 in serologic tests for HSV. Titers are not helpful in guiding management of recurrences.

Oral acyclovir, famciclovir, and valacyclovir are effective **treatments** in reducing the severity and duration of symptoms in primary cases and may reduce recurrences. Once-daily suppressive therapy reduces the frequency of genital herpes recurrences by 70% to 80% among patients who have frequent recurrences (more than six recurrences per year). Local hygiene and sitz baths may relieve some discomfort. The use of condoms provides some protection against sexual transmission of HSV.

TRICHOMONIASIS (*TRICHOMONAS VAGINALIS*)

Trichomoniasis is caused by the protozoan *T. vaginalis*. It often is associated with other STIs, such as gonorrhea and *Chlamydia*. Infected males either are asymptomatic or have nongonococcal urethritis. Infected females have vaginitis with thin, malodorous, frothy yellow-green discharge with vulvar irritation and cervical "strawberry hemorrhages" (see Table 116–3). The diagnosis is based on visualization of motile, flagellated protozoans in the urine or in a saline wet mount, which has a sensitivity of only 60% to 70%. Culture is the most sensitive method of diagnosis. Single-dose **treatment** of both sexual partners with oral metronidazole (2 g) is recommended.

GENITAL WARTS (HUMAN PAPILLOMAVIRUSES)

HPV infections, the cause of genital warts (**condylomata acuminata**), may be the most common STI; most HPV infections are asymptomatic or subclinical. Visible genital warts are associated with HPV types 6 or 11. HPV types 16, 18, 31, 33, and 35 are strongly associated with cervical neoplasia. There is no evidence that the development of symptomatic warts adds to the risk of cancer, or that the treatment or warts, which does not eradicate the virus, reduces the risk.

Genital warts can occur on the squamous epithelium or mucous membranes of the genital and perineal structures of females and males (see Table 116–4). Genital warts are usually multiple, firm, gray-to-pink excrescences. Untreated genital warts may remain unchanged, increase in size or number, or resolve spontaneously. They can become tender if macerated or secondarily infected. The diagnosis usually is established by appearance without biopsy. The differential diagnosis of genital warts includes condylomata lata (secondary syphilis) and tumors.

The goal of **treatment** is removal of symptomatic warts to induce wart-free periods. On cornified skin, patient-applied therapies include podofilox solution or gel or imiquimod cream. Provider-applied therapies include cryotherapy with liquid nitrogen or cryoprobe, topical podophyllin resin, and trichloroacetic acid or dichloroacetic acid, all of which can be applied until the lesions regress. An alternative is surgical removal by tangential scissor excision, tangential shave excision, curettage, or electrosurgery. Intralesional interferon and laser surgery also have been effective. Factors that may influence selection of treatment include wart number, wart size, anatomic sites of wart, wart morphology, patient preference, cost of treatment, convenience, adverse effects, and provider experience. Recurrences after treatment are common and are commonly asymptomatic.

PUBIC LICE (*PHTHIRUS PUBIS*)

Pubic lice, or pediculosis pubis, are caused by infestation with *Phthirus pubis,* the **pubic crab louse**. The louse is predominantly sexually transmitted and lives out its life cycle on pubic hair, where it causes characteristic, intense pruritus (see Table 116–4). Erythematous papules and egg cases (nits) are not seen before puberty. **Treatment** consists of education regarding personal and environmental hygiene and the application of an appropriate pediculicide, such as permethrin 1% cream, lindane 1% shampoo, or pyrethrins with piperonyl butoxide. Bedding and clothing should be decontaminated (machine washed and machine dried using the heat cycle or dry cleaned) or removed from body contact for at least 72 hours.

CHAPTER **117**

Osteomyelitis

ETIOLOGY

Syndromes of pediatric osteomyelitis include acute hematogenous osteomyelitis, which is accompanied by bacteremia; subacute focal disease, which usually follows local inoculation by penetrating trauma and is not associated with systemic symptoms; and chronic osteomyelitis, which is the result of an untreated or inadequately treated bone infection. In children beyond the newborn period and without hemoglobinopathies, bone infections occur almost exclusively in the metaphysis. Sluggish blood flow through tortuous vascular loops unique to this site in long bones is a possible explanation for this phenomenon. Preceding nonpenetrating trauma often is reported and may lead to local bone injury that predisposes to infection. Bone infections in children with sickle cell disease occur in the diaphyseal portion of the long bones, probably as a consequence of antecedent focal infarction. In children younger than 1 year old, the capillaries perforate the epiphyseal growth plate, permitting spread of infection across the epiphysis that can lead to suppurative arthritis (Fig. 117–1A). In older children, the infection is contained in the metaphysis because the vessels no longer cross the epiphyseal plate (see Fig. 117–1B).

S. aureus is responsible for most skeletal infections (Table 117 1). Group B streptococcus and *S. aureus* are major causes in neonates. Sickle cell disease and other hemoglobinopathies predispose to osteomyelitis caused by *Salmonella* and *S. aureus*. *Pasteurella multocida* osteomyelitis usually follows cat or dog bites. Conjugate vaccine has reduced greatly the incidence of Hib

TABLE 117–1. Infectious Causes of Acute Osteomyelitis in Children Beyond the Neonatal Period

Infectious Organism	Frequency (%)
Staphylococcus aureus	25-60
Haemophilus influenzae type b*	4-12
Streptococcus pneumoniae	2-5
Group A streptococcus	2-4
Mycobacterium tuberculosis	<1
Neisseria meningitidis	<1
Salmonella†	<1
None identified	10-15

*The incidence of invasive infections caused by *H. influenzae* type b has diminished greatly since introduction of conjugate vaccine.
†Especially in persons with hemoglobinopathies.

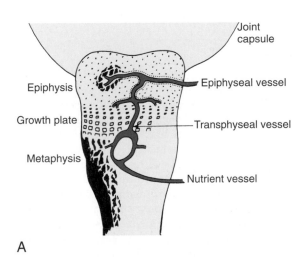

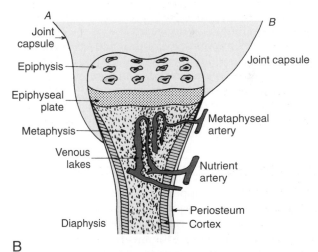

Figure 117–1

A, Major structures of the bone of an infant before maturation of the epiphyseal growth plate. Note the transphyseal vessel, which connects the vascular supply of the epiphysis and metaphysis, facilitating spread of infection between these two areas. **B,** Major structures of the bone of a child. Joint capsule *A* inserts below the epiphyseal growth plate, as in the hip, elbow, ankle, and shoulder. Rupture of a metaphyseal abscess in these bones is likely to produce pyarthrosis. Joint capsule *B* inserts at the epiphyseal growth plate, as in other tubular bones. Rupture of a metaphyseal abscess in these bones is likely to lead to a subperiosteal abscess, but seldom to an associated pyarthrosis. (From Gutman LT: Acute, subacute, and chronic osteomyelitis and pyogenic arthritis in children: Curr Probl Pediatr 15:6, 1985.)

infections; similar reductions of *S. pneumoniae* infections are anticipated with the conjugate pneumococcal vaccine.

Subacute focal bone infections caused by *P. aeruginosa* and *S. aureus* usually occur in ambulatory persons who sustain **puncture wounds** of the foot. *Pseudomonas* **chondritis** is associated strongly with puncture wounds through sneakers, which harbor *Pseudomonas* in the foam insole. *S. aureus* is the most common cause of chronic osteomyelitis. **Multifocal recurrent osteomyelitis** is a poorly understood syndrome characterized by recurrent episodes of fever, bone pain, and radiographic findings of osteomyelitis; no pathogen has been confirmed as the cause of this syndrome.

EPIDEMIOLOGY

Osteomyelitis may occur at any age, but is most common in children 3 to 12 years old. It affects boys twice as frequently as girls. Hematogenous osteomyelitis is the most common form in infants and children. Osteomyelitis from penetrating trauma or peripheral vascular disease is more common in adults. Osteomyelitis from penetrating injuries of the foot is more common in summer months when children are outdoors and exploring.

CLINICAL MANIFESTATIONS

The most common presenting complaints are focal pain, exquisite point tenderness over the bone, warmth, erythema, swelling, and decreased use of the affected extremity. Fever, anorexia, irritability, and lethargy may accompany the focal findings. Weight bearing and active and passive motion are refused, which mimics paralysis (**pseudoparalysis**). Muscle spasm may make the extremity difficult to examine. The adjacent joint space may be involved in young children (see Chapter 118).

Usually only one bone is involved. The femur, tibia, or humerus is affected in two thirds of patients. Infections of the bones of the hands or feet account for an additional 15% of cases. Flat bone infections, including the pelvis, account for approximately 10% of cases. Vertebral osteomyelitis is notable for an insidious onset, vague symptoms, backache, occasional spinal cord compression, and usually little associated fever or systemic toxicity. Patients with osteomyelitis of the pelvis may present with limp; vague abdominal, hip, groin, or thigh pain; and fever.

LABORATORY AND IMAGING STUDIES

The presence of leukocytosis is inconsistent. Elevated acute phase reactants, ESR and CRP, are sensitive but nonspecific findings of osteomyelitis. Serial determinations of ESR and CRP are helpful in monitoring the course of the illness and response to treatment. Direct subperiosteal or metaphyseal needle aspiration is the definitive procedure for establishing the diagnosis of osteomyelitis. Identification of bacteria in aspirated material by Gram stain can establish the diagnosis within hours of clinical presentation. Surgical drainage may be needed after bone aspiration.

Plain radiographs are a useful initial study (Fig. 117–2). The earliest radiographic finding of acute systemic osteomyelitis, at about 9 days, is **loss of the periosteal fat line**. **Periosteal elevation** and **periosteal destruction** are later findings. **Brodie abscess** is a subacute intraosseous abscess that does not drain into the subperiosteal space and is classically located in the distal tibia. **Sequestra**, or portions of avascular bone that have separated from adjacent bone, frequently are covered with a thickened sheath, or an **involucrum**, which are hallmarks of chronic osteomyelitis.

Radionuclide scanning for osteomyelitis has largely been supplanted by MRI, which is sensitive to the inflammatory changes in the marrow even during the earliest stages of osteomyelitis. Technetium-99m bone scans are useful for evaluating multifocal disease. Gallium-67 scans are often positive if the technetium-99m bone scan is negative.

DIFFERENTIAL DIAGNOSIS

Osteomyelitis must be differentiated from infectious arthritis (see Chapter 118), cellulitis, fasciitis, discitis, trauma, juvenile rheumatoid arthritis, and malignancy.

TREATMENT

Initial antibiotic therapy for osteomyelitis is based on knowledge of the likely organism for the age of the child, Gram stain of bone aspirate, and associated diseases (Table 117–2). Initial therapy should be with an antibiotic, such as oxacillin, nafcillin, or clindamycin. Vancomycin should be used if methicillin-resistant *S. aureus* is suspected. For patients with sickle cell disease, initial therapy should include an antibiotic such as cefotaxime and ceftriaxone with activity against *Salmonella*.

There is usually a response to IV antibiotics within 48 hours. Lack of improvement in fever and pain after 48 hours indicates that surgical drainage may be necessary or that an unusual pathogen may be present. Surgical drainage is indicated if **sequestrum** is present, the disease is chronic or atypical, the hip joint is involved, or spinal cord compression is present. Antibiotics are administered for a minimum of 4 to 6 weeks. After initial inpatient treatment and a good clinical response, including decreases in CRP or ESR, consideration may be given for home therapy with IV antibiotics or oral antibiotics, if adherence can be ensured.

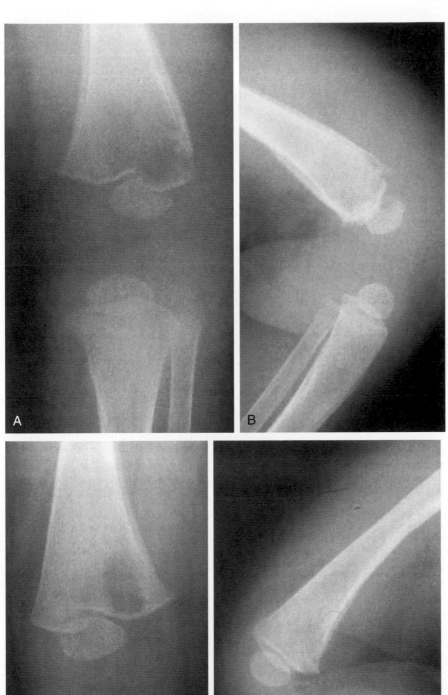

Figure 117-2

Multifocal acute osteomyelitis in a 3-week-old infant with multiple joint swelling and generalized malaise. Frontal **(A)** and lateral **(B)** radiographs of the left knee show focal destruction of the distal femoral metaphysis with periosteal reaction and generalized soft tissue swelling. Frontal **(C)** and lateral **(D)** views of the right knee show an area of focal bone destruction at the distal femoral metaphysis with periosteal reaction and medial soft tissue swelling. Needle aspiration of multiple sites revealed *Staphylococcus aureus*. (From Moffett KS, Aronoff SC: Osteomyelitis. In Jenson HB, Baltimore RS [eds]: Pediatric Infectious Diseases: Principles and Practice, 2nd ed. Philadelphia, WB Saunders, 2002, p 1038.)

TABLE 117–2.   Recommended Antibiotic Therapy for Osteomyelitis in Children

Common Pathogens	Recommended Treatment
Acute Hematogenous Osteomyelitis	
Staphylococcus aureus	Nafcillin (*or* oxacillin) *or* cefazolin
Streptococcus pneumoniae	Penicillin G *or* ceftriaxone (*or* cefotaxime) *or* vancomycin (based on susceptibilities)
Group A streptococcus	Penicillin G
Haemophilus influenzae type b*	Ceftriaxone (*or* cefotaxime)
Subacute Focal Osteomyelitis	
Pseudomonas aeruginosa (puncture wound osteomyelitis)	Ceftazidime *or* piperacillin-tazobactam *and* an aminoglycoside
S. aureus	Nafcillin (*or* oxacillin) *or* cefazolin

*The incidence of invasive infections caused by *H. influenzae* type b has diminished greatly since introduction of conjugate vaccine.

COMPLICATIONS

Complications of acute osteomyelitis are uncommon and usually arise because of inadequate or delayed therapy. Young children are more likely to have spread of infection across the epiphysis, leading to suppurative arthritis (see Chapter 118). Vascular insufficiency, which affects delivery of antibiotics, and trauma are associated with higher rates of complications.

PROGNOSIS

Hematogenous osteomyelitis has an excellent prognosis if treated promptly and if surgical drainage is performed when appropriate. The poorest outcome is in neonates and in infants with involvement of the hip or shoulder joints (see Chapter 118). Recurrent infection occurs in approximately 4% of acute infections despite adequate therapy, and approximately 25% of these fail to respond to extensive surgical débridement and prolonged antimicrobial therapy, ultimately resulting in bone loss, sinus tract formation, and occasionally amputation. Sequelae related to retarded growth are even more common among neonates.

PREVENTION

There are no effective means to prevent hematogenous *S. aureus* osteomyelitis. Universal immunization of infants with conjugate Hib vaccine has practically eliminated serious bacterial infections from this organism, including bone and joint infections. Because the serotypes of *S. pneumoniae* causing joint infections are represented in the conjugate pneumococcal vaccine, the incidence of pneumococcal osteomyelitis should decrease with widespread immunization.

Children with puncture wounds to the foot should receive prompt irrigation, cleansing, débridement, removal of any visible foreign body or debris, and tetanus prophylaxis. The value of oral prophylactic antibiotics for preventing osteomyelitis after penetrating injury is unknown. An oral cephalosporin or amoxicillin-clavulanate may be considered and provides some coverage for *S. aureus*. An oral fluoroquinolone, which also would provide coverage for *P. aeruginosa,* may be an alternative for persons 18 years old or older, especially after puncture wounds of the foot through a sneaker.

CHAPTER 118
Infectious Arthritis

ETIOLOGY

Infectious arthritis, or **suppurative or septic arthritis**, is a serious bacterial infection of the joint space that in children results from hematogenous dissemination of bacteria. Infectious arthritis less often results from contiguous spread of infection from surrounding soft tissues or direct inoculation into the joint (penetrating trauma); spread of osteomyelitis is common and occurs through transphyseal vessels to the epiphysis with rupture into the joint space or rupture of a metaphyseal abscess in the joints where the joint capsule inserts below the epiphysis (see Fig. 117–1). The bacteria causing infectious arthritis are similar to bacteria causing osteomyelitis (Table 118–1). Lyme disease also may cause arthritis as part of the late disease (see Chapter 122).

The arthritis of **disseminated gonococcal infections** includes reactive and suppurative forms of arthritis in early and late gonococcal disease. With untreated genital gonococcal infection, gonococcemia may occur and manifests as a febrile illness with polyarticular, symmetric arthritis and rash, known as the **arthritis-dermatitis syndrome**. Bacterial cultures of the synovium are sterile at this stage despite a relatively high prevalence of bacteremia. Monarticular arthritis of large, weight-bearing joints develops days to weeks later. Cultures of affected synovial fluid at this stage often yield the pathogen.

Reactive arthritis is immune-mediated synovial inflammation that follows a bacterial or viral infection. Reactive arthritis of the hip joints in children 3 to 6

TABLE 118–1.   Infectious Causes of Arthritis

Common	Uncommon
Young Infants (<2 mo)	
Group B streptococcus	*Neisseria gonorrhoeae*
Staphylococcus aureus	*Candida*
Escherichia coli	
Klebsiella pneumoniae	
Older Infants and Children (2 mo to adulthood)	
Streptococcus pneumoniae	Anaerobic bacteria
S. aureus	*Pseudomonas aeruginosa*
Haemophilus influenzae type b*	Group A streptococcus
Kingella kingae	Enterobacteriaceae
N. gonorrhoeae	*Mycobacterium tuberculosis*
Borrelia burgdorferi (Lyme disease)	
Reactive Arthritis	
Yersinia enterocolitica	
Campylobacter jejuni	
Shigella flexneri	
Salmonella	
Group A streptococcus	
Neisseria meningitidis	
Coccidioides immitis	
Rubella virus	

*The incidence of invasive infections caused by *H. influenzae* type b has diminished greatly since introduction of conjugate vaccine.

years old is known as **toxic synovitis** or **transient synovitis** of the hip (see Chapter 198).

EPIDEMIOLOGY

Infectious arthritis occurs most commonly in children younger than 5 years old and adolescents.

CLINICAL MANIFESTATIONS

The typical features of suppurative arthritis include erythema, warmth, swelling, and tenderness over the affected joint, with a palpable effusion and decreased range of movement. The onset may be sudden or insidious, with symptoms noted only when the joint is moved, such as during a diaper change, or if parents become aware of decreased voluntary movement (**pseudoparalysis**) of a joint or limb. Toddlers may have a limp. In septic arthritis of the hip, the lower limb may be preferentially held in external rotation and flexion to minimize pain from pressure on the joint capsule. Similarly, the knee and elbow joints usually are held in flexion. The joints of the lower extremity are most often involved: the knees in 40% of cases, the hips in 20%, and the ankles in 14%. Small joints, such as those of the hand, usually are involved after penetrating trauma and closed fist injuries.

Minor genital tract symptoms that have been ignored may precede development of the early arthritis-dermatitis syndrome associated with disseminated gonococcal infection. A history of febrile illness antedating the development of monarticular arthritis characterizes late gonococcal arthritis.

Reactive arthritis is typically symmetric and polyarticular and usually involves the large joints, especially the hips. Patients may have had a preceding episode of gastroenteritis or urethritis. Urethritis may appear with the arthritis.

LABORATORY AND IMAGING STUDIES

Leukocytosis and an elevated ESR and CRP are common. Arthrocentesis and analysis of the effusion is the test of choice for rapid diagnosis of infectious arthritis (Table 118–2). Adolescents with acute infectious arthritis should have urethral, cervical, rectal, and pharyngeal examination and cultures for *N. gonorrhoeae* (see Chapter 116).

Blood or joint cultures are positive in 70% to 85% of cases. Joint fluid that exhibits the characteristics of pyogenic infection may not reveal bacterial pathogens in 30% of patients, even in the absence of preceding antibiotic therapy, because of the bacteriostatic effects of synovial fluid. Gram stain, acid-fast stain, and KOH preparation for fungi should be performed and are often informative even if the cultures are negative.

Plain radiographs typically add little information to the physical findings. Radiographs may show swelling of the joint capsule, a widened joint space, and displacement of adjacent normal fat lines. Radionuclide scans are of limited use, although technetium-99m bone scans may be helpful to exclude concurrent bone infection, either adjacent or distant from the infected joint. Ultrasound is especially useful for identifying joint effusions and is the diagnostic procedure of choice for evaluation of suppurative infections of the hip. MRI is useful in distinguishing joint infections from cellulitis or deep abscesses.

DIFFERENTIAL DIAGNOSIS

The differential diagnosis of infectious arthritis in infants, children, and adolescents includes other infectious diseases, rheumatoid disorders, rheumatic fever, and trauma. Suppurative arthritis must be distinguished from Lyme disease, osteomyelitis, suppurative bursitis, fasciitis, myositis, cellulitis, and soft tissue abscesses. Psoas muscle abscess often presents with fever and pain on hip flexion and rotation. Juvenile rheuma-

TABLE 118–2. Synovial Fluid Findings in Various Joint Diseases

Condition	Appearance	White Blood Cell Count (µg/L)	Polymorphonuclear Cells (%)	Mucin Clot	Synovial Fluid-to-Blood Glucose Difference (mg/dL)	Comment
Normal	Clear, yellow	0-200 (200)*	<10	Good	No difference	—
Trauma	Clear, turbid, or hemorrhagic	50-4,000 (600)	<30	Good	No difference	Common in hemophilia
Systemic lupus erythematosus	Clear or slightly turbid	0-9,000 (3,000)	<20	Good to fair	No difference	LE cell positive, complement decreased
Rheumatoid arthritis reactive arthritis (Reiter syndrome, inflammatory bowel disease)	Turbid	250-80,000 (19,000)	>70	Poor	30	Decreased complement
Infectious Pyogenic infection	Turbid	10,000-250,000 (80,000)	>90	Poor	50-90	Positive culture, positive Gram stain
Tuberculosis	Turbid	2,500-100,000 (20,000)	>60	Poor	40-70	Positive culture, PPD, and acid-fast stain
Lyme arthritis	Turbid	500-100,000 (20,000)	>60	Poor	70	History of tick bite or erythema chronicum migrans

LE, lupus erythematosus; PPD, purified protein derivative of tuberculin.
*Average in parentheses.

toid arthritis, Kawasaki syndrome, Henoch-Schönlein purpura, other rheumatoid disorders, and Crohn disease must be differentiated from infectious arthritis. In most of these diseases, the presence of symmetric or multiple joint involvement often excludes infectious arthritis. **Suppurative bursitis** with *S. aureus* occurs most often in older boys and men and is usually a consequence of trauma or, less commonly, a complication of bacteremia.

TREATMENT

Initial antibiotic therapy for infectious arthritis is based on knowledge of the likely organism for the age of the child and the Gram stain of joint fluid. Suppurative arthritis of the hip joint especially or shoulder joint necessitates prompt surgical drainage. Because these joints are ball-and-socket joints with insertion of the joint capsule below the epiphysis, the increased pressure in the joint space can affect adversely the vascular supply to the head of the femur or humerus, leading to ischemic injury and necrosis. Infections of the knee may be treated with repeated arthrocenteses in addition to appropriate parenteral antibiotics.

Several antimicrobial agents provide adequate antibiotic levels in joint spaces (Table 118–3). Initial therapy for neonates should include antibiotics, such as nafcillin and cefotaxime, with activity against *S. aureus*, group B streptococcus, and aerobic gram-negative rods. Initial therapy for children 3 months to 5 years old should include antibiotics such as cefotaxime or ampicillin-sulbactam with activity against *S. aureus* and Hib. Confirmed methicillin-susceptible *S. aureus* infections are treated with nafcillin or oxacillin, and methicillin-resistant *S. aureus* infections are treated with vancomycin or clindamycin if susceptible.

The duration of therapy depends on clinical resolution of fever and pain and decline of the ESR. Infection with virulent organisms, such as *S. aureus,* usually

TABLE 118–3. Recommended Antibiotic Therapy for Infectious Arthritis in Children

	Common Pathogens	Recommended Treatment
Infants (<2 mo)	Group B streptococcus	Ampicillin *plus* aminoglycoside
	Escherichia coli	Cefotaxime (*or* ceftriaxone) *plus* aminoglycoside
	Klebsiella pneumoniae	Cefotaxime (*or* ceftriaxone) *plus* aminoglycoside
	Staphylococcus aureus	Nafcillin (*or* oxacillin), vancomycin
Older infants and children	*S. aureus*	Nafcillin (*or* oxacillin), vancomycin
	Streptococcus pneumoniae	Penicillin G *or* cefotaxime (*or* ceftriaxone) *or* vancomycin (based on susceptibilities)
	Group A streptococcus	Penicillin G
	Kingella kingae	Penicillin G *or* nafcillin (*or* oxacillin)
	Haemophilus influenzae type b*	Cefuroxime (*or* cefotaxime *or* ceftriaxone)
Disseminated gonococcal infection	*Neisseria gonorrhoeae*	Ceftriaxone

*The incidence of invasive infections caused by *H. influenzae* type b has diminished greatly since introduction of conjugate vaccine.

necessitates treatment for at least 21 days. Treatment may be changed to oral antibiotics if adherence can be ensured. Oral agents with excellent activity against *S. aureus* that are often used to complete therapy include cephalexin, amoxicillin-clavulanate, dicloxacillin, clindamycin, and ciprofloxacin (in persons ≥18 years old).

COMPLICATIONS

The major complications of neonatal, childhood, and gonococcal arthritis are loss of joint function resulting from damage to the articular surface. The highest incidence of these complications occurs with hip infections, presumably as a result of ischemic injury to the head of the femur. *As a result*, prompt open drainage of infected hip joints and often shoulder joints is recommended. The high incidence of concurrent suppurative arthritis with adjacent osteomyelitis in neonates places the epiphyseal growth plate at high risk for growth abnormalities.

PROGNOSIS

The prognosis for the common forms of infectious arthritis encountered in infants and children is excellent. The poorest outcome is for infectious arthritis of the hip or shoulder. Neonates with concomitant osteomyelitis have an approximately 40% to 50% likelihood of growth disturbances with loss of longitudinal bone growth and ultimate limb shortening.

PREVENTION

There are no effective means to prevent hematogenous *S. aureus* arthritis. Universal immunization of infants with conjugate Hib vaccine has practically eliminated

serious bacterial infections from this organism, including bone and joint infections. Because the serotypes of *S. pneumoniae* causing joint infections are represented in the conjugate pneumococcal vaccine, the incidence of pneumococcal joint infections should decrease with widespread immunization.

CHAPTER 119
Ocular Infections

ETIOLOGY

Acute conjunctivitis, or **red eye**, is usually a bacterial or viral infection of the eye characterized by a rapid onset of symptoms that persists for a few days. The most common causes of bacterial conjunctivitis are nontypable *H. influenzae*, *S. pneumoniae*, and *M. catarrhalis* (Table 119–1). Other causes include *N. gonorrhoeae* and *P. aeruginosa*, which is associated with extended-wear soft contact lenses. Viral conjunctivitis most commonly is caused by adenoviruses, which are the cause of epidemic keratoconjunctivitis, and less frequently by coxsackieviruses and other enteroviruses. **Keratitis**, or inflammation of the cornea, is not commonly associated with conjunctivitis, but does occur with *N. gonorrhoeae*, HSV, and adenovirus infections.

Neonatal conjunctivitis, or **ophthalmia neonatorum**, is purulent conjunctivitis during the first 10 days of life, usually acquired during birth. The common causes of neonatal conjunctivitis, in order of decreasing prevalence, are silver nitrate if used for gonococcal prophylaxis, *C. trachomatis*, common bacterial causes of conjunctivitis, *E. coli*, other gram-negative enteric

TABLE 119–1.   Manifestations of Acute Conjunctivitis in Children

	Common Organisms	
	Bacterial	*Viral*
	Haemophilus influenzae (usually nontypable)	Adenoviruses type 8, 19
	Streptococcus pneumoniae	Enteroviruses
	Moraxella catarrhalis	Herpes simplex virus
Incubation	24-72 hr	1-14 days
Symptoms		
Photophobia	Mild	Moderate to severe
Blurred vision	Common with discharge	If keratitis is present
Foreign body sensation	Unusual	Yes
Signs		
Discharge	Purulent discharge	Watery discharge
Palpebral reaction	Papillary response	Follicular response
Preauricular lymph node	Unusual for acute (<10%)	More common (20%)
Chemosis	Moderate	Mild
Hemorrhagic conjunctivae	Occasionally with *Streptococcus* or *Haemophilus*	Frequent with enteroviruses
Treatment (topical)	Polymyxin B-trimethoprim *or* sulfacetamide 10% *or* erythromycin	Adenovirus: self-limited Herpes simplex virus: trifluridine 1% solution *or* vidarabine 3% ointment; ophthalmologic consultation
End of contagious period	24 hr after start of effective treatment	7 days after onset of symptoms

bacilli, and *N. gonorrhoeae*. Neonatal conjunctivitis also can occur as a part of perinatal HSV infection.

EPIDEMIOLOGY

Conjunctivitis is common in young children, especially if in contact with other children with conjunctivitis. Predisposing factors for bacterial infection include nasolacrimal duct obstruction, sinus disease, ear infection, and allergic children who rub their eyes frequently. Conjunctivitis occurs in 1% to 12% of neonates. A mild to moderate chemical conjunctivitis commonly is present from 24 to 48 hours of age in most newborns who receive ophthalmic silver nitrate as gonococcal prophylaxis. Neonatal acquisition of *C. trachomatis* occurs in approximately 50% of infants born vaginally to infected mothers. In infants with perinatal acquisition of *C. trachomatis,* the risk of chlamydial conjunctivitis, also called **inclusion conjunctivitis**, is 25% to 50% and of chlamydial pneumonia is 5% to 20%.

CLINICAL MANIFESTATIONS

Symptoms include redness, discharge, matted eyelids, and mild photophobia. Physical examination findings include chemosis, injection of the conjunctiva, and edema of the eyelids. Corneal involvement suggests

gonococcal or herpetic infection. Herpetic corneal lesions appear as dendritic or ameboid ulcers or, more commonly, in recurrent infection, as a deep keratitis. Unilateral conjunctivitis with ipsilateral otitis media is often caused by nontypable *H. influenzae*.

The timing and manifestations of neonatal conjunctivitis are helpful in identifying the cause (Table 119–2). *N. gonorrhoeae* causes severe conjunctivitis with profuse purulent discharge. Chlamydial conjunctivitis may appear 3 days to 6 weeks after delivery, but usually occurs in the second week of life. There is mild to moderate inflammation with purulent discharge issuing from one or both eyes.

LABORATORY AND IMAGING STUDIES

Cultures are not routinely obtained because bacterial conjunctivitis is usually self-limited or responds quickly to antibiotic treatment. Gram stain and culture of neonatal conjunctivitis must be obtained, however, if gonococcal conjunctivitis is suspected.

DIFFERENTIAL DIAGNOSIS

Distinguishing bacterial from viral conjunctivitis by presentation and appearance is difficult (see Table 119–1). Vesicular lid lesions, if present, suggest the

TABLE 119–2.   Clinical Manifestations and Treatment of Neonatal Conjunctivitis

Organism	Percentage of Cases	Discharge and External Examination	Typical Age at Onset	Diagnosis	Associated Manifestations	Treatment
Chemical: silver nitrate (1%)	Variable, depending on use of silver nitrate	Watery discharge	1-3 days	No organisms on smear or culture		None
Neisseria gonorrhoeae	<1%	Copious, purulent discharge; severe swelling of lids and conjunctivae; corneal involvement common; risk for perforation and corneal scar	1-7 days	Gram stain (gram-negative intracellular diplococci); culture on chocolate agar	May be associated with disseminated gonococcal infection	Ceftriaxone
Bacterial: *Staphylococcus, Streptococcus, Pseudomonas*	30-50%	Purulent moderate discharge; mild lid and conjunctival swelling; corneal involvement with risk for perforation	2-7 days	Gram stain; culture on blood agar		Topical therapy
Chlamydia trachomatis (inclusion conjunctivitis)	2-40%	Scant discharge; mild swelling; hyperemia; follicular response; late corneal staining	4-19 days	Giemsa stain of scraping (purple intracytoplasmic inclusions near nucleus); direct determination with direct immunofluorescent antibody test; direct determination with PCR	May presage *C. trachomatis* pneumonia (at 3 wk-3 mo of age)	Erythromycin (oral)
HSV	<1%	Clear or serosanguineous discharge; lid swelling; keratitis with cloudy cornea; dendrite formation	3 days-3 wk	Giemsa stain of scraping (multinucleate giant cells with intranuclear inclusions); viral culture; DIF	May be associated with disseminated perinatal HSV infection	Acyclovir IV for systemic involvement

DIF, direct immunofluorescence; HSV, herpes simplex virus; PCR, polymerase chain reaction.

diagnosis of HSV. The differential diagnosis of bacterial and viral conjunctivitis includes allergic conjunctivitis, chemical conjunctivitis (contaminated eye solutions), blepharitis, keratitis, contact lens use, foreign body, nasolacrimal duct obstruction, eye rubbing, corneal abrasion, Kawasaki syndrome, and anterior uveitis (iridocyclitis) associated with juvenile rheumatoid arthritis, Behçet disease, and inflammatory bowel disease (Table 119–3).

Blepharitis is associated with staphylococcal infections, seborrhea, and meibomian gland dysfunction.

The child complains of photophobia, burning, irritation, and a foreign body sensation that causes the child to rub the eyes. Eyelid hygiene with an **eyelid scrub** routine is the initial step in treatment.

Hordeola are acute suppurative nodular inflammatory lesions of the eyelids associated with pain and redness. **External hordeola** or **styes** occur on the anterior eyelid, in the Zeis glands, or in the lash follicles and usually are caused by staphylococci. **Internal hordeola** occur in the meibomian glands and may be infected with staphylococci or may be sterile. If the meibomian

TABLE 119–3. Differential Diagnosis of Ocular Infections

Condition	Etiology	Signs and Symptoms	Treatment
Bacterial conjunctivitis	*Haemophilus influenzae, Haemophilus aegyptius, Streptococcus pneumoniae Neisseria gonorrhoeae*	Mucopurulent unilateral or bilateral discharge, normal vision, photophobia Conjunctival injection and edema (chemosis); gritty sensation	Topical antibiotics, parenteral ceftriaxone for gonococcus, *H. influenzae*
Viral conjunctivitis	Adenovirus, ECHO virus, coxsackievirus	As above; may be hemorrhagic, unilateral	Self-limited
Neonatal conjunctivitis	*Chlamydia trachomatis,* gonococcus, chemical (silver nitrate), *Staphylococcus aureus*	Palpebral conjunctival follicle or papillae; as above	Ceftriaxone for gonococcus and oral erythromycin for *C. trachomatis*
Allergic conjunctivitis	Seasonal pollens or allergen exposure	Itching, incidence of bilateral chemosis (edema) greater than that of erythema, tarsal papillae	Antihistamines, steroids, cromolyn
Keratitis	Herpes simplex, adenovirus, *S. pneumoniae, S. aureus, Pseudomonas, Acanthamoeba,* chemicals	Severe pain, corneal swelling, clouding, limbus erythema, hypopyon, cataracts; contact lens history with amebic infection	Specific antibiotics for bacterial/fungal infections; keratoplasty, acyclovir for herpes
Endophthalmitis	*S. aureus, S. pneumoniae, Candida albicans,* associated surgery or trauma	Acute onset, pain, loss of vision, swelling, chemosis, redness; hypopyon and vitreous haze	Antibiotics
Anterior uveitis (iridocyclitis)	JRA, Reiter syndrome, sarcoidosis, Behçet disease, inflammatory bowel disease	Unilateral/bilateral; erythema, ciliary flush, irregular pupil, iris adhesions; pain, photophobia, small pupil, poor vision	Topical steroids, plus therapy for primary disease
Posterior uveitis (choroiditis)	Toxplasmosis, histoplasmosis, *Toxocara canis*	No signs of erythema, decreased vision	Specific therapy for pathogen
Episcleritis/scleritis	Idiopathic autoimmune disease (e.g., SLE, Henoch-Schönlein purpura)	Localized pain, intense erythema, unilateral; blood vessels bigger than in conjunctivitis; scleritis may cause globe perforation	Episcleritis is self-limiting; topical steroids for fast relief
Foreign body	Occupational or other exposure	Unilateral, red, gritty feeling; visible or microscopic size	Irrigation, removal; check for ulceration
Blepharitis	*S. aureus, Staphylococcus epidermidis,* seborrheic, blocked lacrimal duct; rarely molluscum contagiosum, *Phthirus pubis, Pediculus capitis*	Bilateral, irritation, itching, hyperemia, crusting, affecting lid margins	Topical antibiotics, warm compresses
Dacryocystitis	Obstructed lacrimal sac: *S. aureus, H. influenzae,* pneumococcus	Pain, tenderness, erythema and exudate in areas of lacrimal sac (inferomedial to inner canthus); tearing (epiphora); possible orbital cellulitis	Systemic, topical antibiotics; surgical drainage
Dacryoadenitis	*S. aureus, Streptococcus,* CMV, measles, EBV, enteroviruses; trauma, sarcoidosis, leukemia	Pain, tenderness, edema, erythema over gland area (upper temporal lid); fever, leukocytosis	Systemic antibiotics; drainage of orbital abscesses
Orbital cellulitis (postseptal cellulitis)	Paranasal sinusitis: *H. influenzae, S. aureus, S. pneumoniae,* streptococci Trauma: *S. aureus* Fungi: *Aspergillus, Mucor* if immunodeficient	Rhinorrhea, chemosis, vision loss, painful extraocular motion, proptosis, ophthalmoplegia, fever, lid edema, leukocytosis	Systemic antibiotics, drainage of orbital abscesses
Periorbital cellulitis (preseptal cellulitis)	Trauma: *S. aureus,* streptococci Bacteremia: pneumococcus, streptococci, *H. influenzae*	Cutaneous erythema, warmth, normal vision, minimal involvement of orbit; fever, leukocytosis, toxic appearance	Systemic antibiotics

CMV, cytomegalovirus; EBV, Epstein-Barr virus; JRA, juvenile rheumatoid arthritis; SLE, systemic lupus erythematosus.

gland becomes obstructed, the gland secretions accumulate, and a **chalazion** develops. Hordeola usually respond spontaneously to local treatment measures, but may recur.

Dacryocystitis is an infection or inflammation of the lacrimal sac, which is usually obstructed, and is most commonly caused by *S. aureus* or coagulase-negative staphylococci. A mucopurulent discharge can be expressed with gentle pressure on the nasolacrimal sac. Treatment usually requires probing of the nasolacrimal system to establish communication.

Endophthalmitis is an emergent, sight-threatening infection that usually follows trauma, surgery, or hematogenous spread from a distant focus. Causative organisms include coagulase-negative staphylococci, *S. aureus, S. pneumoniae, B. cereus,* and *Candida albicans.* Examination is difficult because of severe blepharospasm and extreme photophobia. A hypopyon and haze may be visible on examination.

TREATMENT

The lids should be treated as needed with warm compresses to remove the accumulated discharge. Acute bacterial conjunctivitis is frequently self-limited, but topical antibiotics significantly hasten resolution. Antibiotics are instilled between the eyelids four times a day until the discharge subsides, and the chemosis resolves. Recommended treatment includes topical ciprofloxacin solution, trimethoprim–polymyxin B solution, sulfacetamide 10% solution, and erythromycin ointment. Gonococcal conjunctivitis in adults is treated with a single IM dose of ceftriaxone (1 g).

The treatment of ophthalmia neonatorum depends on the cause (see Table 119–2). Gonococcal ophthalmia neonatorum is treated with a single dose of ceftriaxone (25 to 50 mg/kg intravenously or intramuscularly; maximum dose is 125 mg). This treatment also is recommended for newborns to mothers with untreated gonorrhea. The mother and infant should be tested for chlamydial infection. Chlamydial conjunctivitis is treated with oral erythromycin for 14 days, partly to reduce the risk of subsequent chlamydial pneumonia.

PROGNOSIS AND COMPLICATIONS

The prognosis for bacterial and viral conjunctivitis is excellent. The major complication is keratitis, which can lead to ulcerations and perforation. This complication is uncommon except with *N. gonorrhoeae* infection. Complications of neonatal conjunctivitis are uncommon except with *N. gonorrhoeae* and HSV infections. Chlamydial conjunctivitis may progress in infants to chlamydial pneumonia, which typically develops from 4 to 12 weeks of age (see Chapter 110).

PREVENTION

Careful hand washing is important to prevent spread of conjunctivitis. Bacterial conjunctivitis is considered contagious for 24 hours after initiating effective treatment. Children may return to school, but treatment measures must be continued until there is complete clinical resolution.

All infants should receive prophylaxis for gonococcal ophthalmia neonatorum. The traditional **Credé prophylaxis** of instilling silver nitrate 1% is used frequently, but usually causes a chemical conjunctivitis. Alternative methods are equally effective and less irritating and include a single application of erythromycin 0.5% ointment or tetracycline 1% ointment. Prophylaxis is administered to all newborns, whether delivered vaginally or by cesarean section, as soon as possible after delivery.

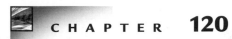

CHAPTER 120

Infection in the Immunocompromised Person

ETIOLOGY

Many diseases or their treatments adversely affect the immune system, including genetic immunodeficiencies, HIV infection and AIDS, cancer, stem cell and organ transplantation, and immunosuppressive drugs used to treat cancer, autoimmune diseases, and transplant patients. These patients are at significant risk of life-threatening infections from invasive **endogenous infection** from bacterial or fungal flora of the oropharynx and gastrointestinal tract, acquisition of **exogenous infection** from infected persons, and reactivation of latent virus until their marrow and immune function recover (Table 120–1).

Episodes of fever and **neutropenia**, defined as an **absolute neutrophil count** of less than 500/mm³ neutrophils and bands, are especially common in cancer and transplant patients. The evaluation of fever in immunocompromised persons differs from that in immunocompetent hosts. The types of infections often can be predicted by which component of the immune system is abnormal. The use of corticosteroids and potent immunosuppressive drugs that impair the activation of T cells increases the risk for pathogens that normally are controlled by T cell–mediated responses, such as *P. jirovecii* (*carinii*) and *T. gondii,* and intracellular pathogens, such as *Salmonella, Listeria,* and *Mycobacterium.*

TABLE 120–1.   Pathogens of Importance in Patients with Cancer

Bacteria	Fungi	Protozoa	Viruses
Bacteroides fragilis	Aspergillus	Cryptosporidium parvum	Adenoviruses
Campylobacter	Blastoschizomyces capitatus	Cyclospora cayetanensis	Cytomegalovirus
Clostridium difficile	Candida	Enterocytozoon bieneusi	Echoviruses
Clostridium septicum,	Chrysosporium	Giardia lamblia	Hepatitis A virus
Clostridium perfringens	Cryptococcus neoformans	Isospora belli	Herpes simplex viruses
Comamonas acidovorans	Cunninghamella bertholletiae	Leishmania donovani	Influenza viruses
Enterobacter cloacae	Fusarium proliferatum,	Septata intestinalis	Parvovirus B19
Enterococcus	Fusarium solani		Human metapneumovirus
Escherichia coli	Geotrichum candidum		Respiratory syncytial virus
Haemophilus influenzae	Hansenula anomala		Varicella-zoster virus
Klebsiella pneumoniae	Malassezia furfur		
Listeria monocytogenes	Scopulariopsis		
Moraxella catarrhalis	Trichosporon beigelii		
Mycobacterium avium complex			
Mycobacterium chelonae			
Mycobacterium haemophilum			
Nocardia asteroides			
Pediococcus acidilactici			
Propionibacterium granulosum			
Pseudomonas aeruginosa			
Pseudomonas pseudomallei			
Coagulase-negative staphylococci			
Staphylococcus aureus			
Vibrio vulnificus			

Bacteria cause most infections in immunocompromised persons (see Table 120–1). *S. aureus, E. coli, P. aeruginosa, K. pneumoniae,* and coagulase-negative staphylococci are the most commonly identified bacterial pathogens. Central indwelling catheters often are associated with coagulase-negative staphylococci, *S. aureus,* and less frequently gram-negative bacteria, *Enterococcus,* and *Candida.*

Fungal pathogens account for approximately 10% of all infections associated with childhood cancer. *Candida* causes 60% of all fungal infections, with *Aspergillus* the second most common pathogen. Besides cancer-associated or therapy-associated cellular immunity defects, risk factors for fungal infections include oropharyngeal and gastrointestinal mucositis facilitating systemic fungal invasion, presence of long-term indwelling intravascular catheters, and broad-spectrum antibacterial therapy that promotes fungal colonization as a precursor to infection.

Infections with *P. jirovecii* (*carinii*) and *T. gondii* represent reactivation of quiescent infection facilitated by cancer-associated or therapy-associated cellular immunodeficiency. *P. jirovecii* (*carinii*) primarily causes pneumonitis in patients with leukemia, lymphoma, or HIV or on long-term corticosteroids, but it also can cause extrapulmonary disease, such as sinusitis and otitis media.

Viral opportunistic infections in patients with cancer usually represent symptomatic reactivation from latency facilitated by cancer-associated or therapy-associated cellular immunodeficiency. HSV can cause severe and prolonged mucocutaneous infection; HSV also can cause disseminated disease. CMV can cause focal disease in immunocompromised persons, especially in stem cell transplant patients. Manifestations of CMV disease include hepatitis, pneumonitis, esophagitis, and enteritis with ulcerations of the gastrointestinal mucosa. VZV can cause serious primary infection in susceptible persons, often with accompanying encephalitis, hepatitis, or, most ominously, pneumonitis. Zoster also can reactivate during chemotherapy and may cause disseminated zoster.

EPIDEMIOLOGY

Chemotherapeutic agents target rapidly dividing cells, especially myeloproliferative cells, which causes myelosuppression. Children receiving allogeneic transplants are at greater risk for infection than children receiving autologous transplants. Prolonged time to hematologic engraftment is a significant risk factor for infection in these patients. Children receiving stem cell or organ transplants have significantly greater immunosuppression as a consequence of the myeloablative conditioning regimens. Foreign bodies (shunts, central venous catheters) interfere with cutaneous barriers against infection and together with neutropenia or immunosuppression increase the risk of bacterial or fungal infections (see Chapter 121).

The relative rate of infection in patients with cancer at the time of admission or during hospitalization is 10% to 15%. The most frequently infected sites, in descending order, are the respiratory tract, the bloodstream, surgical wounds, and the urinary tract.

CLINICAL MANIFESTATIONS

Fever is the most common and sometimes only presenting symptom of serious infection in cancer and transplant patients. The presence of fever with neutropenia, even in the absence of other signs or symptoms, demands prompt evaluation because of the potential for life-threatening infection. Despite being immunocompromised, these patients can develop fever; the typical signs and symptoms that are associated with most infections are usually present. All symptoms and signs should be evaluated thoroughly, in addition to the supplemental evaluation necessitated because of fever in the presence of underlying immunodeficiency.

LABORATORY TESTS AND IMAGING

Assessing fever and neutropenia in immunocompromised persons requires blood cultures for bacterial and fungal pathogens obtained by peripheral venipuncture and from all lumens of any indwelling vascular catheters. Antigen tests, especially for serum cryptococcal antigen, should be considered. Chest radiographs are important to assess for the presence of pulmonary infiltrates. Specialized imaging studies, such as CT or MRI, can be useful in selected cases, such as with suspected sinusitis or intra-abdominal infection. Radionuclide scans such as gallium-67 or indium-111 may be useful in selected cases.

In the absence of neutrophils to localize an infection, it often is difficult to determine the source of infection by physical examination. Chest findings may be absent despite significant infection and revealed only by chest radiograph. Bronchoalveolar lavage is helpful in pulmonary infections. Sinus infection with bacteria, *Aspergillus*, or Zygomycetes is common in neutropenic hosts and may be detected only on CT scan.

DIFFERENTIAL DIAGNOSIS

Initially the patient should have a complete physical examination, including careful scrutiny of the oropharynx, nares, external auditory canals, skin and axilla, groin and perineum, and rectal area. The exit site and subcutaneous tunnel of any indwelling vascular catheter should be examined closely for erythema and palpated for tenderness and expression of purulent material. Perirectal abscess is a potentially serious focus of infection in neutropenic hosts, with tenderness and erythema that may be the only clues to infection. Any presumptive infection identified during the evaluation should help direct appropriate cultures and tailor anti-infective therapy.

TREATMENT

Treatment should be provided as appropriate for focal infections identified by physical examination or diagnostic imaging. Febrile episodes in neutropenic patients without an identifiable focus routinely are treated with broad-spectrum antibiotics until the neutropenia resolves. Empirical treatment of fever and neutropenia without an identified source should include an extended-spectrum penicillin or cephalosporin with activity against gram-negative bacilli, including *P. aeruginosa*, and often is combined with an aminoglycoside (Fig. 120–1). If the patient has an indwelling vascular catheter, vancomycin is added because of the increasing prevalence of methicillin-resistant *S. aureus*, but can be discontinued if it is not isolated after 48 to 72 hours.

If no microbiologic cause is isolated, empirical broad-spectrum antibiotics are continued as long as the patient remains neutropenic, regardless of whether the fever resolves (see Fig. 120–2). Treatment with amphotericin B or another antifungal agent is instituted empirically in patients who have neutropenia and persistent fever without a focus despite broad-spectrum antibacterial therapy for 7 days (Fig. 120–2).

The use of recombinant granulocyte colony-stimulating factor or granulocyte-macrophage colony-stimulating factor stimulates neutrophil production by the bone marrow, reduces the duration and severity of neutropenia, and decreases the risk of infection. Some chemotherapeutic protocols for the treatment of solid tumors that result in prolonged neutropenia incorporate hematopoietic cytokine therapy as part of the treatment protocol.

PREVENTION

Various regimens of prophylactic antibiotics, including oral nonabsorbed antibiotics (erythromycin base, neomycin), have been used in attempts to reduce the

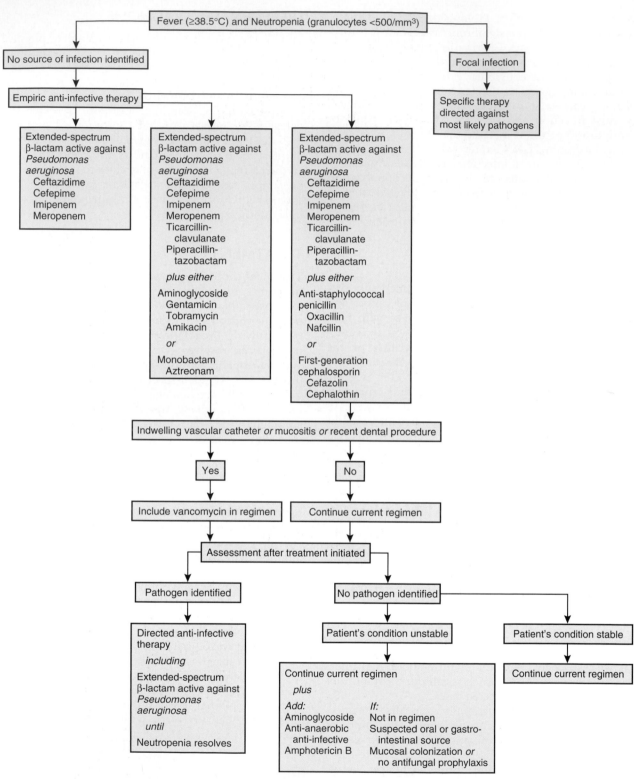

Figure 120–1

Initial management of fever and neutropenia without an identified source in cancer and transplant patients. (From Conrad DA: Patients with cancer. In Jenson HB, Baltimore RS [eds]: Pediatric Infectious Diseases: Principles and Practice, 2nd ed. Philadelphia, WB Saunders, 2002, p 1161.)

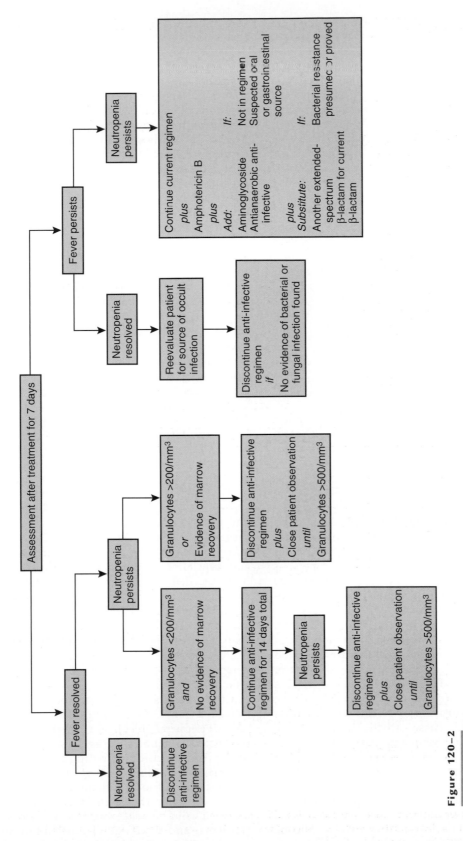

Figure 120–2

Continuing management of possible infection after 7 days of fever without an identified source in cancer and transplant patients. (From Conrad DA: Patients with cancer. In Jenson HB, Baltimore RS [eds]: Pediatric Infectious Diseases: Principles and Practice, 2nd ed. Philadelphia, WB Saunders, 2002, p 1165.)

incidence of gram-negative infections, although no improvement in mortality rates has been shown. Long-term, broad-spectrum prophylaxis also promotes development of antibiotic resistance. Administration of TMP-SMZ to prevent *P. jirovecii* (*carinii*) infection is routine for patients with leukemia or lymphoma and for many patients undergoing intensive chemotherapy for solid tumors. Prophylaxis generally is begun with initiation of anticancer therapy and continued until 6 months after chemotherapy has been completed.

Immunocompromised susceptible persons exposed to chickenpox within 2 days before the onset of rash until 5 days after the onset of rash in the index case should receive VZIG. Modified infection after VZIG may not result in protective immunity, and persons who receive VZIG prophylaxis should be considered to be still at risk with any subsequent exposures.

CHAPTER 121

Infections Associated with Medical Devices

Infections are a common and important complication of medical devices and are a major part of **healthcare-associated infections** (formerly **nosocomial infections**).

VASCULAR DEVICE INFECTIONS

Vascular catheters are inserted in most inpatients and are used in many outpatients. The use of **central catheters** for long-term access to the bloodstream has been an important advance for the care of persons who require parenteral nutrition, chemotherapy, or extended parenteral antibiotic therapy. The major complication of catheters is infection.

Short, peripheral IV catheters used for short-term access in stable patients are associated with a low rate of infection, especially in children. **Peripherally inserted central catheters** are commonly used for short-term central venous access. For extended central venous access, such as for chemotherapy, tunneled silicone elastomer catheters (**Broviac or Hickman catheters**) are commonly placed. These catheters are surgically inserted into a central vein and passed through a subcutaneous tunnel before exiting the skin and are anchored by a subcutaneous cuff. Contamination of the catheter hub or any connection of the IV tubing is common and is a major predisposition to catheter-associated infection. Totally implanted venous access systems (Port-a-Cath, Infuse-a-Port) have a silicone elastomer catheter tunneled beneath the skin to a reservoir implanted in a subcutaneous pocket. Implanted catheters or ports decrease, but do not eliminate the opportunity for microbial entry at the skin site.

Catheter-related thrombosis and catheter-related infection can develop separately or together. Ultrasound or radiographs can identify thrombi, but concomitant infection can be identified only by culture. **Thrombophlebitis** is inflammation with thrombosis. **Septic thrombophlebitis** is thrombosis with organisms embedded in the clot. **Catheter-related bloodstream infection** implies isolation of the same organism from a catheter and from peripheral blood of a patient with clinical symptoms of bacteremia and no other apparent source of infection. Confirmation requires quantitative colony counts of both samples, which is not routinely performed. The source of the bacteremia could be the infusate, contamination via the tubing and catheter connections, or established infection, which may or may not be clinically apparent. Infection may appear as an **exit site infection** limited to the insertion site or may extend along the catheter tunnel of buried catheters to cause a **tunnel infection**.

Many microorganisms cause catheter-related infections, most commonly *S. aureus,* coagulase-negative staphylococci, *Enterococcus,* and *Candida* (Table 121–1). Other skin flora, diphtheroids and *Bacillus,* are often involved. Gram-negative bacilli occur with increased frequency with exit site or tunnel infections (Table 121–2). Fungal catheter infections, usually *C. albicans,* are most common among persons receiving broad-spectrum antibiotics or parenteral nutrition.

The rates of bloodstream infection of peripheral venous catheters are 0 to 2 per 1000 catheter-days and for central catheters less than 2 to 30 per 1000 catheter-days. Risk factors for infection include ICU stay, prematurity, burns and skin disorders that adversely affect the integrity of the skin barrier to infection, neutropenia, and other immunodeficiencies (see Chapter 120). Infection rates are lower for tunneled and implanted catheters. Catheters inserted in emergency settings are more likely to be infected than catheters placed electively. Outbreaks of catheter-related infection have occurred because of contaminated infusion fluids, medications, and in-line attachment devices.

Clinical signs of catheter-associated bacteremia or fungemia range from mild fever to overwhelming sepsis. Peripheral phlebitis or catheter-related infection is classically manifested as a warm, erythematous, tender palpable cord originating at the IV catheter site, but may be subclinical or manifested only by fever without signs of local inflammation. Infection at the site of central catheter entrance is manifested as a localized cellulitis with warmth, tenderness, swelling, erythema, and discharge. Tunnel infection is manifested by similar findings along the tunnel route.

TABLE 121–1.   Percentage of Catheter-Related Infections Caused by Common Microorganisms

Classification of Pathogen	Systemic Infections: Bacteremia and Sepsis (%)*	Local Infections: Exit Site and Tunnel (%)*
Gram-positive cocci	71	52
Gram-negative bacilli	20	40
Fungi	6	2
Candida albicans, other *Candida*		
Malassezia furfur		
Miscellaneous, uncommon bacterial	3	6
Bacillus, Neisseria meningitidis, Micrococcus, others		

*Percentage of total infections for type of infection (septic or local).
From Fisher MC: Infections involving intravascular devices. In Jenson HB, Baltimore RS (eds): Pediatric Infectious Diseases: Principles and Practice, 2nd ed. Philadelphia WB Saunders, p 1246.

The **treatment** of catheter-related infection depends on the site of the infection and the pathogen involved. Catheters that are no longer necessary should be removed if infection is suspected. Catheter removal is indicated with sepsis, septic thrombophlebitis, clinical deterioration despite appropriate therapy, persistently positive blood culture results after 48 to 72 hours of appropriate antimicrobial therapy, embolic lesions, or fungal infection because of poor response to antifungal therapy alone.

Catheter-associated bacteremia can be treated with simple catheter removal, removal plus antibiotics, or,

TABLE 121–2.   Organisms Causing Catheter-Related Infection

Common Isolates

Coagulase-negative staphylococci
Staphylococcus aureus
Enterococcus
Candida albicans

Occasional Isolates

Escherichia coli
Klebsiella
Pseudomonas aeruginosa
Malassezia furfur
Candida parapsilosis
Candida glabrata
Candida tropicalis
Acinetobacter
Enterobacter
Nontuberculous *Mycobacterium*

From Fisher MC: Infections involving intravascular devices. In Jenson HB, Baltimore RS (eds): Pediatric Infectious Diseases: Principles and Practice, 2nd ed. Philadelphia, WB Saunders, 2002, p 1247.

in a stable patient, an attempt of antibiotic therapy alone. Infection with organisms of low virulence may be manifested by fever alone, and removal of the catheter frequently is followed by prompt defervescence and complete resolution of infection. Initial therapy should include antibiotics active against gram-negative organisms, such as a broad-spectrum cephalosporin and aminoglycoside, and against *S. aureus* and coagulase-negative staphylococci, such as oxacillin, nafcillin, or vancomycin. Eradication of infection can be accomplished without removal of the central line in approximately 89% of uncomplicated bacteremic infections, 94% of exit-site infections, and 25% of tunnel infections. If the patient is not critically ill and the pathogen is likely to be susceptible to antibiotic therapy, a trial of antibiotics is given through the infected catheter. The total duration of therapy depends on the pathogen and the duration of positive cultures and is usually 10 to 14 days after sterilization of the bloodstream. Infection of the pocket around an implanted port is unlikely to respond to antibiotics, and removal of the foreign body is usually necessary.

Antibiotic-lock is a method of sterilizing intravascular catheters by using high concentrations of antibiotics infused into the portion of the catheter between the hub and the vessel entry. The solution is allowed to dwell within the catheter segment for several hours. It also may be useful for treatment of catheter-associated infections and for prevention of infection.

Aseptic technique is essential during catheter insertion. Catheters that are placed during emergency situations should be replaced as soon as medically feasible. Care of indwelling catheters involves meticulous attention to sterile technique whenever the system is entered. The use of stopcocks should be minimized. Care of the catheter entry site commonly involves a topical antibiotic or disinfectant. Catheters that are no longer necessary should be removed.

VENTILATOR-ASSOCIATED PNEUMONIA

Intubation of the airway provides direct access to the lungs and bypasses normal host defenses. Organisms enter the lungs directly through the lumen of the tube or by descending around the tube, which may result in ventilator-associated pneumonia. Contaminated respiratory equipment, humidification systems, or condensate introduces bacteria directly into lower airways. The continuously open upper airway increases the risk of aspiration of oropharyngeal flora and reflux of gastric contents and interferes with clearance of the airway by coughing because an effective cough requires a closed glottis. Suctioning of the upper respiratory tract or mouth requires clean technique but does not require aseptic technique. Suction catheters that reach the lower airways must be sterile and usually are designed for single use.

URINARY CATHETERS

The most important risk factors for UTIs are the presence of catheters, instrumentation, and anatomic abnormalities (see Chapter 114). Organisms enter the bladder through the catheter by instillation of contaminated irrigation fluids, backflow of contaminated urine from the drainage bag, or ascent of bacteria around the meatus along the outside of the catheter. Indwelling catheters facilitate direct access to the bladder and should have a closed drainage system. After simple, straight catheterization, the incidence of UTI is 1% to 2%. Organisms that cause catheter-associated UTIs include fecal flora, such as gram-negative enteric bacilli and *Enterococcus. E. coli* is the most common cause of UTIs. With concomitant antibiotic treatment, resistant organisms predominate, and fungi emerge as pathogens.

The most important aspect of prevention is to minimize the duration and use of catheterization. Intermittent catheterization is preferred over indwelling catheter drainage, whenever feasible. Insertion of catheters must be done with aseptic technique, and the drainage system must remain closed at all times, with sterile technique used whenever the system is entered. Drainage bags always should be dependent to avoid backflow of urine into the bladder.

PERITONEAL DIALYSIS–ASSOCIATED INFECTIONS

Peritoneal dialysis requires the placement of an indwelling catheter with possible infectious complications, including exit site infection, tunnel infection, and peritonitis. The usual route of infection is from the skin surface along the tunnel and into the peritoneum. The most common pathogens are skin flora, including *Staphylococcus;* organisms that contaminate water, such as *Pseudomonas* and *Acinetobacter;* enteric flora, such as *E. coli* and *Klebsiella;* and fungi, such as *C. albicans.* Peritonitis may present with fever, vague abdominal pain, and cloudy dialysate. The diagnosis is established on clinical manifestations and confirmed by culture of the dialysate. Prevention of infection requires careful planning of the location of the exit site to minimize contamination, aseptic insertion of the catheter, meticulous care of the catheter site, securing of the catheter to avoid tension and motion, and aseptic technique during dialysis.

CENTRAL NERVOUS SYSTEM SHUNTS

Important risk factors of healthcare-associated CNS infections are surgery, placement of ventriculoperitoneal shunts, and the presence of CSF leaks. Infection of ventriculoperitoneal shunts results from contamination of the system at the time of placement or from hematogenous seeding. Externalized ventricular drains and subdural bolts allow direct access of skin flora to the CSF. For these devices, the rates of infection increase with the duration of catheterization, especially beyond 5 days.

The most common pathogens causing shunt infections are coagulase-negative staphylococci and *S. aureus.* After skull fracture or cranial surgery, a CSF leak may facilitate ascending infection, especially with *S. pneumoniae,* which frequently colonizes the nasopharynx. Patients with shunt infections may present with only fever and headache or may present with typical signs and symptoms of meningitis (see Chapter 100). Coagulase-negative staphylococci typically present with insidious onset of fever, malaise, headache, and vomiting. Initial therapy is usually with vancomycin, with additional antibiotics if gram-negative bacteria are suspected.

Antibiotics frequently are used perioperatively during placement of shunts and other neurosurgical procedures. There is no proof that antibiotics decrease infection rates in these clean procedures. External ventricular drains should be maintained as closed systems with aseptic technique and removed as soon as possible. Drainage bags always should be dependent to avoid backflow.

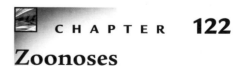

CHAPTER 122

Zoonoses

Zoonoses are infections that are transmitted in nature between vertebrate animals and humans. Many zoonotic pathogens are maintained in nature by means of an **enzootic cycle**, in which mammalian hosts and arthropod vectors reinfect each other. Humans frequently are only incidentally infected. Of the more than 150 different human zoonotic diseases that have been described, Lyme disease (*B. burgdorferi*) accounts for 90% of reported vector borne infections in the U.S. Other common pathogens include *Rickettsia rickettsii* (Rocky Mountain spotted fever), ehrlichiosis (*Ehrlichia chaffeensis*), and anaplasmosis (*Anaplasma phagocytophilum*). The epidemiology of zoonoses is related to the geographic distribution of the hosts and, if vector-borne, the distribution and seasonal life cycle of the vector (Table 122–1).

Many zoonoses are spread by ticks, including Lyme disease, Rocky Mountain spotted fever, ehrlichiosis, tularemia, tick typhus, and babesiosis. Mosquitoes transmit the arboviral encephalitides (see Chapter 101), dengue fever, malaria, and yellow fever. Preventive measures to avoid tick-borne and mosquito-borne diseases include using insect repellants that contain **DEET** (*N, N*-diethyl-*m*-toluamide) on skin and insect repellants that contain **permethrin** on clothing; avoiding tick-infested habitats (thick scrub oak, briar, poison ivy sites); avoiding excretory products of wild animals; wearing shoes or boots and not sandals; wearing long-sleeved shirts and long trousers that cover the arms and legs, with trousers tucked into shoes or socks to prevent ticks from crawling under clothing; wearing light-colored clothing to facilitate detection of crawling ticks; conducting thorough inspections of the body and of pets after returning from the outdoors; and removing ticks promptly.

Ticks are removed using blunt forceps or tweezers to grasp the tick as close to the skin as possible to pull the tick steadily outward. Squeezing, twisting, or crushing the tick should be avoided because the tick's bloated abdomen can act like a syringe if squeezed. Transmission of infection seems to be most efficient after 30 to 36 hours of nymphal tick attachment for human granulocytic ehrlichiosis, after 36 to 48 hours for *B. burgdorferi*, and after 56 to 60 hours for *Babesia*. Prophylactic antimicrobial therapy after a tick bite or exposure is not recommended.

LYME DISEASE (*BORRELIA BURGDORFERI*)

Etiology

Lyme disease is a tick-borne infection caused by the fastidious spirochete, *B. burgdorferi*. The vector in the eastern and midwestern U.S. is *Ixodes scapularis,* the **black-legged tick** that is commonly known as the **deer tick**. The vector on the Pacific Coast is *Ixodes pacificus,* the **western black-legged tick**. Ticks usually become infected by feeding on the white-footed mouse (*Peromyscus leucopus*), which is a natural reservoir for *B.*

burgdorferi. The larvae are dormant over winter and emerge the following spring in the nymphal stage, which is the stage of the tick that is most likely to transmit the infection to humans.

Epidemiology

Approximately 25,000 cases are reported annually in the U.S., with 95% of cases reported from New England and the eastern parts of the Middle Atlantic states and the upper Midwest, with a small endemic focus along the Pacific coast (Fig. 122–1). In Europe, most cases occur in Scandinavian countries and central Europe. Because exposure to ticks is more common in warm months, Lyme disease is noted predominantly in summer. The incidence is highest among children 5 to 10 years old, at almost twice the incidence among adolescents and adults.

Clinical Manifestations

The clinical manifestations are divided into early and late stages. Early infection may be localized or disseminated. **Early localized disease** develops 7 to 14 days after a tick bite as the site forms an erythematous papule that expands to form a red, raised border, often with central clearing. The lesion, **erythema migrans**, harbors *B. burgdorferi* and may be 15 cm wide, pruritic, or painful. Systemic manifestations may include malaise, lethargy, fever, headache, arthralgias, stiff neck, myalgias, and lymphadenopathy. The skin lesions and early manifestations resolve without treatment over 2 to 4 weeks. Not all patients with Lyme disease recall a tick bite or develop erythema migrans.

Approximately 20% of patients develop **early disseminated disease** with multiple secondary skin lesions, aseptic meningitis, pseudotumor, papilledema, cranioneuropathies including Bell palsy, polyradiculitis, peripheral neuropathy, mononeuritis multiplex, or transverse myelitis. Carditis with various degrees of heart block rarely may develop during this stage. Neurologic manifestations usually resolve by 3 months, but may recur or become chronic.

Late disease begins weeks to months after infection. Arthritis is the usual manifestation and may develop in 50% to 60% of untreated patients. The male-to-female ratio is 7:1. The knee is involved in greater than 90% of cases, but any joint may be affected. Symptoms may resolve over 1 to 2 weeks, but often recur in other joints. If untreated, most cases resolve, but chronic erosive arthritis may persist in 10% of patients as the episodes increase in duration and severity. Neuroborreliosis, the late manifestations of Lyme disease involving the CNS, is rarely reported in children.

TABLE 122–1. Major Zoonotic and Vector-Borne Infections*

Disease	Causative Agent	Common Animal Reservoirs	Vectors/Modes of Transmission	Geographic Distribution
Bacterial Diseases				
Anthrax	*Bacillus anthracis*	Cattle, goats, sheep, swine, cats, wild animals	Aerosol inhalation of spores in hides and other animal by-products, direct contact	Worldwide; rare in U.S.
Brucellosis	*Brucella*	Cattle, sheep, goats, swine, horses, dogs	Aerosol inhalation, direct contact, ingestion of contaminated goat cheese and milk	Worldwide
Campylobacteriosis	*Campylobacter jejuni*	Rodents, dogs (puppies), cats, fowl (chickens), swine	Direct contact, ingestion of contaminated food or water	Worldwide
Cat-scratch disease	*Bartonella henselae*	Cats, dogs	Bites and scratches	U.S.
Erysipeloid	*Erysipelothrix rhusiopathiae*	Sheep, swine, turkeys, ducks, fish	Direct contact	Worldwide
Listeriosis	*Listeria monocytogenes*	Cattle, fowl, goats, sheep	Ingestion of contaminated food, unpasteurized cheese and dairy products	Worldwide
Plague	*Yersinia pestis*	Wild and domestic rodents, cats, dogs	Direct contact, flea bite	New Mexico, Arizona, Utah, Colorado, California
Rat-bite fever (bacillary fever)	*Streptobacillus moniliformis*	Mice, rats, hamsters	Bites, ingestion of contaminated food or water	Japan, Asia; rare in U.S.
Salmonellosis	Nontyphoidal *Salmonella*	Fowl, dogs, cats, reptiles, amphibians	Direct contact, ingestion of contaminated food or water	Worldwide
Tularemia	*Francisella tularensis*	Rabbits, squirrels, dogs, cats	Aerosol inhalation, direct contact, ingestion of contaminated meat, tick bite, deerfly bite	California, Utah, Arkansas, Oklahoma
Yersiniosis	*Yersinia enterocolitica, Yersinia pseudotuberculosis*	Rodents, cattle, goats, sheep, swine, fowl, dogs	Direct contact, ingestion of contaminated food or water	Worldwide
Wound infection, bacteremia	*Pasteurella multocida, Capnocytophaga canimorsus*	Cats, dogs, rodents	Direct contact, bites and scratches	Worldwide
Mycobacterial Diseases				
Wound infection	*Mycobacterium marinum, Mycobacterium fortuitum, Mycobacterium kansasii*	Fish, aquarium	Direct contact, scratches	Worldwide
Spirochetal Diseases				
Leptospirosis	*Leptospira interrogans*	Dogs, rodents, livestock	Direct contact, contact with water or soil contaminated by urine of infected animals	Worldwide
Lyme disease	*Borrelia burgdorferi*	Deer, rodents	Tick bite (*Ixodes scapularis, Ixodes pacificus*)	Northeast and Midwest U.S., California

TABLE 122–1.   Major Zoonotic and Vector-Borne Infections*—cont'd

Disease	Causative Agent	Common Animal Reservoirs	Vectors/Modes of Transmission	Geographic Distribution
Rat-bite fever (Haverhill fever)	*Spirillum minus*	Mice, rats, hamsters	Bites, ingestion of contaminated food or water	Japan, Asia; rare in U.S.
Relapsing fever	*Borrelia*	Rodents, fleas	Louse bite, flea bite, transplacental transmission	Western and southern U.S.
Southern tick-associated rash illness	*Borrelia lonestari*	Deer, rodents	Tick bite (*I. scapularis*)	Southeastern and south-central U.S.

Rickettsial Diseases

Spotted Fever Group				
Rocky Mountain spotted fever	*Rickettsia rickettsii*	Dogs, rodents	Tick bite (*Dermacentor variabilis*, the American dog tick; *Dermacentor andersoni*, the wood tick; *Rhipicephalus sanguineus*, the brown dog tick; *Amblyomma cajennense*)	Western hemisphere
Mediterranean spotted fever (boutonneuse fever)	*Rickettsia conorii*	Dogs, rodents	Tick bite	Africa, Mediterranean region, India, Middle East
African tick-bite fever	*Rickettsia africae*	Cattle, goats (?)	Tick bite	Sub-Saharan Africa, Caribbean
Rickettsialpox	*Rickettsia akari*	Mice	Mite bite	North America, Russia, Ukraine, Adriatic region, Korea, South Africa
Murine typhus–like illness	*Rickettsia felis*	Opossums, cats, dogs	Flea bite	Western hemisphere, Europe
Typhus Group				
Murine typhus	*Rickettsia typhi*	Rats	Rat flea or cat flea feces	Worldwide
Epidemic typhus	*Rickettsia prowazekii*	Humans	Louse feces	Africa, South America, Central America, Mexico, Asia
Brill-Zinsser disease (recrudescent typhus)	*R. prowazekii*	Humans	Reactivation of latent infection	Potentially worldwide; U.S., Canada, Eastern Europe
Flying squirrel (sylvatic) typhus	*R. prowazekii*	Flying squirrels	Lice or fleas of flying squirrel	U.S.
Scrub Typhus				
Scrub typhus	*Orientia tsutsugamushi*	Rodents (?)	Chigger bite	Southern Asia, Japan, Indonesia, Australia, Korea, Asiatic Russia, India, China
Ehrlichiosis and Anaplasmosis				
Human monocytic ehrlichiosis	*Ehrlichia chaffeensis*	Deer, dogs	Tick bite (*Amblyomma americanum*)	U.S., Europe, Africa
Anaplasmosis (human granulocytic ehrlichiosis)	*Anaplasma phagocytophilum*	Rodents, deer, ruminants	Tick bite (*I. scapularis*)	U.S., Europe
Ehrlichiosis ewingii	*Ehrlichia ewingii*	Dogs	Tick bite	U.S.

Continued

TABLE 122–1. Major Zoonotic and Vector-Borne Infections*–cont'd

Disease	Causative Agent	Common Animal Reservoirs	Vectors/Modes of Transmission	Geographic Distribution
Sennetsu ehrlichiosis	*Neorickettsia sennetsu*	Unknown	Ingestion of helminth-contaminated fish (?)	Japan, Malaysia
Q Fever				
Q fever	*Coxiella burnetii*	Cattle, sheep, goats, cats, rabbits	Inhalation of infected aerosols, ingestion of contaminated dairy products, ticks (?)	Worldwide
Viral Diseases				
Colorado tick fever	Orbivirus	Rodents, ticks	Aerosol inhalation, tick bite, blood transfusion, ingestion of contaminated food	Rocky Mountains, Pacific Northwest, western Canada
Dengue fever	Dengue viruses (types 1-4)	Humans	Mosquito bite (*Aedes aegypti, Aedes albopictus*)	Tropical areas of the Caribbean, the Americas, and Asia
Hantavirus cardiopulmonary syndrome	Hantavirus	Rodents, mice, cats	Aerosol inhalation	Southwestern U.S.
Herpesvirus B infection	Herpesvirus B	Old World primates (rhesus, *Macaca cynomolgus*)	Animal bite	Africa, Asia (and primate centers worldwide)
Lymphocytic choriomeningitis	Lymphocytic choriomeningitis virus	Rodents, hamsters, mice	Aerosol inhalation, direct contact, bite	Worldwide
Rabies	Rabies virus	Dogs, skunks, bats, raccoons, foxes, cats	Bites and scratches	Worldwide
Vesicular stomatitis	Vesicular stomatitis virus	Horses, cattle, swine	Direct contact	Americas
Protozoan Diseases				
African trypanosomiasis				
East African sleeping sickness	*Trypanosoma brucei rhodesiense*	Wild and domestic animals	Insect bite (tsetse fly)	East Africa
West African sleeping sickness	*Trypanosoma brucei gambiense*	Wild and domestic animals	Insect bite (tsetse fly)	West Africa
American trypanosomiasis (Chagas disease)	*Trypanosoma cruzi*	Wild and domestic animals	Insect bite (reduviid bug); contact with fecal material of reduviid bug	South America, Central America, South Texas
Babesiosis	*Babesia*	Cattle, wild and domestic rodents	Tick bite (*I. scapularis*), blood transfusion	Worldwide
Leishmaniasis, mucocutaneous and cutaneous	*Leishmania*	Domestic and wild dogs	Sandfly bite	Tropics
Leishmaniasis, visceral	*Leishmania donovani* complex	Domestic and wild dogs	Sandfly bite	Tropics
Malaria	*Plasmodium*	Humans	Mosquito bite (*Anopheles*)	Usually imported to the U.S., Southern California
Toxoplasmosis	*Toxoplasma gondii*	Cats, livestock, pigs	Ingestion of oocysts in fecally contaminated material or ingestion of tissue cysts in undercooked meat	Worldwide

*Many helminths are also zoonotic (see Tables 123-4 and 123-5).

Adapted from Christenson JC: Epidemiology of infectious diseases. In Jenson HB, Baltimore RS (eds): Pediatric Infectious Diseases: Principles and Practice, 2nd ed. Philadelphia, WB Saunders, 2002, pp 18-20.

Areas of predicted Lyme disease transmission

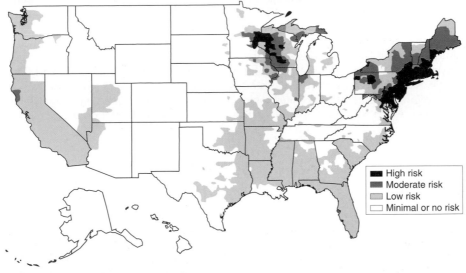

High risk
Moderate risk
Low risk
Minimal or no risk

Figure 122–1

The approximate distribution of predicted risk for Lyme disease in the U.S. The risk varies by the distribution of *Ixodes scapularis* and *Ixodes pacificus,* the proportion of infected ticks for each species at each stage of the tick's life cycle, and the presence of grassy or wooded locations favored by white-tailed deer. (From Centers for Disease Control and Prevention: National Lyme Disease Risk Map. Fort Collins, Colo, Division of Vector-Borne Diseases, National Center for Infectious Diseases, 2003.)

Laboratory and Imaging Studies

In late disease, the ESR is elevated, and complement may be reduced. The joint fluid shows an inflammatory response with total WBC count of 25,000 to 125,000 cells/mm³, often with a polymorphonuclear predominance (see Table 118–1). The rheumatoid factor and antinuclear antibody are negative, but the VDRL test may be falsely positive. With CNS involvement, the CSF shows a lymphocytic pleocytosis with normal glucose and slightly elevated protein.

Antibody tests during early, localized Lyme disease may be negative and are not useful. The diagnosis of late disease is confirmed by serologic tests specific for *B. burgdorferi*. The sensitivity and specificity of serologic tests for Lyme disease vary substantially. A positive ELISA or immunofluorescence assay result must be confirmed by immunoblot showing antibodies against at least either two or three (for IgM) or five (for IgG) proteins of *B. burgdorferi* (at least one of which is one of the more specific, low-molecular-weight, outer-surface proteins).

Differential Diagnosis

A history of a tick bite and the classic rash are helpful, but are not always present. Erythema migrans of early,

localized disease may be confused with nummular eczema, tinea corporis, granuloma annulare, an insect bite, or cellulitis. **Southern tick-associated rash illness**, which is similar to erythema migrans, has been described in southeastern and south-central states and is associated with the bite of *Amblyomma americanum,* the lone star tick. A spirochete, which has been named *Borrelia lonestari,* has been detected by DNA analysis, but has not yet been cultured.

During early, disseminated Lyme disease, multiple lesions may appear as erythema multiforme or urticaria. The aseptic meningitis is similar to viral meningitis, and the seventh nerve palsy is indistinguishable from herpetic or idiopathic Bell palsy. The carditis is similar to viral myocarditis. Monarticular or pauciarticular arthritis of late Lyme disease may mimic suppurative arthritis, juvenile rheumatoid arthritis, or rheumatic fever (see Chapter 89). The differential diagnosis of neuroborreliosis includes degenerative neurologic illness, encephalitis, and depression.

Treatment

Early, localized disease and early, disseminated disease, including facial nerve palsy (or other cranial nerve palsy) and carditis with first-degree or second-degree heart block, is treated with doxycycline or amoxicillin for 14 to 21 days. Early disease with carditis with third-degree heart block or meningitis and late neurologic disease (neurologic disease other than facial nerve or other cranial nerve palsy) are treated with IV or IM ceftriaxone or IV penicillin G for 14 to 28 days. Arthritis is treated with doxycycline (≥9 years old) or amoxicillin for 28 days. If there is recurrence, treatment should be with a repeated oral regimen or as for late neurologic disease.

Complications

Carditis, especially conduction disturbances, and arthritis are the major complications of Lyme disease. Even untreated, most cases eventually resolve without sequelae, including cases with multiple recurrences of arthritis that were documented before Lyme disease was described and treatment was available.

Prognosis

Lyme disease is readily treatable and curable. The long-term prognosis is excellent for early and late disease. Early treatment may prevent progression to carditis and meningitis. Recurrences of arthritis are rare after recommended treatment. A community-based study of children with Lyme disease found no evidence of impairment 4 to 11 years later.

Prevention

Measures to minimize exposure to tick-borne diseases are the most reasonable means of preventing Lyme disease. Postexposure prophylaxis is not routinely recommended because the overall risk of acquiring Lyme disease after a tick bite is only 1% to 2% even in endemic areas, and treatment of the infection, if it develops, is highly effective. Nymphal stage ticks must feed for 36 to 48 hours, and adult ticks must feed for 48 to 72 hours before the risk of transmission of *B. burgdorferi* from infected ticks becomes substantial. In hyperendemic regions, prophylaxis of adults with doxycycline, 200 mg as a single dose, within 72 hours of a nymphal tick bite is effective in preventing Lyme disease.

ROCKY MOUNTAIN SPOTTED FEVER (*RICKETTSIA RICKETTSII*)

Etiology

The cause of Rocky Mountain spotted fever is *R. rickettsii*. Rickettsiae are gram-negative coccobacillary organisms that resemble bacteria, but have incomplete cell walls and require an intracellular site for replication. The organism invades and proliferates within the endothelial cells of the blood vessels causing vasculitis, resulting in increased vascular permeability, edema, and, eventually, decreased vascular volume, altered tissue perfusion, and widespread organ failure. Many tick species are capable of transmitting *R. rickettsii*. The principal ticks are *Dermacentor variabilis* (the American dog tick) in the eastern U.S. and Canada, *Dermacentor andersoni* (the wood tick) in the western U.S. and Canada, *Rhipicephalus sanguineus* (the brown dog tick) in Mexico, and *Amblyomma cajennense* in Central and South America.

Epidemiology

Rocky Mountain spotted fever is the most common rickettsial illness in the U.S., occurring primarily in the eastern coastal, southeastern, and western states. Most cases occur from May to October after outdoor activity in wooded areas, with peak incidence among children 1 to 14 years old. Approximately 40% of infected persons are unable to recall a tick bite.

Clinical Manifestations

The incubation period of Rocky Mountain spotted fever is 2 to 14 days, with an average of 7 days. The onset is nonspecific with headache, malaise, and fever. A pale, rose-red macular or maculopapular rash appears in 90% of cases that begins peripherally and spreads to involve the entire body, including palms and soles. The early rash blanches on pressure and is accentuated by warmth. It progresses over hours or days to a petechial and purpuric eruption that appears first on the feet and ankles, then the wrists and hands, and progresses centripetally to the trunk and head. Myalgias, especially of the lower extremities, and intractable headaches are common. Severe cases progress with splenomegaly, myocarditis, renal impairment, pneumonitis, and shock.

Laboratory and Imaging Studies

Thrombocytopenia (usually <100,000/mm³), anemia, hyponatremia, and elevated hepatic transaminase levels are common laboratory findings. Organisms can be detected in skin biopsy specimens by fluorescent antibodies, although this test is not widely available. Serologic testing usually is used to confirm the diagnosis, although treatment is begun before laboratory confirmation.

Differential Diagnosis

The differential diagnosis includes meningococcemia, bacterial sepsis, toxic shock syndrome, leptospirosis, ehrlichiosis, measles, enteroviruses, infectious mononucleosis, collagen vascular diseases, Henoch-Schönlein purpura, and idiopathic thrombocytopenic purpura. The diagnosis of Rocky Mountain spotted fever should be suspected with fever and petechial rash, especially with a history of a tick bite or outdoor activities during spring and summer in endemic regions. Fever, headache, and myalgias lasting longer than 1 week in patients in endemic areas indicate Rocky Mountain spotted fever. Delayed diagnosis and late treatment usually result from atypical initial symptoms and late appearance of the rash.

Treatment

Therapy for suspected Rocky Mountain spotted fever should not be postponed pending results of diagnostic tests. Doxycycline is the drug of choice, even for young children despite the theoretical risk of dental staining in children younger than 9 years old. Fluoroquinolones also are active against *R. rickettsii* and may be an alternative treatment for adults.

Complications

In severe infections, capillary leakage results in noncardiogenic pulmonary edema (acute respiratory distress syndrome), hypotension; disseminated intravascular coagulation, circulatory collapse, and multiple organ failure including encephalitis, myocarditis, hepatitis, and renal failure.

Prognosis and Prevention

Untreated illness may persist for 3 weeks before progressing to multisystem involvement. The mortality rate is 25% without treatment, which is reduced to 3.4% with treatment. Permanent sequelae are common after severe disease. Preventive measures to avoid tick-borne infections and careful removal of ticks are recommended.

EHRLICHIOSIS (*EHRLICHIA CHAFFEENSIS*) AND ANAPLASMOSIS (*ANAPLASMA PHAGOCYTOPHILUM*)

Etiology

The term **ehrlichiosis** often is used to refer to all forms of infection with *Ehrlichia*. **Human monocytic ehrlichiosis** is caused by *E. chaffeensis,* which infects predominantly monocytic cells and is transmitted by the tick *A. americanum.* **Human anaplasmosis,** formerly named **granulocytic ehrlichiosis,** is caused by *A. phagocytophilum* and is transmitted by the tick *I. scapularis.* Disease caused by *Ehrlichia ewingii* has been identified by various names, including **ehrlichiosis ewingii.**

Epidemiology

Ehrlichiosis occurs commonly in the U.S. Human monocytic ehrlichiosis occurs in broad areas across the southeastern, south central, and mid-Atlantic U.S. in a distribution that parallels that of Rocky Mountain spotted fever. Anaplasmosis is the most frequently recognized ehrlichiosis and is found mostly in the northeastern and upper midwestern U.S., but infections have now been identified in northern California, the mid-Atlantic, and broadly across Europe.

Clinical Manifestations

Human monocytic ehrlichiosis, anaplasmosis, and ehrlichiosis ewingii cause similar acute febrile illness characterized by fever, malaise, headache, myalgias, anorexia, and nausea, but often without a rash. In contrast to adult patients, nearly two thirds of children with human monocytic ehrlichiosis present with a macular or maculopapular rash, although petechial lesions may occur. Symptoms usually last 4 to 12 days.

Laboratory and Imaging Studies

Characteristic laboratory findings include leukopenia, lymphocytopenia, thrombocytopenia, anemia, and elevated hepatic transaminases. Morulae are found infrequently in circulating monocytes of persons with human monocytic ehrlichiosis, but are found in 40% of circulating neutrophils in 20% to 60% of persons with anaplasmosis (Fig. 122–2). Seroconversion or fourfold rise in antibody titer confirms the diagnosis.

Differential Diagnosis

Ehrlichiosis is clinically similar to other arthropod-borne infections, including Rocky Mountain spotted fever, tularemia, babesiosis, early Lyme disease, murine typhus, relapsing fever, and Colorado tick fever. The differential diagnosis also includes infectious mononucleosis, Kawasaki disease, endocarditis, viral infections, hepatitis, leptospirosis, Q fever, collagen vascular diseases, and leukemia.

Treatment

As with Rocky Mountain spotted fever, therapy for suspected ehrlichiosis should not be postponed pending results of diagnostic tests. Ehrlichiosis and anaplasmosis are treated with tetracyclines, primarily doxycycline.

Complications

Severe pulmonary involvement with acute respiratory distress syndrome has been reported in several cases.

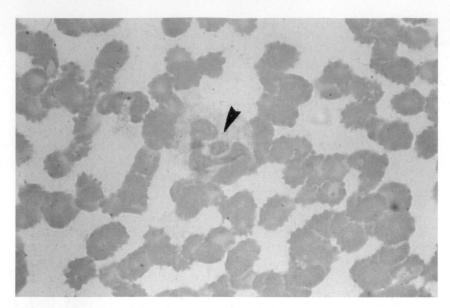

Figure 122–2

A morula *(arrowhead)* containing *Anaplasma phagocytophilum* in a neutrophil. *Ehrlichia chaffeensis* and *A. phagocytophilum* have similar morphologies, but are serologically and genetically distinct. (Wright stain, original magnification ×1200.)

Other reported severe complications include meningoencephalitis and myocarditis.

Prognosis and Prevention

Most patients improve within 48 hours. Preventive measures to avoid tick-borne infections and careful removal of ticks are recommended.

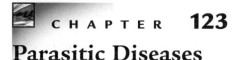

CHAPTER 123
Parasitic Diseases

PROTOZOAL DISEASES

Protozoa are the simplest organisms of the animal kingdom. They are unicellular, and most are free living, but some have a commensal or parasitic existence. Protozoal diseases include malaria, toxoplasmosis, babesiosis, and the intestinal protozoal diseases, amebiasis, cryptosporidiosis, and giardiasis (see Chapter 112).

MALARIA
Etiology

Malaria is caused by obligate intracellular protozoa of the genus *Plasmodium,* including *P. falciparum, P. malariae, P. ovale,* and *P. vivax. Plasmodium* exists in a variety of forms and has a complex life cycle that enables survival in different cellular environments in the human host and in the mosquito vector. There are two major phases in the life cycle, an **asexual phase (schizogony)** in humans and a **sexual phase (sporogony)** in mosquitoes. The **erythrocytic phase** of *Plasmodium* asexual development begins when the merozoites released from exoerythrocytic schizonts in the liver penetrate erythrocytes. When inside the erythrocyte, the parasite transforms into the **ring form**, which enlarges to become a **trophozoite**. These latter two forms can be identified with Giemsa stain on blood smear, which is the primary means of confirming the diagnosis of malaria.

The parasites usually are transmitted to humans by female *Anopheles* mosquitoes. Malaria also can be transmitted through blood transfusion, via contaminated needles, and transplacentally to a fetus.

Epidemiology

Malaria is a worldwide problem with transmission in more than 100 countries with a combined population of more than 1.6 billion people. Malaria is the most important cause of fever and morbidity in the tropical world. The principal areas of transmission are sub-Saharan Africa, southern Asia, South East Asia, Mexico, Haiti, the Dominican Republic, Central and South America, Papua New Guinea, and the Solomon Islands. Approximately 1000 to 2000 imported cases are recognized annually in the U.S., with most cases occurring among infected foreign civilians from endemic areas who travel to the U.S. and among U.S. citizens who travel to endemic areas without appropriate chemoprophylaxis.

Clinical Manifestations

The clinical manifestations of malaria range from asymptomatic infection to fulminant illness and death depending on the virulence of the infecting malaria species and the host immune response. The incubation period ranges from 6 to 30 days depending on the *Plasmodium* species (Table 123–1). The most characteristic clinical feature of malaria, which is seldom noted with other infectious diseases, is **febrile paroxysms** alternating with periods of fatigue but otherwise relative wellness. The classic symptoms of the febrile paroxysms of malaria include high fever, rigors, sweats, and headache. Paroxysms coincide with the rupture of schizonts that occur every 48 hours with *P. vivax* and *P. ovale* (**tertian periodicity**) and every 72 hours with *P. malariae* (**quartan periodicity**).

Short-term relapse describes the recurrence of symptoms after a primary attack that is due to the survival of erythrocyte forms in the bloodstream. **Long-term relapse** describes the renewal of symptoms long after the primary attack, usually due to release of merozoites from an exoerythrocytic source in the liver. Long-term relapse occurs with *P. vivax* and *P. ovale* because of persistence in the liver and with *P. malariae* because of persistence in the erythrocyte.

Laboratory and Imaging Studies

The diagnosis of malaria is established by identification of organisms on stained smears of peripheral blood. In nonimmune persons, symptoms typically occur 1 to 2 days before parasites are detectable on blood smear. Although *P. falciparum* is most likely to be identified from blood during a febrile paroxysm, the timing of the smears is less important than their being obtained several times each day over 3 successive days. Thick and thin blood smears should be examined. The concentration of erythrocytes on a **thick smear** is approximately 20 to 40 times greater than on a **thin smear**. Thick smears are used to scan large numbers of erythrocytes quickly. Thin smears allow for positive identification of the malaria species and determination of the percentage of infected erythrocytes, which also is useful in following the response to therapy.

TABLE 123–1.   Characteristics of Plasmodia Causing Malaria

Characteristic	*P. falciparum*	*P. vivax*	*P. ovale*	*P. malariae*
Exoerythrocytic cycle	5.5-7 days	6-8 days	9 days	12-16 days
Erythrocytic cycle	48 hr	42-48 hr	49-50 hr	72 hr
Prepatent period	9-10 days	11-13 days	10-14 days	15 days
Usual incubation period (range)	12 days (9-14 days)	13 days (12-17 days; may be 6-12 mo)	17 days (16-18 days; may be longer)	28 days (18-40 days; may be longer)
Merozoites per hepatic schizont	30,000	10,000	15,000	2,000
Erythrocyte preference	Young erythrocytes, but can infect all	Reticulocytes	Reticulocytes	Older erythrocytes
Usual parasite load (% erythrocytes infected)	≥1-5	1-2	1-2	1-2
Secondary exoerythrocytic cycle (hypnozoites) and relapses	Absent	Present	Present	Absent
Duration of untreated infection	1-2 yr	1.5-4 yr (includes liver stage)	1.5-4 yr (includes liver stage)	3-50 yr
Severity of primary attack	Severe in nonimmune patients—**a medical emergency**—failure to recognize and treat can lead to death	Mild to severe—danger of splenic rupture, relapse related to persistence of latent exoerythrocytic forms	Mild—danger of splenic rupture, relapse related to persistence of latent exoerythrocytic forms	Can be chronic in subclinical and subpatent forms; can cause nephritis in children
Usual periodicity of febrile attacks	None	48 hr	48 hr	72 hr
Duration of febrile paroxysm	16-36 hr (may be longer)	8-12 hr	8-12 hr	8-10 hr

Adapted from Strickland GT: Malaria. In Strickland GT (ed): Hunter's Tropical Medicine, 7th ed. Philadelphia, WB Saunders, 1991, p 589.

Differential Diagnosis

The most important aspect of diagnosis of malaria in children is to consider the possibility of malaria in any child who has fever, chills, splenomegaly, anemia, or decreased level of consciousness with a history of recent travel or residence in an endemic area, regardless of the use of chemoprophylaxis. The differential diagnosis is broad and includes many infectious diseases, such as tuberculosis, typhoid fever, brucellosis, relapsing fever, infective endocarditis, influenza, polio, yellow fever, trypanosomiasis, kala-azar, and amebic liver abscess.

Treatment

Chloroquine is the recommended treatment except for chloroquine-resistant *P. falciparum* (Table 123–2). Patients with malaria usually require hospitalization and may require ICU admission.

Complications

Cerebral malaria is a complication of *P. falciparum* infection and a frequent cause of death (20% to 40%), especially among children and nonimmune adults. Similar to other complications, cerebral malaria is more likely to occur among patients with intense parasitemia (>5%). Other complications include splenic rupture, renal failure, severe hemolysis (**blackwater fever**), pulmonary edema, hypoglycemia, thrombocytopenia, and **algid malaria** (sepsis syndrome with vascular collapse).

Prognosis

Death may occur with any of the malarial species, but is most frequent with complicated *P. falciparum* malaria. The likelihood of death is increased in children with preexisting health problems, such as measles, intestinal parasites, schistosomiasis, anemia, and malnutrition. Death is much more common in poor developing countries.

Prevention

There are two components of malaria prevention: reduction of exposure to infected mosquitoes and chemoprophylaxis. Mosquito protection is necessary because no prophylactic regimen can guarantee protection in every instance because of the widespread development of resistant organisms.

Chemoprophylaxis is necessary for all visitors to and residents of the tropics who have not lived there since infancy. Children of nonimmune women should have chemoprophylaxis from birth. Children of women from endemic areas have passive immunity until 3 to 6 months of age, after which they are increasingly likely to acquire malaria. Chemoprophylaxis should be started 1 to 2 weeks before a person enters the endemic area except for doxycycline, which can be started 1 to 2 days before, and should continue for at least 4 weeks after the person leaves. In the few remaining areas of the world that are free of chloroquine-resistant malaria strains, chloroquine is given once per week on the same day of the week. In areas where chloroquine-resistant *P. falciparum* exists, mefloquine is recommended for all ages except for travelers to the Thai-Cambodian and Thai-Myanmar (Burma) border areas, where mefloquine resistance is common, and doxycycline is recommended. Atovaquone-proguanil is recommended for travelers to the Amazon River basin, South East Asia, and some countries in Africa because of sulfadoxine-pyrimethamine resistance. Mefloquine should not be used for self-treatment because of the frequency of serious adverse effects at treatment doses. There have been several reports of mefloquine and pyrimethamine-sulfadoxine resistance.

TOXOPLASMOSIS

Toxoplasmosis is a zoonosis caused by *T. gondii,* an intracellular protozoan parasite. Infection is acquired by infectious oocysts, such as those excreted by newly infected cats, which play an important role in amplifying the organism in nature, or from ingesting cysts in contaminated, undercooked meat. Less commonly, transmission occurs transplacentally during acute infection of pregnant women. In the U.S., the incidence of congenital infection is 1 to 2 per 1000 live births.

Acquired toxoplasmosis is usually an asymptomatic infection. Symptomatic infection is characterized as a heterophil-negative mononucleosis syndrome that includes lymphadenopathy, fever, and hepatosplenomegaly. Disseminated infection, including myocarditis, pneumonia, and CNS toxoplasmosis, is more common among immunocompromised persons, especially persons with AIDS. Among women infected during pregnancy, 40% to 60% give birth to an infected infant. The later in pregnancy that infection occurs, the more likely it is that the fetus will be infected, but the less severe the illness (see Chapter 66). Serologic diagnosis can be established by a fourfold increase in antibody titer or seroconversion, a positive IgM antibody titer, or positive PCR for *T. gondii* in peripheral WBCs, CSF, serum, or amniotic fluid.

Treatment includes pyrimethamine and sulfadiazine, which act synergistically against *Toxoplasma.* Because these compounds are folic acid inhibitors, they are used in conjunction with folinic acid. Spiramycin, which is not licensed in the U.S., also is used in therapy of pregnant women with toxoplasmosis. Corticosteroids are reserved for patients with acute CNS or ocular infection.

TABLE 123–2.   Treatment of Malaria

Drug[1]	Adult Dosage	Pediatric Dosage
All *Plasmodium* Species Except Chloroquine-Resistant *P. Falciparum*		
Oral Drug of Choice		
Chloroquine phosphate[2]	600 mg base (1 g), then 300 mg base (500 mg) 6 hr later, followed by 300 mg base (500 mg) at 24 and 48 hr	10 mg/kg base (maximum 600 mg) followed by 5 mg/kg base (maximum 300 mg) 6 hr later and 5 mg/kg base daily (maximum 300 mg) at 24 and 48 hr
Parenteral Drug of Choice		
Quinidine gluconate[3]	10 mg/kg loading dose IV (maximum 600 mg) in normal saline solution slowly over 1-2 hr followed by a continuous infusion of 0.02 mg/kg/min until oral therapy can be started	Same as adult dose
Chloroquine-Resistant *P. Falciparum*		
Oral Drug of Choice		
Quinine sulfate[4]	650 mg tid for 3-7 days	25 mg/kg/day (maximum 650 mg per dose) divided tid for 3-7 days
plus Tetracycline[5]	250 mg qid for 7 days	25 mg/kg/day (maximum 250 mg per dose) divided qid for 7 days
Alternative Oral Regimens[6]		
Quinine sulfate *plus* pyrimethamine-sulfadoxine (Fansidar)[7]	Same as above	Same as above
or	Single dose of 3 tablets on the last day of quinine	<1 yr: single dose of $^1/_4$ tablet 1-3 yr: single dose of $^1/_2$ tablet 4-8 yr: single dose of 1 tablet 9-14 yr: single dose of 2 tablets >14 yr: single dose of 3 tablets
Mefloquine	Single dose of 1250 mg	>15 kg: 25 mg/kg (maximum 1250 mg) in a single dose
or		
Atovaquone *plus* proguanil (Malarone)[8]	2 tablets (500 mg atovaquone, 200 mg proguanil) bid for 3 days	11-20 kg: $^1/_2$ tablet bid for 3 days 21-30 kg: 1 tablet bid for 3 days 31-40 kg: $1^1/_2$ tablets bid for 3 days >40 kg: 2 tablets bid for 3 days
Parenteral Drug of Choice		
Quinidine gluconate	Same as above	Same as above
Prevention of Relapses: **P. vivax** *and* **P. ovale** *Only*		
Primaquine phosphate[9] (after completion of chloroquine)	15 mg base (26.3 mg salt) once a day for 14 days or 45 mg base (79 mg salt) once a wk for 8 wk	0.3 mg/kg base (maximum 15 mg base [26.3 mg salt]) once a day for 14 days

[1]Review contraindications and adverse effects before use.
[2]If chloroquine phosphate is not available, hydroxychloroquine sulfate is as effective (400 mg of hydroxychloroquine sulfate is equivalent to 500 mg of chloroquine phosphate).
[3]Quinine dihydrochloride is an alternative parenteral drug for treatment of non–chloroquine-resistant *Plasmodium*, but is not available in the U.S.
[4]Quinine sulfate should be given for 7 days for treatment of *P. falciparum* infections acquired in Thailand.
[5]Physicians must weigh the benefits of the tetracycline therapy against the possibility of dental staining in children <9 years old.
[6]Quinine sulfate *plus* clindamycin or halofantrine alone are other alternative oral regimens. Data on efficacy of clindamycin for treatment of malaria in children are limited. Quinine sulfate *plus* clindamycin is a treatment choice for pregnant women. Halofantrine is not available in the U.S.
[7]Fansidar should be avoided for treatment of *P. falciparum* infections acquired in Thailand, Myanmar (Burma), Cambodia, or the Amazon basin because of Fansidar resistance in these areas.
[8]Available as a combination tablet (Malarone) containing atovaquone (250 mg) and proguanil (100 mg).
[9]Primaquine can cause hemolytic anemia in patients with glucose-6-dehydrogenase deficiency, which should be tested before administration. Primaquine should not be given during pregnancy.
From Krause PJ: Malaria. In Jenson HB, Baltimore RS (eds): Pediatric Infectious Diseases: Principles and Practice, 2nd ed. Philadelphia, WB Saunders, 2002, p 371.

Ingesting only well-cooked meat and avoiding cats or soil in areas where cats defecate are prudent measures for pregnant or immunocompromised persons. Administration of spiramycin to infected pregnant women has been associated with lower risks of congenital infection in their offspring.

HELMINTHIASES

Helminths are divided into three groups: roundworms, or nematodes, and two groups of flatworms, the trematodes (flukes) and the cestodes (tapeworms).

Hookworm Infections

Hookworm infection is caused by **several species of hookworms**, with *Ancylostoma duodenale* and *Necator americanus* being the most important (Table 123–3). More than 9 million humans are infected with hookworms. *A. duodenale* is the predominant species in Europe, the Mediterranean region, northern Asia, and the west coast of South America. *N. americanus* predominates in the Western hemisphere, sub-Saharan Africa, South East Asia, and the Pacific Islands. Optimal soil conditions and fecal contamination are found in many agrarian tropical countries and in the southeastern U.S. Infection typically occurs in young children, especially during the first decade of life. The larvae are found in warm, damp soil and infect humans by penetrating the skin. They migrate to the lungs, ascend the trachea, are swallowed, and reside in the intestine. The worms mature and attach to the intestinal wall, where they suck blood and shed eggs.

Infections are usually asymptomatic. Intense pruritus ("**ground itch**") occurs at the site of larval penetration, usually the soles of the feet or between the toes, and may include papules and vesicles. Migration of larvae through the lungs usually is asymptomatic. Symptoms of abdominal pain, anorexia, indigestion, fullness, and diarrhea occur with hookworm infestation. The major manifestation of infection is anemia. Examination of fresh stool for hookworm eggs is diagnostic. Therapy includes anthelmintic treatment with albendazole, mebendazole, or pyrantel pamoate and treatment for anemia. Eradication depends on sanitation of the patient's environment and chemotherapy.

TABLE 123–3. Major Pediatric Syndromes Caused by Parasitic Nematodes

Syndrome	Etiologic Agent	Transmission	Treatment
Hookworm iron deficiency	*Ancylostoma duodenale*	Larval ingestion and penetration	Albendazole *or* mebendazole *or* pyrantel pamoate
	Necator americanus	Larval penetration	
Cutaneous larva migrans	*Ancylostoma braziliense* (a zoonotic hookworm)	Larval penetration (and failure to migrate)	Albendazole *or* ivermectin *or* thiabendazole topically
Infant ancylostomiasis	*A. duodenale*	Perinatal (?)	Albendazole *or* mebendazole *or* pyrantel pamoate
Trichuris dysentery or colitis	*Trichuris trichiura*	Egg ingestion	Mebendazole *or* albendazole *or* pyrantel pamoate and oxantel pamoate
Intestinal ascariasis	*Ascaris lumbricoides*	Ingestion of ascaris eggs	Albendazole *or* mebendazole *or* pyrantel pamoate
Neonatal ascariasis		Transplacental	
Visceral larva migrans Ocular larva migrans	*Toxocara canis* *Toxocara cati* *Baylisascaris procyonis*	Egg ingestion	Albendazole *or* mebendazole
Diarrhea, malabsorption ("celiac-like")	*Strongyloides stercoralis*	Larval penetration	Ivermectin *or* thiabendazole
Swollen belly syndrome	*Strongyloides fuelleborni*	Perinatal	Ivermectin *or* thiabendazole
Pinworm	*Enterobius vermicularis*	Ingestion of embryonated eggs	Albendazole *or* mebendazole *or* pyrantel pamoate
Trichinellosis	*Trichinella spiralis*	Ingestion of infected undercooked meat	Mebendazole *or* albendazole *plus* corticosteroids for severe symptoms
Abdominal angiostrongyliasis	*Angiostrongylus costaricensis*	Ingestion of contaminated food	Mebendazole *or* thiabendazole
Eosinophilic meningitis	*Angiostrongylus cantonensis* (rat lungworm)	Ingestion of undercooked contaminated seafood	Mebendazole

Ascariasis

Ascariasis is caused by *Ascaris lumbricoides,* a large nematode. It is the most prevalent helminthiasis, affecting 1 billion people (see Table 123–3). After humans ingest the eggs, larvae are released and penetrate the intestine, migrate to the lungs, ascend the trachea, and are reswallowed. On entering the intestines again, they mature and produce eggs that are excreted in the stool and are deposited in the soil, where they survive for prolonged periods.

Manifestations may be the result of migration of the larvae to other sites of the body or the presence of adult worms in the intestine. **Pulmonary ascariasis** occurs as the larvae migrate through the lung, producing cough, blood-stained sputum, eosinophilia, and transient infiltrates on chest x-ray films. Adult larvae in the small intestine may cause abdominal pain and distention. Intestinal obstruction from adult worms rarely occurs. Migration of worms into the bile duct may rarely cause acute biliary obstruction. Examination of fresh stool for characteristic eggs is diagnostic. Effective control depends on adequate sanitary treatment and disposal of infected human feces.

Visceral Larva Migrans

Visceral larva migrans is a systemic nematodiasis caused by ingestion of the eggs of the dog tapeworm, *Toxocara canis,* or, less commonly, the cat tapeworm, *Toxocara cati,* or the raccoon tapeworm, *Baylisascaris procyonis* (see Table 123–3). These organisms also cause **ocular larva migrans**.

Visceral larva migrans is most common in young children with pica who have dogs or cats as pets. Ocular toxocariasis occurs in older children. The eggs of these roundworms are produced by adult worms residing in the dog and cat intestine. Ingested eggs hatch into larvae that penetrate the gastrointestinal tract and migrate to the liver, lung, eye, CNS, and heart, where they die and calcify.

Symptoms of visceral larva migrans are the result of the number of migrating worms and the associated immune response. Light infections are often asymptomatic. Symptoms include fever, cough, wheezing, and seizures. Physical findings may include hepatomegaly, crackles, rash, and lymphadenopathy. Visual symptoms may include decreased acuity, strabismus, periorbital edema, or blindness. Eye examination may reveal granulomatous lesions near the macula or disc. Ocular larva migrans is characterized by isolated, unilateral ocular disease and no systemic findings. Larvae probably enter the anterior vitreous of the eye from a peripheral branch of the retinal artery and elicit granulomas in the posterior and peripheral poles that cause vision loss.

Eosinophilia and hypergammaglobulinemia associated with elevated isohemagglutinin levels suggest the diagnosis, which may be confirmed by serology (ELISA) or, less commonly, by biopsy. This is usually a self-limiting illness. In severe disease, albendazole or mebendazole is used. Deworming puppies and kittens, the major excreters of eggs, decreases the risk of infection.

Enterobiasis (Pinworm)

Pinworm is caused by *Enterobius vermicularis,* a nematode that is distributed worldwide. Enterobiasis affects individuals at all socioeconomic levels, especially children. Crowded living conditions predispose to infection. Humans ingest the eggs carried on hands or present in house dust or on bedclothes. The eggs hatch in the stomach, and the larvae migrate to the cecum and mature. At night, the females migrate to the perianal area to lay their eggs, which are viable for 2 days.

The most common symptoms are nocturnal anal pruritus (**pruritus ani**) and sleeplessness, presumably resulting from the migratory female worms. Vaginitis and salpingitis may develop secondary to aberrant worm migration. The eggs are detected by microscopically examining adhesive cellophane tape pressed against the anus in the morning to collect eggs. Less commonly, a worm may be seen in the perianal region. Treatment is with albendazole (400 mg), mebendazole (100 mg), or pyrantel pamoate (11 mg/kg, maximum 1 g) each given as a single oral dose and repeated in 2 weeks.

Schistosomiasis

Schistosomiasis (bilharziasis) is caused by flukes that parasitize the bloodstream, including *Schistosoma haematobium, Schistosoma mansoni, Schistosoma japonicum,* and, rarely, *Schistosoma intercalatum* and *Schistosoma mekongi* (Table 123–4). Schistosomiasis affects more than 2 million people, mainly children and young adults with a peak age range of 10 to 20 years. Humans are infected by cercariae in contaminated water that emerge in an infectious form from snails and penetrate intact skin. Each adult worm migrates to specific sites: *S. haematobium* to the **bladder plexus** and *S. intercalatum* and *S. mekongi* to the **mesenteric vessels**. The eggs are deposited by the adult flukes in urine (*S. haematobium*) or stool (*S. mansoni* and *S. japonicum*). Intermediate hosts for these complex parasites are freshwater snails that are infected by miracidia, which hatch from eggs in freshwater. *S. haematobium* is prevalent in Africa and the Middle East; *S. mansoni* in Africa, the Middle East, the Caribbean, and South America; *S. japonicum* in China, the Philippines, and Indonesia; *S. mekongi* in the Far East; and *S. intercalatum* in West Africa.

TABLE 123–4.   Major Pediatric Syndromes Caused by Parasitic Trematodes

Syndrome	Etiologic Agent	Transmission	Treatment
Schistosomes		Freshwater contact with penetration through the skin	
Intestinal or hepatic schistosomiasis	*Schistosoma mansoni*		Praziquantel *or* oxamniquine
Intestinal or hepatic schistosomiasis	*Schistosoma japonicum*		Praziquantel
Intestinal or hepatic schistosomiasis	*Schistosoma mekongi*		Praziquantel
Urinary schistosomiasis	*Schistosoma haematobium*		Praziquantel
Other trematodes		Ingestion of raw or inadequately cooked foods	
Clonorchiasis (Chinese liver fluke)	*Clonorchis sinensis*		Praziquantel *or* albendazole
Fascioliasis (sheep liver fluke)	*Fasciola hepatica*		Triclabendazole *or* bithionol
Fasciolopsiasis	*Fasciolopsis buski*		Praziquantel
Heterophyiasis	*Heterophyes heterophyes*		Praziquantel
Metagonimiasis	*Metagonimus yokogawai*		Praziquantel
Metorchiasis (North American liver fluke)	*Metorchis conjunctus*		Praziquantel
Nanophyetiasis (Salmon fluke)	*Nanophyetus salmincola*		Praziquantel
Opisthorchiasis (Southeast Asian liver fluke)	*Opisthorchis viverrini*		Praziquantel
Paragonimiasis (lung fluke)	*Paragonimus pulmonalisa, P. westermani, P. mexicaa, P. kellicotti, P. uterobilateralis*		Praziquantel *or* bithionol

The manifestations of schistosomiasis result from eggs that are trapped at the site of deposition or at metastatic locations. Within 3 to 12 weeks of infection, while the worms are maturing, a syndrome of fever, malaise, cough, abdominal pain, and rash can occur. This syndrome is followed by a resultant inflammatory response that leads to further symptoms. **Katayama fever** is an acute condition, with fever, weight loss, hepatosplenomegaly, and eosinophilia. Eggs may be found in the urine (*S. haematobium*) or stool (*S. mansoni* and *S. japonicum*) of infected individuals. Sanitary measures, molluscacides, and therapy for infected individuals may help control the illness.

Echinococcosis

Echinococcosis includes **hydatid or unilocular cyst disease**, caused by *Echinococcus granulosus* (the **minute dog tapeworm**) or *Echinococcus vogeli,* and **alveolar cyst disease**, caused by *Echinococcus multilocularis* (Table 123–5). Dogs become infected with tapeworms by eating infected sheep or cattle viscera and excrete eggs in their stools. Humans acquire echinococcosis by ingesting eggs and become an intermediate host.

The eggs hatch in the intestinal tract, and the larva (**oncospheres**) penetrate the mucosa and enter the circulation to pass to the liver and other visceral organs, forming cysts 2 cm in diameter.

E. granulosus has a worldwide distribution, but is endemic in sheep-raising and cattle-raising areas of Australia, South America, South Africa, the former Soviet Union, and the Mediterranean region. The prevalence is highest in children. Symptoms caused by *E. granulosus* result from space-occupying cysts. Pulmonary cysts may cause hemoptysis, cough, dyspnea, and respiratory distress. Brain cysts appear as tumors; liver cysts cause problems as they compress and obstruct blood flow. Ultrasonography confirms the cystic nature of the lesion. Serologic tests are helpful. Large or asymptomatic granulosa cysts are removed surgically. Treatment with albendazole has shown some benefit.

Neurocysticercosis

Neurocysticercosis is caused by infection with the larval stages (**cysticerci**) of the **pork tapeworm**, *Taenia solium,* and is the most frequent helminthic infection of the CNS (see Table 123–5). Human cysticercosis is

TABLE 123–5. Major Pediatric Syndromes Caused by Parasitic Cestodes

Syndrome	Etiologic Agent	Transmission	Treatment
Echinococcosis		Ingestion of *Echinococcus* eggs	
Unilocular echinococcosis	*Echinococcus granulosus*		Surgical resection *plus* albendazole
Unilocular echinococcosis	*Echinococcus granulosus* var. *canadensis*		Expectant observation
Alveolar echinococcosis	*Echinococcus multilocularis*		Surgical resection is the only reliable means of treatment. Some reports suggest adjunct use of albendazole or mebendazole
Neurocysticercosis	Larval stage of *Taenia solium* (cysticerci)	Ingestion of infected raw/undercooked pork	Albendazole *or* praziquantel
Adult tapeworm infections	*T. solium* (pork tapeworm)	Ingestion of contaminated raw/undercooked pork	Praziquantel
	Taenia saginata (beef tapeworm)	Ingestion of contaminated raw/undercooked beef	Praziquantel
	Dipylidium caninum	Ingestion of infected fleas	Praziquantel
	Diphyllobothrium latum	Ingestion of contaminated raw fish	Praziquantel
	Hymenolepis diminuta	Fecal-oral transmission	Praziquantel
	Hymenolepis nana	Fecal-oral transmission	Praziquantel

a biologic "dead end" infection. Humans are infected after consuming cysticerci in raw or undercooked larva-containing pork. *T. solium* is endemic in Asia, Africa, and Central and South America.

Cysts typically enlarge slowly, causing no or minimal symptoms for years or decades until the organism begins to die. The cyst then begins to swell, and leakage of antigen incites an inflammatory response, resulting in the presenting signs of focal or generalized seizures and calcified cerebral cysts identified by CT or MRI. The CSF shows lymphocytic or eosinophilic pleocytosis. The diagnosis can be confirmed by serologic testing. Neurocysticercosis is treated with albendazole or praziquantel, corticosteroids for concomitant cerebral inflammation from cyst death, and anticonvulsant drugs.

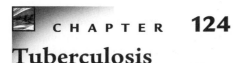

CHAPTER 124
Tuberculosis

ETIOLOGY

The agent of human tuberculosis is *M. tuberculosis*. The tubercle bacilli are pleomorphic, weakly gram-positive curved rods about 2 to 4 μm long. A hallmark of all mycobacteria is **acid fastness**: the capacity to form stable mycolate complexes with arylmethane dyes. The term **acid-fast bacilli** is practically synonymous with mycobacteria. Mycobacteria grow slowly. Isolation from clinical specimens on solid synthetic media usually takes 3 to 6 weeks, and drug-susceptibility testing requires an additional 4 weeks. Growth can be detected in 1 to 3 weeks in selective liquid media using radiolabeled nutrients and PCR technology that allow almost immediate diagnosis in many laboratories.

EPIDEMIOLOGY

Susceptibility to infection with *M. tuberculosis* disease depends on the likelihood of exposure to an individual with infectious tuberculosis (primarily determined by the individual's environment) and the ability of the person's immune system to control the initial infection and keep it latent. An estimated 10 to 15 million persons in the U.S. have latent tuberculosis infection. Without treatment, tuberculosis *disease* develops in 5% to 10% of immunologically normal adults with tuberculosis *infection* at some time during their lives. An estimated 8 million new cases of tuberculosis occur each year among adults, and 3 million deaths are attributed to the disease annually. In developing countries, 1.3 million new cases of the disease occur in children younger than 15 years of age, and 450,000 children die each year of tuberculosis. Most children with tuberculosis infection and disease acquire *M. tuberculosis* from an adult with tuberculosis.

Transmission of *M. tuberculosis* is from person to person, usually by **respiratory droplets** that become airborne when the ill individual coughs, sneezes, laughs, sighs, or breathes. Infected droplets dry and become **droplet nuclei**, which may remain suspended in the air for hours, long after the infectious person has left the environment. Only particles less than 10 μm in diameter can reach the alveoli and establish infection.

Several patient-related factors have been associated with an increased chance of transmission. Of these, a positive acid-fast smear of the sputum is most closely correlated with infectivity. Children with primary pulmonary tuberculosis disease rarely, if ever, infect other children or adults. Tubercle bacilli are relatively sparse in the endobronchial secretions of children with primary pulmonary tuberculosis, and a significant cough is usually lacking. When young children do cough, they rarely produce sputum, and they lack the tussive force necessary to project and suspend infectious particles of the correct size. Nevertheless, hospitalized children with suspected pulmonary tuberculosis are kept in respiratory isolation initially if their parents or adult visitors have not been evaluated fully for tuberculosis. Most initially infectious patients become noninfectious within 2 weeks of starting effective treatment, and many become noninfectious within several days.

In North America, tuberculosis rates are highest in foreign-born persons from high-prevalence countries, residents of prisons, residents of nursing homes, homeless persons, users of illegal drugs, persons who are poor and medically indigent, healthcare workers, and children exposed to adults in high-risk groups. Among U.S. urban dwellers with tuberculosis, persons with AIDS and racial minorities are overrepresented. Most children are infected with *M. tuberculosis* from household contacts, but outbreaks of childhood tuberculosis centered in elementary and high schools, nursery schools, family daycare homes, churches, school buses, and stores still occur. A high-risk adult working in the area has been the source of the outbreak in most cases.

CLINICAL MANIFESTATIONS

Tuberculosis infection describes the asymptomatic stage of infection with *M. tuberculosis,* also termed **latent tuberculosis**. The tuberculin skin test (TST) is positive, but the chest radiograph is normal, and there are no signs or symptoms of illness. **Tuberculosis disease** occurs when there are clinical signs and symptoms or abnormal chest radiographs or extrapulmonary tuberculosis becomes apparent. The term *tuberculosis* usually refers to the disease. The interval between latent tuberculosis and the onset of disease may be several weeks or many decades in adults. In young children, tuberculosis usually develops as an immediate complication of the primary infection, and the distinction between infection and disease may be less obvious.

Primary pulmonary tuberculosis in older infants and children is usually an asymptomatic infection. Often the disease is manifested by a positive TST with minimal abnormalities on the chest radiograph, such as an infiltrate with hilar lymphadenopathy or **Ghon complex**. Malaise, low-grade fever, erythema nodosum, or symptoms resulting from lymph node enlargement may occur after the development of delayed hypersensitivity.

Progressive primary disease is characterized by a primary pneumonia that develops shortly after initial infection. Progression of the primary complex to pulmonary disease or disseminated miliary disease or progression of CNS granulomas to meningitis occurs most commonly in the first year of life. Hilar lymphadenopathy may compress the bronchi or trachea.

Tuberculous pleural effusion, which may accompany primary infection, generally represents the immune response to the organisms. Pleurocentesis reveals lymphocytes and an increased protein level, but usually does not contain bacilli. A pleural biopsy may be necessary to obtain tissue to confirm the diagnosis by showing the expected granuloma formation and acid-fast organisms.

Reactivation pulmonary tuberculosis, common in adolescents and typical in adults with tuberculosis, usually is confined to apical segments of upper lobes or superior segments of lower lobes. There is usually little lymphadenopathy and no extrathoracic infection as a result of established hypersensitivity. This is a manifestation of a secondary expansion of infection at a site seeded years previously during primary infection. Advanced disease is associated with cavitation and endobronchial spread of bacilli. Symptoms include fever, night sweats, malaise, and weight loss. A productive cough and hemoptysis often herald cavitation and bronchial erosion.

Tuberculous pericarditis usually occurs when organisms from the lung or pleura spread to the contiguous surfaces of the pericardium. There is an accumulation of fluid with lymphocytic infiltration in the pericardial space. Persistent inflammations may result in a cellular immune response, with rupture of granulomas into the pericardial space and the development of constrictive pericarditis. In addition to antimycobacterial therapy, tuberculous pericarditis is managed with corticosteroids to decrease inflammation.

Lymphadenopathy is common in primary pulmonary disease. The most common extrathoracic sites of lymphadenitis are the cervical, supraclavicular, and submandibular areas (**scrofula**). Enlargement may cause compression of adjacent structures. **Miliary tuberculosis** refers to widespread hematogenous dissemination with infection of multiple organs. The lesions are of roughly the same size as that of a millet seed, from which the name *miliary* is derived. **Miliary tuberculosis** is characterized by fever, general malaise, weight loss, lymphadenopathy, night sweats, and hepatosplenomegaly. Diffuse bilateral pneumonitis is common, and meningitis may be present. The chest radiograph reveals bilateral miliary infiltrates, showing overwhelming infection. The TST may be nonreactive as a result of **anergy**. Liver or bone marrow biopsy is useful for the diagnosis.

Tuberculous meningitis most commonly occurs in children younger than 5 years old and often within 6 months of primary infection. Tubercle bacilli that seed the meninges during the primary infection replicate, triggering an inflammatory response. This condition may have an insidious onset, initially characterized by low-grade fever, headache, and subtle personality change. Progression of the infection results in basilar meningitis with impingement of the cranial nerves and is manifested by meningeal irritation and eventually increased intracranial pressure, deterioration of mental status, and coma. CT scans show hydrocephalus, edema, periventricular lucencies, and infarctions. CSF analysis reveals increased cell number (50 to 500/mm^3 leukocytes), which early in the course of disease may be either lymphocytes or polymorphonuclear leukocytes. Glucose is low, and protein is significantly elevated. Acid-fast bacilli are not detected frequently in the CSF by either routine or fluorescent staining procedures. Although culture is the gold standard for diagnosis, PCR for *M. tuberculosis* is useful to make this diagnosis. Treatment regimens for tuberculous meningitis generally include four antituberculous drugs and corticosteroids.

Skeletal tuberculosis with mycobacterial infection of the bone results from either hematogenous seeding or direct extension from a **caseous lymph node**. This is usually a chronic disease with an insidious onset that may be mistaken for chronic osteomyelitis caused by *S. aureus*. Radiographs reveal cortical destruction; biopsy and culture are essential for proper diagnosis. Tuberculosis of the spine, **Pott disease**, is the most common skeletal site, followed by the hip and the fingers and toes (**dactylitis**).

Other forms of tuberculosis include **abdominal tuberculosis** that occurs from swallowing infected material. This is a relatively uncommon complication in developed nations, where dairy herds are inspected for bovine tuberculosis. **Tuberculous peritonitis** is associated with abdominal tuberculosis and presents as fever, anorexia, ascites, and abdominal pain. **Urogenital tuberculosis** is a late reactivation complication and is rare in children. Symptomatic illness presents as dysuria, frequency, urgency, hematuria, and "sterile" pyuria.

LABORATORY AND IMAGING STUDIES
Tuberculin Skin Test

The most important diagnostic tool for tuberculosis is the TST. The TST response to tuberculin antigen is a manifestation of a T cell–mediated delayed hypersensitivity. It is usually positive 2 to 6 weeks after onset of infection (occasionally 3 months) and at the time of symptomatic illness. The **Mantoux test**, an intradermal injection of 5 TU (tuberculin units) (intermediate test strength) of Tween-stabilized purified tuberculous antigen (purified protein derivative standard [PPD-S]) usually on the volar surface of the forearm, is the standard for screening high-risk populations and for diagnosis in all ill patients or contacts. False-negative responses may occur early in the illness, with use of inactivated antigen (as a result of poor storage practice or inadequate administration), or as a result of immunosuppression (secondary to underlying illness, AIDS, malnutrition, or overwhelming tuberculosis). Tests with questionable results should be repeated after several weeks of therapy and adequate nutrition.

The only TST that should be used in ordinary practice is the 5-TU test (Mantoux test) that is interpreted based on the host status and size of induration (Table 124–1). Only persons at high risk should be offered a Mantoux test (Table 124–2). When persons at low risk are given the TST, the positive predictive value of a positive test decreases, and persons with active tuberculosis (mainly persons with asymptomatic infection with atypical mycobacteria) are subjected to unnecessary treatment.

Culture

The ultimate diagnostic confirmation relies on culture of the organism, a process that usually is more successful when tissue is used (pleural biopsy, pericardial membrane), rather than only the pleural or pericardial fluid. Sputum is an excellent source for diagnosis in adults, but is difficult to obtain in young children. Therefore gastric fluid taken before or immediately on waking containing swallowed sputum may yield positive results. Induced sputum may be another method for young children. Large volumes of fluid (CSF, pericardial fluid) yield a higher rate of recovery of organisms, but slow growth of the mycobacteria makes culture less helpful in very ill children. When the organism is grown, the drug susceptibilities should be determined because of the increasing incidence of resistant organisms. Antigen detection and DNA probes have expedited diagnosis, especially in CNS disease.

Diagnostic Imaging

Because many cases of pulmonary tuberculosis in children are clinically relatively silent, radiography is a

TABLE 124–1. Definitions of Positive Tuberculin Skin Test Results in Infants, Children, and Adolescents*

Induration ≥5 mm

Children in close contact with known or suspected contagious cases of tuberculosis disease
Children suspected to have tuberculosis disease
  Findings on chest radiograph consistent with active or previously active tuberculosis
  Clinical evidence of tuberculosis disease[†]
Children receiving immunosuppressive therapy[‡] or with immunosuppressive conditions, including HIV infection

Induration ≥10 mm

Children at increased risk of disseminated disease
  Children <4 years old
  Children with other medical conditions, including Hodgkin disease, lymphoma, diabetes mellitus, chronic renal failure, or malnutrition
Children with increased exposure to tuberculosis disease
  Children born, or whose parents were born, in high-prevalence regions of the world
  Children frequently exposed to adults who are HIV-infected, homeless, users of illicit drugs, residents of nursing homes, incarcerated or institutionalized, or migrant farm workers
  Children who travel to high-prevalence regions of the world

Induration ≥15 mm

Children ≥4 years old without any risk factors

---

*These definitions apply regardless of previous bacille Calmette-Guérin immunization. Erythema at tuberculin skin test site does not indicate a positive test result. Tuberculin skin tests should be read at 48 to 72 hours after placement.
[†]Evidence by physical examination or laboratory assessment that would include tuberculosis in the working differential diagnosis (e.g., meningitis).
[‡]Including immunosuppressive doses of corticosteroids.

TABLE 124–2. Tuberculin Skin Test Recommendations for Infants, Children, and Adolescents

Children for whom immediate TST is indicated
  Contacts of people with confirmed or suspected contagious tuberculosis (contact investigation)
  Children with radiographic or clinical findings suggesting tuberculosis disease
  Children emigrating from endemic countries (e.g., Asia, Middle East, Africa, Latin America)
  Children with travel histories to endemic countries or significant contact with indigenous people from such countries
Children who should have annual TST[†]
  Children infected with HIV
  Incarcerated adolescents
Some experts recommend children should be tested every 2-3 yr[‡]
  Children with ongoing exposure to HIV-infected people, homeless people, residents of nursing homes, institutionalized adolescents or adults, users of illicit drugs, incarcerated adolescents or adults, and migrant farm workers; foster children with exposure to adults in the preceding high-risk groups are included
Some experts recommend children should be considered for TST at 4-6 and 11-16 years old
  Children whose parents emigrated (with unknown TST status) from regions of the world with high prevalence of tuberculosis; continued potential exposure by travel to the endemic areas or household contact with people from the endemic areas (with unknown TST status) should be an indication for a repeated TST
Children at increased risk of progression of infection to disease
  Children with other medical conditions, including diabetes mellitus, chronic renal failure, malnutrition, and congenital or acquired immunodeficiencies, warrant special consideration. Without recent exposure, children are not at increased risk of acquiring tuberculosis infection. Underlying immunodeficiencies associated with these conditions theoretically would enhance the possibility for progression to severe disease. Initial histories of potential exposure to tuberculosis should be included for all of these patients. If these histories or local epidemiologic factors suggest a possibility of exposure, immediate and periodic TST should be considered. **An initial TST should be performed before initiation of immunosuppressive therapy, including prolonged steroid administration, for any child with an underlying condition that necessitates immunosuppressive therapy**

---

*Recommendations from the American Thoracic Society, Centers for Disease Control and Prevention, Infectious Diseases Society of America, and the American Academy of Pediatrics. Am J Respir Crit Care Med 61:S221-247, 2000.
[†]Bacille Calmette-Guérin immunization is not a contraindication to TST.
[‡]Initial TST is at the time of diagnosis or circumstance, beginning at 3 months of age.
TST, tuberculin skin test.

cornerstone for the diagnosis of disease. The initial parenchymal inflammation that follows deposition of infected droplet nuclei in the alveoli of the lung usually is not visible radiographically. A localized, nonspecific infiltrate with an overlying pleural reaction may be seen, however. This lesion usually resolves within 1 to 2 weeks. All lobar segments of the lung are at equal risk of being the focus of the initial infection. In 25% of cases, two or more lobes of the lungs are involved, although disease usually occurs at only one site. Spread of infection to regional lymph nodes occurs early.

The hallmark of childhood pulmonary tuberculosis is the relatively large size and importance of the hilar lymphadenitis compared with the less significant size of the initial parenchymal focus, together historically referred to as the **Ghon complex** (with or without calcification of the lymph nodes). Hilar lymphadenopathy is inevitably present with childhood tuberculosis, but it may not be detected on a plain radiograph when calcification is not present. Partial bronchial obstruction caused by external compression from the enlarging nodes can cause air trapping, hyperinflation, and lobar emphysema. Occasionally, children have a picture of lobar pneumonia without impressive hilar lymphadenopathy. If the infection is progressively destructive, liquefaction of the lung parenchyma leads to formation of a thin-walled primary tuberculous cavity. Adolescents with pulmonary tuberculosis may develop segmental lesions with hilar lymphadenopathy or the apical infiltrates, with or without cavitation, that are typical of adult reactivation tuberculosis.

Radiographic studies aid greatly in the diagnosis of **extrapulmonary tuberculosis** in children. Plain radiographs, CT, and MRI of the **tuberculous spine** usually show collapse and destruction of the vertebral body with narrowing of the involved disc spaces. Radiographic findings in bone and joint tuberculosis range from mild joint effusions and small lytic lesions to massive destruction of the bone.

In tuberculosis of the CNS, CT or MRI of the brains of patients with tuberculous meningitis may be normal during early stages of the infection. As the disease progresses, basilar enhancement and communicating hydrocephalus with signs of cerebral edema or early focal ischemia are the most common findings. In children with **renal tuberculosis**, IV pyelograms may reveal mass lesions, dilation of the proximal ureters, multiple small filling defects, and hydronephrosis if ureteral stricture is present.

DIFFERENTIAL DIAGNOSIS

The differential diagnosis of tuberculosis includes a multitude of diagnoses because tuberculosis may affect any organ, and in early disease the symptoms and signs may be nonspecific. In pulmonary disease, tuberculosis may appear similar to pneumonia, malignancy, and any systemic disease in which generalized lymphadenopathy occurs. The diagnosis of tuberculosis should be suspected if the TST is positive or if there is history of tuberculosis in a contact. Otherwise, culture of respiratory secretions or of biopsied pulmonary tissue may be required.

The differential diagnosis of tuberculous lymphadenopathy includes infections caused by atypical mycobacteria, cat-scratch disease, fungal infection, viral or bacterial disease, toxoplasmosis, sarcoidosis, drug reactions, and malignancy. The diagnosis may be confirmed by fine needle aspiration, but may necessitate excisional biopsy accompanied by appropriate histologic and microbiologic studies.

TREATMENT

The treatment of tuberculosis is affected by the presence of naturally occurring drug-resistant organisms in large bacterial populations, even before chemotherapy is initiated, and the fact that mycobacteria replicate slowly and can remain dormant in the body for prolonged periods. Although a population of bacilli as a whole may be considered drug susceptible, a subpopulation of drug-resistant organisms occurs at fairly predictable frequencies of 10^{-5} to 10^{-7}, depending on the drug. Cavities may contain 10^9 tubercle bacilli with thousands of organisms resistant to any one drug, but only rare organisms resistant to multiple drugs. The chance that an organism is naturally resistant to two drugs is on the order of 10^{-11} to 10^{-13}. Because populations of this size rarely occur in patients, organisms naturally resistant to two drugs are essentially nonexistent.

For patients with large populations of bacilli, such as adults with cavities or extensive infiltrates, at least two antituberculous drugs must be given, but for patients with tuberculosis infection but no disease, the bacterial population is small, and a single drug, such as isoniazid, can be given. Therapy for latent infection is aimed at eradicating the presumably small inoculum of organisms sequestered within macrophages and suppressed by normal T cell activity. To prevent reactivation of these latent bacilli, therapy with a single agent (usually isoniazid for 9 months) is suggested. Children with primary pulmonary tuberculosis and patients with extrapulmonary tuberculosis have medium-sized populations in which significant numbers of drug-resistant organisms may or may not be present. In general, these patients are treated with at least two drugs (Table 124–3).

Antibiotics

Isoniazid and rifampin are bactericidal for *M. tuberculosis* and are effective against all populations of mycobacteria. Along with pyrazinamide, they form the backbone of the antimicrobial treatment of tuberculosis. Other drugs are used in special circumstances, such as tuberculous meningitis and antibiotic-resistant tuberculosis. Ethambutol, ethionamide, streptomycin, and cycloserine are bacteriostatic and are used with bactericidal antituberculous agents to prevent emergence of resistance.

Treatment Duration

A 9-month regimen of isoniazid and rifampin cures more than 98% of cases of drug-susceptible pulmonary

TABLE 124–3. Recommended Treatment Regimens for Drug-Susceptible Tuberculosis in Infants, Children, and Adolescents

Infection or Disease Category	Regimen	Comments
Latent tuberculosis infection (positive TST result, no disease)		
Isoniazid-susceptible	9 mo of isoniazid, once a day	If daily therapy is not possible, DOT twice a week can be used for 9 mo
Isoniazid-resistant	6 mo of rifampin, once a day	
Isoniazid-rifampin-resistant	Consult a tuberculosis specialist	
Pulmonary and extrapulmonary (except meningitis and bone/joint)	2 mo of isoniazid, rifampin, and pyrazinamide daily, followed by 4 mo of isoniazid and rifampin twice weekly under DOT	If possible drug resistance is a concern, another drug (ethambutol or an aminoglycoside) is added to the initial 3-drug therapy until drug susceptibilities are determined. DOT is highly desirable
If hilar lymphadenopathy only, a 6-mo course of isoniazid and rifampin is sufficient
Drugs can be given 2 or 3 times/wk under DOT in the initial phase if nonadherence is likely
Meningitis, bone/joint	2 mo of isoniazid, rifampin, pyrazinamide, and an aminoglycoside or ethionamide, once a day, followed by 7-10 mo of isoniazid and rifampin, once a day or twice a week (9-12 mo total)	A fourth drug, usually an aminoglycoside, is given with initial therapy until drug susceptibility is known
For patients who may have acquired tuberculosis in geographic areas where resistance to streptomycin is common, capreomycin, kanamycin, or amikacin may be used instead of streptomycin

Recommendations from the American Thoracic Society, Centers for Disease Control and Prevention, and Infectious Diseases Society of America. Am J Respir Crit Care Med 167:603-662, 2003.

DOT, directly observed therapy; TST, tuberculin skin test.

tuberculosis in adults. After daily administration for the first 1 to 2 months, both drugs can be given daily or twice weekly for the remaining 7 to 8 months with equivalent results and low rates of adverse reactions. The addition of pyrazinamide at the beginning of the regimen reduces the duration of necessary treatment to 6 months. Therapy with isoniazid, rifampin, pyrazinamide, and streptomycin during the initial 2 months of treatment followed by isoniazid and rifampin in the remaining 4 months routinely yields cure rates of more than 98% with relapse rates less than 4% in adults. In children with drug-susceptible pulmonary tuberculosis, a 9-month regimen of isoniazid and rifampin is highly successful. Medications should be given daily at first, but may be administered twice weekly during the final 7 to 8 months of treatment. The AAP has endorsed a regimen of 6 months of isoniazid and rifampin supplemented during the first 2 months by pyrazinamide as standard therapy for intrathoracic tuberculosis in children (see Table 124–3). Noncompliance, or nonadherence, is a major problem in tuberculosis control because of the long-term nature of treatment and the sometimes difficult social circumstances of the patients. As treatment regimens become shorter, adherence assumes an even greater importance. Improvement in compliance occurs with **directly observed therapy**, which means that the healthcare worker is physically present when the medications are administered.

COMPLICATIONS

Tuberculosis of the spine may result in angulation or **gibbus** formation that requires surgical correction after the infection is cured. With extrapulmonary tuberculosis, the major problem is often delayed recognition of the cause of disease and delayed initiation of treatment. Most childhood tuberculous meningitis occurs in developing countries, where the prognosis is poor.

PROGNOSIS

In general, the prognosis of tuberculosis in infants, children, and adolescents is excellent with early recognition and effective chemotherapy. In most children with pulmonary tuberculosis, the disease completely resolves, and ultimately radiographic findings are normal. The prognosis for children with bone and joint tuberculosis and tuberculous meningitis depends directly on the stage of disease at the time antituberculous medications are started.

PREVENTION

Tuberculosis control programs involve case finding and treatment, which interrupts secondary transmission of infection from close contacts. Infected close contacts are identified by positive TST reactions and can be started on appropriate treatment to prevent transmission.

Prevention of transmission in healthcare settings involves appropriate physical ventilation of the air around the source case. Offices, clinics, and hospital rooms used by adults with possible tuberculosis should have adequate ventilation, with air exhausted to the outside (**negative-pressure ventilation**). Healthcare providers should have annual TSTs.

Bacille Calmette-Guérin Vaccine

The only available vaccine against tuberculosis is the BCG. The original vaccine organism was a strain of *Mycobacterium bovis* attenuated by subculture every 3 weeks for 13 years. The preferred route of administration is intradermal injection with a syringe and needle because this is the only method that permits accurate measurement of an individual dose. The official recommendation of the World Health Organization is a single dose administered during infancy. In the United Kingdom, a single dose is administered during adolescence. In many countries, the first dose is given in infancy, then one or more additional vaccinations are given during childhood. In some countries, repeat vaccination is universal; in others, it is based either on tuberculin negativity or on the absence of a typical scar. Some studies showed a great deal of protection from BCG, but others showed no efficacy at all. BCG vaccine is not used frequently in the U.S. Many infants who receive BCG vaccine never have a positive tuberculin reaction. When a reaction does occur, the induration size is usually less than 10 mm, and the reaction wanes after several years.

CHAPTER 125

HIV and AIDS

ETIOLOGY

The cause of AIDS is HIV, a single-stranded RNA virus of the retrovirus family that produces a reverse transcriptase enabling the viral RNA to act as a template for DNA transcription and integration into the host genome. HIV-1 causes 99% of all human cases. HIV-2, which is less virulent, causes 1% to 9% of cases in parts of Africa and is very rare in the U.S.

HIV infects human helper T cells (CD4 cells) and cells of monocyte-macrophage lineage via interaction of viral protein gp120 with the CD4 molecule and chemokines that serve as coreceptors, permitting membrane fusion and cell entry. Because helper T cells are important for delayed hypersensitivity, T cell–dependent B cell antibody production, and T cell–mediated lymphokine activation of macrophages, their destruction produces a profound combined (B and T cell) immunodeficiency. A lack of T cell regulation and unrestrained antigenic stimulation result in polyclonal hypergammaglobulinemia with nonspecific and ineffective globulins. Other cells bearing CD4, such as microglia, astrocytes, oligodendroglia, and placental tissues, also may be infected with HIV.

HIV infection is a continuously progressive process with a variable period of clinical latency before development of AIDS-defining conditions. All untreated patients have evidence of ongoing viral replication. There are no overt manifestations of immunodeficiency until the host can no longer maintain replacement of the CD4 cells destroyed by infection, then CD4 cell numbers progressively decline to critical threshold levels. Quantitation of the viral load has become an important parameter in management.

Horizontal transmission of HIV is by unprotected heterosexual or homosexual contact and IV drug use. Transmission by contaminated blood and blood products has been eliminated in developed countries, but still occurs in developing countries. **Vertical transmission** of HIV from mother to infant may occur transplacentally in utero, during birth, or by breastfeeding. Risk factors for perinatal transmission include prematurity, rupture of membranes more than 4 hours, and high maternal circulating levels of HIV at delivery. Perinatal transmission can be decreased from approximately 25% to less than 8% with antiretroviral treatment of the mother before and during delivery and postnatal treatment of the infant. Breastfeeding by HIV-infected mothers increases the risk of vertical transmission by 50% to 100%. In untreated infants, the mean incubation interval for development of an AIDS-defining condition after vertical transmission is 5 months (range 1 to 24 months) compared with an incubation period after horizontal transmission of generally 7 to 10 years.

EPIDEMIOLOGY

Worldwide, as of 2003, more than 38 million persons have been infected with HIV, including more than 20 million persons who have died of AIDS, with 80% of the deaths in Africa. More than 16,000 persons become newly infected with HIV each day. An estimated 5 million persons acquired HIV in 2003, the greatest number in any single year since the beginning of the epidemic. In areas of Africa and Asia, infection rates of 40% are largely the result of heterosexual transmission. There are approximately 900,000 persons who have been diagnosed with AIDS in the U.S., including approximately 9300 children younger than 13 years old. There are approximately 40,000 new HIV infections annually in the U.S.

Vertical transmission has accounted for greater than 90% of all cases of AIDS in children in the U.S. Before perinatal prophylaxis, approximately 1000 to 2000 infants were born with HIV infection each year in the U.S. The effectiveness of perinatal prophylaxis has reduced dramatically the numbers of new cases of pediatric AIDS in developed countries. Most pediatric cases now occur in adolescents who engage in unprotected sexual activities.

CLINICAL MANIFESTATIONS

In adolescents and adults, primary infection results in the **acute retroviral syndrome**, which develops after an incubation period of 2 to 6 weeks and consists of fever, malaise, weight loss, pharyngitis, lymphadenopathy, and often a maculopapular rash. The risk of oppor-

tunistic infections and other AIDS-defining conditions is related to the depletion of CD4 T cells. A combination of CD4 cell count and percentage and clinical manifestations is used to classify HIV infection in children (Tables 125–1, 125–2, and 125–3). Initial symptoms with vertical transmission vary and may include failure to thrive, neurodevelopmental delay, lymphadenopathy, hepatosplenomegaly, chronic or recurrent diarrhea, interstitial pneumonia, or oral thrush. These findings may be subtle and remarkable only by their persistence. Manifestations that are more common in children than adults with HIV infection include recurrent bacterial infections, lymphoid hyperplasia, chronic parotid swelling, lymphocytic interstitial pneumonitis, and earlier onset of progressive neurologic deterioration. Pulmonary manifestations of HIV infection are common and include *P. jirovecii* (*carinii*) pneumonia, which can present early in infancy as a primary pneumonia characterized by hypoxia, tachypnea, retractions, elevated serum lactate dehydrogenase, and fever.

In the U.S., most pregnant women are screened and, if indicated, treated for HIV infection. Infants born to HIV-infected mothers receive prophylaxis and are prospectively tested for infection. The diagnosis of HIV infection in most infants born in the U.S. is confirmed before development of clinical signs of infection.

LABORATORY AND IMAGING STUDIES

HIV infection can be diagnosed definitively by 1 month of age and in virtually all infected infants by 6 months of age using viral diagnostic assays (RNA PCR, DNA PCR, or virus culture). Maternal antibodies may be detectable until 12 to 15 months of age, and a positive serologic test is not considered diagnostic until 18 months of age.

Diagnostic viral testing should be performed by 48 hours of age, at 1 to 2 months of age, and at 3 to 6 months of age. An additional test at 14 days of age is often performed because the diagnostic sensitivity

TABLE 125–1.   1994 Revised HIV Pediatric Classification System: Immunologic Categories*

Immune Category	<12 mo		1-5 yr		6-12 yr	
	No./mm³	(%)	No./mm³	(%)	No./mm³	(%)
Category 1: no suppression	≥1500	(≥25)	≥1000	(≥25)	≥500	(≥25)
Category 2: moderate suppression	750-1499	(15-24)	500-999	(15-24)	200-499	(15-24)
Category 3: severe suppression	<750	(<15)	<500	(<15)	<200	(<15)

*Based on age-specific CD4 T cell count and percentage of total lymphocytes.
From Centers for Disease Control and Prevention: 1994 revised classification system for human immunodeficiency virus infection in children less than 13 years of age. MMWR Morb Mortal Wkly Rep 43(RR-12):1-10, 1994.

TABLE 125–2.   1994 Revised HIV Pediatric Classification System: Clinical Categories

Category N: Not Symptomatic

Children who have no signs or symptoms considered to be the result of HIV infection or who have only one of the conditions listed in category A

Category A: Mildly Symptomatic

Children with ≥2 of the following conditions, but none of the conditions listed in categories B and C
Lymphadenopathy (≥0.5 cm at >2 sites; bilateral = 1 site)
Hepatomegaly
Splenomegaly
Dermatitis
Parotitis
Recurrent or persistent upper respiratory infection, sinusitis, or otitis media

Category B: Moderately Symptomatic

Children who have symptomatic conditions, other than those listed for category A or category C, that are attributed to HIV infection. Examples of conditions in clinical category B include, but are not limited to, the following:
Anemia (<8 g/dL), neutropenia (<1000/mm^3), or thrombocytopenia (<100,000/mm^3) persisting ≥30 days
Bacterial meningitis, pneumonia, or sepsis (single episode)
Candidiasis, oropharyngeal (i.e., thrush) persisting for >2 mo in children aged >6 mo
Cardiomyopathy
Cytomegalovirus infection with onset before age 1 mo
Diarrhea, recurrent or chronic
Hepatitis
HSV stomatitis, recurrent (i.e., >2 episodes within 1 yr)
HSV bronchitis, pneumonitis, or esophagitis with onset before age 1 mo
Herpes zoster (i.e., shingles) involving at least 2 distinct episodes or >1 dermatome
Leiomyosarcoma
LIP or pulmonary lymphoid hyperplasia complex
Nephropathy
Nocardiosis
Fever lasting >1 mo
Toxoplasmosis with onset before age 1 mo
Varicella, disseminated (i.e., complicated chickenpox)

Category C: Severely Symptomatic

Children who have any condition listed in the 1987 surveillance case definition for acquired immunodeficiency syndrome, with the exception of LIP (which is a category B condition)

HSV, herpes simplex virus; LIP, lymphoid interstitial pneumonia.
From Centers for Disease Control and Prevention: 1994 revised classification system for human immunodeficiency virus infection in children less than 13 years of age. MMWR Morb Mortal Wkly Rep 43(RR-12):1-10, 1994.

TABLE 125–3.   Centers for Disease Control and Prevention Classification of Pediatric HIV Infection Based on Immunologic and Clinical Categories*

	Clinical Categories			
Immune Categories	*N—No Signs/Symptoms*	*A—Mild Signs/Symptoms*	*B—Moderate Signs/Symptoms*†	*C—Severe Signs/Symptoms*†
1. No evidence of suppression	N1	A1	B1	C1
2. Evidence of moderate suppression	N2	A2	B2	C2
3. Severe suppression	N3	A3	B3	C3

*Children whose HIV infection status is not confirmed are classified by using the above grid with a letter *E* (for perinatally exposed) placed before the appropriate classification code (e.g., EN2).
†Category C and lymphoid interstitial pneumonitis in category B are reportable to state and local health departments as AIDS.
From Centers for Disease Control and Prevention: 1994 revised classification system for human immunodeficiency virus infection in children less than 13 years of age. MMWR Morb Mortal Wkly Rep 43(RR-12):1-10, 1994.

increases rapidly by 2 weeks of age. HIV DNA PCR is the preferred virologic method for diagnosing HIV infection during infancy and identifies 38% of infected infants at 48 hours and 96% at 28 days. HIV RNA PCR has 25% to 40% sensitivity during the first weeks of life, increasing to 90% to 100% by 2 to 3 months of age. HIV culture is complicated and not routinely performed.

HIV infection of an exposed infant is confirmed if virologic tests are positive on two separate occasions. HIV infection can be reasonably excluded in nonbreast-fed infants with at least two virologic tests performed at older than 1 month of age, with one test being performed at older than 4 months of age, or at least two negative antibody tests performed at older than 6 months of age, with an interval of at least 1 month between the tests. Loss of HIV antibody combined with negative HIV DNA PCR confirms the absence of HIV infection. Persistence of a positive HIV antibody test at older than 18 months of age indicates HIV infection.

DIFFERENTIAL DIAGNOSIS

The differential diagnosis of AIDS in infants includes primary immunodeficiency syndromes and intrauterine infection. Prominence of individual symptoms, such as diarrhea, may suggest other etiologies.

TREATMENT

Management of HIV infection in children and adolescents is rapidly evolving and becoming increasingly complex and should be directed by a specialist in the treatment of HIV infection. Therapy is initiated based on the severity of HIV disease, as indicated by AIDS-defining conditions, and the risk of disease progression, as indicated by CD4 cell count and plasma HIV RNA level. The timing of initiation of antiretroviral therapy for HIV-infected children is controversial. Initiation while the patient is still asymptomatic may preserve immune function and prevent clinical progression, but incurs the adverse effects of therapy and may facilitate emergence of drug-resistant virus. Because the risk of HIV progression is fourfold to sixfold greater in infants and very young children, treatment recommendations for children are more aggressive than for adults. All age groups show rapid increases in risk as CD4 cell percentage declines to less than 15%.

Initiation of therapy is recommended for infants younger than 12 months old who have clinical or immunologic symptoms of HIV disease, regardless of HIV RNA level, and should be considered for HIV-infected infants who are asymptomatic and have normal immune parameters. Initiation of therapy is recommended for all children older than 12 months of age with AIDS (clinical category C) or severe immunosuppression (immune category 3) and should be consid-

ered for children who have mild to moderate clinical symptoms (clinical category A or B), moderate immunologic suppression (immune category 2), or confirmed plasma HIV RNA levels greater than 100,000 copies/mL. Indications for treatment of adolescents and adults include CD4 cell count less than 200 to 350/mm^3 or plasma HIV RNA levels greater than 55,000 copies/mL.

Combination therapy with **highly active antiretroviral therapy (HAART)** is recommended (Table 125–4). Antiretroviral drugs include nucleoside analogue or nucleoside reverse transcriptase inhibitors, nonnucleoside reverse transcriptase inhibitors, protease inhibitors, and fusion inhibitors. Viral loads are reduced significantly with effective combination therapy, leading to the amelioration of clinical symptoms and opportunistic infections. Combination therapy with dual nucleoside reverse transcriptase inhibitor combinations (zidovudine-lamivudine, zidovudine-didanosine, or stavudine-lamivudine) and a protease inhibitor is a common initial regimen for children.

The ability of HIV to become resistant to antiretroviral agents rapidly and the development of cross-resistance to several classes of agents simultaneously are major problems. Determination of HIV RNA, CD4 cell count, and HIV phenotype and genotype is essential for monitoring and modifying antiretroviral treatment.

Routine immunizations are recommended to prevent vaccine-preventable infections, but may result in suboptimal immune responses. In addition to heptavalent pneumococcal conjugate vaccine, 23-valent pneumococcal polysaccharide vaccine is recommended for HIV-infected children at 2 years of age and adolescents and adults with CD4 counts 200/mm^3 or more. Because of the risk of fatal measles in children with AIDS, children without severe immunosuppression should receive their first dose of MMR at 12 months of age with the second dose of MMR 1 month later. MMR should not be administered to severely immunocompromised (clinical category 3) children. VZV vaccine should be given only to asymptomatic, nonimmunosuppressed children beginning at 12 months of age as two doses of vaccine at least 3 months apart. Inactivated split influenza virus vaccine should be administered annually to all HIV-infected children 6 months old or older. HIV-infected children exposed to varicella or measles should receive VZIG or immunoglobulin prophylaxis.

COMPLICATIONS

The approach to the numerous opportunistic infections in HIV-infected patients involves treatment for infections and prophylaxis for infections likely to occur as CD4 cells are depleted. With potent antiretroviral therapy and immune reconstitution, routine prophylaxis for the common opportunistic infections depends

TABLE 125–4. Recommended Antiretroviral Regimens for Initial Therapy for HIV Infection in Children

Protease Inhibitor–Based Regimens

Strongly recommended:	Two NRTIs[1] *plus* lopinavir/ritonavir *or* nelfinavir *or* ritonavir
Alternative recommendation:	Two NRTIs[1] *plus* amprenavir (child ≥4 years old)[2] *or* indinavir

Non-Nucleoside Reverse Transcriptase Inhibitor-Based Regimens

Strongly recommended:	Children >3 years old: Two NRTIs[1] *plus* efavirenz[3] (with or without nelfinavir)
	Children ≤3 years old or who cannot swallow capsules: Two NRTIs[1] *plus* nevirapine[3]
Alternative recommendation:	Two NRTIs[1] *plus* nevirapine[3] (children >3 years old)

Nucleoside Analogue–Based Regimens

Strongly recommended:	None
Alternative recommendation:	Zidovudine *plus* lamivudine *plus* abacavir
Use in special circumstances:	Two NRTIs[1]

Regimens That Are Not Recommended

Monotherapy[4]
Certain two NRTI combinations[1]
Two NRTIs *plus* saquinavir soft or hard gel capsule as a sole protease inhibitor[5]

Insufficient Data to Recommend

Two NRTIs[1] *plus* delavirdine
Dual protease inhibitors, including saquinavir soft or hard gel capsule with low-dose ritonavir, with the exception of lopinavir/ritonavir[4]
NRTI *plus* NNRTI *plus* protease inhibitor[6]
Tenofovir-containing regimens
Enfuvirtide (T-20)-containing regimens
Emtricitabine (FTC)-containing regimens
Atazanavir-containing regimens
Fosamprenavir-containing regimens

[1]Dual NRTI combination recommendations:
  Strongly recommended choices: zidovudine plus didanosine or lamivudine; or stavudine plus lamivudine
  Alternative choices: abacavir plus zidovudine or lamivudine; or didanosine plus lamivudine
  Use in special circumstances: stavudine plus didanosine; or zalcitabine plus zidovudine
  Insufficient data: tenofovir- or emtricitabine-containing regimens
  Not recommended: zalcitabine plus didanosine, stavudine, or lamivudine; or zidovudine plus stavudine
[2]Amprenavir should not be administered to children under age 4 years due to the propylene glycol and vitamin E content of the oral liquid preparation and lack of pharmacokinetic data in this age group.
[3]Efavirenz is currently available only in capsule form, although a liquid formulation is currently under study to determine appropriate dosage in HIV-infected children <3 years old; nevirapine would be the preferred NNRTI for children <3 years old or who require a liquid formulation.
[4]Except for zidovudine chemoprophylaxis administered to HIV-exposed infants during the first 6 wk of life to prevent perinatal HIV transmission; if an infant is confirmed as HIV-infected while receiving zidovudine prophylaxis, therapy should either be discontinued or changed to a combination antiretroviral drug regimen.
[5]With the exception of lopinavir/ritonavir, data on the pharmacokinetics and safety of dual protease inhibitor combinations (e.g., low-dose ritonavir pharmacologic boosting of saquinavir, indinavir, or nelfinavir) are limited; use of dual protease inhibitors as a component of initial therapy is not recommended, although such regimens may have utility as secondary treatment regimens for children who have failed initial therapy. Saquinavir soft and hard gel capsules require low dose ritonavir boosting to achieve adequate levels in children, but pharmacokinetic data on appropriate dosing not yet available.
[6]With the exception of efavirenz plus nelfinavir plus 1 or 2 NRTIs, which has been studied in HIV-infected children and shown to have virologic and immunologic efficacy in a clinical trial.
NRTI, nucleoside analogue reverse transcriptase inhibitor; NNRTI, non-nucleoside analogue reverse transcriptase inhibitor.
From Working Group on Antiretroviral Therapy and Medical Management of HIV-Infected Children: Guidelines for the Use of Antiretroviral Agents in Pediatric HIV Infection. http://AIDSinfo.nih.gov. May 1, 2005.

TABLE 125–5.   Prophylaxis to Prevent First Episode of Opportunistic Disease in Infants and Children Infected with HIV

Pathogens and Indications	Prophylaxis
Strongly Recommended as Standard of Care	
Vaccine-preventable pathogens	Routine immunizations (see Figure 94-1)
Pneumocystis jirovecii (*carinii*)(PCP)	TMP-SMZ
HIV-infected or HIV-indeterminate, infants 1-12 months old	Alternatives: dapsone, aerosolized pentamidine, atovaquone
HIV-infected children 1-5 years old with CD4 count <500/µL or CD4 percentage <15%	
HIV-infected children 6-12 years old with CD4 count <200/µL or CD4 percentage <15%	
Mycobacterium tuberculosis	Isoniazid-sensitive: isoniazid
TST reaction, ≥5mm *or* prior positive TST result without treatment; or contact with any case of active tuberculosis regardless of TST result	Isoniazid-resistant: rifampin Multidrug resistance: consult public health authorities
Mycobacterium avium complex	Clarithromycin or azithromycin
<1 year old: CD4 count <750/µL	
1-2 years old: CD4 count <500/µL	
2-6 years old: CD4 count <75/µL	
≥6 years old: CD4 count <50/µL	
Varicella-zoster virus	Varicella-zoster immunoglobulin
Significant exposure to varicella or zoster with no history of chickenpox or zoster	
Generally Recommended	
Toxoplasma gondii	TMP-SMZ
IgG antibody to *Toxoplasma* and severe immunosuppression	Alternatives: dapsone *plus* pyrimethamine *plus* leucovorin or atovaquone
Varicella-zoster virus	Varicella-zoster vaccine
HIV-infected children who are asymptomatic and not immunosuppressed	
Influenza virus	Inactivated split trivalent influenza vaccine
All HIV-infected persons (annually, before influenza season)	Alternative: oseltamivir during outbreaks for children ≥13 years old
Not Recommended for Most Children—Indicated for Use Only in Unusual Circumstances	
Invasive bacterial infections	IVIG (400 mg/kg every 2-4 wk)
Hypogammaglobulinemia (IgG <400 mg/dL)	
Cryptococcus neoformans	Fluconazole
Severe immunosuppression	Alternative: itraconazole
Histoplasma capsulatum	Itraconazole
Severe immunosuppression, endemic geographic area	
Cytomegalovirus	Ganciclovir (oral)
Cytomegalovirus antibody positivity and severe immunosuppression	

IVIG, IV immunoglobulin; PCP, *Pneumocystis carinii* pneumonia; TMP-SMZ, trimethoprim-sulfamethoxazole; TST, tuberculin skin test.

on the child's age and CD4 count (Table 125–5). Infants born to HIV-infected mothers receive prophylaxis for *P. jirovecii* (*carinii*) pneumonia with TMP-SMZ beginning at 4 to 6 weeks of age and continued for the first year of life or discontinued if HIV infection is subsequently excluded. TMP-SMZ prophylaxis for *P. jirovecii* (*carinii*) pneumonia for older children and adolescents is provided if CD4 cell counts are less than 200/mm³ or there is history of oropharyngeal candidiasis. Rifabutin prophylaxis for *M. avium* complex infection is provided if CD4 cell counts are less than 50/mm³. Pneumococcal sepsis is common, and some patients may benefit from immunization or IV immunoglobulin because normal B cell function is often impaired.

P. jirovecii (*carinii*) pneumonia is treated with high-dose TMP-SMZ and corticosteroids. Oral and gastrointestinal candidiasis is common in children and usually responds to imidazole therapy. VZV infection may be severe and should be treated with acyclovir or other antivirals. Recurrent HSV infections also may require antiviral prophylaxis. Other common infections in HIV-infected patients are toxoplasmosis, CMV, EBV, salmonellosis, and tuberculosis.

Children and adults with HIV are prone to malignancies, especially non-Hodgkin lymphomas, with the gastrointestinal tract being the most common site. Leiomyosarcomas are the second most common tumors among HIV-infected children. Kaposi sarcoma, caused by HHV-8, is distinctly rare in children with HIV. It was once common among adults with AIDS but has become infrequent with HAART.

PROGNOSIS

The availability of HAART has improved the prognosis for HIV and AIDS dramatically. Children with opportunistic infections (*P. jirovecii* [*carinii*] pneumonia), encephalopathy, or wasting syndrome have the poorest prognosis, with 75% dying before 3 years of age.

PREVENTION

Identification of HIV-infected women before or during pregnancy is crucial to providing optimal therapy for infected women and their infants and to preventing perinatal transmission. Prenatal HIV counseling and testing with consent should be provided for all pregnant women in the U.S. Women who use drugs during pregnancy pose special concerns because they are least likely to obtain prenatal care.

The rate of vertical transmission is reduced to less than 8% by chemoprophylaxis with a regimen of zidovudine to the mother (100 mg five times/24 hr orally) started by 4 weeks' gestation and continued during delivery (2 mg/kg loading dose intravenously followed by 1 mg/kg/hr intravenously) and to the newborn for the first 6 weeks of life (2 mg/kg every 6 hours orally). Other regimens incorporating single-dose nevirapine for infants have been shown to be similarly effective and are used in developing countries. The additional benefit of elective cesarean section to prevent vertical transmission is negligible, especially if the mother's viral load is less than 500 copies/mL.

Preventing HIV infection in adults decreases the incidence of infection in children. Adult prevention results from behavior changes ("safe sex," decrease in IV drug use, needle exchange). Prevention of pediatric AIDS includes avoidance of pregnancy and breast-feeding (in developed countries) in high-risk women. Screening of blood donors has reduced markedly the risk of HIV transmission from blood products. HIV infection almost never is transmitted in a casual or nonsexual household setting.

SUGGESTED READING

American Academy of Pediatrics, Committee on Infectious Diseases, Pickering LK (ed): Red Book: Report of the Committee on Infectious Diseases, 26th ed. Elk Grove Village, Ill, American Academy of Pediatrics, 2003.

Behrman RE, Kliegman RB, Jenson HB (eds): Nelson Textbook of Pediatrics, 17th ed. Philadelphia, WB Saunders, 2004.

Feigin RD, Cherry J, Demmler GJ, Kaplan S (eds): Textbook of Pediatric Infectious Diseases, 5th ed. Philadelphia, WB Saunders, 2004.

Glauser M, Pizzo PA (eds): Management of Infections in Immunocompromised Patients. Philadelphia, WB Saunders, 2000.

Guerrant RL, Walker DH, Weller PF (eds): Tropical Infectious Diseases: Principles, Pathogens, and Practice. Philadelphia, Churchill Livingstone, 1999.

Jenson HB, Baltimore RS (eds): Pediatric Infectious Diseases: Principles and Practice, 2nd ed. Philadelphia, WB Saunders, 2002.

Kliegman RM, Greenbaum LA, Lye PS (eds): Practical Strategies in Pediatric Diagnosis and Therapy, 2nd ed. Philadelphia, WB Saunders, 2004.

Mandell GL, Bennett JE, Dolin R (eds): Mandell, Douglas, and Bennett's Principles and Practice of Infectious Diseases, 6th ed. Philadelphia, Churchill Livingstone, 2005.

Plotkin SA, Orenstein WA (eds): Vaccines, 4th ed. Philadelphia, WB Saunders, 2004.

Remington JS, Klein JO (eds): Infectious Diseases of the Fetus and Newborn Infant, 5th ed. Philadelphia, WB Saunders, 2001.

THE DIGESTIVE SYSTEM

Warren P. Bishop

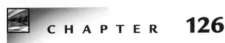

CHAPTER 126

Assessment

Children commonly present with symptoms originating in the digestive tract. Before carefully examining common gastrointestinal (GI) disorders, the pediatrician must be able to evaluate the techniques used to investigate digestive disorders and common manifestations. The following chapters describe in detail disorders affecting each organ or region of the gut. The pediatrician needs to be able to evaluate a child's symptoms quickly using knowledge, careful history, physical examination, and appropriate diagnostic tests.

HISTORY

The process of investigating and diagnosing an illness is a challenging and stimulating search for clues, followed by gathering of evidence, deducing the cause, and treating the patient. Because younger children may not be able to describe their symptoms accurately, the reports of "witnesses," usually the parents, are important. Proper assessment of the history before moving on to physical examination and diagnostic testing helps narrow the possibilities; this allows a focused examination and precise use of diagnostic studies.

Onset and **progression** of the major symptom should be determined. Is it getting worse, better, or staying the same? What appears to aggravate and alleviate the symptom? Are there associated symptoms, such as fever or weight loss? Have family members or other contacts been sick? Has the child been traveling, or have there been any environmental exposures?

Next, the pediatrician should ask about the child's **current status**, what **investigations** have been performed, and whether **therapies** have been used. How often do symptoms occur, and what is their duration? What is the relationship to meals and defecation? Is the child attending school or staying home? Have blood tests, x-rays, or other imaging studies been performed? If medications have been used, which ones, and at what dose? Have the medications yielded any therapeutic effect? Finally, the initial visit should include a thorough **review of systems, family history, social history**, and **past medical history.**

PHYSICAL EXAMINATION

The history may provide some initial ideas about the diagnosis and what to look for on examination. Children with GI complaints need a full examination and a thorough abdominal examination. Extraintestinal disorders may produce GI manifestations (e.g., emesis and group A streptococcal pharyngitis, abdominal pain and lower lobe pneumonia). The examination should begin with a careful external inspection for abdominal distention, bruising or discoloration, abnormal veins, jaundice, surgical scars, and ostomies. The pediatrician should listen to bowel sounds for abnormalities of intensity and pitch. He or she should assess carefully for tenderness, noting location, facial expression, guarding, and rebound tenderness. The liver and spleen should be examined, measuring enlargement with a tape measure and noting abnormal firmness or contour. Assessment for the presence of palpable feces and mass lesions should occur. A rectal examination needs to be done when it is indicated. Children with history suggesting constipation, GI bleeding, abdominal pain, chronic diarrhea, and suspicion of inflammatory bowel disease (IBD) may have important findings on rectal examination. The examination includes external inspection for fissures, skin tags, abscesses, and fistulous openings. Digital rectal examination should include assessment of anal sphincter tone, anal canal size and elasticity, tenderness, extrinsic masses, presence of fecal impaction, and caliber of the rectum. Stool obtained on the glove should be tested for occult blood.

SCREENING TESTS

After the history and physical examination, laboratory testing may be needed to guide the diagnosis or treatment. Careful selection of tests minimizes cost, discomfort, and risk to the patient, while not excluding studies important to the assessment.

A **complete blood count** is useful in evaluation of many GI symptoms because it provides evidence for inflammation (white blood cell [WBC] and platelet count), poor nutrition or bleeding (hemoglobin, red blood cell volume, reticulocyte count), and infection (WBC number and differential, presence of toxic granulation). Serum electrolytes, BUN, and creatinine help define the patient's hydration status. Tests of liver function include total and direct bilirubin, alanine aminotransferase, aspartate aminotransferase, and γ-glutamyltransferase or alkaline phosphatase for more specific evidence of bile duct injury. Hepatic synthetic function can be assessed by coagulation factor levels, coagulation times, and albumin level. Pancreatic enzyme tests (amylase, lipase, trypsinogen) give evidence of pancreatic injury or inflammation. Tests also are available to **screen** for specific conditions, such as celiac disease, viral hepatitis, α_1-antitrypsin deficiency, Wilson disease, ulcerative colitis (UC), Crohn disease (CD), and metabolic conditions. Urinalysis can be helpful in gauging dehydration and assessing effects of digestive system disease on the urinary tract.

DIAGNOSTIC IMAGING

Radiology

Plain abdominal radiographs and barium studies have great utility. There is no reason to start with CT or MRI to evaluate a patient with abdominal pain and vomiting. In choosing an imaging study, consultation with a radiologist is often advisable not only to discuss which imaging method might be best, but also to decide what variants of the technique should be used and how to prepare the patient for the study. In some cases, it is important for the patient to be fasting (ultrasound examination of the gallbladder). An IV catheter may be needed for contrast or radionuclide administration, or a preparatory enema may be required.

It is not necessary always to obtain a plain abdominal x-ray to document excessive retained stool in a child whose history is consistent with constipation and encopresis. When the examination confirms the presence of a fecal mass in the left lower quadrant and rectal examination discloses a fecal impaction, the results of the study are not likely to change the treatment plan. Similarly, if a simple barium upper GI series is planned to diagnose small bowel CD, a CT scan may not be needed, unless there are other concerns, such as abscess or lymphoma.

Endoscopy

Endoscopy permits the direct visualization of the interior of the gut. Nearly all GI endoscopes are **video endoscopes** with high-quality electronic optics. Endoscopes are small and safe and applicable to very small infants. The design of endoscopes permits a great deal of control of tip movement, illumination, image acquisition, and endoscope advancement through the gut. Endoscopes also allow for suction of intestinal contents and air and water insufflation; they have a separate channel for introducing instruments, such as biopsy forceps, snares, foreign body retrievers, electocoagulators, injection needles, and other specialized tools. **Capsule endoscopy** extends the diagnostic capabilities and the reach of endoscopy by telemetry.

COMMON MANIFESTATIONS OF GASTROINTESTINAL DISORDERS
Abdominal Pain
General Considerations

Abdominal pain can result from injury to the intraabdominal organs, injury to overlying somatic structures in the abdominal wall, or extra-abdominal diseases. **Visceral pain** results when nerves within the gut detect injury. The nerve fibers responsible for visceral sensation are nonmyelinated and mediate pain sensation, which is vague, dull, slow in onset, and poorly localized. A variety of stimuli, including normal peristalsis and various chemical and osmotic states, activate these fibers to some degree, allowing some sensation of normal activity. Regardless of the stimulus, visceral pain is perceived when a threshold of intensity or duration is crossed. Lower degrees of activation may result in perception of nonpainful or perhaps vaguely uncomfortable sensations, whereas more intensive stimulation of these fibers results in pain. Overactive sensation may be the basis of some kinds of abdominal pain, such as functional abdominal pain.

In contrast to visceral pain, **somatic pain** results when overlying body structures are injured. Somatic structures include the parietal peritoneum, fascia, muscles, and skin of the abdominal wall. In contrast to the vague, poorly localized pain emanating from visceral injury, somatic nociceptive fibers are myelinated and are capable of rapid transmission of well-localized painful stimuli. When intra-abdominal processes extend to cause inflammation or injury to the parietal peritoneum or other somatic structures, poorly local-ized visceral pain becomes well-localized somatic pain. In acute appendicitis, visceral nociceptive fibers are activated initially by the early phases of the infection. When the inflammatory process extends to involve the overlying parietal peritoneum, the pain becomes more acute and localizes generally to the right lower quad-rant. This is called **somatoparietal pain**.

Referred pain is a painful sensation in a body region distant from the true source of pain. The phys-iologic cause is the activation of spinal cord somatic sensory cell bodies by intense signaling from visceral afferent nerves, located at the same level of the spinal cord. The location of referred pain is predictable based on the locus of visceral injury. Cardiac visceral pain is referred to left-sided T1-5 somatic segments, causing left shoulder and arm pain. Stomach pain is referred to the epigastric and retrosternal regions, and liver and pancreas pain is referred to the epigastric region. Gall-bladder pain often is referred to the region below the right scapula. Somatic pathways stimulated by small bowel visceral afferents affect the periumbilical area, and a noxious event in the colon results in infraumbil-ical referred pain.

Acute Abdominal Pain

Distinguishing Features. Acute abdominal pain can signal the presence of a dangerous intra-abdominal process, such as appendicitis or bowel obstruction, or may originate from extraintestinal sources, such as lower lobe pneumonia or urinary tract stone. Not all episodes of acute abdominal pain require emergency intervention. Appendicitis must be ruled out as quickly as possible; the evaluation must be efficient, properly focused, and rapid. Only a few children presenting with acute abdominal pain actually have a surgical emer-gency. These surgical cases must be separated from cases that can be managed conservatively.

Initial Diagnostic Evaluation. Table 126-1 lists a diagnostic approach to acute abdominal pain in chil-dren. Important clues to the diagnosis can be deter-mined by history and physical examination. The **onset of pain** can provide some clues. Events that occur with a discrete, abrupt onset, such as passage of a stone, per-foration of a viscus, or infarction, result in a sudden onset. Gradual onset of pain is common with infec-tious or inflammatory causes, such as appendicitis and IBD.

A standard group of laboratory tests usually is per-formed for abdominal pain (see Table 126-1). An abdominal x-ray series also is usually obtained. Further imaging studies may be warranted to identify specific causes. CT can visualize the appendix if the examina-tion and laboratory findings suggest a possibility of appendicitis but the diagnosis remains in doubt. If the

history and other features suggest intussusception, a barium or pneumatic (air) enema may be the first choice to diagnose and treat this condition with hydro-static reduction (see Chapter 129).

Differential Diagnosis. Table 126-2 lists the dif-ferential diagnosis of acute abdominal pain in children. With acute pain, the urgent task of the clinician is to rule out surgical emergencies. In young children, malrotation, incarcerated hernia, congenital anomalies, and intussusception are common concerns. In older children and teenagers, appendicitis is more common. An acute surgical abdomen is characterized by signs of peritonitis, including tenderness, abdominal wall rigid-ity, guarding, and absent or diminished bowel sounds. Helpful characteristics of onset, location, referral, and quality of pain are noted in Table 126-3.

Recurrent (Chronic) Abdominal Pain

Recurrent abdominal pain is defined as the occurrence of multiple episodes of abdominal pain over at least 3 months that are severe enough to cause some limita-tion of activity. Recurrent abdominal pain is a common problem in children, affecting more than 10% of chil-dren at some time during childhood. The peak inci-dence occurs between ages 7 and 12 years. Although the differential diagnosis of recurrent abdominal pain is fairly extensive (Table 126-4), most children with this condition are not found to have a serious (or even iden-tifiable) underlying illness causing the pain.

Differential Diagnosis. The most common disor-der to consider is **functional abdominal pain**. Children with functional pain have pain that charac-teristically occurs daily or nearly every day, is not asso-ciated with or relieved by eating or defecation, and is associated with significant loss of the ability to func-tion normally. These children typically have personal-ity traits that include a tendency toward anxiety and perfectionism, which result in stress at school and in novel social situations. The parents typically state that the child enjoys going to school, but the pain often is worst at the start of the school day and before return-ing to school after vacations. A child with suspected functional pain must be evaluated carefully to exclude other causes of discomfort. Functional abdominal pain differs from **irritable bowel syndrome (IBS)** in minor ways. Children with IBS have pain beginning with a change in stool frequency or consistency, a stool pattern fluctuating between diarrhea and constipation, and relief of pain with defecation. Symptoms in IBS are linked to gut motility. Pain is commonly accompanied in both groups of children by school avoidance, sec-ondary gains, anxiety about imagined causes, lack of coping skills, and disordered peer relationships.

Distinguishing Features. One needs to distin-guish between functional pain and IBS and more

TABLE 126–1.   Diagnostic Approach to Acute Abdominal Pain

History

Onset	Sudden or gradual, prior episodes, association with meals, history of injury
Nature	Sharp versus dull, colicky or constant, burning
Location	Epigastric, periumbilical, generalized, right or left lower quadrant, change in location over time
Fever	Presence suggests appendicitis or other infection
Extraintestinal symptoms	Cough, dyspnea, dysuria, urinary frequency, flank pain
Course of symptoms	Worsening or improving, change in nature or location of pain

Physical Examination

General	Growth and nutrition, general appearance, hydration, degree of discomfort, body position
Abdominal	Tenderness, distention, bowel sounds, rigidity, guarding, mass
Genitalia	Testicular torsion, hernia, pelvic inflammatory disease, ectopic pregnancy
Surrounding structures	Breath sounds, rales, rhonchi, wheezing, flank tenderness, tenderness of abdominal wall structures, ribs, costochondral joints
Rectal examination	Perianal lesions, stricture, tenderness, fecal impaction, blood

Laboratory

CBC, C-reactive protein, ESR	Evidence of infection or inflammation
AST, ALT, GGT, bilirubin	Biliary or liver disease
Amylase, lipase	Pancreatitis
Urinalysis	Urinary tract infection, bleeding due to stone, trauma, or obstruction
Pregnancy test (older females)	Ectopic pregnancy

Radiology

Plain flat and upright abdominal films	Bowel obstruction, appendiceal fecalith, free intraperitoneal air, kidney stones
CT scan	Rule out abscess, appendicitis, Crohn disease, pancreatitis, gallstones, kidney stones
Barium enema	Intussusception, malrotation
Ultrasound	Gallstones, appendicitis, intussusception, pancreatitis, kidney stones

Endoscopy

Upper endoscopy	Suspected peptic ulcer or esophagitis

ALT, alanine aminotransferase; AST, aspartate aminotransferase; CBC, complete blood count; ESR, erythrocyte sedimentation rate; GGT, γ-glutamyltransferase.

serious underlying disorders. When taking the history, the pediatrician should ask about the **warning signs** for underlying illness listed in Table 126–5. If any warning signs are present, further investigation is necessary. Even if the warning signs are absent, some laboratory evaluation is warranted. The physician and the parents must feel assured that no serious illness is being missed; a judicious laboratory evaluation after a careful history and complete physical examination can accomplish this. One mistake that must be avoided in treating recurrent pain is performing too many tests. When the physician responds to each normal test with an order for another one, the parents and child may think that there is a serious illness that is being missed. Instead of being reassured by normal tests, the child's parents are made to believe that the mystery is deepening with every subsequent normal test result. The initial evaluation recommended in Table 126–6 avoids these problems. While waiting for laboratory and ultrasound results, a 3-day trial of a lactose-free diet should be instituted to rule out lactose intolerance. If tests are normal and no warning signs are present, testing should be stopped. If there are warning signs, worrisome symptoms, progression of symptoms, or laboratory abnormalities that suggest a specific diagnosis, additional investigation may be necessary. If antacids consistently relieve pain, an upper GI endoscopy is indicated. If the child is losing weight, a barium upper GI series with a small bowel follow-through or contrast CT is a good idea to look for

TABLE 126–2. Differential Diagnosis of Acute Abdominal Pain

Traumatic

Duodenal hematoma
Ruptured spleen
Perforated viscus

Functional

Constipation*
Irritable bowel syndrome*
Dysmenorrhea*
Mittelschmerz (ovulation)*
Infantile colic*

Infectious

Appendicitis*
Viral or bacterial gastroenteritis/adenitis*
Abscess
Spontaneous bacterial peritonitis
Pelvic inflammatory disease
Cholecystitis
Urinary tract infection*
Pneumonia
Bacterial typhlitis
Hepatitis

Genital

Testicular torsion
Ovarian torsion
Ectopic pregnancy

Genetic

Sickle cell crisis*
Familial Mediterranean fever
Porphyria

Metabolic

Diabetic ketoacidosis

Inflammatory

Inflammatory bowel disease
Vasculitis
Henoch-Schönlein purpura*
Pancreatitis

Obstructive

Intussusception*
Malrotation with volvulus
Ileus*
Incarcerated hernia
Postoperative adhesion
Meconium ileus equivalent (cystic fibrosis)
Duplication cyst, congenital stricture

Biliary

Gallstone
Gallbladder hydrops
Biliary dyskinesia

Peptic

Gastric or duodenal ulcer
Gastritis*
Esophagitis

Renal

Kidney stone
Hydronephrosis

*Common.

evidence of CD. Celiac disease (see Chapter 129) also should be considered.

Treatment of Recurrent Abdominal Pain. A child who is kept home or sent home from school because of pain receives a lot of attention for the symptoms, is excused from responsibilities, and withdraws from full social functioning. This situation rewards complaints and increases the child's anxiety about health. When the child observes that the adults are worried, the child worries too. To break this cycle of pain and disability, the child must **return to normal activities** immediately, even before all test results are available. The child should not be sent home from school with stomachaches; rather, the child may be allowed to take a short break from class in the nurse's office until the cramping abates. It is useful to inform the child and the parents that the pain is likely to be worse on the day the child returns to school. Anxiety worsens dysmotility and pain perception. Sometimes, medications can be helpful. **Fiber supplements** are useful to manage symptoms of IBS. In difficult and persistent cases, amitriptyline or a selective serotonin reuptake inhibitor may be beneficial.

Vomiting

Vomiting is a coordinated, sequential series of events that leads to forceful oral emptying of gastric contents. It is a common problem in children and has many causes. Vomiting should be distinguished from **regurgitation** of stomach contents, also known as gastroesophageal reflux (GER), chalasia, or "spitting up." Although the end result of vomiting and regurgitation is similar, they have completely different characteris-

TABLE 126–3.   Distinguishing Features of Abdominal Pain in Children

Disease	Onset	Location	Referral	Quality	Comments
Functional: irritable bowel syndrome	Recurrent	Periumbilical, splenic and hepatic flexures	None	Dull, crampy, intermittent; duration 2 hr	Family stress, school phobia, diarrhea and constipation; hypersensitive to pain from distention
Esophageal reflux	Recurrent, after meals, at bedtime	Substernal	Chest	Burning	Sour taste in mouth; Sandifer syndrome
Duodenal ulcer	Recurrent, before meals, at night	Epigastric	Back	Severe burning, gnawing	Relieved by food, milk, antacids; family history important; GI bleeding
Pancreatitis	Acute	Epigastric-hypogastric	Back	Constant, sharp, boring	Nausea, emesis, marked tenderness
Intestinal obstruction	Acute or gradual	Periumbilical-lower abdomen	Back	Alternating cramping (colic) and painless periods	Distention, obstipation, bilious emesis, increased bowel sounds
Appendicitis	Acute	Periumbilical or epigastric; localizes to right lower quadrant	Back or pelvis if retrocecal	Sharp, steady	Nausea, emesis, local tenderness, ± fever, avoids motion
Meckel diverticulum	Recurrent	Periumbilical-lower abdomen	None	Sharp	Hematochezia; painless unless intussusception, diverticulitis, or perforation
Inflammatory bowel disease	Recurrent	Depends on site of involvement		Dull cramping, tenesmus	Fever, weight loss, ± hematochezia
Intussusception	Acute	Periumbilical-lower abdomen	None	Cramping, with painless periods	Guarded position with knees pulled up, currant jelly stools, lethargy
Lactose intolerance	Recurrent with milk products	Lower abdomen	None	Cramping	Distention, gaseousness, diarrhea
Urolithiasis	Acute, sudden	Back	Groin	Severe, colicky pain	Hematuria
Pyelonephritis	Acute, sudden	Back	None	Dull to sharp	Fever, costochondral tenderness, dysuria, urinary frequency, emesis
Cholecystitis and cholelithiasis	Acute	Right upper quadrant	Right shoulder	Severe, colicky pain	Hemolysis ± jaundice, nausea, emesis

Adapted from Andreoli TE, Carpenter CJ, Plum F, et al: Cecil Essentials of Medicine. Philadelphia, WB Saunders, 1986.

tics. Vomiting is manifested by nausea with pallor and diaphoresis, followed by forceful gagging and retching. Regurgitation is effortless and not preceded by nausea. Occasionally the unpleasant sensation of gastric contents in the mouth during regurgitation may trigger gagging and true vomiting. The history must include sufficient detail about the events to distinguish between vomiting and regurgitation.

Differential Diagnosis

In neonates with vomiting, congenital obstructive lesions should be considered. Allergic reactions to formula also are common in the first 2 months of life. **Infantile GER** ("spitting up") is present to some degree in most infants and can be large in volume, occasionally mimicking true vomiting. **Pyloric stenosis** can develop in the neonatal period and is characterized by marked hunger, vomiting forcefully immediately after feedings, an accelerating pattern of vomiting, and a visibly distended stomach in an otherwise flat abdomen, often with visible peristaltic waves. Pyloric stenosis is more common in male infants, and there may be a positive family history. Other structural defects, such as intestinal atresias, webs, and stenosis or midgut malrotation, must be ruled out. Metabolic disorders (organic

TABLE 126–4. Differential Diagnosis of Recurrent Abdominal Pain

Functional abdominal pain*
Irritable bowel syndrome*
Chronic pancreatitis
Gallstones
Peptic disease
    Duodenal ulcer
    Gastric ulcer
    Esophagitis
Lactose intolerance*
Fructose malabsorption
Inflammatory bowel disease*
    Crohn disease
    Ulcerative colitis
Constipation*
Obstructive uropathy
Congenital intestinal malformation
    Malrotation
    Duplication cyst
    Stricture or web
Celiac disease*

*Common.

TABLE 126–5. Warning Signs of Underlying Illness in Recurrent Abdominal Pain

Vomiting
Abnormal screening laboratory study
Fever
Bilious emesis
Growth failure
Pain awakening child from sleep
Weight loss
Location away from periumbilical region
Blood in stools or emesis
Delayed puberty

Distinguishing Features

Is there fever, diarrhea, abdominal pain, or distention? Is the vomited material bilious (dark green), or does it contain bright red blood, dark red blood, or coffee-ground material? Are there accompanying symptoms, such as vertigo, headache, lethargy, stiff neck, cough, or sore throat? Is the child taking medications, or has the child been exposed to any potential toxins? Table 126–7 lists common diagnoses that must be considered and important historical features. Physicians caring for children see hundreds of children with viral gastroenteritis for every one with a less common diagnosis. It is important to be alert for unusual features that suggest another diagnosis. Viral gastroenteritis usually is not associated with severe abdominal pain or headache and does not recur at frequent intervals.

Physical examination should include a rapid assessment of the child's hydration status, including

acidemias, galactosemia, urea cycle defects, adrenogenital syndrome) can cause vomiting in infants. In older children, acquired conditions, such as viral or bacterial gastroenteritis or food poisoning, lead the list. Other infections, especially streptococcal pharyngitis, urinary tract infections, and otitis, commonly result in vomiting. CNS causes (increased intracranial pressure, migraine), anatomic anomalies such as intussusception and malrotation, and peptic disorders must be considered.

TABLE 126–6. Suggested Evaluation of Recurrent Abdominal Pain

Initial Evaluation	Follow-up Evaluation*
Complete history and physical examination	CT scan of the abdomen and pelvis with oral, rectal, and intravenous contrast
Ask about "warning signs" (see Table 126–5)	Celiac disease serology—endomysial antibody or tissue transglutaminase antibody
Determine degree of functional impairment (e.g., missing school)	Barium upper GI series with small bowel follow-through
CBC	Endoscopy of the esophagus, stomach, and duodenum
ESR	Colonoscopy
Amylase, lipase	
Urinalysis	
Abdominal ultrasound—examine liver, bile ducts, gallbladder, pancreas, kidneys, ureters	
Trial of 3-day lactose-free diet	

*Consider using one or more of these to investigate warning signs, abnormal laboratory tests, or specific or persistent symptoms.
CBC, complete blood count; ESR, erythrocyte sedimentation rate; GI, gastrointestinal.

TABLE 126–7.   Differential Diagnosis and Historical Features of Vomiting

Differential Diagnosis	Historical Clues
Viral gastroenteritis	Fever, diarrhea, sudden onset, absence of pain
Gastroesophageal reflux	Effortless, not preceded by nausea, chronic
Hepatitis	Jaundice, history of exposure
Extra-gastrointestinal infections	
Otitis media	Fever, ear pain
Urinary tract infection	Dysuria, unusual urine odor, frequency, incontinence
Pneumonia	Cough, fever, chest discomfort
Allergic	
Milk or soy protein intolerance (infants)	Associated with particular formula or food, blood in stools
Other food allergy (older children)	
Peptic ulcer or gastritis	Epigastric pain, blood or coffee-ground material in emesis, pain relieved by acid blockade
Appendicitis	Fever, abdominal pain migrating to the right lower quadrant, tenderness
Anatomic obstruction	
Intestinal atresia	Neonate, usually bilious, polyhydramnios
Midgut malrotation	Pain, bilious vomiting, GI bleeding, shock
Intussusception	Colicky pain, lethargy, vomiting, currant jelly stools, mass occasionally
Duplication cysts	Colic, mass
Pyloric stenosis	Nonbilious vomiting, postprandial, <4 mo old, hunger
Bacterial gastroenteritis	Fever, often with bloody diarrhea
CNS	
Hydrocephalus	Large head, altered mental status
Meningitis	Fever, stiff neck
Migraine syndrome	Attacks scattered in time, relieved by sleep; headache
Cyclic vomiting syndrome	Similar to migraine, usually no headache
Brain tumor	Morning vomiting, accelerating over time, headache, diplopia
Motion sickness	Associated with travel in vehicle
Labyrinthitis	Vertigo
Metabolic disease	Presentation early in life, worsens when catabolic or exposure to substrate
Pregnancy	Morning, sexually active, cessation of menses
Drug reaction or side effect	Associated with increased dose or new medication
Cancer chemotherapy	Temporally related to administration of chemotherapeutic drugs

assessment of capillary refill, moistness of mucous membranes, and skin turgor (see Chapter 38). The chest should be auscultated for evidence of rales or other signs of pulmonary involvement. The abdomen must be examined carefully for distention, organomegaly, bowel sounds, tenderness, and guarding. A rectal examination and testing stool for occult blood should be performed.

Laboratory evaluation of vomiting should include serum electrolytes, tests of renal function, complete blood count, amylase, lipase, and liver function tests. Additional testing may be required immediately when history and examination suggest a specific etiology. Ultrasound is useful to look for pyloric stenosis, gallstones, renal stones, hydronephrosis, biliary obstruction, malrotation, intussusception, and other anatomic abnormalities. CT may be indicated to rule out appendicitis or to observe structures that cannot be visualized well by ultrasound. Barium studies can show obstructive or inflammatory lesions of the gut and can be therapeutic, as in the use of contrast enemas for intussusception (see Chapter 129).

Treatment of vomiting needs to address the consequences and the causes of the vomiting. In the vomiting child, dehydration must be treated with fluid resuscitation. This can be accomplished in most cases with oral fluid-electrolyte solutions, but IV fluids also commonly are required. Electrolyte imbalances should be corrected by appropriate choice of fluids. Underlying causes should be treated when possible.

The use of **antiemetic medications** is controversial. These drugs should not be prescribed until the etiology of the vomiting is known and then only for severe symptoms. Phenothiazines, such as prochlorperazine, may be useful for reducing symptoms in food poisoning and motion sickness. Their side-effect profile must be considered carefully, however, and the dose prescribed should be conservative. Anticholinergics, such as scopolamine, and antihistamines, such as dimenhydrinate, are useful for the prophylaxis and treatment of motion sickness. Drugs that block serotonin 5-HT$_3$ receptors, such as ondansetron and granisetron, are not considered useful for viral gastroenteritis, but are helpful for chemotherapy-induced vomiting. These drugs can be extremely effective, especially when combined with dexamethasone. No antiemetic should be used in patients with surgical emergencies or when a specific treatment of the underlying condition is possible. Therapy of dehydration, ketosis, and acidosis by fluid resuscitation is helpful to reduce vomiting in most patients with viral gastroenteritis.

Acute and Chronic Diarrhea

Diarrhea is a major cause of childhood morbidity and mortality worldwide. Deaths from diarrhea are rare in industrialized countries, but are common elsewhere. **Acute diarrhea** is a major problem when it occurs with malnutrition or in the absence of basic medical care (see Chapter 30). In North America, most acute diarrhea is viral and is self-limited, requiring no diagnostic testing or specific intervention. Bacterial agents tend to cause much more severe illness and typically are seen in outbreaks or in regions with poor public sanitation. Bacterial enteritis should be suspected when there is **dysentery** (bloody, mucous stools with fever) and whenever severe symptoms are present. These infections can be diagnosed by stool culture or other assays for specific pathogens. **Chronic diarrhea** lasts more than 2 weeks and has a wide range of possible causes, including more difficult to diagnose serious and benign conditions.

What Is Diarrhea?

Parents use the word *diarrhea* to describe loose or watery stools, excessively frequent stools, or stools that are large in volume. Constipation with overflow incontinence (see later) can be mislabeled as diarrhea. A more exact definition is excessive daily stool liquid volume (>10 mL stool/kg body weight/day). When assessing a child with diarrhea, the pediatrician should ask about stool texture, volume, and frequency. Liquid stool that overflows an infant's diaper multiple times per day is an example of obvious diarrhea. One runny stool per day is less likely to meet the criterion.

Differential Diagnosis

Diarrhea may be classified by etiology or by physiologic mechanisms (secretory or osmotic). Etiologic agents include viruses, bacteria or their toxins, chemicals, parasites, malabsorbed substances, and inflammation. Table 126-8 lists common causes of diarrhea in childhood. **Secretory diarrhea** occurs when the intestinal mucosa directly secretes fluid and electrolytes into the stool. This secretion may be the result of inflammation, as in Crohn's disease or UC, or a chemical stimulus. Cholera is a secretory diarrhea stimulated by the enterotoxin of *Vibrio cholerae*. This toxin causes increased levels of cAMP within enterocytes, leading to secretion into the small bowel lumen. Secretion also is stimulated by mediators of inflammation and by various hormones, such as vasoactive intestinal peptide secreted by a neuroendocrine tumor (neuroblastoma).

Osmotic diarrhea occurs after malabsorption of ingested substances, which pull water into the bowel lumen. A classic example is lactose intolerance. When dairy products are ingested in the absence of sufficient lactase activity in the small intestinal brush border, malabsorption of the undigested lactose creates an osmotic effect. Osmotic diarrhea also can result from maldigestion, such as that seen with pancreatic insufficiency, or with malabsorption caused by intestinal injury. Certain nonabsorbable laxatives, such as polyethylene glycol and magnesium hydroxide (milk of magnesia) also cause osmotic diarrhea. The end result is osmotically active solute in the stool with excessive fecal water content. Fermentation of some of these malabsorbed substances (e.g., lactose) often can occur in the colon, resulting in gas production, cramps, and acidic stools. The most common cause of loose stools in early childhood is chronic nonspecific diarrhea, commonly known as **toddler's diarrhea**. This condition is defined by frequent watery stools in the setting of normal growth and weight gain and is caused by excessive intake of fruit juices that contain nondigestible carbohydrates. Diarrhea typically improves tremendously when the child's beverage intake is reduced or changed.

Distinguishing Features

Normal stools are isosmotic—that is, they have the same osmolarity as body fluids. Stools are isosmotic because of the relatively free exchange of water across the intestinal mucosa. Osmoles present in the stool are a mixture of electrolytes and other osmotically active solutes. To determine whether the diarrhea is osmotic or secretory, the **osmotic gap** is calculated:

$$\text{Osmotic gap} = 290 - 2([Na^+] + [K^+])$$

The formula for the osmotic gap assumes that the stool is isosmotic (an osmolarity of 290 mOsm/L). Stool sodium and potassium are measured, added together, and multiplied by 2 to account for their associated anions. This result is subtracted from 290. Secretory diarrhea is characterized by an osmotic gap of less than 50 because most of the dissolved substances in the stool are electrolytes. A number significantly higher

TABLE 126–8. Differential Diagnosis of Diarrhea

	Infant	Child	Adolescent
Acute			
Common	Gastroenteritis* Systemic infection Antibiotic associated Overfeeding	Gastroenteritis* Food poisoning Systemic infection Antibiotic associated	Gastroenteritis* Food poisoning Antibiotic associated
Rare	Primary disaccharidase deficiency Hirschsprung toxic colitis Adrenogenital syndrome	Toxic ingestion	Hyperthyroidism
Chronic			
Common	Postinfectious secondary lactase deficiency Cow's milk/soy protein intolerance Chronic nonspecific diarrhea of infancy (toddler's diarrhea) Celiac disease Cystic fibrosis AIDS enteropathy	Postinfectious secondary lactase deficiency Irritable bowel syndrome Celiac disease Lactose intolerance Giardiasis Inflammatory bowel disease AIDS enteropathy	Irritable bowel syndrome Inflammatory bowel disease Lactose intolerance Giardiasis Laxative abuse (anorexia nervosa) AIDS enteropathy
Rare	Primary immune defects Familial villous atrophy Secretory tumors Congenital chloridorrhea Acrodermatitis enteropathica Lymphangiectasia Abetalipoproteinemia Eosinophilic gastroenteritis Short bowel syndrome Intractable diarrhea syndrome Autoimmune enteropathy Factitious	Acquired immune defects Secretory tumor Pseudo-obstruction Factitious	Secretory tumors Primary bowel tumor

*Gastroenteritis includes viral (rotavirus, norovirus, astrovirus) and bacterial (*Salmonella, Shigella, E. coli, C. difficile, Yersinia, Campylobacter*, other) agents.

than 50 defines osmotic diarrhea and indicates that malabsorbed substances other than electrolytes account for fecal osmolarity.

Another way to differentiate between osmotic and secretory diarrhea is to stop all feedings and observe. This observation must be done only in a hospitalized patient receiving IV fluids to prevent dehydration. If the diarrhea stops completely while the patient is receiving nothing by mouth (NPO), the patient has osmotic diarrhea. A child with cholera, a pure secretory diarrhea, would continue to have massive stool output. Neither of these methods for classifying diarrhea works perfectly because most diarrheal illnesses are a mixture of secretory and osmotic components. Viral enteritis damages the intestinal lining, causing malabsorption and osmotic diarrhea. The associated inflammation results in release of mediators that cause excessive secretion. A child with viral enteritis may have decreased stool volume while NPO, but the secretory component of the diarrhea would not stop completely until the inflammation receded.

The **history** should include the onset of diarrhea, number and character of stools, estimates of stool volume, and presence of other symptoms, such as blood in the stool, fever, and weight loss. Recent travel should be documented, dietary factors should be investigated, and a list of medications being used should be obtained. Factors that seem to worsen or improve the diarrhea should be determined. **Physical examination** should be thorough, with a focus on the abdominal examination. Is there abdominal distention or tenderness? Are bowel sounds hyperactive? Is there blood in the stool on rectal examination? Is the anal sphincter tone adequate?

Laboratory testing should include stool culture and complete blood count if bacterial enteritis is suspected; additional stool testing is tailored to the patient's presentation. If diarrhea occurs after a course of antibiotics, a *Clostridium difficile* toxin assay should be ordered; if stools are reported to be oily or fatty, fecal fat content should be checked. Tests for specific diagnoses should be sent when appropriate, such as serum antibody tests for celiac disease or colonoscopy for suspected UC. A trial of lactose restriction for several days is helpful to rule out lactose intolerance, or a more specific test, such as lactose breath hydrogen analysis, can be performed.

Constipation and Encopresis

Constipation is a common problem in childhood, accounting for a significant percentage of visits to primary care providers and 25% of consultations by gastroenterologists. Parents may have different descriptions about what is constipation. They may be referring to straining with defecation, a hard stool consistency, large stool size, decreased stool frequency, fear of passing stools, or any combination. **Constipation** is defined as *two or fewer stools per week or passage of hard, pellet-like stools for at least 2 weeks*. Infants may experience symptoms of straining for prolonged periods and crying, followed by passage of soft stool. This pattern of difficult defecation is called **infantile dyschezia** and is present only in the first 3 months of life. Another common pattern of constipation is **functional fecal retention**, which is voluntary withholding of stool with "retentive posturing" (standing or sitting with legs extended and stiff or crossed legs) and infrequent passage of large diameter, often painful, stools. Children with functional fecal retention often have associated fecal soiling as a result of overflow of excessive colonic contents.

Differential Diagnosis

The differential diagnosis is listed in Table 126–9. Young children are vulnerable to **habit constipation**, also known as functional fecal retention, whenever they ignore the need to defecate and delay the passage of stool. Habit constipation commonly occurs during toilet training, when the child may not be wearing a diaper but is unwilling to sit on the toilet. The child may be afraid of the flushing toilet noise or be fearful of falling into the toilet. Retained stool becomes harder and larger over time. When the child finally passes a stool, it is large, hard, and painful, leading to more fear of defecation, voluntary withholding of stool, and perpetuation of the constipation. Colonic motility commonly forces pasty, watery stool around the impacted stool. This soils the underwear when sphincter pressure is exceeded, causing **encopresis**.

Hirschsprung disease is characterized by delayed meconium passage in newborns, abdominal distention, vomiting, occasional fever, and foul-smelling stools. This condition is caused by failure of ganglion cells to migrate into the distal bowel, resulting in spasm and functional obstruction of the aganglionic segment. Only about 6% of infants with Hirschsprung disease pass meconium in the first 24 hours of life compared with 95% of normal infants. Most infants rapidly become ill with enterocolitis or obstruction. Affected older children do not have large caliber stools because of rectal spasm, and they do not have encopresis. When evaluating a 3-year-old with fear of defecation, large stools, fecal soiling, and no history of neonatal constipation, Hirschsprung disease is not a likely etiology. Other causes of constipation include spinal cord abnormalities, hypothyroidism, drugs, cystic fibrosis, and anorectal malformations (see Table 126–9). A variety of systemic disorders affecting metabolism or muscle function can result in constipation. Children with **developmental disabilities** have a great propensity for constipation because of diminished capacity to cooperate with toileting, reduced effort or control of pelvic floor muscles during defecation, and diminished perception of the need to pass stool.

Distinguishing Features

Table 126–9 includes typical characteristics of the common causes of constipation. Congenital malformations usually cause symptoms from birth. Functional constipation is overwhelmingly the most common diagnosis in older patients and typically occurs around the time of toilet training. Another common time of onset for constipation is after starting school, when free and private access to toilets may be significantly restricted. Use of some drugs, especially opiates and some psychotropic medications, also is associated with constipation.

For a few specific causes of constipation, directed diagnostic testing can make the diagnosis. Hirschsprung disease is characterized by neonatal-onset constipation and can be diagnosed by barium enema, which shows a narrowed, aganglionic distal bowel and dilated proximal bowel. Rectal suction biopsy confirms the absence of ganglion cells in the rectal submucosal plexus, with hypertrophy of nerve fibers. Lack of internal anal sphincter relaxation can be shown by anorectal manometry. Hypothyroidism is diagnosed by examination and by thyroid function testing. Anorectal malformations are shown easily by direct examination. Cystic fibrosis (meconium ileus) is diagnosed by sweat chloride determination or *CFTR* gene mutation analysis (see Chapter 137). Most children with constipation have functional fecal retention and do not have any laboratory abnormality. Examination

TABLE 126–9. Common Causes of Constipation and Characteristic Features

Causes of Constipation	Clinical Features
Hirschsprung disease	*History:* Failure to pass stool in first 24 hr, abdominal distention, vomiting, symptoms of enterocolitis (fever, foul-smelling diarrhea, megacolon). Not associated with large caliber stools or encopresis *Examination:* Snug anal sphincter, empty, contracted rectum. May have explosive release of stool as examiner's finger is withdrawn *Laboratory:* Absence of ganglion cells on rectal suction biopsy specimen, absent relaxation of the internal sphincter, "transition zone" from narrow distal bowel to dilated proximal bowel on barium enema
Functional constipation	*History:* No history of significant neonatal constipation, onset at potty training, large caliber stools, retentive posturing, may have encopresis *Examination:* Normal or reduced sphincter tone, dilated rectal vault, fecal impaction, soiled underwear, palpable fecal mass in left lower quadrant *Laboratory:* No abnormalities, barium enema would show dilated distal bowel

Anorectal and colonic malformations
  Anal stenosis
  Anteriorly displaced anus
  Imperforate anus
  Colonic stricture
	History: Constipation from birth due to abnormal anatomy
	Examination: Anorectal abnormalities are shown easily on physical examination. Anteriorly displaced anus is found chiefly in females, with a normal-appearing anus located close to the posterior fourchette of the vagina
	Laboratory: Barium enema shows the anomaly

Multisystem disease
  Muscular dystrophy
  Cystic fibrosis
  Diabetes mellitus
  Developmental delay
  Celiac disease
	History: Presence of other symptoms or prior diagnosis
	Examination: Specific abnormalities may be present that directly relate to the underlying diagnosis
	Laboratory: Tests directed at suspected disorder confirm the diagnosis

Spinal cord abnormalities
  Meningomyelocele
  Tethered cord
  Sacral teratoma or lipoma
	History: History of swelling or exposed neural tissue in the lower back, history of urinary incontinence
	Examination: Lax sphincter tone due to impaired innervation, visible or palpable abnormality of lower back usually (but not always) present
	Laboratory: Bony abnormalities often present on plain x-ray. MRI of spinal cord reveals characteristic abnormalities

Drugs
  Narcotics
  Psychotropics
	History: Recent use of drugs known to cause constipation
	Examination: Features suggest functional constipation
	Laboratory: No specific tests available

reveals normal or reduced anal sphincter tone (owing to stretching by passage of large stools). Fecal impaction is usually present, but a large caliber, empty rectum may be found if a stool has just been passed.

Evaluation and Treatment of Functional Constipation

In most cases of constipation, the history is consistent with functional constipation—no neonatal constipation, active fecal retention, and infrequent, large stools. In these patients, no testing is necessary other than a good physical examination. The pediatrician should emphasize to the parents that young children with painful defecation must have a prolonged course of stool softener therapy to alleviate fear of defecation before

they stop withholding stool. The child should be asked to sit on the toilet for a few minutes on awakening in the morning and after meals. These are the times when the colon is maximally active, and it is easiest to pass a stool. Use of a positive reinforcement system for taking medication and sitting on the toilet is a good idea for younger children with constipation. The stool softener chosen should be non–habit forming, safe, and palatable; choices include electrolyte-free polyethylene glycol, milk of magnesia, and mineral oil. Polyethylene glycol is safe, effective, and well accepted by children and parents.

Gastrointestinal Bleeding

GI tract bleeding can be an emergency when large volume bleeding is present, but the presence of small amounts of blood in stool or emesis is sufficient to cause concern. Evaluation of bleeding should include confirmation that blood truly is present, estimation of the amount of bleeding, stabilization of the patient's intravascular blood volume, localization of the source of bleeding, and appropriate treatment of the underlying cause. When bleeding is massive, it is crucial that the patient receive adequate resuscitation with fluid and blood products before moving ahead with diagnostic testing.

Differential Diagnosis

GI bleeding has different causes at different ages (Table 126–10). In newborns, blood in emesis or stool may be maternal blood swallowed during delivery or during breastfeeding. Blood-streaked stools are particularly associated with allergic colitis or necrotizing enterocolitis in this age group, but small streaks of bright red blood also can be seen in the diaper of infants with anal fissure. Coagulopathy, peptic disease, and arteriovenous malformations can cause upper or lower GI tract bleeding in neonates.

In infants up to 2 years of age, peptic disease or nonsteroidal anti-inflammatory drug (NSAID)–induced gastric injury causes hematemesis; esophageal varices occur in this age group with severe congenital liver disease, such as biliary atresia. After this age, peptic disease and esophageal varices continue to be common causes of

TABLE 126–10.   Causes and Distinguishing Characteristics of Gastrointestinal Bleeding

Age	Type of Bleeding	Characteristics
Newborn		
Ingested maternal blood*	Hematemesis or rectal, large amount	Apt test indicates adult hemoglobin is present
Peptic disease	Hematemesis, amount varies	Blood found in stomach on lavage
Coagulopathy	Hematemesis or rectal, bruising, other sites	History of home birth (no vitamin K)
Allergic colitis*	Streaks of bloody mucus in stool	Eosinophils in feces and in rectal mucosa
Necrotizing enterocolitis	Rectal	Sick infant with tender and distended abdomen
Duplication cyst	Hematemesis	Cystic mass in abdomen on imaging study
Volvulus	Hematemesis, hematochezia	Acute tender distended abdomen
Infancy to 2 Years Old		
Peptic disease	Usually hematemesis, rectal possible	Epigastric pain, coffee-ground emesis
Esophageal varices	Hematemesis	History or evidence of liver disease
Intussusception*	Rectal bleeding	Crampy pain, distention, mass
Meckel diverticulum*	Rectal	Massive, bright red bleeding; no pain
Bacterial enteritis*	Rectal	Bloody diarrhea, fever
NSAID injury	Usually hematemesis, rectal possible	Epigastric pain, coffee-ground emesis
>2 Years Old		
Peptic disease	See above	See above
Esophageal varices	See above	See above
NSAID injury*	See above	See above
Inflammatory bowel disease	Usually rectal	Crampy pain, poor weight gain, diarrhea
Bacterial enteritis*	Rectal	Fever, bloody stools
Pseudomembranous colitis	Rectal	History of antibiotic use, bloody diarrhea
Juvenile polyp	Rectal	Painless, bright red blood in stool; not massive
Meckel diverticulum*	See above	See above
Nodular lymphoid hyperplasia	Rectal	Streaks of blood in stool, no other symptoms
Mallory-Weiss syndrome*	Hematemesis	Bright red or coffee-ground, follows retching
Hemolytic uremic syndrome	Rectal	Thrombocytopenia, anemia, uremia

*Common.
NSAID, nonsteroidal anti-inflammatory drug.

hematemesis. Rectal bleeding in older children is likely to be caused by a juvenile polyp, IBD, Meckel diverticulum, or nodular lymphoid hyperplasia. The presence of diarrhea and mucus in the stool particularly suggests IBD or bacterial dysentery. When rectal bleeding is massive and painless, Meckel diverticulum is a common etiology. The bleeding caused by polyps or lymphoid hyperplasia can be significant, but seldom is profuse enough to result in changes in pulse or blood pressure.

Distinguishing Features

Is It Blood? Red substances in foods or beverages occasionally can be mistaken for blood. A test for occult blood is worth performing whenever the diagnosis is in doubt.

Where Is the Bleeding? Blood may not be coming from the GI tract. The clinician should ask about cough, look in the mouth and nostrils, and examine the lungs carefully to exclude these as a source of bleeding. Blood in the toilet or diaper may be coming from the urinary tract, vagina, or a severe diaper rash. If the bleeding is GI, the clinician needs to determine whether it is originating high in the GI tract or distal to the ligament of Treitz. Vomited blood is always proximal. Rectal bleed-

ing may be coming from anywhere in the gut. When dark clots or melena are seen mixed with stool, a higher location is suspected, whereas bright red blood on the surface of stool probably is coming from lower in the colon. If the child has passed voluminous dark blood in stools, has a history of burning epigastric pain, or has been taking NSAIDs or aspirin, a gastric or duodenal ulcer is likely to be present. When upper GI tract bleeding is suspected in a child with bloody stools, a nasogastric tube may be placed and gastric contents aspirated. This simple test determines whether or not there has been recent bleeding in the proximal gut.

The location and hemodynamic significance of the bleeding should be assessed by history and examination. The parents should be asked to quantify the bleeding: Is it streaks of blood? How much bleeding is present? Is it a few teaspoons, a few streaks of bloody mucus, or much more? Details of associated symptoms should be sought. The pediatrician should look carefully at the vital signs and assess for orthostatic changes when bleeding volume is large. The pediatrician should examine pulses and capillary refill and check for pallor of the mucous membranes. Laboratory assessment and imaging studies should be ordered as indicated (Table 126–11).

TABLE 126–11. Evaluation of Gastrointestinal Bleeding

Laboratory Investigation	Initial Radiologic Evaluation
All Patients	**All Patients**
CBC and platelet count Coagulation tests: prothrombin time, partial thromboplastin time Liver function tests: AST, ALT, GGT, bilirubin Occult blood test of stool or vomitus Blood type and crossmatch	Abdominal x-ray series
	Evaluation of Hematemesis
	Upper endoscopy Barium upper GI series if endoscopy not available
Evaluation of Bloody Diarrhea	**Evaluation of Bleeding with Pain and Vomiting (Bowel Obstruction)**
Stool culture, *Clostridium difficile* toxin Sigmoidoscopy or colonoscopy—rule out inflammatory bowel disease Barium enema or CT with contrast	Abdominal x-ray series Pneumatic or contrast enema—rule out intussusception Upper GI series or ultrasound—rule out malrotation, volvulus
Evaluation of Rectal Bleeding with Formed Stools	
External and digital rectal examination Sigmoidoscopy or colonoscopy—rule out fissures, polyps Meckel scan—rule out Meckel diverticulum Mesenteric arteriogram or capsule endoscopy—rule out arteriovenous malformation	

ALT, alanine aminotransferase; AST, aspartate aminotransferase; CBC, complete blood count; GGT, γ-glutamyltransferase; GI, gastrointestinal.

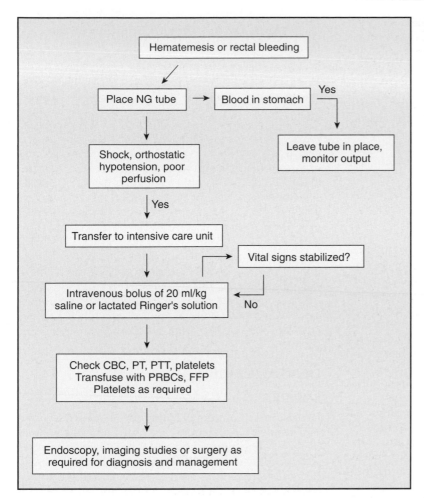

Figure 126–1

Initial management of gastrointestinal bleeding. CBC, complete blood count; FFP, fresh frozen plasma; NG, nasogastric; PRBCs, packed red blood cells; PT, prothrombin time; PTT, partial thromboplastin time.

Treatment

Treatment of GI bleeding should begin with an initial assessment, rapid stabilization of the hemodynamic status of the patient, and logical and rapid sequence of diagnostic tests. When a treatable cause is identified, specific therapy should be started. In many cases, the amount of blood is small, and no resuscitation is required. For children with large volume bleeds, the **ABCs** of resuscitation (airway, breathing, circulation) should be addressed first (see Chapters 38 and 40). Oxygen should be administered and the airway protected with an endotracheal tube if massive hematemesis is present. The pediatrician should start two large bore IV lines, restore adequate circulation with fluid boluses, transfuse with packed red blood cells as required, and continue to reassess frequently as time passes (Fig. 126–1).

CHAPTER 127
Oral Cavity

The oral cavity is a complex structure including the lips, gums, tongue, teeth, and surrounding structures involved in the functions of chewing and swallowing. The health of oral tissues has a significant impact on the ability of children to take adequate nourishment and to protect their airway from foreign body aspiration. Systemic disorders often may have manifestations in the oral cavity that are readily detectable on examination.

EFFECTS OF SYSTEMIC DISEASE ON THE ORAL CAVITY

Medications taken for a variety of conditions may cause oral abnormalities. Drugs with anticholinergic properties diminish saliva production and increase the risk of dental caries and parotitis. Tetracyclines taken before the eruption of the permanent teeth stain the enamel. Excessive fluoride in vitamin preparations or in drinking water can result in mottled teeth. Gingival hypertrophy may be caused by cyclosporine, phenytoin, and calcium channel blockers.

GER can lead to substantial enamel erosion and caries. Neonatal hyperbilirubinemia can result in bluish black discoloration of the deciduous teeth. Renal failure is associated with mottled enamel of the permanent teeth. Congenital syphilis causes marked abnormalities in the shape of teeth, especially incisors and molars. CD and Behçet disease are associated with oral ulcers. Abnormal pigmentation of the lips and buccal mucosa is seen with Peutz-Jeghers syndrome and Addison disease. Candidiasis is seen commonly with immunodeficiency disorders and diabetes. Leukemic infiltrates result in gum hyperplasia and bleeding; treatment of neoplastic conditions can cause severe mucositis. Some tumors, including lymphoma, may present as mass lesions of the buccal cavity.

Osteogenesis imperfecta is associated with abnormal dentin and risk of caries. Children with *ectodermal dysplasias* commonly have malformed or missing teeth. Pierre Robin syndrome is associated with micrognathia and cleft palate. Disorders resulting in facial dysmorphism can have a profound effect on dental occlusion and mandibular function. Examples include mandibulofacial dysostosis, Crouzon syndrome, conditions associated with dwarfism, and others.

DECIDUOUS AND PRIMARY TEETH

Most infants are born without teeth. *Natal teeth* are present at birth, are usually supernumerary, and may be poorly attached. Usually no treatment is necessary, but these sometimes need to be removed by a dentist if they are causing difficulties with feeding or injuries to the tongue. Table 127–1 presents the ages when normal **deciduous teeth** are acquired. The lower central incisors are the first to erupt, followed by the upper central incisors, lateral incisors, first molars, and bicuspids. **Delayed eruption** may occur in association with hypopituitarism, hypothyroidism, osteopetrosis, Gaucher disease, Down syndrome, cleidocranial dysplasia, and rickets. Deciduous teeth begin to be replaced by the permanent teeth at around age 6 years. The sequence of replacement is similar to that of the appearance of deciduous teeth.

TABLE 127–1. Time of Eruption of the Primary and Permanent Teeth

Tooth Type	Primary, Age (mo)		Permanent, Age (yr)	
	Upper	Lower	Upper	Lower
Central incisor	6 ± 2	7 ± 2	7-8	6-7
Lateral incisor	9 ± 2	7 ± 2	8-9	7-8
Cuspids	18 ± 2	16 ± 2	11-12	9-10
First bicuspids	—	—	10-11	10-12
Second bicuspids	—	—	10-12	11-12
First molars	14 ± 4	12 ± 4	6-7	6-7
Second molars	24 ± 4	20 ± 4	12-13	11-13
Third molars	—	—	17-21	17-21

DENTAL CARIES

Etiology

Dental caries, commonly referred to as "cavities," occur as a result of interactions between the tooth enamel, dietary carbohydrates, and oral flora. There is increased susceptibility if the enamel is abnormal or hypoplastic. Bacteria (*Streptococcus mutans*) that can adhere to and colonize the teeth, survive at low pH, and produce acids during fermentation of carbohydrates cause dental caries. The diet has a significant role. A classic example is "bottle mouth," or **baby bottle caries**. This condition results from the practice of allowing an infant to have a bottle in the mouth for prolonged periods, especially during sleep, and with sweet beverages or milk in the bottle. This practice allows bacteria to have continuous substrate for acid production and can result in destruction of multiple teeth, especially the upper incisors. Sticky sweet foods, such as many candies, also offer a mechanism for prolonged presence of carbohydrate at the surface of the tooth.

Epidemiology and Treatment

Risk of caries is associated with lack of dental care and poor socioeconomic status and predictably is greatest in developing countries. Baby bottle caries are seen in 50% to 70% of low-income infants. Treatment of caries is with dental restorative surgery. The carious portion is removed and filled with silver amalgam or plastic. If the damage is severe, a protective crown may be required; extraction of the tooth may be necessary when not salvageable. When not properly treated, dental decay results in inflammation and infection of the dental pulp and surrounding alveolar bone, which can lead to abscess and facial space infections.

Prevention

Avoiding inappropriate use of bottles and excessive sweets is a commonsense remedy for baby bottle caries. Oral hygiene offers some protection, but young children (<8 years old) do not have the ability to brush their own teeth adequately; brushing should be done by the parents. Fluoride supplementation of community water supplies to a concentration of 1 ppm is highly effective in reducing dental caries. Home water supplies, such as from a well, should have the fluoride content tested before prescribing supplements. If the child spends part of the day at another location, the total fluoride concentration from all sources must be considered before prescribing any oral supplements. Excessive fluoride supplementation causes fluorosis, a largely cosmetic defect of chalky white marks and brown staining of the teeth.

CLEFT LIP AND PALATE

Epidemiology

Cleft lip and palate occur separately or together and affect approximately 1 in 700 infants. It is more common in Asians (1:500) and least common in Africans (1:2500). Clefting occurs with two possible patterns: isolated soft tissue cleft palate or cleft lip with or without associated clefts of the hard palate. Isolated cleft palate is associated with a higher risk of other congenital malformations. The combined cleft lip/palate type has a male predominance.

Etiology

Cleft lip is due to hypoplasia of the mesenchymal tissues with subsequent failure of fusion. There is a strong genetic component; the risk is higher in children with affected first-degree relatives. Monozygotic twins are affected with only 60% concordance, suggesting other nongenomic factors. Environmental factors during gestation also increase risk, including drugs (phenytoin, valproic acid, thalidomide), maternal alcohol and tobacco use, dioxins and other herbicides, and possibly high altitude. Chromosomal and nonchromosomal syndromes are associated with clefting as are specific genes in some families.

Clinical Manifestations and Treatment

Cleft lip can be unilateral or bilateral and associated with cleft palate and defects of the alveolar ridge and dentition. When present, palatal defects allow direct communication between the nasal and oral cavities, creating problems with speech and swallowing. Feeding is a significant problem. Management includes squeeze-bottle feedings, special nipples, nipples with attached shields to seal the palate, and gastrostomy in severe cases. Surgical closure of the cleft lip is usually done by 3 months of age. Closure of the palate follows, usually before 1 year of age. Missing teeth are replaced by prostheses. Cosmetic results are often good, but depend on the severity of the defect.

Complications

Speech is nasal as a result of the cleft palate. Surgical treatment is effective, but sometimes does not restore palatal function completely. Speech therapy or occasionally the use of a speech-assisting appliance may help. Frequent episodes of otitis media are common, as are defects of teeth and the alveolar ridge.

TEETHING

Clinical Manifestations

Parents link the eruption of teeth to health problems. Fussiness, sleep disturbance, gum inflammation, and drooling are the most common symptoms observed, but fevers, diarrhea, and a multitude of other complaints have been popularly blamed on teething without justification. Symptoms other than minor fussiness and localized mild discomfort should not be attributed to teething.

Treatment

Teething is best treated conservatively. Nonpharmacologic management includes the use of rubbery teething toys that help the child "chew" the tooth through the gums, teething biscuits, and even frozen bananas. Some teething devices are liquid-filled and are designed to be cooled in the freezer to provide a numbing effect. Topical anesthetics can be used in small amounts with good effect. In some cases, use of acetaminophen or NSAIDs to reduce pain or inflammation may be helpful. There is no evidence that bronchitis, ear infections, or pulmonary infections are causally related to teething.

THRUSH

Epidemiology

Oropharyngeal *Candida albicans* infection, or thrush, is common in healthy neonates. The organism may be acquired in the birth canal or from the environment. Persistent infection is common in breastfed infants as a result of colonization or infection of the mother's nipples. Thrush can occur in otherwise normal older patients, but should suggest the possibility of an immunodeficiency, broad-spectrum antibiotic use, or diabetes. Common conditions associated with severe thrush include innate immunodeficiency, AIDS, anti–transplant rejection drug therapy, and cancer chemotherapy.

Clinical Manifestations

Thrush is easily visible as white plaques, often with a "fuzzy" appearance, on oral mucous membranes. When scraped with a tongue depressor, the plaques are difficult to remove, and the underlying mucosa is inflamed and friable. Clinical diagnosis is usually adequate, but may be confirmed by fungal culture or potassium hydroxide smear. Oropharyngeal candidiasis is sometimes painful (especially if associated with esophagitis) and can interfere with feeding.

Treatment

Thrush is treated with topical nystatin or azole antifungal agents. Nystatin therapy is started first, but treatment response is slow and often incomplete. Fluconazole and itraconazole, taken orally, have a systemic effect and an excellent response rate. When the mother's breasts are infected and painful, consideration should be given to treating her at the same time. Because thrush is commonly self-limited in newborns, withholding therapy in asymptomatic infants and treating only persistent or severe cases is a reasonable approach.

CHAPTER 128
Esophagus and Stomach

GASTROESOPHAGEAL REFLUX
Etiology and Epidemiology

GER is defined as the effortless retrograde movement of gastric contents upward into the esophagus or oropharynx. In infancy, GER is not always an abnormality. **Physiologic GER** ("spitting up") is normal in infants younger than 8 to 12 months old. Nearly half of all infants are reported to spit up at 2 months of age. Infants who regurgitate stomach contents meet the criteria for physiologic GER so long as they maintain adequate nutrition and have no signs of respiratory or peptic complications. Factors involved in GER include

liquid diet; horizontal body position; short, narrow esophagus; small, noncompliant stomach; frequent, relatively large volume feedings; and an immature lower esophageal sphincter (LES). As infants grow, they spend more time upright, eat more solid foods, develop a longer and larger diameter esophagus, have a larger and more compliant stomach, and experience lower caloric needs per unit of body weight. As a result, most infants stop spitting up by 9 to 12 months of age.

Clinical Manifestations

The presence of GER is easy to observe in an infant who spits up. In some cases, especially in older children, the refluxate is kept down by reswallowing, but GER may be suspected by associated symptoms, such as heartburn, cough, dysphagia (trouble swallowing), wheezing, aspiration pneumonia, hoarse voice, failure to thrive, and recurrent otitis media or sinusitis. In severe cases of esophagitis, there may be laboratory evidence of anemia and hypoalbuminemia secondary to esophageal bleeding and inflammation.

Pathologic GER is diagnosed after 18 months of age or if there are complications, such as esophagitis, respiratory symptoms, or failure to thrive, in younger infants. In older children, normal protective mechanisms against GER include antegrade esophageal motility, tonic contraction of the LES, and the geometry of the gastroesophageal junction. Abnormalities that cause GER in older children and adults include reduced tone of the LES, transient relaxations of the LES, esophagitis (which impairs esophageal motility), increased intra-abdominal pressure, cough, respiratory difficulty (asthma or cystic fibrosis), and hiatal hernia. When esophagitis develops as a result of acid reflux, esophageal motility and LES function are impaired further, creating a cycle of reflux and esophageal injury.

Laboratory and Imaging Studies

A clinical diagnosis is often sufficient in children with classic effortless regurgitation and no complications. Diagnostic studies are indicated if there are persistent symptoms or complications or if other symptoms suggest the possibility of GER in the absence of regurgitation. A child with recurrent pneumonia, chronic cough, or apneic spells without overt emesis may have occult GER. A **barium upper GI series** helps to rule out gastric outlet obstruction, malrotation, or other anatomic contributors to GER. Because of the brief nature of the examination, a negative barium study does *not* rule out GER. Another study, **24-hour esophageal pH probe monitoring**, uses a pH electrode placed transnasally into the distal esophagus, with continuous recording of esophageal pH. Data typically are gathered for 24 hours, following which the number and temporal pattern of acid reflux events are analyzed. A similar test, which does not require the presence of acid in the stomach, is **esophageal impedance monitoring**, which records the migration of electrolyte-rich gastric fluid in the esophagus. **Endoscopy** is useful to rule out esophagitis, esophageal stricture, and anatomic abnormalities.

Treatment

In otherwise healthy young infants ("well-nourished, happy spitters"), no treatment is necessary, other than a towel on the shoulder of the caretaker. For infants with complications of GER, pharmacologic therapy with a proton-pump inhibitor should be offered (Table 128–1). Lesser benefits are obtained with H_2 receptor antagonists. Prokinetic drugs, such as metoclopramide, occasionally may be helpful by enhancing gastric emptying and increasing LES tone, but are seldom very effective. When severe symptoms persist despite medication, or if life-threatening aspiration is present, surgical intervention may be required. Fundoplication procedures, such as the Nissen operation, are designed to enhance the antireflux anatomy of the LES. In children with a severe neurologic defect who cannot tolerate oral or gastric tube feedings, placement of a feeding jejunostomy should be considered as an alternative to fundoplication.

ESOPHAGEAL ATRESIA AND TRACHEOESOPHAGEAL FISTULA

Etiology and Epidemiology

The esophagus and trachea develop in close proximity to each other during 4 to 6 weeks of fetal life. Defects in the mesenchyme separating these two structures result in a tracheoesophageal fistula (TEF), often in association with other anomalies (renal, heart, spine, limbs). This defect occurs in about 1:3000 live births. TEF is not thought to be a genetic defect because concordance between monozygotic twins is poor.

Clinical Manifestations

The most common forms of TEF occur with esophageal atresia; the "H-type" TEF without atresia is uncommon, as is esophageal atresia without TEF (Fig. 128–1). Associated defects include the **VACTERL** association—**v**ertebral anomalies (70%), **a**nal atresia (imperforate anus) (50%) **c**ardiac anomalies (30%), **TEF** (70%), **r**enal anomalies (50%), and **l**imb anomalies (polydactyly, forearm defects, absent thumbs, syndactyly) (70%). A single artery umbilical cord is often present at birth. Infants with esophageal atresia have a history of polyhydramnios and exhibit drooling and have mucus and saliva bubbling from the nose and mouth. Patients with a TEF are vulnerable to aspiration pneumonia. When TEF is suspected, the first

TABLE 128–1.   Treatment of Gastroesophageal Reflux

Therapies	Comments
Conservative Therapies	
Towel on caregiver's shoulder	Cheap, effective. Useful only for physiologic reflux
Thickened feedings	Reduces number of episodes, enhances nutrition
Smaller, more frequent feedings	Can help some. Be careful not to *underfeed* child
Avoidance of tobacco smoke and alcohol	Always a good idea. May help reflux symptoms
Abstaining from caffeine	Inexpensive, offers some benefit
Positional therapy—upright in seat, elevate head of crib or bed	Prone positioning with head up is helpful, but *not* for young infants due to risk of SIDS
Medical Therapy	
Proton-pump inhibitor	Effective medical therapy for heartburn and esophagitis
H_2 receptor antagonist	Reduces heartburn, less effective for healing esophagitis
Metoclopramide	Enhances stomach emptying and LES tone. Real benefit is often minimal
Surgical Therapy	
Nissen or other fundoplication procedure	For life-threatening or medically unresponsive cases
Feeding jejunostomy	Useful in child requiring tube feeds. Delivering feeds downstream eliminates GERD

GERD, gastroesophageal reflux disease; LES, lower esophageal sphincter; SIDS, sudden infant death syndrome.

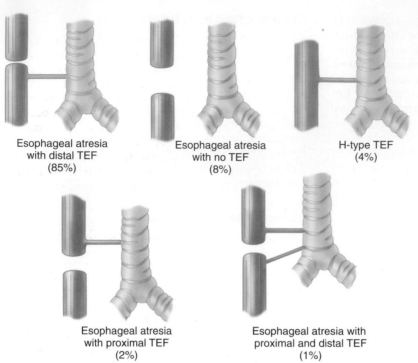

Figure 128–1

Various types of tracheoesophageal fistulas (TEF) with relative frequency (%).

Esophageal atresia
with distal TEF
(85%)

Esophageal atresia
with no TEF
(8%)

H-type TEF
(4%)

Esophageal atresia
with proximal TEF
(2%)

Esophageal atresia with
proximal and distal TEF
(1%)

feeding should be delayed until a diagnostic study is performed.

Laboratory and Imaging Studies

The simplest test for TEF is to attempt gently to place a 10F or larger tube via the mouth into the stomach. The passage of the tube is blocked at the level of the atresia. Confirmation is by chest x-ray with the tube coiled in the esophageal pouch. Air can be injected through the tube to outline the atretic pouch. Barium should not be used because of extreme risk of aspiration, but a tiny amount of dilute water-soluble contrast agent can be given carefully, then aspirated when the defect is clearly shown.

Treatment and Prognosis

The treatment of TEF is surgical. A thoracotomy provides access to the mediastinum via extrapleural dissection. The fistula is divided and ligated. The esophageal ends are approximated and anastomosed. In some cases, primary anastomosis cannot be performed because of a long gap between the proximal and distal esophagus. Various techniques have been described to deal with this problem, including pulling up the stomach, elongating the esophagus by myotomy, and simply delaying esophageal anastomosis and providing continuous suction to the upper pouch and allowing for growth.

Complications

The surgically reconstructed esophagus is not normal and is prone to poor motility, GER, anastomotic stricture, recurrent fistula, and leakage. The trachea also is malformed; tracheomalacia is common.

ESOPHAGEAL FOREIGN BODIES
Etiology and Epidemiology

Young children often place nonfood items in their mouths. When these items are swallowed, they may become lodged in the upper esophagus at the thoracic inlet. The most common objects are coins. Smaller coins may pass harmlessly into the stomach, where they rarely cause symptoms. Other common esophageal foreign bodies include food items, small toys or toy parts, disc batteries, and other small household items. Children with a prior history of esophageal atresia or with poor motility secondary to GER are more prone to food impactions, which seldom occur in the normal esophagus.

Clinical Manifestations

Some children are asymptomatic, but most exhibit some degree of drooling, food refusal, or chest discomfort. Older children usually can point to the region of the chest where they feel the object to be lodged. Respiratory symptoms tend to be minimal, but cough may be present, especially when the esophagus is completely blocked by a large object, such as a piece of meat, which presses on the trachea.

Diagnosis

Plain chest and abdominal radiographs should be taken when foreign body ingestion is suspected. Metallic objects are easily visualized. A plastic object often can be seen if the child is given a small amount of dilute x-ray contrast material to drink, although endoscopy is probably safer and more definitive.

Treatment

Endoscopy is ultimately necessary in most cases to remove an esophageal foreign body. Various devices can be used to remove the object, depending on its size, shape, and location. Coins usually are grasped with a special-purpose forceps and removed. Nets, baskets, and snares also are available. Whenever objects that may threaten the airway are being recovered, endoscopy should be performed with endotracheal intubation and under general anesthesia.

Complications

Sharp objects may lacerate or perforate the esophagus; smooth objects present for a long time also may result in perforation. Corrosive objects, such as zinc-containing pennies and disc batteries, can cause considerable local tissue injury and esophageal perforation.

CAUSTIC INJURIES AND PILL ULCERS
Etiology and Epidemiology

In adolescents, caustic ingestion injuries are usually the result of suicide attempts. In toddlers, the accidental ingestion of household cleaning products is common. Typical injurious agents include drain cleaners, toilet bowl cleaners, dishwasher detergents, and powerful bleaching agents. Childproof lids for commercial products offer some protection, but have not eliminated the problem. Lye-based drain cleaners, especially liquid products, cause the worst injuries because they are swallowed easily and liquefy tissue rapidly. Full-thickness burns can occur in seconds. Granular products are less likely to cause esophageal injury during accidental exposures because they burn the tongue and lips and often are expelled before swallowing. Less caustic agents, such as bleach and detergents, cause less serious injury. **Pill ulcers** occur when certain medications (tetracyclines and NSAIDs) are swallowed without sufficient liquids, allowing prolonged direct contact of the pill with the esophageal mucosa.

Clinical Manifestations

Caustic burns cause immediate and severe mouth pain. The child cries out, drools, spits, and usually drops the container immediately. Burns of the lips and tongue are visible almost immediately. These burns clearly indicate the possibility of esophageal involvement, although esophageal injury can occur in the absence of oral burns. Symptoms may not be present; further evaluation by endoscopy usually is indicated with any significant history of caustic ingestion. Pill injury causes severe chest pain and often prominent odynophagia (painful swallowing) and dysphagia.

Laboratory and Imaging Studies

A chest x-ray should be obtained to rule out aspiration and to inspect for mediastinal air. The child should be admitted to the hospital and given IV fluids until endoscopy. The true extent of burns may not be endoscopically apparent immediately, but delayed endoscopy can increase the risk of perforation. Most endoscopists perform the initial endoscopy soon after injury, when the patient has been stabilized. The extent of injury and severity of the burn should be carefully determined. Risk of subsequent esophageal strictures is related to the degree of burn and whether the injury is circumferential.

Treatment

A nasogastric tube can be placed over a guidewire at the time of the initial endoscopy to provide a route for feeding and to stent the esophagus. Systemic steroid use does not always reduce the risk of stricture. Broad-spectrum antibiotics should be prescribed if infection is suspected.

Complications

Esophageal strictures, if they occur, usually develop within 1 to 2 months and are treated with balloon dilation. The risk of perforation during dilation is significant. When esophageal destruction is severe, surgical reconstruction of the esophagus using stomach or intestine may be necessary.

PYLORIC STENOSIS
Etiology and Epidemiology

Pyloric stenosis is an acquired condition caused by hypertrophy and spasm of the pyloric muscle, resulting in gastric outlet obstruction. It occurs in 6 to 8 per 1000 live births and has a 5:1 male predominance and is more common in first-born children. Its cause is unknown, but it seems that a deficiency in inhibitory neuronal signals, mediated by nitric oxide, is likely.

Clinical Manifestations

Infants with pyloric stenosis typically begin vomiting during the first month of life, but onset of symptoms may be delayed. The emesis becomes increasingly more frequent and forceful as time passes. Vomiting in pyloric stenosis differs from spitting up because of its extremely forceful and often projectile nature. The vomited material never contains bile because the gastric outlet obstruction is proximal to the duodenum. This feature differentiates pyloric stenosis from most other obstructive lesions of early childhood. Affected infants are ravenously hungry early in the course of the illness, but become more lethargic with increasing malnutrition and dehydration. The stomach becomes massively enlarged with retained food and secretions, and gastric **peristaltic waves** are often visible in the left upper quadrant. A hypertrophied pylorus (the "olive") may be palpated. As the illness progresses, very little of each feeding is able to pass through the pylorus, and the child becomes progressively thinner and more dehydrated.

Laboratory and Imaging Studies

Repetitive vomiting of purely gastric contents results in loss of hydrochloric acid; the classic laboratory finding is a **hypochloremic hypokalemic metabolic alkalosis** with elevated BUN secondary to dehydration. Jaundice with unconjugated hyperbilirubinemia also occurs. Plain abdominal x-rays typically show a huge stomach and diminished or absent gas in the intestine (Fig. 128–2). Ultrasound examination of the pylorus shows marked elongation and thickening of the pylorus (Fig. 128–3). A barium upper GI series also may be obtained whenever doubt about the diagnosis exists; this shows a "string sign" caused by barium moving through an elongated, constricted pyloric channel.

Treatment

Treatment of pyloric stenosis includes IV fluid and electrolyte resuscitation followed by surgical pyloromyotomy. Before surgery, dehydration and hypochloremic alkalosis must be corrected, generally with an initial normal saline fluid bolus followed by infusions of half-normal saline containing 5% dextrose and potassium chloride when urine output is observed. For pyloromyotomy, a small incision is made, usually directly over the pylorus or at the umbilicus, and the pyloric muscle is incised longitudinally to release the constriction. Care is taken not to cut into the mucosa itself.

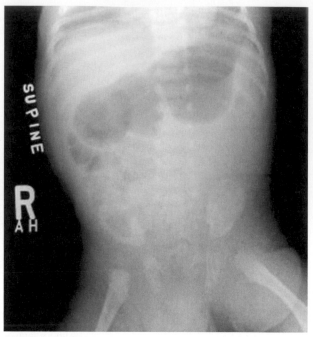

Figure 128–2

Pyloric stenosis. Note the huge, gas-filled stomach extending across the midline, with minimal air in the intestine downstream. (Courtesy of Warren Bishop, MD.)

PEPTIC DISEASE

Etiology and Epidemiology

Acid-related injury can occur in the esophagus, stomach, or duodenum. Table 128–2 lists risk factors for **peptic ulcer disease** in children. *Helicobacter pylori* is responsible for more than half of ulcers in the stomach and the duodenum in adults. *H. pylori* plays a

TABLE 128–2. Risk Factors for Peptic Ulcer Disease
Helicobacter pylori infection
Drugs
NSAIDs, including aspirin
Tobacco use
Bisphosphonates
Potassium supplements
Family history
Sepsis
Head trauma
Burn injury
Hypotension

NSAIDs, nonsteroidal anti-inflammatory drugs.

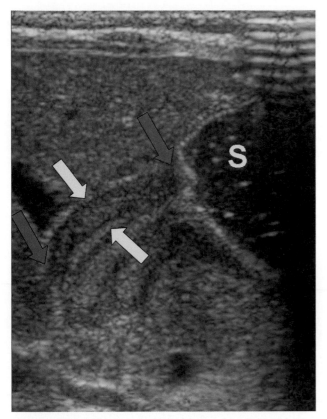

Figure 128-3

Ultrasound image of infant with pyloric stenosis. Large, fluid-filled stomach (S) is seen at right, with an elongated, thickened pylorus. The length of the pylorus is marked by the red arrows; the wall thickness is marked by the yellow arrows.

significant but lesser role in childhood ulcer disease. Risk factors for acquisition of *H. pylori* are low socio-economic status and poor sanitation, with the highest incidence in developing countries. **Nonulcer dyspepsia** includes upper abdominal symptoms (pain, bloating, nausea, early satiety) in the absence of gastric or duodenal ulceration. Nonulcer dyspepsia is *not* associated with *H. pylori* infection of the stomach. GER (see Chapter 126) allows acidic gastric contents to injure the esophagus, resulting in **esophagitis**. Esophagitis is characterized by retrosternal and epigastric burning pain and is best diagnosed by endoscopy. It can range from minimal, with only erythema and microscopic inflammation on biopsy, to superficial erosions and finally to frank ulceration.

Clinical Manifestations

Typical symptoms are listed in Table 128–3. The presence of burning epigastric and retrosternal pain strongly suggests esophagitis. With duodenal ulcers, pain typically occurs several hours after meals and often awakens patients at night. Eating tends to relieve the pain. Gastric ulcers differ in that pain is commonly aggravated by eating, resulting in weight loss. GI bleeding from either can occur. Many patients report significant symptom relief with antacids or acid blockers.

Laboratory and Imaging Studies

Whenever symptoms are localized to the upper abdomen or the retrosternal region, upper GI

TABLE 128–3. Peptic Disorders, Symptoms, and Clinical Investigation	
Syndrome and Associated Symptoms	**Clinical Investigation**
Esophagitis	
Retrosternal and epigastric location	Endoscopy
Burning pain	Therapeutic trial of acid-blocker therapy
Sensation of regurgitation	pH probe study
Dysphagia, odynophagia	
Nonulcer Dyspepsia	
Upper abdominal location	Endoscopy
Fullness	Therapeutic trial of acid-blocker therapy
Bloating	Upper GI series to ligament of Treitz—rule out malrotation
Nausea	CBC, ESR, amylase, lipase, abdominal ultrasound
Peptic Ulcer Disease	
"Alarm" symptoms	Endoscopy—mandatory with alarm symptoms
Weight loss	Test for *Helicobacter pylori*
Hematemesis	CBC, ESR, amylase, lipase, abdominal ultrasound
Melena, heme-positive stools	
Chronic vomiting	
Microcytic anemia	
Nocturnal pain	
Other symptoms—same as for esophagitis and nonulcer dyspepsia	

CBC, complete blood count; ESR, erythrocyte sedimentation rate; GI, gastrointestinal.

endoscopy is indicated. Empirical therapy with a proton-pump inhibitor may be considered, but has the risk of not diagnosing the underlying condition. The possibilities of IBD, anatomic abnormality such as malrotation, pancreatitis, and biliary disease should be ruled out by appropriate testing when suspected (see Chapter 126 and Table 128–3 for recommended studies). Testing for *H. pylori* should be performed by biopsy during every endoscopy. If endoscopy is not done, noninvasive tests for infection can be done with reasonable accuracy with *H. pylori* antibodies, ^{13}C urea breath tests (urea is metabolized into ^{13}CO$_2$ by the organism), and stool *H. pylori* antigen tests.

Treatment

If *H. pylori* is present in association with ulcers, it should be treated with a multidrug regimen, such as omeprazole-clarithromycin-metronidazole, omeprazole-amoxicillin-clarithromycin, or omeprazole-amoxicillin-metronidazole, given twice daily for 1 to 2 weeks. Other proton-pump inhibitors may be substituted when necessary. Bismuth compounds are effective against *H. pylori* and can be considered. In North America, only the subsalicylate salt is available, the use of which raises some concerns about Reye syndrome and potential salicylate toxicity. Tetracycline is useful in adults, but should be avoided in children (see Chapter 127). In the absence of *H. pylori,* esophagitis and peptic ulcer disease are treated with a proton-pump inhibitor, which yields higher rates of healing than H$_2$ receptor antagonists. Gastric and duodenal ulcers heal in 4 to 8 weeks in at least 80% of patients. Esophagitis requires 4 to 5 months of proton-pump inhibitor treatment for optimal healing.

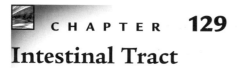

CHAPTER 129
Intestinal Tract

MIDGUT MALROTATION
Etiology and Epidemiology

During early fetal life, the midgut is attached to the yolk sac and loops outward into the umbilical cord. Beginning at around 10 weeks' gestation, the bowel reenters the abdomen and rotates counterclockwise around the superior mesenteric artery until the cecum arrives in the right lower quadrant. The duodenum rotates behind the artery and terminates at the **ligament of Treitz** in the left upper quadrant. The base of the mesentery becomes fixed along a broad attachment posteriorly, running from the cecum to the

ligament of Treitz (Fig. 129–1A). When rotation is incomplete or otherwise abnormal, "malrotation" is present. Incomplete rotation occurs when the cecum stops near the right upper quadrant, and the duodenum fails to move behind the mesenteric artery; this results in an extremely narrow mesenteric root (see Fig. 129–1B) that makes the child susceptible to midgut **volvulus** (Fig. 129–2). It is common for abnormal mesenteric attachments (Ladd bands) to extend from the cecum across the duodenum, causing partial obstruction.

Clinical Manifestations

About 60% of children with malrotation present with symptoms of bilious vomiting during the first month of life. The remaining 40% present later in infancy or childhood. The emesis initially may be due to obstruction by Ladd bands without volvulus. When midgut volvulus occurs, the venous drainage of the gut is impaired, and congestion results in ischemia, pain, tenderness, and often bloody emesis and stools. The bowel undergoes ischemic necrosis, and the child may appear septic. Physicians caring for children must be alert to the possibility of volvulus in patients with vomiting and fussiness or abdominal pain.

Laboratory and Imaging Studies

Plain abdominal x-rays generally show evidence of obstruction. Abdominal ultrasound may show evidence of malrotation. An upper GI series shows the absence of a typical duodenal "C-loop," with the duodenum instead remaining on the right side of the abdomen. When doubt exists about the normalcy of the duodenal course, the contrast material can be followed until it reaches the cecum. Abnormal placement of the cecum on follow-through (or by contrast enema) confirms the diagnosis. Laboratory studies are nonspecific, showing evidence of dehydration, electrolyte loss, or evidence of sepsis. A decreasing platelet count is a common indicator of bowel ischemia.

Treatment

Treatment is surgical. The bowel is untwisted, and Ladd bands and other abnormal membranous attachments are divided. The mesentery is spread out and flattened against the posterior wall of the abdomen by moving the cecum to the left side of the abdomen. Sutures may be used to hold the bowel in position, but postoperative adhesions tend to hold the mesentery in place, resulting in a broad attachment and eliminating the risk of recurrent volvulus. Necrotic bowel is resected and at times results in short gut syndrome.

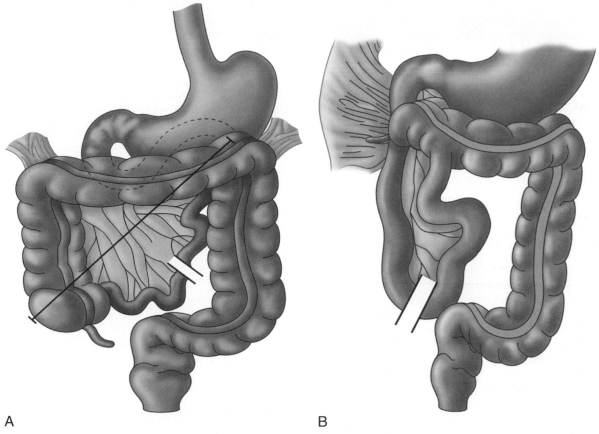

Figure 129–1

A, Normal rotation of the midgut. Note the long axis of mesenteric attachment *(line)*. **B,** Midgut malrotation. Note the narrow mesentery, which predisposes to volvulus, and the presence of Ladd bands extending across the duodenum from the abnormally elevated cecum. (From Donellan WJ [ed]: Abdominal Surgery of Infancy and Childhood. Luxembourg, Harwood Academic Publishers, 1996, pp 43/6, 43/8.)

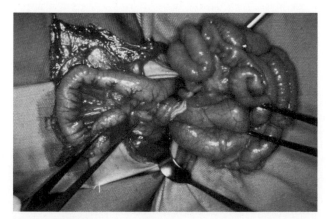

Figure 129–2

Malrotation with volvulus. Midgut is twisted around the mesentery, with an area of darker, ischemic intestine visible. (Courtesy of Robert Soper, MD.)

INTESTINAL ATRESIA

Etiology and Epidemiology

Congenital partial or complete blockage of the intestine is a developmental defect that occurs in about 1:1500 live births. Atresia occurs in several forms (Fig. 129–3). One or more segments of bowel may be missing completely, there may be varying degrees of obstruction caused by webs or stenosis, or there may be obliteration of the lumen in cordlike bowel remnants. The end result is obstruction with upstream dilation of the bowel and small, disused intestine distally. When obstruction is complete or high grade, bilious vomiting and abdominal distention are present in the newborn period. In lesser cases, as in "windsock" types of intestinal webs, the obstruction is partial, and symptoms are more subtle.

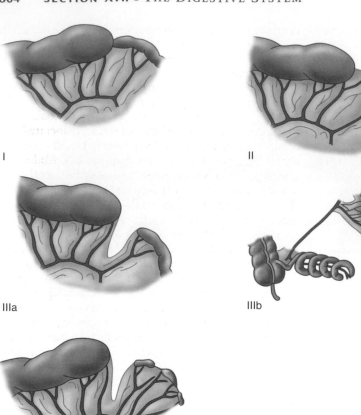

I

II

IIIa

IIIb

IV

Figure 129–3

Types of intestinal atresia. I, internal web; II, cordlike remnant connecting proximal and distal bowel; IIIa, interrupted bowel with V-shaped mesenteric defect; IIIb, "apple peel" atresia with surviving bowel spiraling around a marginal artery; IV, multiple atresias. (From Grosfeld JL, Ballantine TVN, Shoemaker R: Operative management of intestinal atresia based on pathologic findings. J Pediatr Surg 14:368, 1979.)

Clinical Manifestations

Intestinal atresia presents with a history of poly-hydramnios and with abdominal distention and bilious vomiting in the neonatal period. If intestinal perforation is present, peritonitis and sepsis are inevitable.

Laboratory and Imaging Studies

Plain abdominal x-rays may localize the area of atresia and identify evidence of perforation, such as free air or calcifications typical of meconium peritonitis. Duodenal atresia appears as a double-bubble sign (gas in the stomach and enlarged proximal duodenum), with no gas distally. Atresias of the distal intestine are characterized by longer segments of dilated, air-filled bowel. Contrast studies are helpful if plain films are not sufficient. Atresia may be a complication of **meconium ileus** associated with cystic fibrosis. Laboratory evaluation for **cystic fibrosis** (see Chapter 137) is indicated in cases of small bowel atresia. Other laboratory studies are not specific for atresia, but a complete blood count, serum electrolytes, liver functions, and amylase should be measured to identify dehydration, pancreatitis, and other complications.

Treatment

The treatment of intestinal atresia is surgical, but surgery must be preceded by adequate stabilization of the patient. IV fluids, nasogastric suction, and broad-spectrum antibiotics should be given.

OTHER CONGENITAL DISORDERS

Gastroschisis is an abdominal wall defect not involving the umbilicus, through which intestinal contents have herniated. In contrast to omphalocele (see later), the bowel is not covered by peritoneum or amniotic membrane. As a result, prolonged contact with the amniotic fluid typically causes a thick, exudative covering (a "peel") on the exposed bowel. Gastroschisis is not associated with extraintestinal anomalies, but segments of intestinal atresia are common. After surgical reduction of the defect, return of normal bowel function may be slow and requires prolonged parenteral nutrition for infants with long atretic segments (short bowel syndrome) and infants with a thick peel.

Omphalocele is an abdominal wall defect at the umbilicus caused by failure of the intestine to return to the abdomen during fetal life. The bowel remains within the umbilical cord and is covered by peritoneum and amniotic membranes. This defect is associated with other congenital anomalies, especially cardiac defects, **Beckwith-Wiedemann syndrome** (somatic overgrowth, hyperinsulinemic hypoglycemia, risk for Wilms tumor), and intestinal complications. Treatment is surgical closure, which sometimes must be performed in stages to fit the bowel into a congenitally small abdominal cavity.

Duplication cysts are abnormal fluid-filled structures lined with intestinal or gastric mucosa. They are found within the mesentery and lie adjacent to normal bowel. These cysts generally do not communicate with the adjacent bowel lumen. Although some cysts may cause symptoms in early infancy, cysts may grow slowly for years, eventually causing problems secondary to perforation, bowel obstruction, intussusception, or volvulus. Duplication cysts are diagnosed by ultrasound, CT scan, or contrast studies. Treatment is surgical excision.

Anorectal malformations, including imperforate anus and its variants, are embryologic defects recognized at birth by the absence of a normal anal opening. Evaluation of these infants should include observation for emergence of meconium from the urethra or fistulas on the perineum. A urinary catheter should be placed if urinary distention is present. In low lesions, a fistulous opening that drains meconium is present on the perineum. Low lesions commonly are associated with fistulization between the bowel and bladder, vagina, or urethra. Lateral plain x-rays show the level of the defect and show gas in the bladder caused by a fistula. These children are treated initially by colostomy to divert the fecal flow, with subsequent anogenital reconstruction. The internal sphincter muscle is functionally absent in high lesions, and continence after repair is difficult to achieve. All children with imperforate anus require MRI of the lumbosacral spinal cord because of high incidence of tethered spinal cord. Urologic dysfunction is common and should be evaluated appropriately.

Hirschsprung disease is a motility defect caused by failure of ganglion cell precursors to migrate into the distal bowel during fetal life. The aganglionic distal segment does not exhibit normal motility and is functionally obstructed secondary to spasm. In 75% of cases, the involved segment is limited to the rectosigmoid, but total colonic involvement is seen in 8%. Rarely, long segments of small bowel also are aganglionic. "Ultrashort" segment involves only a few centimeters of distal rectum. Hirschsprung disease typically presents in the newborn period with failure to pass meconium by 24 hours of age. About 95% of normal infants pass stool spontaneously by this age; 95% of infants with Hirschsprung disease do not. Symptoms of distal bowel obstruction occur with distention and bilious vomiting. If the diagnosis is not made quickly, **enterocolitis** can result, associated with a high rate of mortality. Diagnosis is based on examination and one or more diagnostic studies. Abdominal distention is present in most cases. Digital rectal examination reveals an empty rectum that clenches around the examiner's finger, giving the impression of an elongated sphincter. When the finger is withdrawn, a powerful gush of retained stool is often expelled. A deep **rectal biopsy** specimen obtained surgically or by using a suction biopsy instrument is required for diagnosis. When no ganglion cells are shown in the submucosal plexus, accompanied by nerve trunk hyperplasia, the diagnosis is certain. **Barium enema** and **anorectal manometry** may be used before biopsy, but false-negative and false-positive results can occur. Therapy is surgical. When the bowel is markedly distended or inflamed, an initial colostomy usually is performed above the aganglionic segment, followed weeks later by one of several definitive repair procedures. The transanal pull-through excises the aganglionic bowel and creates a primary colorectal anastomosis without laparotomy. This procedure can be considered in patients with uncomplicated involvement limited to the rectosigmoid region.

Meckel diverticulum is a remnant of the fetal omphalomesenteric duct and is an outpouching of the distal ileum present in 1% to 2% of the population. Although most diverticula are asymptomatic throughout life, some cause massive, painless GI bleeding. Ectopic gastric tissue within the diverticulum causes ulceration of mucosa in the adjacent ileum. Meckel diverticulum may be a lead point for intussusception (see later) or may enable twisting (volvulus) of neighboring bowel around its vascular supply. Diverticulitis mimics appendicitis. Diagnosis may be made in most cases by technetium scan (Meckel scan), which labels the acid-producing mucosa. Because not all diverticula are seen, ultrasound and barium enteroclysis may be useful. When the level of suspicion is high, surgical or laparoscopic investigation is warranted. The treatment is surgical excision.

INFLAMMATORY BOWEL DISEASE
Epidemiology and Etiology

The peak incidence of IBD in children is in the second decade of life. IBD includes CD, which can involve the entire gut, and UC, which affects only the colon. The incidence of IBD is increasing, especially in industrialized countries, for reasons that are unclear. IBD is uncommon in tropical and Third World countries. It is more common in Jewish than in other ethnic populations. Genetic factors play a role in susceptibility, with significantly higher risk if there is a family history of IBD. Having a first-degree relative with IBD increases the risk about 30-fold. Susceptibility has been linked to some HLA subtypes, and linkage analysis has identified multiple other susceptibility loci on several chromosomes. Environmental factors also seem to play a role because there is often nonconcordance among monozygotic twins. The environmental agents responsible have not been identified. It is possible that viral infections can initiate the inflammatory process. Dietary triggers are unproven. Smoking doubles the risk of CD and halves the risk for UC.

Clinical manifestations depend on the region of involvement. UC involves only the colon, whereas CD can include the entire gut from mouth to anus. **Colitis** from either condition results in diarrhea, blood, and mucus in the stool; urgency; and *tenesmus,* a sensation of incomplete emptying after defecation. When colitis is severe, the child often awakens from sleep to pass stool. **Toxic megacolon** is a life-threatening complication characterized by fever, abdominal distention and pain, massively dilated colon, anemia, and low serum albumin owing to fecal protein losses. Symptoms of colitis always are present in UC and usually suggest the diagnosis early in its course. Extraintestinal manifestations of UC occur in a few patients and may include primary sclerosing cholangitis, arthritis, uveitis, and pyoderma gangrenosum (Table 129–1).

Symptoms can be subtle in CD. **Small bowel involvement** in CD is associated with loss of appetite, crampy postprandial pain, poor growth, delayed puberty, anemia, and lethargy. Some symptoms may be present for some time before the diagnosis is made. Severe CD may cause partial or complete small bowel obstruction. Perineal abnormalities, including skin tags and fistulas, are another feature distinguishing CD from UC. Other extraintestinal manifestations of CD include arthritis, erythema nodosum, and uveitis or iritis.

Laboratory and Imaging Studies

Blood tests should include complete blood count, erythrocyte sedimentation rate, and C-reactive protein and possibly serologic tests for IBD (Table 129–2). Anemia and elevated platelet counts are typical. Testing for abnormal serum antibodies can be helpful in diagnosing IBD and in discriminating between the colitis of CD and UC. **Atypical perinuclear staining by antineutrophil cytoplasmic antibody** is found in about 66% of UC patients and in only a few

TABLE 129–1. Comparison of Crohn Disease and Ulcerative Colitis

Feature	Crohn Disease	Ulcerative Colitis
Malaise, fever, weight loss	Common	Common
Rectal bleeding	Sometimes	Usual
Abdominal mass	Common	Rare
Abdominal pain	Common	Common
Perianal disease	Common	Rare
Ileal involvement	Common	None (backwash ileitis)
Strictures	Common	Unusual
Fistula	Common	Very rare
Skip lesions	Common	Not present
Transmural involvement	Usual	Not present
Crypt abscesses	Variable	Usual
Intestinal granulomas	Common	Rarely present
Risk of cancer*	Increased	Greatly increased
Erythema nodosum	Common	Less common
Mouth ulceration	Common	Rare
Osteopenia at onset	Yes	No
Autoimmune hepatitis	Rare	Yes
Sclerosing cholangitis	Rare	Yes

*Colonic cancer, cholangiocarcinoma.

CD cases. **Anti-*Saccharomyces cerevisiae* antibody** is present in most CD patients and is uncommon in UC. Another IBD-specific antibody is anti-OmpC, directed against an *Escherichia coli* membrane protein. Because there is overlap between CD and UC, none of these tests can discriminate absolutely between the two conditions.

In patients with suspected IBD, an **upper GI series with small bowel follow-through** is needed to detect small bowel involvement. **Colonoscopy** is preferred over contrast enema because biopsy specimens can be obtained and because visual features can be diagnostic. Findings in UC include diffuse carpeting of the distal or entire colon with tiny ulcers and loss of haustral folds. Within the involved segment, no skip areas are present. In CD, ulcerations tend to be much larger with a linear, branching, or aphthous appearance; skip areas are usually present. **Upper endoscopy** cannot evaluate the jejunum and ileum, but is more sensitive than contrast studies in identifying proximal CD involvement. The capsule endoscope, a swallowed device that can visualize the entire small bowel, is potentially useful to visualize subtle small bowel disease.

TABLE 129–2. Diagnostic Studies for Inflammatory Bowel Disease

Studies	Interpretation
Blood Tests	
CBC with WBC differential	Anemia, elevated platelets suggest IBD
ESR	Elevated in many, but not all, IBD patients
C-reactive protein	Elevated in many, but not all, IBD patients
ASCA	Found in most CD patients and few UC patients
Atypical p-ANCA	Found in most UC patients and few CD patients
Anti-OmpC	Found in some UC and CD patients, rare in non-IBD
Imaging Studies	
Upper GI series with SBFT	Essential to rule out ileal and jejunal CD
CT scan	Used to detect abscess, small bowel involvement
Tagged WBC scan	Sometimes helpful in determining extent of disease
Endoscopy	
Upper endoscopy	Evaluate for CD of esophagus, stomach, and duodenum; obtain tissue for histologic diagnosis
Colonoscopy	Show presence or absence of colitis and terminal ileal CD; obtain tissue for histology
Capsule endoscopy	Emerging role in diagnosis of small bowel CD, more sensitive than upper GI series with SBFT

Anti-OmpC, antibody to outer membrane protein C; ASCA, anti-*Saccharomyces cerevisiae* antibody; atypical p-ANCA, atypical perinuclear staining by antineutrophil cytoplasmic antibody; CBC, complete blood count; CD, Crohn disease; ESR, erythrocyte sedimentation rate; GI, gastrointestinal; IBD, inflammatory bowel disease; SBFT, small bowel follow-through; WBC, white blood cell.

Treatment

Ulcerative Colitis

UC is treated with the aminosalicylate drugs, which deliver **5-aminosalicylic acid** (5-ASA) to the distal gut. Because it is rapidly absorbed, pure 5-ASA (mesalamine) must be specially packaged in coated capsules or pills or taken as a suppository to be effective in the colon. Other aminosalicylates (sulfasalazine, olsalazine, and balsalazide) use 5-ASA covalently linked to a carrier molecule. Sulfasalazine is the least expensive, but side effects resulting from its sulfapyridine component are common. When aminosalicylates alone cannot control the disease, steroid therapy may be required to induce remission. Whenever possible, steroids should not used for long-term therapy. An immunosuppressive drug, such as **6-mercaptopurine** or **azathioprine**, is useful to spare excessive steroid use in difficult cases. More potent immunosuppressives, such as cyclosporine or tacrolimus, are under investigation as rescue therapy when other treatments fail. Surgical colectomy with ileoanal anastomosis is an option for unresponsive severe disease or electively to end chronic symptoms and to reduce the risk of colon cancer, which is high in patients with UC.

Crohn Disease

Inflammation in CD typically responds less well to aminosalicylates; oral or IV steroids are more important in inducing remission. To avoid the need for repetitive steroid therapy, immunosuppressive drugs, usually either azathioprine or 6-mercaptopurine, are started soon after diagnosis. CD that is difficult to control also may be treated with methotrexate or with agents that block the action of tumor necrosis factor-α. **Infliximab** is the most effective such drug; thalidomide also blocks tumor necrosis factor action, but its use must be supervised carefully because of teratogenicity. Other antibodies that inhibit WBC migration or action, such as natalizumab, also show promise. As with UC, surgery is sometimes necessary, usually because of obstructive symptoms, abscess, or severe, unremitting symptoms. Because surgery is not curative in CD, its use must be limited, and the length of bowel resection must be minimized.

CELIAC DISEASE

Etiology and Epidemiology

Celiac disease, or celiac sprue, is an injury to the mucosa of the small intestine caused by the ingestion of **gluten** (a toxic protein component) from wheat, rye, barley, and related grains. Rice does not contain toxic gluten and can be eaten freely, as can special pure preparations of oats not contaminated by other grains. In its severe form, celiac disease causes malabsorption and malnutrition. Diagnosis was based on the presence of typical symptoms, followed by small bowel biopsy. The availability of more sensitive and specific serologic testing has revealed a "celiac iceberg" of many patients with few or no symptoms who have early, attenuated, or latent disease. Approximately 1 in 250 persons in the U.S. have celiac disease, only a few of which have been diagnosed. The disease is seen in association with diabetes and trisomy 21.

Clinical Manifestations

Symptoms can begin at any age when gluten-containing foods are given. Diarrhea, abdominal bloating, failure to thrive, irritability, decreased appetite, and ascites caused by hypoproteinemia are classic. Children may be minimally symptomatic or may be severely malnourished. Constipation is found in a few patients, probably because of reduced intake. A careful inspection of the child's growth curve and determination of reduced subcutaneous fat and abdominal distention are crucial. Celiac disease should be considered in any child with chronic abdominal complaints.

Laboratory and Imaging Studies

Serologic markers include IgA antiendomysial antibody and IgA tissue transglutaminase antibody. Because IgA deficiency is common in celiac disease, total serum IgA also must be measured to document the accuracy of these tests. In the absence of IgA deficiency, either test yields a sensitivity and specificity of 95%. An endoscopic **small bowel biopsy** is essential to confirm the diagnosis and should be performed while the patient is still taking gluten. The biopsy specimen shows various degrees of villous atrophy (short or absent villi), mucosal inflammation, crypt hyperplasia, and increased numbers of intraepithelial lymphocytes. When there is any question about response to treatment, a repeat biopsy specimen may be obtained several months later. Other laboratory studies should be performed to rule out complications, including complete blood count, calcium, phosphate, total protein and albumin, and liver function tests. Mild elevations of the transaminases are common and should normalize with dietary therapy.

Treatment

Treatment is complete elimination of gluten from the diet. The role of gluten in causing intestinal injury must be explained carefully. Consultation with a dietitian experienced in celiac disease is helpful, as is membership in a celiac disease support group. Lists of prepared foods that contain hidden gluten are particularly important for patients to use. Starchy foods that are safe include rice, soy, tapioca, buckwheat, potatoes, and (pure) oats. Many resources also are available via the Internet to help families cope with the large changes in diet and cooking that are required. Most patients respond clinically within a few weeks with weight gain, improved appetite, and improved sense of well-being. Histologic improvement lags behind clinical response, requiring several months to normalize.

MILK AND SOY PROTEIN INTOLERANCE (ALLERGIC COLITIS)
Etiology and Epidemiology

Dietary proteins are a common cause of intestinal inflammation with rectal bleeding in infants. The most commonly implicated agents are cow's milk and less often soy proteins. Other dietary antigens are possible in breastfed infants; breast milk also contains a sampling of protein fragments from the entire range of foods consumed by the mother. Symptoms can appear from 1 to 2 weeks of age to 12 months.

Clinical Manifestations

Most infants with dietary protein intolerance appear healthy despite the presence of streaks of bloody mucus in their stools. This presentation often leads to an erroneous diagnosis of anal fissure. Careful examination of the anus is essential. There is no abdominal tenderness or distention and no vomiting. If these are present, other diagnoses, such as intussusception or volvulus, should be considered. Some children develop severe anemia; intestinal protein loss produces edema and a **protein-losing enteropathy**.

Laboratory and Imaging Studies

No blood test is particularly helpful. Peripheral eosinophilia generally is not present on complete blood count, which nevertheless should be performed to rule out an associated iron deficiency anemia. Most children are diagnosed clinically and treated empirically. For children with persistent symptoms or other concerns, the diagnosis can be confirmed safely and easily by rectal mucosal biopsy; this shows eosinophilic inflammation of the mucosa. Visual findings at proctoscopy usually include mucosal friability and **lymphoid hyperplasia**, giving a lumpy, "mosquito-bitten" appearance to the rectal mucosa.

Treatment

Infants who are bottle-fed should be switched to a **hydrolyzed protein formula** (e.g., Nutramigen, Pregestamil, or Alimentum). Breastfed infants may continue breastfeeding, but the mother should restrict soy and dairy products from her diet. Visible blood in the stools typically resolves within a few days, although occult blood persists for several weeks. For infants with persistent bleeding, an amino acid–based formula is occasionally necessary. Nearly all of these infants lose their sensitivity to the offending protein by 1 year of age. The first intentional exposure to cow's milk should be performed in the physician's office because of a small risk of anaphylaxis. Treatment of iron deficiency also is indicated (see Chapter 150).

INTUSSUSCEPTION

Etiology and Epidemiology

Intussusception is the "telescoping" of a segment of proximal bowel (the intussusceptum) into downstream bowel (the intussuscipiens). Most cases occur in infants 1 to 2 years old. In infants younger than 2 years old, nearly all cases are idiopathic. Viral-induced lymphoid hyperplasia may produce a lead point in these children. In older children, the proportion of cases caused by a pathologic lead point increases. In young children, **ileocolonic** intussusception is common; the ileum invaginates into the colon, beginning at or near the ileocecal valve. When pathologic lead points are present, the intussusception may be ileoileal, jejunoileal, or jejunojejunal. There is a slight male predominance.

Clinical Manifestations

An infant with intussusception has sudden onset of crampy abdominal pain; the infant's knees draw up, and the infant cries out and exhibits pallor with a colicky pattern occurring every 15 to 20 minutes. Feedings are refused. As the intussusception progresses, and obstruction becomes prolonged, bilious vomiting becomes prominent, and the dilated, fatigued intestine generates less pressure and less pain. As the intussuscepted bowel moves further and further into the downstream intestine by its native motility, the mesentery is pulled with it and becomes stretched and compressed. The venous outflow from the intussusceptum is obstructed, leading to edema, weeping of fluid, and congestion with bleeding. Third space fluid losses and "currant jelly" stools result. Another unexpected feature of intussusception is **lethargy**. Between episodes of pain, the infant is glassy-eyed and groggy and appears to have been sedated. A sausage-shaped mass caused by the swollen, intussuscepted bowel may be palpable in the right upper quadrant or epigastrium.

Laboratory and Imaging Studies

The diagnosis depends on the direct demonstration of bowel-within-bowel. A simple and direct way of showing this is by abdominal ultrasound. If the ultrasound is positive, or if good visualization has not been achieved, a pneumatic or contrast enema under fluoroscopy is indicated. This is the most direct and potentially useful way to show and **treat** intussusception. Air and barium can show the intussusception quickly and, when administered with controlled pressure, usually can reduce it completely. The success rate for pneumatic reduction is probably a bit higher than hydrostatic reduction with barium and approaches 90% if done when symptoms have been present for less than 24 hours. The pneumatic enema has the additional advantage over barium of not preventing subsequent radiologic studies, such as upper GI series or CT scan. Nonoperative reduction should not be attempted if the patient is unstable or has evidence of perforation or peritonitis.

Treatment

Therapy must begin with placement of an IV catheter and a nasogastric tube. Before radiologic intervention is attempted, the child must have adequate **fluid resuscitation** to correct the often severe dehydration caused by vomiting and third space losses. Ultrasound may be performed before the fluid resuscitation is complete. Surgical consultation should be obtained early because the surgeon often prefers to be present during nonoperative reduction. If pneumatic or hydrostatic reduction is successful, the child should be admitted to the hospital for overnight observation of possible recurrence (risk is 5% to 10%). If reduction is not complete, emergency surgery is required. The surgeon attempts gentle manual reduction, but may need to resect the involved bowel after failed radiologic reduction because of severe edema, perforation, a pathologic lead point (polyp, Meckel diverticulum), or necrosis.

APPENDICITIS

Etiology and Epidemiology

Appendicitis is the most common surgical emergency in childhood. The incidence peaks in the late teenage years, with only 5% of cases occurring in children younger than 5 years old. There is a slight male predominance. Appendicitis begins with obstruction of the lumen, most commonly by fecal matter (fecalith), but appendiceal obstruction also can occur secondary to hyperplasia of lymphoid tissue associated with viral infections or the presence of neoplastic tissue, commonly an appendiceal carcinoid tumor. Trapped bacteria proliferate and begin to invade the appendiceal wall, inducing inflammation and secretion. The obstructed appendix becomes engorged, its blood supply is compromised, and it finally ruptures. The entire process is rapid, with appendiceal rupture usually occurring within 48 hours of the onset of symptoms.

Clinical Manifestations

Classic appendicitis begins with **visceral pain**, localized to the periumbilical region. Nausea and vomiting occur soon after, triggered by the appendiceal distention. As the inflammation begins to irritate the parietal peritoneum adjacent to the appendix, **somatic pain** fibers are activated, and the pain localizes to the right lower quadrant. Examination of the patient reveals a tender right lower quadrant. Voluntary guarding is present initially, progressing to rigidity, then to rebound tenderness with rupture and peritonitis. These classic findings may not be present, however, especially in young children, if the appendix is retrocecal, covered by omentum, or in another unusual location. When classic history and physical examination findings are present, the patient is taken to the operating room. When doubt exists, imaging is helpful to rule out complications (right lower quadrant abscess, liver disease) and other disorders, such as mesenteric adenitis and ovarian or fallopian tube disorders. If the workup is negative but some doubt remains, the child should be admitted to the hospital for close observation and serial examinations.

Laboratory and Imaging Studies

The history and examination are often enough to make the diagnosis, but laboratory and imaging studies are helpful when the diagnosis is uncertain (Table 129–3). A WBC count greater than 10,000/mm³ is found in 89% of patients with appendicitis and 93% with perforated appendicitis. This criterion is met by 62% of abdominal pain patients without appendicitis, however. The specificity of an elevated WBC count is low. Urinalysis is done to rule out urinary tract infection, and the chest x-ray rules out pneumonia masquerading as abdominal pain. Amylase, lipase, and liver enzymes are done to look for pancreatic or liver and gallbladder disease. The plain abdominal x-ray may reveal a calcified fecalith, which strongly suggests the diagnosis. When these studies are inconclusive, imaging is indicated with a CT scan or abdominal ultrasound, which may reveal the presence of an enlarged, thick-walled appendix with surrounding

---

TABLE 129–3.   Diagnostic Studies in Suspected Appendicitis
Initial Laboratory Testing
CBC with differential
Urinalysis
Amylase and lipase
ALT, AST, GGT
Flat and upright abdominal radiographs
Chest x-ray
Follow-up Studies*
CT scan of abdomen
Abdominal ultrasound

*Perform when diagnosis remains in doubt.
ALT, alanine aminotransferase; AST, aspartate aminotransferase; CBC, complete blood count; GGT, γ-glutamyltransferase.

---

fluid. A diameter of more than 6 mm is considered diagnostic.

Treatment

Treatment of appendicitis is surgical. Simple appendectomy is curative if performed before perforation. With perforation, a course of postoperative IV antibiotics is required. Broad-spectrum coverage is necessary to cover the mixed bowel flora.

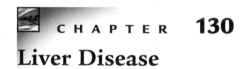

CHAPTER **130**

Liver Disease

CHOLESTASIS

Etiology and Epidemiology

Cholestasis is defined as reduced bile flow and is characterized by elevation of the conjugated, or direct, bilirubin fraction. This condition must be distinguished from ordinary neonatal jaundice, in which the direct bilirubin is never elevated (see Chapter 62). Neonatal jaundice that is secondary to unconjugated hyperbilirubinemia is the result of immature hepatocellular excretory function or hemolysis, which increases the production of bilirubin. When direct bilirubin is elevated, many potentially serious disorders must be considered (Fig. 130–1). Emphasis must be placed on the rapid diagnosis of treatable disorders, especially biliary atresia and metabolic disorders, such as galactosemia or tyrosinemia.

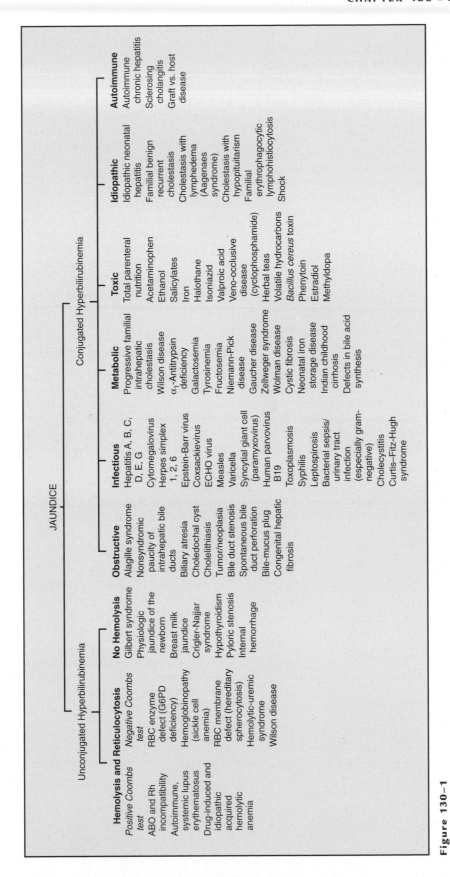

Figure 130-1

Differential diagnosis of jaundice in childhood. G6PD, glucose-6-phosphate dehydrogenase; RBC, red blood cell.

Clinical Manifestations

Cholestasis is caused by many different disorders, the common characteristic of which is cholestatic jaundice. Clinical features of several of the most common causes are given.

The jaundice of **extrahepatic biliary atresia** (biliary atresia) usually is not evident immediately at birth, but develops in the first week or two of life. The reason is that extrahepatic bile ducts are usually present at birth, but are then destroyed by an idiopathic inflammatory process. Aside from jaundice, these infants do not initially appear ill. The liver injury progresses rapidly to cirrhosis; symptoms of portal hypertension with splenomegaly, ascites, muscle wasting, and poor weight gain are evident by a few months of age. If surgical drainage is not performed successfully early in the course (ideally by 2 months), progression to liver failure is inevitable.

Neonatal hepatitis is characterized by an ill-appearing infant with an enlarged liver and jaundice. There is no specific diagnostic test, but if liver biopsy is performed, the presence of hepatocyte giant cells is characteristic. Cytomegalovirus and syphilis must be ruled out. Hepatobiliary scintigraphy typically shows slow hepatic uptake with eventual excretion of isotope into the intestine. These infants have a good prognosis overall, with spontaneous resolution occurring in most.

α_1-**Antitrypsin deficiency** presents with clinical findings indistinguishable from neonatal hepatitis.

Only about 20% of all infants with the genetic defect exhibit neonatal cholestasis. Of these affected infants, about 30% go on to have severe chronic liver disease resulting in cirrhosis and liver failure. α_1-Antitrypsin deficiency is the leading metabolic disorder requiring liver transplantation.

Alagille syndrome is characterized by chronic cholestasis with the unique liver biopsy finding of paucity of bile ducts in the portal triads. Associated abnormalities in some (syndromic) types include peripheral pulmonic stenosis or other cardiac anomalies; hypertelorism; unusual facies with deep-set eyes, prominent forehead, and a pointed chin; butterfly vertebrae; and a defect of the limbus (*posterior embryotoxon*). Cholestasis is variable but is usually lifelong and associated with hypercholesterolemia and severe pruritus. Progression to end-stage liver disease is uncommon. Liver transplantation sometimes is performed electively to relieve severe and uncontrollable pruritus.

Laboratory and Imaging Studies

The laboratory approach to diagnosis of a neonate with cholestatic jaundice is presented in Table 130–1. Noninvasive studies are performed immediately in hopes of making a rapid diagnosis. Imaging studies also are performed early to rule out biliary obstruction and other anatomic lesions that may be surgically

---

TABLE 130–1.　Laboratory and Imaging Evaluation of Neonatal Cholestasis

Evaluation	Rationale
Initial Tests	
Total and direct bilirubin	Elevated direct fraction confirms cholestasis
AST, ALT	Hepatocellular injury
GGT	Biliary obstruction/injury
RBC galactose-1-phosphate uridyltransferase	Galactosemia
α_1-Antitrypsin level	α_1-Antitrypsin deficiency
Urinalysis and urine culture	Urinary tract infection can cause cholestasis in neonates
Blood culture	Sepsis can cause cholestasis
Serum amino acids	Aminoacidopathies
Urine organic acids	Zellweger syndrome, lysosomal disorders
Sweat chloride or CF mutation analysis	Cystic fibrosis
Urine culture for cytomegalovirus	Congenital cytomegalovirus infection
Initial Imaging Study	
Abdominal ultrasound	Choledochal cyst, gallstones, mass lesion, Caroli disease
Secondary Imaging Study	
Hepatobiliary scintigraphy	Rule out biliary atresia

ALT, alanine aminotransferase; AST, aspartate aminotransferase; CF, cystic fibrosis; GGT, γ-glutamyltransferase; RBC, red blood cell.

Figure 130–2

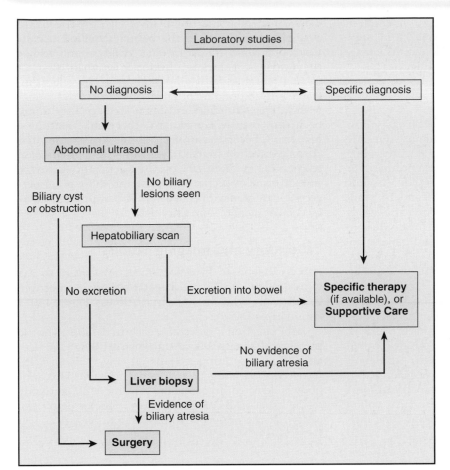

Flow chart for evaluation of neonatal cholestasis.

treatable. When necessary to rule out biliary atresia or to obtain prognostic information, liver biopsy is a final option (Fig. 130–2).

Treatment

Treatment of extrahepatic biliary atresia is the surgical **Kasai procedure**, in which the damaged bile duct remnant is removed and replaced with a roux-en-Y loop of jejunum. This operation must be performed before 3 months of age to have the best chance of success. Even so, the success rate is low; many children require liver transplantation. Some metabolic causes of neonatal cholestasis are treatable by dietary manipulation (galactosemia) or medication (tyrosinemia); all affected patients require supportive care. This includes fat-soluble vitamin supplements (vitamins A, D, E, and K) and formula containing medium-chain triglycerides, which can be absorbed without bile salt–induced micelles. Choleretic agents, such as ursodeoxycholic acid and phenobarbital, may improve bile flow in some conditions.

VIRAL HEPATITIS

Etiology and Epidemiology

Transient biochemical evidence of hepatitis may be found in many viral infections, even in the absence of jaundice. The term *hepatitis* usually is applied, however, to infections with predominantly hepatic involvement. Hepatitis A, B, C, D, and E viruses meet this criterion; many other viruses cause hepatitis with jaundice and elevated transaminases (see Fig. 130–1). Hepatitis A virus (HAV) is transmitted by the fecal-oral route and is highly infectious. Hepatitis B and C viruses (HBV, HCV) are less infectious under ordinary circumstances, but can be transmitted in infected blood products and body fluids, vertically from mother to child, and by sexual contact, especially homosexual activity and with multiple partners. HBV is highly prevalent in parts of Asia and Africa, where 13% of the population is chronically infected. In the U.S., the prevalence of chronic HBV is about 0.5%. The incidence of new infections has declined 10-fold since routine immunization began in 1990. Transmission is decreasing since testing of blood products for HBV and HCV, but still occurs in children by vertical transmission (HBV) in about 5% of pregnancies of infected mothers and in adolescents engaging in high-risk sexual behavior or IV drug use.

Clinical Manifestations

HAV has an average incubation period of 30 days. Most cases are self-limited and relatively minor, but rare cases can manifest as fulminant liver failure. In young children, the illness is mild, either asymptomatic or manifesting with malaise and vomiting, but usually without jaundice. Between the ages of 6 and 14, jaundice is evident in about half of cases. After the age of 14 years, 70% to 80% of cases present with jaundice. In this older age group, headache, fever, and malaise are followed by jaundice that persists for a few weeks. Symptoms tend to diminish as the jaundice peaks, heralding recovery.

HBV has a longer incubation period of 1 to 3 months. A prodrome of malaise, fatigue, low-grade fever, and arthralgias is followed by jaundice, pruritus, nausea, and vomiting. In some cases, the prodromal illness resembles serum sickness, with prominent migrating polyarticular arthritis, urticaria, macropapular rash, and glomerulonephritis. Prodromal symptoms subside as active hepatitis begins. As with HAV, young children may not develop clinical hepatitis. The inci-

dence of chronic infection is inversely proportional to age. Infants infected in the perinatal period usually develop chronic illness. In older children and adults, the incidence of chronic infection is less than 10%.

HCV has an incubation period of 6 to 7 weeks. Clinical manifestations are often absent early in the course, with fatigue, jaundice, and other signs of liver injury occurring later. In contrast to other viral hepatitides, hepatitis C becomes chronic in about 80% of cases. The chronic infection is characterized by slow progression to cirrhosis in about 20% of cases, generally occurring over 30 years. A higher incidence and more rapid progression are seen with concurrent liver injury caused by HIV, HBV, alcohol, and fatty liver.

Laboratory and Imaging Studies

HAV is diagnosed by detection of antibodies to the virus. IgM antibodies are detectable early in infection, usually before the onset of clinical illness. Figure 130–3 summarizes these events.

HBV infection is detectable early in the illness by the presence of hepatitis B early antigen (HBeAg) and hepatitis B surface antigen (HBsAg) (Fig. 130–4). With recovery, these antigens are cleared, and anti-HBs antibody is detected. In acute and chronic HBV, antibody to the hepatitis B core protein (anti-HBc) is detectable as IgM at the onset of symptoms and persists as IgG

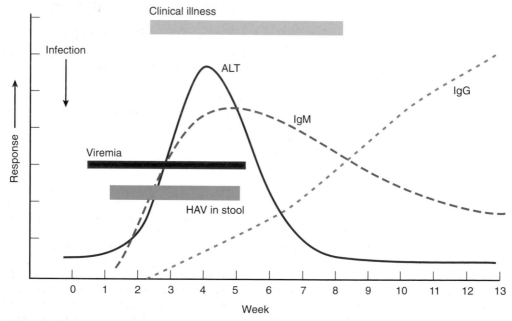

Figure 130–3

Serology of acute hepatitis A. ALT, alanine aminotransferase; HAV, hepatitis A virus. (From Centers for Disease Control and Prevention: http://www.cdc.gov/ncidod/diseases/hepatitis/slideset/index.htm.)

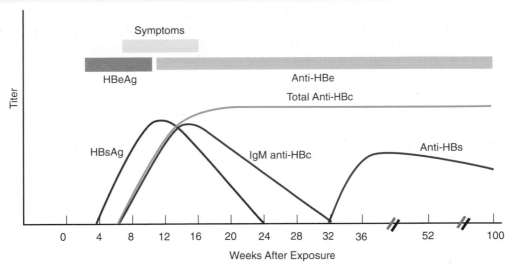

Figure 130-4

Acute hepatitis B virus infection with recovery. Typical serologic course. HBc, hepatitis B core antigen; HBe, HBeAg, hepatitis B early antigen; HBs, HBsAg, hepatitis B surface antigen. (From Centers for Disease Control and Prevention: http://www.cdc.gov/ncidod/diseases/hepatitis/slideset/index.htm.)

for years afterward. If the infection persists as chronic HBV, HBsAg and HBeAg persist, and anti-HBs antibodies do not appear (Fig. 130-5).

Acute HCV infection is best diagnosed by measurement of HCV RNA in the blood by polymerase chain reaction. Within 2 to 3 months of infection, anti-HCV antibodies appear. Most cases result in chronic infection, which is characterized by persistence of anti-HCV and HCV RNA (Fig. 130-6).

Transaminases (alanine aminotransferase, aspartate aminotransferase), serum total and direct bilirubin, serum albumin, and tests of blood clotting (prothrombin time, partial thromboplastin time) should be measured serially in acute and chronic hepatitis. These tests give an idea of the degree of liver injury and adequacy of hepatocellular synthetic function.

Treatment

There is no specific treatment for HAV. Supportive care with IV fluids is occasionally necessary with severe symptoms. In fulminant cases, multisystem support is provided. HBV is currently treated only when transaminases are elevated because response to treatment in individuals without hepatic inflammation is poor. Currently available treatments include interferon alfa and the DNA polymerase–inhibiting agents lamivudine and adefovir. HCV is best treated by a combination of interferon alfa and ribavirin. In contrast to HBV, persistent elevation of transaminases is not associated with increased efficacy of treatment. The response to treatment in HCV corresponds well to viral genotype, which should be determined before starting therapy.

FULMINANT LIVER FAILURE
Etiology and Epidemiology

Fulminant liver failure is defined as severe liver disease with onset of hepatic encephalopathy within 8 weeks after initial symptoms, in the absence of chronic liver disease. Etiology includes viral hepatitis, metabolic disorders, ischemia, neoplastic disease, and toxins (Table 130-2).

Clinical Manifestations

Liver failure is a multisystem disorder with complex interactions among the liver, kidneys, vascular structures, gut, CNS, and immune function. Hepatic encephalopathy is characterized by varying degrees of impairment (Table 130-3). Respiratory compromise occurs as severity of the failure increases and requires early institution of ventilatory support. Hypoglycemia resulting from impaired glycogenolysis and gluconeogenesis must be prevented. Renal function is impaired, and frank renal failure, or **hepatorenal syndrome**, may occur. This syndrome is characterized by low urine output, azotemia, and low urine sodium content. Ascites develops secondary to hypoalbuminemia and disordered regulation of fluid and electrolyte

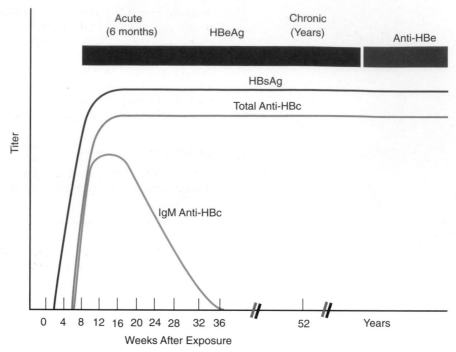

Figure 130–5

Progression to chronic hepatitis B virus infection. Typical serologic course. HBc, hepatitis B core antigen; HBe, HBeAg, hepatitis B early antigen; HBsAg, hepatitis B surface antigen.

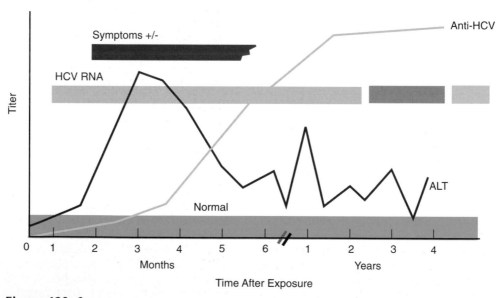

Figure 130–6

Serologic pattern of acute hepatitis C infection with progression to chronic infection. ALT, alanine aminotransferase; HCV, hepatitis C virus. (From Centers for Disease Control and Prevention: http://www.cdc.gov/ncidod/diseases/hepatitis/slideset/index.htm.)

TABLE 130-2.   Causes of Fulminant Liver Failure in Childhood

Metabolic

Neonatal hemochromatosis
Electron chain transport defects
Disorders of fatty acid oxidation
Galactosemia
Hereditary fructose intolerance
Bile acid synthesis disorders
Wilson disease

Cardiovascular

Shock, hypotension
Congestive heart failure
Budd-Chiari syndrome

Infectious

Echovirus
Coxsackievirus
Adenovirus
Parvovirus
Cytomegalovirus
Sepsis
Herpes simplex

Neoplastic

Acute leukemia
Lymphoproliferative disease

Toxic

Acetaminophen
Valproic acid
Phenytoin
Isoniazid
Halothane
Amanita mushrooms

measure factor V serially as a sensitive index of synthetic function. Renal function tests, electrolytes, serum ammonia, blood counts, and urinalysis also should be followed. In the setting of acute liver failure, liver biopsy may be indicated to ascertain the nature and degree of injury and estimate the likelihood of recovery. In the presence of coagulopathy, biopsy must be done using a transjugular or surgical approach.

Treatment

Because of the life-threatening and complex nature of this condition, management must be carried out in an

TABLE 130-3.   Stages of Hepatic Encephalopathy

Stage I

Alert and awake
Agitated and distractible
Infants and young children—irritable and fussy
Normal reflexes
Tremor, poor handwriting
Obeys age-appropriate commands

Stage II

Confused and lethargic
Combative or inappropriate euphoria
Hyperactive reflexes
Asterixis present
Purposeful movements, but may not obey commands

Stage III

Stuporous but arousable
Sleepy
Incoherent speech
Motor response to pain
Hyperreflexic
Hyperventilation
Asterixis present

Stage IV

Unconscious, not arousable
Unresponsive or responds nonpurposefully to pain
Reflexes hyperactive
Irregular respirations
Pupil response sluggish

Stage V

Unconscious
Hypoactive reflexes
Flaccid muscle tone
Apneic
Pupils fixed

homeostasis. Increased risk of infection occurs and may cause death. Esophageal varices may cause significant hemorrhage, whereas hypersplenism from portal hypertension may produce thrombocytopenia.

Laboratory and Imaging Studies

Laboratory studies are used to follow the severity of the liver injury and to monitor the response to therapy. Coagulation tests and serum albumin are used to follow hepatic synthetic function. These tests are confounded by administration of blood products and clotting factors. Vitamin K should be administered to maximize the liver's ability to synthesize factors II, VII, IX, and X. In addition to monitoring prothrombin time and partial thromboplastin time, many centers

TABLE 130–4. Treatment of Fulminant Liver Failure	
Hepatic encephalopathy	Avoid sedatives
	Lactulose via nasogastric tube—start with 1-2 mL/kg/day, adjust dose to yield several loose stools per day
	Enemas if constipated
	Mechanical ventilation if stage III or IV
Coagulopathy	Fresh frozen plasma only if active bleeding, monitor coagulation studies frequently
	Platelet transfusions as required
Hypoglycemia	IV glucose supplied with ≥10% dextrose solution, electrolytes as appropriate
Ascites	Restrict fluid intake to 50%-60% maintenance
	Restrict sodium intake to 0.5-1 mEq/kg/day
	Monitor central venous pressure to maintain adequate intravascular volume (avoid renal failure)
Renal failure	Maintain adequate intravascular volume, give albumin if low
	Diuretics
	Vasoconstrictors
	Dialysis or hemofiltration
	Exchange transfusion
	Liver transplantation

ICU at a liver transplant center. Treatment of acute liver failure is supportive; the definitive lifesaving therapy is liver transplantation. Supportive measures are listed in Table 130-4. Efforts are made to treat metabolic derangements, avoid hypoglycemia, support respiration, minimize hepatic encephalopathy, and support renal function.

CHRONIC LIVER DISEASE

Etiology and Epidemiology

Chronic liver disease in childhood is characterized by the development of cirrhosis and its complications and by progressive hepatic failure. Causative conditions may be congenital or acquired. Major congenital disorders leading to chronic disease include biliary atresia, tyrosinemia, untreated galactosemia, and α_1-antitrypsin deficiency. In older children, HBV, HCV, autoimmune hepatitis, Wilson disease, primary sclerosing cholangitis, cystic fibrosis, and biliary obstruction secondary to choledochal cyst are leading causes.

Clinical Manifestations

Chronic liver disease is characterized by the consequences of portal hypertension, impaired hepatocellular function, and cholestasis. **Portal hypertension** caused by cirrhosis results in risk of GI bleeding, ascites, and reduced hepatic blood flow. Blood entering the portal vein from the splenic and mesenteric veins is diverted to collateral circulation that bypasses the liver, enlarging these previously tiny vessels in the esophagus, stomach, and abdomen. **Esophageal varices** are particularly prone to bleed, but bleeding also can occur from hemorrhoidal veins, engorged gastric mucosa, and gastric varices. **Ascites** develops as a result of weeping of a high-pressure ultrafiltrate from the surfaces of the viscera and is at risk of infection (spontaneous bacterial peritonitis); ascites often becomes quite massive and interferes with patient comfort and respiration. The spleen enlarges secondary to impaired splenic vein outflow, causing excessive scavenging of platelets and WBCs; this increases the patient's susceptibility to bleeding and infection.

Impaired hepatocellular function is associated with coagulopathy unresponsive to vitamin K, low serum albumin, elevated ammonia, and **hepatic encephalopathy**. The diversion of portal blood away from the liver via collateral circulation worsens this process. Malaise develops and contributes to poor nutrition, leading to muscle wasting and other consequences.

Chronic cholestasis causes debilitating pruritus and deepening jaundice, and the reduced excretion of bile acids impairs absorption of fat calories and fat-soluble vitamins. This impaired absorption contributes to the poor nutritional state. Deficiency of vitamin K impairs production of clotting factors II, VII, IX, and X and increases the risk of bleeding. Vitamin E deficiency leads to hematologic and neurologic consequences unless corrected.

Laboratory and Imaging Studies

Laboratory studies include specific tests for diagnosis of the underlying illness and testing to monitor the status of the patient. Children presenting for the first time with evidence of chronic liver disease should have a standard investigation (Table 130–5). Monitoring should include coagulation tests, electrolytes and renal function testing, complete blood count with platelet count, transaminases, alkaline phosphatase, and γ-glutamyltransferase at appropriate intervals. Frequency of testing should be tailored to the pace of the patient's illness. Ascites fluid can be tested for infection by culture and cell count and generally is found to have an albumin concentration lower than that of serum.

Treatment

Treatment of chronic liver disease is complex. The clinician is faced with a long struggle against a host of worsening problems. Supportive care for each of the many problems encountered in these patients is outlined in Table 130–6. Ultimately, survival depends on the availability of a donor liver and the patient's candidacy for transplantation. When transplantation is not possible or is delayed, palliative procedures, such as portosystemic shunts, can be considered. Transjugular intrahepatic portosystemic shunt has an expandable stent placed between the hepatic vein and a branch of the portal vein within the hepatic parenchyma. This procedure is performed using catheters inserted via the jugular vein and is entirely nonsurgical. All portosystemic shunts carry increased risk of hepatic encephalopathy.

SELECTED CHRONIC HEPATIC DISORDERS

Wilson Disease

Wilson disease is characterized by abnormal storage of copper in the liver, leading to hepatocellular injury, CNS dysfunction, and hemolytic anemia. It is an autosomal recessive trait caused by mutations in the *ATP7B* gene. The encoded protein of this gene functions as an ATP-driven copper pump. The **diagnosis** is made by identifying depressed serum levels of ceruloplasmin, elevated 24-hour urine copper excretion, the presence of Kayser-Fleischer rings in the iris, evidence of hemolysis, and elevated hepatic copper content. In any single patient, one or more of these measures may be normal. **Clinical presentation** also varies, but seldom occurs before age 3 years. Neurologic abnormalities may predominate, including tremor, decline in school performance, worsening handwriting, and psychiatric disturbances. Anemia may be the first noted symptom. Hepatic presentations include appearance of jaundice, spider hemangiomas, portal hypertension and its consequences, and fulminant hepatic failure. **Treatment**

TABLE 130–5. Laboratory and Imaging Investigation of Chronic Liver Disease

Metabolic Testing

Serum α₁-antitrypsin level
α₁-Antitrypsin phenotype if low serum level
Serum ceruloplasmin
Sweat chloride, CF gene tests if CF suspected
Testing for other specific conditions as indicated by clinical/laboratory findings

Viral Hepatitis

HBsAg
Hepatitis B viral DNA, HBeAg if HBsAg positive
Hepatitis C antibody
Hepatitis C antibody confirmatory test if positive
Hepatitis C viral RNA, genotype if antibody confirmed

Autoimmune Hepatitis

Antinuclear antibody
Liver-kidney microsomal antibody
Anti–smooth muscle antibody
Antineutrophil cytoplasmic antibody
Total serum IgG (usually elevated)

Tests to Evaluate Liver Function and Injury

Prothrombin time and partial thromboplastin time
Serum ammonia
CBC with platelet count
Serum albumin
AST, ALT, GGT, alkaline phosphatase
Total and direct bilirubin
Serum cholylglycine or bile acids
Serum cholesterol
Ultrasound examination of liver and bile ducts
Doppler ultrasound of hepatic vessels*
Magnetic resonance cholangiography*
Magnetic resonance angiography of hepatic vessels*
Percutaneous or endoscopic cholangiography*
Liver biopsy*

Anatomic Evaluation

Ultrasound of liver, pancreas, and biliary tree
Consider magnetic resonance cholangiography or ERCP if evidence of biliary process
Liver biopsy—as required for diagnosis or prognosis

Tests to Evaluate Nutritional Status

Height, weight, skinfold thickness
25-Hydroxyvitamin D level
Vitamin A level
Prothrombin time and partial thromboplastin time before and after vitamin K administration
Serum albumin and prealbumin

*Perform when indicated to obtain specific anatomic information.
ALT, alanine aminotransferase; AST, aspartate aminotransferase; CBC, complete blood count; CF, cystic fibrosis; ERCP, endoscopic retrograde cholangiopancreatography; GGT, γ-glutamyltransferase; HBeAg, hepatitis B early antigen; HBsAg, hepatitis B surface antigen.

TABLE 130–6.   Management of Chronic Liver Disease

Problem	Clinical Manifestations	Diagnostic Testing	Treatment
Gastrointestinal variceal bleeding*	Hematemesis, rectal bleeding, melena, anemia	CBC, coagulation tests, Doppler ultrasound, magnetic resonance angiography, endoscopy	Somatostatin (octreotide) infusion, variceal band ligation or sclerotherapy, propranolol to reduce portal pressure, acid-blocker therapy, TIPSS or surgical portosystemic shunt if transplant not possible
Ascites	Abdominal distention, shifting dullness and fluid wave, respiratory compromise, spontaneous bacterial peritonitis	Abdominal ultrasound, diagnostic paracentesis; measure ascites fluid albumin (and serum albumin), cell count, WBC differential, culture fluid in blood culture bottles	Restrict sodium intake to 0.5-1 mEq/kg/day, restrict fluids, monitor renal function, treat peritonitis and portal hypertension. Central portosystemic shunt may be required
Nutritional compromise	Muscle wasting, fat-soluble vitamin deficiencies, poor or absent weight gain, fatigue	Coagulation studies, serum albumin, 25-hydroxyvitamin D level, vitamin E level, vitamin A level	Fat-soluble vitamin supplements: vitamins A, D, E, and K; use water-soluble form of vitamins. Supplemental feedings—nasogastric or parenteral if necessary
Hepatic encephalopathy	Irritability, confusion, lethargy, somnolence, coma	Serum ammonia	Lactulose orally or via nasogastric tube, avoid narcotics and sedatives, liver transplantation

*May also have peptic ulcerations.
CBC, complete blood count; TIPSS, transjugular intrahepatic portosystemic shunt; WBC, white blood cell.

consists of administration of copper chelating drugs (penicillimine or trientine), with monitoring of urine copper excretion at intervals. Zinc salts occasionally may be used in place of chelating agents, especially when urine copper excretion declines, indicating successful reduction of the excessive body copper stores. Adequate therapy must be continued for life to prevent liver and CNS deterioration.

Autoimmune Hepatitis

Immune-mediated liver injury may be primary or occur in association with other autoimmune disorders, such as IBD or systemic lupus erythematosus. **Diagnosis** is made on the basis of elevated serum total IgG and the presence of an autoantibody, most commonly antinuclear, anti–smooth muscle, or anti–liver-kidney microsomal antibody. Liver biopsy specimen shows the presence of a plasma cell–rich portal infiltrate with piecemeal necrosis. **Treatment** consists of corticosteroids initially, usually with the addition of an immunosuppressive drug after remission is achieved. Steroids are tapered gradually as tolerated to minimize glucocorticoid side effects. Many patients require lifelong immunosuppressive therapy, but some may be able to stop medications after several years under careful monitoring for recurrence.

Primary Sclerosing Cholangitis

Primary sclerosing cholangitis occurs by itself or more often in association with UC. It may be accompanied by evidence of autoimmune hepatitis; when this occurs, *overlap syndrome* is diagnosed. Antineutrophil cytoplasmic antibody is present in many cases. **Diagnosis** is by liver biopsy and cholangiography, generally performed as endoscopic retrograde cholangiopancreatography (ERCP). These studies show inflammation and fibrosis surrounding bile ducts in biopsy specimens and varying degrees of segmental stricturing of larger bile ducts by cholangiography. Treatment consists of ursodiol administration, which seems to slow progression and improves indices of hepatic injury; dilation of major biliary strictures during ERCP; and liver transplantation for end-stage liver disease.

Steatohepatitis, also known as *nonalcoholic fatty liver disease* or *nonalcoholic fatty hepatitis,* is characterized by the presence of macrovesicular fatty change in hepatocytes on biopsy. Varying degrees of inflammation and portal fibrosis may be present. This disorder occurs in obese children, sometimes in association with insulin-resistant (type 2) diabetes and hyperlipidemia. Children with marked obesity, with or without type 2 diabetes, who have elevated liver enzymes and no other identifiable liver disease, are likely to have this condition. Nonalcoholic fatty liver disease can progress to significant fibrosis. Treatment is with diet and exercise. Vitamin E may have some benefit. Efforts should be made to control blood glucose and hyperlipidemia and promote weight loss. In general, the rate of progression to end-stage liver disease is slow.

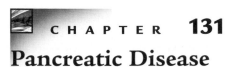

CHAPTER 131
Pancreatic Disease

PANCREATIC INSUFFICIENCY
Etiology and Epidemiology

The cause of inadequate pancreatic digestive function in 95% of cases is **cystic fibrosis** (see Chapter 137). The defect in *CFTR* chloride channel function results in thick secretions in the lungs, intestines, pancreas, and bile ducts. In the pancreas, there is destruction of pancreatic function, often before birth. Some mutations result in less severe defects in *CFTR* function and later onset of lung disease and pancreatic insufficiency. Less common causes of pancreatic insufficiency are Shwachman-Diamond syndrome and Pearson syndrome in developed countries and severe malnutrition in developing countries.

Clinical Manifestations

Children with pancreatic exocrine insufficiency have many bulky, foul-smelling stools each day, usually with visible oil or fat. They typically have voracious appetites because of massive malabsorption of calories from fat, complex carbohydrates, and proteins. Failure to thrive is uniformly present if diagnosis and treatment are not accomplished rapidly. It is important to distinguish children with malabsorption due to pancreatic disease from children with intestinal disorders that interfere with digestion or absorption. Appropriate testing should be performed to rule out conditions such as celiac disease and IBD if any doubt about the state of pancreatic sufficiency exists.

Laboratory and Imaging Studies

Testing of pancreatic function is difficult. Direct measurement of enzyme concentrations in aspirated pancreatic juice is not routine and is technically difficult. Stools can be tested for the presence of maldigested fat. The presence of fecal fat usually indicates poor fat digestion. Measuring fecal fat is relatively simple and, depending on method, can give either a qualitative assessment of fat absorption (fecal Sudan stain) or a semiquantitative measurement (72-hour fecal fat

determination) of fat maldigestion. Another way to assess pancreatic function is to test for the presence of pancreatic enzymes in the stool. Of these, measuring fecal elastase-1 seems to be the most accurate method of assessment. Elastase-1 is resistant to digestion, and its presence in the stool is easy to measure by immunoassay. Depressed fecal elastase-1 concentration correlates well with the presence of pancreatic insufficiency.

Treatment

Replacement of missing pancreatic enzymes is the best available therapy. Pancreatic enzymes are available as enzyme powder, which can be mixed with formula for infants, and capsules containing enteric-coated microspheres for older children. The coating on these spheres is designed to protect the enzymes from gastric acid degradation. For children unable to swallow capsules, the contents may be sprinkled on a spoonful of soft food, such as applesauce. Excessive use of enzymes must be avoided because high doses (usually >6000 U/kg/meal) can cause colonic fibrosis. In infants, typical dosing is 2000 to 4000 U of lipase/120 mL of formula. In children younger than 4 years old, 1000 U/kg/meal is given. For older children, 500 U/kg/meal is usual. This dose may be adjusted upward as required to control steatorrhea, but a dose of 2500 U/kg/meal should not be exceeded. Use of H_2 receptor antagonists or proton-pump inhibitors can increase the efficacy of pancreatic enzymes by enhancing their release from the microspheres and reducing inactivation by acid.

ACUTE PANCREATITIS
Etiology and Epidemiology

The exocrine pancreas produces numerous proteolytic enzymes, including trypsin, chymotrypsin, and carboxypeptidase. These are produced as inactive proenzymes to protect the pancreas from autodigestion. Trypsin is activated after leaving the pancreas by enterokinase, an intestinal brush border enzyme. After activation, trypsin cleaves other proteolytic proenzymes into their active states. Protease inhibitors found in pancreatic juice inhibit early activation of trypsin; the presence of self-digestion sites on the trypsin molecule allows for feedback inactivation. Pancreatitis occurs when digestive enzymes are activated inside the pancreas, causing injury. Triggers for acute pancreatitis differ between adults and children. In the adult patient, most episodes are related to alcohol abuse or gallstones. In children, most cases are idiopathic. Some cases are caused by drugs, hypertriglyceridemia, biliary microlithiasis, trauma, or viral infection. Collagen vascular disorders and parasite infestations are responsible for the remainder.

Clinical Manifestations

Acute pancreatitis presents with relatively rapid onset of pain, usually in the epigastric region. The pain may radiate to the back and is nearly always aggravated by eating. The patient moves frequently to find a position of comfort. Nausea and vomiting occur in most cases. Pain is typically continuous and quite severe, usually requiring narcotics. Severe pancreatitis can lead to hemorrhage, visible as ecchymoses in the flanks (Grey Turner sign) or periumbilical region (Cullen sign). Rupture of a minor pancreatic duct can lead to development of a pancreatic pseudocyst, characterized by persistent severe pain and tenderness and a palpable mass. With necrosis and fluid collections, patients experiencing severe pancreatitis are prone to infectious complications, and the clinician must be alert for fever and signs of sepsis.

Laboratory and Imaging Studies

Acute pancreatitis can be surprisingly difficult to diagnose. Elevations in total serum amylase or lipase support the diagnosis. These pancreatic enzymes are released into the blood during pancreatic injury. Nonspecific elevations of the enzymes are common, however. As acute pancreatitis progresses, the amylase level tends to decline faster than lipase, making the latter a good choice for diagnostic testing late in the course of the disease.

Serial measurement of laboratory studies is important to monitor for severe complications. At diagnosis, baseline complete blood count, C-reactive protein, electrolytes, BUN, creatinine, glucose, calcium, and phosphorus should be obtained. These should be measured at least daily, along with amylase and lipase, until the patient has recovered.

Because enzyme levels are not 100% sensitive or specific, imaging studies are important for the diagnosis of pancreatitis. In acute pancreatitis, edema is present in all but the mildest cases. Ultrasound is capable of detecting this edema and should be performed as part of the overall diagnostic approach. If overlying bowel gas obscures the pancreas, a CT scan allows complete visualization of the gland. CT scans should be done with oral and IV contrast agents to facilitate interpretation. Ultrasound and CT also can be used to monitor for the development of **pseudocysts** and for evidence of ductal dilation secondary to obstruction. The other important reason to perform imaging studies early in the course of pancreatitis is to rule out gallstones; the liver, gallbladder, and common bile duct all should be visualized.

Treatment

There are no proven specific therapies for acute pancreatitis. If a predisposing etiology is found, such as a drug reaction or a gallstone obstructing the sphincter of Oddi, this should be specifically treated. Otherwise, the old maxim of "rest the gland" is accomplished by prohibiting oral intake, use of an acid-blocking drug, and (except in mild cases) nasogastric suction. Fluid resuscitation is necessary because of vomiting and third space losses. Pain relief should be provided, avoiding morphine because of its tendency to cause spasm of the sphincter of Oddi. Meperidine is the traditional narcotic of choice, but neurotoxicity of its metabolites limits long-term high-dose use; fentanyl is used frequently. Nutritional support should be provided early in the course because the patient may be NPO for extended periods. Feedings administered downstream from the duodenum via a nasojejunal tube are generally well tolerated. If this is not possible, parenteral nutrition is an option. Fewer complications and more rapid recovery occur with jejunal feedings compared with parenteral nutrition. Antibiotics should be considered if the patient is febrile, has extensive pancreatic necrosis, or has laboratory evidence of infection. A broad-spectrum antibiotic, such as imipenem, is considered the best choice.

CHRONIC PANCREATITIS

Etiology and Epidemiology

Chronic pancreatitis is defined as recurrent or persistent attacks of pancreatitis, which have resulted in irreversible morphologic changes in pancreatic structure. These include scarring of the ducts with irregular areas of narrowing and dilation (beading), fibrosis of parenchyma, and loss of acinar and islet tissue. Pancreatic exocrine insufficiency and diabetes mellitus may result from unremitting chronic pancreatitis. Most patients have discrete attacks of acute symptoms occurring repeatedly, but chronic pain may be present. The causes of chronic pancreatitis include hereditary pancreatitis and milder phenotypes of cystic fibrosis associated with pancreatic sufficiency. Familial disease is caused by one of several known mutations in the trypsinogen gene. These mutations obliterate autodigestion sites on the trypsin molecule, inhibiting feedback inhibition of trypsin digestion. Genetic testing is readily available for these mutations. Genetic testing for cystic fibrosis can be performed, but must include screening for the less common mutations associated with pancreatic sufficiency. Sweat chloride testing is less expensive and is abnormal in most. Less commonly, mutations in the *SPINK1* gene, which codes for pancreatic trypsin inhibitor, have been found.

Clinical Manifestations

Children with chronic pancreatitis initially present with recurring attacks of acute pancreatitis. Injury to the pancreatic ducts predisposes these children to continued attacks owing to scarring of small and large pancreatic ducts, stasis of pancreatic secretions, stone formation, and inflammation. Loss of pancreatic exocrine and endocrine tissue over time can lead to exocrine and endocrine deficiency. More than 90% of the pancreatic mass must be destroyed before exocrine deficiency becomes clinically apparent; this is a late complication that does not occur in all cases. Chronic pain is a serious problem in most affected individuals. These patients have many episodes; many do not require hospitalization.

Laboratory and Imaging Studies

Laboratory diagnosis of chronic pancreatitis is similar to acute pancreatitis. Monitoring also should include looking for consequences of chronic injury, including diabetes mellitus and compromise of the pancreatic and biliary ducts. Pancreatic and biliary imaging has been accomplished by ERCP. ERCP offers the possibility of therapeutic intervention to remove gallstones, dilate strictures, and place stents to enhance flow of pancreatic juice. Magnetic resonance cholangiopancreatography is an alternative to ERCP. Plain abdominal x-rays may show pancreatic calcifications. Diagnostic testing for the etiology of chronic pancreatitis should include genetic testing for hereditary pancreatitis and cystic fibrosis and sweat chloride determination.

Treatment

Treatment is largely supportive. Potential but unproven therapies include the use of daily pancreatic enzyme supplements, octreotide (somatostatin) to abort early attacks, low-fat diets, and daily antioxidant therapy. Care must be taken that extreme diets do not result in nutritional deprivation. Interventional ERCP to dilate large strictures and remove stones and surgical pancreatic drainage procedures to decompress dilated pancreatic ducts by creating a side-to-side pancreaticojejunostomy may have some value.

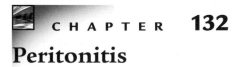

CHAPTER 132
Peritonitis

ETIOLOGY AND EPIDEMIOLOGY

The peritoneum consists of a single layer of mesothelial cells that covers all intra-abdominal organs. The portion that covers the abdominal wall is derived from the underlying somatic structures and is innervated by somatic nerves. The portion covering the viscera is derived from visceral mesoderm and is innervated by nonmyelinated visceral afferents. Inflammation of the peritoneum, or peritonitis, usually is caused by infection, but may result from exogenous irritants introduced by penetrating injuries or surgical procedures, radiation, and endogenous irritants, such as meconium. Infectious peritonitis can be an acute complication of intestinal inflammation and perforation, as in appendicitis, or it can occur secondary to contamination of preexisting ascites associated with renal, cardiac, or hepatic disease. In this setting, when there is no other intra-abdominal source, it is referred to as **spontaneous bacterial peritonitis**. Spontaneous bacterial peritonitis is usually due to pneumococcus and less often to *E. coli*.

CLINICAL MANIFESTATIONS

Peritonitis is characterized on examination by marked abdominal tenderness. Rebound tenderness also generally is quite pronounced. The patient tends to move very little owing to intense peritoneal irritation and pain. Fever is not always present, and absence of fever should not be regarded as contradictory to the diagnosis. Patients who are taking corticosteroids for an underlying condition, such as nephrotic syndrome, are likely to have little fever and reduced tenderness.

LABORATORY AND IMAGING STUDIES

Blood tests should focus on identifying the nature of the inflammation and its underlying cause. An elevated WBC count, erythrocyte sedimentation rate, and C-reactive protein suggest infection. In children older than 5 years, appendicitis is the leading cause. Total serum protein, albumin, and urinalysis should be ordered to rule out nephrotic syndrome. Liver function tests should be performed to rule out chronic liver disease causing ascites. The best way to diagnose suspected peritonitis is to sample the peritoneal fluid with a needle or catheter (paracentesis). Peritoneal fluid in spontaneous bacterial peritonitis has a high neutrophil count of greater than 250 cells/mm^3. Other tests that should be run on the peritoneal fluid include amylase (to rule out pancreatic ascites), culture, albumin, and lactate dehydrogenase concentration. For culture, a large sample of fluid should be placed into aerobic and anaerobic blood culture bottles immediately on obtaining the sample.

As discussed in Chapter 129, appendicitis may be identified by ultrasound or CT scan. When other intra-abdominal emergencies are suspected, such as midgut volvulus, meconium ileus, peptic disease, or any other condition predisposing to intestinal perforation, specific testing should be performed.

TREATMENT

Peritonitis caused by an intra-abdominal surgical process, such as appendicitis or a penetrating wound, must be managed surgically. Spontaneous bacterial peritonitis should be treated with a broad-spectrum antibiotic with good coverage of resistant pneumococcus and enteric bacteria. Cefotaxime is generally effective as initial therapy while awaiting culture and sensitivity results. Anaerobic coverage with metronidazole should be added whenever a perforated viscus is suspected.

SUGGESTED READING

Altschuler S, Liacouras CA (eds): Clinical Pediatric Gastroenterology. Philadelphia, Churchill Livingstone, 1998.

Behrman RE, Kliegman RM, Jenson HB (eds): Nelson Textbook of Pediatrics, 17th ed. Philadelphia, WB Saunders, 2004.

Feldman M, Friedman LS, Sleisenger MH (eds): Gastrointestinal and Liver Disease: Pathophysiology/Diagnosis/Management. Philadelphia, WB Saunders, 2002.

Kliegman RM, Greenbaum LA, Lye PS (eds): Practical Strategies in Pediatric Diagnosis and Therapy, 2nd ed. Philadelphia, WB Saunders, 2004.

Suchy FJ, Sokol RJ, Balistreri WF (eds): Liver Disease in Children. Philadelphia, Lippincott Williams & Wilkins, 2001.

Walker WA, Durie PR, Hamilton JR, et al (eds): Pediatric Gastrointestinal Disease. Hamilton, Ontario, BC Decker, 2000.

THE RESPIRATORY SYSTEM

Susan G. Marshall and Jason S. Debley

CHAPTER **133**

Assessment

ANATOMY OF THE RESPIRATORY SYSTEM

Air enters the **nose** and passes over the **turbinates** (bony protrusions into the nasal cavity) covered by **ciliated respiratory epithelium**, which increases the total surface area within each nostril. The large surface area and the convoluted patterns the airflow makes as it passes over the turbinates create a high resistance and serve to warm, humidify, and filter the inspired air. Secretions draining from the paranasal sinuses are carried from the nasal cavity to the **pharynx** by the mucociliary action of the epithelium. The eustachian tubes open from the middle ear into the posterior aspect of the nasopharynx. Lymphoid tissue at this location (**adenoids**) may obstruct the orifice of the eustachian tubes.

The **epiglottis** helps protect the larynx during swallowing by deflecting swallowed material toward the esophagus. The epiglottis of children has a contour like an *omega* (Ω). The **arytenoid cartilages**, which assist in opening and closing the glottis, usually are not prominent in children. The **vocal cords** form a V-shaped opening (the glottis), with the apex of the V being anterior, at the base of the epiglottis. Beneath the cords, the walls of the **subglottic space** converge toward the **cricoid ring**, a complete ring of cartilage. In children younger than 2 or 3 years old, the cricoid ring (first tracheal ring) is the narrowest portion of the airway. In older children and adults, the glottis is the smallest part of the airway.

Rings of cartilage extending about 320 degrees around the airway circumference support the **trachea** and main **bronchi**. The posterior wall is membranous. Beyond the lobar bronchi, the cartilaginous support for the airways becomes discontinuous. The more peripheral airways are supported entirely by elastic forces within the **lung parenchyma**.

The right lung normally has three lobes (upper, middle, and lower) and occupies about 55% of the total lung volume. The left lung normally has two lobes (upper and lower). The left upper lobe has an inferior division (the lingula) that is analogous to the right middle lobe.

The lung has a tremendous capacity for growth. At birth, a full-term infant has approximately 25 million alveoli; this number increases to nearly 300 million in adulthood. Most of the growth occurs by 8 years of age. The greatest growth is in the first 3 to 4 years.

PULMONARY PHYSIOLOGY
Pulmonary Mechanics

The major function of the lungs is to **exchange oxygen** (O_2) and **carbon dioxide** (CO_2) between the atmosphere and the blood. Factors that influence this exchange are the anatomy and mechanics of the airways, mechanics of the respiratory muscles and rib cage, structure of the blood-gas interface (alveolar surface), pulmonary circulation, tissue metabolic demands, and central mechanisms for neuromuscular control of ventilation.

Air enters the lungs via the upper airway whenever the pressure in the thorax is less than that of the surrounding atmosphere. During inspiration at rest, the negative intrathoracic pressure is caused by contraction (and lowering) of the **diaphragm**. Accessory muscles of respiration may be recruited during labored breathing. The **external intercostal, scalene,** and **sternocleidomastoid muscles** lift the rib cage and function as muscles of inspiration. During quiet breathing, most exhalation is passive, but during forced exhalation or lower airway obstruction, intrathoracic pressure is increased by the **abdominal muscles** and by the **internal intercostal muscles**, which pull the ribs together.

The diameter of the conducting airway, its length, the viscosity of the gas, and the nature of the airflow determine the **airway resistance**. During quiet breathing, airflow (especially in the smaller airways) may be laminar, in which case the resistance is inversely proportional to the fourth power of the radius of the airway. At higher flow rates (exercise), the flow becomes turbulent, and the resistance increases. Relatively small changes in airway diameter (increases with normal growth or decreases resulting from mucosal edema or bronchoconstriction) may produce large changes in airway resistance. This phenomenon is shown more dramatically in infants, where the same degree of airway narrowing in the smaller airways of an infant produces proportionately greater physiologic effects than it does in the larger airways of an older child or an adult.

When all mechanical forces acting on the lung are at equilibrium (at the end of a normal relaxed breath), the lung contains a volume of gas known as the **functional residual capacity (FRC)** (Fig. 133–1). This gas volume is important in maintaining exchange of O_2 across the alveolar surface during exhalation. Alterations in **lung compliance** that lead to decreased FRC include surfactant deficiency (neonatal respiratory distress syndrome), acute respiratory distress syndrome,

and restrictive lung diseases. Obstructive lung diseases, including asthma and cystic fibrosis (CF), may increase FRC secondary to gas trapping in the lungs.

Normal tidal breathing uses the middle range of lung volumes, reaching neither residual volume (RV) nor total lung capacity (TLC) (see Fig. 133–1). **RV** is the volume of gas in the lungs at the end of a maximal exhalation. **TLC** is the volume of gas in the lungs at the end of maximal inhalation. **Vital capacity (VC)** is the difference between TLC and RV.

With partial **airway obstruction**, airways collapse during exhalation, preventing normal emptying and increasing RV and decreasing VC. An increase in obstruction increases FRC. Another manifestation of obstruction is decreased expiratory flow rates.

Alveolar ventilation is defined as the exchange of gas between the alveoli and external environment. Not all of the air inspired during each breath reaches the alveoli. Normally, about 30% of each tidal breath fills the **anatomic dead space** (non–gas exchanging parts of the respiratory system). Because dead space is relatively constant, increasing tidal volume may enhance the efficiency of ventilation. If tidal volume is decreased (central depression of respiratory drive or neuromuscular disease), the ratio of dead space to tidal volume increases, and alveolar ventilation decreases.

The most common forms of lung disease in children result in **airway obstruction**. Excess secretions, bronchospasm, mucosal edema, inflammation, stenosis, foreign bodies, excessively compliant extrathoracic airways, and airway compression (intraluminal or extraluminal masses or blood vessels) all may produce symptomatic airway obstruction. **Restrictive disease** is less common and is characterized by normal to low FRC and RV, low TLC and VC, decreased lung compliance, and relatively normal flow rates. Restrictive lung disease can result from neuromuscular weakness, an intrathoracic space-filling process (lobar pneumonia, pleural effusion, or mass), distorted thoracic anatomy (scoliosis, severe pectus excavatum), or abdominal distention.

Respiratory Gas Exchange

Gas exchange depends on **alveolar ventilation**, **pulmonary capillary blood flow**, and **diffusion** of the gases across the alveolar-capillary surfaces. CO_2 diffuses 20 times more readily than O_2. Hypercapnia is a relatively late manifestation of disordered gas exchange, whereas hypoxemia occurs earlier.

A significant percentage of the capillary bed is not open under normal resting conditions. The flow to the pulmonary circulation is capable of increasing at least fivefold. Under normal circumstances, physiologic matching of ventilation and blood flow is maintained by anatomic mechanisms and **hypoxic pulmonary**

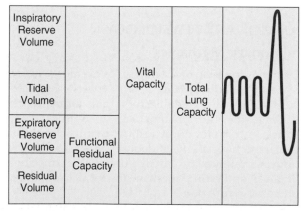

Figure 133–1

Lung volumes and capacities. Although vital capacity and its subdivisions can be measured by spirometry, calculation of residual volume requires measurement of functional residual capacity by body plethysmography, helium dilution technique, or nitrogen washout. (From Andreoli TE, Bennett JC, Carpenter CJ, et al [eds]: Cecil Essentials of Medicine, 4th ed. Philadelphia, WB Saunders, 1997, p 127.)

TABLE 133–1. Causes of Hypoxemia

Cause	Examples	PaO$_2$	PaCO$_2$	PaO$_2$ Improves with Supplemental Oxygen
Ventilation-perfusion mismatch	Asthma Bronchopulmonary dysplasia Cystic fibrosis Pneumonia	↓	Normal, ↓, or ↑	Yes
Hypoventilation	Apnea Narcotic overdose Neuromuscular disease	↓	↑	Yes
Extrapulmonary pure shunt	Cyanotic heart disease (tetralogy of Fallot)	↓	Normal or ↑	No
Intrapulmonary pure shunt	Pulmonary arteriovenous malformation	↓	Normal or ↑	No
Low FIO$_2$	Mountain climbing	↓	↓	Yes
Diffusion defect (rare)	Scleroderma	↓	Normal	Yes

vasoconstriction (local constriction of the pulmonary vessels in areas that are hypoventilated). If hypoxic pulmonary vasoconstriction fails, however, the underventilated lung continues to be perfused, and the blood returning from that area is deoxygenated, producing an **intrapulmonary shunt** with **hypoxemia**. This hypoxemia usually leads to an increased minute volume and a decrease in PaCO$_2$ as the shunt increases. Disorders of unequal **ventilation-perfusion matching** are much more common causes of hypoxemia than are abnormalities of diffusion, especially in children (Table 133–1).

Lung Defense Mechanisms

The airways are a direct connection between the lungs and the atmosphere, which is not typically clean or sterile. The **nose** is the primary filter for large particles. The paranasal sinuses and the nasal turbinates are lined with **ciliated epithelium**, which carries these filtered particles to the pharynx. Particles smaller than 10 μm in diameter may reach the trachea and bronchi, where they are deposited on the mucosa. Particles smaller than 1 μm may reach the alveoli, where they either remain or are exhaled without being deposited. Ciliated cells line the airways from the larynx to the bronchioles. The cilia continuously move a thin layer of mucus toward the mouth, carrying inhaled particulates. Normally, **mucociliary transport** in the larger airways is fast, with rates averaging 10 mm/min. **Alveolar macrophages** and **polymorphonuclear cells** can engulf particles or pathogens opsonized by locally secreted IgA antibodies or transudated serum

antibodies. Additional immunologically active proteins include the collectins (surfactant-associated proteins), β defensins, and cathelicidins.

Reflex mechanisms also protect the lungs. The most important of these mechanisms is **cough**, a forceful expiration that removes foreign or infected material from the airways. A cough may be voluntary or may be generated by reflex irritation of the nose, sinus, pharynx, larynx, trachea, bronchi, or bronchioles. During a cough, the person inspires deeply to 60% to 80% of TLC. The glottis closes, the expiratory muscles contract to increase intrathoracic pressure (approximately 100 cm H$_2$O), and the glottis opens suddenly, forcefully releasing air from the system. Loss of the cough reflex leads to aspiration and pneumonia. In infants and young children, secretions may be swallowed rather than expectorated. Nasal irritation may produce reflex bronchoconstriction to limit the penetration of noxious vapors.

HISTORY

Characterization of signs and symptoms of respiratory disease should include information about the presence or absence of a **prodrome**, **onset** of symptoms including any triggers, **work of breathing**, ability to **swallow**, and history of **exposure** to others with respiratory illness. A description of respiratory sounds (**wheezing, stridor**) may direct further questions. The signs or symptoms in children with respiratory disease are often different during eating and sleeping. Inquiry about the impact of these activities on symptoms is important. Concurrent signs and symptoms of infection (fever, malaise) are often present, given the prevalence of infection as the etiology of respiratory disease. Questioning a 3- or 4-year-old child may reveal information unknown to the parents ("last week I choked on a peanut"). A **family history** may identify hereditary causes of respiratory disease. An **environmental history** includes exposure to smoke, pets, and other toxins that may cause or exacerbate pulmonary pathology.

PHYSICAL EXAMINATION

Examining the young child in a parent's lap decreases anxiety. Clothing should be removed from the upper half of the child's body so that the thorax may be inspected. Observation of the respiratory pattern, rate, and work of breathing while the child is quiet (and not crying) is optimal. The shape of the chest wall, symmetry of the chest and of the back, and anterior-to-posterior diameter also should be noted.

The **respiratory rate** is an important indicator of respiratory status. Any factor that impairs respiratory mechanics is likely to result in more rapid breathing. Fever frequently results in tachypnea. Because anxiety or excitement also increases respiratory rates, the sleeping respiratory rate is most reliable. Infants younger than 1 year old may have sleeping rates ranging from 25 to 35 breaths/min. While awake, the same infants may take 40 to 60 breaths/min. With increasing maturity, sleeping rates gradually decline toward the adult range of 10 to 15 breaths/min (Table 133–2).

In addition to the rate of respiration, its **pattern**, **depth**, and **degree of effort** (work of breathing) are important observations. **Hyperpnea** (increased depth of respiration) may occur with fever, metabolic acidosis, salicylism, pulmonary and cardiac disease, or extreme anxiety (hyperventilation syndrome, panic attack). Hyperpnea without signs of respiratory distress suggests a nonpulmonary etiology (acidosis, fever, salicylism). When the degree of effort is increased because of airway obstruction or decreased pulmonary compliance, the intrathoracic pressure may be more negative than usual, and **intercostal retractions** can be observed. Use of accessory muscles, such as the sternocleidomastoids, should alert the physician to the presence of a pathologic pulmonary condition. In children, increased inspiratory effort also results in **nasal flaring**, which is a relatively reliable sign of dyspnea. **Grunting** (forced expiration against a partially closed glottis) suggests hypoxia, atelectasis, pneumonia, or pulmonary edema. Identification of increased respiratory effort during a particular phase of respiration is helpful in identifying the affected respiratory compartment. Causes of increased work of breathing during inspiration include upper airway obstruction (croup), fixed central airway tracheal obstruction (tracheal stenosis), or decreased pulmonary compliance (pneumonia, pulmonary edema). Increased expiratory work of breathing usually indicates airway obstruction at or below the glottis (asthma) (see Table 133–2).

The **sounds of breathing** warrant careful documentation. **Stridor**, usually heard on inspiration, is a harsh sound that emanates from the upper airway and is caused by a partially obstructed extrathoracic airway.

A **wheeze** is produced by partial obstruction of the lower airways and is heard on exhalation. Wheezes may be harsh, monophonic, and low pitched (usually from large, central airways) or high pitched and almost musical (from small peripheral airways). Secretions in the intrathoracic airways may result in wheezing, but

TABLE 133–2. Breathing Patterns

Pattern	Features
Normal rate (breaths/min)	Preterm: 40-60 Term: 30-40 5 yr: 25 10 yr: 20 15 yr: 16 Adult: 12
Obstructed	
Mild	Reduced rate, increased tidal volume
Severe	Increased rate, increased retraction of accessory muscles, anxiety, cyanosis
Restrictive	Rapid rate, decreased tidal volume
Kussmaul respiration	Increased rate, increased tidal volume, regular deep respiration; consider metabolic acidosis or diabetes mellitus
Cheyne-Stokes respiration	Gradually increasing tidal volume followed sequentially by gradually decreasing tidal volume and apnea; consider CNS injury, depressant drugs, heart failure, uremia, or prematurity
Biot respiration	Ataxic or periodic breathing with a respiratory effort followed by apnea; consider brainstem injury or posterior fossa mass
Gasping	Slow rate, variable tidal volume; consider hypoxia, shock, sepsis, or asphyxia

more commonly result in irregular sounds called **rhonchi**. Fluid or secretions in small airways may produce a sound that is characteristic of crumpling cellophane (**rales** or **crackles**). This sound may disappear after a few deep inspirations or a cough, but its persistence suggests airway secretions, pneumonitis, or pulmonary edema. Children may not take a breath deep enough to produce audible crackles, rhonchi, or wheezes. With patience, most infants can be listened to during at least one deep inspiration, however, and older children can be asked to take a deep breath and "pretend to blow out a candle" or asked to "blow away a paper" held 8 to 12 inches away.

The quality of breath sounds may be **bronchial**, normally heard over the trachea, with inspiration and expiration clearly auscultated. More peripheral breath sounds are **vesicular**, with a greater proportion of inspiration heard as the expiratory component lessens. Bronchial breath sounds in the lung periphery suggest consolidation or the interface of a pleural effusion. Decreased breath sounds when respiratory effort is adequate may suggest atelectasis, lobar consolidation (pneumonia), or a pleural effusion.

The physical findings, when combined with inspection for tracheal or cardiac deviation, chest wall motion, percussion, fremitus, voice signs, and the presence or absence of breath sounds, help identify the intrathoracic pathology (Table 133–3). **Digital clubbing** is seen in CF and in some patients with chronic pulmonary disease, but may be noted in other chronic diseases (cyanotic congenital heart disease, endocarditis, celiac disease, inflammatory bowel disease, chronic active hepatitis, biliary cirrhosis, thalassemia, and Hodgkin disease) or, rarely, as a benign familial trait.

Cough is a common respiratory complaint. Cough results from stimulation of irritant receptors in the airway mucosa. Acute cough generally is associated with respiratory infections (rhinitis, bronchitis, pneumonia, sinusitis) or irritant exposure (smoke) and subsides as the infection resolves or exposure is eliminated. Sudden onset of coughing after a choking episode suggests foreign body aspiration. The characteristics of the cough and the circumstances under which the cough occurs may help in understanding the etiology. Morning cough usually is associated with excess production of secretions and may be seen with asthma, bronchitis, bronchiectasis, or CF. Nocturnal cough suggests asthma, allergy, gastroesophageal reflux, or sinusitis. Coughing with exercise often is caused by exercise-induced asthma. Paroxysmal cough suggests pertussis or foreign body aspiration. A repetitive, staccato cough is heard in chlamydial infections in infants.

TABLE 133–3. Physical Signs of Pulmonary Disease

Disease Process	Mediastinal Deviation	Chest Motion	Vocal Fremitus	Percussion	Breath Sounds	Adventitious Sounds	Voice Signs
Consolidation	No	Reduced over area	Increased	Dull	Bronchial or reduced	None or rales	Egophony,* whispering pectoriloquy increased†
Bronchospasm	No	Hyperexpansion with limited motion	Normal or decreased	Hyperresonant	Normal to decreased	Wheezes, rales	Normal to decreased
Atelectasis	Shift toward lesion	Reduced over area	Decreased	Dull	Reduced	None or rales	None
Pneumothorax	Tension deviates trachea and PMI to opposite side	Reduced over area	None	Resonant	None	None	None
Pleural effusion	Deviation to opposite side	Reduced over area	None or reduced	Dull	None	Friction rub; splash if hemopneumothorax	None
Interstitial process	No	Reduced	Normal to increased	Normal	Normal	Rales	None

*Egophony is present when *e* sounds like *a*.
†Whispering pectoriloquy produces clearer sounding whispered words.
PMI, point of maximum impulse.
Adapted from Andreoli TE, Bennett JC, Carpenter CJ, et al (eds): Cecil Essentials of Medicine, 4th ed. Philadelphia, WB Saunders, 1997, p 115.

A harsh, brassy, or "seal-like" cough suggests croup, tracheomalacia, or habit cough. Habit cough disappears with sleep.

Chronic cough is a daily cough lasting longer than 6 weeks. It occurs for diverse reasons, including allergy (asthma, postnasal drip, rhinitis), anatomic abnormalities (tracheoesophageal fistula, gastroesophageal reflux, swallowing dysfunction), chronic infection (CF, sinusitis, recurrent aspiration pneumonia, tuberculosis, AIDS-related infection), environmental exposure to irritants (tobacco smoke, wood stove smoke), foreign body aspiration, psychogenic causes (habit cough, cough tic, Tourette syndrome), and neurologic dysfunction.

During the first several years of life, children may experience frequent viral respiratory infections, especially if they are exposed to other young children (daycare or preschool). Cough that resolves promptly and is clearly associated with a viral infection does not require further diagnostic workup. Cough that persists longer than 4 to 6 weeks in a child (and even shorter than that in an infant) warrants more attention.

DIAGNOSTIC MEASURES

Imaging Techniques

Chest radiographs are extremely useful in diagnosing respiratory disease in children. Failure to obtain satisfactory inspiration, the most common problem, may lead to the erroneous impression of cardiomegaly or of the presence of infiltrates. External skin folds, rotation or other improper position of the chest, or motion also may produce a distorted or unclear image. Chest radiographs should be obtained in the posteroanterior and the lateral projections because lesions may be apparent on only one of the two views. Estimation of lung hyperinflation based on a single posteroanterior view is unreliable, whereas flattened diaphragms and an increased anterior-posterior diameter on a lateral projection suggest hyperinflation secondary to diffuse lower airway obstruction. Expiratory views and fluoroscopy are helpful in detecting the presence of partial bronchial obstruction resulting from an aspirated foreign body, where a lung or lobe that does not empty on expiration appears hyperinflated.

A **barium esophagogram** is valuable in the diagnosis of chest disease. Disorders of swallowing or esophageal motility, vascular rings, tracheoesophageal fistulas, or gastroesophageal reflux may lead to aspiration and recurrent or persistent pulmonary disease. When the esophagogram reveals that abnormal vascular structures are compressing the esophagus, the same vessels may be compressing the airways. The search for an H-type tracheoesophageal fistula requires injection of contrast material under pressure through a catheter while the injection sites are observed in the lateral projection (see Chapter 128). Simple barium swallows are much less likely to show the often small connection between the trachea and the esophagus. Although the presence of gastroesophageal reflux on a barium esophagogram may be helpful in establishing this diagnosis, it is an insensitive test that should not be used to rule out gastroesophageal reflux definitively.

CT is useful in diagnosing chest disease, especially in evaluating parenchymal disease and lesions in the mediastinum or hilum. Rapid, fine-cut, high-resolution CT provides information about the lumen size or presence of masses within the central intrathoracic airways. Bronchiectasis also may be detected. Chest CT may be useful in the evaluation of pulmonary embolism, pleural effusion, pulmonary abscess, and interstitial pneumonitis.

MRI can identify pathologic conditions in the trachea and large central airways. MRI may be helpful in visualizing the relationships between the great vessels and central airways.

Ultrasonography can determine the nature of some intrathoracic masses, determine the presence of pleural fluid, and identify loculated fluid collections, such as those occurring with empyema or complicated pleural effusion. Diaphragmatic dysfunction (paralysis or paresis) also may be assessed by ultrasound.

Measures of Respiratory Gas Exchange

A properly performed **arterial blood gas** analysis is one of the most useful measures of lung function; it provides information about the effectiveness of oxygenation and ventilation. Given a constant CO_2 production, P_{CO_2} is regulated almost entirely by ventilation (tidal volume × respiratory rate). The ratio of bicarbonate concentration (regulated by the kidneys) to P_{CO_2} governs the pH, as determined by the Henderson-Hasselbach equation:

$$pH = 6.1 + \log([HCO_3]/0.03\ P_{CO_2})$$

A distinction should be made between metabolic and respiratory causes of acidosis or alkalosis (see Chapter 37). At the normal pH of 7.4, the Pa_{CO_2} should be about 40 mm Hg, and the bicarbonate should be about 25 mEq/L. Metabolic acidosis, which exhibits low bicarbonate, can be compensated by hyperventilation, which lowers the P_{CO_2}. Respiratory acidosis, which is due to elevated P_{CO_2}, can be compensated by renal retention of bicarbonate. Respiratory compensation is a much faster process than renal compensation, which generally requires several days to reach equilibrium.

Pulse oximetry (measurement of O_2 saturation using light absorption) provides a painless, noninvasive, relatively easy and reliable means of measuring oxygenation. A small probe consisting of a light source and sensor is clipped to a finger or toe, and continuous or single O_2 saturation measurements are obtained. Because of the shape of the oxyhemoglobin dissociation curve, O_2 saturation does not decrease appreciably until the PaO_2 reaches approximately 60 mm Hg.

The measurement of CO_2 is accomplished most reliably by blood gas analysis. Noninvasive monitoring of CO_2 samples expired air at end expiration (**end-tidal CO_2**) or averaged over the respiratory cycle. These methods provide an approximate measure of alveolar PCO_2. Although they are most commonly used in intubated and mechanically ventilated patients, capnography units that monitor CO_2 content in expired air at the nares are available. Similarly, **transcutaneous electrodes** may be used to monitor PO_2 and PCO_2 at the skin surface. Each of these techniques to monitor PCO_2 is best suited for continuous monitoring in an ICU and for detecting trends rather than for providing absolute numbers.

Pulmonary Function Testing

The simplest clinically useful measures of ventilatory function are **VC** and **expiratory flow rates**, which can be measured with a **spirometer**. Predicted values for lung functions are based on the patient's age, height, and gender. Simple spirometry can be performed in most children 6 years old or older. Even an older child cannot be expected to perform reproducibly without training and experience with the technique, and great care must be taken in interpreting the results of testing.

Airway resistance, FRC, and RV (among other measures) require the use of a **plethysmograph** and a spirometer. Flow rates at lower lung volumes are relatively independent of effort and reflect the function of more peripheral airways. Full forced expiratory maneuvers in sedated infants can be obtained using an inflatable jacket to produce a rapid, thoracoabdominal compression.

Pulmonary function studies may be useful in evaluating an older child's functional status, although they rarely yield an etiologic diagnosis. Abnormal results may be described in terms of **obstructive disease** (low flow rates and increased RV or FRC) or **restrictive disease** (low VC and TLC, with relative preservation of flow rates and FRC). The extent of functional impairment often can be estimated.

Airway obstruction can be defined clinically through measurement of the volume of air exhaled during the first second of a forced vital capacity maneuver (**forced expiratory volume in 1 second [FEV_1]**). The **forced expiratory flow rate (FEF_{25-75})** is the volume of air exhaled per second during the forced expiratory maneuver between 25% and 75% of forced vital capacity. It is more sensitive to obstruction in peripheral airways than is FEV_1, but also is more variable. VC, FEV_1, and FEF_{25-75} are clinically useful measures and can be determined with a simple spirometer. **Peak expiratory flow rate (PEFR)** measures the most rapid rate of airflow (in L/sec or L/min) during a forced expiratory maneuver. It is largely a measure of airflow in central airways and is highly dependent on patient effort. PEFR is best measured with a **peak flowmeter**, a simple hand-held device readily available in the office or emergency department setting. Pulmonary function testing can also be used to detect reversible airway obstruction characteristic of asthma. A significant improvement in pulmonary function after the inhalation of a bronchodilator generally indicates reactive airway disease. These tests are useful not only for determining the diagnosis, but also for managing therapy. Inhalational **challenge testing** with methacholine or cold, dry air is used for the diagnosis of reactive airway disease; such tests require sophisticated equipment and special expertise and should be performed in a pulmonary function laboratory.

Endoscopic Evaluation of the Airways

Diagnostic **bronchoscopy** is indicated whenever necessary information about the lungs or airways can be obtained most definitively, safely, or rapidly by this method. No absolute contraindications to bronchoscopy exist, provided that the proper equipment is available and the physician's skill is adequate. Airway structure can be examined, the dynamics of the airways during breathing can be documented, and specimens can be obtained for a variety of diagnostic purposes. Flexible instruments are advantageous for most diagnostic purposes, whereas rigid instruments must be used for foreign body extraction and for most operative procedures. An airway mucosal biopsy also is possible through pediatric-sized flexible bronchoscopes. Bronchoscopy accompanied by **bronchoalveolar lavage** assists in the diagnosis of pulmonary infection, particularly in an immunocompromised patient. **Laryngoscopy** is often useful in the diagnosis of stridor and should be performed carefully under appropriate conditions and with the use of sedation, anesthesia, or both.

Examination of Sputum

Sputum specimens, although important in evaluating inflammatory processes in the lower airways, are often difficult to obtain in young children. An expectorated specimen may not provide a representative sample of the lower airway secretions. Microscopic examination helps determine the source of a putative sputum specimen. Sputum should contain macrophages.

Ciliated cells also are often seen. Specimens containing large numbers of squamous epithelial cells either are most likely not from the lower airways or are heavily contaminated. Diagnostic tests performed on such specimens may yield misleading results. Infected sputum should have many polymorphonucleated leukocytes and one predominant organism in large numbers present on Gram stain. If sputum cannot be obtained, bronchoalveolar lavage (lung washings obtained by bronchoscopy) specimens may be used for microbiologic or cytologic diagnosis in selected situations. In patients with CF, special throat cultures may be done to reflect and help to follow lower airway microbiology.

Lung Biopsy

When less invasive methods have failed in the diagnosis of pulmonary disease, lung biopsy may be required. Although **transbronchial lung biopsy** through a bronchoscope is useful in adults, it is seldom done in children. Either a **thoracoscopic procedure** or a **thoracotomy** for open biopsy is preferred in children. Thoracotomy allows the surgeon to inspect and palpate the lung and, combined with imaging studies, to choose the best site for performing the biopsy. Open biopsy provides sufficient material for a variety of diagnostic tests. In most cases, infants and children tolerate lung biopsy well.

THERAPEUTIC MEASURES

Oxygen Administration

Any child in respiratory distress should be given **supplemental O_2** as soon as feasible. Although depressing the respiratory drive is possible if the patient's central chemoreceptors are blunted by chronic hypercapnia, patients in such a state are rare in pediatric practice and should be readily recognized as having chronic, severe respiratory disease (CF, bronchopulmonary dysplasia). Even in these patients, O_2 therapy may be lifesaving without producing apnea.

In an acute situation, an appropriately sized **mask** is often the most useful technique for administering O_2. For a child frightened by a mask, a high-flow O_2 source may be held near the child's face until a more satisfactory method can be arranged. For long-term administration of O_2, a **nasal cannula** may be helpful, freeing the face and mouth, allowing the patient to eat and speak unhindered by the O_2 delivery system.

The concentration of administered O_2 should be high enough to relieve hypoxemia, yet as low as possible to prevent O_2 toxicity. Inspired O_2 concentrations less than 40% are usually safe for long-term use. Determining the concentration of inspired O_2 is more difficult in patients receiving O_2 by nasal cannula. Titrating the delivery (in L/min.) according to measurements of PaO_2 or by pulse oximetry is best in these patients.

The safe, acceptable range of O_2 saturation is 92% to 95%. It is unnecessary to achieve 100% saturation, especially if it requires potentially toxic levels of inspired O_2. O_2, as obtained from tanks or wall sources, is dry and must be humidified to avoid dehydration of the respiratory tract.

Aerosol Therapy

Delivering therapeutic agents to the lower respiratory tract often is accomplished by having the patient inhale the agents in aerosol form. The use of **aerosol generators** that deliver relatively small particles is necessary to achieve optimal deposition in the lower airways. The pattern of the patient's breathing greatly influences deposition of the particles. Slow, deep inspirations are needed for maximal effect, but most children, especially infants, cannot perform inspirations in this fashion. Inhaling aerosols from a facemask or mouthpiece for several minutes during quiet tidal breathing usually achieves the desired therapeutic effect, however. **Metered-dose inhalers** produce a high-pressure stream of particles that, with proper technique, can deposit an amount of medication in the lower airways equivalent to that of an aerosol generator. Administration of inhaled medications to infants and toddlers via a metered-dose inhaler with a facemask and **spacer device** is frequently preferable to aerosol treatments delivered via a nebulizer because they are portable, do not require electricity, and are much faster than traditional nebulizers. The drugs most often given by aerosol are bronchodilators and inhaled steroids. In certain situations, antibiotics (tobramycin for CF) may be given by aerosol.

Chest Physiotherapy and Clearance Techniques

When disease processes impair clearance of pulmonary secretions, certain clearance techniques may help maintain airway patency. **Percussion** of the thorax over the pulmonary segments while the patient is positioned so that the airways of the percussed segments are directed downward may move secretions toward the central airways, from which they can be expectorated. **Chest physiotherapy** also may be performed effectively with techniques and devices, such as **autogenic drainage**, the **flutter valve**, **Acapella device**, and **percussive vests**. A typical therapy session may require 15 to 30 minutes. Most children with lung disease requiring chest physiotherapy need one to three such sessions daily. These sessions may be increased in frequency during acute exacerbations of disease. In older children, sustained exercise (for 5 to 15 minutes) that produces hyperpnea also can be helpful. Chest physiotherapy is most beneficial for children with CF, but may be useful for individuals with neuromuscular disease and atelectasis. It generally is not beneficial for pneumonia or asthma.

Intubation

When the natural upper airway is obstructed or when assisted ventilation is needed because of disease or anesthesia, providing an **artificial airway** for the patient may be necessary. Intubation alters the physiology of the respiratory tract in many ways, not all of which are beneficial. It interferes with the humidification, warming, and filtration of inspired air; with phonation; and with transport of secretions. Intubation also stimulates increased production of secretions. Depending on the reason for intubation, the airway resistance may be increased or decreased and the physiologic dead space may be increased.

Endotracheal tubes can damage the larynx and the airways easily if the tubes are of improper size or are not carefully maintained. The cricoid ring is the smallest portion of a child's airway and is completely surrounded by cartilage; this makes it vulnerable to damage, which can lead to subglottic stenosis. If the pressure created by the tube against the airway mucosa exceeds capillary filling pressure (roughly 35 cm H_2O), mucosal ischemia develops, and, within hours, mucosal necrosis results. A small air leak around the endotracheal tube minimizes the risk of this necrosis.

Artificial airways of all types must be kept clear of secretions. Mucous plugs in artificial airways can be fatal. Providing adequate humidification of the inspired air and suctioning the tube help reduce the probability of occlusion by secretions.

Tracheostomy

Tracheostomy is the surgical placement of an artificial airway into the trachea below the larynx. If prolonged intubation is anticipated, elective tracheostomy should be considered to prevent laryngeal trauma and subsequent subglottic stenosis and to increase the patient's comfort and the ease of nursing care. No clear guidelines are available as to how long a particular patient is likely to tolerate an endotracheal tube or when a tracheostomy is indicated.

Children with severe chronic upper airway obstruction or who need long-term mechanical ventilation may require a tracheostomy for a prolonged period. Because the tracheostomy tube typically prevents the child from effectively phonating and from communicating distress, the child must be monitored carefully at all times. As with endotracheal tubes, tracheostomy tubes must be kept clear and clean, and vigilant care

must be taken to reduce complications. Occlusion of the tube with secretions or accidental dislodgment of the tube can be fatal. Children with tracheostomies may be cared for successfully at home if the caregivers are well trained and adequately equipped.

Mechanical Ventilation

Patients who are unable to maintain adequate gas exchange because of airway obstruction, an intrapulmonary pathologic condition, neuromuscular disease, or other factors are candidates for mechanical ventilation. Techniques for mechanical ventilation involve inflation of the lungs with compressed gas (see Chapter 61). Exhalation is passive.

Positive-pressure ventilation most often requires endotracheal intubation or tracheostomy. Some patients use "noninvasive" ventilation, which delivers pressure and flow of air/O_2 via mask or other device Noninvasive ventilation is particularly useful in patients with neuromuscular disease, such as muscular dystrophy.

No method of mechanical ventilation accurately mimics natural breathing, and all methods have their drawbacks and complications. Positive pressure is transmitted to the entire thorax and may impede venous return to the heart during inspiration (venous return increases during spontaneous inspiration). The airways and lung parenchyma may be damaged by high inflation pressures and by high concentrations of inspired O_2. In general, inflation pressures should be limited to pressures necessary to provide sufficient lung expansion for adequate ventilation and prevention of atelectasis. Pressure-cycled and volume-cycled ventilators are used in pediatrics. Other modes of ventilation are high-frequency jet ventilation and very high frequency oscillation. These techniques are used to reduce mean airway pressure and the probability of barotrauma.

C H A P T E R   134
Control of Breathing

CONTROL OF VENTILATION

Ventilation is controlled by **central chemoreceptors** in the medulla that respond to the intracellular pH (PCO_2) (Fig. 134–1). To a lesser extent, ventilation also is controlled by **peripheral receptors** in the carotid and aortic bodies, which respond predominantly to PO_2. The central receptors are quite sensitive. Small changes in $PaCO_2$ normally result in significant changes

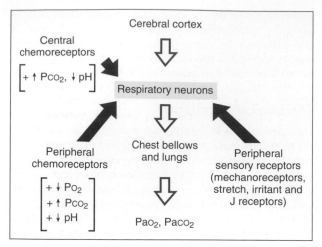

Figure 134–1

Schematic representation of the respiratory control system. The respiratory neurons in the brainstem receive information from the chemoreceptors, peripheral sensory receptors, and cerebral cortex. This information is integrated, and the resulting neural output is transmitted to the chest bellows and lungs. +, stimulation. (From Andreoli TE, Bennett JC, Carpenter CJ, et al [eds]: Cecil Essentials of Medicine, 4th ed. Philadelphia, WB Saunders, 1997, p 171.)

in **minute ventilation**. If $PaCO_2$ is elevated for some time, equilibration of the cerebral intracellular space to a higher bicarbonate level may result in relative hypoventilation for the degree of CO_2 elevation. The peripheral receptors do not affect ventilation until the PaO_2 decreases to approximately 50 mm Hg. These receptors may become important when lung disease results in chronic elevation of $PaCO_2$.

The output of the central respiratory center also is modulated by reflex mechanisms. Full lung inflation inhibits inspiratory effort (**Hering-Breuer reflex**) through vagal afferent fibers. Other reflexes from the airways and intercostal muscles may influence the depth and frequency of respiratory efforts (see Fig. 134–1).

DISORDERS OF CONTROL OF BREATHING

Acute Life-Threatening Events

Etiology

An acute life-threatening event is defined as an unexpected and frightening change in behavior characterized by apnea, color change, limpness, choking, or gagging. The incidence of such events is 0.05% to 1%. Specific causes can be identified in more than 50% of the cases. CNS causes account for 15% of cases. Cardiovascular causes, metabolic causes, airway obstruction, and child abuse account for smaller percentages.

Diagnostic Studies

The evaluation of a child with an acute life-threatening event includes a chest radiograph, ECG, blood gas analysis, blood chemistry evaluations (including measurements of glucose, calcium, BUN, and electrolytes), evaluation for gastroesophageal reflux (barium swallow or pH probe study), 12- to 24-hour recording of heart and respiratory activity (pneumogram), and perhaps an electroencephalogram.

Treatment and Prevention

Parents of infants ascertained to be at high risk for recurrence of acute life-threatening events may be offered home monitoring with an electronic monitor. Clear objective guidelines do not exist, however, for instituting or terminating the monitoring. The ability to predict which infant is at high risk for sudden infant death syndrome (SIDS) on the basis of a pneumogram is not established, but infants with a high percentage of periodic breathing or with apneic spells lasting longer than 15 seconds may be at high risk. Many infants with previously normal pneumograms have subsequently died of SIDS, whereas most infants with abnormal pneumograms have not. The parents of infants who have had acute life-threatening events should be instructed in basic cardiac pulmonary resuscitation.

Sudden Infant Death Syndrome

Etiology and Epidemiology

SIDS is defined as the **unexpected death** of an infant younger than 1 year of age, the cause of which remains unexplained after an autopsy, death scene investigation, and review of clinical history. The incidence of SIDS has decreased dramatically since the 1980s. The rates are highest in boys, in infants of young, impoverished mothers who smoke cigarettes, in premature and low birth weight infants, in African American and Native American infants, and in infants whose mothers have abused drugs. Incidence rates are highest during the winter. SIDS is rare before 4 weeks or after 6 months of age and is most common between 2 and 4 months of age. The risk of SIDS is increased three to five times in siblings of infants who have died of SIDS.

TABLE 134–1. Differential Diagnosis of Sudden Infant Death Syndrome

Fulminant infection*‡
Infant botulism†
Seizure disorder‡
Brain tumor*
Hypoglycemia†‡
Medium-chain acyl-coenzyme A dehydrogenase deficiency†
Carnitine deficiency*†
Urea cycle defect†
Child abuse*‡
Hemosiderosis/pulmonary hemorrhage syndrome
Exposure to toxic environmental fungus
Drug intoxication†
Cardiac arrhythmia
Gastroesophageal reflux*‡
Midgut volvulus/shock*
Laryngospasm

*Obvious or suspected at autopsy.
†Diagnostic test required.
‡Common.

The etiology of the increased risk is unknown. Monitoring of siblings may be indicated.

A variety of mechanisms have been proposed to explain SIDS, although none have been proved. Leading theories include cellular brainstem abnormalities or maturational delay related to neural or cardiorespiratory control. A portion of SIDS deaths may be attributed to prolongation of the Q-T interval, abnormal CNS control of respiration, CO_2 rebreathing from sleeping face down (especially in soft bedding), and possibly vascular compression of the vertebral arteries in some positions of the infant head.

Differential Diagnosis

See Table 134–1 for the differential diagnosis of SIDS.

Prevention

Because infants who sleep in the prone position are at increased risk for SIDS, current recommendations are that otherwise normal infants **sleep supine**. The decline in SIDS deaths seen in recent years is correlated with supine sleeping. Other recommended measures are prevention of maternal cigarette smoking and avoidance of use of polystyrene and other soft cushions for infant bedding. Because SIDS strikes without warning in an infant previously thought to be healthy, the effect on families is especially devastating, and psychological support is needed.

Apnea

Etiology

Apnea is defined as the cessation of breathing resulting from the lack of respiratory effort (**central apnea**) or total airway obstruction (**obstructive apnea**). In many patients, apneic episodes may have central and obstructive components (**mixed apnea**). Brief respiratory pauses lasting 10 seconds, during which no respiratory effort can be detected, are common in normal infants and children, especially after a sigh. Pauses lasting longer than 15 seconds are considered abnormal, however. Normally when a child whose airway is occluded tries to breathe, respiratory centers in the brain recruit a progressively greater amount of motor output from the respiratory center until the obstruction is overcome. If this output fails to overcome the obstruction, however, an arousal impulse is triggered in the brain that causes the child to move his or her head or body involuntarily to relieve the obstruction. If any individual component of this final arousal response system fails, the apneic child dies.

The etiology of apnea is diverse and not well understood. Premature infants commonly exhibit episodes of apnea, which may be associated with cyanosis and bradycardia. Apnea occurring in older infants warrants thorough investigation (Table 134–2).

Obstructive sleep apnea syndrome affects 1% to 2% of children and presents with snoring and distress during sleep because of complete or partial upper airway obstruction. Episodes of respiratory pauses, gasping, and hypoxia may lead to cor pulmonale, failure to thrive, and poor school performance. Tonsil and adenoid hypertrophy, obesity, craniofacial malformations, glossoptosis, and neuromuscular diseases are risk factors. Polysomnography is required because not all children who snore have obstructive sleep apnea syndrome. In contrast to adults, daytime hypersomnolence is uncommon in children with obstructive sleep apnea syndrome. Surgical intervention (removal of tonsils, adenoids, or other obstructing tissue) may be necessary in children who are symptomatic with obstructive apnea. Nighttime use of noninvasive mask ventilation may be beneficial.

Central alveolar hypoventilation leads to apnea and respiratory arrest, usually during sleep. Symptoms of congenital hypoventilation usually develop in the first several weeks to months of life. Secondary causes of central hypoventilation include medications impairing central respiratory drive (narcotics), Arnold-Chiari malformation, dysautonomia, increased intracranial pressure, some tumors, and mitochondrial metabolic disorders.

TABLE 134–2. Categories of Apnea

Disease	Example	Mechanism	Signs	Treatment
Apnea of prematurity	Premature (<36 wk)	Central control, airway obstruction	Apnea, bradycardia	Theophylline, caffeine, nasal CPAP, intubation
Ondine curse	Congenital central hypoventilation syndrome	Central control	Apnea	Mechanical ventilation
Obesity hypoventilation	Obesity, Prader-Willi syndrome	Airway obstruction, central control	Obesity, somnolence, polycythemia, cor pulmonale	Theophylline, weight loss
Obstructive sleep apnea	Chronic tonsil hypertrophy, Pierre Robin syndrome, Down syndrome, cerebral palsy, myotonic dystrophy, myopathy	Airway obstruction by enlarged tonsils or adenoids, choanal stenosis or atresia, large tongue, temporomandibular joint dysfunction, micrognathia, velopharyngeal incompetence; also may be central	Daytime sleepiness, snoring, night insomnia and enuresis, hyperactivity, poor school performance, behavioral problems, mouth breathing, inspiratory stridor	Tonsillectomy, adenoidectomy, nasal trumpets, CPAP, uvuloveloplasty
Cyanotic "breath-holding spells"	Breath holder <3 yr old	Prolonged expiratory apnea; hyperventilation; cerebral anoxia	Cyanosis, syncope, brief tonic-clonic movements	Reassurance that the condition is self-limiting; must exclude seizure disorder
Pallid "breath-holding spells"	Breath holder	Asystole; reflex anoxic seizures	Rapid onset, with or without crying; pallor; bradycardia; opisthotonos; seizures; follows painful stimuli	Atropine (?); must exclude seizure disorder; less benign than cyanotic breath holding
SIDS	Previously normal child; increased incidence with prematurity, SIDS in sibling, maternal drug abuse, cigarette smoking, males; may have preceding minor URI	Central respiratory control; cardiac arrhythmia (prolonged QT syndrome) (?); central cardiac control (?); prolonged expiratory apnea (?) Rebreathing (?) Other: Parental-induced airway obstruction–suffocation (accidental or abuse) Chemoreceptor dysfunction Overheating	2- to 4-mo-old child found cyanotic, apneic, and pulseless in bed	No treatment; prevention with home apnea monitor unproven; supine sleep position reduces risk

(?), unproven contributing factor; CPAP, continuous positive airway pressure by facial mask or nasal prongs; SIDS, sudden infant death syndrome; URI, upper respiratory infection.

Data from Southall D: Role of apnea in the sudden infant death syndrome. Pediatrics 81:73, 1988; Mark J, Brooks J: Sleep-associated airway problems in children. Pediatr Clin North Am 31:907, 1984; Gordon N: Breath-holding spells. Dev Med Child Neurol 29:811, 1987.

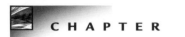

CHAPTER 135

Upper Airway Obstruction

ETIOLOGY

An upper airway obstruction is defined as blockage of the portion of the airways located above the thoracic inlet. Upper airway obstruction ranges from nasal obstruction associated with the common cold to life-threatening obstruction of the larynx or upper trachea. Nasal obstruction is usually more of a nuisance than a danger because the mouth can be used as an airway; it may be a serious problem for neonates, who breathe predominantly through the nose. The etiology of airway obstruction varies with the age of the child (Tables 135–1 and 135–2). A careful history and physical examination are essential to determine the correct diagnosis. The differential diagnosis of airway obstruction in children can be divided between entities causing obstruction above (upper airway) versus below (lower airway) the thoracic inlet. The differential diagnosis of upper airway obstruction can be divided further into **supraglottic** and **subglottic** causes (Table 135–3).

CLINICAL MANIFESTATIONS

Upper airway obstruction is manifested during inspiration because the pressure within the upper airway is negative relative to the atmosphere. This negative pressure tends to collapse the upper airway, producing the characteristic sounds associated with upper airway obstruction. The clinical manifestation most commonly associated with upper airway obstruction is inspiratory **stridor**, a harsh sound produced usually at or near the larynx by the vibration of upper airway structures. Less commonly, stridor may be present on expiration. **Hoarseness** suggests involvement of the **vocal cords**. Stridor that changes with position of the child's head or neck suggests a supraglottic etiology. Children with **laryngomalacia** or pharyngeal hypotonia may exhibit much less stridor while crying because their parapharyngeal muscle tone increases. In contrast, an obstructing lesion below the glottis usually produces more stridor during crying because the inspiratory flow rates increase. In many children, stridor decreases during sleep because inspiratory flow rates are lowest at that time. Positional stridor suggests an anatomic problem.

A child with upper airway obstruction usually has some degree of **suprasternal retraction** as a result

TABLE 135–1. Age-Related Differential Diagnosis of Upper Airway Obstruction

Newborn

Foreign material (e.g., meconium or amniotic fluid)
Congenital subglottic stenosis (uncommon)
Choanal atresia
Micrognathia (Pierre Robin syndrome, Treacher Collins syndrome, DiGeorge syndrome)
Macroglossia (Beckwith-Wiedemann syndrome, hypothyroidism, Pompe disease, trisomy 21, hemangioma)
Laryngeal web, clefts, atresia
Laryngospasm (intubation, aspiration, transient)
Vocal cord paralysis (weak cry; unilateral or bilateral, with or without increased intracranial pressure from Arnold-Chiari malformation or other CNS pathology)
Tracheal web, stenosis, malacia, atresia
Pharyngeal collapse (cause of apnea in preterm infant)
Dislocated nasal cartilage
Nasal piriform aperture stenosis
Nasal encephalocele

Infancy

Laryngomalacia (most common etiology)
Subglottic stenosis (congenital, acquired after intubation)
Hemangioma
Tongue tumor (dermoid, teratoma, ectopic thyroid)
Laryngeal dyskinesis
Laryngeal papillomatosis
Vascular rings/slings
Rhinitis

Toddlers

Viral croup (most common etiology in children 6 mo to 4 yr old)
Bacterial tracheitis (toxic, high fever)
Foreign body (sudden cough; airway or esophageal)
Spasmodic (recurrent) croup
Laryngeal papillomatosis
Retropharyngeal abscess
Hypertrophied tonsils and adenoids
Diphtheria (rare)

>2-3 Years Old

Epiglottitis (infection, uncommon)
Inhalation injury (burns, toxic gas, hydrocarbons)
Foreign bodies
Rhinitis medicamentosa
Angioedema (familial history, cutaneous angioedema)
Anaphylaxis (allergic history, wheezing, hypotension)
Trauma (tracheal or laryngeal fracture)
Peritonsillar abscess (adolescents)
Mononucleosis
Ludwig angina
Diphtheria (rare)

TABLE 135–2. Differential Diagnosis of Acute Upper Airway Obstruction

	Laryngotracheobronchitis (Croup)	Laryngitis	Spasmodic Croup	Epiglottitis	Membranous Croup (Bacterial Tracheitis)
Age	6 mo-3 yr	5 yr-teens	3 mo-3 yr	2-6 yr	Any age (3-10 yr)
Location	Subglottic	Subglottic	Subglottic	Supraglottic	Trachea
Etiology	Parainfluenza virus, influenza virus, RSV; rarely *Mycoplasma*, measles, adenovirus	As per croup	Unknown	*Haemophilus influenzae* b and a	Prior croup or influenza virus with secondary bacterial infection by *Staphylococcus aureus, Moraxella catarrhalis, H. influenzae*
Prodrome onset	Insidious, URI	As per croup	Sudden onset at night; prior episodes	Rapid, short prodrome	Biphasic illness with sudden deterioration
Stridor	Yes	None	Yes	Yes—soft inspiratory	Yes
Retractions	Yes	None	Yes	Yes	Yes
Voice	Hoarse	Hoarse; whispered	Hoarse	Muffled	Normal or hoarse
Position and appearance	Normal	Normal	Normal	Tripod sitting leaning forward; agitation	Normal
Swallowing (dysphagia)	Normal	Normal	Normal	Drooling	Normal
Barking cough	Yes	Rare	Yes	No	Yes
Toxicity	Rare	No	No	Severe	Severe; may also manifest toxic shock syndrome
Fever	<101°F	<101°F	None	>102°F	>102°F
X-ray	Subglottic narrowing; steeple sign	Normal	Subglottic narrowing	Thumb sign of thickened epiglottis	Ragged irregular tracheal border; as per croup
WBC count	Normal	Normal	Normal	Leukocytosis with left shift	Leukocytosis with left shift
Therapy	Racemic epinephrine aerosol, systemic steroids, aerosolized steroids, cold mist	None	Cool mist; occasionally as for croup	Endotracheal intubation, ceftriaxone	Antibiotics; intubation if needed
Prevention	None	None	None	*H. influenzae* b conjugated vaccine	None

FFP, fresh frozen plasma; HPV, human papillomavirus; RSV, respiratory syncytial virus; URI, upper respiratory tract infection, coryza, sneezing; WBC, white blood cell.

Modified from Arnold JE: Airway obstruction in children. In Kliegman RM, Nieder ML, Super DM (eds): Practical Strategies in Pediatric Diagnosis and Therapy. Philadelphia, WB Saunders, 1996, p 126.

Retropharyngeal Abscess	Foreign Body	Angioedema	Peritonsillar Abscess	Laryngeal Papillomatosis
<6 yr	6 mo-5 yr	All ages	>10 yr	3 mo-3 yr
Posterior pharynx	Supraglottic, subglottic, variable	Variable	Oropharynx	Larynx, vocal cords, trachea
S. aureus, anaerobes	Small objects, vegetables, toys, coins	Congenital C1-esterase deficiency; acquired anaphylaxis	Group A streptococci, anaerobes	HPV
Insidious to sudden	Sudden	Sudden	Biphasic with sudden worsening	Chronic
None	Yes	Yes	No	Possible
Yes	Yes—variable	Yes	No	No
Muffled	Complete obstruction—aphonic; other variable	Hoarse, may be normal	"Hot potato," muffled	Hoarse
Arching of neck or normal	Normal	Normal; may have facial edema, anxiety	Normal	Normal
Drooling	Variable, usually normal	Normal	Drooling, trismus	Normal
No	Variable; brassy if tracheal	Possible	None	Variable
Severe	No, but dyspnea	No, unless anaphylactic shock or severe anoxia	Dyspnea	None
>101°F	None	None	>101°F	None
Thickened retropharyngeal space	Radiopaque object may be seen	As per croup	None needed	May be normal
Leukocytosis with left shift	Normal	Normal	Leukocytosis with left shift	Normal
Antibiotics; surgical drainage if abscess	Endoscopic removal	Anaphylaxis—epinephrine, IV fluids, steroids; C1-esterase deficiency—danazol, C1-esterase infusion	Antibiotics; aspiration	Laser therapy, repeated excision, interferon
None	Avoid small objects; supervision	Avoid allergens; FFP for congenital angioedema; danazol	Treat group A streptococci early	Treat maternal genitourinary lesions; possible cesarean section?

TABLE 135–3.　Differentiating Supraglottic from Subglottic Causes of Airway Obstruction

	Supraglottic	Subglottic
Example	Epiglottitis, peritonsillar and retropharyngeal abscess	Croup, angioedema, foreign body, tracheitis
Stridor	Quiet	Loud
Voice	Muffled	Hoarse
Dysphagia	Yes	No
Sitting-up or arching posture	Yes	No
Barking cough	No	Yes
Fever	High (40°C [104°F])	Low grade (38°-39°C [100.4°-102.2°F])
Toxic	Yes	No, unless tracheitis is present
Trismus	Yes	No
Drooling	Yes	No
Facial edema	No	No, unless angioedema is present

Adapted from Davis H, Gartner JC, Galvis AG, et al: Acute upper airway obstruction: Croup and epiglottitis. Pediatr Clin North Am 28:859-880, 1981.

of the pressure gradient between the trachea and the atmosphere. Obstruction below the thoracic inlet seldom leads to suprasternal retraction because the major pressure drop occurs below the sternal notch.

DIAGNOSTIC STUDIES

Radiographic evaluation of a child with stridor should include views of the lateral neck and nasopharynx and an anteroposterior view of the neck taken with the head in extension. The subglottic space on the anteroposterior view should be symmetric, and the lateral walls of the airway should fall away steeply. Asymmetry suggests subglottic stenosis or a mass lesion, whereas narrow tapering suggests subglottic edema. CT scans help delineate the lesion further. It is important to differentiate between supraglottic and subglottic obstruction. Bronchoscopy may be used to visualize the areas of obstruction and the dynamic changes in the airway during inspiration and exhalation.

DIFFERENTIAL DIAGNOSIS
Adenoidal and Tonsillar Hypertrophy
Etiology

The most common chronic obstructive lesion of the airway in children is due to adenoidal and tonsillar hypertrophy. The adenoids consist of lymphoid tissue arising from the posterior and superior wall of the nasopharynx in the region of the choanae. Lymphoid hyperplasia may result from recurrent infection, allergy, or nonspecific stimuli and may cause partial or total obstruction of the nasopharynx.

Clinical Manifestations

The signs of adenoidal hypertrophy are persistent mouth breathing, snoring, and, in some patients, obstructive sleep apnea (see Chapter 134). The eustachian tube enters the nasopharynx at the choanae and may be obstructed by enlarged adenoids, promoting recurrent or persistent otitis media.

Diagnostic Studies

Adenoidal hypertrophy is confirmed by a lateral radiograph of the nasopharynx or by nasopharyngoscopy.

Treatment

Airway obstruction often is treated by surgical excision. Because the adenoids are not a discrete organ, but consist merely of lymphoid tissue, regrowth after adenoidectomy is common. Tonsils also may enlarge to the point of producing airway obstruction. Obstruction sufficient to produce sleep apnea, retractions, or cor pulmonale may necessitate tonsillectomy.

Choanal Stenosis (Atresia)

Choanal stenosis (atresia) may be bilateral or unilateral and is a relatively rare cause of respiratory distress in newborns. Neonates are generally obligate nose breathers; nasal obstruction may be fatal. Crying relieves the obstruction, which is worse during quiet activity. Inability to pass a small catheter through the nostrils easily should raise the suspicion of choanal atresia. The diagnosis is confirmed by CT or by inspecting the area directly with a nasopharyngoscope or bronchoscope. An oral airway may be lifesaving, but the definitive treatment is surgery (see Chapter 61).

Croup (Laryngotracheobronchitis)

▶ SEE CHAPTER 107.

Epiglottitis

▶ SEE CHAPTER 107.

Bacterial Tracheitis

▶ SEE CHAPTER 107.

Laryngomalacia

Etiology

Stridor beginning at birth or shortly thereafter should raise the suspicion of laryngomalacia (see Table 135–1). This relatively common condition involves the collapse of the **epiglottis** or **arytenoid cartilages** during inspiration and usually is benign and self-limiting. In some infants, the epiglottis alone is involved; these patients tend to become asymptomatic during the first year of life. Other infants have large arytenoid cartilages that prolapse into the glottis during inspiration; in these patients, stridor tends to last longer, sometimes for several years.

Clinical Manifestations

An infant with laryngomalacia has **inspiratory stridor**, but should have no evidence of significant expiratory obstruction. The stridor typically is loudest when the infant is feeding or quietly relaxing or is in a supine or neck flexion position. Stridor usually diminishes during sleep or when the infant is crying (when increased muscle tone may hold the supraglottic structures out of the air stream). Viral infections may exacerbate laryngomalacia. Symptoms usually disappear by 18 to 24 months of age.

Diagnostic Studies

Establishing a definitive diagnosis in suspected laryngomalacia is important for its appropriate management and to exclude other, more serious lesions. Bronchoscopy provides information about the patency and collapse of the larynx and bronchi.

Treatment

No therapy is needed unless the infant has hypoxia or growth failure resulting from the airway obstruction. Tracheostomy or epiglottoplasty may be required.

Subglottic Stenosis

Etiology

Subglottic stenosis may be congenital or, more commonly, iatrogenic. Aggressive management of premature infants with intubation and mechanical ventilation may produce residual damage to the larynx. Infants with Down syndrome seem to have a smaller larynx than normal and are more susceptible to subglottic stenosis.

Clinical Manifestations

Subglottic obstruction produces stridor that is frequently biphasic (present on expiration and on inspiration). With increasing degrees of respiratory effort, the stridor worsens (in contrast to laryngomalacia, in which the stridor may lessen with increasing respiratory efforts). Viral infection may exacerbate subglottic stenosis.

Diagnostic Studies

Definitive diagnosis requires endoscopic evaluation.

Treatment

A tracheostomy and reconstructive surgery may be necessary, although milder congenital cases often improve with age as the larynx grows and require no intervention.

Mass Lesions

Numerous mass lesions affect the larynx, but the most common laryngeal tumor in childhood is the **hemangioma**, which usually is found in the subglottic space. Most patients come to the physician's attention before 6 months of age. Infants with stridor should be examined carefully for cutaneous hemangiomas, which may occur in 50% of children with a laryngeal hemangioma. Subglottic lesions produce asymmetric narrowing of the subglottic space and may be detected on anteroposterior radiographs of the larynx. Definitive diagnosis requires endoscopy. The airway obstruction, which usually worsens with crying, eventually may produce pulmonary hypertension and cor pulmonale. Treatment of hemangiomas is controversial, but in some patients tracheostomy is required. **Laser therapy** and **steroids** have been used with moderate success. As with cutaneous hemangiomas, spontaneous regression is the rule, but this may require many months to several years.

Juvenile laryngeal papillomatosis, benign tumors caused by human papillomavirus acquired at birth from maternal genital warts, occurs in infants younger than 2 years old. Treatment involves laser therapy and interferon, but response to therapy is often poor.

Vocal Cord Paralysis

Etiology

Vocal cord paralysis is an important cause of laryngeal dysfunction. Paralysis may be unilateral or bilateral and more often is caused by damage to the recurrent laryngeal nerves than by a central lesion. The left recurrent laryngeal nerve passes around the arch of the aorta and is more susceptible to damage than the right laryngeal nerve. Trauma, such as neck traction during delivery, and lesions in the mediastinum are common causes of vocal cord paralysis. Central causes include Arnold-Chiari malformation, hydrocephalus, intracranial hemorrhage, and dysgenesis of the nucleus ambiguus.

Clinical Manifestations

The symptoms of vocal cord paralysis are stridor, a weak cry (in infants), hoarseness, and aphonia. Unilateral paralysis may be relatively asymptomatic. Rarely the cords are paralyzed in the abducted position, and aspiration results.

Treatment and Prognosis

Patients with vocal cord paralysis resulting in severe airway obstruction may require tracheostomy. No other specific treatment exists. The prognosis for return of vocal cord function depends on the nature of the injury and whether or not the recurrent laryngeal nerve has been disrupted. Patients with traumatic injury to the recurrent laryngeal nerve may have spontaneous improvement over time, in part as a result of compensatory movement by the nonparalyzed cord.

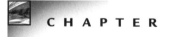

CHAPTER **136**

Lower Airway, Parenchymal, and Pulmonary Vascular Diseases

ETIOLOGY

Lower airway obstruction has multiple causes (Table 136–1), the most common of which is diffuse bronchial obstruction resulting from airway inflammation, constriction of bronchial smooth muscle, or excessive secretions (**asthma**). Although it often is useful to administer a bronchodilator to determine whether the

TABLE 136–1.   Causes of Wheezing in Childhood
Acute
Reactive airway disease
Asthma
Exercise-induced asthma
Hypersensitivity reactions
Bronchial edema
Infection (e.g., bronchiolitis)
Inhalation of irritant gases or particulates
Increased pulmonary venous pressure
Bronchial hypersecretion
Infection
Inhalation of irritant gases or particulates
Cholinergic drugs
Aspiration
Foreign body
Aspiration of gastric contents
Chronic or Recurrent
Reactive airway disease (see under Acute)
Hypersensitivity reactions, allergic aspergillosis
Dynamic airway collapse
Bronchomalacia/Tracheomalacia
Vocal cord adduction
Airway compression by mass or blood vessel
Vascular ring/sling
Anomalous innominate artery
Pulmonary artery dilation (absent pulmonary valve)
Bronchial or pulmonary cysts
Lymph nodes or tumors
Aspiration
Foreign body
Gastroesophageal reflux
Swallowing dysfunction
Tracheoesophageal fistula
Bronchial hypersecretion or failure to clear secretions
Bronchitis, bronchiectasis
Cystic fibrosis
Dysmotile cilia syndrome
Intrinsic airway lesions
Endobronchial tumors
Endobronchial granulation tissue
Bronchial or tracheal stenosis
Bronchiolitis obliterans
Sequelae of bronchopulmonary dysplasia
Congestive heart failure

wheezing is acutely reversible, reversibility does not establish a diagnosis of asthma, and it does not eliminate anatomic causes of wheezing. Conversely the most common cause of wheezing in childhood is reactive airway disease (asthma).

Because of their small airways, children younger than 2 to 3 years old are more likely to wheeze in response to **viral infections**. Wheezing that begins in the first weeks or months of life or that is persistent despite maximal bronchodilator therapy is more likely to be the result of some other cause, and more extensive diagnostic evaluation may be warranted. Wheezing that is localized to one area of the chest warrants especially close diagnostic attention (foreign body or compressing lymph node).

CLINICAL MANIFESTATIONS

In contrast to upper airway obstruction, obstruction of the airways below the thoracic inlet produces more **expiratory symptoms** than inspiratory symptoms. During inspiration, intrathoracic pressure becomes negative relative to the atmosphere. The airways tend to increase their diameter during inspiration, and unless substantial, relatively fixed obstruction (vascular ring/sling or significant lower airway wall inflammation and edema) is present, few or no abnormal noises may be generated during inspiration. Intrathoracic pressure is increased relative to atmospheric pressure during exhalation, which tends to collapse the intrathoracic airways and produce wheezing. A **wheeze** is a relatively continuous expiratory sound that is produced by turbulent airflow and generally has a more musical quality than stridor. Partial airway obstruction may produce wheezing only during the later phase of exhalation.

DIAGNOSTIC STUDIES

Although children known to have asthma do not need **radiographic evaluation** with each episode of wheezing, other children with significant respiratory distress, fever, history of aspiration, localizing signs, or persistent wheezing should have posterior and lateral chest films as part of their diagnostic evaluation. Generalized **hyperinflation**, with flattening of the diaphragm and an increased anteroposterior diameter of the chest, suggests diffuse obstruction of small airways. Localized hyperinflation, especially on expiratory films, suggests localized bronchial obstruction, such as a foreign body or an anatomic anomaly. Infants with persistent wheezing may require a **videofluoroscopic swallowing study** to rule out a primary swallowing abnormality causing aspiration or a **barium swallow** to rule out reflux resulting in aspiration, or both. For a full discussion of asthma, see Chapter 78.

DIFFERENTIAL DIAGNOSIS
Tracheomalacia
Etiology

Tracheomalacia is the most common anomaly of tracheal structure and dynamics, but it is an uncommon cause of airway obstruction. The tracheal cartilage rings normally extend through an arc of approximately 300 degrees, maintaining rigidity of the trachea during changes in intrathoracic pressure. With tracheomalacia, the cartilage rings do not extend nearly so far around the circumference, and a larger portion of the tracheal wall is membranous. This anatomy results in collapse of the lumen of the intrathoracic portion of the trachea during expiration. Tracheomalacia is invariably present in children who have had esophageal atresia and a tracheoesophageal fistula. Tracheomalacia must be differentiated from extrinsic compressing lesions. In some patients, localized tracheomalacia may persist after the trachea has been relieved of compression by a mass lesion or an abnormal blood vessel. Viral infections may exacerbate the airway obstruction of tracheomalacia.

Clinical Manifestations

Tracheal collapse may be apparent only during forced exhalation or with cough. Coarse, persistent stridor or wheezing may be a prominent symptom in other patients. The voice is normal, as is inspiratory effort. Tracheomalacia localized to the cervical trachea may lead to inspiratory obstruction.

Treatment

Mild tracheomalacia usually requires no intervention. Rarely, patients with severe tracheomalacia may require long-term tracheostomy and ventilatory support.

Tracheoesophageal Fistula

▶ SEE CHAPTER 128.

Tracheal Compression

Compression of the trachea by abnormal or aberrant vessels may produce persistent wheezing or stridor or both, cough, and dyspnea. The most common cause of tracheal compression is anterior compression resulting from an **anomalous innominate artery**, which arises more distally than normal along the arch of the aorta. Surgical treatment generally is required only for the most severe cases, particularly cases complicated by apnea.

A more serious lesion involves complete encirclement of the trachea at and just above the carina by a **vascular ring**. This anomaly may be caused by a double aortic arch or by a right aortic arch with a persisting left-sided ligamentum arteriosum and an aberrant left subclavian artery (most common). Both lesions have a right-sided aortic arch visible on chest x-ray. The rarest lesion is the **pulmonary sling** (aberrant left pulmonary artery arising from the right pulmonary artery). In addition to respiratory symptoms, emesis or dysphagia may be present as a result of esophageal compression. Complications include tracheomalacia and lower airway compression. The diagnosis can often be made by a barium swallow test. A vascular dye contrast study or magnetic resonance angiography may be required before surgical repair. Less common causes of extrinsic tracheal compression are enlarged mediastinal lymph nodes or masses and cystic hygromas.

Foreign Body Aspiration

Epidemiology

Aspiration of foreign bodies into the tracheobronchial tree is common. Young children put virtually anything into their mouths and momentarily manage to be out of sight of even the most diligent caregiver. Most patients are younger than 4 years old, and most deaths secondary to foreign body aspiration occur in this age group. Because the right main bronchus is a more direct continuation of the trachea than the left main bronchus, foreign bodies tend to enter the right lung preferentially. Some foreign bodies, especially nuts or seeds, may migrate from place to place in the airways and lodge in the larynx on coughing, totally occluding the airway. Such migratory foreign bodies often are not associated with radiographic abnormalities and are difficult to detect. Younger children most commonly aspirate food, small toys, balloons, and other small objects. Coins tend to go down the esophagus, although they rarely are found in the trachea.

Clinical Manifestations

A high percentage of children who aspirate foreign bodies have a clear-cut history of choking (or witnessed aspiration) or exhibit physical or radiographic evidence of the foreign body. A small percentage of patients with foreign body aspiration have a negative history because events have gone unobserved or unrecognized. Physical findings consistent with acute foreign body aspiration include cough, localized wheezing, unilateral absence of breath sounds, stridor, and rarely bloody sputum.

Most foreign bodies are small and quickly coughed out, but some may remain in the lung for long periods before diagnosis and may come to medical attention because of symptoms of fever, cough, sputum production, or chest pain. In patients with persistent wheezing unresponsive to bronchodilator therapy, persistent atelectasis, recurrent or persistent pneumonia, or persistent cough without other explanation, the presence of a foreign body should be suspected.

Foreign bodies also may lodge in the esophagus and compress the trachea, producing respiratory symptoms. An esophageal foreign body should be included in the differential diagnosis of infants or young children with persistent stridor or wheezing, particularly if the conditions are associated with dysphagia.

Diagnostic Studies

Radiographic studies may reveal the presence of a radiopaque object (rare) or evidence of air trapping on exhalation. When aspiration is suspected, expiratory or lateral decubitus chest films should be requested. Fluoroscopy may also be helpful.

If good evidence exists for a bronchial foreign body (by history, physical examination, or radiograph), the patient should undergo rigid bronchoscopy. Flexible bronchoscopy may be a useful diagnostic technique when the presentation is not straightforward; however, foreign body removal should not be attempted during flexible bronchoscopy.

Prevention

The best approach to foreign body aspiration is to educate parents and caregivers in preventing the event. Before molar teeth have developed, infants and children should not have nuts, uncooked carrots, and other foods that may be easily broken into small pieces and aspirated. Additionally, tiny toys are at risk for being aspirated by young children. Sound parental judgment is required to determine at what age and stage of development tiny objects should be easily accessible to small children.

Bronchiolitis

▶ SEE CHAPTER 109.

Bronchopulmonary Dysplasia

▶ SEE CHAPTER 61.

Endobronchial Mass Lesions

Endobronchial mass lesions are relatively uncommon in children, but when they occur, they most commonly consist of **granulation tissue** and are the result of localized inflammatory lesions. Partial obstruction of an airway by either an intrinsic or an extrinsic mass may result in wheezing or obstructive emphysema. If the airways become totally obstructed, atelectasis results.

Chest radiographs, CT scans, bronchoscopy, or vascular contrast studies may be required for diagnosis.

Primary tumors of the lungs and airways, such as non-secreting carcinoid tumor and congenital bronchial cysts, are rare in children. Metastatic tumors, such as osteogenic sarcoma, may spread to the endobronchial airways from other areas of the body.

Emphysema

Emphysema, a condition that results when alveolar septa are disrupted or destroyed, is relatively uncommon in children. Generalized or localized **overinflation** is seen as the result of airway obstruction from a variety of causes and is common. In pediatrics, the term *emphysema* often is used to refer to overinflation or to leakage of air into the lung's interstitial tissues or the subcutaneous tissue. True emphysema develops in the absence of antiproteases (α_1-**antitrypsin deficiency**), but rarely appears before adulthood.

Congenital lobar overdistention (formally referred to as congenital lobar emphysema) consists of overinflation of one lobe during the neonatal period, most often the left upper lobe, which may produce respiratory distress because the surrounding lung tissue has become compressed. Mediastinal shift may result. Lobectomy may be required if respiratory distress is severe and progressive.

Immotile (Dysmotile) Cilia Syndrome

Etiology

Immotile (dysmotile) cilia syndrome is an inherited disorder in which ultrastructural abnormalities in the cilia result in absent or disordered movement. The disorder affects 1:19,000 persons. In **Kartagener syndrome**, the cilia lack dynein arms, ultrastructural features that represent an ATPase necessary for ciliary motility. Many other variants of the syndrome exist that have a variety of ultrastructural abnormalities of the cilia. In some patients, cilia may move, but their beat is abnormal, usually uncoordinated, and ineffective.

Clinical Manifestations

The most classic form of the syndrome, Kartagener syndrome, is an autosomal recessive disorder characterized by **situs inversus**, **pansinusitis**, and **bronchiectasis**. Otitis media also is common; male infertility is universal (as a result of immotile sperm). Because respiratory tract cilia fail to beat normally, secretions accumulate in the airways, and bacterial infection occurs. Chronic infection leads to bronchiectasis by early adulthood. The diagnosis should be suspected in patients with early-onset chronic bronchitis or bronchiectasis; in patients with chronic, recurrent, or persistent pneumonia; and especially in patients with pulmonary symptoms and pansinusitis or chronic otitis media.

Diagnostic Studies

Ciliary dysfunction is confirmed by electron microscopy of respiratory cilia. The cilia may be obtained from nasal scrapings, but because chronic infection and inflammation may lead to ultrastructural abnormalities in nasal cilia, care must be taken in validating the diagnosis. Bronchoscopy may be required for ciliary samples and to confirm the diagnosis. CF should be excluded by appropriate testing.

Treatment

Pulmonary therapy, similar to that used for patients with CF, is directed toward improving clearance of respiratory secretions and controlling infection. Chest physiotherapy, immunoprophylaxis of viral infections (influenza), and prompt treatment of bacterial infections are helpful, but the course of the disease tends to be slowly progressive.

Pneumonia

▶ SEE CHAPTER 110.

Pulmonary Edema

Etiology

At the alveolar-capillary interface, capillary hydrostatic forces and tissue osmotic pressures tend to push fluid into the airspaces, whereas plasma osmotic pressures and tissue mechanical forces tend to force fluid away from the airspaces. Under normal circumstances, the vectorial sum of these forces favors absorption so that the alveolar spaces remain dry. Any fluid entering the alveolus normally is removed by the pulmonary lymphatics. Pulmonary edema forms when transcapillary fluid flux exceeds lymphatic drainage. Reduced left ventricular function accompanied by pulmonary venous hypertension increases capillary hydrostatic pressure, which floods the interstitial space and alveoli with fluid, producing pulmonary edema. Fluid initially enters the interstitial space around the terminal bronchioles, alveoli, and arteries (**interstitial edema**), causing increased lung stiffness, premature closure of bronchioles on expiration, dyspnea, and tachypnea as a result of stimulation of lung receptors. If the process continues, fluid enters the alveolar space, reducing compliance and creating a perfused but unventilated area called an **intrapulmonary shunt**, which produces hypoxia.

Pulmonary hypertension, as occurs in cor pulmonale, rarely produces pulmonary edema because the increased vascular resistance is proximal to the capillary bed. Pulmonary edema may be seen, however, when intrathoracic pressure becomes excessively negative (in upper airway obstruction from hypertrophied tonsils). Pulmonary edema also may occur in patients with decreased serum oncotic pressure, receiving large volumes of IV fluid after capillary damage (from smoke inhalation or hydrocarbon aspiration), with ascent to high altitude, and with a history of CNS injury (neurogenic).

Clinical Manifestations

Pulmonary edema typically produces **dyspnea**, cough (often with frothy, pink-tinged sputum), tachypnea, signs of increased respiratory effort, and diffuse rales or crackles.

Diagnostic Studies

Chest radiographs reveal a diffuse infiltrate that classically is in a perihilar pattern, but may be obscured by underlying lung disease. Signs of interstitial edema (**Kerley B lines**) may be seen, especially at the lung bases.

Treatment and Prognosis

Therapy should include positioning of the patient in an upright posture and administration of O_2, but is otherwise directed toward relieving the underlying problem. Morphine may relieve dyspnea and, by dilating central veins, reduce venous return to the heart. Diuretic therapy (furosemide) and rapid-acting IV inotropic agents may also be helpful. In severe cases, continuous positive airway pressure or intubation with positive end-expiratory pressure may be required. The prognosis for patients with pulmonary edema depends on the nature of the underlying cause and on the response to therapy.

Acute Respiratory Distress Syndrome

▶ SEE CHAPTER 39.

Pulmonary Hypertension and Cor Pulmonale

Etiology

Diffuse lung disease, upper airway obstruction (hypertrophied tonsils or adenoids), pulmonary thromboembolism, or exposure to high altitude may produce pulmonary hypertension. Pulmonary hypertension also may result from **excessive pulmonary blood flow** when there is a left-to-right cardiac shunt (see Chapter 143). With prolonged hypertension, resulting from either increased flow or hypoxic vasoconstriction, permanent changes occur in the intima and media of the pulmonary artery, making the increased vascular resistance irreversible.

Primary pulmonary hypertension is idiopathic, occurs in the absence of parenchymal lung or cardiac disease, may be associated with autoimmune disease (systemic lupus erythematosus, scleroderma) or anorectic antiobesity drugs, or may be inherited (autosomal dominant with incomplete penetrance; female predominance) because of mutations in the bone morphogenetic receptor gene. Pulmonary hypertension resulting from lung disease leads to hypertrophy and eventually to dilation of the right ventricle. In advanced states, right heart failure may occur, with limitation of exercise capacity, hepatic congestion, fluid retention, and signs of tricuspid insufficiency, a condition known as **cor pulmonale**. In severe disease, the ventricular septum may be displaced toward the left ventricle, reducing its volume and reducing left ventricular function.

The most common causes of cor pulmonale in children are diffuse chronic lung diseases, such as CF and bronchopulmonary dysplasia. In these conditions, airway obstruction leads to alveolar hypoxia, and parenchymal scarring may increase pulmonary vascular resistance. Severe untreated obstructive sleep apnea also may lead to cor pulmonale.

Clinical Manifestations and Diagnostic Studies

The diagnosis of pulmonary hypertension should be suspected whenever there is prolonged hypoxemia or severe left-to-right shunting. In addition to the other physical findings associated with pulmonary or cardiac disease, an accentuated pulmonic component of the second heart sound may be heard in the left second interspace. Definitive diagnosis is made by cardiac catheterization, but echocardiography may confirm the presence of significant right ventricular hypertrophy, ventricular dysfunction, and tricuspid insufficiency indicative of increased pulmonary artery pressure.

Treatment and Prognosis

Therapy directed at the underlying condition should be provided. The relief of hypoxemia is essential and usually requires supplemental O_2 therapy. Heart failure may necessitate administration of diuretics and restriction of salt and fluid intake. Vasodilator therapy is helpful in some patients. IV infusions of vasodilators, such as prostacyclin or sildenafil, either acutely or chronically, can help reduce pulmonary artery pressures. Inhaled nitric oxide may be valuable in acute severe cases. Lung or heart-lung transplantation is the treatment for end-stage cor pulmonale. The prognosis is poor when chronic cor pulmonale is present. If left ventricular failure is evident, the prognosis is further guarded.

Pulmonary Hemorrhage

Etiology

Pulmonary hemorrhage is a rare but potentially life-threatening condition in children presenting with **hemoptysis**. When evaluating a child with a history of hemoptysis, it is imperative to rule out more common extrapulmonary sources of bleeding, including hematemesis and bleeding from the nasopharynx or mouth.

Pulmonary hemosiderosis is characterized by the accumulation of hemosiderin in the lungs as a result of bleeding into the lungs. Red blood cells are phagocytosed by alveolar macrophages. The hemoglobin is converted to hemosiderin, which, with the use of special iron-staining techniques, can be identified microscopically within the alveolar macrophages. Hemosiderin-laden macrophages may be found in sputum, gastric aspirate, bronchoalveolar lavage fluid, or a lung biopsy. Although the term *hemosiderosis* sometimes is used interchangeably with pulmonary hemorrhage, it is a pathologic state that may result from bleeding anywhere in the lung, airway, pharynx, nasopharynx, or mouth leading to hemosiderin accumulation in the lung. *Pulmonary hemorrhage* is a preferable term for bleeding from an intrathoracic source.

Clinical Manifestations

In addition to hemoptysis, presenting symptoms and signs of pulmonary hemorrhage include cough, wheezing, shortness of breath, pallor, fatigue, cyanosis, or fever. Episodic pulmonary hemorrhage frequently manifests with a history of recurrent pulmonary infiltrates on chest x-ray. Symptomatic pulmonary hemorrhage may be associated with minimal radiographic changes, however. Some patients experience a localized bubbling sensation in the chest, which can be helpful in differentiating local from diffuse sources of pulmonary bleeding. Physical examination findings may include locally or diffusely decreased breath sounds, cyanosis, crackles, or wheezes. The **differential diagnosis** of pulmonary hemorrhage includes Heiner syndrome (milk allergy), diffuse alveolitis secondary to collagen vascular diseases (Goodpasture syndrome, Wegener granulomatosis, systemic lupus erythemato-

sus, Henoch-Schönlein purpura), clotting disorders or veno-occlusive disease, diffuse alveolar injury (smoke inhalation, acid aspiration), heart disease associated with increased pulmonary venous and capillary pressures (mitral stenosis), infection, and focal sources of bleeding (including bronchiectasis, arteriovenous malformations, foreign body, or endobronchial tumor) (Table 136–2).

Diagnostic Studies

If extrapulmonary sources of bleeding have been excluded, diagnostic workup may require serial chest x-rays, chest CT scan, bronchoscopy, echocardiogram, urinalysis and serum creatinine to look for evidence of

TABLE 136–2.   Differential Diagnosis of Hemoptysis–Pulmonary Hemorrhage
Cardiovascular
Heart failure Eisenmenger syndrome Mitral stenosis Veno-occlusive disease Arteriovenous malformation (Osler-Weber-Rendu syndrome) Pulmonary embolism
Pulmonary
Respiratory distress syndrome Bronchogenic cyst Sequestration Pneumonia (bacterial, mycobacterial, fungal, or parasitic) Cystic fibrosis Tracheobronchitis Bronchiectasis Abscess Tumor (adenoma, carcinoid, hemangioma, metastasis) Foreign body retention Contusion-trauma
Immune
Henoch-Schönlein purpura Heiner syndrome Goodpasture syndrome Wegener granulomatosis Systemic lupus erythematosus Allergic bronchopulmonary aspergillosis
Other
Hyperammonemia Kernicterus Intracranial hemorrhage (preterm infant) Toxins Diffuse alveolar injury (smoke inhalation)

nephritis (Goodpasture syndrome, Wegener granulo-matosis, systemic lupus erythematosus), and serologic screens for collagen vascular disease (antinuclear antibody, antineutrophilic cytoplasmic antibody, antibodies to basement membrane).

Treatment

The management of the acute episodes of pulmonary bleeding may involve administration of O_2, blood transfusions, intratracheal epinephrine, and, if necessary, mechanical ventilation accompanied by positive end-expiratory pressure to tamponade the bleeding. Attempts should be made to identify the cause of the bleeding. An open lung biopsy may be necessary. Idiopathic pulmonary hemosiderosis may respond to corticosteroids. Other immunosuppressant agents, such as azathioprine and cyclophosphamide, have been used when the condition has not responded to the administration of corticosteroids over 2 to 3 months. Pulmonary hemorrhage that responds quickly to therapy in previously healthy infants is often a self-limited illness of unknown etiology.

Pulmonary Embolism

Etiology

Pulmonary embolism is rare in childhood and may be associated with indwelling vascular catheters, oral contraceptive pills, lupus anticoagulant or other hypercoagulable states, trauma, abortion, or malignancy.

Clinical Manifestations

Because the pulmonary vascular bed is very distensible, small emboli, even if multiple, are usually not detected unless they are infected and cause pulmonary infection. Large emboli may lead to acute dyspnea, pleuritic chest pain, cough, hemoptysis, and death, however. **Hypoxia** is common, as are nonspecific ST segment and T wave changes on the ECG, an increased P_2 heart sound, or presence of S_4.

Diagnostic Studies

Although the chest x-ray is usually negative, atelectasis or cardiomegaly may be seen. **Ventilation-perfusion scans** are useful in diagnosis by revealing defects in perfusion without matching ventilation defects. Other diagnostic tests, such as measurement of D dimers in circulating blood, helical chest CT scan, and venous ultrasonography for patients with suspected leg venous thrombosis, can be useful adjuncts. For definitive diagnosis, however, a **pulmonary angiogram** is the procedure of choice.

Treatment

Supportive therapy (**O_2 administration**) of proven pulmonary embolism is provided. Therapy should be directed toward the predisposing factors. **Heparin** may be useful in preventing the development of further emboli. Thrombolytic therapy or surgery may be helpful in treating massive embolization.

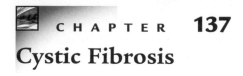

CHAPTER **137**

Cystic Fibrosis

ETIOLOGY AND EPIDEMIOLOGY

CF, an autosomal recessive disorder, is the most common life-limiting recessive genetic disease in whites. In the U.S., 1 in 3200 white newborns is born with CF. CF is less common in African Americans (1 : 15,000), Asians (1 : 31,000), and other populations.

The gene for CF, localized to the long arm of chromosome 7, is a large gene that encodes a polypeptide termed **cystic fibrosis transmembrane regulator (CFTR)**. The most common mutation is a specific deletion of three base pairs resulting in a deletion of phenylalanine at position ΔF508. Hundreds of mutations of the *CFTR* gene have been identified. Dysfunctional epithelial transport is associated with the *CFTR* mutation, leading to the clinical manifestations of CF.

The secretory and absorptive characteristics of epithelial cells are affected. The *CFTR* is a chloride channel and substantially regulates epithelial chloride and possibly sodium transport. The CFTR involvement with chloride ion conductance is responsible for the elevated sweat chloride in 99% of CF patients. How the abnormal chloride conductance accounts for the clinical manifestations of CF is not completely understood. It may reduce the function of airway defenses or promote bacterial adhesion to the airway epithelium.

CLINICAL MANIFESTATIONS

CF is a chronic, insidiously progressive disease exhibiting multiple complications related to viscous mucus, malabsorption, and infection (Table 137–1). The respiratory epithelium of patients with CF exhibits marked impermeability to chloride and an excessive reabsorption of sodium. These alterations in the bioelectrical properties of the epithelium lead to a relative dehydration of the airway secretions, resulting in impaired mucociliary transport and airway obstruction. **Chronic bronchial infection** then develops. Most

TABLE 137–1. Complications of Cystic Fibrosis

Respiratory

Bronchiectasis, bronchitis, bronchiolitis, pneumonia
Atelectasis
Hemoptysis
Pneumothorax
Nasal polyps
Sinusitis
Reactive airway disease
Cor pulmonale
Respiratory failure
Mucoid impaction of the bronchi
Allergic bronchopulmonary aspergillosis

Gastrointestinal

Meconium ileus
Meconium peritonitis
Distal intestinal obstruction syndrome (non-neonatal obstruction)
Rectal prolapse
Intussusception
Volvulus
Fibrosing colonopathy (strictures)
Appendicitis
Intestinal atresia
Pancreatitis
Biliary cirrhosis (portal hypertension: esophageal varices, hypersplenism)
Neonatal obstructive jaundice
Hepatic steatosis
Gastroesophageal reflux
Cholelithiasis
Inguinal hernia
Growth failure (malabsorption)
Vitamin deficiency states (vitamins A, K, E, D)
Insulin deficiency, symptomatic hyperglycemia, diabetes
Malignancy (rare)

Other

Infertility
Delayed puberty
Edema-hypoproteinemia
Dehydration–heat exhaustion
Hypertrophic osteoarthropathy–arthritis
Clubbing
Amyloidosis

patients are colonized with *Haemophilus influenzae, Staphylococcus aureus,* or *Pseudomonas aeruginosa* (which predominates in older patients with advanced disease). Chronic bronchial infection leads to cough (the most common initial pulmonary manifestation), sputum production, hyperinflation, bronchiectasis, and eventually pulmonary insufficiency and death. **Digital clubbing** is common in patients with CF, even without significant lung disease. **Chronic sinusitis** is nearly universal, and nasal polyposis is common.

Most patients with CF have exocrine **pancreatic insufficiency** early in life (if not at birth) as a result of inspissation of mucus in the pancreatic ducts. Maldigestion with secondary malabsorption results in **steatorrhea** (large, fatty, floating, foul-smelling stools) and many secondary deficiency states (vitamins A, D, E, and K) in untreated patients. Nutrient malabsorption also results in failure to thrive despite a ravenous appetite. Approximately 10% of patients are born with intestinal obstruction resulting from inspissated meconium (**meconium ileus**). In older patients, intestinal obstruction may occur because of maldigestion and thick mucus in the intestinal lumen (**distal intestinal obstruction syndrome**). Such events may occur after dietary indiscretions or with inadequate pancreatic enzyme replacement. In adolescent or adult patients, **relative insulin deficiency** may develop. Hyperglycemia and CF-related diabetes may become symptomatic; ketoacidosis is rare.

Inspissation of mucus in the reproductive tract leads to dysfunction. Secondary amenorrhea is often present as a result of chronic illness and markedly reduced body weight. Women with CF have given birth, however. Males are almost universally azoospermic, with atrophy or absence of the vas deferens. The failure of the sweat ducts to conserve salt may lead to heat exhaustion or to unexplained hypochloremic alkalosis in infants.

Pulmonary infections with certain virulent strains of *Burkholderia cepacia* are particularly difficult to treat and may be associated with an accelerated clinical deterioration. **Allergic bronchopulmonary aspergillosis** also may complicate CF lung disease and necessitate treatment with steroids and antifungal agents. Other potential pulmonary complications of CF include atelectasis, progressive bronchiectasis, hemoptysis, and pneumothorax.

DIAGNOSTIC STUDIES

The diagnosis of CF should be considered seriously in any patient with chronic or recurring respiratory or gastrointestinal symptoms. Indications for performing a **sweat test** are listed in Table 137–2. The following criteria must be met for the diagnosis to be established: the presence of one or more typical phenotypic features of CF (chronic sinopulmonary disease, characteristic gastrointestinal and nutritional abnormalities, salt loss syndromes, and obstructive azoospermia), a sibling with a history of CF or a positive result from a newborn screening test, a positive result obtained from a sweat test on two or more occasions (positive if >60 mEq/L with adequate sweat collection of at least 75 mg,

TABLE 137–2. Indications for Sweat Testing

Respiratory

Chronic or recurrent cough
Chronic or recurrent pneumonia
Recurrent bronchiolitis
Recurrent or persistant atelectasis
Hemoptysis
Staphylococcal pneumonia
Pseudomonas aeruginosa in the respiratory tract (in the
  absence of such circumstances as tracheostomy or
  prolonged intubation)
Mucoid *P. aeruginosa* in the respiratory tract

Gastrointestinal

Meconium ileus
Neonatal intestinal obstruction (meconium plug, atresia)
Steatorrhea, malabsorption
Hepatic cirrhosis in childhood (including any
  manifestations such as esophageal varices or portal
  hypertension)
Pancreatitis
Rectal prolapse
Vitamin deficiency states (A, D, E, K)
Prolonged, direct-reacting neonatal jaundice

Miscellaneous

Digital clubbing
Failure to thrive
Family history of cystic fibrosis (sibling or cousin)
Salty taste when kissed; salt crystals on skin after
  evaporation of sweat
Heat prostration, especially under seemingly
  inappropriate circumstances
Hyponatremic hypochloremic alkalosis in infants
Nasal polyps
Recurrent sinusitis
Aspermia
Absent vas deferens

Heterozygote detection and prenatal diagnosis of children with ΔF508 and more than 70 other deletions is easily accomplished. Present testing identifies greater than 90% of carriers. Prenatal detection of a known CF genotype may be accomplished by amniotic fluid or chorionic villus sampling.

TREATMENT

Lung disease is treated by combining several therapies. **Clearance techniques** (chest physiotherapy, exercise) are used to help remove mucus from the airways. **Pharmacologic measures** (aerosolized DNase and bronchodilators) thin and clear mucus and improve airway patency. **Antibiotic therapy** controls chronic infection. Monitoring pulmonary bacterial flora and providing aggressive therapy with appropriate antibiotics in full therapeutic doses (oral, aerosolized, and parenteral) help slow the progression of the lung disease. Patients are hospitalized for high-dose IV antibiotic therapy and aggressive chest physiotherapy whenever necessary, especially when they have pulmonary infections with organisms resistant to oral agents (*Pseudomonas*). Under normal circumstances, therapy should last at least 2 weeks. Even when the most aggressive therapy is used, it is difficult to sterilize the lungs.

TABLE 137–3. Causes of False-Positive and False-Negative Sweat Test

False Positive

Adult age
Adrenal insufficiency
Eczema
Ectodermal dysplasia
Nephrogenic diabetes insipidus
Hypothyroidism
Fucosidosis
Mucopolysaccharidosis
Dehydration
Malnutrition
Poor technique
Type I glycogen storage disease
Panhypopituitarism
Pseudohypoaldosteronism
Hypoparathyroidism
Prostaglandin E_1 administration

False Negative

Edema
Poor technique
Atypical cystic fibrosis (uncommon)

borderline if 40 to 60 mEq/L, and negative if <40 mEq/L), two mutations known to cause CF identified, or a characteristic abnormality in ion transport across nasal epithelium shown in vivo.

Although highly specific for CF, the sweat test is subject to numerous technical problems. False-positive and false-negative (less common) sweat test results occur in a few well-defined clinical states (Table 137–3). Other supportive tests, such as measurement of bioelectrical potential differences across nasal epithelium, low levels of stool elastase, and detection of a known CF mutation by DNA analysis, may be useful. Conventional commercial CF genotyping testing for many mutations identifies 95% of all alleles. A patient without identified alleles still can have CF.

Pancreatic insufficiency is treated by replacing pancreatic enzymes, preferably in enteric-coated form, and by encouraging higher caloric intake than normal. Despite the best enzyme replacement, stool losses of fat and protein may be high. Fat is not withheld from the diet, even when significant steatorrhea exists. Instead, enzyme doses are increased to enhance absorption as much as possible. Lipase concentrations exceeding 2500 U/kg/meal are contraindicated, however, because these concentrations have been associated with intestinal obstruction caused by **fibrosing colonopathy**. Fat-soluble vitamins are given in twice-normal doses, preferably in water-miscible form.

Meconium ileus in a newborn may require surgical intervention, but sometimes can be managed with contrast (Gastrografin) enemas. Intestinal obstruction occurring in CF patients beyond the neonatal period (known as meconium ileus equivalent or distal intestinal obstruction syndrome) may respond to a balanced intestinal lavage solution (GoLYTELY) via nasogastric tube or enemas of Gastrografin or *N*-acetylcysteine. Pancreatic enzyme dosage adjustment, lactulose, adequate hydration, and dietary fiber may help prevent recurrent episodes. Patients with CF-related diabetes are treated with insulin, primarily to improve nutrition and prevent dehydration, as ketoacidosis is very rare. Although transaminase elevation is common in patients with CF, only 1% to 3% of patients have progressive cirrhosis resulting in portal hypertension. Cholestasis may be treated with ursodiol or endoscopic dilation of the ampulla of Vater if stenosis is present.

The complex management of CF is best coordinated by a tertiary CF accredited referral center. As in the treatment of any chronic disease, physicians, patients, families, and other caregivers, including nurses, dietitians, and social workers, must work together to maintain an optimistic, aggressive approach to life and treatment. Efforts to prevent the occurrence of complications and the progression of lung disease are vital.

CHAPTER 138
Chest Wall and Pleura

SCOLIOSIS

Marked curvature of the thoracic spine is associated with chest wall deformity and limitation of chest wall movement, which decreases lung volumes (restrictive lung disease). In advanced scoliosis, bronchial obstruction may develop when the bronchi become kinked or compressed by the great vessels that shift to abnormal positions in relation to the airways. Significant loss of inspiratory capacity often leads to pulmonary hypertension, recurrent infection, atelectasis, and respiratory insufficiency (see Chapter 202).

PECTUS EXCAVATUM AND CARINATUM

Pectus Excavatum

Sternal concavity may be seen in children of all ages. It is predominant in children with obstructive lung disease, but is often present in children with no underlying pulmonary problem. Although the pectus excavatum may be significant, it seldom interferes with pulmonary function. It may create great cosmetic concern for the patients and family. In a child or adolescent with a more severe pectus deformity, careful exercise history should be elicited. Resting spirometry is often done for these patients. Exercise tolerance testing also may be indicated. Surgical correction, if necessary, is often delayed until adolescence. It is generally done for cosmetic reasons, but much less commonly is performed to improve function.

Pectus Carinatum

This chest wall shape, where the sternum bows out, is frequently know as "pigeon breast." Underlying pulmonary disease may contribute to the deformity, but the chest wall shape itself does not produce ventilation difficulties. Surgery for this condition is less common than for pectus excavatum and is usually done for cosmetic purposes after adolescence.

PNEUMOTHORAX

Etiology

Pneumothorax is the accumulation of air in the pleural space that may result from external trauma or from leakage of air from the lungs or airways. **Spontaneous pneumothoraces** may occur in teenagers and young adults, more commonly in tall, thin males and smokers. Predisposing conditions include mechanical ventilation, asthma, CF, trauma, disorders of collagen (**Marfan syndrome**), idiopathic subpleural bullae (common and often bilateral), and exertion with a Valsalva maneuver.

Clinical Manifestations

The symptoms of pneumothorax often begin while the patient is at rest (if spontaneous). Symptoms are pain, dyspnea, and cyanosis. If the air leak communicates with the mediastinum, subcutaneous emphysema may become apparent. Physical findings may include decreased breath sounds, a tympanitic percussion note, signs of mediastinal shift, and subcutaneous crepitus (see Table 133–3). If the amount of air collection is small, few or no physical signs of pneumothorax may be present. Symptoms may progress rapidly if the air in the pleural space is under pressure (known as **tension pneumothorax**), with death resulting if the tension is not relieved.

Diagnostic Studies

The diagnosis is confirmed by chest radiograph. In infants, transillumination of the chest wall may help in the rapid diagnosis of pneumothorax.

Treatment

Intervention depends on the amount of intrapleural air and the nature of the underlying disease. Small (<20%) pneumothoraces often resolve spontaneously. Inhaling high concentration O_2 for 12 to 24 hours can speed reabsorption. Larger pneumothoraces (and tension pneumothoraces) necessitate immediate drainage of the air. In an emergency situation, a simple needle aspiration may suffice, but placement of a chest tube may be required for resolution. Sclerosing the pleural surfaces to obliterate the pleural space (pleurodesis) may benefit patients with recurrent pneumothoraces.

PNEUMOMEDIASTINUM

Pneumomediastinum results from the dissection of air from a leak in the pulmonary parenchyma into the mediastinum. The most common cause in children is acute asthma. Symptoms are pain and dyspnea. Physical findings may be absent or may include a crunching noise over the sternum on auscultation. Frequently, subcutaneous emphysema is present in the neck. The diagnosis is confirmed by radiograph. Treatment is directed toward the underlying lung disease.

PLEURAL EFFUSION
Etiology

Fluid accumulates in the pleural space whenever the local hydrostatic forces pushing fluid out of the vascular space exceed osmotic forces, pulling fluid back into the vascular space. The underlying causes of pleural effusion are inflammation or infection of the pleura, congestive heart failure, hypoproteinemia, obstruction of lymphatic drainage, malignancy, and collagen vascular disease. Infection producing a reactive **parapneumonic effusion** or a more serious purulent **empyema** is the most common cause of pleural effusion in children. Empyema often is caused by *Streptococcus pneumoniae,* group A streptococci, or *S. aureus*

(and rarely by *Mycobacterium tuberculosis, Mycoplasma,* or adenovirus). Anaerobic bacteria produce empyema associated with aspiration pneumonia and dental, lung, or subdiaphragmatic abscesses. *H. influenzae* frequently causes parapneumonic effusion but is rare in immunized populations.

Clinical Manifestations

Pleural effusion commonly accompanies inflammatory processes in the lungs and may be heralded by pain, dyspnea, and signs of respiratory insufficiency resulting from compression of the underlying lung. Physical findings include tachypnea, dullness to percussion, decreased breath sounds, mediastinal shift, and decreased tactile fremitus (see Table 133–3). The diagnosis is confirmed radiographically. Decubitus views, ultrasonography, or CT may help to determine size, location, and presence or absence of loculations of fluid.

Diagnostic Studies

Thoracentesis can help establish the cause of the effusion and exclude infection. The diagnostic culture yield of thoracentesis is low, however, in children with obvious infection who have received antibiotics for greater than 24 hours. In the absence of inflammation, pleural fluid should have a low specific gravity (<1.015) and protein content (<2.5 g/dL), low lactic dehydrogenase activity (<200 IU/L), and a low cell count with few polymorphonuclear cells (a transudate). In contrast, exudative pleural effusions resulting from inflammation have a high specific gravity, high protein (>3 g/dL) and lactic dehydrogenase (>250 IU/L) content, low pH (<7.2), low glucose (<40 mg/dL) level, and a high cell count with many polymorphonuclear leukocytes.

Treatment

Therapy is directed at the underlying condition causing the effusion and at relief of the mechanical consequences of the fluid collection. For small effusions, especially if they are transudative, no drainage therapy is usually required. For large effusions, drainage with a **chest tube**, especially if the fluid is purulent (empyema), is often needed. In this latter case, the fluid is often thick and may be loculated, which makes simple drainage difficult. In cases of empyema and parapneumonic effusion, in which drainage is complicated by a loculated pleural collection, **video-assisted thoracoscopic surgical débridement** is useful and may reduce morbidity and length of hospital stay. Many small to moderate sized parapneumonic effusions can be managed conservatively with IV antibiotics. If the underlying condition is treated successfully, the prognosis for pediatric patients with pleural effusions, including empyema, is excellent.

SUGGESTED READING

Austin J, Ali T: Tracheomalacia and bronchomalacia in children: Pathophysiology, assessment, treatment and anaesthesia management. Pediatr Anaesth 13:3-11, 2003.

Behrman RE, Kliegman RM (eds): Nelson Essentials of Pediatrics, 4th ed. Philadelphia, WB Saunders, 2002.

Byard RW, Krous HF: Sudden infant death syndrome: Overview and update. Pediatr Dev Pathol 6:112-127, 2003.

Chernick V, Boat TF, Kendig EL (eds): Kendig's Disorders of the Respiratory Tract in Children, 6th ed. Philadelphia, WB Saunders, 1998.

Harty MP, Kramer SS: Recent advances in pediatric pulmonary imaging. Curr Opin Pediatr 10:227-235, 1998.

Hodson ME, Geddes DM (eds): Cystic Fibrosis, 2nd ed. London, Arnold Publishers, 2000.

Kliegman RM, Greenbaum LA, Lye PS (eds): Practical Strategies in Pediatric Diagnosis and Therapy, 2nd ed. Philadelphia, WB Saunders, 2004.

Lewis RA, Feign RD: Current issues in the diagnosis and management of pediatric empyema. Semin Pediatr Infect Dis 13:280-288, 2002.

Rovin JD, Rodgers BM: Pediatric foreign body aspiration. Pediatr Rev 21:86-89, 2000.

Taussig LM, Landau LI (eds): Pediatric Respiratory Medicine. St. Louis, Mosby, 1999.

Wilmott RW, Khurana-Hershey G, Stark JM: Current concepts on pulmonary host defense mechanisms in children. Curr Opin Pediatr 12:187-193, 2000.

CHAPTER **139**

Assessment

HISTORY

Heart disease in children originates from a combination of genetic and environmental causes. The focus of the cardiovascular history depends on the age of the patient and is directed by the chief complaint. The **prenatal history** may identify evidence of a maternal infection early in pregnancy (possibly teratogenic) or later in pregnancy (causing myocarditis or myocardial dysfunction in infants). A **maternal history** of medication, drug, or alcohol use or excessive smoking may contribute to cardiac and other systemic findings. **Growth** is an extremely valuable sign of cardiovascular health. The birth weight is an indicator of the prenatal health of the fetus and the mother. Infants with **congestive heart failure (CHF)** grow poorly, with weight being more significantly affected than height and head circumference.

CHF may present with a history of **fatigue** or **diaphoresis** with feeds or fussiness. Breastfeeding or formula-feeding may be difficult and prolonged because of tachypnea and dyspnea. **Tachypnea** without significant dyspnea may be present. Older children with CHF may have easy fatigability, **shortness of breath** on exertion, and sometimes orthopnea. **Exercise intolerance** may be determined by asking how well children keep up playing with their friends or in physical education class. Before diagnosis of CHF, patients may have been diagnosed with recurrent "pneumonia," "bronchitis," wheezing, or asthma.

A history of a heart **murmur** is important, but many well children have a normal or innocent heart murmur at some time in their life. Other cardiac symptoms include cyanosis, palpitations, chest pain, syncope, and near-syncope. A review of systems should assess for possible systemic diseases or congenital malformation syndromes that may cause cardiac abnormalities (Tables 139-1 and 139-2). Current and past medication use is important. A history of drug use is important in older children and adolescents. **Family history** should be reviewed for hereditary diseases, early atherosclerotic heart disease, congenital heart disease, sudden unexplained deaths, thrombophilia, rheumatic fever, hypertension, and hypercholesterolemia.

PHYSICAL EXAMINATION

A complete cardiovascular examination starts in the supine position and includes evaluation in the sitting and standing positions. This examination is impossible in infants and may be difficult in toddlers. Much information regarding the cardiovascular status can be gained by observation and **inspection**, which is supplemented by **palpation** and **auscultation**.

The examination starts with vital signs, focusing on heart rate, respiratory rate, and blood pressure. The normal **heart rate** varies with age and activity (Fig. 139-1). Tachycardia may be a manifestation of anemia, dehydration, shock, heart failure, or dysrhythmia. Bradycardia can be a normal finding in patients with high vagal tone (athletes), but may be a manifestation of atrioventricular block. The **respiratory rate** of infants is best assessed while observing the infant sitting quietly with the parent. Respiratory rate may be increased when there is a left-to-right shunt or pulmonary venous congestion.

The normal **blood pressure** also varies with age. A properly sized cuff should have a bladder width that is at least 90% of the arm circumference and a length that is 80% to 100% of the arm circumference. Initially, blood pressure in the right arm is measured. If elevated,

TABLE 139–1.   Cardiac Manifestations of Systemic Diseases

Systemic Disease	Cardiac Complications
Hunter-Hurler syndrome	Valvular insufficiency, heart failure, hypertension
Fabry disease	Mitral insufficiency, coronary artery disease with myocardial infarction
Pompe disease	Short P-R interval, cardiomegaly, heart failure, arrhythmias
Friedreich ataxia	Cardiomyopathy, arrhythmias
Duchenne dystrophy	Cardiomyopathy, heart failure
Juvenile rheumatoid arthritis	Pericarditis
Systemic lupus erythematosus	Pericarditis, Libman-Sacks endocarditis, congenital AV block
Marfan syndrome	Aortic and mitral insufficiency, dissecting aortic aneurysm
Homocystinuria	Coronary thrombosis
Kawasaki disease	Coronary artery aneurysm, thrombosis, myocardial infarction, myocarditis
Lyme disease	Arrhythmias, myocarditis, heart failure
Graves disease (hyperthyroidism)	Tachycardia, arrhythmias, heart failure
Tuberous sclerosis	Cardiac rhabdomyoma
Neurofibromatosis	Pulmonic stenosis, coarctation of aorta

AV, atrioventricular.

TABLE 139–2.   Congenital Malformation Syndromes Associated with Congenital Heart Disease

Syndrome	Cardiac Features
Trisomy 21 (Down syndrome)	Endocardial cushion defect, VSD, ASD, PDA
Trisomy 18	VSD, ASD, PDA, PS
Trisomy 13	VSD, ASD, PDA, dextrocardia
XO (Turner syndrome)	Coarctation of aorta, aortic stenosis
CHARGE association (coloboma, heart, atresia choanae, retardation, genital and ear anomalies)	TOF, aortic arch and conotruncal anomalies*
22q11 (DiGeorge) syndrome	Aortic arch anomalies, conotruncal anomalies*
VACTERL association† (vertebral, anal, cardiac, tracheoesophageal, radial, renal, limb anomalies)	VSD
Congenital rubella	PDA, peripheral pulmonic stenosis, mitral regurgitation (in infancy)
Marfan syndrome	Dilated and dissecting aorta, aortic valve regurgitation, mitral valve prolapse
Williams syndrome	Supravalvular aortic stenosis, peripheral pulmonary stenosis
Infant of diabetic mother	Hypertrophic cardiomyopathy, VSD, conotruncal anomalies
Holt-Oram syndrome	ASD, VSD
Asplenia syndrome	Complex cyanotic heart lesions, anomalous pulmonary venous return, dextrocardia, single ventricle, single AV valve
Polysplenia syndrome	Azygos continuation of inferior vena cava, pulmonary atresia, dextrocardia, single ventricle
Fetal alcohol syndrome	VSD, ASD
Ellis–van Creveld syndrome	Single atrium
Zellweger syndrome	PDA, VSD, ASD
Fetal hydantoin syndrome	TGA, VSD, TOF

ASD, atrial septal defect; AV, atrioventricular; PDA, patent ductus arteriosus; PS, pulmonic stenosis; TGA, transposition of great vessels; TOF, tetralogy of Fallot; VSD, ventricular septal defect.
*Conotruncal—tetralogy of Fallot, pulmonary atresia, truncus arteriosus, transposition of great arteries.
†VACTERL association is also known as VATER (vertebral, anal, tracheoesophageal, radial, renal anomalies) association.

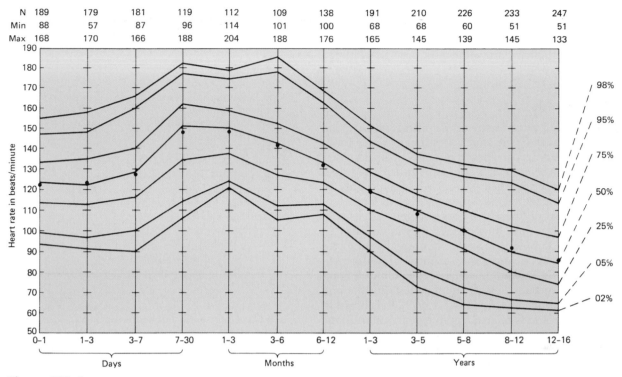

N	189	179	181	119	112	109	138	191	210	226	233	247
Min	88	57	87	96	114	101	100	68	68	60	51	51
Max	168	170	166	188	204	188	176	165	145	139	145	133

Figure 139–1

Heart rate versus age (• = mean). (From Davignon A, Rautaharju P, Boiselle E: Pediatr Cardiol 1:123, 1980.)

measurements in the left arm and leg are indicated to evaluate for possible coarctation of the aorta. The **pulse pressure** is determined by subtracting the diastolic pressure from the systolic pressure. It is normally less than 50 mm Hg or half the systolic pressure, whichever is less. A wide pulse pressure usually is seen with aortopulmonary connections (patent ductus arteriosus [PDA], truncus arteriosus), arteriovenous malformations, aortic insufficiency, or relative intravascular volume depletion (anemia, vasodilation with fever or sepsis). A narrow pulse pressure is seen with pericardial tamponade, aortic stenosis, or CHF. The blood pressure cuff needs to be the proper size to obtain reliable information.

Inspection or observation includes the general appearance, nutritional status, circulation, and respiratory effort. Many chromosomal abnormalities and syndromes associated with cardiac defects have dysmorphic features or failure to thrive (see Table 139–2). Skin color must be assessed for **cyanosis** and pallor. Cyanosis may be central (tongue, lips) or peripheral (hands, feet). Central cyanosis is associated with arterial desaturation, whereas isolated peripheral cyanosis is associated with normal arterial saturation and increased peripheral extraction of oxygen. Perioral cyanosis is a common finding, especially in pale infants

or when infants and toddlers become cold. Chronic arterial desaturation results in **clubbing** of the fingernails and toenails. Inspection of the chest may reveal asymmetry or a prominent left precordium suggesting chronic cardiac enlargement.

After inspection, **palpation** of pulses in all four extremities, the precordial activity, and the abdomen is performed. Pulses should be assessed for rate, regularity, intensity, symmetry, and timing between upper and lower extremities. The presence of a good pedal pulse effectively rules out coarctation of the aorta if the right arm blood pressure is normal. Precordial palpation is important and often suggests significant cardiovascular disease in the absence of obvious auscultatory findings. The precordium should be assessed for apical impulse, **point of maximum impulse**, hyperactivity, and presence of a **thrill**. Abdominal palpation is primarily for assessment of liver and spleen size. The liver size provides a good assessment of intravascular volume and is enlarged with systemic venous congestion. The spleen is rarely enlarged with heart failure, but may be enlarged with infective endocarditis.

Auscultation is the most important part of the cardiovascular examination, but should supplement what already has been found by observation, inspection, and palpation. It requires systematic listening in a quiet room with assessment of each portion of the cardiac cycle. In addition to the heart rate and regularity, the heart sounds, clicks, and murmurs need to be timed and characterized.

Heart Sounds

S₁ is associated with closure of the mitral and tricuspid valves, is usually single, and is best heard at the lower left sternal border or apex (Fig. 139–2). Although it can normally be split, if a split S₁ is heard, the possibility of an ejection click or, much less commonly, S₄ should be considered. **S₂** is associated with closure of the aortic and pulmonary valves and generally is considered an important and valuable portion of the cardiovascular examination. S₂ should normally split with inspiration and be single with expiration. Abnormalities of the splitting and intensity of the pulmonic component are associated with significant anatomic and physiologic abnormalities (Table 139–3). **S₃** is heard in early diastole and is related to rapid ventricular filling. It is best heard at the lower left sternal border or apex and may be a normal sound. A loud S₃ is abnormal and heard in conditions with dilated ventricles. **S₄** occurs late in diastole just before S₁. It is best heard at the lower left sternal border/apex and is associated with

TABLE 139–3. Abnormal Second Heart Sound
Single S_2
Pulmonary hypertension (severe)
One semilunar valve (aortic atresia, pulmonary atresia, truncus arteriosus)
Malposed great arteries (d-TGA, l-TGA)
Severe aortic stenosis
Widely split S_2
Increased flow across valve (ASD, PAPVR)
Prolonged flow across valve (pulmonary stenosis)
Electrical delay (right bundle branch block)
Early aortic closure (severe mitral regurgitation)
Paradoxically split S_2
Severe aortic stenosis
Abnormal intensity of P_2
Increased in pulmonary hypertension
Decreased in severe pulmonary stenosis, tetralogy of Fallot

ASD, atrial septal defect; d-TGA, dextroposed transposition of the great arteries; l-TGA, levotransposed transposition of the great arteries; PAPVR, partial anomalous pulmonary venous return.

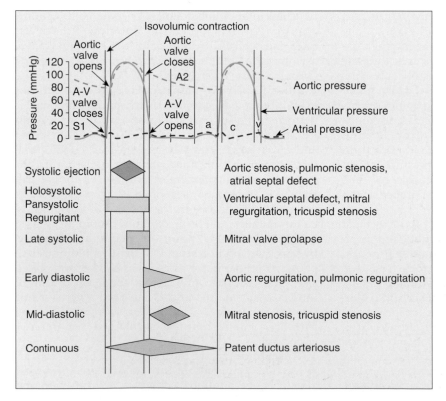

Figure 139–2

Timing of heart murmurs. A-V, atrioventricular.

decreased ventricular compliance. It is rare and is always abnormal.

Clicks

A click implies a valvular abnormality or dilated great artery and may be ejection or mid-systolic in timing. A mid-systolic click is associated with mitral valve prolapse. There may or may not be an associated murmur. **Ejection clicks** occur early in systole. Pulmonary ejection clicks are best heard at the left upper sternal border and vary in intensity with respiration. Aortic clicks are often louder at the apex, left mid-sternal border, or right upper sternal border. They do not vary with respiration.

Murmurs

Murmur evaluation should determine timing and duration of the murmur, location, intensity, radiation, and frequency or pitch of the murmur. The timing is most important in determining a murmur's significance and can be used to develop a differential diagnosis and to determine the need for further evaluation (see Fig. 139–2). Murmurs should be classified as **systolic**, **diastolic**, or **continuous** (Fig. 139–3). Most murmurs are systolic and can be divided further into systolic ejection murmurs or holosystolic (also called *pansystolic* or *regurgitant*) murmurs. **Ejection murmurs** are crescendo-decrescendo with a short time between S_1

and the onset of the murmur (isovolumic contraction). Systolic ejection murmurs require the ejection of blood from the ventricle and may occur with aortic stenosis, pulmonic stenosis, atrial septal defects (ASDs), and coarctation of the aorta. **Holosystolic murmurs** have their onset with S_1, and there is flow during isovolumic contraction. The murmur has a plateau quality. Holosystolic murmurs may be heard with ventricular septal defects (VSDs), mitral regurgitation, or tricuspid regurgitation. A "late regurgitant" murmur may be heard after the mid-systolic click in mitral valve prolapse.

Murmurs are often heard along the path of blood flow. Ejection murmurs usually are best heard at the base of the heart, whereas holosystolic murmurs are louder at the lower left sternal border and apex. Pulmonary ejection murmurs radiate to the back and axilla, whereas aortic ejection murmurs radiate to the neck. The **intensity** or loudness of a heart murmur is graded I through VI (Table 139–4). The **frequency** or pitch of a murmur provides information regarding the hemodynamics or pressure gradient. The higher the pressure gradient across a narrowed area (valve, vessel, or defect), the faster the flow and higher the frequency of the murmur. Low-frequency murmurs imply low pressure gradients and mild obstruction.

Diastolic murmurs are much less common than systolic murmurs, and all should be considered abnormal. Early diastolic murmurs occur when there is regurgitation through the aortic or pulmonary valves.

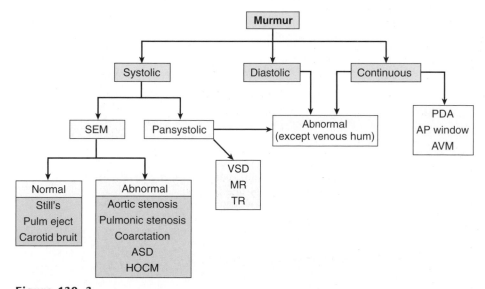

Figure 139–3

Differential diagnosis of heart murmur based on timing. AP, aortic pulmonary; ASD, atrial septal defect; AVM, arteriovenous malformation; HOCM, hypertrophic obstructed cardiomyopathy; MR, mitral regurgitation; PDA, patent ductus arteriosus; Pulm eject, pulmonary ejection murmur; SEM, systolic ejection murmur; TR, tricuspid regurgitation; VSD, ventricular septal defect.

TABLE 139–4. Heart Murmur Intensity	
Grade I	Very soft, heard in quiet room with cooperative patient
Grade II	Easily heard but not loud
Grade III	Loud but no thrill
Grade IV	Loud with palpable thrill
Grade V	Loud with thrill, audible with stethoscope at 45-degree angle
Grade VI	Loud with thrill, audible with stethoscope off chest 1 cm

Mid-diastolic murmurs are heard when there is increased flow across the mitral or tricuspid valves (VSD, ASD), or when there is anatomic stenosis at these valves.

Continuous murmurs are heard when there is flow throughout the entire cardiac cycle and are abnormal with one common exception, the **venous hum** (Table 139–5). A PDA is the most common abnormal continuous murmur. Continuous murmurs can also be heard with coarctation of the aorta when collateral vessels are present.

Normal physiologic or **innocent murmurs** are common, occurring in at least 80% of normal infants and children at some time in life. They have also been called *benign, functional, vibratory,* and *flow murmurs.*

These normal murmurs are heard most often during the first 6 months of life, from 3 to 6 years of age, and in early adolescence. Characteristic findings of innocent murmurs include the quality of the sound, lack of significant radiation, and significant alteration in the intensity of the murmur with positional changes (see Table 139–5). Most importantly, the cardiovascular history and examination are otherwise normal. The presence of symptoms, including failure to thrive or dysmorphic features, should make one more cautious about diagnosing a "normal" murmur. Diastolic, holosystolic, late systolic, and continuous (except for the venous hum) murmurs and the presence of a thrill are not normal.

LABORATORY AND IMAGING TESTS
Pulse Oximetry

Pulse oximetry is a painless, inexpensive, and valuable tool to assess oxygen saturation in a patient with possible congenital heart disease. The ability to recognize cyanosis varies depending on experience and the patient's hemoglobin. Mild desaturation that is not clinically apparent may be the only early finding in complex congenital heart defects. Comparing pulse oximetry between the right arm and a lower extremity

TABLE 139–5. Normal or Innocent Heart Murmurs		
Murmur	**Timing/Location/Quality**	**Usual Age**
Still murmur/vibratory murmur	Systolic ejection murmur LLSB or between LLSB and apex Grade I-III/VI Vibratory, musical quality Intensity decreases in upright position	3-6 yr
Venous hum	Continuous murmur Infraclavicular region (right > left) Grade I-III/VI Louder in upright position Changes with compression of jugular vein or turning head	3-6 yr
Carotid bruit	Systolic ejection murmur Neck, over carotid artery Grade I-III/VI	Any age
Adolescent ejection murmur	Systolic ejection murmur LUSB Grade I-III/VI Usually softer when upright position Does not radiate to back	8-14 yr
Peripheral pulmonic stenosis Murmur of infancy	Systolic ejection murmur Axilla and back, LUSB/RUSB Grade I-II/VI Harsh, short, high frequency	Newborn-6 mo

LLSB, left lower scapular border; LUSB, left upper scapular border; RUSB, right upper scapular border.

may allow diagnosis of a ductal dependent lesion where desaturated blood flows right to left across a PDA to perfuse the lower body.

Electrocardiography

The ECG is a valuable, noninvasive screening tool to assess cardiac disease. The 12-lead ECG provides information about the **rate**, **rhythm**, **depolarization**, and **repolarization** of the cardiac cells and the size and wall thickness of the chambers. It should be assessed for rate, rhythm, axis (P wave, QRS, and T wave), intervals (P-R, QRS, Q-Tc) (Fig. 139–4), and voltages (left atrial, right atrial, left ventricular, right ventricular) adjusted for the child's age.

The **P wave** represents atrial depolarization. A criterion for right atrial enlargement is an increase of the amplitude of the P wave, reflected best in lead II. The diagnosis of left atrial enlargement is made by prolongation of the second portion of the P wave, exhibited best in the chest leads.

The **P-R interval** is measured from the beginning of the P wave to the beginning of the QRS complex. It represents the time it takes for electricity to travel from the high right atrium to the ventricular myocardium. The P-R interval increases with age. Conduction time is shortened when the conduction velocity is increased (glycogen storage disease) or when the atrioventricular node is bypassed (Wolff-Parkinson-White syndrome). A prolonged P-R interval usually indicates slow conduction through the atrioventricular node. Diseases in the atrial myocardium, bundle of His, or Purkinje system may also contribute to prolonged P-R intervals.

The **QRS complex** represents ventricular depolarization. A specific sequence of activation is present and can be observed on the ECG. A greater volume or mass of the ventricles causes a greater magnitude of the complex. The proximity of the right ventricle to the chest surface accentuates that ventricle's contribution to the complex. Changes in the normal ECG occur with age, and normative data for each age group must be known to make a diagnosis from the ECG.

The **Q-T interval** is measured from the beginning of the QRS complex to the end of the T wave. The corrected Q-T interval (corrected for rate) should be less than 0.45 second ($QTc = QT/\sqrt{RR}$). The interval may be prolonged in children with hypocalcemia or hypokalemia. It is also prolonged in a group of children at risk for severe ventricular arrhythmias and sudden death (**prolonged Q-T syndrome**). Drugs such as quinidine and erythromycin may prolong the Q-T interval.

Chest Radiography

A systematic approach to reading a chest radiograph includes assessment of extracardiac structures, the shape and size of the heart, and the size and position of the pulmonary artery and aorta (Fig. 139–5). Abnormalities of the thoracic skeleton, diaphragms, lungs, or upper abdomen may be associated with congenital heart defects. Assessment of the location and size of the heart and **cardiac silhouette** may suggest a cardiac defect. On a good inspiratory film, the cardiothoracic ratio should be less than 55% in infants younger than 1 year of age and less than 50% in older children and adolescents. An enlarged heart may be due to an increased volume load (large left-to-right shunt from a VSD) or may be due to myocardial dysfunction (dilated cardiomyopathy). A normal heart size virtually rules out CHF; however, a large heart is not diagnostic of

Figure 139–4

Nomenclature of ECG waves and intervals.

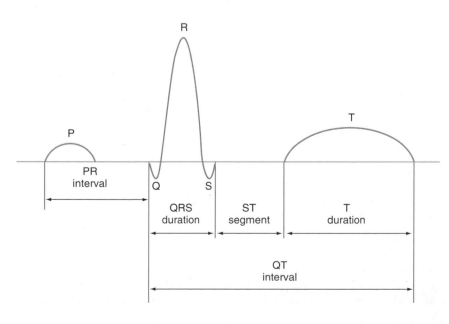

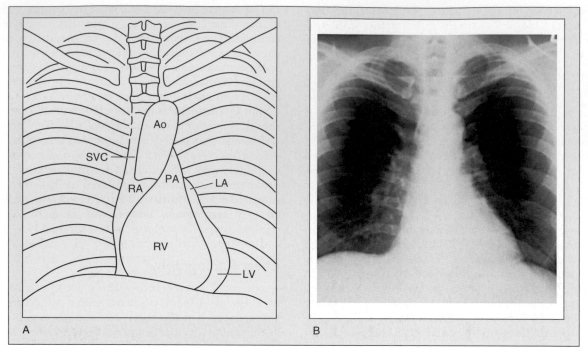

Figure 139–5

A, Parts of the heart whose outlines can be identified on a routine chest x-ray. **B,** Routine posteroanterior x-ray of the normal cardiac silhouette. Ao, aorta; LA, left atrium; LV, left ventricle; PA, pulmonary artery; RA, right atrium; RV, right ventricle; SVC, superior vena cava. (From Andreoli TE, Carpenter CCJ, Plum F, et al [eds]: Cecil Essentials of Medicine, 2nd ed. Philadelphia, WB Saunders, 1990.)

CHF. The shape of the heart may suggest specific congenital heart defects. The most common examples are the "boot-shaped" heart seen with tetralogy of Fallot, the "egg-on-a-string" seen with dextroposed transposition of the great arteries, and the "snowman" seen with supracardiac total anomalous pulmonary venous return. The chest x-ray can be helpful in the assessment of **pulmonary blood flow**. Defects associated with left-to-right shunting have increased pulmonary blood flow or "shunt vascularity" on x-ray, whereas right-to-left shunts have decreased pulmonary blood flow.

Echocardiography

Echocardiography has become the most important noninvasive tool in the diagnosis and management of cardiac disease. Using ultrasound, two-dimensional echocardiography provides a full **anatomic evaluation** in most congenital heart defects (Fig. 139–6). **Physiologic data** on the direction of blood flow can be obtained with the use of pulsed, continuous wave, and color flow Doppler. Imaging from multiple views provides an assessment of the **three-dimensional spatial relationships**. Prenatal or fetal echocardiography can diagnose congenital heart disease by 18 weeks of gestation. Prenatal diagnosis allows for delivery of the infant at a tertiary care hospital, eliminating the need to transport critically ill newborns and improving the timeliness of therapy. Many congenital heart defects now are surgically repaired based on the echocardiogram without need for cardiac catheterization.

Transesophageal echocardiography provides better imaging in patients when transthoracic imaging is inadequate. It is also used intraoperatively to assess results and cardiac function after surgery. Transesophageal echocardiography and intracardiac echocardiography are used to guide interventional catheterization and radiofrequency ablation of dysrhythmias. Three-dimensional echocardiography now is being used to provide even more precise noninvasive imaging.

Cardiac Catheterization

Cardiac catheterization is performed in patients who need additional anatomic information or precise **hemodynamic information** before operating or establishing a management plan. After gaining access to the vascular system, a catheter is advanced to the heart, and pressures, oxygen saturations, and oxygen content are measured in each chamber and blood vessel entered (Fig. 139–7).

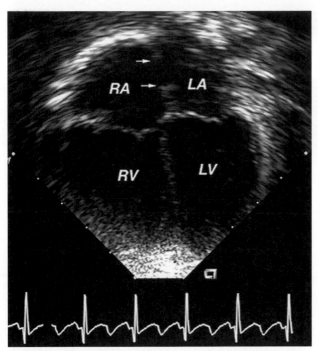

Figure 139–6

Four-chamber echocardiogram of an atrial septal defect. The defect margins are identified by the two arrows. LA, left atrium; LV, left ventricle; RA, right atrium; RV, right ventricle.

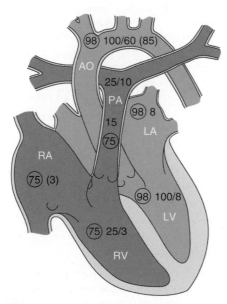

Figure 139–7

The normal heart. AO, aorta; LA, left atrium; LV, left ventricle; PA, pulmonary artery; RA, right atrium; RV, right ventricle. Circled values are oxygen saturations.

This information is used to calculate systemic and pulmonary blood flow and systemic and pulmonary vascular resistance. **Angiography** is performed by injecting contrast material into selected sites to define anatomy and supplement noninvasive information. An increasing percentage of cardiac catheterizations are done to perform an intervention. **Interventional cardiac catheterization** includes balloon dilation of stenotic valves and vessels, stenting of stenotic lesions, closure of collateral vessels by coil embolization, and device closure of PDAs, secundum ASDs, patent foramen ovales, and muscular VSDs. Catheterization is also done to assess the electrical system of the heart. **Electrophysiologic studies** allow precise mapping of the electrical activity, can assess the risk of abnormal heart rhythms, and often are done in anticipation of **radiofrequency ablation**. With radiofrequency ablation, the site of a dysrhythmia is altered so that it no longer can cause the dysrhythmia.

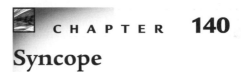

CHAPTER 140

Syncope

ETIOLOGY

Syncope is the transient loss of consciousness and muscle tone that, by history, does not suggest other altered states of consciousness. Presyncope or near-syncope has many or all of the prodromal symptoms without loss of consciousness. Syncope is relatively common and has many causes (Table 140–1). The frequency of episodes and amount of stress and functional impairment caused by syncope vary. Most syncopal events are relatively benign, but can represent a serious cardiac condition that may lead to sudden death.

CLINICAL MANIFESTATIONS

It is useful to divide syncope into typical versus atypical events. **Typical syncopal events** usually occur in the upright position or are related to changing position. Syncope may be associated with anxiety, pain, blood drawing or the sight of blood, fasting, a hot environment, or crowded places. There is a prodrome consisting of "dizziness," lightheadedness, nausea, diaphoresis, visual changes (blacking out), or possibly palpitations. The patient often is described as being pale. Because there is a prodrome or warning, the patient is rarely hurt if he or she falls to the ground. Unconsciousness lasts for less than 1 minute, and a gradual return to normal consciousness occurs

TABLE 140–1. Syncope and Dizziness: Etiology

Diagnosis	History	Symptoms	Description	Heart Rate/ Blood Pressure	Duration	Postsyncope	Recurrence
Neurocardiogenic (vasodepressor)	At rest	Pallor, nausea, visual changes	Brief ± convulsion	↓/↓	<1 min	Residual pallor, sweaty, hot; recurs if child stands	Common
Other vagal							
Vasovagal	Needle stick	Pallor, nausea	Brief ± convulsion	↓/↓	<1 min	Residual pallor; may recur if child stands	Situational
Micturition	Postvoiding	Pallor, nausea	Brief; convulsions rare	↓/↓	<1 min		(+)
Cough (deglutition)	Paroxysmal cough	Cough	Abrupt onset	May not change	<5 min	Fatigue or baseline	(+)
Carotid sinus	Tight collar, turned head	Vague, visual changes	Sudden onset, pallor	Usually ↓/↓	<5 min	Fatigue or baseline	(+)
Metabolic							
Hypoglycemia	Fasting, insulin use	Gradual hunger	Pallor, sweating; loss of consciousness rare	No change or mild tachycardia	Variable	Relieved by eating only	(+)
Neuropsychiatric							
Hyperventilation	Anxiety	SOB, fear, claustrophobia	Agitated, hyperpneic	Mild ↓/↓	<5 min	Fatigue or baseline	(+)
Syncopal migraine	Headache	Aura, migraine, nausea	± Pallor	No change	<10 min	Headache, often occipital	(+)
Seizure disorder	Anytime	± Aura	Convulsion ± incontinence	No change or mild tachycardia	Any duration	Postictal lethargy + confusion	(+)
Hysterical	Always an "audience" present	Psychological distress	Gentle, graceful swoon	No change	Any duration	Normal baseline	(+)
Breath holding (hypoxic)	Agitation or injury	Crying	Cyanosis ± brief convulsion	↓/↓ Frequent asystole	<10 min	Fatigue, residual pallor	(+)
Cardiac syncope							
LVOT obstruction	Exercise	± Chest pain, SOB	Abrupt during or after exertion, pallor	↑/↓	Any duration	Fatigue, residual pallor, and sweating	(+)
Pulmonary hypertension	Anytime, especially exercise	SOB	Cyanosis and pallor	↑/↓	Any duration	Fatigue, residual cyanosis	(+)
Myocarditis	Postviral exercise	SOB, chest pain, palpitations	Pallor	↑/↓	Any duration	Fatigue	(+)
Tumor or mass	Recumbent, paroxysmal	SOB ± chest pain	Pallor	↑/↓	Any duration	Baseline	(+)
Coronary artery disease	Exercise	SOB ± chest pain	Pallor	↑/↓	Any duration	Fatigue, chest pain	(+)
Dysrhythmia	Anytime	Palpitations ± chest pain	Pallor	↑ or ↑/↓	Usually <10 min	Fatigue or baseline	(+)

LVOT, left ventricular outflow obstruction; SOB, shortness of breath; ±, with or without; (+), yes but not consistent or predictable.
From Lewis DA: Syncope and dizziness. In Kliegman RM (ed): Practical Strategies in Pediatric Diagnosis and Therapy. Philadelphia, WB Saunders, 1996.

relatively quickly. Most of these syncopal episodes are vasovagal or neurocardiogenic in origin. The physical examination is normal.

Atypical syncope is syncope during exercise without prodromal symptoms or syncope preceded by palpitations or chest pain. Because there is no warning, significant injury may occur. A family history of unexplained sudden death or an abnormal cardiovascular physical examination also warrants more extensive cardiac evaluation. Seizure activity or loss of bowel or bladder control warrants more extensive neurologic evaluation.

DIAGNOSTIC STUDIES

Depending on the number, frequency, and amount of functional impairment, syncopal episodes may require no more than reassurance to the patient and family. If the episodes have a significant impact on daily activities, further evaluation may be indicated. It is appropriate to do an ECG on any patient presenting with a chief complaint of syncope with attention to the Q-Tc and P-R intervals (see Chapter 142). Additional testing may include **tilt-table testing** before considering medical therapy.

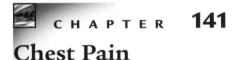

CHAPTER 141
Chest Pain

ETIOLOGY

Chest pain is a common chief complaint in pediatric patients, often generating a significant amount of patient and parental concern. Although chest pain is rarely cardiac in origin in children, common knowledge about atherosclerotic heart disease raises concerns about a child experiencing chest pain. Most chest pain in childhood is musculoskeletal in origin. A significant amount remains idiopathic, however. Knowledge of the complete differential diagnosis is necessary to make an accurate assessment (Table 141–1).

CLINICAL MANIFESTATIONS

Assessment of a patient with chest pain must include a thorough history to determine what the child is doing at the onset; the location, radiation, quality, and duration of the pain; what makes the pain better and worse during the time that it is present; and any associated symptoms. A good family history and assessment of how much anxiety the symptom is causing are important and often revealing. Although the history

---

TABLE 141–1. Differential Diagnosis of Pediatric Chest Pain

Common

Musculoskeletal
  Costochondritis
  Trauma or muscle overuse/strain
Pulmonary
  Asthma (often exercise induced)
  Severe cough
  Pneumonia
Gastrointestinal
  Reflux esophagitis
Psychogenic
  Anxiety, hyperventilation
Miscellaneous
  Precordial catch syndrome (Texidor's twinge)
  Sickle cell vaso-occlusive crisis
  Idiopathic

Uncommon/Rare

Cardiac
  Ischemia (coronary artery abnormalities, severe AS or PS, HOCM, cocaine)
  Infection/inflammation (myocarditis, pericarditis, Kawasaki disease)
  Dysrhythmia
  Mitral valve prolapse
Musculoskeletal
  Abnormalities of rib cage/thoracic spine
  Tietze syndrome
  Slipping rib
  Tumor
Pulmonary
  Pleurisy
  Pneumothorax, pneumomediastinum
  Pleural effusion
  Pulmonary embolism
Gastrointestinal
  Esophageal foreign body
  Esophageal spasm
Psychogenic
  Conversion symptoms
  Somatization disorders
  Depression

AS, aortic stenosis; HOCM, hypertrophic obstructive cardiomyopathy; PS, pulmonic stenosis.

---

alone often determines the etiology, a careful general physical examination should focus on the chest wall, heart, lungs, and abdomen. A history of chest pain associated with exertion, syncope, or palpitations, or acute onset associated with fever suggests a cardiac etiology. Cardiac causes of chest pain are generally ischemic, inflammatory, or arrhythmic in origin.

DIAGNOSTIC STUDIES

Tests rarely may be indicated based on the history or the need to supplement clinical findings and reassure the patient and family. A chest x-ray, ECG, 24-hour Holter monitoring, echocardiogram, and exercise stress testing may be obtained based on history and examination. Referral to a pediatric cardiologist is based on the history, physical examination findings, family history, and frequently the high level of anxiety in the patient or family members regarding the pain.

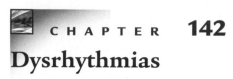

CHAPTER 142
Dysrhythmias

ETIOLOGY AND DIFFERENTIAL DIAGNOSIS

Cardiac dysrhythmias or abnormal heart rhythms are uncommon in pediatrics, but may be caused by infection and inflammation, structural lesions, metabolic abnormalities, and intrinsic conduction abnormalities (Table 142–1). Many pediatric dysrhythmias are normal variants that do not require treatment or even further evaluation.

Sinus rhythm originates in the sinus node and has a normal-axis P wave (upright in leads I and AVF) preceding each QRS complex. Because normal rates vary with age, sinus bradycardia and sinus tachycardia are defined based on age. **Sinus arrhythmia** is a common finding in children and represents a normal variation in the heart rate associated with breathing. The heart rate increases with inspiration and decreases with expiration, producing a recurring pattern on the ECG tracing. Sinus arrhythmia does not require further evaluation or treatment.

Atrial Dysrhythmias

A **wandering atrial pacemaker** (Table 142–2) is a change in the morphology of the P waves with variable P-R interval and normal QRS complex. This is a benign finding, requiring no further evaluation or treatment.

Premature atrial contractions are relatively common prenatally and in infants. A premature P wave, usually with an abnormal axis consistent with its ectopic origin, is present. The premature atrial activity may be blocked (no QRS following it), conducted normally (normal QRS present), or conducted aberrantly (a widened, altered QRS morphology). Premature atrial contractions are usually benign and, if present around the time of delivery, often disappear during the first few weeks of life.

TABLE 142–1. Etiology of Arrhythmias
Drugs
Intoxication (cocaine, tricyclic antidepressants, and others)
Antiarrhythmic agents (proarrhythmic agents [quinidine])
Sympathomimetic agents (caffeine, theophylline, ephedrine, and others)
Digoxin
Infection and Postinfection
Endocarditis
Lyme disease
Diphtheria
Myocarditis
Guillain-Barré syndrome
Rheumatic fever
Metabolic-Endocrine
Cardiomyopathy
Electrolyte disturbances ($\downarrow\uparrow K^+$, $\downarrow\uparrow Ca^{2+}$, $\downarrow Mg^{2+}$)
Uremia
Thyrotoxicosis
Pheochromocytoma
Porphyria
Mitochondrial myopathies
Structural Lesions
Mitral valve prolapse
Ventricular tumor
Ventriculotomy
Pre-excitation and aberrant conduction system (Wolff-Parkinson-White syndrome)
Congenital heart defects
Arrhythmogenic right ventricle (dysplasia)
Other Causes
Adrenergic-induced
Prolonged Q-T interval
Maternal SLE
Idiopathic
Central venous catheter

SLE, systemic lupus erythematosus.

Atrial flutter and **atrial fibrillation** are uncommon dysrhythmias in pediatrics and usually present after surgical repair of complex congenital heart disease. They may also be seen in patients with myocarditis or in association with drug toxicity.

Supraventricular tachycardia (SVT) is the most common symptomatic arrhythmia in pediatric patients. The rhythm is a rapid, regular rate with a narrow complex QRS. The rate of SVT varies with age. SVT in infants is often 280 to 300 beats/min with slower rates for older children and adolescents. The tachycardia has an abrupt onset and termination. In a

TABLE 142–2. Arrhythmias in Children

Type	ECG Characteristics	Treatment
Supraventricular tachycardia	Rate usually >200 beats/min (180-320 beats/min); abnormal atrial rate for age; ventricular rate may be slower because of AV block; P waves usually present and are related to QRS complex; normal QRS complexes unless aberrant conduction is present	Increase vagal tone (bag of ice water to face, Valsalva maneuver); adenosine; digoxin; sotalol; electrical cardioversion if acutely ill; catheter ablation
Atrial flutter	Atrial rate usually 300 beats/min, with varying degrees of block; sawtooth flutter waves	Digoxin, sotalol, cardioversion
Premature ventricular contraction	Premature, wide, unusually shaped QRS complex, with large inverted T wave	None if normal heart and if premature ventricular contractions disappear on exercise; lidocaine, procainamide
Ventricular tachycardia	≥3 Premature ventricular beats; AV dissociation; fusion beats, blocked retrograde AV conduction; sustained if >30 sec; rate 120-240 beats/min	Lidocaine, procainamide, propranolol, amiodarone, cardioversion
Ventricular fibrillation	No distinct QRS complex or T waves; irregular undulations with varied amplitude and contour, no conducted pulse	Nonsynchronized cardioversion
Complete heart block	Atria and ventricles have independent pacemakers; AV dissociation; escape-pacemaker is at atrioventricular junction if congenital	Awake rate <55 beats/min in neonate or <40 beats/min in adolescent or hemodynamic instability requires permanent pacemaker
First-degree heart block	Prolonged P-R interval for age	Observe, obtain digoxin level if on therapy
Mobitz type I (Wenckebach) second-degree heart block	Progressive lengthening of P-R interval until P wave is not followed by conducted QRS complex	Observe, correct underlying electrolyte or other abnormalities
Mobitz type II second-degree heart block	Sudden nonconduction of P wave with loss of QRS complex without progressive P-R interval lengthening	Consider pacemaker
Sinus tachycardia	Rate <240 beats/min	Treat fever, remove sympathomimetic drugs

AV, atrioventricular.

child with a structurally normal heart, most episodes are relatively asymptomatic other than a pounding heart beat. If there is structural heart disease or the episode is prolonged (>12 hours), there may be alteration in the cardiac output and development of symptoms of CHF. Although most patients with SVT have structurally normal hearts and normal baseline ECGs, some children have Wolff-Parkinson-White syndrome or pre-excitation as the cause of the dysrhythmia.

Ventricular Dysrhythmias

Premature ventricular contractions are less common than premature atrial contractions in infancy but more common in older children and adolescents (see Table 142-2). The premature beat is not preceded by a P wave, and the QRS complex is wide and bizarre. If the heart is structurally normal, and the premature ventricular contractions are singleton, are uniform in focus, and disappear with increased heart rate, they are usually benign and require no treatment. Any deviation from this presentation, including a history of syncope or a family history of sudden death, requires further investigation and possibly treatment with antiarrhythmic medications.

Ventricular tachycardia, defined as three or more consecutive premature ventricular contractions, is also relatively rare in pediatric patients. Although there are multiple causes of ventricular tachycardia, it usually is a sign of serious cardiac dysfunction or pathology. Rapid rate ventricular tachycardia results in decreased cardiac output and cardiovascular instability. Treatment in symptomatic patients is synchronized cardioversion. Medical management with lidocaine or amiodarone may be appropriate in a conscious asymptomatic patient. Complete evaluation of the etiology is necessary, including electrophysiologic study.

TABLE 142–3. Classification of Drugs for Antiarrhythmia

Class	Action	Examples
I	Depresses phase o depolarization (velocity of upstroke of action potential); sodium channel blockers	
Ia	Prolongs QRS complex and Q-T interval	Quinidine, procainamide, disopyramide
Ib	Significant effect on abnormal conduction	Lidocaine, mexiletine, phenytoin, tocainide
Ic	Prolongs QRS complex and P-R interval	Flecainide, propafenone, moricizine?
II	β blockade, slows sinus rate, prolonged P-R interval	Propranolol, atenolol, acebutolol
III	Prolonged action potential; prolonged P-R, Q-T intervals, QRS complex; sodium and calcium channel blocker	Bretylium, amiodarone, sotalol
IV	Calcium channel blockade; reduced sinus and AV node pacemaker activity and conduction; prolonged P-R interval	Verapamil and other calcium channel blocking agents

AV, atrioventricular.

Heart Block

First-degree heart block is the presence of a prolonged P-R interval. It is asymptomatic and when present in otherwise normal children requires no evaluation or treatment. **Second-degree heart block** is when some, but not all, of the P waves are followed by a QRS complex. Mobitz type I (also known as *Wenckebach*) is characterized by a progressive prolongation of the P-R interval until a QRS is dropped. It usually does not progress to other forms of heart block and does not require further evaluation or treatment in otherwise normal children. Mobitz type II is present when the P-R interval does not change, but a QRS is intermittently dropped. This form may progress to complete heart block and may require pacemaker placement. **Third-degree heart block**, which may be congenital or acquired, is present when there is no relationship between the atrial and ventricular activity. The ventricular rate is much slower than the atrial rate. **Congenital complete heart block** is associated with maternal collagen vascular disease (systemic lupus erythematosus) or congenital heart disease. The acquired form most often occurs after cardiac surgery, but may be secondary to infection, inflammation, or drugs.

TREATMENT

Most atrial dysrhythmias require no intervention. Treatment of SVT depends on presentation and symptoms. Acute treatment of SVT in infants usually consists of **vagal maneuvers**, such as application of cold (ice bag) to the face. IV **adenosine** usually converts the dysrhythmia because the atrioventricular node forms a part of the reentry circuit in most patients with SVT. In patients with cardiovascular compromise at the time of presentation, **synchronized cardioversion** is indicated using 1 to 2 J/kg. In patients with a complaint of palpitations, it is important to document heart rate and rhythm during their symptoms before considering therapeutic options. The frequency, length, and associated symptoms of the episodes and what is required to convert the rhythm determines the need for treatment. Some patients may not require anything more than education regarding the dysrhythmia and follow-up. Ongoing pharmacologic management with either **digoxin** or a **β-blocker** is usually the first choice. However, digoxin is contraindicated in patients with Wolff-Parkinson-White syndrome. Additional antiarrhythmic medications rarely may be needed. In difficult-to-manage cases, patients who are symptomatic, and patients not wanting to take daily medications, **radiofrequency ablation** may be performed.

A variety of antiarrhythmic agents are used to treat ventricular dysrhythmias that require intervention (Table 142–3). Management of third-degree heart block depends on the ventricular rate and presence of symptoms. Treatment, if needed, often requires placement of a pacemaker.

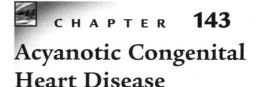

CHAPTER **143**

Acyanotic Congenital Heart Disease

ETIOLOGY AND EPIDEMIOLOGY

Congenital heart disease occurs in 8 per 1000 births. The spectrum of lesions ranges from asymptomatic to fatal. Although most cases of congenital heart disease are multifactorial, some lesions are associated with chromosomal disorders, single gene defects,

TABLE 143–1. Classification of Congenital Cardiac Defects

| Stenotic | Shunting | | Mixing |
	Right→Left	Left→Right	
Aortic stenosis	Tetralogy	Patent ductus arteriosus	Truncus
Pulmonic stenosis	Transposition	Ventricular septal defect	TAPVR
Coarctation of the aorta	Tricuspid atresia	Atrial septal defect	HLH

HLH, hypoplastic left heart syndrome; TAPVR, total anomalous pulmonary venous return.

teratogens, or maternal metabolic disease (see Table 139–2). Congenital heart defects can be divided into three broad pathophysiologic groups: (1) **left-to-right shunts**, (2) **right-to-left shunts**, and (3) **obstructive stenotic lesions** (Table 143–1). Acyanotic congenital heart disease includes left-to-right shunts resulting in an increase in pulmonary blood flow and obstructive lesions, which usually have normal pulmonary blood flow. The most common left-to-right shunts are VSD, ASD, and PDA. All three lesions have normal systemic oxygen saturations in the presence of excessive pulmonary blood flow.

VENTRICULAR SEPTAL DEFECT
Etiology and Epidemiology

The ventricular septum is a complex structure that can be divided into four components. The largest component is the **muscular septum**. The inlet or posterior septum comprises **endocardial cushion** tissue. The subarterial or **supracristal septum** comprises conotruncal tissue. The **membranous septum** is below the aortic valve and is relatively small. VSDs occur when any of these components fails to develop normally (Fig. 143–1). VSDs are the most common congenital heart defect, accounting for 25% of all congenital heart disease. **Perimembranous VSDs** are the most common of all VSDs (67%).

Although the location of the VSD is important prognostically and in approach to repair, physiologically, the amount of flow crossing a VSD depends on the size of the defect and the pulmonary vascular resistance. Even large VSDs are not symptomatic at birth because the pulmonary vascular resistance is normally elevated at this time. As the pulmonary vascular resistance normally decreases over the first 6 to 8 weeks of life, however, the amount of shunt increases, and symptoms may develop.

Clinical Manifestations

The size of the VSD affects the clinical presentation. Small VSDs, with little shunt, are often asymptomatic, other than a loud murmur. Moderate to large VSDs result in pulmonary overcirculation and CHF, presenting as fatigue, diaphoresis with feedings, and poor growth. The typical physical finding with a VSD is a **pansystolic murmur** usually heard best at the lower left sternal border. There may be a thrill in the same region. Larger shunts result in increased flow across the mitral valve causing a **mid-diastolic murmur** at the apex. The splitting of S_2 and intensity of P_2 depend on the pulmonary artery pressure.

Imaging Studies

ECG and chest x-ray findings depend on the size of the VSD. Small VSDs may have normal studies. Larger VSDs cause volume overload to the left side of the heart resulting in ECG findings of left atrial and ventricular enlargement and hypertrophy. A chest radiograph may reveal cardiomegaly, enlargement of the left ventricle, and an increase in the pulmonary artery silhouette and increased pulmonary blood flow. Pulmonary hypertension due to either increased flow or increased

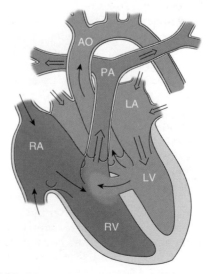

Figure 143–1

Ventricular septal defect. AO, aorta; LA, left atrium; LV, left ventricle; PA, pulmonary artery; RA, right atrium; RV, right ventricle.

pulmonary vascular resistance may lead to right ventricular enlargement and hypertrophy.

Treatment

Approximately 35% of all VSDs close spontaneously. Small VSDs usually close spontaneously; if they do not close, surgical closure may not be required, but **prophylactic antibiotics** are needed to prevent subacute bacterial endocarditis. Initial treatment for moderate to large VSDs includes **diuretics** and **digoxin**. Continued poor growth or pulmonary hypertension despite therapy requires closure of the defect. Most VSDs are closed in **surgery**, but some VSDs, especially muscular defects, can be closed with **devices** placed at cardiac catheterization.

ATRIAL SEPTAL DEFECT

Etiology and Epidemiology

During the embryologic development of the heart, a septum grows toward the endocardial cushions to divide the atria. **Failure of septal growth or excessive reabsorption** of tissue leads to ASDs (Fig. 143–2). ASDs represent approximately 10% of all congenital heart defects. A **secundum defect**, with the hole being in the region of the foramen ovale, is the most common ASD. A **primum ASD**, located near the endocardial cushions, may be part of a complete atrioventricular canal defect, but can be present with an intact ventricular septum. The least common ASD is the **sinus**

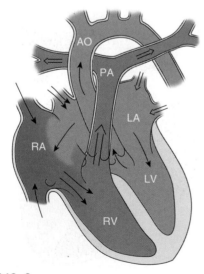

Figure 143–2

Atrial septal defect. AO, aorta; LA, left atrium; LV, left ventricle; PA, pulmonary artery; RA, right atrium; RV, right ventricle.

venosus defect, which may be associated with anomalous pulmonary venous return.

Clinical Manifestations

Regardless of the site of the ASD, the pathophysiology and amount of shunting depend on the size of the defect and the relative compliance of the right and left ventricles. Even with large ASDs and significant shunts, infants and children are rarely symptomatic. A prominent left precordium with a **right ventricular impulse** at the left lower sternal border often can be palpated. A soft (grade I or II) **systolic ejection murmur** in the region of the right ventricular outflow tract and a **fixed split S₂** (owing to overload of the right ventricle with prolonged ejection into the pulmonary circuit) are often audible. A larger shunt may result in a mid-diastolic murmur at the left lower sternal border as a result of the increased volume passing across the tricuspid valve.

Imaging Studies

ECG and chest x-ray findings reflect the **increased blood flow** through the right atrium, right ventricle, pulmonary arteries, and lungs. The ECG may show **right axis deviation** and **right ventricular hypertrophy**. A chest radiograph may show cardiomegaly, right atrial enlargement, and a prominent pulmonary artery.

Treatment

Medical management is rarely indicated; **prophylaxis** for subacute bacterial endocarditis is warranted for nonsecundum ASDs. If a significant shunt is still present at around 3 years of age, **closure** is usually recommended. Many secundum ASDs can be closed with an ASD **closure device** in the catheterization laboratory. Primum and sinus venosus defects require **surgical closure**.

PATENT DUCTUS ARTERIOSUS

Etiology and Epidemiology

The ductus arteriosus allows blood to flow from the pulmonary artery to the aorta during fetal life. Failure of the normal closure of this vessel results in a PDA (Fig. 143–3). With a falling pulmonary vascular resistance after birth, left-to-right shunting of blood and increased pulmonary blood flow occur. Excluding premature infants, PDAs represent approximately 5% to 10% of congenital heart disease.

Clinical Manifestations

Symptoms depend on the amount of extra blood flow to the lungs. The magnitude of the shunt, which can

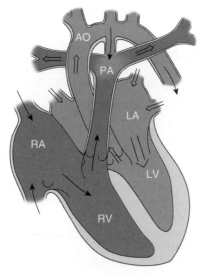

Figure 143–3

Patent ductus arteriosus. AO, aorta; LA, left atrium; LV, left ventricle; PA, pulmonary artery; RA, right atrium; RV, right ventricle.

be similar to a VSD, depends on the size of the PDA (including diameter, length, and tortuosity) and the pulmonary vascular resistance. Patients with small PDAs are asymptomatic. Moderate to larger shunts produce the symptoms of CHF as the pulmonary vascular resistance decreases over the first 6 to 8 weeks of life.

The physical examination depends on the size of the shunt. A **widened pulse pressure** is often present due to the runoff of blood into the pulmonary circulation during diastole. A **continuous machine-like murmur** can be heard at the left infraclavicular area, and a thrill may be palpable. The murmur radiates along the pulmonary arteries and is often well heard over the left back. Larger shunts with increased flow across the mitral valve may result in a mid-diastolic murmur at the apex and a **hyperdynamic precordium**. Splitting of S₂ and the intensity of the P₂ depend on the pulmonary artery pressure. Higher pulmonary pressures result in greater intensity of P₂ and may result in an earlier closing of the pulmonary valve.

Imaging Studies

ECG and chest x-ray findings are normal with small PDAs. Moderate to large shunts may result in a **full pulmonary artery silhouette** and **increased pulmonary vascularity**. ECG findings vary from normal to evidence of left ventricular hypertrophy. If pulmonary hypertension is present, there is also right ventricular hypertrophy.

Treatment

Spontaneous closure of a PDA after a few weeks of age is uncommon in full-term infants. Moderate and large PDAs may be managed initially with **diuretics** and **digoxin**, but eventually require closure. Closure of small PDAs also is recommended because of the risk of subacute bacterial endocarditis. Most PDAs can be closed in the catheterization laboratory by either **coil embolization** or a **PDA closure device**.

ENDOCARDIAL CUSHION DEFECT
Etiology and Epidemiology

Endocardial cushion defects, also referred to as **atrioventricular canal defects**, may be complete or partial (Fig. 143–4). The defect occurs as the result of abnormal development of the endocardial cushion tissue, resulting in failure of the septum to fuse with the endocardial cushion; this results in **abnormal atrioventricular valves** as well. The complete defect results in a primum ASD, a posterior or inlet VSD, and clefts in the anterior leaflet of the mitral and septal leaflet of the tricuspid valves. In addition to left-to-right shunting at both levels, there may be **atrioventricular valvular insufficiency**.

Clinical Manifestations

The symptoms of **CHF** usually develop as the pulmonary vascular resistance decreases over the first 6 to

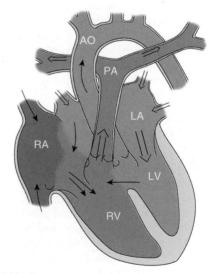

Figure 143–4

Atrioventricular canal defects. AO, aorta; LA, left atrium; LV, left ventricle; PA, pulmonary artery; RA, right atrium; RV, right ventricle.

8 weeks of life. Symptoms may be earlier and more severe if significant atrioventricular valve insufficiency is present. Pulmonary hypertension resulting from increased pulmonary circulation often develops early; this results in a **prominent S₂**. The presence of murmurs varies depending on the balance of flows. If intracardiac dynamics are balanced, there is little shunting and no significant murmur. If dynamics are less balanced, murmurs consistent with an ASD, VSD, or valvular insufficiency may be heard. Growth is usually poor. Many children with Down syndrome have complete endocardial cushion defects.

Imaging Tests

The diagnosis usually is made with echocardiography. A chest radiograph reveals **cardiomegaly** with enlargement of all chambers and the presence of **increased vascularity**. An ECG reveals **left axis deviation** and **combined ventricular hypertrophy** and may show combined atrial enlargement.

Treatment

Initial management includes digoxin and diuretics for treatment of CHF. **Surgical repair** of the entire defect ultimately is required, however.

PULMONARY STENOSIS
Etiology

Pulmonary stenosis accounts for approximately 10% of all congenital heart disease and can be **valvular**, **subvalvular**, or **supravalvular** in nature. The valve develops early in gestation as the truncus arteriosus develops. Pulmonary stenosis results from the failure of the development of the three leaflets of the valve, insufficient resorption of infundibular tissue, or insufficient canalization of the peripheral pulmonary arteries.

Clinical Manifestations

Regardless of the site of obstruction, symptoms depend on the degree of obstruction present. Infants and children with mild pulmonary stenosis are asymptomatic. Moderate to severe stenosis results in **exertional dyspnea** and easy **fatigability**. Newborns with severe stenosis may be more symptomatic and even cyanotic because of right-to-left shunting at the atrial level.

Pulmonary stenosis causes a **systolic ejection murmur** at the second left intercostal space (P₂), which radiates to the back. A **thrill** may be present. S₂ may be widely split with a quiet pulmonary component. With more severe pulmonary stenosis, an impulse at the left lower sternal border results from **right ventricular hypertrophy**. Valvular stenosis may result in a **click**

that varies with respiration. Worsening stenosis causes an increase in the duration of the murmur and a higher frequency of the sound. Murmurs of **peripheral pulmonary stenosis** vary with the location of the lesions. The systolic ejection murmur is heard distal to the obstruction along the course of blood flow in the pulmonary circulation.

Imaging Tests

ECG and chest x-ray findings are normal in mild stenosis. Moderate to severe stenosis results in **right axis deviation** and **right ventricular hypertrophy**. The heart size is usually normal on chest x-ray, although the main pulmonary artery segment may be prominent because of **poststenotic dilation**. Echocardiography provides assessment of the site of stenosis, degree of hypertrophy, and valve morphology and an estimate of the pressure gradient.

Treatment

Valvular pulmonary stenosis usually does not progress, especially if it is mild. **Balloon valvuloplasty** is usually successful in reducing the gradient to acceptable levels for more significant or symptomatic stenosis. **Surgical repair** is required if balloon valvuloplasty is unsuccessful or when subvalvular (muscular) stenosis is present. **Subacute bacterial endocarditis prophylaxis** is recommended for appropriate indications.

AORTIC STENOSIS
Etiology and Epidemiology

Valvular, **subvalvular**, or **supravalvular aortic stenosis** represents approximately 5% of all congenital heart disease. The valve forms early in gestation, and lesions result from failure of development of the three leaflets or failure of resorption of tissue around the valve.

Clinical Manifestations

Symptoms depend on the degree of stenosis. Mild to moderate obstructions cause no symptoms. More severe stenosis results in symptoms of easy fatigability, exertional chest pain, and syncope. Infants with critical aortic stenosis may present with symptoms of CHF.

A **systolic ejection murmur** is heard at the right second intercostal space along the sternum and radiating into the neck. The murmur increases in length and becomes higher in frequency as the degree of stenosis increases. With valvular stenosis, a **systolic ejection click** often is heard, and a thrill may be present at the right upper sternal border or in the suprasternal notch. The aortic component of S₂ may be decreased in intensity.

Imaging Studies

ECG and chest x-ray findings are normal with mild degrees of stenosis. **Left ventricular hypertrophy** develops with moderate to severe stenosis and is detected on the ECG and chest x-ray. **Poststenotic dilation** of the ascending aorta or aortic knob may be seen on chest radiographs. Echocardiography shows the site of stenosis, valve morphology, and presence of left ventricular hypertrophy and allows estimate of the pressure gradient.

Treatment

The degree of stenosis frequently progresses with growth. Aortic insufficiency often develops or progresses. Serial follow-up with echocardiography is indicated because of the likelihood of progressive obstruction. **Balloon valvuloplasty** is usually the first interventional procedure for significant stenosis. It is not as successful as pulmonary balloon valvuloplasty and has a higher risk of significant valvular insufficiency. **Surgical management** is necessary when balloon valvuloplasty is unsuccessful, or significant valve insufficiency develops. **Subacute bacterial endocarditis prophylaxis** is indicated throughout the child's life.

COARCTATION OF THE AORTA

Etiology and Epidemiology

Coarctation of the aorta occurs in approximately 10% of all congenital heart defects. It is almost always **juxtaductal** in position. During development of the aortic arch, the area near the insertion of the ductus arteriosus fails to develop correctly, resulting in a narrowing of the aortic lumen.

Clinical Manifestations

Timing of presentation depends primarily on the severity of obstruction and associated cardiac defects. Infants presenting with coarctation of the aorta frequently have hypoplastic aortic arches, abnormal aortic valves, and VSDs. They may be **dependent on a patent ductus** to provide flow to the descending aorta. Symptoms develop when the aortic ampulla of the ductus closes. Less severe obstruction causes no symptoms because blood flow into the descending aorta is not dependent on the ductus.

Symptoms, including poor feeding, respiratory distress, and shock, may develop before 2 weeks of age. Classically the **femoral pulses** are weaker and delayed compared with the radial pulses. The blood pressure in the lower extremities is lower than that in the upper extremities. If cardiac function is poor, however, these differences may not be apparent until appropriate resuscitation is accomplished. There may be no murmur, but an S_3 is usually present.

Older children presenting with coarctation of the aorta are usually asymptomatic, although there may be a history of **leg discomfort** with exercise, headache, or epistaxis. Decreased or absent lower extremity pulses, **hypertension** (upper extremity), or a murmur may be present. The murmur of coarctation is typically best heard in the left interscapular area of the back. If significant collaterals have developed, continuous murmurs may be heard throughout the chest. An abnormal aortic valve is present approximately 50% of the time, causing a systolic ejection click and systolic ejection murmur of aortic stenosis.

Imaging Studies

The ECG and chest x-ray show evidence of right ventricular hypertrophy in infantile coarctation with marked **cardiomegaly** and **pulmonary edema**. Echocardiography shows the site of coarctation and associated lesions. In older children, the ECG and chest x-ray usually show left ventricular hypertrophy and a mildly enlarged heart. **Rib notching** may also be seen in older children (>8 years old) with large collaterals. Echocardiography shows the site and degree of coarctation, presence of left ventricular hypertrophy, and aortic valve morphology and function.

Treatment

Management of an infant presenting with cardiac decompensation includes IV infusions of **prostaglandin E_1** (chemically opens the ductus arteriosum), inotropic agents, diuretics, and other supportive care. **Balloon angioplasty** has been done, especially in critically ill infants, but **surgical repair** of the coarctation is most commonly performed.

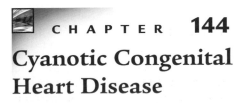

CHAPTER **144**

Cyanotic Congenital Heart Disease

ETIOLOGY

Cyanotic congenital heart disease occurs when some of the systemic venous return crosses from the right heart to the left and goes back to the body without going through the lungs (**right-to-left shunt**). **Cyanosis**, the visible sign of this shunt, occurs when approximately 5 g/100 mL of reduced hemoglobin is present in systemic blood. The patient's hemoglobin level determines the

TABLE 144-1.　Categories of Presenting Symptoms in the Neonate

Symptom	Physiologic Category	Anatomic Cause	Lesion
Cyanosis with respiratory distress	Increased pulmonary blood flow	Transposition	d-Transposition with or without associated lesions
Cyanosis without respiratory distress	Decreased pulmonary blood flow	Right heart obstruction	Tricuspid atresia Ebstein anomaly Pulmonary atresia Pulmonary stenosis Tetralogy of Fallot
Hypoperfusion	Poor cardiac output	Left heart obstruction	Total anomalous pulmonary venous return with obstruction Aortic stenosis Hypoplastic left heart syndrome
	Poor cardiac function	Normal anatomy	Cardiomyopathy Myocarditis
Respiratory distress with desaturation (not visible cyanosis)	Bidirectional shunting	Complete mixing	Truncus arteriosus AV canal Complex single ventricle (including heterotaxias) without pulmonary stenosis
Respiratory distress with normal saturation	Left-to-right shunting	Simple intracardiac shunt	ASD VSD PDA Aortopulmonary window AVM

ASD, atrial septal defect; AV, atrioventricular; AVM, arteriovenous malformation; PDA, patent ductus arteriosus; VSD, ventricular septal defect.

presentation of clinical cyanosis. A polycythemic patient appears cyanotic with a lower percentage of reduced hemoglobin, whereas a patient with anemia requires a higher percentage of reduced hemoglobin for the recognition of cyanosis.

The most common cyanotic congenital heart defects are the 5 "Ts": tetralogy of Fallot, transposition of the great arteries, tricuspid atresia, truncus arteriosus, and total anomalous pulmonary venous return. Other congenital heart defects that allow complete mixing of systemic and pulmonary venous return can present with cyanosis depending on how much pulmonary blood flow is present. Many cyanotic heart lesions present in the neonatal period (Table 144-1).

TETRALOGY OF FALLOT
Etiology and Epidemiology

Tetralogy of Fallot is the most common cyanotic congenital heart defect, representing about 10% of all congenital heart defects (Fig. 144-1). Anatomically, there are four structural defects: **VSD**, **pulmonary stenosis**, **overriding aorta** and **right ventricular hypertrophy**. Tetralogy of Fallot is believed to be due to abnormalities in the septation of the truncus arteriosus into the aorta and pulmonary arteries that occur early in

gestation (3 to 4 weeks). The VSD is large and the pulmonary stenosis is most commonly subvalvular or infundibular. It may also be valvular, supravalvular, or, frequently, a combination of levels of obstruction.

Clinical Manifestations

The degree of cyanosis depends on the amount of pulmonary stenosis. Infants initially may be acyanotic. A **pulmonary stenosis murmur** is the usual initial abnormal finding. If the pulmonary stenosis is more severe, or as it becomes more severe over time, the amount of right-to-left shunting at the VSD increases, and the patient becomes more cyanotic. With increasing severity of pulmonary stenosis, the murmur becomes shorter and softer. In addition to varying degrees of cyanosis and a murmur, a **single S_2** and **right ventricular impulse** at the left sternal border are typical findings.

When **hypoxic ("Tet") spells** occur, they are usually progressive. During a spell, the child typically becomes restless and agitated and may cry inconsolably. An ambulatory toddler may squat. Hyperpnea occurs with gradually increasing cyanosis and loss of the murmur. In severe spells, prolonged unconsciousness and convulsions, hemiparesis, or death may occur. Indepen-

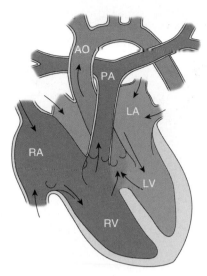

Figure 144–1

Tetralogy of Fallot. AO, aorta; LA, left atrium; LV, left ventricle; PA, pulmonary artery; RA, right atrium; RV, right ventricle.

dent of hypoxic spells, patients with tetralogy are at increased risk for cerebral thromboembolism and cerebral abscesses resulting in part from their right-to-left intracardiac shunt.

Imaging Studies

The ECG usually has **right axis deviation** and **right ventricular hypertrophy**. The classic chest x-ray finding is a **boot-shaped heart** created by the small main pulmonary artery and upturned apex secondary to right ventricular hypertrophy. Echocardiography shows the anatomic features, including the levels of pulmonary stenosis, and provides quantification of the degree of stenosis. Coronary anomalies, specifically a left coronary artery crossing the anterior surface of the right ventricular outflow tract, are present in 5% of patients with tetralogy of Fallot.

Treatment

The natural history of tetralogy of Fallot is progression of pulmonary stenosis and cyanosis. Treatment of hypoxic spells consists of oxygen administration, placing the child in the knee-chest position (to increase venous return), and giving morphine sulfate (to relax the pulmonary infundibulum and for sedation). If necessary, the systemic vascular resistance can be increased acutely through the administration of an α-adrenergic agonist (phenylephrine). If spells are frequent, β-adrenergic antagonists (propranolol) decrease muscular spasm.

Complete surgical repair with closure of the VSD and removal or patching of the pulmonary stenosis can be performed in infancy. Occasionally, **palliative shunt surgery** between the subclavian artery and pulmonary artery is performed for complex forms of tetralogy of Fallot with more complete repair at a later time. **Subacute bacterial endocarditis prophylaxis** is indicated.

TRANSPOSITION OF THE GREAT ARTERIES

Etiology and Epidemiology

Although **dextroposed transposition of the great arteries** represents only about 5% of congenital heart defects, it is the most common cyanotic lesion to present in the newborn period (Fig. 144–2). Transposition of the great arteries is ventriculoarterial discordance secondary to abnormalities of septation of the truncus arteriosus. In dextroposed transposition, the aorta arises from the right ventricle, anterior and to the right of the pulmonary artery, which arises from the left ventricle. This transposition results in desaturated blood returning to the right heart and being pumped back out to the body, while well-oxygenated blood returning from the lungs enters the left heart and is pumped back to the lungs. Without mixing of the two circulations, death occurs quickly. Mixing can occur at the atrial (patent foramen ovale/ASD), ventricular (VSD), or great vessel (PDA) level.

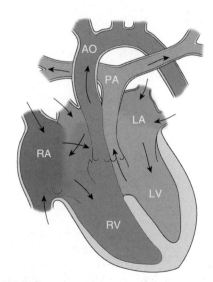

Figure 144–2

Transposition of the great vessels. AO, aorta; LA, left atrium; LV, left ventricle; PA, pulmonary artery; RA, right atrium; RV, right ventricle.

Clinical Manifestations

A history of **cyanosis** is always present, although it may not be profound and depends on the amount of mixing. **Quiet tachypnea** and a **single S₂** are typically present. If the ventricular septum is intact, there may be no murmur.

Children with transposition and a large VSD have improved intracardiac mixing. They may present with signs of CHF. The heart is hyperdynamic, with palpable left and right ventricular impulses. A loud VSD murmur is heard. S₂ is single.

Imaging Studies

ECG findings typically include **right axis deviation** and **right ventricular hypertrophy**. The chest x-ray reveals **increased pulmonary vascularity**, and the cardiac shadow is classically **an egg on a string** created by the narrow superior mediastinum. Echocardiography shows the transposition of the great arteries, the sites and amount of mixing, and any associated lesions.

Treatment

Initial medical management includes **prostaglandin E₁** to maintain ductal patency. If the infant remains significantly hypoxic on prostaglandin therapy, a **balloon atrial septostomy** is performed to improve mixing between the two circulations. Complete surgical repair is most often an **arterial switch**; the atrial switch is rarely done. The arterial switch usually is performed within the first 2 weeks of life, when the left ventricle still can maintain a systemic pressure.

TRICUSPID ATRESIA
Etiology and Epidemiology

Tricuspid atresia accounts for approximately 2% of all congenital heart defects (Fig. 144–3). It occurs when the normal development of the valve from endocardial cushions and septal tissue fails. The absence of the tricuspid valve results in a **hypoplastic right ventricle**. All systemic venous return must cross the atrial septum into the left atrium. The presence of a PDA or VSD also is necessary for pulmonary blood flow and survival.

Clinical Manifestations

Infants with tricuspid atresia are usually **severely cyanotic** and have a **single S₂**. If a VSD is present, there may be a murmur. A diastolic murmur across the mitral valve may be audible. Frequently there is no significant murmur.

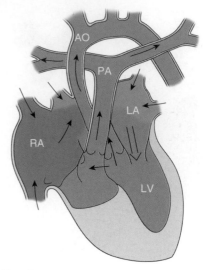

Figure 144–3

Tricuspid atresia. AO, aorta; LA, left atrium; LV, left ventricle; PA, pulmonary artery; RA, right atrium.

Imaging Studies

The ECG shows **left ventricular hypertrophy** and a **superior QRS axis** (between 0 and −90 degrees). The chest x-ray reveals a normal or mildly enlarged cardiac silhouette with **decreased pulmonary blood flow**. Echocardiography shows the anatomy, associated lesions, and source of pulmonary blood flow.

Treatment

Management initially depends on the presence of a VSD and the amount of blood flow across the VSD to the lungs. If there is no VSD, or it is small, prostaglandin E₁ is used to maintain pulmonary blood flow until surgery. Surgery is staged with an initial subclavian artery–to–pulmonary shunt (**Blalock-Taussig procedure**) typically followed by a two-stage procedure (**bidirectional Glenn** and **Fontan procedure**), which directs systemic venous return directly to the pulmonary arteries.

TRUNCUS ARTERIOSUS
Etiology and Epidemiology

Truncus arteriosus occurs in less than 1% of all cases of congenital heart disease (Fig. 144–4). It results from the failure of septation of the truncus, which normally occurs during the first 3 to 4 weeks of gestation. Anatomically a single arterial trunk arises from the heart with a large VSD immediately below the

VSD closure and placement of a conduit between the right ventricle and pulmonary arteries.

TOTAL ANOMALOUS PULMONARY VENOUS RETURN

Etiology and Epidemiology

Total anomalous pulmonary venous return accounts for about 1% of congenital heart disease (Fig. 144–5). Disruption of the development of normal pulmonary venous drainage during the third week of gestation results in one of four abnormalities. Anatomically, all of the pulmonary veins fail to connect to the left atrium and return abnormally via the right heart. They may have **supracardiac**, **cardiac**, **infracardiac**, or **mixed drainage**. An atrial level communication is necessary for systemic cardiac output and survival.

Clinical Manifestations

The most important determinant of presentation is the presence or absence of **obstruction** to the pulmonary venous drainage. Infants without obstruction have minimal cyanosis and may be asymptomatic. The pulmonary blood flow creates a **continuous murmur** and reenters the right atrium and right ventricle. There is a hyperactive **right ventricular impulse** with a **widely split S$_2$** (owing to increased volume ejected from the right ventricle) and a **systolic ejection**

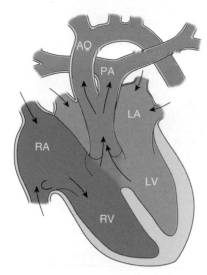

Figure 144–4

Truncus arteriosus. AO, aorta; LA, left atrium; LV, left ventricle; PA, pulmonary artery; RA, right atrium; RV, right ventricle.

truncal valve. The pulmonary arteries arise from the single arterial trunk either as a single vessel that divides or individually from the arterial trunk to the lungs.

Clinical Manifestations

Varying degrees of **cyanosis** depend on the amount of pulmonary blood flow. If not diagnosed at birth, the infant may develop signs of **CHF** as pulmonary vascular resistance decreases. The signs include tachypnea and cough. Peripheral pulses are usually bounding as a result of the diastolic runoff into the pulmonary arteries. A **single S$_2$** is due to the single valve. There may be a systolic ejection click, and there is often a **systolic murmur** at the left sternal border.

Imaging Studies

ECG findings include **combined ventricular hypertrophy** and **cardiomegaly**. **Increased pulmonary blood flow** is usually seen on chest x-ray. Pulmonary arteries may appear displaced. Echocardiography defines the anatomy, including the VSD, truncal valve function, and origin of the pulmonary arteries.

Treatment

Medical management is usually needed and includes **anticongestive medications**. **Surgical repair** includes

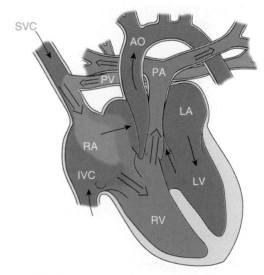

Figure 144–5

Total anomalous pulmonary venous return. AO, aorta; IVC, inferior vena cava; LA, left atrium; LV, left ventricle; PA, pulmonary artery; PV, pulmonary vein; RA, right atrium; RV, right ventricle; SVC, superior vena cava.

murmur at the left upper sternal border. Growth is relatively poor. Infants with **obstruction** present with cyanosis, marked tachypnea and dyspnea, and signs of right heart failure including hepatomegaly. The obstruction results in little, if any, increase in right ventricular volume. There may be no murmur or changes in S_2.

Imaging Studies

For infants without obstruction, the ECG is consistent with **right ventricular volume overload**. Cardiomegaly with increased pulmonary blood flow is seen on chest x-ray. Infants with obstructed veins have **right axis deviation** and **right ventricular hypertrophy** on ECG. On chest x-ray, the heart is normal or mildly enlarged with varying degrees of pulmonary edema that can appear similar to hyaline membrane disease or pneumonia. Echocardiography shows the volume-overloaded right heart, right-to-left atrial level shunting, and common pulmonary vein including site of drainage and degree of obstruction.

Treatment

At **surgery**, the common pulmonary vein is opened into the left atrium, and there is ligation of any vein or channel that had been draining the common vein.

HYPOPLASTIC LEFT HEART SYNDROME

Etiology and Epidemiology

Hypoplastic left heart syndrome accounts for 1% of all congenital heart defects (Fig. 144–6). It is the most common cause of death from cardiac defects in the first month of life. Hypoplastic left heart syndrome occurs when there is failure of development of the mitral or aortic valve or the aortic arch. A small left ventricle that is unable to support normal systemic circulation is a central finding of hypoplastic left heart syndrome, regardless of etiology. Associated degrees of hypoplasia of the ascending aorta and aortic arch are present. Left-to-right shunting occurs at the atrial level.

Clinical Manifestations

After delivery, the infant is dependent on right-to-left shunting at the ductus arteriosus for systemic blood flow. As the ductus arteriosus constricts, the infant becomes critically ill with signs and symptoms of **CHF** from excessive pulmonary blood flow and obstruction of pulmonary venous return. Pulses are diffusely weak

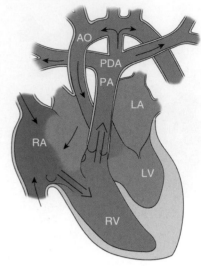

Figure 144–6

Hypoplastic left heart. AO, aorta; LA, left atrium; LV, left ventricle; PA, pulmonary artery; PDA, patent ductus arteriosus; RA, right atrium; RV, right ventricle.

or absent. S_2 is single and loud. There is usually no heart murmur. Cyanosis may be minimal, but **low cardiac output** gives a grayish color to the cool, mottled skin.

Imaging Studies

ECG findings include **right ventricular hypertrophy** with **decreased left ventricular forces**. The chest x-ray reveals **cardiomegaly** (with right-sided enlargement) and pulmonary venous congestion or pulmonary edema. Echocardiography shows the small left heart, the degree of stenosis of the aortic and mitral valves, the hypoplastic ascending aorta, and the adequacy of left-to-right atrial flow.

Treatment

Medical management includes **prostaglandin E_1** to open the ductus arteriosus, **correction of acidosis**, and ventilatory and blood pressure support as needed. **Surgical repair** is staged with the first surgery (Norwood procedure) done in the newborn period. Subsequent procedures create a systemic source for the pulmonary circulation (bidirectional Glenn and Fontan procedures), leaving the right ventricle to supply systemic circulation. There have been and continue to be many modifications to all three stages of the surgical repair.

TABLE 144–2. Extracardiac Complications of Cyanotic Congenital Heart Disease

Problem	Etiology	Therapy
Polycythemia	Persistent hypoxia	Phlebotomy
Relative anemia	Nutritional deficiency	Iron replacement
CNS abscess	Right-to-left shunting	Antibiotics, drainage
CNS thromboembolic stroke	Right-to-left shunting or polycythemia	Phlebotomy
Gingival disease	Polycythemia, gingivitis, bleeding	Dental hygiene
Gout	Polycythemia, diuretic agents	Allopurinol
Arthritis, clubbing	Hypoxic arthropathy	None
Pregnancy	Poor placental perfusion, poor ability to increase cardiac output	Bed rest
Infectious disease	Associated asplenia, DiGeorge syndrome	Antibiotics
	Fatal RSV pneumonia with pulmonary hypertension	Ribavirin, RSV immune globulin
Growth	Failure to thrive, increased oxygen consumption, decreased nutrient intake	Treat heart failure; correct defect early
Psychosocial adjustment	Limited activity, peer pressure; chronic disease, multiple hospitalizations, cardiac surgical techniques	Counseling

RSV, respiratory syncytial virus.

COMPLICATIONS OF CONGENITAL HEART DISEASE

Extracardiac complications are summarized in Table 144–2.

BACTERIAL ENDOCARDITIS

Bacterial endocarditis is infrequent in pediatric patients and occurs on native valves; valves damaged by congenitally abnormal valves, rheumatic fever, and acquired valvular lesions (mitral valve prolapse); and prosthetic replacement valves. The condition is a potential consequence of jet streams of turbulent blood (from PDA, VSD, or systemic-to-pulmonary shunts). Predisposing factors for the preceding bacteremia, laboratory tests, and clinical manifestations of bacterial endocarditis are listed in Table 144–3. Because of the endovascular nature of endocarditis, bacteremia is usually of a continuous nature, may be low grade (few bacteria per milliliter of blood), and may not be altered during episodes of fever or chills. The pathogens responsible for endocarditis depend on the status of the heart valve and the presence or absence of a predisposing procedure. Because some bacterial agents have unusual nutritional requirements, and others may need longer than the usual incubation period to show growth in vitro, the blood samples should be labeled when endocarditis is suspected; the sample can be observed for a longer time. Despite adequate blood culture techniques, 5% to 10% of endocarditis cases are culture negative.

Treatment of a culture-negative patient requires knowledge of the epidemiology and historical risk factors for the patient. Treatment of a culture-positive patient is directed against the particular bacterium (*Staphylococcus aureus*, viridans group streptococcus, enterococcus, or HACEK [*Haemophilus, Actinobacillus, Cardiobacterium, Eikenella, Kingella*] group bacteria), using bactericidal antibiotics. Therapy is continued for 4 to 8 weeks. Surgery is indicated if medical treatment is unsuccessful or for an unusual pathogen, myocardial abscess formation, refractory heart failure, serious embolic complications, or refractory prosthetic valve disease.

Antibiotic prophylaxis to prevent endocarditis has a pathophysiologic justification, carries a very low risk, and prevents a potentially life-threatening disease. Prophylaxis is recommended for all patients with most structural congenital heart disease, including unoperated, palliated or repaired defects; rheumatic valve lesions; prosthetic heart valves; mitral valve prolapse with a regurgitant valve; idiopathic hypertrophic subaortic stenosis; transvenous pacemaker leads; or previous endocarditis. Antimicrobial prophylaxis is not indicated for an isolated secundum ASD, a repaired secundum ASD or VSD 6 months after patch placement, or a divided and ligated PDA 6 months after repair. The antibiotic regimen to prevent endocarditis during dental or respiratory procedures is oral amoxicillin. Preventive treatment for gastrointestinal or genitourinary manipulation includes oral amoxicillin or parenteral ampicillin and gentamicin. The latter recommendation is for high-risk patients, such as patients with prosthetic heart valves, systemic-to-pulmonary shunts, or previous endocarditis. Clindamycin is indicated for most patients allergic to penicillin.

TABLE 144–3. Manifestations of Infective Endocarditis

History

Prior congenital or rheumatic heart disease
Preceding dental, urinary, or intestinal procedure
IV drug abuse
Central venous catheter
Prosthetic heart valve

Symptoms

Fever
Chills
Chest pain
Arthralgia and myalgia
Dyspnea
Malaise

Signs

Fever
Tachycardia
Embolic phenomena (Roth spots, petechiae, Osler nodes, and CNS lesion)
Janeway lesions
New or changing murmur
Splenomegaly
Arthritis
Heart failure
Arrhythmias

Laboratory Tests

Positive blood culture
Elevated ESR, C-reactive protein
Leukocytosis
Immune complexes
Rheumatoid factor
Hematuria
Echocardiographic evidence of valve vegetations

ESR, erythrocyte sedimentation rate.

CHAPTER 145
Congestive Heart Failure

ETIOLOGY AND EPIDEMIOLOGY

Myofibril contraction is summated and translated into cardiac work or pump performance. The force generated by the muscle fiber depends on its contractile status and its basal length, which is equivalent to the preload. As the preload (fiber length, left ventricular filling pressure or volume) increases, the myocardial performance (stroke volume and wall tension) increases up to a point (the normal Starling curve). The relationship is the **ventricular function curve** (Fig. 145–1). Alterations in the contractile state of the muscle lower the relative position of the curve, but retain the relationship of fiber length to muscle work.

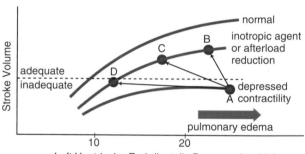

Figure 145–1

Ventricular function curve illustrating the effect of inotropic agents or arterial vasodilators. In contrast to diuretics, the effect of digitalis or arterial vasodilator therapy in a patient with heart failure is movement onto another ventricular function curve intermediate between the normal and the depressed curves. When the patient's ventricular function moves from *A* to *B* by the administration of one of these agents, the left ventricular end-diastolic pressure may also decrease because of improved cardiac function; further administration of diuretics or venodilators may shift the function further to the left along the same curve from *B* to *C* and eliminate the risk of pulmonary edema. A vasodilating agent that has arteriolar and venous dilating properties (e.g., nitroprusside) would shift this function directly from *A* to *C*. If this agent shifts the function from *A* to *D* because of excessive venodilation or administration of diuretics, the cardiac output may decrease too much, even though the left ventricular end-diastolic pressure would be normal (10 mm Hg) for a normal heart. Left ventricular end-diastolic pressures of 15 to 18 mm Hg are usually optimal in the failing heart to maximize cardiac output, but to avoid pulmonary edema. (From Andreoli TE, Carpenter CCJ, Griggs RC, Loscalzo J [eds]: Cecil Essentials of Medicine, 5th ed. Philadelphia, WB Saunders, 2001.)

TABLE 145–1. Factors Affecting Cardiac Performance

Preload (Left Ventricular Diastolic Volume)

Total blood volume
Venous tone (sympathetic tone)
Body position
Intrathoracic and intrapericardial pressure
Atrial contraction
Pumping action of skeletal muscle

Afterload (Impedance Against Which the Left Ventricle Must Eject Blood)

Peripheral vascular resistance
Left ventricular volume (preload, wall tension)
Physical characteristics of the arterial tree (elasticity of vessels or presence of outflow obstruction)

Contractility (Cardiac Performance Independent of Preload or Afterload)

Sympathetic nerve impulses*
Circulating catecholamines*
Digitalis, calcium, other inotropic agents*
Increased heart rate or postextrasystolic augmentation*
Anoxia, acidosis[†]
Pharmacologic depression[†]
Loss of myocardium[†]
Intrinsic depression[†]

Heart Rate

Autonomic nervous system
Temperature, metabolic rate

*Increases contractility.
[†]Decreases contractility.
From Andreoli TE, Carpenter CCJ, Griggs RC, Loscalzo J: Cecil Essentials of Medicine, 5th ed. Philadelphia, WB Saunders, 2001.

TABLE 145–2. Etiology of Heart Failure

Fetus

Severe anemia (hemolysis, fetal-maternal transfusion, hypoplastic anemia)
Supraventricular tachycardia
Ventricular tachycardia
Complete heart block
Atrioventricular valve insufficiency
High-output cardiac failure (arteriovenous malformation, teratoma)

Premature Neonate

Fluid overload
PDA
VSD
Cor pulmonale (BPD)

Full-Term Neonate

Asphyxial cardiomyopathy
Arteriovenous malformation (vein of Galen, hepatic)
Left-sided obstructive lesions (coarctation of aorta, hypoplastic left heart, critical aortic stenosis)
Transposition of great arteries
Large mixing cardiac defects (single ventricle, truncus arteriosus)
Viral myocarditis
Anemia
Supraventricular tachycardia
Complete heart block

Infant-Toddler

Left-to-right cardiac shunts (VSD)
Hemangioma (arteriovenous malformation)
Anomalous left coronary artery
Metabolic cardiomyopathy
Acute hypertension (hemolytic-uremic syndrome)
Supraventricular tachycardia
Kawasaki disease
Postoperative repair of congenital heart disease

Child-Adolescent

Rheumatic fever
Acute hypertension (glomerulonephritis)
Viral myocarditis
Thyrotoxicosis
Hemochromatosis-hemosiderosis
Cancer therapy (radiation, doxorubicin)
Sickle cell anemia
Endocarditis
Cor pulmonale (cystic fibrosis)
Arrhythmias
Chronic upper airway obstruction (cor pulmonale)
Unrepaired or palliated congenital heart disease
Cardiomyopathy

BPD, bronchopulmonary dysplasia; PDA, patent ductus arteriosus; VSD, ventricular septal defect.

Heart rate is another important determinant of cardiac work because the cardiac output equals stroke volume times the heart rate. Additional factors also affect cardiac performance (Table 145–1).

CHF is defined as the pathophysiologic state in which the heart is unable to pump blood at a rate commensurate with the body's metabolic needs (oxygen delivery). This state may be due to a change in **myocardial contractility** that results in low cardiac output or to **abnormal loading conditions** being placed on the myocardium. The abnormal loading conditions may be **afterload** (pressure overload, such as with aortic stenosis, pulmonary stenosis, or coarctation of the aorta) or **preload** (volume overload, such as in VSD, PDA, or valvular insufficiency). Volume overload is the most common cause of CHF in children.

It is helpful to approach the differential diagnosis of CHF based on age of presentation (Table 145–2). In the first weeks of life, CHF is most commonly due to an excessive afterload being placed on the myocardium. CHF presenting around 2 months of age is usually due to increasing left-to-right shunts of congenital heart defects that become apparent as the pulmonary vascular resistance decreases. Acquired heart disease, such as myocarditis and cardiomyopathy, can present at any age.

CLINICAL MANIFESTATIONS

Clinical presentation of CHF in infants includes poor feeding, failure to thrive, tachypnea, and diaphoresis with feeding. Older children may present with shortness of breath, easy fatigability, and edema. The physical examination findings depend on whether pulmonary venous congestion, systemic venous congestion, or both are present. Tachycardia, a gallop rhythm, and thready pulses may be present with either cause. If left-sided failure is predominant, tachypnea,

orthopnea, wheezing, and pulmonary edema are seen. If right-sided failure is present, hepatomegaly, edema, and distended neck veins are present.

IMAGING STUDIES

Noninvasive studies, such as chest radiography, are not specific, but the absence of cardiomegaly on a chest x-ray usually rules out the diagnosis of CHF. An echocardiogram assesses the heart chamber sizes, measures myocardial function accurately, and diagnoses congenital heart defects when present.

TREATMENT

Initial treatment is directed at improving myocardial function and optimizing preload and afterload. **Diuretics**, **inotropic support**, and, often, **afterload reduction** are employed (Table 145–3). Long-term therapy is

TABLE 145–3. Treatment of Heart Failure

Therapy	Mechanism
General Care	
Rest	Reduces cardiac output
Oxygen	Improves oxygenation in presence of pulmonary edema
Sodium, fluid restrictions	Decreases vascular congestion; decreases preload
Diuretics	
Furosemide	Salt excretion by ascending loop of Henle; reduces preload; afterload reduced if hypertension improves; may also cause venodilation
Combination of distal tubule and loop diuretics	Greater sodium excretion
Inotropic Agents	
Digitalis	Inhibits membrane Na^+, K^+-ATPase and increases intracellular Ca^{2+}, improves cardiac contractility, increases myocardial oxygen consumption
Dopamine	Releases myocardial norepinephrine plus direct effect on β-receptor, may increase systemic blood pressure; at low infusion rates, dilates renal artery, facilitating diuresis
Dobutamine	β_1-receptor agent; often combined with dopamine
Amrinone/milrinone	Nonsympathomimetic, noncardiac glycosides with inotropic effects; may produce vasodilation
Afterload Reduction	
Hydralazine	Arteriolar vasodilator
Nitroprusside	Arterial and venous relaxation; venodilation reduces preload
Captopril/enalapril	Inhibition of angiotensin-converting enzyme; reduces angiotensin II production
Other	
Mechanical counterpulsation	Improves coronary flow, afterload
Transplantation	Removes diseased heart
Extracorporeal membrane oxygenation	Bypasses heart
Carvedilol	β-blocking agent

usually **digoxin** and diuretics. Depending on the etiology of failure, afterload reduction frequently is added. Long-term therapy with **β-blockers** also may be beneficial.

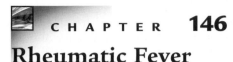

CHAPTER 146
Rheumatic Fever

ETIOLOGY AND EPIDEMIOLOGY

Although uncommon in the United States, acute rheumatic fever remains an important preventable cause of cardiac disease. It is most common in children 6 to 15 years old. It is due to an immunologic reaction that is a delayed sequela of group A beta-hemolytic streptococcal infections of the pharynx (see Chapter 103). A family history of rheumatic fever and lower socioeconomic status are additional factors.

CLINICAL MANIFESTATIONS

Acute rheumatic fever is diagnosed using the **revised Jones criteria**, which consist of clinical and laboratory findings (Table 146–1). The presence of either two **major criteria** or one major and two **minor criteria**, along with evidence of an antecedent **streptococcal infection**, confirm a diagnosis of acute rheumatic fever. The infection often precedes the presentation of rheumatic fever by 2 to 6 weeks. Streptococcal antibody tests, such as the antistreptolysin O titer, are the most reliable laboratory evidence of prior infection.

Arthritis is the most common major manifestation. It usually involves the large joints and is migratory. Arthralgia cannot be used as a minor manifestation if arthritis is used as a major manifestation. **Carditis** occurs in about 50% of patients. Tachycardia, a new murmur (mitral or aortic regurgitation), pericarditis, cardiomegaly, and signs of CHF are evidence of carditis. **Erythema marginatum**, a serpiginous, nonpruritic, and evanescent rash, is uncommon, occurs on the trunk, and is brought out by warmth. **Subcutaneous nodules** are seen predominantly with chronic or recurrent disease. They are firm, painless, nonpruritic, mobile nodules found on the extensor surfaces of the large and small joints, the scalp, and the spine. **Chorea** (Sydenham chorea or St. Vitus dance) consists of neurologic and psychiatric signs. It also is uncommon and often presents long after the infection.

TREATMENT AND PREVENTION

Management of acute rheumatic fever consists of **benzathine penicillin** to eradicate the beta-hemolytic streptococcus, anti-inflammatory therapy with **salicylates** after the diagnosis is established, and **bed rest**. Additional supportive therapy for CHF or chorea may be necessary during the acute presentation. **Long-term penicillin prophylaxis**, preferably with IM benzathine penicillin G, 1.2 million U every 28 days, is required. Oral regimens for prophylaxis generally are not as effective. The prognosis of acute rheumatic fever depends on the degree of permanent cardiac damage. Cardiac involvement may resolve completely, especially if it is the first episode and the prophylactic regimen is followed. The severity of cardiac involvement worsens with each recurrence of rheumatic fever.

TABLE 146–1.   Major Criteria in the Jones System for Acute Rheumatic Fever*†

Sign	Comments
Polyarthritis	Common; swelling, limited motion, tender, erythema
	Migratory; involves large joints but rarely small or unusual joints, such as vertebrae
Carditis	Common; pancarditis, valves, pericardium, myocardium
	Tachycardia greater than explained by fever; new murmur of mitral or aortic insufficiency; Carey-Coombs mid-diastolic murmur; heart failure
Chorea (Sydenham disease)	Uncommon; presents long after infection has resolved; more common in females; antineuronal antibody positive
Erythema marginatum	Uncommon; pink macules on trunk and proximal extremities, evolving to serpiginous border with central clearing; evanescent, elicited by application of local heat; nonpruritic
Subcutaneous nodules	Uncommon; associated with repeated episodes and severe carditis; present over extensor surface of elbows, knees, knuckles, and ankles or scalp and spine; firm, nontender

*Minor criteria include fever (101°F to 102°F [38.2°C to 38.9°C]), arthralgias, previous rheumatic fever, leukocytosis, elevated erythrocyte sedimentation rate/C-reactive protein, and prolonged P-R interval.
†One major and two minor, or two major, criteria with evidence of recent group A streptococcal disease (e.g., scarlet fever, positive throat culture, or elevated antistreptolysin O or other antistreptococcal antibodies) strongly suggest the diagnosis of acute rheumatic fever.

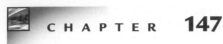

CHAPTER 147

Cardiomyopathies

ETIOLOGY

A cardiomyopathy is an intrinsic disease of the heart muscle and is not associated with other forms of heart disease (Table 147–1). There are three types of cardiomyopathy based on anatomic and functional features: (1) **dilated**, (2) **hypertrophic**, or (3) **restrictive** (Table 147–2). Dilated cardiomyopathies are the most common. They are often idiopathic, but may be due to infection (echovirus or coxsackie B virus) or be post-infectious, familial, secondary to systemic disease, or secondary to cardiotoxic drugs. Hypertrophic cardiomyopathies are usually familial with autosomal dominant inheritance, but may occur sporadically. Restrictive cardiomyopathies are rare. They may be idiopathic, but can be associated with systemic disease.

CLINICAL MANIFESTATIONS

Dilated cardiomyopathies result in enlargement of the left ventricle only or both ventricles. Myocardial contractility is variably decreased. Clinically, children with

---

TABLE 147–1. Etiology of Myocardial Disease

Familial-Hereditary	**Connective Tissue—Granulomatous Disease**
Duchenne muscular dystrophy	SLE
Other muscular dystrophies (Becker, limb girdle)	Scleroderma
Myotonic dystrophy	Churg-Strauss syndrome
Kearns-Sayre syndrome (progressive external ophthalmoplegia)	Rheumatoid arthritis
Friedreich ataxia	Rheumatic fever
Hemochromatosis	Sarcoidosis
Fabry disease	Amyloidosis
Pompe disease (glycogen storage)	Dermatomyositis
Carnitine deficiency syndromes	**Drugs-Toxins**
Endocardial fibroelastosis	
Mitochondrial myopathy syndromes	Doxorubicin (Adriamycin)
Familial restrictive cardiomyopathy	Ipecac
Familial hypertrophic cardiomyopathy	Iron overload (hemosiderosis)
Familial dilated cardiomyopathy (dominant, recessive, X-linked)	Irradiation
	Cocaine
Infections (Myocarditis)	Amphetamines
	Coronary Arteries
Viral (e.g., coxsackievirus, mumps, Epstein-Barr virus, influenza, parainfluenza, measles, varicella, HIV)	Anomalous left coronary artery
Rickettsiae (e.g., psittacosis, *Coxiella*, Rocky Mountain spotted fever)	Kawasaki disease
Bacterial (e.g., diphtheria, *Mycoplasma*, meningococcus, leptospirosis, Lyme disease)	**Other**
Parasitic (e.g., Chagas disease, toxoplasmosis, *Loa loa*)	Sickle cell anemia
Metabolic, Nutritional, Endocrine	Hypereosinophilic syndrome
	Endomyocardial fibrosis
Beriberi (thiamine deficiency)	Asymmetric septal hypertrophy
Keshan disease (selenium deficiency)	Right ventricular dysplasia
Hypothyroidism	Idiopathic
Hyperthyroidism	
Carcinoid	
Pheochromocytoma	
Mitochondrial myopathies and oxidative respiratory chain defects	
Type II, X-linked 3-methylglutaconic aciduria	

SLE, systemic lupus erythematosus.

TABLE 147–2. Anatomic and Functional Features of Cardiomyopathies

	Dilated	Hypertrophic	Restrictive
Etiology	Infectious Metabolic Toxic Idiopathic	Sporadic Inherited (autosomal dominant)	Infiltrative Myocardial hypertrophy Myocardial fibrosis Idiopathic
Hemodynamics	Decreased systolic function	Diastolic dysfunction (impaired ventricular filling)	Diastolic dysfunction (impaired ventricular filling)
Treatment	Positive inotropes Diuretics Afterload reduction β-Blockers Antiarrhythmics Anticoagulants Cardiac transplantation	β-Blockers Calcium channel blockersation	Diuretics Anticoagulants Corticosteroids Cardiac transplantation

dilated cardiomyopathy present with signs and symptoms of inadequate cardiac output and **CHF**. Tachypnea and tachycardia are present on examination. Peripheral pulses are often weak owing to a **narrow pulse pressure**. Rales may be audible on pulmonary auscultation. Heart sounds may be muffled, and S_3 is often present. Concurrent infectious illness may result in circulatory collapse and shock in children with dilated cardiomyopathies.

Hypertrophic cardiomyopathy is initially difficult to diagnose. Infants, but not older children, frequently present with signs of CHF. Older children may be asymptomatic, with sudden death as the initial presentation. Dyspnea, fatigue, chest pain, syncope or near-syncope, and palpitations may be present. A murmur is heard in more than 50% of children referred after identification of an affected family member.

Restrictive cardiomyopathies are relatively rare in pediatrics. Presenting symptoms usually include dyspnea exacerbated by a respiratory illness, syncope, hepatomegaly, and S_3.

IMAGING STUDIES

Cardiomegaly usually is seen on chest radiographs for all three types of cardiomyopathies. The ECG in dilated cardiomyopathy may have nonspecific ST-T wave changes and left ventricular hypertrophy. Twenty-five percent of children also have ECG evidence of right ventricular hypertrophy. The ECG in infants and children with hypertrophic cardiomyopathy is universally abnormal, but changes are nonspecific. Primary hypertrophic cardiomyopathy is associated with a prolonged Q-T interval. Children with restrictive cardiomyopathies may show atrial enlargement on the ECG.

Echocardiography features vary by type of cardiomyopathy. Dilated cardiomyopathies result in dilation of the left atrium and ventricle, a decreased shortening fraction, and globally depressed contractility. Asymmetric septal hypertrophy and obstruction of the left ventricular outflow tract are seen in hypertrophic cardiomyopathies. Massive atrial dilation is seen in restrictive cardiomyopathies.

Endomyocardial biopsy specimens may be obtained when the patient is hemodynamically stable to identify histology or test for mitochondrial or infiltrative diseases.

TREATMENT

Supportive therapy, including **diuretics**, **inotropic medications**, and **afterload reduction**, is provided for all three types of cardiomyopathy and depends on the degree of symptoms and severity of cardiovascular compromise. If a specific etiology can be identified, treatment is directed at the etiology. Symptomatic therapy with close monitoring and follow-up is crucial. Because of the high mortality rate associated with all forms of cardiomyopathy, **cardiac transplantation** must be considered.

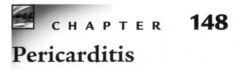

CHAPTER **148**

Pericarditis

ETIOLOGY AND EPIDEMIOLOGY

Pericarditis is inflammation of the parietal and visceral surfaces of the pericardium. It is most often viral in origin with many viruses identified as causative agents. A bacterial etiology is rare, but usually causes a much more serious and symptomatic pericarditis. *S. aureus* and *Streptococcus pneumoniae* are the most likely bacterial causes. Pericarditis is associated with collagen vascular diseases, such as rheumatoid arthritis, and is seen with uremia (Table 148-1). **Postpericardiotomy syndrome** is a relatively common form of pericarditis that follows heart surgery.

CLINICAL MANIFESTATIONS

The symptoms of pericarditis (Table 148-2) depend on the amount of fluid in the pericardial space and how fast it accumulates. A small effusion usually is well tolerated. A large effusion may be remarkably well

---

TABLE 148-1.   Etiology of Pericarditis and Pericardial Effusion

Idiopathic (Presumed Viral) Infectious Agents

Bacteria
Group A streptococcus
Staphylococcus aureus
Pneumococcus, meningococcus*
*Haemophilus influenzae**
Salmonella
Mycoplasma pneumoniae
Borrelia burgdorferi
Mycobacterium tuberculosis
Rickettsia
Tularemia

Viral[†]
Coxsackievirus (group A, B)
Echovirus
Mumps
Influenza
Epstein-Barr
Cytomegalovirus
Herpes simplex
Herpes zoster
Hepatitis B

Fungal
Histoplasma capsulatum
Coccidioides immitis
Blastomyces dermatitidis
Cryptococcus neoformans
Candida
Aspergillus

Parasitic
Toxoplasma gondii
Entamoeba histolytica
Schistosomes

Collagen Vascular–Inflammatory and Granulomatous Diseases

Rheumatic fever
Systemic lupus erythematosus (idiopathic and drug-induced)
Rheumatoid arthritis
Kawasaki disease
Scleroderma
Mixed connective tissue disease

Reiter syndrome
Inflammatory bowel disease
Wegener granulomatosis
Dermatomyositis
Behçet syndrome
Sarcoidosis
Vasculitis
Familial Mediterranean fever
Serum sickness
Stevens-Johnson syndrome

Traumatic

Cardiac contusion (blunt trauma)
Penetrating trauma
Postpericardiotomy syndrome
Radiation

Contiguous Spread

Pleural disease
Pneumonia
Aortic aneurysm (dissecting)

Metabolic

Hypothyroidism
Uremia
Gaucher disease
Fabry disease
Chylopericardium

Neoplastic

Primary
Contiguous (lymphoma)
Metastatic
Infiltrative (leukemia)

Others

Drug reaction
Pancreatitis
After myocardial infarction
Thalassemia
Central venous catheter perforation
Heart failure
Hemorrhage (coagulopathy)
Biliary-pericardial fistula

*Infectious or immune complex.
[†]Common (viral pericarditis or myopericarditis is probably the most common cause of acute pericarditis in a previously normal host).
From Sigman G: Chest pain. In Kliegman RM, Nieder ML, Super DM (eds): Practical Strategies in Pediatric Diagnosis and Therapy. Philadelphia, WB Saunders, 1996.

TABLE 148–2.   Manifestations of Pericarditis

Symptoms

Chest pain (worsened if lying down or with inspiration)
Dyspnea
Malaise
Patient assumes sitting position

Signs

Nonconstrictive

Fever
Tachycardia
Friction rub (accentuated by inspiration, body position)
Enlarged heart by percussion and x-ray examination
Distant heart sounds

Tamponade

As above, plus:
Distended neck veins
Hepatomegaly
Pulsus paradoxus (>10 mm Hg with inspiration)
Narrow pulse pressure
Weak pulse, poor peripheral perfusion

Constrictive Pericarditis

Distended neck veins
Kussmaul sign (inspiratory increase of jugular venous pressure)
Distant heart sounds
Pericardial knock
Hepatomegaly
Ascites
Edema
Tachycardia

TABLE 148–3.   Laboratory Evidence of Pericarditis

Test	Evidence Seen
ECG	Elevated ST segments, T wave inversion (late), tachycardia, reduced QRS voltage, electrical alternans (variable QRS amplitudes)
Chest radiograph	Cardiomegaly ("water bottle heart")
Echocardiogram	Pericardial fluid
Pericardiocentesis	Gram and acid-fast stains, culture, PCR (virus, bacteria, mycobacteria, fungus), cytology, cell count, glucose, protein, pH
Blood tests	ESR, viral titers, ANA, ASO titers, EBV titers

ANA, antinuclear antibodies; ASO, antistreptolysin O; EBV, Epstein-Barr virus; ESR, erythrocyte sedimentation rate; PCR, polymerase chain reaction.

tolerated if it accumulates slowly. The faster the fluid accumulates, the sooner the patient is hemodynamically compromised.

IMAGING AND LABORATORY STUDIES

Echocardiography is the most specific and useful diagnostic test for detection of pericardial effusion. A chest x-ray may reveal cardiomegaly. A large effusion creates a rounded, globular cardiac silhouette. The ECG may show tachycardia, elevated ST segments, and changes in the QRS complex. The causative organism may be identified through blood tests or diagnostic testing of the pericardial fluid (Table 148–3).

TREATMENT

Pericardiocentesis is indicated not only for treatment of hemodynamically significant effusions, but also provides valuable information with regards to the etiology of the pericarditis. Additional treatment is directed at the specific etiology. There is no specific treatment for viral pericarditis other than **anti-inflammatory medications**.

SUGGESTED READING

Behrman RE, Kliegman RM, Jenson HB (eds): Nelson Textbook of Pediatrics, 17th ed. Philadelphia, WB Saunders, 2004.

Bernstein D: Evaluation of the cardiovascular system: Laboratory evaluation. In Behrman RE, Kliegman RM, Jenson HB (eds): Nelson Textbook of Pediatrics, 17th ed. Philadelphia, WB Saunders, 2004, pp 1488-1499.

Dreyer WJ, Fisher DJ: Clinical recognition and management of chronic congestive heart failure. In: Garson A Jr., Bricker JT, Fisher DJ, Neish SR (eds): The Science and Practice of Pediatric Cardiology, 2nd ed. Baltimore, Williams & Wilkins, 1998, pp 2309-2325.

Gessner IH: Physical examination. In: Gessner IH, Victorica BE (eds): Pediatric Cardiology: A Problem Oriented Approach. Philadelphia, WB Saunders, 1993, pp 3-22.

Kay JD, Colan SD, Graham TP: Congestive heart failure in pediatric patients. Am Heart J 142:923-928, 2001.

Park MK: Syncope. In: Park MK, George R, Troxler MPH (eds): Pediatric Cardiology for Practitioners, 4th ed. St. Louis, Mosby, 2002, pp 449-459.

Park MK: Pathophysiology of left-to-right shunt lesions, pathophysiology of obstructive and valvular regurgitant lesions, pathophysiology of cyanotic congenital heart defects. In: Park MK, George R, Troxler MPH (eds): Pediatric Cardiology for Practitioners, 4th ed. St. Louis, Mosby, 2002, pp 98-128.

Stewart JM: Orthostatic intolerance in pediatrics. J Pediatr 140:404-411, 2002.

Tingelstad J: Consultation with the specialist: Cardiac dysrhythmias. Pediatr Rev 22:91-94, 2001.

CHAPTER **149**

Assessment

HISTORY

A detailed, careful history of the onset of a hematologic problem, severity, progression, associated symptoms, presence of systemic complaints, and exacerbating factors is crucial to the diagnosis of a blood disorder. A key question clarifies whether this is the initial episode of a disease process or a recurring problem. In many blood disorders, a **detailed pedigree** is crucial because a pattern of inheritance can point to the diagnosis of hemophilia, Wiskott-Aldridge syndrome, chronic granulomatous disease, or glucose-6-phosphate dehydrogenase (G6PD) deficiency (X-linked traits); sickle cell disease, pyruvate kinase deficiency, or certain storage diseases (autosomal recessive); or hereditary spherocytosis or von Willebrand disease (usually autosomal dominant).

PHYSICAL EXAMINATION AND COMMON MANIFESTATIONS

The physical examination of patients with blood disorders first focuses on the child's hemodynamic stability. Acute episodes of anemia may be life-threatening, with the person presenting with impairment of perfusion and impairment of cognitive status. The two most common findings of anemia include **pallor** and **jaundice**. The presence of petechiae, purpura, or deeper sites of **bleeding**, including generalized hemorrhage, indicates abnormalities of platelets, coagulation factors, or consumptive coagulopathy. **Growth parameters** can point to whether anemia is an acute or a chronic process. Severe types of anemia, thrombocy-

topenia, and pancytopenia are associated with congenital anomalies and often a pattern of growth delay. The presence or absence of other organ system involvement or systemic illness, especially findings of **hepatosplenomegaly** and **lymphadenopathy**, points to a generalized illness as the cause for hematologic abnormalities (Table 149–1).

INITIAL DIAGNOSTIC EVALUATION

The history and physical examination provide important clues to the diagnosis of blood diseases (see Table 149–1). Nevertheless, the basis for the diagnosis of blood disorders is laboratory testing. Diagnosis of pediatric blood disorders requires a detailed knowledge of normal hematologic values during infancy and childhood. These values vary according to age and, after puberty, according to sex. Clinicians who interpret data must know what is normal and what is not for the age of a child (Table 149–2). From the history, physical examination, and screening laboratory studies, the astute clinician proceeds in an orderly manner to the diagnosis using specific diagnostic testing to confirm the diagnosis.

DEVELOPMENTAL HEMATOLOGY

Hematopoiesis begins by 3 weeks of gestation with **erythropoiesis** in the yolk sac. By 2 months' gestation, the primary site of hematopoiesis has migrated to the liver. Red blood cells (RBCs), platelets, and leukocytes are synthesized at this site. By 5 to 6 months' gestation, the process of hematopoiesis shifts from the liver to the bone marrow. An extremely premature infant may have significant **extramedullary hematopoiesis** with limited bone marrow hematopoiesis. During infancy, virtually all marrow cavities are actively hematopoietic, and the proportion of hematopoietic to stromal

TABLE 149–1. Presentation of Hematologic Disorders

Condition	Symptoms and Signs	Common Examples
Anemia	Pallor, fatigue, heart failure, jaundice	Iron deficiency, hemolytic anemia
Polycythemia	Irritability, cyanosis, seizures, jaundice, stroke, headache	Cyanotic heart disease, infant of diabetic mother, cystic fibrosis
Neutropenia	Fever, pharyngitis, oral ulceration, cellulitis, lymphadenopathy, bacteremia	Congenital or drug-induced agranulocytosis, leukemia
Thrombocytopenia	Petechiae, ecchymosis, gastrointestinal hemorrhage, epistaxis	ITP, leukemia
Coagulopathy	Bruising, hemarthrosis, mucosal bleeding	von Willebrand disease, hemophilia, DIC
Thrombosis	Pulmonary embolism, deep venous thrombosis	Lupus anticoagulant; protein C, protein S, or antithrombin III deficiency, factor V Leiden, prothrombin 20210

DIC, disseminated intravascular coagulation; ITP, idiopathic thrombocytopenic purpura.

elements is quite high. As the child grows, hematopoiesis moves to the central bones of the body (vertebrae, sternum, ribs, and pelvis), and the marrow of the extremities and the skull is replaced with fat. This replacement of marrow with fat is a gradual and partially reversible process. Hemolysis or marrow damage may lead to marrow repopulation of cavities where hematopoiesis previously had ceased or may cause a delay in the shift of hematopoiesis. Children with thalassemia and other chronic hemolytic diseases may have large head circumferences and prominent skull bones as a result of increased erythropoiesis within the medullary cavities of the skull. Hepatosplenomegaly in patients with chronic hemolysis may signify extramedullary hematopoiesis. Because of the extensive use of all bone marrow cavities, very young children do not have the marrow reserves of older children and adults. When a patient with cytopenia is being evaluated, a **bone marrow examination** provides valuable information about processes that lead to underproduction of circulating cells. Additionally, bone marrow infiltration by neoplastic elements or storage cells often occurs in concert with similar infiltration in the spleen, liver, and lymph nodes.

The hematopoietic cells consist of (1) a small compartment of **pluripotential progenitor stem cells** that morphologically resemble small lymphocytes and are capable of forming all myeloid elements; (2) a large compartment of committed, **proliferating cells of myeloid, erythroid, and megakaryocytic lineage**; and (3) a large compartment of **postmitotic maturing cells** (Fig. 149–1). Hematopoiesis is controlled by numerous cytokines. The bone marrow is the major storage organ for mature neutrophils and contains about seven times the intravascular pool of neutrophils. It contains 2.5 to 5 times as many cells of myeloid lineage as cells of erythroid lineage. Smaller numbers of megakaryocytes, plasma cells, histiocytes, lymphocytes, and stromal cells are stored in the marrow.

Erythropoiesis (RBC production) is controlled by erythropoietin, a hormone made by the juxtaglomerular apparatus of the kidney in response to local tissue hypoxia. The normally high hemoglobin level of the fetus is a result of fetal erythropoietin production in the liver in response to low PO_2 in utero. Control of erythropoiesis by erythropoietin begins at the time of hepatic hematopoiesis in early gestation. Erythropoietin is a glycoprotein that stimulates the primitive pluripotential stem cell to differentiate along the erythroid line, leading to production of what is recognized in vitro as the **erythroid colony-forming unit**. The earliest recognizable erythroid cell in vivo is the erythroblast, which forms eight or more daughter cells. The immature RBC nucleus becomes gradually pyknotic as the cell matures and eventually is extruded before being released from the marrow as a **reticulocyte**. The reticulocyte maintains residual mitochondrial and protein synthetic capacity. These highly specialized RBC precursors are engaged primarily in the production of **globin chains**, **glycolytic enzymes**, and **heme**. Iron is taken up via transferrin receptors and incorporated into the heme ring, which combines with globin chains synthesized within the immature RBC. When the messenger RNA and mitochondria are gone from the RBC, it is no longer capable of heme or protein synthesis; however, the RBC continues to function for its normal life span of about 120 days in older children and adults.

During embryonic and fetal life, the globin genes are sequentially activated and inactivated. Embryonic hemoglobins are produced during yolk sac erythropoiesis, then are replaced by **fetal hemoglobin** (hemoglobin F-$\alpha_2\gamma_2$) during the hepatic phase. During the

TABLE 149–2. Hematologic Values During Infancy and Childhood

Age	Hemoglobin (g/dL) Mean	Range	Hematocrit (%) Mean	Range	Reticulocytes (%) Mean	Leukocytes (per mm³) Mean	Range	Differential Counts							
								Neutrophils (%) Mean	Range	Lymphocytes (%) Mean	Eosinophils (%) Mean	Monocytes (%) Mean	Nucleated Red Cells/ 100 WBCs		
Cord blood	16.8	13.7-20.1	55	45-65	5	18,000	9,000-30,000	61	40-80	31	2	6	7
2 wk	16.5	13-20	50	42-66	1	12,000	5,000-21,000	40		48	3	9	3-10
3 mo	12.0	9.5-14.5	36	31-41	1	12,000	6,000-18,000	30		63	2	5	0
6 mo-6 yr	12.0	10.5-14	37	33-42	1	10,000	6,000-15,000	45		48	2	5	0
7-12 yr	13.0	11-16	38	34-40	1	8,000	4,500-13,500	55		38	2	5	0
Adult													
Female	14.0	12-16	42	37-47	1.6	7,500	5,000-10,000	55	35-70	35	3	7	0
Male	16.0	14-18	47	42-52									

WBCs, white blood cells.
From Behrman RE (ed): Nelson Textbook of Pediatrics, 14th ed., Philadelphia, WB Saunders, 1992.

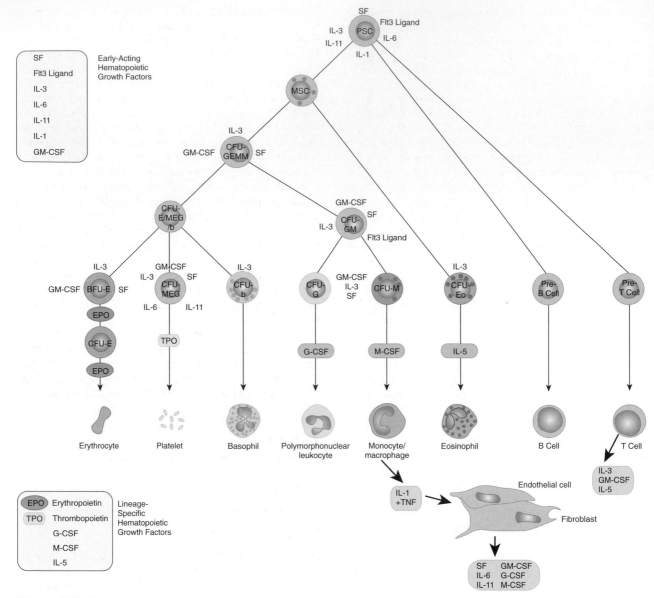

Figure 149–1

Major cytokine sources and actions to promote hematopoiesis. Cells of the bone marrow microenvironment, such as macrophages, endothelial cells, and reticular fibroblasts, produce macrophage colony-stimulating factor (M-CSF), granulocyte-macrophage colony-stimulating factor (GM-CSF), and granulocyte colony-stimulating factor (G-CSF) after stimulation. These cytokines and others as listed in the text have overlapping interactions during hematopoietic differentiation, as indicated; for all lineages, optimal development requires a combination of early and late acting factors. BFU, burst-forming unit; CFU, colony-forming unit; EPO, erythropoietin; MSC, myeloid stem cells; PSC, pluripotent stem cells; TNF, tumor necrosis factor; TPO, thrombopoietin. (From Sieff CA, Nathan DG, Clark SC: The anatomy and physiology of hematopoiesis. In Orkin SH, Nathan DG [eds]: Hematology of Infancy and Childhood, 5th ed. Philadelphia, WB Saunders, 1998, p 168.)

third trimester, gamma chain production gradually diminishes, and gamma chains are replaced by beta chains, resulting in **hemoglobin A** ($\alpha_2\beta_2$). Some fetal factors (e.g., infant of a diabetic mother) delay onset of beta chain production, but premature birth does not. Just after birth, with the expansion of the lungs and establishment of normal neonatal cardiorespiratory function, the oxygen saturation rapidly increases from 65% in utero to nearly 100%. Erythropoietin production ceases and shuts down erythropoiesis. Fetal RBCs have a short survival time compared with the survival time of RBCs of older children (60 days versus 120 days).

Fetal RBCs have less deformable membranes and have enzymatic differences from the cells of older children. Senescent RBCs are destroyed in the liver and spleen, where they are recognized as abnormal by changes in their membrane sialic acid content and by the metabolic depletion that occurs as they age. During the first few months of postnatal life, rapid growth, shortened RBC survival, and shutting down of erythropoiesis cause a gradual decline in hemoglobin levels, with a nadir at 8 to 10 weeks of life. This so-called **physiologic nadir** is accentuated in premature infants. Erythropoietin is produced in response to the decline in hemoglobin and decreased oxygen delivery. Erythropoiesis subsequently resumes with an increase in the reticulocyte count. The hemoglobin level gradually increases, accompanied by the synthesis of increasing amounts of hemoglobin A. By 6 months of age in healthy infants, only trace gamma chain synthesis occurs.

Production of **neutrophil precursors** is controlled predominantly by two different colony-stimulating factors (see Fig. 149–1). The most immature neutrophil precursors are controlled by **granulocyte-monocyte colony-stimulating factor** (GM-CSF), which is produced by monocytes and lymphocytes. GM-CSF increases the entry of primitive precursor cells into the myeloid line of differentiation. **Granulocyte colony-stimulating factor** (G-CSF) augments the production of more mature granulocyte precursors. GM-CSF and G-CSF, working in concert, can augment production of neutrophils, shorten the usual baseline 10- to 14-day production time from stem cell to mature neutrophil, and stimulate functional activity. The rapid increase in neutrophil count that occurs with infection is caused by release of stored neutrophils from the bone marrow. This activity also is under the control of GM-CSF. During maturation, a mitotic pool of neutrophil precursors exists—myeloblasts, promyelocytes, and myelocytes possessing primary granules. The postmitotic pool consists of metamyelocytes, bands, and mature polymorphonuclear leukocytes containing secondary or specific granules that define the cell type. Only bands and mature neutrophils are fully functional with regard to phagocytosis, chemotaxis, and bacterial killing. Neutrophils migrate from the bone marrow, circulate for 6 to 7 hours, and enter the tissues, where they become end-stage cells that do not recirculate. Eosinophil production is under the control of a related glycoprotein hormone, interleukin-3. Eosinophils, which play a role in host defense against parasites, also are capable of living in tissues for prolonged periods.

Megakaryocytes are giant, multinucleated cells that derive from the primitive stem cell and are polyploid (16 to 32 times the normal DNA content) because of nuclear but not cytoplasmic cell division. Platelets form by invagination of the megakaryocytic cell membrane and bud off from the periphery. **Thrombopoietin** is the primary regulator of platelet production. Platelets function by adhering to damaged endothelium and subendothelial surfaces via specific receptors for the adhesive proteins, von Willebrand factor (vWF), and fibrinogen. Platelets also have specific granules that readily release their contents after stimulation and trigger the process of platelet aggregation. Platelets circulate for 7 to 10 days and, similar to RBCs, have no nucleus.

Lymphocytes are particularly abundant in the bone marrow of young children, although they are a significant component of normal bone marrow at all ages. These are primarily B lymphocytes arising in the spleen and lymph nodes, but T lymphocytes also are present.

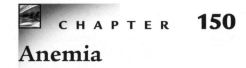

CHAPTER 150

Anemia

ETIOLOGY

Anemia may be defined either quantitatively or functionally (physiologically). The diagnosis of anemia is determined by comparison of the patient's **hemoglobin level** with age-specific and sex-specific normal values (see Table 149–2). A normal newborn has a hemoglobin value of 17 g/dL that decreases at 2 months of age to its nadir of 11 g/dL, then gradually increases to the normal infant value of 12.7 g/dL by 1 year of age. The normal hemoglobin value increases slightly as the child approaches adolescence. The onset of puberty in boys with the production of androgens causes males to maintain a normal hemoglobin value about 1.5 to 2 g/dL higher than girls with average values of 15.5 g/dL for boys and 14 g/dL for girls in late adolescence. The easiest quantitative definition of anemia is any value for the hemoglobin or hematocrit that is 2 SDs (95% confidence limits) below the mean for age and sex. Nevertheless, in certain pathologic states, anemia may be present when the hemoglobin level is within the "normal range," such as in cyanotic cardiac or pulmonary disease or when a hemoglobin with an abnormally high affinity for oxygen is present. In these circumstances, the physiologic definition is more appropriate. Anemia is often not a disease per se, but rather a manifestation of some other primary process. Anemia is a common complication of many disorders and may accentuate other organ dysfunction.

Anemias are classified based on the size and hemoglobin content of the cells (Fig. 150–1). **Hypochromic, microcytic anemia** is caused by an inadequate production of hemoglobin. The most common causes of this type of anemia are iron deficiency and thalassemia. Most **normocytic anemias** are associated with a systemic illness that impairs adequate marrow synthesis of RBCs. Vitamin B_{12} and folic acid deficiencies lead to **macrocytic anemia**.

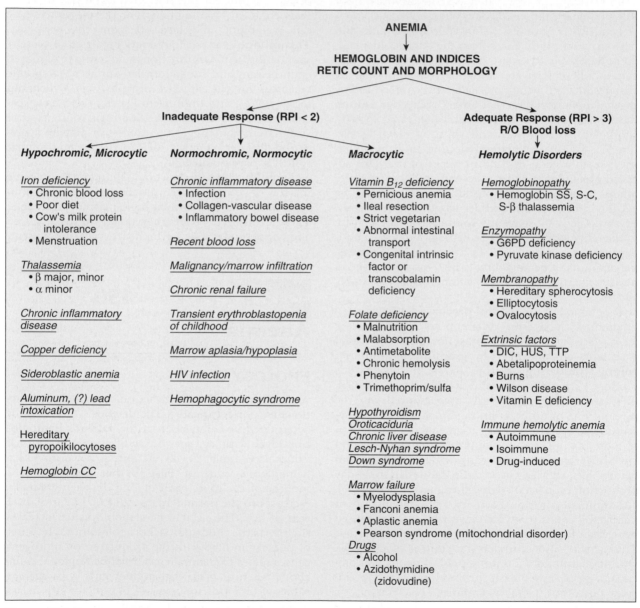

Figure 150–1

Use of the complete blood count, reticulocyte count, and blood smear in the diagnosis of anemia. DIC, disseminated intravascular coagulation; G6PD, glucose-6-phosphate dehydrogenase; HUS, hemolytic uremic syndrome; R/O, rule out; RPI, reticulocyte production index; TTP, thrombotic thrombocytopenic purpura.

Anemias may also occur from increased destruction. **Hemolytic diseases** are mediated either by intrinsic disorders of the RBC or by disorders extrinsic to the RBC itself. The most common RBC membrane disorders are **hereditary spherocytosis** and **hereditary elliptocytosis**. In both of these disorders, abnormalities of proteins within the cytoskeleton lead to abnormal RBC shape and function. Numerous RBC enzyme deficiencies may lead to hemolysis, but only two are common: G6PD deficiency and pyruvate kinase deficiency. Immune-mediated hemolysis may be extravascular when RBCs coated with antibodies or complement are phagocytosed by the reticuloendothelial system. The hemolysis may be intravascular when antibody binding leads to complement fixation and lysis of RBCs.

CLINICAL MANIFESTATIONS

The physiologic consequences of anemia can be determined from the history and physical examination. Acute onset of anemia is often poorly compensated for and may be manifested as an elevated pulse rate, hemic flow cardiac murmur, poor exercise tolerance, headache, excessive sleeping (especially in infants), poor feeding, and syncope. In contrast, chronic anemia often is exceptionally well tolerated in children because of their cardiovascular reserve. Anemia that would induce angina in an adult may not produce symptoms in a young child. The urgency of diagnostic and therapeutic intervention, especially the use of packed RBC transfusion, should be dictated by the extent of cardiovascular or functional impairment more than the absolute level of hemoglobin.

The causes of anemia often can be suspected from a careful history adjusted for the patient's age (Tables 150–1 and 150–2). Anemia at any age demands a search for **blood loss**. A history of jaundice, pallor, previously affected siblings, drug ingestion by the mother, or excessive blood loss at the time of birth provides important clues to the diagnosis in newborns. When the patient is a young infant, a careful **dietary history** is crucial. A history of jaundice suggests hemolytic disease, whereas systemic complaints suggest acute or chronic illnesses as probable causes of anemia. In later childhood and in teenagers, the presence of constitutional symptoms, unusual diets, drug ingestion, or blood loss, especially from menstrual bleeding, often points to a diagnosis. **Congenital hemolytic disorders** (enzyme deficiencies and membrane problems) often present in the first 6 months of life and frequently are associated with neonatal jaundice, although these disorders often go undiagnosed. A careful **drug history** is essential for detecting problems that may be drug induced (hemolysis in G6PD deficiency, bone marrow suppression, or antibody-mediated hemolysis). Pure dietary iron deficiency is rare except in infancy, when cow's milk protein intolerance causes gastrointestinal blood loss and further complicates an already inadequate iron intake.

The physical examination also suggests the presence of anemia and may point to the potential causes (see Table 150–2). The first step in the physical examination of an anemic patient is to assess the **physiologic stability** of the patient. Acute blood loss and acute hemolysis may manifest with tachycardia, blood pressure changes, and, most ominously, an altered state of consciousness. The presence of **jaundice** suggests hemolysis. **Petechiae** and **purpura** indicate a bleeding tendency. **Hepatosplenomegaly** and **adenopathy** suggest infiltrative disorders. **Growth failure** or poor weight gain suggests an anemia of chronic disease or organ failure. An essential element of the physical examination in a patient with anemia is the investigation of the stool for the presence of **occult blood**.

LABORATORY STUDIES

The initial laboratory evaluation of anemia involves a hemoglobin or hematocrit test to indicate the severity of the anemia. When the diagnosis of anemia has been substantiated, the workup should include a **complete blood count** with differential, platelet count, indices, and reticulocyte count. Examination of the peripheral blood smear is crucial to assess the number and **morphology** of RBCs (Fig. 150–2), white blood cells (WBCs), and platelets. All cell lines should be scrutinized to determine whether anemia is the result of a process limited to the erythroid line or of a process that affects other marrow elements. Using data obtained from the indices and **reticulocyte count**, the workup for anemia can be organized on the basis of whether RBC production is adequate or inadequate and whether the cells are microcytic, normocytic, or macrocytic (see Fig. 150–1).

The **reticulocyte production index** (RPI), which corrects the reticulocyte count for the degree of anemia, indicates whether the bone marrow is responding appropriately to the anemia. Reticulocytes routinely are counted per 1000 RBCs. A reduction in the denominator, which occurs in anemia, falsely increases the reticulocyte count. The formula for calculating the RPI is as follows:

$$RPI = \text{reticulocyte count} \times \text{hemoglobin}_{observed}/\text{hemoglobin}_{normal} \times 0.5$$

An RPI of greater than 3 suggests increased production and implies either hemolysis or blood loss, whereas an index less than 2 suggests decreased or ineffective production for the degree of anemia. Reticulocytopenia in the face of anemia signifies that the anemia is so acute in onset that the marrow has not had adequate time to respond, that reticulocytes are being destroyed in the

TABLE 150–1.   Historical Clues in Evaluation of Anemia

Variable	Comments
Age	Iron deficiency rare in the absence of blood loss before 6 mo in term or before doubling birth weight in preterm infants
	Neonatal anemia with reticulocytosis suggests hemolysis or blood loss; with reticulocytopenia, suggests bone marrow failure
	Sickle cell anemia and β-thalassemia appear as fetal hemoglobin disappears (4-8 mo of age)
Family history and genetic considerations	X-linked: G6PD deficiency
	Autosomal dominant: spherocytosis
	Autosomal recessive: sickle cell anemia, Fanconi anemia
	Family member with early age of cholecystectomy (bilirubin stones) or splenectomy
	Ethnicity (thalassemia in individuals of Mediterranean origin; G6PD deficiency in blacks, Greeks, and Middle Eastern individuals)
	Race (β-thalassemia in individuals of Mediterranean, African, or Asian descent; α-thalassemia in blacks and those of Asian descent; SC and SS in blacks)
Nutrition	Cow's milk diet: iron deficiency
	Strict vegetarian: vitamin B_{12} deficiency
	Goat's milk: folate deficiency
	Pica: plumbism, iron deficiency
	Cholestasis, malabsorption: vitamin E deficiency
Drugs	G6PD: oxidants (e.g., nitrofurantoin, antimalarials)
	Immune-mediated hemolysis (e.g., penicillin)
	Bone marrow suppression (e.g., chemotherapy)
	Phenytoin, increasing folate requirements
Diarrhea	Malabsorption of vitamins B_{12} or E or iron
	Inflammatory bowel disease and anemia of chronic disease with or without blood loss
	Milk protein intolerance–induced blood loss
	Intestinal resection: vitamin B_{12} deficiency
Infection	*Giardia:* iron malabsorption
	Intestinal bacterial overgrowth (blind loop): vitamin B_{12} deficiency
	Fish tapeworm: vitamin B_{12} deficiency
	Epstein-Barr virus, cytomegalovirus: bone marrow suppression, hemophagocytic syndromes
	Mycoplasma: hemolysis
	Parvovirus: bone marrow suppression
	HIV
	Chronic infection
	Endocarditis
	Malaria: hemolysis
	Hepatitis: aplastic anemia

G6PD, glucose-6-phosphate dehydrogenase.

marrow (antibody-mediated), or that intrinsic bone marrow disease is present. Some machines that perform complete blood counts report an absolute reticulocyte number that corrects the artifact caused by the degree of anemia.

DIFFERENTIAL DIAGNOSIS

Hypochromic, Microcytic Anemia with Inadequate Red Blood Cell Production

Iron Deficiency Anemia

Etiology. Infants fed large volumes of cow's milk and menstruating teenage girls who are not receiving supplemental iron are at high risk for iron deficiency. **Dietary** iron deficiency anemia is most common in bottle-fed infants who are receiving large volumes of cow's milk. They ingest little in the way of dietary substances high in iron, such as meat and green vegetables (see Chapters 28 and 31). Iron deficiency anemia also may be found in children with chronic inflammatory diseases, even without **chronic blood loss**.

Epidemiology. The prevalence of iron deficiency, the most common cause of anemia in the world, is about 9% in toddlers, 9% to 11% in adolescent girls, and less than 1% in teenage boys. Iron deficiency anemia occurs in about one third of children who are iron deficient. Some underprivileged minority populations in

TABLE 150–2. Physical Findings in the Evaluation of Anemia

System	Observation	Significance
Skin	Hyperpigmentation	Fanconi anemia, dyskeratosis congenita
	Café-au-lait spots	Fanconi anemia
	Vitiligo	Vitamin B_{12} deficiency
	Partial oculocutaneous albinism	Chédiak-Higashi syndrome
	Jaundice	Hemolysis
	Petechiae, purpura	Bone marrow infiltration, autoimmune hemolysis with autoimmune thrombocytopenia, hemolytic uremic syndrome, hemophagocytic syndromes
	Erythematous rash	Parvovirus, Epstein-Barr virus
	Butterfly rash	SLE antibodies
Head	Frontal bossing	Thalassemia major, severe iron deficiency, chronic subdural hematoma
	Microcephaly	Fanconi anemia
Eyes	Microphthalmia	Fanconi anemia
	Retinopathy	Hemoglobin SS, SC disease
	Optic atrophy	Osteopetrosis
	Blocked lacrimal gland	Dyskeratosis congenita
	Kayser-Fleischer ring	Wilson disease
	Blue sclera	Iron deficiency
Ears	Deafness	Osteopetrosis
Mouth	Glossitis	Vitamin B_{12} deficiency, iron deficiency
	Angular stomatitis	Iron deficiency
	Cleft lip	Diamond-Blackfan syndrome
	Pigmentation	Peutz-Jeghers syndrome (intestinal blood loss)
	Telangiectasia	Osler-Weber-Rendu syndrome (blood loss)
	Leukoplakia	Dyskeratosis congenita
Chest	Shield chest or widespread nipples	Diamond-Blackfan syndrome
	Murmur	Endocarditis: prosthetic valve hemolysis; severe anemia
Abdomen	Hepatomegaly	Hemolysis, infiltrative tumor, chronic disease, hemangioma, cholecystitis, extramedullary hematopoiesis
	Splenomegaly	Hemolysis, sickle cell disease, (early) thalassemia, malaria, lymphoma, Epstein-Barr virus, portal hypertension
	Nephromegaly	Fanconi anemia
	Absent kidney	Fanconi anemia
Extremities	Absent thumbs	Fanconi anemia
	Triphalangeal thumb	Diamond-Blackfan syndrome
	Spoon nails	Iron deficiency
	Beau line (nails)	Heavy metal intoxication, severe illness
	Mees line (nails)	Heavy metals, severe illness, sickle cell anemia
	Dystrophic nails	Dyskeratosis congenita
Rectal	Hemorrhoids	Portal hypertension
	Heme-positive stool	Gastrointestinal bleeding
Nerves	Irritable, apathy	Iron deficiency
	Peripheral neuropathy	Deficiency of vitamins B_1, B_{12}, and E, lead poisoning
	Dementia	Deficiency of vitamins B_{12} and E
	Ataxia, posterior column signs	Vitamin B_{12} deficiency
	Stroke	Sickle cell anemia, paroxysmal nocturnal hemoglobinuria
General	Small stature	Fanconi anemia, HIV, malnutrition

SLE, systemic lupus erythematosus.

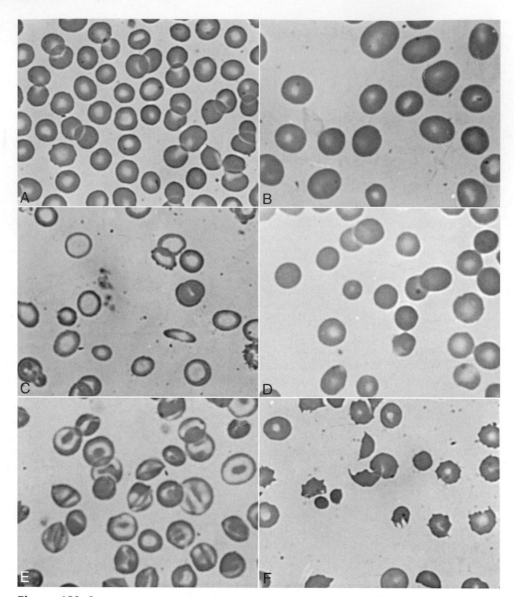

Figure 150–2

Morphologic abnormalities of the red blood cell. A, Normal. **B,** Macrocytes (folic acid deficiency). **C,** Hypochromic microcytes (iron deficiency). **D,** Spherocytes (hereditary spherocytosis). **E,** Target cells (hemoglobin CC disease). **F,** Schistocytes (hemolytic uremic syndrome). (From Behrman RE [eds]: Nelson Textbook of Pediatrics, 14th ed. Philadelphia, WB Saunders, 1992, p 1237.)

the U.S. may be at increased risk for iron deficiency because of poor dietary intake (see Chapter 31). Breast-fed infants are less likely to have iron deficiency than bottle-fed infants because although there is less iron in breast milk, this iron is more effectively absorbed. Menstruating adolescents also are at increased risk of iron deficiency because of dietary insufficiency and blood loss. The laboratory findings vary because the hemoglobin decreases secondary to iron deficiency anemia (Table 150–3).

Clinical Manifestations. In addition to the manifestations of anemia, CNS abnormalities (**apathy, irritability, poor concentration**) have been linked to iron deficiency, presumably resulting from alterations of iron-containing enzymes (monoamine oxidase) and cytochromes. Poor muscle endurance, gastrointestinal

TABLE 150–3. Stages in Development of Iron Deficiency Anemia

Hemoglobin (g/dL)	Peripheral Smear	Serum Iron (µg/dL)	Bone Marrow	Serum Ferritin (ng/mL)
13+ (normal)	nc/nc	50/150	Fe^{2+}	40-340 (male) 40-150 (female)
10-12	nc/nc	↓	Fe^{2+} absent, erythroid hyperplasia	<12
8-10	hypo/nc	↓	Fe^{2+} absent, erythroid hyperplasia	<12
<8	hypo/micro*	↓	Fe^{2+} absent, erythroid hyperplasia	<12

*Microcytosis, determined by a mean corpuscular volume (in fL) <2 SD below the mean, must be adjusted for age (e.g., −2 SD at 3-6 mos = 74; at 0.5-2 yr = 70; at 2-6 yr = 75; at 6-12 yr = 77; and at 12-18 yr = 78).

Hypo/micro, Hypochromic, microcytic; Hypo/nc, hypochromic, normocytic; nc/nc, normochromic, normocytic.

From Andreoli TE, Bennett JC, Carpenter CC, et al: Cecil Essentials of Medicine, 4th ed. Philadelphia WB Saunders, 1997.

dysfunction, and impaired WBC and T cell function also have been noted in association with iron deficiency. Iron deficiency in infancy may be associated with later **cognitive deficits** and poor school performance.

Treatment. If the dietary history in an appropriate-age child suggests iron deficiency, a **therapeutic trial of iron** is appropriate with or without laboratory confirmation. In an otherwise healthy child, a therapeutic trial is the best diagnostic study for iron deficiency as long as the child is re-examined, and a response is documented. The response to oral iron includes rapid subjective improvement, especially in neurologic function (in 24 to 48 hours) and reticulocytosis (in 48 to 72 hours); an increase in hemoglobin levels (in 4 to 30 days); and repletion of iron stores (in 1 to 3 months). A usual therapeutic dose of 4 to 6 mg/day of elemental iron induces an increase in hemoglobin of 0.25 to 0.4 g/dL/day (a 1%/day increase in hematocrit). If the hemoglobin level fails to increase within 2 weeks after the institution of iron treatment, the clinician should re-evaluate the patient carefully for ongoing blood loss, development of infection, poor compliance, or other causes of microcytic anemia (Table 150–4; see also Fig. 150–1).

Prevention. Iron deficiency is easily prevented. In infancy, bottle-fed infants should receive an iron-containing formula until 12 months of age, and breastfed infants older than 6 months of age should receive an iron supplement. Teen-age girls who are menstruating should receive iron supplements in the form of a woman's vitamin with iron.

TABLE 150–4. Differentiating Features of Microcytic Anemias*

Tests	Iron Deficiency Anemia	Thalassemia Minor[†]	Anemia of Chronic Disease[‡]
Serum iron	Low	Normal	Low
Serum iron-binding capacity	High	Normal	Low or normal
Serum ferritin	Low	Normal or high	Normal or high
Marrow iron stores	Low or absent	Normal or high	Normal or high
Marrow sideroblasts	Decreased or absent	Normal or increased	Normal or increased
Free erythrocyte protoporphyrin	High	Normal or slightly increased	High
Hemoglobin A_2 or F	Normal	High β-thalassemia; normal α-thalassemia	Normal
Red blood cell distribution width[§]	High	Normal	Normal/↑

*See Table 150–3 for definition of microcytosis.

[†]α-thalassemia minor can be diagnosed by the presence of Bart hemoglobin on newborn screening.

[‡]Usually normochromic; 25% are microcytic.

[§]Red blood cell distribution width quantitates the degree of anisocytosis (different sizes) of red blood cells.

Thalassemia Minor

Etiology and Epidemiology. α-Thalassemia is common in South East Asia. Individuals of South East Asian descent are also at risk of having three or four α genes deleted, resulting in hemoglobin H disease (β_4) or hydrops fetalis with only Bart (γ_4) hemoglobin. α-Thalassemia occurs in 1.5% of African Americans and is a common cause of microcytosis, either without anemia or with a mild hypochromic, microcytic anemia. **β-Thalassemia minor** is prevalent throughout the Mediterranean region, the Middle East, India, and South East Asia.

Laboratory Testing. The thalassemia minor syndromes are characterized by a mild hypochromic, microcytic anemia with a low reticulocyte production index (Table 150–5). The blood smear is normal with the α-thalassemia trait except for microcytosis. No basophilic stippling is present. Outside of the neonatal period, when Bart hemoglobin is detectable, hemoglobin electrophoresis usually is normal in α-thalassemia minor (Fig. 150–3). Blood smears of patients with β-thalassemia minor show microcytic RBCs. Target cells and basophilic stippled RBCs also may be present. The stippling is caused by precipitation of alpha chain tetramers. The diagnosis is based on an elevation of hemoglobin A_2 and F levels.

Lead Poisoning

Lead poisoning may be associated with a hypochromic, microcytic anemia. Most patients have concomitant iron deficiency. The history of a child with **pica** who lives in an older home (built before 1980) with chipped paint or lead dust should raise suspicion of lead poisoning. **Basophilic stippling** on the blood smear is common. Detection by routine screening, removal from exposure, chelation therapy, and correction of iron deficiency are crucial to the potential development of affected children. Lead intoxication rarely may also cause hemolytic anemia.

TABLE 150–5. Comparison of the Thalassemia Syndromes

Genetic Abnormality	Percent Hemoglobin			Other	Clinical Syndrome
	Hb A	Hb A_2	Hb F		
Normal αβ	90-98	2-3	2-3		None
β-Thalassemias					
Thalassemia major					
$\beta^0\,\beta^0$	0	2-5	95	—	Severe anemia, abnormal growth, iron overload, needs transfusion, Cooley anemia
$\beta^0\,\beta^+$	Very low	2-5	20-80	—	
Thalassemia intermedia					
$\beta^+\,\beta^+$	20-40	5	60-80		Severe hypo/micro anemia with Hb 7-9 g/dL, hepatosplenomegaly, bone changes, iron overload, less need for transfusion
Thalassemia minor					
$\beta\,\beta^0$ or $\beta\,\beta^+$	90-95	5-7	2-10	Stippled RBCs	Hypo/micro blood smear, mild to no anemia
α-Thalassemias					
Homozygous α-thalassemia ––/––	—	—	—	Hb H (B4) Hb Bart (γ4)	Hydrops fetalis, stillborn
Hemoglobin H disease ––/–α	60-70	2-5	2-5	Hb H 30-40	Hypo/micro anemia, Hb 7-10 g/dL, Heinz bodies
α-Thalassemia trait –α/–α, αα/––	90-98	2-3	2-3		Hypo/micro smear, no anemia
Silent carrier –α/αα	90-98	2-3	2-3		Normal
Hemoglobin Lepore (δβ fusion)					
Heterozygote	70-80	1-2	5-20	Hb Lepore 5-15	Mild hypo/micro anemia
Homozygote	0	0	70-90	Hb Lepore 10-30	Severe thalassemia major

Hypo/micro, hypochromic, microcytic; RBCs, red blood cells.
From Andreoli TE, Bennett JC, Carpenter CC, et al: Cecil Essentials of Medicine, 4th ed. Philadelphia, WB Saunders, 1997.

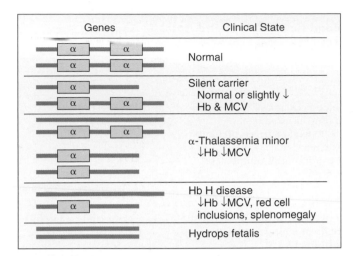

Figure 150-3

Schematic illustration of α-globin gene deletions and their clinical consequences. Hb, hemoglobin; MCV, mean corpuscular volume. (From Beutler E: The common anemias. JAMA 259:2433, 1988.)

Normocytic Anemia with Inadequate Red Blood Cell Production

Etiology and Treatment

Anemia is a common component of **chronic inflammatory disease**. Elevated cytokine levels cause a reticuloendothelial blockade within the marrow mediated by the protein hepcidin, causing iron to be taken up by the reticuloendothelial cells but not released for erythroid synthesis. The anemia may be normocytic or, less often, microcytic. At times, this situation poses a clinical challenge, when children with inflammatory disorders that may be associated with blood loss (inflammatory bowel disease) exhibit a microcytic anemia. In these circumstances, the only specific diagnostic test that can differentiate the two entities clearly is a bone marrow aspiration with staining of the sample for iron (see Table 150-4). Low ferritin levels indicate concurrent iron deficiency. A trial of iron therapy is not indicated without a specific diagnosis in children who appear to be systemically ill.

Bone marrow **infiltration by malignant cells** commonly leads to a normochromic, normocytic anemia. The mechanism by which neoplastic cells interfere with RBC and other marrow cell synthesis is multifactorial. The reticulocyte count is low. Immature myeloid elements may be released into the peripheral blood as a result of the presence of the offending tumor cells. An examination of the peripheral blood may reveal lymphoblasts; when solid tumors metastasize to the marrow, these cells are seldom seen in the peripheral blood. Teardrop cells may be seen in the peripheral blood. Performance of a bone marrow examination is frequently necessary in the face of normochromic, normocytic anemia.

Congenital pure RBC aplasia (Diamond-Blackfan syndrome), a lifelong disorder, usually presents in the first few months of life or at birth (Table 150-6). Congenital anomalies are common. Many patients (50% to 66%) respond to corticosteroid treatment, but must receive therapy indefinitely. At the time of presentation, the patient may have mild macrocytosis or may be normocytic. Patients who do not respond to corticosteroid treatment are transfusion-dependent and are at risk of the multiple complications of long-term transfusion therapy, especially iron overload.

In contrast to the congenital hypoplastic anemias, **transient erythroblastopenia of childhood**, a normocytic anemia caused by suppression of RBC synthesis, usually appears after 6 months of age in an otherwise normal infant. Viral infections are thought to trigger transient erythroblastopenia of childhood, although the mechanism leading to RBC aplasia is poorly understood. The onset is gradual, but the anemia may become severe. Recovery usually is spontaneous. Transfusion of packed RBCs may be necessary if the anemia becomes symptomatic before recovery. Differentiation from Diamond-Blackfan syndrome, in which erythroid precursors also are absent or diminished in the bone marrow, is necessary.

Aplastic crises, which may complicate any chronic hemolytic anemia, are periods of reticulocytopenia during which the usual high rate of RBC destruction leads to an acute exacerbation of the anemia, potentially precipitating cardiovascular decompensation. Human parvovirus B19 (the cause of fifth disease) infects erythroid precursors and shuts down erythropoiesis. Transient erythroid aplasia is without consequence in individuals with normal RBC survival. Recovery from parvovirus infection in hemolytic disease is spontaneous, but patients may need transfusion if the anemia is severe.

TABLE 150–6.   Differentiation of Red Blood Cell Aplasias and Aplastic Anemias

Disorder	Age of Onset	Characteristics	Treatment
Congenital			
Diamond-Blackfan syndrome (congenital hypoplastic anemia)	Newborn-1 mo; 90% are <1 yr of age	Pure red blood cell aplasia, autosomal recessive trait, elevated fetal hemoglobin, fetal i antigen present, macrocytic, short stature, web neck, cleft lip, triphalangeal thumb; late onset leukemia	Prednisone, transfusion
Acquired			
Transient erythroblastopenia	6 mo-5 yr of age; 85% are >1 yr of age	Pure red cell defect; no anomalies, fetal hemoglobin, or i antigen; spontaneous recovery, normal MCV	Expectant transfusion for symptomatic anemia
Idiopathic aplastic anemia (s/p hepatitis, drugs, unknown)	All ages	All cell lines involved; exposure to chloramphenicol, phenylbutazone, radiation	Bone marrow transplant, antithymocyte globulin, cyclosporine, androgens
Familial			
Fanconi syndrome	Before 10 yr of age; mean is 8 yr	All cell lines; microcephaly, absent thumbs, café au lait spots, cutaneous hyperpigmentation, short stature; chromosomal breaks, high MCV and hemoglobin F; horseshoe or absent kidney; leukemic transformation; autosomal recessive trait	Androgens, corticosteroids, bone marrow transplant
Paroxysmal nocturnal hemoglobinuria	After 5 yr	Initial hemolysis followed by aplastic anemia; increased complement-mediated hemolysis; thrombosis; iron deficiency	Iron, bone marrow transplant, androgens, steroids
Dyskeratosis congenita	Mean 10 yr for skin; mean 17 yr for anemia	Pancytopenia; hyperpigmentation, dystrophic nails, leukoplakia; X-linked recessive; lacrimal duct stenosis; high MCV and fetal hemoglobin	Androgens, splenectomy, bone marrow transplant
Familial hemophagocytic lymphohistiocytosis	Before 2 yr	Pancytopenia; fever, hepatosplenomegaly, hypertriglyceridemia, CSF pleocytosis	Transfusion; often lethal; VP-16, bone marrow transplantation, IVIG, cyclosporine
Infectious			
Parvovirus	Any age	Any chronic hemolytic anemia, typically sickle cell; new-onset reticulocytopenia	Transfusion
Epstein-Barr virus (EBV)	Any age; usually <5 yr of age	X-linked immunodeficiency syndrome, pancytopenia	Transfusion, bone marrow transplantation
Viral-associated hemophagocytic syndrome (CMV, HHV-6, EBV)	Any age	Pancytopenia; hemophagocytosis present in marrow, fever, hepatosplenomegaly	Transfusion, antiviral therapy, IVIG

CMV, cytomegalovirus; CSF, cerebrospinal fluid; HHV-6, human herpesvirus 6; IVIG, IV immunoglobulin; MCV, mean corpuscular volume; VP-16, etoposide.

Macrocytic Anemia (See Figure 150-1)

Hemolytic Anemias

Clinical Manifestations. The key findings in patients with hemolytic anemias are **jaundice**, **pallor**, and **splenomegaly**. Because of increased bilirubin production, **gallstones** (bilirubinate), a result of chronic hemolysis, are a common complication. Patients who are candidates for splenectomy for hemolytic disease should be immunized against *Streptococcus pneumoniae* and *Haemophilus influenzae* before surgery.

Laboratory Studies. The best indicators of the severity of hemolysis are the hemoglobin level and the elevation of the **reticulocyte count**. Biochemical evidence of hemolysis includes an increase in levels of bilirubin and lactate dehydrogenase and decrease in haptoglobin.

Hemolytic Anemia Caused by Intrinsic Red Blood Cell Disorders

Membrane Disorders

Etiology. The biochemical bases of **hereditary spherocytosis** and **hereditary elliptocytosis** are similar. Both conditions appear to have a defect in the protein lattice (spectrin, ankyrin, protein 4.2, band 3) that underlies the RBC lipid bilayer and provides stability of the membrane shape. In hereditary spherocytosis, pieces of membrane bud off as microvesicles because of abnormal vertical interaction of the cytoskeletal proteins and uncoupling of the lipid bilayer from the cytoskeleton. When the RBC loses membrane, the shape changes from a biconcave disc to a spherocyte, which has the lowest ratio of surface area to volume. The RBC is less deformable when passing through narrow passages in the spleen. Hereditary elliptocytosis is a disorder of spectrin dimer interactions that occurs primarily in individuals of African descent. The transmission of the two variants is usually autosomal dominant, but spontaneous mutations causing hereditary spherocytosis are common.

Clinical Manifestations. Hereditary spherocytosis varies greatly in clinical severity, ranging from an asymptomatic, well-compensated, mild hemolytic anemia that may be discovered incidentally to a severe hemolytic anemia with growth failure, splenomegaly, and chronic transfusion requirements in infancy necessitating early splenectomy. The most common variant of hereditary elliptocytosis is a clinically insignificant, morphologic abnormality without shortened RBC survival. The less common variant is associated with spherocytes, ovalocytes, and elliptocytes and with a moderate, usually compensated, hemolysis. Far more significant hemolysis occurs in a small percentage of patients with elliptocytes, spherocytes, fragmented RBCs, and striking microcytosis. This disorder is termed **hereditary pyropoikilocytosis** and is the result of a structural abnormality of spectrin. Such patients may have particularly bizarre blood smears in the newborn period with small fragmented RBCs. The term *pyropoikilocytosis* refers to the unusual instability of the erythrocytes when they are exposed to heat (45°C).

Laboratory Testing. The diagnosis of hereditary spherocytosis should be suspected in patients with even a few spherocytes found on the blood smear because the spleen preferentially removes spherocytes. An incubated **osmotic fragility test** confirms the presence of spherocytes and increases the likelihood of the diagnosis of hereditary spherocytosis. The osmotic fragility test result is abnormal in any hemolytic disease in which spherocytes are present, however, especially antibody-mediated hemolysis.

Treatment. **Splenectomy** corrects the anemia and normalizes the RBC survival, but the morphologic abnormalities persist. Splenectomy should be considered for any child with symptoms referable to anemia or growth failure, but should be deferred until age 5 years, if possible, to minimize the risk of overwhelming postsplenectomy sepsis and to maximize the antibody response to the polyvalent pneumococcal vaccine. In several reports, partial splenectomy seems to improve the hemolytic anemia and maintain splenic function in host defense.

Red Blood Cell Enzyme Deficiencies

Glucose-6-Phosphate Dehydrogenase Deficiency

Etiology. G6PD deficiency is an abnormality in the **hexose monophosphate shunt pathway** of glycolysis that results in the depletion of reduced nicotinamide adenine dinucleotide phosphate (NADPH) and the inability to regenerate reduced glutathione. Reduced glutathione protects sulfhydryl groups in the RBC membrane from oxidation. When a patient with G6PD is exposed to significant oxidant stress, hemoglobin is oxidized, forming precipitates of sulfhemoglobin (Heinz bodies). **Heinz bodies** are visible on specially stained preparations. The gene for G6PD is on the X chromosome.

The severity of the hemolysis depends on the enzyme variant. In many G6PD variants, the enzymes become unstable with aging. Young RBCs have normal G6PD activity that is lost as the cell ages. The activity cannot be replaced because the cell is anucleated. Older cells are most susceptible to oxidant-induced hemolysis. In other variants, the enzyme is kinetically abnormal.

Epidemiology. The most common variants of G6PD have been found in areas where malaria is endemic. G6PD deficiency protects against parasitism of the erythrocyte. The most common variant with normal activity is termed **type B** and is defined by its electrophoretic mobility. The approximate gene frequencies in African Americans are 70% type B, 20% type A^+, and 10% type A^-. Only the A^- **variant** is unstable. The A^- variant is termed the *African variant*. Ten percent of black males are affected. A group of variants found in Sardinians, Sicilians, Greeks, Sephardic and Oriental Jews, and Arabs is termed the **Mediterranean variant** and is associated with chronic hemolysis and potentially life-threatening hemolytic disease. Because the gene for G6PD is carried on the X chromosome, clinical hemolysis is most common in males. Heterozygous females who have randomly inactivated a higher percentage of the normal gene may become symptomatic, as may homozygous females with the A^- variant, which occurs in 0.5% to 1% of females of African descent.

Clinical Manifestations. G6PD deficiency has two common presentations. Individuals with the A^- variant have normal hemoglobin values when well, but develop an **acute episode of hemolysis** triggered by serious (bacterial) infection or ingestion of an oxidant drug. The RBC morphology during episodes of acute hemolysis is striking. RBCs appear to have "bites" (cookie cells) taken out of them. These are areas of absent hemoglobin that are produced by phagocytosis of Heinz bodies by splenic macrophages; as a result, the RBCs appear blistered. Clinically evident jaundice, dark urine resulting from bilirubin pigments, hemoglobinuria when hemolysis is intravascular, and decreased haptoglobin levels are common during hemolytic episodes. Early on, the hemolysis usually exceeds the ability of the bone marrow to compensate, so the reticulocyte count may be low for 3 to 4 days.

Laboratory Studies. The diagnosis of G6PD deficiency is based on decreased NADPH formation. G6PD levels may be normal, however, in the setting of acute, severe hemolysis because the most deficient cells have been destroyed. Repeating the test at a later time when the patient is in a steady-state condition, testing the mothers of boys with suspected G6PD deficiency, or performing electrophoresis to identify the precise variant present facilitates diagnosis.

Treatment and Prevention. The treatment of G6PD deficiency is supportive, including transfusion when significant cardiovascular compromise is present and protecting the kidneys against damage from precipitated free hemoglobin by maintaining hydration and urine alkalization. Hemolysis is prevented by avoidance of known oxidants, particularly long-acting sulfonamides, nitrofurantoin, primaquine, dimercaprol and moth balls (naphthalene). Fava beans (favism) have triggered hemolysis, particularly in patients with the Mediterranean variant. Infection also is a major precipitant of hemolysis in G6PD-deficient young children.

Pyruvate Kinase Deficiency. Pyruvate kinase deficiency is much less common than G6PD deficiency and represents a clinical spectrum of disorders caused by the functional deficiency of pyruvate kinase. Some individuals have a true deficiency state, and others have abnormal enzyme kinetics. This enzyme in the Embden-Meyerhof pathway of glycolysis is important for the production of two moles of ATP per mole of glucose metabolized. The metabolic consequence of pyruvate kinase deficiency is ATP depletion, impairing RBC survival.

Pyruvate kinase deficiency is usually an autosomal disorder, and most children who are affected (and are not products of consanguinity) are double heterozygotes for two abnormal enzymes. Hemolysis is not aggravated by oxidant stress because patients with this condition tend to have a profound reticulocytosis. Aplastic crises are potentially life-threatening. The spleen is the site for RBC removal in pyruvate kinase deficiency. Most patients have amelioration of the anemia and a reduction of transfusion requirements after splenectomy.

Major Hemoglobinopathies

Etiology

Because alpha chains are needed for fetal erythropoiesis and production of hemoglobin F ($\alpha_2\gamma_2$), **alpha chain hemoglobinopathies** are present in utero. Four alpha genes are present on the two number 16 chromosomes (see Fig. 150–3 and Table 150–5). Single gene deletions produce no disorder (the silent carrier state), but can be detected by measuring the rates of α and β synthesis or by using molecular biologic techniques. Deletion of two genes produces **α-thalassemia minor** with mild or no anemia and microcytosis. In individuals of African origin, the gene deletions occur on different chromosomes (*trans*), and the disorder is benign because few individuals of African descent have more than two genes deleted. In the Asian population, deletions may occur on the same chromosome (*cis*), and infants may inherit two number 16 chromosomes lacking three or even four genes. Deletion of all four genes leads to hydrops fetalis, severe intrauterine anemia, and death, unless intrauterine transfusions are administered. Deletion of three genes produces moderate hemolytic anemia with γ_4 tetramers (**Bart hemoglobin**) in the fetus and β_4 tetramers (hemoglobin H) in older children and adults (see Table 150–5).

Beta chain hemoglobinopathies are more common than alpha chain disorders because these abnormalities are not symptomatic in utero. The major beta hemoglobinopathies include those that alter hemoglobin function, including **hemoglobins S, C, E, and D**, and those that alter beta chain production, the β-thalassemias. Because each RBC has two copies of chromosome 11 and the β-globin genes are both expressed, most of the disorders of beta chains are not clinically severe, unless both beta chains are abnormal. By convention, when describing β-thalassemia genes, β^0 indicates a thalassemic gene resulting in absent beta chain synthesis, whereas β^+ indicates a thalassemic gene that permits reduced but not absent synthesis of normal β chains. Disorders of the beta chain usually manifest themselves clinically between 4 and 12 months of age, unless they have been detected prenatally or by cord blood screening.

β-Thalassemia Major (Cooley Anemia)

Etiology and Epidemiology. β-Thalassemia major is a hemoglobinopathy caused by mutations that impair **beta chain synthesis**. Excess gamma and beta chains do not damage the RBCs, whereas excess alpha chain tetramers are toxic. Because of unbalanced synthesis of alpha and beta chains, alpha chains precipitate within the cells, resulting in RBC destruction either in the bone marrow or in the spleen when the cell is released. Beta-Thalassemia major is seen most commonly in individuals of Mediterranean or Asian descent. The clinical severity of the illness varies on the basis of the molecular defect.

Clinical Manifestations. Signs and symptoms of β-thalassemia major result from the combination of chronic hemolytic disease, decrease in or absent production of normal hemoglobin A, and ineffective erythropoiesis in the marrow. The anemia is severe and leads to growth failure and high output heart failure. **Ineffective erythropoiesis** causes increased expenditure of energy and expansion of the bone marrow cavities of all bones, leading to osteopenia, pathologic fractures, extramedullary erythropoiesis, and an increase in the rate of iron absorption. Patients usually are transfusion dependent before 12 months old. Adolescents are subject to complications from transfusion-related iron overload (**hemochromatosis**), including nonimmune diabetes mellitus, cirrhosis, heart failure, bronzing of the skin, and multiple endocrine abnormalities (of the thyroid or gonad).

Treatment. Treatment of β-thalassemia major is based on a **hypertransfusion program** that corrects the anemia and suppresses the patient's own ineffective erythropoiesis, limiting the stimulus for increased iron absorption. This suppression permits the bones to heal, decreases the metabolic expenditures, increases growth, and limits dietary iron absorption. Splenectomy may reduce the transfusion volume, but adds to the risk of serious infection. Chelation therapy with deferoxamine, which removes excess iron and prolongs life, should start when laboratory evidence of **iron overload** is present and before there are clinical signs of iron overload. The amount of iron the patient acquires from transfusion may be estimated by the formula stating that each milliliter of packed RBCs contains approximately 1 mg of iron. Hematopoietic stem cell transplantation in childhood, before organ dysfunction induced by iron overload, has had a high success rate in β-thalassemia major and is the treatment of choice.

Sickle Cell Disease

Etiology and Epidemiology. The common sickle cell syndromes are **hemoglobin SS disease, hemoglobin S-C disease, hemoglobin S-β thalassemia**, and rare variants (Table 150–7). The specific hemoglobin phenotype must be identified because the clinical complications differ in frequency, type, and severity. As a result of a single **amino acid substitution** (valine for glutamic acid at the β6 position), hemoglobin S cells change from a normal biconcave disc (when oxygenated) to a sickled form, with resultant decreased deformability in deoxygenated conditions. Sickle hemoglobin crystallizes and forms a gel in the deoxygenated state. When reoxygenated, the sickle hemoglobin is normally soluble. The so-called reversible sickle cell is capable of entering the microcirculation where oxygen is extracted. As the oxygen saturation declines, however, sickling may occur, with resultant occlusion of the microvasculature. The surrounding tissue undergoes infarction, inducing pain and dysfunction. This sickling phenomenon is exacerbated by hypoxia, acidosis, increased or decreased temperature, and dehydration.

Clinical Manifestations and Treatment. A child with sickle cell anemia is vulnerable to **life-threatening infection** by 4 months of age. By that time, **splenic dysfunction** is caused by sickling of the RBCs within the spleen, resulting in an inability to filter microorganisms from the bloodstream. Splenic dysfunction is followed eventually by **splenic infarction**, usually by 2 to 4 years of age. In the absence of normal splenic function, the patient is susceptible to overwhelming infection by encapsulated organisms, especially *S. pneumoniae* and other pathogens (Table 150–8). The hallmark of infection is fever. A patient with a sickle cell syndrome who has a temperature greater than 38.5°C (>101.5°F) must be evaluated immediately (see Chapter 96). Current precautions to prevent infections include prophylactic daily oral penicillin begun at diagnosis and vaccinations against pneumococcus, *H. influenzae* type b, hepatitis B virus, and influenza virus.

The anemia of SS disease is usually a chronic, moderately severe, compensated anemia that is not

TABLE 150–7. Comparison of Sickle Cell Syndromes

Genotype	Clinical Condition	Percent Hemoglobin					Other Findings
		Hb A	Hb S	Hb A_2	Hb F	Hb C	
SA	Sickle cell trait	55-60	40-45	2-3	—	—	Usually asymptomatic
SS	Sickle cell anemia	0	85-95	2-3	5-15	—	Clinically severe anemia; Hb F heterogeneous in distribution
S-β^0 thalassemia	Sickle cell–β^0 thalassemia	0	70-80	3-5	10-20	—	Moderately severe anemia; splenomegaly in 50%; smear: hypochromic, microcytic anemia
S-β^+ thalassemia	Sickle cell–β^+ thalassemia	10-20	60-75	3-5	10-20		Hb F distributed heterogeneously; mild microcytic anemia
SC	Hb SC disease	0	45-50	—	—	45-50	Moderately severe anemia; splenomegaly; target cells
S-HPFH	Sickle-hereditary persistence of Hb F	0	70-80	1-2	20-30	—	Asymptomatic; Hb F is uniformly distributed

From Andreoli TE, Bennett JC, Carpenter CC, et al: Cecil Essentials of Medicine, 4th ed. Philadelphia, WB Saunders, 1997.

routinely transfusion dependent. The severity depends in part on the patient's phenotype. Manifestations of chronic anemia include jaundice, pallor, variable splenomegaly in infancy, a cardiac flow murmur, and delayed growth and sexual maturation. Decisions about transfusion should be made on the basis of the patient's clinical condition, the hemoglobin level, and the reticulocyte count.

Sickle cell disease is a chronic hemolytic anemia complicated by sudden, occasionally severe and life-threatening events caused by the acute intravascular sickling of the RBCs, with resultant pain or organ dysfunction (so-called crisis). In three different clinical situations, an acute, potentially life-threatening decline in the hemoglobin level may be superimposed on the chronic compensated anemia. **Splenic sequestration crisis** is a life-threatening, hyperacute decline in the hemoglobin level (blood volume) secondary to splenic pooling of the patient's RBCs and sickling within the spleen. The spleen is moderately to markedly enlarged, and the reticulocyte count is elevated. In an **aplastic crisis**, parvovirus B19 infects RBC precursors in the bone marrow and induces transient RBC aplasia with reticulocytopenia and a rapid worsening of anemia. In the **hyperhemolytic crisis**, there may be an acute decrease in hemoglobin, associated with medications or infection. The level of bilirubin increases, and reticulocytosis and accentuated jaundice may occur. Patients with these conditions usually have G6PD deficiency. For sequestration, aplastic, and hemolytic crises, simple transfusion therapy is indicated when the anemia is symptomatic.

Vaso-occlusive crises may occur in any organ of the body and are manifested by pain or significant dysfunction (see Table 150–8). The **acute chest syndrome** is a vaso-occlusive crisis within the lungs, often associated with infection and infarction. The patient may first complain of pain but within a few hours develops cough, increasing respiratory and heart rates, hypoxia, and progressive respiratory distress. Physical examination of the chest reveals areas of decreased breath sounds and dullness to percussion. Treatment involves early recognition and prevention of arterial hypoxemia. Oxygen, fluids, judicious use of analgesic medications, antibiotics, bronchodilators, and RBC transfusion (rarely exchange transfusion) usually are indicated in therapy for acute chest syndrome. *Incentive spirometry* reduces the incidence of acute chest crisis in patients presenting with pain in the chest or abdomen.

Vaso-occlusive events also may develop in patients within the CNS, causing clinical or "silent" **stroke**. These events may present as the sudden onset of an altered state of consciousness, seizures, or focal paralysis. **Priapism** occurs most typically in boys between 6 and 20 years old. The child experiences a sudden, painful onset of a tumescent penis that will not relax. Therapeutic steps for stroke, priapism, and other potentially life-threatening complications include the administration of oxygen, fluids, transfusion to achieve a hemoglobin S less than 30% (often by partial exchange transfusion), and analgesia when appropriate. Fluid management requires recognition that renal medullary infarction results in loss of the ability to concentrate urine. Vaso-occlusive crises within the

Manifestation	Comments
Anemia	Chronic, onset 3-4 mo of age; may require folate therapy for chronic hemolysis; hematocrit usually 18-26%
Aplastic crisis	Parvovirus infection, reticulocytopenia; acute and reversible; may need transfusion
Sequestration crisis	Massive splenomegaly (may involve liver), shock; treat with transfusion
Hemolytic crisis	May be associated with G6PD deficiency
Dactylitis	Hand-foot swelling in early infancy
Painful crisis	Microvascular painful vaso-occlusive infarcts of muscle, bone, bone marrow, lung, intestines
Cerebrovascular accidents	Large and small vessel occlusion → thrombosis/bleeding (stroke); requires chronic transfusion
Acute chest syndrome	Infection, atelectasis, infarction, fat emboli, severe hypoxemia, infiltrate, dyspnea, absent breath sounds
Chronic lung disease	Pulmonary fibrosis, restrictive lung disease, cor pulmonale, pulmonary hypertension
Priapism	Causes eventual impotence; treated with tranfusion, oxygen, or corpora cavernosa–to–spongiosa shunt
Ocular	Retinopathy
Gallbladder disease	Bilirubin stones; cholecystitis
Renal	Hematuria, papillary necrosis, renal-concentrating defect; nephropathy
Cardiomyopathy	Heart failure
Skeletal	Osteonecrosis (avascular) of femoral or humeral head
Leg ulceration	Seen in older patients
Infections	Functional asplenia, defects in properdin system; pneumococcal bacteremia, meningitis, and arthritis; deafness from meningitis; *Salmonella* and *Staphylococcus aureus* osteomyelitis; severe *Mycoplasma* pneumonia
Growth failure, delayed puberty	May respond to nutritional supplements
Psychological problems	Narcotic addiction (rare), dependence unusual; chronic illness, chronic pain

TABLE 150–8. Clinical Manifestations of Sickle Cell Anemia*

*Clinical manifestations with sickle cell trait are unusual, but include renal papillary necrosis (hematuria), sudden death on exertion, intraocular hyphema extension, and sickling in unpressurized airplanes.
G6PD, glucose-6-phosphate dehydrogenase.

femur may lead to avascular necrosis of the femoral head and chronic hip disease.

Pain crisis is the most common type of vaso-occlusive event. The pain usually localizes to the long bones of the arms or legs, but may occur in smaller bones of the hands or feet in infancy (hand-foot syndrome). These painful crises usually last 2 to 7 days. The treatment of a pain crisis includes administration of fluids, analgesia (usually with narcotics or non-steroidal anti-inflammatory drugs), oxygen if the patient is hypoxic, and monitoring of arterial oxygen saturation. The clinician must maintain a sympathetic attitude toward the patient in pain crisis because pain is impossible to quantitate, and the risk for drug dependency is highly overrated.

Laboratory Diagnosis. The diagnosis is made by identifying the precise amount and type of hemoglobin present using **hemoglobin electrophoresis**, **isoelectric focusing**, or **high-performance liquid chromatography**. Every member of an at-risk population should have a precise hemoglobin phenotype performed at birth (preferably) or during early infancy.

Most states perform newborn screening for sickle cell disease.

Treatment. Direct therapy of sickle cell anemia is evolving. **Hydroxyurea**, which increases hemoglobin F, has been shown in adults and children to decrease the number and severity of vaso-occlusive events. **Hematopoietic stem cell transplantation** has cured many children with sickle cell disease.

Methemoglobinemia

Methemoglobinemia, in which ferrous (Fe^{2+}) iron has been oxidized to the ferric (Fe^{3+}) state, may be either congenital or acquired. **Congenital methemoglobinemia** may be a result of abnormalities in either the alpha or the beta chain. Homozygosity is lethal, whereas heterozygotes usually have a level of 20% to 30% methemoglobin and are cyanotic in the face of normal PaO2. Homozygous deficiency of reduced nicotinamide adenine dinucleotide reductase (diaphorase) is common in Navajo Indians and results in chronic methemoglobinemia. Infants younger than

3 months, whose antioxidant mechanisms are poorly developed, are especially vulnerable.

Acquired methemoglobinemia is seen with ingestion of certain oxidants. **Nitrates** and **nitrites**, derived from fertilizer and disinfectants in well water and foods or from enteric bacteria during diarrhea, are major etiologic factors. If sufficiently severe, this condition may be life-threatening. Methemoglobinemia should be suspected in a deeply cyanotic infant without cardiopulmonary disease in whom metabolic acidosis, a high PaO_2, and unsaturated hemoglobin are present. When drawn to measure methemoglobin levels, blood is often described as chocolate colored. Treatment with methylene blue or ascorbate usually rapidly reduces Fe^{3+} to Fe^{2+}, correcting this condition.

Hemolytic Anemia Caused by Disorders Extrinsic to the Red Blood Cell

Etiology and Clinical Manifestations. **Isoimmune hemolysis** is caused by active maternal immunization against fetal antigens that the mother's erythrocytes do not express (see Chapter 62). Examples are antibodies to the A, B, and Rh D antigens; other Rh antigens; and the Kell, Duffy, and other blood groups. Anti-A and anti-B hemolysis is caused by the placental transfer of naturally occurring maternal antibodies from mothers who lack A or B antigen (usually blood type O). Positive results of the direct antiglobulin (**Coombs**) test on the infant's RBCs (Fig. 150–4), the indirect antiglobulin test on the mother's serum and

the presence of spherocytes and immature erythroid precursors (erythroblastosis) on the infant's blood smear confirm this diagnosis. Isoimmune hemolytic disease varies in its clinical severity. No clinical manifestations may be present, or the infant may exhibit jaundice, severe anemia, and hydrops fetalis.

Autoimmune hemolytic anemia is usually an acute, self-limited process that develops after an infection (*Mycoplasma,* Epstein-Barr, or other viral infections). Autoimmune hemolytic anemia may also be the presenting symptom of a chronic autoimmune disease (systemic lupus erythematosus, lymphoproliferative disorders, or immunodeficiency). Drugs may also induce a Coombs-positive hemolytic anemia by forming a hapten on the RBC membrane (penicillin). Alternatively, drugs may form immune complexes (quinidine) that attach to the RBC membrane. Antibodies then activate complement-induced intravascular hemolysis. The third type of drug-induced immune hemolysis occurs during treatment with α-methyldopa and a few other drugs. In this type, prolonged exposure to the drug alters the RBC membrane, inducing neoantigen formation. Antibodies are produced that bind to the neoantigen; this produces a positive antiglobulin test result far more commonly than it actually induces hemolysis. In each of these conditions, the erythrocyte acts as an "innocent bystander."

A second form of acquired hemolytic disease that is not antibody mediated is caused by mechanical damage to the membrane of the RBCs during circulation. In **thrombotic microangiopathy**, the RBCs are

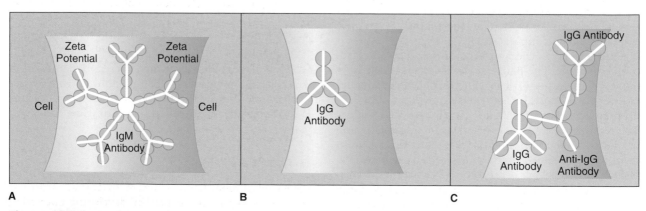

A   **B**   **C**

Figure 150–4

Coombs or direct antiglobulin test (DAT). In the DAT, so-called Coombs sera that recognizes human immunoglobulin (Ig) or complement (C) is used to detect the presence of antibody or C on the surface of the red blood cells (RBCs) by agglutination. **A,** An IgM antibody can bind two RBCs simultaneously because of its multiple antigen-binding sites. The great size of the IgM allows it to bridge the surface repulsive forces (zeta potential) between RBCs and cause agglutination. **B,** An IgG antibody is too small to bridge the zeta potential and cause agglutination. **C,** On the addition of Coombs sera, the zeta potential is bridged successfully, and RBCs agglutinate. (Modified from Ware RE, Rosse WF: Autoimmune hemolytic anemia. In Orkin SH, Nathan DG et al [eds]: Hematology of Infancy and Childhood, 6th ed. Philadelphia, WB Saunders, 2003, p 530.)

trapped by fibrin strands in the circulation and physically broken by shear stress as they pass through these strands. Hemolytic uremic syndrome, disseminated intravascular coagulation (DIC), thrombotic thrombocytopenic purpura, malignant hypertension, toxemia, and hyperacute renal graft rejection all produce thrombotic microangiopathy. The platelets are usually large, indicating that they are young. These platelets have a decreased survival even if the numbers are normal. Consumption of clotting factors is more prominent in DIC than in the other forms of thrombotic microangiopathy. The smear shows RBC fragments (schistocytes), microspherocytes, teardrop forms, and polychromasia. Other examples of mechanical injury to RBCs include damage by exposure to nonendothelialized surfaces (as in artificial heart valves—the "Waring blender" syndrome) or as a result of high flow and shear rates in giant hemangiomas (**Kasabach-Merritt syndrome**).

Alterations in the plasma lipids, especially cholesterol, may lead to damage to the RBC membrane and shorten RBC survival. Lipids in the plasma are in equilibrium with lipids in the RBC membrane. High cholesterol levels increase the membrane cholesterol and the total membrane surface without affecting the volume of the cell. This condition produces **spur cells**. The spur cells are seen in abetalipoproteinemia and liver diseases. Hemolysis occurs in the spleen, where poor RBC deformability results in erythrocyte destruction. **Circulating toxins**, such as snake venoms and heavy metals (copper or arsenic), that bind sulfhydryl groups may damage the RBC membrane and induce hemolysis. Irregularly spiculated RBCs (burr cells) are seen in renal failure. **Vitamin E deficiency** can also cause an acquired hemolytic anemia as a result of abnormal sensitivity of membrane lipids to oxidant stress. Vitamin E deficiency may occur in premature infants who are not being supplemented with vitamin E or who have insufficient nutrition, in infants with severe malabsorption syndromes (including cystic fibrosis), and in infants with transfusional iron overload, which can lead to severe oxidant exposure.

Laboratory Diagnosis. The peripheral blood smear in autoimmune hemolytic anemia usually reveals spherocytes and occasionally nucleated RBCs. The reticulocyte count varies because some patients have relatively low reticulocyte counts as a result of autoantibody that cross-reacts with RBC precursors.

Treatment and Prognosis. Transfusion for the treatment of autoimmune hemolysis is challenging because crossmatching is difficult, as the autoantibodies react with virtually all RBCs. In addition to **transfusion**, which may be lifesaving, management of autoimmune hemolytic anemia depends on antibody type. Management may involve administration of **corticosteroids** and, at times, **IV immunoglobulin**.

The corticosteroids reduce the clearance of the sensitized RBCs in the spleen. In drug-induced hemolysis, withdrawal of the drug usually leads to resolution of the hemolytic process. More than 80% of children with autoimmune hemolytic anemia recover spontaneously.

PANCYTOPENIA

Etiology

Pancytopenia is a quantitative decrease in the formed elements of the blood—erythrocytes, leukocytes, and platelets. Patients more often exhibit symptoms of infection or bleeding than anemia because of the relatively short life span of WBCs and platelets compared with the life span of RBCs. Causes of pancytopenia include failure of production (implying intrinsic bone marrow disease), sequestration (as in hypersplenism), or increased peripheral destruction.

Differential Diagnosis

Features that suggest **bone marrow failure** and mandate an examination of bone marrow include a low reticulocyte count, teardrop forms of RBCs (implying marrow replacement, not just failure), presence of abnormal forms of leukocytes or myeloid elements less mature than band forms, small platelets, and an elevated mean corpuscular volume in the face of a low reticulocyte count. Pancytopenia resulting from bone marrow failure is usually a gradual process. Patients initially may have one or two involved cell lines, but later progress to involvement of all three cell lines. Features suggesting **increased destruction** are reticulocytosis, jaundice, immature erythroid or myeloid elements on the blood smear, large platelets, and increased serum bilirubin and lactic dehydrogenase.

Pancytopenia Resulting from Bone Marrow Failure

Aplastic Anemia

Etiology and Epidemiology. In a child with aplastic anemia, pancytopenia evolves as the hematopoietic elements of the bone marrow disappear and the marrow is replaced by fat. In developed countries, aplastic anemia is most often idiopathic. Alternatively, this disorder may be induced by drugs such as chloramphenicol and felbamate or by toxins such as benzene. Aplastic anemia also may follow infections, particularly hepatitis and infectious mononucleosis (see Table 150–6). Immunosuppression of hematopoiesis is postulated to be an important mechanism in patients with postinfectious and idiopathic aplastic anemia.

Laboratory Studies. A **bone marrow biopsy** is crucial to determine the extent of depletion of the hematopoietic elements.

Treatment. Survival is only about 20% in severe aplastic anemia with supportive care alone, although the duration of survival may be years when vigorous blood product and antibiotic support is provided. For children with severe aplastic anemia—defined by an RPI less than 1%, absolute neutrophil count less than 500/mm^3, platelet count less than 20,000/mm^3, and bone marrow cellularity on biopsy specimen less than 10% of normal—the treatment of choice is **hematopoietic stem cell transplantation** from a sibling with identical HLA and compatible mixed lymphocytes. When hematopoietic stem cell transplantation occurs before the recipient is sensitized to blood products, the survival rate is greater than 80%. The treatment of aplastic anemia without an HLA-matched donor for transplantation is evolving, with two major options: potent immunosuppressive therapy or either unrelated or partially matched hematopoietic stem cell transplantation. Results of trials using antithymocyte globulin, cyclosporine, and corticosteroids in combination with hematopoietic growth factors have been encouraging. Such therapy is often toxic, and relapses often occur when therapy is stopped.

Fanconi Anemia

Etiology and Epidemiology. Fanconi anemia is a constitutional form of aplastic anemia that usually presents in the latter half of the first decade of life and may evolve over years. A group of genetic defects in proteins involved in **DNA repair** have been identified in Fanconi anemia. Fanconi anemia is inherited in an autosomal recessive manner. A diagnosis of Fanconi anemia is based on demonstration of increased chromosomal breakage after exposure of cells to agents that damage DNA. The repair mechanism for DNA damage is abnormal in all cells in Fanconi anemia, which may contribute to the development of malignancies (terminal acute leukemia develops in 10% of cases).

Clinical Manifestations. Patients with Fanconi anemia have numerous characteristic clinical findings (see Table 150–6).

Treatment. Hematopoietic stem cell transplantation can cure the pancytopenia caused by bone marrow aplasia. Many patients with Fanconi anemia and about 20% of children with aplastic anemia seem to respond for a time to **androgenic therapy**, which induces masculinization and may cause liver injury and liver tumors. Androgenic therapy increases RBC synthesis and may diminish transfusion requirements. The effect on granulocytes, and especially the platelet count, is less impressive.

Marrow Replacement

Marrow replacement may occur as a result of **leukemia**, **solid tumors** (especially neuroblastoma), **storage diseases**, **osteopetrosis** in infants, and **myelofibrosis**, which is rare in childhood. The mechanisms by which malignant cells impair marrow synthesis of normal hematopoietic elements are complex and incompletely understood. Bone marrow aspirate and biopsy are needed for precise diagnosis of the etiology of marrow synthetic failure.

Pancytopenia Resulting from Destruction of Cells

Pancytopenia resulting from destruction of cells may be caused by **intramedullary destruction** of hematopoietic elements (myeloproliferative disorders, deficiencies of folic acid and vitamin B$_{12}$) or by the **peripheral destruction** of mature cells. The usual site of peripheral destruction of blood cells is the spleen, although the liver and other parts of the reticuloendothelial system may participate. **Hypersplenism** may be the result of anatomic causes, such as portal hypertension or splenic hypertrophy from thalassemia; infections (including malaria); storage diseases, such as Gaucher disease; lymphomas; or histiocytosis. Splenectomy is indicated only when the pancytopenia is of clinical significance. An example is seen when the condition causes the patients to have increased susceptibility to bleeding or infection or produces high transfusion requirements.

DISORDERS OF LEUKOCYTES

▶ SEE CHAPTER 74.

CHAPTER 151
Hemostatic Disorders

NORMAL HEMOSTASIS

Hemostasis is the dynamic process of **coagulation** as it occurs on areas of vascular injury. The clot is limited to areas of injury and does not extend beyond the initial site of vascular damage. This process involves the carefully modulated interaction of platelets, vascular wall, and procoagulant and anticoagulant proteins. After an injury to the vascular endothelium, subendothelial collagen induces a conformational change in von Willebrand factor (**vWF**), an adhesive protein to which platelets bind via their glycoprotein Ib receptor.

After adhesion, platelets undergo activation and release numerous intracellular contents, including ADP. These **activated platelets** subsequently induce aggregation of additional platelets. Simultaneously, tissue factor, collagen, and other matrix proteins in the tissue activate the coagulation cascade, leading to the formation of the enzyme **thrombin** (Fig. 151–1). Thrombin has multiple effects on the coagulation mechanism, such as further aggregation of platelets, a positive feedback activation of factors V and VIII, the conversion of fibrinogen to fibrin, and the activation of factor XIII. A **platelet plug** forms, and bleeding ceases, usually within 3 to 7 minutes. The generation of thrombin leads to formation of a permanent clot by the activation of factor XIII, which cross-links fibrin forming a stable thrombus. As a final element to this process, contractile elements within the platelet mediate **clot retraction**. Thrombin also contributes to the eventual limitation of clot size by binding to the protein thrombomodulin on intact endothelial cells, converting protein C into activated protein C. Thrombin contributes to the eventual lysis of the thrombus by activating plasminogen to plasmin. All of the hemostatic processes are closely interwoven and occur on the biologic surfaces that mediate coagulation: the platelet, the endothelial cell, and the subendothelium.

Although it is convenient to think of coagulation as having **intrinsic and extrinsic pathways**, the reality is that these pathways are closely interactive and do not react independently (Fig. 151–2). In vivo, factor VII

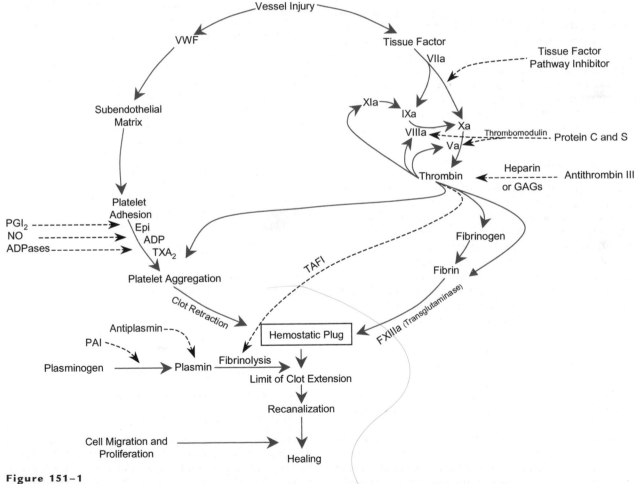

Figure 151–1

Diagram of the multiple interactions of the hemostatic mechanism. Solid lines indicate reactions that favor coagulation, and dashed lines indicate reactions that inhibit clotting. Epi, epinephrine; GAGs, glycosaminoglycans; NO, nitric oxide; PAI, plasminogen activator inhibitor; PGI$_2$, prostaglandin I$_2$ (prostacyclin); TAFI, thrombin-activated fibrinolytic inhibitor; TXA$_2$, thromboxane A$_2$; VWF, von Willebrand factor. (Modified from Montgomery RR, Scott JP: Hemostasis. In Behrman RE, Kliegman RM, Jenson HB [eds]: Nelson Textbook of Pediatrics, 17th ed. Philadelphia, WB Saunders, 2004, p 1653.)

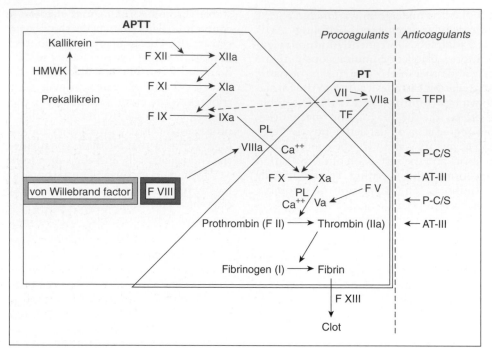

Figure 151–2

Simplified pathways of blood coagulation. The area inside the solid black line is the intrinsic pathway measured by the activated partial thromboplastin time (APTT). The area inside the green line is the extrinsic pathway, measured by the prothrombin time (PT). The area encompassed by both lines is the common pathway. AT-III, antithrombin III; F, factor; HMWK, high-molecular-weight kininogen; P-C/S, protein C/S; PL, phospholipid; TFPI, tissue factor pathway inhibitor. (Adapted from Montgomery RR, Scott JP: Hemostasis. In Behrman RE, Kliegman RM, Jenson HB [eds]: Nelson Textbook of Pediatrics, 16th ed. Philadelphia, WB Saunders, 2000.)

autocatalyzes, forming small amounts of factor VIIa. When tissue is injured, **tissue factor** is released and causes a burst of factor VIIa generation. In vivo, tissue factor, in combination with calcium and factor VIIa, activates factor IX and factor X. The major physiologic pathway is the activation of factor IX by factor VIIa, with eventual generation of thrombin. Thrombin then feeds back on factor XI, generating factor XIa, and accelerates thrombin formation. This process explains why deficiency of factor VIII or factor IX leads to severe bleeding disorders, whereas deficiency of factor XI is usually mild, and deficiency of factor XII is asymptomatic.

As the procoagulant proteins are activated, a series of inhibitory factors serve to tightly regulate the activation of coagulation. **Antithrombin III** inactivates thrombin and factors Xa, IXa, and XIa. The **protein C and protein S** system inactivates the activated factors V and VIII, which are cofactors localized in the "tenase" and "prothrombinase" complexes. The **tissue factor**

pathway inhibitor, an anticoagulant protein, limits the activation of the coagulation cascade by factor VIIa and factor Xa. **Fibrinolysis** is initiated by the action of tissue plasminogen activator on plasminogen, producing plasmin, the active enzyme that degrades fibrin into split products. Fibrinolysis eventually dissolves the clot and allows normal flow to resume.

DEVELOPMENTAL HEMOSTASIS

In the fetus, fibrinogen, factor V, factor VIII, and platelets approach normal levels during the second trimester. Levels of other clotting factors and anticoagulant proteins increase gradually throughout gestation. The premature infant is simultaneously at increased risk of bleeding or clotting complications that are exacerbated by many of the medical interventions needed for care and monitoring, especially indwelling arterial or venous catheters. Most children attain normal levels of procoagulant and anticoagulant proteins by 1 year of age, although levels of protein C lag and normalize in adolescence.

HEMOSTATIC DISORDERS

Etiology and Epidemiology

A detailed **family history** is crucial for bleeding and thrombotic disorders. **Hemophilia** is X-linked, and almost all affected children are boys. **von Willebrand disease** usually is inherited in an autosomal dominant fashion. In the investigation of thrombotic disorders, a personal or family history of blood clots in the legs or lungs, early-onset stroke, or heart attack suggests a hereditary predisposition to thrombosis. The causes of bleeding may be hematologic in origin or due to vascular, nonhematologic causes (Fig. 151–3). Thrombotic disorders can be congenital or acquired (Table 151–1) and frequently present after an initial event (central catheter, major trauma, infections, treatment with hormonal contraceptive agents) provides a

nidus for clot formation or provides a procoagulant stimulus.

Clinical Manifestations

Patients with hemostatic disorders may have complaints of either bleeding or clotting. A careful history and physical examination are crucial to the diagnosis of a bleeding or clotting disorder (see Fig. 151–3). Age at onset of bleeding indicates whether the problem is congenital or acquired. The **sites of bleeding** (mucocutaneous or deep) and **degree of trauma** (spontaneous or significant) required to induce injury suggest the type and severity of the disorder. Certain medications (aspirin and valproic acid) are known to exacerbate preexisting bleeding disorders by interfering with platelet function.

The **physical examination** should characterize the presence of skin or mucous membrane (mucocutaneous) bleeding and deeper sites of hemorrhage into

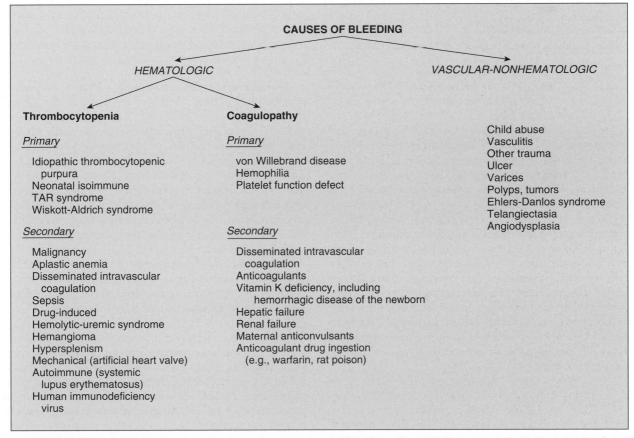

Figure 151–3

Common causes of bleeding. TAR, thrombocytopenia with absence of radius (syndrome).

TABLE 151–1. Common Hypercoagulable States

Congenital Disorders

Factor V leiden (activated protein C resistance)
Prothrombin 20210
Protein C deficiency
Protein S deficiency
Antithrombin III deficiency
Plasminogen deficiency
Dysfibrinogenemia
Homocystinuria

Acquired Disorders

Indwelling catheters
Lupus anticoagulant/antiphospholipid syndrome
Nephrotic syndrome
Malignancy
Pregnancy
Birth control pills
Autoimmune disease
Immobilization/surgery
Trauma
Infection
Inflammatory bowel disease

From Scott JP: Bleeding and thrombosis. In Kliegman RM (ed): Practical Strategies in Pediatric Diagnosis and Therapy. Philadelphia, WB Saunders, 1996.

the muscles and joints or internal bleeding sites. The term **petechia** refers to a nonblanching lesion less than 2 mm in size. **Purpura** is a group of adjoining petechiae, **ecchymoses** (bruises) are isolated lesions larger than petechiae, and **hematomas** are raised, palpable ecchymoses.

Because systemic disorders may induce either hemorrhagic or thrombotic disorders, the physical examination should search for manifestations of an underlying disease, lymphadenopathy or hepatosplenomegaly, vasculitic rash, or chronic hepatic or renal disease. **Deep venous thrombi** cause warm, swollen (distended), tender, purplish-discolored extremities or organs. **Arterial clots** cause acute, painful, pale, and poorly perfused extremities. Arterial thrombi of the internal organs present with signs and symptoms of infarction.

Laboratory Testing

Screening laboratory studies for bleeding patients include a **platelet count**, **prothrombin time**, **partial thromboplastin time**, **fibrinogen**, and **bleeding time** or other screening test of platelet function. No single laboratory test can screen for all bleeding disorders.

The findings on screening tests for bleeding vary with the specific disorder (Table 151–2).

Differential Diagnosis

Disorders of Platelets

Thrombocytopenia. Platelet counts less than $150,000/mm^3$ constitute thrombocytopenia. **Mucocutaneous bleeding** is the hallmark of platelet disorders, including thrombocytopenia. The risk of bleeding correlates imperfectly with the platelet count. Children with platelet counts greater than $80,000/mm^3$ are able to withstand all but the most extreme hemostatic challenges, such as surgery or major trauma. Children with platelet counts less than $20,000/mm^3$ are at risk for spontaneous bleeding. These generalizations are modified by factors such as the age of the platelets (young, large platelets usually function better than old ones) and the presence of inhibitors of platelet function, such as antibodies, drugs (especially aspirin), fibrin degradation products, and toxins formed in the presence of hepatic or renal disease. The size of platelets is now routinely measured as the mean platelet volume. The etiology of thrombocytopenia may be organized into disorders of (1) decreased platelet production, (2) increased destruction, and (3) sequestration (Fig. 151–4).

Thrombocytopenia Resulting from Decreased Platelet Production. Primary disorders of megakaryopoiesis are rare in childhood, other than as part of an aplastic syndrome. **Thrombocytopenia with absent radii syndrome** is characterized by severe thrombocytopenia in association with orthopedic abnormalities, especially of the upper extremity. The thrombocytopenia usually improves over time. **Amegakaryocytic thrombocytopenia** presents at birth or shortly thereafter with findings of severe thrombocytopenia, but no other congenital anomalies. The marrow is devoid of megakaryocytes.

Acquired thrombocytopenia as a result of decreased production is rarely an isolated finding. It is seen more often in the context of **pancytopenia resulting from bone marrow failure** caused by infiltrative or aplastic processes. Certain chemotherapeutic agents may affect megakaryocytes selectively more than other marrow elements. **Cyanotic congenital heart disease with polycythemia** often is associated with thrombocytopenia, but this is rarely severe or associated with significant clinical bleeding. Congenital (TORCH [toxoplasmosis, other (congenital syphilis and viruses), rubella, cytomegalovirus, and herpes simplex virus]) and acquired **viral infections** (HIV, Epstein-Barr virus, and measles) and some **drugs** (anticonvulsants, antibiotics, cytotoxic agents, heparin, and quinidine) may induce thrombocytopenia. Postnatal infections and

TABLE 151–2. Screening Tests for Bleeding Disorders

Test	Mechanism Tested	Normal Values	Disorder
Prothrombin time	Extrinsic and common pathway	<12 sec beyond neonate; 12-18 sec in term neonate	Defect in vitamin K–dependent factors; hemorrhagic disease of newborn, malabsorption, liver disease, DIC, oral anticoagulants, ingestion of rat poison
Activated partial thromboplastin time	Intrinsic and common pathway	25-40 sec beyond neonate; 70 sec in term neonate	Hemophilia; von Willebrand disease, heparin; DIC; deficient factors XII and XI; lupus anticoagulant
Thrombin time	Fibrinogen to fibrin conversion	10-15 sec beyond neonate; 12-17 sec in term neonate	Fibrin split products, DIC, hypofibrinogenemia, heparin, uremia
Bleeding time	Hemostasis, capillary and platelet function	3-7 min beyond neonate	Platelet dysfunction, thrombocytopenia, von Willebrand disease, aspirin
Platelet count	Platelet number	150,000-450,000/mm³	Thrombocytopenia differential diagnosis (Fig. 151–4)
Blood smear	Platelet number and size; RBC morphology	—	Large platelets suggest peripheral destruction; fragmented, bizarre RBC morphology suggests microangiopathic process (e.g., hemolytic uremic syndrome, hemangioma, DIC)

DIC, disseminated intravascular coagulation; RBC, red blood cell.

drug reactions usually cause transient thrombocytopenia, whereas congenital infections may produce prolonged suppression of bone marrow function.

Thrombocytopenia Resulting from Peripheral Destruction

Etiology. In a child who appears well, **immune-mediated mechanisms** are the most common cause of thrombocytopenia. Thrombocytopenia results from increased rates of antibody-dependent platelet destruction. **Neonatal alloimmune thrombocytopenic purpura** (NATP) occurs as a result of sensitization of the mother to antigens present on fetal platelets during gestation. Antibodies cross the placenta and attack the fetal platelet (see Chapter 59). Many platelet alloantigens have been identified and sequenced, permitting prenatal diagnosis of the condition in an at-risk fetus. Mothers with idiopathic thrombocytopenic purpura (**maternal ITP**) or with a history of ITP may have passive transfer of antiplatelet antibodies that react with fetal platelets, with resultant neonatal thrombocytopenia (see Chapter 59). The maternal platelet count is sometimes a useful indicator of the probability that the infant will be affected. If the mother has had a splenectomy, the maternal platelet count may be normal and is a poor predictor of the likelihood of severe neonatal thrombocytopenia because maternal antibody triggers destruction of the fetal platelets in the fetal spleen.

Clinical Manifestations. The infant with NATP is at risk for **intracranial hemorrhage** in utero and during the immediate delivery process. In ITP, the greatest risk seems to be present during passage through the birth canal, during which molding of the head may induce intracranial hemorrhage. Fetal scalp sampling or percutaneous umbilical blood sampling may be performed to measure the fetal platelet count.

Treatment. Administration of IV immunoglobulin before delivery has been shown to be effective in increasing fetal platelet counts and may alleviate thrombocytopenia in the infant in cases of NATP and ITP. Delivery by cesarean section is recommended to prevent CNS bleeding (see Chapter 59). Neonates with severe thrombocytopenia (platelet counts <20,000/mm³) may be treated with IV immunoglobulin or corticosteroids or both until the period of thrombocytopenia remits. If necessary, infants with NATP may receive washed maternal platelets.

Idiopathic Thrombocytopenic Purpura

Etiology. Autoimmune thrombocytopenic purpura of childhood (**childhood ITP**) is a common disorder in children that usually follows an acute viral infection. Childhood ITP is caused by an antibody (IgG or IgM) that binds to the platelet membrane. The condition results in splenic destruction of antibody-coated platelets. Rarely, ITP may be the presenting symptom of an autoimmune disease, such as systemic lupus erythematosus.

Clinical Manifestations. Young children typically exhibit ITP 1 to 4 weeks after viral illness, with abrupt onset of petechiae, purpura, and epistaxis. The throm-

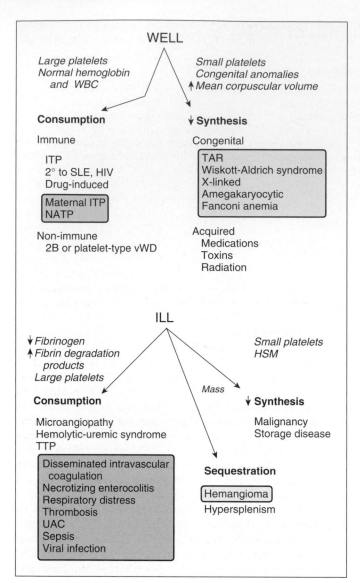

Figure 151–4

Differential diagnosis of childhood thrombocytopenic syndromes. The syndromes initially are separated by their clinical appearances. Clues leading to the diagnosis are presented in italics. The mechanisms and common disorders leading to these findings are shown in the lower part of the figure. Disorders that commonly affect neonates are listed in the shaded boxes. HSM, hepatosplenomegaly; ITP, idiopathic immune thrombocytopenic purpura; NATP, neonatal alloimmune thrombocytopenic purpura; SLE, systemic lupus erythematosus; TAR, thrombocytopenia with absence of radius (syndrome); TTP, thrombotic thrombocytopenic purpura; UAC, umbilical artery catheter; WBC, white blood cell. (From Scott JP: Bleeding and thrombosis. In Kliegman RM [ed]: Practical Strategies in Pediatric Diagnosis and Therapy. Philadelphia, WB Saunders, 1996, p 849.)

bocytopenia usually is severe. Significant adenopathy or hepatosplenomegaly is unusual, and the RBC and WBC counts are normal.

Laboratory Diagnosis. Diagnosis of ITP usually is made based on clinical presentation and the platelet count and often does not require a bone marrow examination. If atypical findings are noted, however, marrow examination is indicated to rule out an infiltrative disorder (leukemia) or an aplastic process (aplastic anemia). In ITP, an examination of the bone marrow reveals increased megakaryocytes and normal erythroid and myeloid elements.

Treatment and Prognosis. Therapy seldom is indicated for platelet counts greater than 30,000/mm³. Therapy does not affect the long-term outcome of ITP but is intended to increase the platelet count acutely. For clinical bleeding or severe thrombocytopenia (platelet count <20,000/mm³), therapeutic options include **prednisone**, 2 to 4 mg/kg/ 24 hours for 2 weeks; IV immunoglobulin, 1 g/kg/24 hours for 1 to 2 days; or **IV anti-D** (WinRho SD), 50 to 75 µg/kg/dose for Rh-positive individuals. All of these approaches seem to work by decreasing the rate of clearance of sensitized platelets, rather than decreasing production of antibody. The optimal choice for therapy (if any) is controversial. Splenectomy is indicated in acute ITP only for life-threatening bleeding. Approximately 80% of children have a spontaneous resolution of ITP within 6 months after diagnosis. Serious bleeding, especially intracranial bleeding, occurs in less than 1% of patients with ITP.

ITP that persists for 6 to 12 months is classified as **chronic ITP**. Repeated treatments with IV immunoglobulin or IV anti-D or high-dose pulse steroids have been effective in delaying the need for splenectomy. Secondary causes of chronic ITP, especially systemic lupus erythematosus and HIV infection, should be ruled out. Splenectomy is effective in inducing a remission in 70% to 80% of childhood chronic ITP cases. The risks of splenectomy (surgery or sepsis from encapsulated bacteria, such as pneumococcus) must be weighed against the risk of severe bleeding.

Other Disorders. Wiskott-Aldrich syndrome is an X-linked disorder characterized by hypogammaglobinemia, eczema, and thrombocytopenia caused by a molecular defect in a cytoskeletal protein common to lymphocytes and platelets (see Chapter 74). Small platelets are seen on a peripheral blood smear. Nevertheless, thrombocytopenia often is improved by splenectomy. Hematopoietic stem cell transplantation cures the immunodeficiency and thrombocytopenia. Familial X-linked thrombocytopenia is a variant of Wiskott-Aldrich syndrome.

Thrombotic microangiopathy causes thrombocytopenia, anemia secondary to intravascular RBC destruction, and, in some cases, depletion of clotting factors. Children with thrombotic microangiopathy usually are quite ill. In a child with **DIC**, the deposition of fibrin strands within the vasculature and activation of thrombin and plasmin result in a wide-ranging hemostatic disorder with activation and clearance of platelets. **Hemolytic uremic syndrome** occurs as a result of exposure to a toxin that induces endothelial injury, fibrin deposition, and platelet activation and clearance (see Chapter 164). In **thrombotic thrombocytopenic purpura**, platelet consumption, precipitated by a congenital or acquired deficiency of a metalloproteinase that cleaves vWF, seems to be the primary process, with a modest deposition of fibrin and RBC destruction.

Disorders of Platelet Function

Etiology. Primary disorders of platelet function may involve receptors on the platelet membrane for the adhesive proteins. Deficiency of glycoprotein Ib complex (vWF receptor) causes **Bernard-Soulier syndrome**. A deficiency of glycoprotein IIb-IIIa (the fibrinogen receptor) causes **Glanzmann thrombasthenia**. Mild abnormalities of platelet aggregation and release, detectable by platelet aggregometry, are far more common. Secondary disorders caused by toxins and drugs (uremia, valproic acid, aspirin, nonsteroidal anti-inflammatory drugs, and infections) may cause a broad spectrum of platelet dysfunction.

Clinical Manifestations. Disorders of platelet function present with mucocutaneous bleeding and a prolonged bleeding time and may be primary or secondary.

Laboratory Diagnosis. The bleeding time is an insensitive screen for mild and moderate platelet function disorders, but is usually prolonged in severe platelet function disorders, such as Bernard-Soulier syndrome or Glanzmann thrombasthenia.

Disorders of Clotting Factors

Etiology. Hereditary deficiencies of most procoagulant proteins lead to bleeding. The genes for factor VIII and factor IX are on the X chromosome, whereas virtually all the other clotting factors are coded on autosomal chromosomes and are inherited autosomally. **Factor VIII and factor IX deficiencies** are the most common severe inherited bleeding disorders. **von Willebrand disease** is the most common congenital bleeding disorder. Of the procoagulant proteins, only deficiencies of the so-called contact factors (prekallikrein, high molecular weight kininogen, and Hageman factor [XII]) are not associated with a predisposition to bleeding.

Hemophilia

Etiology. **Hemophilia A** (factor VIII deficiency) occurs in 1 in 5000 males. **Hemophilia B** (factor IX deficiency) occurs in approximately 1 in 25,000. Clinically the two disorders are indistinguishable other than by their therapy (Table 151–3). Because of a lack of factor VIII or factor IX, a delay occurs in the generation of thrombin, which is crucial to forming a normal, functional fibrin clot and solidifying the platelet plug that has formed in areas of vascular injury. The severity of the disorder is determined by the degree of clotting factor deficiency.

Clinical Manifestations. Patients with less than 1% (severe hemophilia) factor VIII or factor IX may have **spontaneous bleeding** or bleeding with minor trauma. Patients with 1% to 5% (moderate hemophilia) factor VIII or factor IX usually require moderate trauma to induce bleeding episodes. In mild hemophilia (>5% factor VIII or factor IX), significant trauma is necessary to induce bleeding; spontaneous bleeding does not occur. Mild hemophilia may go undiagnosed for many years, whereas severe hemophilia manifests in infancy when the child reaches the toddler stage. In severe hemophilia, spontaneous bleeding occurs, usually in the muscles or joints (**hemarthroses**).

Laboratory Studies. The diagnosis of hemophilia is based on a **prolonged activated partial thromboplastin time**. In the activated partial thromboplastin time, a surface-active agent activates the intrinsic system of coagulation, of which factors VIII and IX are crucial components. In factor VIII or factor IX deficiency, the activated partial thromboplastin time is quite prolonged, but should correct to normal when the patient's plasma is mixed 1:1 with normal plasma. When an abnormal activated partial thromboplastin

TABLE 151–3.   Comparison of Hemophilia A, Hemophilia B, and von Willebrand Disease

	Hemophilia A	Hemophilia B	von Willebrand Disease
Inheritance	X-linked	X-linked	Autosomal dominant
Factor deficiency	Factor VIII	Factor IX	von Willebrand factor and VIIIC
Bleeding site(s)	Muscle, joint, surgical	Muscle, joint, surgical	Mucous membranes, skin, surgical, menstrual
Prothrombin time	Normal	Normal	Normal
Activated partial thromboplastin time	Prolonged	Prolonged	Prolonged or normal
Bleeding time	Normal	Normal	Prolonged or normal
Factor VIII coagulant activity	Low	Normal	Low or normal
von Willebrand factor antigen	Normal	Normal	Low
von Willebrand factor activity	Normal	Normal	Low
Factor IX	Normal	Low	Normal
Ristocetin-induced platelet agglutination	Normal	Normal	Normal, low, or increased at low-dose ristocetin
Platelet aggregation	Normal	Normal	Normal
Treatment	DDAVP* or recombinant VIII	Recombinant IX	DDAVP* or vWF concentrate

*Desmopressin (DDAVP) for mild to moderate hemophilia A or type 1 von Willebrand disease.

time is obtained, **specific factor assays** are needed to make a precise diagnosis (see Table 151–2), which is crucial for deciding on the appropriate factor replacement therapy. Prenatal diagnosis and carrier diagnosis now are possible, using either coagulation-based methods or (preferably) molecular techniques.

Treatment. Early, appropriate **replacement therapy** is the aim of optimal hemophilia care. Acute bleeding episodes are best treated in the home when the patient has attained the appropriate age, and the parents have learned home treatment. Bleeding associated with surgery, trauma, or dental extraction often can be anticipated, and excessive bleeding can be prevented with appropriate replacement therapy. For life-threatening bleeding, levels of 80% to 100% of normal factor VIII or factor IX are necessary. For mild to moderate bleeding episodes (hemarthroses), a 40% level for factor VIII or a 30% to 40% level for factor IX is appropriate. The dose can be calculated using the knowledge that 1 U/kg body weight of factor VIII increases the plasma level 2%, whereas 1.5 U/kg of recombinant factor IX increases the plasma level 1%:

$$\text{Dose for factor VIII} = \text{desired level (\%)} \times \text{weight (kg)} \times 0.5$$

or

$$\text{Dose for recombinant factor IX} = \text{desired level (\%)} \times \text{weight (kg)} \times 1.5$$

Desmopressin acetate is a synthetic vasopressin analogue with minimal vasopressor effect. Desmopressin triples or quadruples the initial factor VIII level of a patient with mild or moderate (not severe) hemophilia A, but has no effect on factor IX levels. When adequate hemostatic levels can be attained, desmopressin is the treatment of choice for individuals with mild and moderate hemophilia A. Aminocaproic acid is an inhibitor of fibrinolysis that may be useful for oral bleeding.

Complications and Prevention. Patients treated with older factor VIII or IX concentrates derived from large pools of plasma donors were at high risk for **hepatitis B**, **C**, and **D** and **HIV**. Recombinant factor VIII and factor IX concentrates are safe from virally transmitted illnesses. Older patients who were exposed to factor concentrates or cryoprecipitate or both before modern viral testing for HIV and hepatitis viruses have a high prevalence of HIV infection. AIDS is the most common cause of death in older patients with hemophilia. Many older patients also have chronic hepatitis C.

Inhibitors are IgG antibodies directed against transfused factor VIII or factor IX in congenitally deficient patients. Inhibitors arise in 15% of severe factor VIII hemophiliacs and less commonly in factor IX hemophiliacs. They may be high or low titer and show an anamnestic response to treatment. The treatment of bleeding patients with an inhibitor is difficult. For low titer inhibitors, options include continuous factor VIII infusions or administration of porcine factor VIII. For high titer inhibitors, it is usually necessary to administer a product that bypasses the inhibitor, preferably recombinant factor VIIa. Activated prothrombin complex concentrates, used in the past to treat inhibitor patients, paradoxically increased the risks of thrombosis, resulting in fatal complications, such as myocardial infarction. For long-term treatment of inhibitor patients, induction of immune tolerance by repeated infusion of the deficient factor plus immunosuppression may be beneficial.

Prevention of long-term crippling orthopedic abnormalities is a major goal of hemophilic care. Early institution of factor replacement and continuous prophylaxis beginning in early childhood should prevent the chronic joint disease associated with hemophilia.

von Willebrand Disease

Etiology. von Willebrand disease is a common disorder (found in 1% of the population) caused by a deficiency of **vWF**. vWF is an adhesive protein that serves two functions: to act as a bridge between subendothelial collagen and platelets and to bind circulating factor VIII and protect factor VIII from rapid clearance from circulation. von Willebrand disease usually is inherited as an autosomal dominant trait and rarely as an autosomal recessive trait. vWF may be either quantitatively deficient (partial = type 1 or absolute = type 3) or qualitatively abnormal (type 2 = dysproteinemia). Approximately 80% of patients with von Willebrand disease have classic (type 1) disease (i.e., a mild to moderate deficiency of vWF). Several other subtypes are clinically important, each requiring different therapy.

Clinical Manifestations. Mucocutaneous bleeding, epistaxis, gingival bleeding, cutaneous bruising, and menorrhagia occur in patients with von Willebrand disease. In severe disease, factor VIII deficiency may be profound, and the patient may have manifestations similar to hemophilia A (hemarthrosis). Findings in classic von Willebrand disease differ from findings in hemophilia A and B (see Table 151–3).

Laboratory Diagnosis. vWF testing involves measurement of the amount of protein, usually measured immunologically as the **vWF antigen** (vWF:Ag). vWF activity (vWF:Act) is measured functionally in the **ristocetin cofactor assay** (vWFR:Co), which uses the antibiotic ristocetin to induce vWF to bind to platelets.

Treatment. The treatment of von Willebrand disease depends on the severity of the bleeding. **Desmopressin** is the treatment of choice for most bleeding episodes in patients with type 1 disease and some patients with type 2 disease. When high levels of vWF are needed but cannot be achieved satisfactorily with desmopressin, treatment with a virally attenuated, **vWF-containing concentrate** (Humate P) may be appropriate. The dosage can be calculated as for factor VIII in hemophilia. Cryoprecipitate should not be used because it is not virally attenuated. Hepatitis B vaccine should be given before the patient is exposed to plasma-derived products. As in all bleeding disorders, aspirin should be avoided for patients with von Willebrand disease.

Vitamin K Deficiency

▶ SEE CHAPTERS 27 AND 31.

Disseminated Intravascular Coagulation

Etiology. DIC is a disorder in which a severely ill patient sustains widespread activation of the coagulation mechanism, usually associated with shock. Bleeding and clotting manifestations may be present. Normal hemostasis is a balance between hemorrhage and thrombosis. In DIC, this balance is altered by the severe illness, so the patient has activation of coagulation mediated by thrombin and fibrinolysis mediated by plasmin. Coagulation factors, especially platelets, fibrinogen, and factors II, V, and VIII, are consumed, as are the anticoagulant proteins, especially antithrombin, protein C, and plasminogen. Endothelial injury, tissue release of thromboplastic procoagulant factors, or, rarely, exogenous factors (snake venoms) directly activate the coagulation mechanism (Table 151–4).

Clinical Manifestations. The diagnosis of DIC usually is suspected clinically and is confirmed by laboratory findings of a **decline in platelets and fibrinogen** associated with elevated prothrombin time, partial thromboplastin time, and levels of fibrin(ogen) degradation products (Table 151–5). In some patients, DIC may evolve more slowly, and there may be a degree of compensation. In a severely ill patient, the sudden occurrence of bleeding from a venipuncture or incision site, gastrointestinal or pulmonary hemorrhage, petechiae, or ecchymosis or evidence of peripheral gangrene or thrombosis suggests the diagnosis of DIC.

Treatment. The treatment of DIC is challenging. General guidelines include the following: treat the disorder inducing the DIC first; **support** the patient by correcting hypoxia, acidosis, and poor perfusion; and replace depleted blood clotting factors, platelets, and anticoagulant proteins by transfusion. **Heparin** may be used to treat significant arterial or venous thrombotic disease unless sites of life-threatening bleeding coexist. **Drotrecogin alfa** (recombinant activated protein C) reduces mortality in adults with DIC and sepsis.

Thrombosis

Etiology. A hereditary predisposition to thrombosis (see Table 151–1) may be caused by a deficiency of an anticoagulant protein (**protein C or S**, **antithrombin**, or **plasminogen**) (Fig. 151–5), by an abnormality of a

TABLE 151–4.   Causes of Disseminated Intravascular Coagulation

Infectious

Meningococcemia (purpura fulminans)
Other gram-negative bacteria (*Haemophilus, Salmonella, Escherichia coli*)
Rickettsia (Rocky Mountain spotted fever)
Virus (cytomegalovirus, herpes, hemorrhagic fevers)
Malaria
Fungus

Tissue Injury

CNS trauma (e.g., massive head injury)
Multiple fractures with fat emboli
Crush injury
Profound shock or asphyxia
Hypothermia or hyperthermia
Massive burns

Malignancy

Acute promyelocytic leukemia
Acute monoblastic or myelocytic leukemia
Widespread malignancies (neuroblastoma)

Venom or Toxin

Snake bites
Insect bites

Microangiopathic Disorders

"Severe" thrombotic thrombocytopenic purpura or hemolytic uremic syndrome
Giant hemangioma (Kasabach-Merritt syndrome)

Gastrointestinal Disorders

Fulminant hepatitis
Severe inflammatory bowel disease
Reye syndrome

Hereditary Thrombotic Disorders

Antithrombin III deficiency
Homozygous protein C deficiency

Newborn

Maternal toxemia
Group B streptococcal infections
Abruptio placentae
Severe respiratory distress syndrome
Necrotizing enterocolitis
Congenital viral disease (e.g., cytomegalovirus or herpes)
Erythroblastosis fetalis

Miscellaneous

Severe acute graft rejection
Acute hemolytic transfusion reaction
Severe collagen vascular disease
Kawasaki disease
Heparin-induced thrombosis
Infusion of "activated" prothrombin complex concentrates
Hyperpyrexia/encephalopathy, hemorrhagic shock syndrome

From Scott JP: Bleeding and thrombosis. In Kliegman RM (ed): Practical Strategies in Pediatric Diagnosis and Therapy. Philadelphia, WB Saunders, 1996.

TABLE 151–5.   Differential Diagnosis of Coagulopathies That Can Be Confused with Disseminated Intravascular Coagulation

	Prothrombin Time	Partial Thromboplastin Time	Fibrinogen	Platelets	Fibrinogen Degradation Products	Clinical Keys
DIC	↑	↑	↓	↓	↑	Shock
Liver failure	↑	↑	↓	Normal or ↓	↑	Jaundice
Vitamin K deficiency	↑	↑	Normal	Normal	Normal	Malabsorption, liver disease
Sepsis without shock	↑	↑	Normal	Normal	↑ or normal	Fever

DIC, disseminated intravascular coagulation.
From Scott JP: Bleeding and thrombosis. In Kliegman RM (ed): Practical Strategies in Pediatric Diagnosis and Therapy. Philadelphia, WB Saunders, 1996.

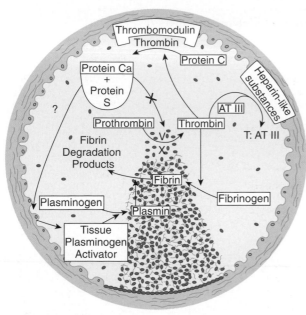

Figure 151–5

Formation of the hemostatic plug at the site of vascular injury. Three major physiologic anticoagulant mechanisms—antithrombin III (AT III), protein C, and the fibrinolytic system—are activated to limit clot formation to the site of damage and to prevent generalized thrombosis. T, thrombin. (From Schafer A: The hypercoaguable state. Ann Intern Med 102:814-828, 1985.)

procoagulant protein that makes such protein resistant to proteolysis by its respective inhibitor (**factor V Leiden**), by a mutation resulting in an increased level of a procoagulant protein (prothrombin 20210), or by damage to endothelial cells (**homocysteinemia**). Neonates with deficiency syndromes may be particularly vulnerable to thrombosis (neonates with homozygous protein C deficiency present with purpura fulminans or thrombosis of the major arteries and veins or both). Many individuals with an inherited predisposition to thrombosis exhibit symptoms in adolescence or early adulthood. Protein C deficiency presenting in adulthood usually is inherited as an autosomal dominant trait, whereas the homozygous form usually is autosomal recessive. Protein S and antithrombin III deficiencies are inherited as autosomal dominant traits. Factor V Leiden is the most common hereditary cause of a predisposition to thrombosis, appearing in 3% to 5% of whites. **Acquired antiphospholipid antibodies** (anticardiolipin and lupus anticoagulant) also predispose to thrombosis.

Clinical Manifestations. Neonates and adolescents are the most likely pediatric patients to present with thromboembolic disease. Indwelling catheters, vasculi-

tis, sepsis, immobilization, nephrotic syndrome, coagulopathy, trauma, infection, surgery, inflammatory bowel disease, oral contraceptive agents, pregnancy, and abortion all predispose to thrombosis. The manifestations of pulmonary emboli may vary, from no findings to findings of chest pain, diminished breath sounds, increased pulmonic component of S_2, cyanosis, tachypnea, and hypoxemia.

Diagnostic and Imaging Studies. Venous thrombosis can be detected noninvasively by Doppler flow compression studies or plethysmography. The gold standard for diagnosis is the venogram. Findings of pulmonary embolism on a chest radiograph vary, but an abnormal ("high probability") ventilation-perfusion scan or detection of an intravascular thrombus on helical CT is diagnostic of pulmonary emboli. There are no appropriate screening studies for thrombotic disorders. Diagnosis of a congenital or acquired predisposition to thrombosis requires a battery of specific assays.

Treatment. Therapy of thrombotic disorders depends on the underlying condition and usually involves **heparin** and then longer term anticoagulation with **warfarin**. Major vessel thrombosis or life-threatening thrombosis may necessitate treatment with **fibrinolytic agents** (recombinant tissue plasminogen activator). In newborns, inherited deficiency syndromes may present as emergencies and necessitate **replacement** with plasma, antithrombin-III concentrates, or protein C concentrates. Symptomatic individuals with an inherited predisposition to thrombosis are usually given warfarin for long-term anticoagulation.

CHAPTER 152

Blood Component Therapy

Transfusion of RBCs, granulocytes, platelets, and coagulation factors can be lifesaving or life maintaining (Table 152–1). **Whole blood** is indicated only when acute hypovolemia and reduced oxygen carrying capacity are present. Otherwise, **packed RBCs** are indicated to treat anemia by increasing oxygen carrying capacity. Blood cell transfusions should not be used to treat asymptomatic nutritional deficiencies that can be corrected by administering the appropriate deficient nutrient (iron or folic acid). Blood component therapy requires proper anticoagulation of the blood, screening for a variety of infectious agents, and blood group compatibility testing before administration. Typical **transfusion reactions** are listed in Table 152–2. Filtering of

TABLE 152–1. Commonly Used Transfusion Products

Component	Content	Indication	Dose	Expected Outcome
Packed RBCs	250-300 mL RBCs/u	↓ Oxygen-carrying capacity*	10-15 mL/kg	4 mL/kg → 1 g/dL ↑ in Hgb
Platelet concentrate	$5\text{-}7 \times 10^{10}$ platelets/ unit	Severe thrombocytopenia ± bleeding	1 u/10 kg	↑ Platelet count by 50,000/μL
Fresh frozen plasma	1 unit/mL of each clotting factor	Multiple clotting factor deficiency	10-15 mL/kg	Improvement in prothrombin and partial thromboplastin times
Cryoprecipitate	Fibrinogen, factor VIII, vWF, factor XIII	Hypofibrinogenemia, factor XIII deficiency	1 bag/5 kg	↑ Fibrinogen by 50-100 mg/dL
Recombinant factor concentrates	Units as labeled	Hemophilic bleeding or prophylaxis	FVIII: 20-50 units/kg* FIX: 40-120 units/kg*	FVIII: 2%/unit/kg FIX: 0.7/unit/kg
Recombinant factor VIIa (NovoSeven)	μg	Hemophilic bleeding in inhibitor patient; uncontrolled post operative hemorrhage	90 μg/kg q3 h	Cessation of bleeding

*Should be clinically significant.
Hgb, hemoglobin; RBCs, red blood cells; vWF, von Willebrand factor.

blood products to remove WBCs may prevent febrile reactions. Long-term complications of transfusions are iron overload, alloimmunization to RBCs and WBCs or platelets and plasma proteins (1:100), graft-versus-host disease, and **infectious diseases (hepatitis B and C [<1:250,000], HIV [<1:1 million], malaria, syphilis, babesiosis, brucellosis, Chagas disease).** Transfusion therapy also may result in circulatory overload, especially in the presence of chronic cardiopulmonary deficiency.

TABLE 152–2. Evaluation of Transfusion Reactions

Type of Reaction	Clinical Signs	Management of Problems
Major hemolytic (1:100,000) (incompatibility)	Acute shock, back pain, flushing, early fever, intravascular hemolysis, hemoglobinemia, hemoglobinuria; may be delayed 5-10 days and less severe if anamnestic response is present	1. Stop transfusion; return blood to bank with fresh sample of patient's blood 2. Hydrate IV; support blood pressure, maintain high urine flow, alkalinize urine 3. Check for hemoglobinemia, hemoblobinuria, hyperkalemia 4. Jaundice, anemia if delayed
Delayed hemolytic transfusion reaction	Onset 7-14 days after transfusion: pain, fever, jaundice, hemoglobinuria; fall in hemoglobin; reticulocytopenia	Corticosteroids; erythropoietin?; avoid transfusion if possible
Febrile (1:100)	Fever at end of transfusion, urticaria (usually because of sensitization to WBC HLA antigens), chills	Pretreat with hydrocortisone, antipyretics, diphenhydramine (Benadryl), or all three; use leukocyte-poor RBCs, washed RBCs, filtered or frozen RBCs
Allergic	Fever, urticaria, anaphylactoid reaction (often because of sensitivity to donor plasma proteins)	Benadryl, hydrocortisone; use washed RBCs or frozen RBCs

RBCs, red blood cells; WBC, white blood cell.
Adapted from Andreoli TE, Bennett JC, Carpenter CC, Plum F, et al: Cecil Essentials of Medicine, 4th ed. Philadelphia, WB Saunders, 1997.

SUGGESTED READING

Behrman RE, Kliegman RM (eds): Nelson Essential of Pediatrics, 4th ed. Philadelphia, WB Saunders, 2002, pp 605-644

Behrman RE, Kliegman RM, Jenson HB (eds): Nelson Textbook of Pediatrics, 17th ed. Philadelphia, WB Saunders, 2004.

Lusher JM: Clinical and laboratory approach to the bleeding patient. In Nathan DG, Orkin SH, Ginsburg D, Look AT (eds): Hematology of Infancy and Childhood, 6th ed. Philadelphia, WB Saunders, 2003, pp 1515-1526.

Oski FA, Brugnara C, Nathan DG: A diagnostic approach to the anemic patient. In Nathan DG, Orkin SH, Ginsburg D, Look AT (eds): Hematology of Infancy and Childhood, 6th ed. Philadelphia, WB Saunders, 2003, pp 409-419.

Scott JP: Bleeding and thrombosis. In Kliegman RM, Nieder ML, Super DM (eds): Practical Strategies in Pediatric Diagnosis and Therapy. Philadelphia, WB Saunders, 1996, pp 839-857.

Thomas W. McLean and Marcia M. Wofford

CHAPTER 153

Assessment

HISTORY

The history is the first and most important aspect of evaluating a child with suspected cancer. Childhood cancer is rare; only about 1% of new cancer cases in the U.S. occur among children 19 years old or younger. Hematopoietic tumors (leukemia, lymphoma) are the most common childhood cancers, followed by brain/CNS tumors and sarcomas of soft tissue and bone (Fig. 153–1). There is wide variability in the age-specific incidence of childhood cancers. Embryonal tumors, such as neuroblastoma and retinoblastoma, peak during the first 2 years of life; acute lymphoblastic leukemia peaks during early childhood (age 2 to 5 years); osteosarcoma peaks during adolescence; and Hodgkin disease peaks during late adolescence with a transition to the risk of adult malignancies (Fig. 153–2). The overall incidence of cancer among white children is higher than among other ethnic groups.

Many signs and symptoms of childhood cancer are nonspecific. Most children with fever, fatigue, weight loss, or limp do not have cancer. Each of these symptoms may be a manifestation of an underlying malignancy, however. Uncommonly a child may have no symptoms at all. An abdominal mass may be palpated on routine examination, or a complete blood count may be unexpectedly abnormal. Most children with cancer have some symptom or sign that ultimately leads to a diagnosis. Some children have a genetic susceptibility to cancer and should be screened appropriately (Table 153–1).

The chief complaint is usually the most important part of the history. It is important to explore quality, duration, location, severity, and precipitating events. A prominent lymph node that does not resolve over weeks to months (with or without antibiotics) may warrant a biopsy. A limp that does not improve within days to weeks should prompt a complete blood count and probably a radiograph or a bone scan. Persistent headaches or morning vomiting should prompt a CT scan of the head. Fever, night sweats, or weight loss should raise the concern for lymphoma. In addition to the history of present illness, it is important to obtain the birth history, past medical and surgical history, growth history, developmental history, family history, and social history.

PHYSICAL EXAMINATION

The physical examination is the next step in assessing a child with suspected cancer. Growth (height, weight, head circumference) and vital signs are important to obtain. Pulse oximetry should be obtained if respiratory symptoms are prominent. The overall appearance of the patient should be noted, particularly for ill appearance, pain, cachexia, pallor, and respiratory distress. If a mass is palpable, measurements should be obtained. Lymphadenopathy and organomegaly should be sought and quantified, if present. The skin should be examined thoroughly for the presence of rashes, bruises, and petechiae. Careful neurologic, ophthalmologic, and endocrine examinations are crucial if headache or vomiting is present; most patients with CNS tumors have abnormal neurologic examinations.

COMMON MANIFESTATIONS

The types of cancer that occur in childhood differ significantly from cancers that occur in adults. Carcinomas that develop in solid organs are the most common adult cancers, whereas carcinomas are rare in children. Acute leukemias, lymphomas, and brain tumors are the

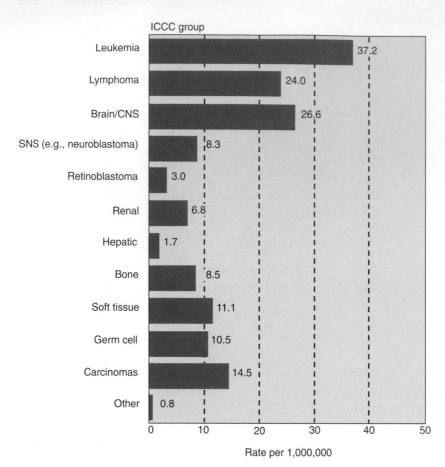

ICCC group

Figure 153–1

Childhood cancer incidence rates.
Childhood cancer incidence rates,
1975-1995, from the Surveillance,
Epidemiology, and End Results (SEER)
program of the National Cancer
Institute, according to the 12 tumor
groups of the International
Classification of Childhood Cancer
(ICCC), for persons younger than 20
years of age, including both sexes and
all races. SNS, sympathethic nervous
system (e.g., neuroblastoma). (From
Ries LAG, Eisner MP, Kosary CL,
et al [eds]: SEER Cancer Statistics
Review, 1975-2000. Bethesda, Md,
National Cancer Institute.
http://seer.cancer.gov/csr/1975_2000.)

most common pediatric and young adult cancers (see Fig. 153–1). Leukemia and various embryonal tumors, such as Wilms tumor, neuroblastoma, retinoblastoma, and hepatoblastoma, are more common in infancy and early childhood, whereas Hodgkin disease, bone cancers, and gonadal malignancies are more common in adolescents. The **most common manifestations** of childhood cancer are fatigue, anorexia, malaise, pain, fever, abnormal lump or mass, pallor, bruising, petechiae, bleeding, headache, vomiting, visual changes, weight loss, and night sweats (Table 153–2).

DIFFERENTIAL DIAGNOSIS

Distinguishing a malignant process from another disease may be difficult. Ultimately a tissue diagnosis (from bone marrow or solid tumor) with pathologic confirmation is required to confirm a malignancy. Infection commonly masquerades as a potential malignancy. In particular, Epstein-Barr virus, cytomegalovirus, and mycobacterial infections can mimic leukemia or lymphoma by causing fever, lymphadenopathy, organomegaly, or abnormal blood counts. Trauma may

produce swelling that can mimic solid tumors. Idiopathic thrombocytopenic purpura and iron deficiency can produce thrombocytopenia and anemia. Immunodeficiencies or autoimmune diseases (autoimmune hemolytic anemia or neutropenia) also can produce cytopenias. Juvenile rheumatoid arthritis and other collagen vascular diseases can cause musculoskeletal pain, mimicking leukemia. Benign tumors are relatively common in children and include mature germ cell tumors/hamartomas, hemangiomas or other vascular tumors, mesoblastic nephromas, and bone cysts.

DISTINGUISHING FEATURES

Patients with leukemia or a tumor that has infiltrated the bone marrow typically have one or more of the following: fever, pallor, bruising, petechiae, and bleeding. Lymphadenopathy and organomegaly also are common in leukemia, particularly with T cell acute lymphoblastic leukemia (ALL) or non-Hodgkin lymphoma (NHL). Patients with solid tumors usually have a palpable or measurable mass. Other signs and symptoms include pain, limp, cough, dyspnea, headache,

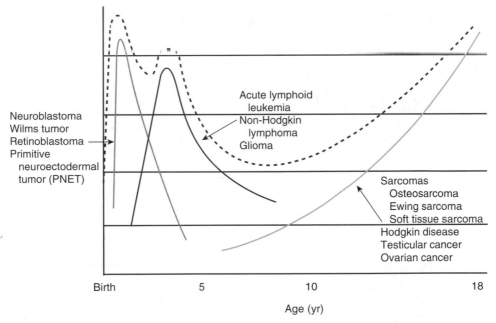

Figure 153–2

Incidence of the most common types of cancer in children by age. The cumulative incidence is shown as a dashed line. (From Behrman RE, Kliegman RM, Jenson HB [eds]: Nelson Textbook of Pediatrics, 17th ed. Philadelphia, WB Saunders, 2004, p 1680.)

vomiting, cranial nerve palsies, and papilledema. Malignant masses are usually firm, fixed, and nontender, whereas masses that are infectious or inflammatory in nature are relatively softer, mobile, and tender to palpation.

INITIAL DIAGNOSTIC EVALUATION

Screening Tests

A complete blood count with differential and review of the peripheral blood smear is the best screening test for many pediatric malignancies. Leukopenia (with or without neutropenia), anemia, or thrombocytopenia may be present in leukemia or any cancer that invades the bone marrow, such as neuroblastoma, rhabdomyosarcoma, and Ewing sarcoma. Leukemia also may produce leukocytosis, usually with blasts present on the peripheral blood smear. An isolated cytopenia (neutropenia, anemia, or thrombocytopenia) widens the differential diagnosis, but still could be the only abnormal laboratory finding. Patients with leukemia may have a normal complete blood count. Serum lactate dehydrogenase and uric acid levels often are elevated in fast-growing tumors, especially leukemia and lymphoma and occasionally in sarcomas and neuroblastoma. In many cases, it is appropriate to assess electrolytes and to screen renal and hepatic function.

Palpation of an abdominal mass or an elevated blood pressure, confirmed by repeat measurement, should prompt obtaining a urinalysis.

Diagnostic Imaging

When a diagnosis of cancer is confirmed, diagnostic imaging is important for assessment of the primary tumor and for metastases, although the needs in individual cases may vary (Table 153–3). A chest x-ray (posterior-anterior and lateral) is the best screening radiographic study for a patient with fever, weight loss, or suspicious cervical lymphadenopathy. Most mediastinal masses can be detected on chest x-ray. Some malignancies also produce a pleural effusion. Abdominal signs or symptoms may warrant an ultrasound or CT scan; persistent headache, vomiting, or abnormal neurologic findings warrant a head CT scan. For suspected bone tumors, plain radiographs are indicated and usually reveal the lesion, if present. If a bony pelvic lesion is suspected, radiographs may be normal, and a CT scan or MRI should be obtained. Other imaging studies should be obtained to better delineate a mass and to search for suspected metastases. The use of total body MRI for detection of metastases in pediatric malignancies and positron emission tomography scans for lymphomas is under investigation.

TABLE 153–1.　Familial or Genetic Susceptibility to Malignancy

Disorder	Tumor or Cancer	Comment
Chromosomal Syndromes		
Chromosome 11p– (deletion)	Wilms tumor	Associated with genitourinary anomalies, mental retardation; sporadic aniridia
Chromosome 13q– (deletion)	Retinoblastoma	Associated with mental retardation, skeletal malformations
Trisomy 21	Lymphocytic or nonlymphocytic leukemia	Risk is 15 times normal
Klinefelter syndrome (47, XXY)	Breast cancer, germ cell tumors	
Gonadal dysgenesis (XO/XY)	Gonadoblastoma	Gonads must be removed; 25% chance of gonadal malignancy
DNA Fragility		
Xeroderma pigmentosum	Basal, squamous cell skin cancers	Autosomal recessive; failure to repair solar-damaged DNA
Fanconi anemia	Leukemia	Autosomal recessive; 10% risk for AML; chromosome fragility, positive diepoxybutane test
Bloom syndrome	Leukemia, lymphoma	Autosomal recessive; chromosome fragility, immunodeficiency; high risk for malignancy
Ataxia-telangiectasia	Lymphoma, leukemia	Autosomal recessive; sensitive to x-radiation, radiomimetic drugs; chromosome fragility, immunodeficiency
Dysplastic nevus syndrome	Melanoma	Autosomal dominant
Immunodeficiency Syndromes		
Wiskott-Aldrich syndrome	Lymphoma	Immunodeficiency; X-linked recessive
X-linked immunodeficiency (Duncan syndrome)	Lymphoma	Epstein-Barr virus is inciting agent
Severe combined immunodeficiency	Leukemia, lymphoma	Immunodeficiency; X-linked recessive
Other Single-Gene Defects		
Neurofibromatosis	Neurofibroma, peripheral nerve sheath, optic glioma, acoustic neuroma, astrocytoma, meningioma, pheochromocytoma	Autosomal dominant
Tuberous sclerosis	Fibroangiomatous nevi, myocardial rhabdomyoma	Autosomal dominant
Retinoblastoma, genetic form	Sarcoma	Autosomal dominant
Wilms tumor, genetic form	Wilms tumor	Autosomal dominant
Familial adenomatous polyposis coli	Adenocarcinoma of colon, hepatoblastoma, thyroid cancer	Autosomal dominant
Gardner syndrome	Adenocarcinoma of colon; skull and soft tissue tumors	Autosomal dominant
Peutz-Jeghers syndrome	Gastrointestinal carcinoma	Autosomal dominant
Tyrosinemia, galactosemia	Hepatic carcinoma	Nodular cirrhosis; autosomal recessive
Multiple endocrine neoplasia syndrome I (Wermer syndrome)	Parathyroid adenoma, pancreatic islet tumor, pituitary adenoma, carcinoid	Autosomal dominant; Zollinger-Ellison syndrome
Multiple endocrine neoplasia syndrome II (Sipple syndrome)	Medullary carcinoma of the thyroid, hyperparathyroidism, pheochromocytoma	Autosomal dominant; monitor calcitonin and calcium levels
Multiple endocrine neoplasia III (multiple mucosal neuroma syndrome)	Mucosal neuroma, pheochromocytoma, medullary thyroid carcinoma; Marfan habitus; neuropathy	Autosomal dominant

CHAPTER 153 ● Assessment   729

TABLE 153–1. Familial or Genetic Susceptibility to Malignancy—cont'd

Disorder	Tumor or Cancer	Comment
von Hippel–Lindau disease	Hemangioblastoma of the cerebellum and retina, pheochromocytoma	Autosomal dominant; mutation of tumor suppressor gene
Cancer family syndrome	Colonic, uterine carcinoma	Autosomal dominant
Li-Fraumeni syndrome	Bone, soft tissue sarcoma, breast	Autosomal dominant mutation of p53
Other Congenital Conditions		
Hemihypertrophy ± Beckwith syndrome	Wilms tumor, hepatoblastoma, adrenal carcinoma	25% develop tumor, most in first 5 yr of life

AML, acute myelogenous leukemia.

TABLE 153–2. Common Manifestations of Childhood Malignancies

Signs and Symptoms	Significance	Example
Hematologic		
Pallor, anemia	Bone marrow infiltration	Leukemia, neuroblastoma
Petechiae, thrombocytopenia	Bone marrow infiltration	Leukemia, neuroblastoma
Fever, pharyngitis, neutropenia	Bone marrow infiltration	Leukemia, neuroblastoma
Systemic		
Bone pain, limp, arthralgia	Primary bone tumor, metastasis to bone	Osteosarcoma, Ewing sarcoma, leukemia, neuroblastoma
Fever of unknown origin, weight loss, night sweats	Lymphoreticular malignancy	Hodgkin disease, non-Hodgkin lymphoma
Painless lymphadenopathy	Lymphoreticular malignancy, metastatic solid tumor	Leukemia, Hodgkin disease, non-Hodgkin lymphoma, Burkitt lymphoma, thyroid carcinoma
Cutaneous lesion	Primary or metastatic disease	Neuroblastoma, leukemia, Langerhans cell histiocytosis, melanoma
Abdominal mass	Adrenal-renal tumor	Neuroblastoma, Wilms tumor, lymphoma
Hypertension	Sympathetic nervous system tumor	Neuroblastoma, pheochromocytoma, Wilms tumor
Diarrhea	Vasoactive intestinal polypeptide	Neuroblastoma, ganglioneuroma
Soft tissue mass	Local or metastatic tumor	Ewing sarcoma, osteosarcoma, neuroblastoma, thyroid carcinoma, rhabdomyosarcoma, eosinophilic granuloma
Diabetes insipidus, galactorrhea, poor growth	Neuroendocrine involvement of hypothalamus or pituitary gland	Adenoma, craniopharyngioma, prolactinoma, Langerhans cell histiocytosis
Emesis, visual disturbances, ataxia, headache, papilledema, cranial nerve palsies	Increased intrathecal pressure	Primary brain tumor; metastasis
Ophthalmologic Signs		
Leukokoria	White pupil	Retinoblastoma
Periorbital ecchymosis	Metastasis	Neuroblastoma
Miosis, ptosis, heterochromia	Horner syndrome: compression of cervical sympathetic nerves	Neuroblastoma
Opsomyoclonus, ataxia	Neurotransmitters? Autoimmunity?	Neuroblastoma
Exophthalmos, proptosis	Orbital tumor	Rhabdomyosarcoma, lymphoma
Thoracic Mass		
Anterior mediastinal	Cough, stridor, pneumonia, tracheal-bronchial compression	Germ cell tumor, T cell lymphoma, Hodgkin disease
Posterior mediastinal	Vertebral or nerve root compression; dysphagia	Neuroblastoma, neuroenteric cyst

TABLE 153–3. Minimum Workup Required for Common Pediatric Malignancies to Assess Primary Tumor and Potential Metastases*

	Bone Marrow Aspirate/ Biopsy	Chest X-ray	CT Scan	MRI	Bone Scan	CSF Analysis	Specific Markers	Other Tests
Leukemia	Yes	Yes				Yes		
Non-Hodgkin lymphoma	Yes	Yes	Yes		Yes	Yes		
Hodgkin disease	Yes	Yes	Yes		Yes			Gallium scan
CNS tumors				Yes		Yes		
Neuroblastoma	Yes		Yes		Yes		VMA, HVA	MIBG scan
Wilms tumor		Yes	Yes					
Rhabdomyosarcoma	Yes	Yes	Yes		Yes	Yes (for parameningeal tumors only)		
Osteosarcoma		Yes	Yes (of chest)	Yes (for primary tumors)	Yes			
Ewing sarcoma	Yes	Yes	Yes (of chest)	Yes (for primary tumors)	Yes			
Germ cell tumors		Yes	Yes	Consider MRI of brain			AFP, HCG	
Liver tumors		Yes	Yes				AFP	
Retinoblastoma	±		Yes, if MRI not available	Yes (of brain)	±	Yes		Retinoblastoma gene analysis

*Individual cases may require additional studies.
AFP, alpha-fetoprotein; HVA, homovanillic acid; MIBG, metaiodobenzylguanidine; VMA, vanillylmandelic acid.

CHAPTER **154**

Principles of Cancer Treatment

The overall goal of pediatric oncology is to cure all patients with minimal toxicity. The 5-year survival probability for children with cancer has increased from 56% in 1974 to greater than 75%. Eligible patients should be offered participation in a clinical trial because outcomes are superior for patients treated in clinical trials compared with patients not treated in clinical trials. Treatment for children with cancer may involve surgery, radiation therapy, or chemotherapy. Surgery and radiation usually are local treatment modalities (an exception is total body irradiation as part of a stem cell transplantation), whereas chemotherapy has local and systemic effects.

Primary prevention strategies are unknown for most pediatric malignancies. In contrast to many adult malignancies, childhood malignancies are not associated with tobacco or alcohol use, dietary factors, sun exposure, or preventable infection. A notable exception is the lowered rates of hepatocellular carcinoma from the use of hepatitis B vaccine in high endemicity areas, such as Taiwan. Exposure to certain chemotherapy agents and radiation therapy increase the rate of **second malignant neoplasms**. Secondary prevention may be accomplished by screening an at-risk child, such as a patient with Beckwith-Wiedemann syndrome (Wilms tumor) or the twin of a patient with leukemia or neuroblastoma, but these circumstances are rare.

ONCOLOGIC EMERGENCIES

Adverse effects of tumors and treatments may result in oncologic emergencies in children and adolescents (Table 154–1). Mediastinal masses from lymphoma can cause life-threatening airway obstruction. Tumors with

TABLE 154–1.   Oncologic Emergencies

Condition	Manifestations	Etiology	Malignancy	Treatment
Metabolic				
Hyperuricemia	Uric acid nephropathy; gout	Tumor lysis syndrome	Lymphoma, leukemia	Allopurinol, alkalinize urine; hydration and diuresis, rasburicase
Hyperkalemia	Arrhythmias, cardiac arrest	Tumor lysis syndrome	Lymphoma, leukemia	Kayexalate; sodium bicarbonate, glucose, and insulin; check for pseudohyperkalemia from leukemic cell lysis in test tube
Hyperphosphatemia	Hypocalcemic tetany; metastatic calcification, photophobia, pruritus	Tumor lysis syndrome	Lymphoma, leukemia	Hydration, forced diuresis; stop alkalinization; oral aluminum hydroxide to bind phosphate
Hyponatremia	Seizure, lethargy, asymptomatic	SIADH; fluid, sodium losses in vomiting	Leukemia, CNS tumor	Restrict free water for SIADH; replace sodium if depleted
Hypercalcemia	Anorexia, nausea, polyuria, pancreatitis, gastric ulcers; prolonged PR, shortened QT interval	Bone resorption; ectopic parathormone, vitamin D, or prostaglandins	Metastasis to bone, rhabdomyosarcoma	Hydration and furosemide diuresis; corticosteroids; mithramycin; calcitonin, diphosphonates
Hematologic				
Anemia	Pallor, weakness, heart failure	Bone marrow suppression or infiltration; blood loss	Any with chemotherapy	Packed red blood cell transfusion
Thrombocytopenia	Petechiae, hemorrhage	Bone marrow suppression or infiltration	Any with chemotherapy	Platelet transfusion
Disseminated intravascular coagulation	Shock, hemorrhage	Sepsis, hypotension, tumor factors	Promyelocytic leukemia, others	Fresh frozen plasma; platelets, treat infection
Neutropenia	Infection	Bone marrow suppression or infiltration	Any with chemotherapy	If febrile, administer broad-spectrum antibiotics, and G-CSF if appropriate
Hyperleukocytosis (>50,000/mm^3)	Hemorrhage, thrombosis; pulmonary infiltrates, hypoxia; tumor lysis syndrome	Leukostasis; vascular occlusion	Leukemia	Leukapheresis; chemotherapy
Graft-versus-host disease	Dermatitis, diarrhea, hepatitis	Immunosuppression and nonirradiated blood products; bone marrow transplantation	Any with immunosuppression	Corticosteroids; cyclosporine; antithymocyte globulin

Continued

TABLE 154–1. Oncologic Emergencies—cont'd

Condition	Manifestations	Etiology	Malignancy	Treatment
Space-Occupying Lesions				
Spinal cord compression	Back pain ± radicular *Cord above T10:* symmetric weakness, increased deep tendon reflex; sensory level present; toes up *Conus medullaris (T10-L2):* symmetric weakness, increased knee reflexes, decreased ankle reflexes; saddle sensory loss; toes up or down *Cauda equina (below L2):* asymmetric weakness, loss of deep tendon reflex and sensory deficit; toes down	Metastasis to vertebra and extramedullary space	Neuroblastoma; medulloblastoma	MRI or myelography for diagnosis; corticosteroids; radiotherapy; laminectomy; chemotherapy
Increased intracranial pressure	Confusion, coma, emesis, headache, hypertension, bradycardia, seizures, papilledema, hydrocephalus; III and VI nerve palsies	Primary or metastatic brain tumor	Neuroblastoma, astrocytoma; glioma	CT or MRI for diagnosis; corticosteroids; phenytoin; ventriculostomy tube; radiotherapy; chemotherapy
Superior vena cava syndrome	Distended neck veins, plethora, edema of head and neck, cyanosis, proptosis; Horner syndrome	Superior mediastinal mass	Lymphoma	Chemotherapy; radiotherapy
Tracheal compression	Respiratory distress	Mediastinal mass compressing trachea	Lymphoma	Radiation, corticosteroids

G-CSF, granulocyte colony-stimulating factor; SIADH, syndrome of inappropriate antidiuretic hormone secretion.

a large tumor burden, notably Burkitt lymphoma or germ cell tumors, may affect renal function adversely from tubular deposition of uric acid crystals. Serum levels of uric acid and creatinine should be measured, and allopurinol or uric acid oxidase can be administered before chemotherapy. A common metabolic emergency is **tumor lysis syndrome**, often seen in treatment of leukemia and lymphoma as large amounts of phosphates and potassium are released into the circulation from lysed cells. Overwhelming infection and neurologic compromise are other oncologic emergencies (Table 154–2).

SURGERY

Patients with solid tumors usually have a palpable mass lesion or symptoms related to a mass lesion (pain, respiratory distress, abdominal obstruction). Appro-priate imaging (usually with CT or MRI) should be obtained followed by resection when possible or a biopsy if complete resection is not feasible. An exception is a suspected lymphoma, for which a biopsy may be needed but resection is not because most pediatric lymphomas are chemosensitive and do not require surgical resection. Many pediatric solid tumors (NHL, neuroblastoma, Ewing sarcoma, rhabdomyosarcoma) may have similar appearances on light microscopic examination and as a group are referred to as **small, round, blue cell tumors**. To diagnose the particular tumor type adequately, additional pathologic studies, such as surface marker analysis, immunohistochemistry, and electron microscopy, may be required. Cytogenetic evaluations should be performed in most cases of childhood cancer. Many types of leukemia and certain solid tumors show either specific chromosomal translocations or recurring cytogenetic abnormalities

TABLE 154–2. Infectious Complications of Malignancy

Predisposing Factor	Etiology	Site of Infection	Infectious Agents
Neutropenia	Chemotherapy, bone marrow infiltration	Sepsis, shock, pneumonia, soft tissue, proctitis, mucositis	*Staphylococcus aureus, Staphylococcus epidermidis, Escherichia coli, Pseudomonas aeruginosa, Candida, Aspergillus,* anaerobic oral and rectal bacteria
Immunosuppression, lymphopenia, lymphocyte-monocyte dysfunction	Chemotherapy, prednisone	Pneumonia, meningitis, disseminated viral infection	*Pneumocystis carinii, Cryptococcus neoformans, Mycobacterium, Nocardia, Listeria monocytogenes, Candida, Aspergillus, Strongyloides, Toxoplasma,* varicella-zoster virus, cytomegalovirus, herpes simplex
Splenectomy	Staging of Hodgkin disease	Sepsis, shock, meningitis	Pneumococcus, *Haemophilus influenzae,* meningococcus
Indwelling central venous catheter	Nutrition, administration of chemotherapy	Line sepsis, tract of tunnel, exit site	*S. epidermidis, S. aureus, Candida albicans, P. aeruginosa, Aspergillus, Corynebacterium* JK, *Streptococcus faecalis, Mycobacterium fortuitum, Propionibacterium acnes*

or gene alterations that can lead to the correct diagnosis. It is crucial to determine the amount of tissue required and the appropriate distribution of the tissue so that all of the necessary studies may be performed. A general oncologic surgery principle is to resect the tumor and a surrounding margin of normal tissue if possible to ensure the entire tumor has been resected.

CHEMOTHERAPY

Because most pediatric solid tumors have a high risk for micrometastatic disease at the time of diagnosis, chemotherapy is used in almost all cases (Table 154–3). Exceptions include low-stage neuroblastoma (particularly in infants) and low-grade CNS tumors. Chemotherapy for localized solid tumors administered after removal of the primary tumor is referred to as **adjuvant** therapy, and chemotherapy administered while the primary tumor is still present is referred to as **neoadjuvant** chemotherapy. Neoadjuvant chemotherapy has many potential benefits, including an early attack on presumed micrometastatic disease, shrinkage of the primary tumor to facilitate local control, and additional time to plan for definitive surgery. In addition, in patients with osteosarcoma or Ewing sarcoma who undergo surgical removal of the primary tumor after neoadjuvant chemotherapy, the higher the degree of necrosis induced in the primary tumor, the better the prognosis. Anticancer drugs act at different sites (Fig. 154–1).

Resistance to a particular chemotherapeutic agent can develop in many ways: decreased influx or increased efflux of the chemotherapeutic agent from the malignant cell, mutation in the target of a chemotherapeutic drug so that it cannot be inhibited by the drug, amplification of a drug target to overcome inhibition, and blockade of normal cellular processes, which leads to programmed cell death or apoptosis. Because mutation is an ongoing process in a malignant tumor, it follows that certain subpopulations of tumor cells within a tumor may be more or less sensitive to any particular chemotherapy drug. Given this fact, combinations of chemotherapy drugs are used (as opposed to sequential single agents) to treat the various forms of childhood cancer.

Certain areas of the body may be inaccessible to chemotherapeutic agents given orally, intravenously, or intramuscularly. The blood-brain barrier prevents the penetration of chemotherapeutic drugs into the CNS; instillation of the chemotherapeutic agent directly into the CSF (by lumbar puncture) may be necessary.

RADIATION THERAPY

Radiation therapy is the process of delivering ionizing radiation to malignant cells to kill them directly or, more commonly, prevent them from dividing by interfering with DNA replication. Conventional radiation therapy uses photons, but atomic particles, such as electrons, protons, and neutrons, also are used. Not all

TABLE 154–3.   Cancer Chemotherapy

Drug*	Action	Metabolism	Excretion	Indication	Toxicity
Antimetabolites					
Methotrexate	Folic acid antagonist; inhibits dihydrofolate reductase	Hepatic	Renal, 50%-90% excreted unchanged; biliary	ALL, lymphoma, medulloblastoma, osteosarcoma	Myelosuppression (nadir 7-10 days), mucositis, stomatitis, dermatitis, hepatitis, renal and CNS with high-dose administration; prevent with leucovorin, monitor levels
6-Mercaptopurine	Purine analogue	Hepatic; allopurinol inhibits metabolism	Renal	ALL	Myelosuppression; hepatic necrosis; mucositis; allopurinol increases toxicity
Cytosine arabinoside (Ara-C)	Pyrimidine analogue; inhibits DNA polymerase	Hepatic	Renal	ALL, lymphoma, sarcoma	Myelosuppression, conjunctivitis, mucositis, CNS dysfunction
Alkylating Agents					
Cyclophosphamide (Cytoxan)	Alkylates guanine; inhibits DNA synthesis	Hepatic	Renal	ALL, lymphoma, sarcoma	Myelosuppression; hemorrhagic cystitis; pulmonary fibrosis, inappropriate ADH secretion, bladder cancer, anaphylaxis
Ifosfamide	Similar to Cytoxan	Hepatic	Renal	Lymphoma, Wilms tumor, sarcoma, germ cell and testicular tumors	Similar to Cytoxan; CNS dysfunction, cardiac toxicity
Antibiotics					
Doxorubicin (Adriamycin) and daunorubicin (Cerubidine)	Binds to DNA, intercalation	Hepatic	Biliary, renal	ALL, AML, osteosarcoma, Ewing sarcoma, lymphoma, neuroblastoma	Cardiomyopathy, red urine, tissue necrosis on extravasation, myelosuppression, conjunctivitis, radiation dermatitis, arrhythmia
Dactinomycin	Binds to DNA, inhibits transcription	—	Renal, stool, 30% excreted unchanged drug	Wilms tumor, rhabdomyosarcoma, Ewing sarcoma	Tissue necrosis on extravasation, myelosuppression, radiosensitizer, stomatitis
Bleomycin	Binds to DNA, cuts DNA	Hepatic	Renal	Hodgkin disease, lymphoma, germ cell tumors	Pneumonitis, stomatitis, Raynaud phenomenon, pulmonary fibrosis, dermatitis
Vinca Alkaloids					
Vincristine (Oncovin)	Inhibits microtubule	Hepatic	Biliary	ALL, lymphoma, Wilms tumor, Hodgkin disease, Ewing sarcoma, neuroblastoma, rhabdomyosarcoma, brain tumors	Local cellulitis, peripheral neuropathy, constipation, ileus, jaw pain, inappropriate ADH secretion, seizures, ptosis, minimal myelosuppression
Vinblastine (Velban)	Inhibits microtuble formation	Hepatic	Biliary	Hodgkin disease, Langerhans cell histiocytosis	Local cellulitis, leukopenia

TABLE 154–3.   Cancer Chemotherapy—cont'd

Drug*	Action	Metabolism	Excretion	Indication	Toxicity
Enxymes					
Asparaginase	Depletion of asparagine	–	Reticuloendothelial system	ALL	Allergic reaction; pancreatitis, hyperglycemia, platelet dysfunction and coagulopathy, encephalopathy
Hormones					
Prednisone	Direct lymphocyte cytotoxicity	Hepatic	Renal	ALL; Hodgkin disease, lymphoma	Cushing syndrome, cataracts, diabetes, hypertension, myopathy, osteoporosis, infection, peptic ulceration, psychosis
Miscellaneous					
BCNU (carmustine, nitrosourea)	Carbamylation of DNA; inhibits DNA synthesis	Hepatic; phenobarbital increases metabolism, decreases activity	Renal	CNS tumors, lymphoma, Hodgkin disease	Delayed myelosuppression (4-6 wk); pulmonary fibrosis, carcinogenic, stomatitis
Cisplatin	Inhibits DNA synthesis	–	Renal	Gonadal tumors; osteosarcoma, neuroblastoma, CNS tumors, germ cell tumors	Nephrotoxic; myelosuppression, ototoxicity, tetany, neurotoxicity, hemolytic-uremic syndrome; aminoglycosides may increase nephrotoxicity, anaphylaxis
Carboplatin	Inhibits DNA synthesis	–	Renal	Same as cisplatin	Myelosuppression
Etoposide (VP-16)	Topoisomerase inhibitor	–	Renal	ALL, lymphoma, germ cell tumor	Myelosuppression, secondary leukemia
Etretinate (vitamin A analogue) and tretinoin	Enhances normal differentiation	Liver	Liver	Some leukemias; neuroblastoma	Dry mouth, hair loss, pseudo-tumor cerebri, premature epiphyseal closure

*Many drugs produce nausea and vomiting during administration, and many cause alopecia with repeated doses.
ADH, Antidiuretic hormone; ALL, acute lymphoblastic leukemia; AML, acute myelogenous leukemia.

tumors are radiosensitive, and radiation therapy is not necessary in all tumors that are radiosensitive.

OTHER THERAPIES

Certain cancers have been treated with cytokines, biologic response modifiers, or monoclonal antibodies in addition to standard treatments. **Targeted therapies** specifically target the tumor cells, and normal host cells are spared. Imatinib mesylate is a protein kinase inhibitor that targets the effects of the t(9;22) translocation of chronic myelogenous leukemia. Supportive care also plays an important role in pediatric oncology, including the use of appropriate antimicrobials, blood products, nutritional support, intensive care, and possibly alternative therapies.

ADVERSE EFFECTS

Because chemotherapy agents are cellular toxins, numerous adverse effects are associated with their use. Bone marrow suppression, immunosuppression, nausea, vomiting, and alopecia are general adverse effects of commonly used chemotherapy drugs. Each chemotherapy drug has specific toxicities. Doxorubicin can cause cardiac damage, cisplatin can cause renal damage and ototoxicity, bleomycin can cause pulmonary fibrosis, cyclophosphamide and ifosfamide can cause hemorrhagic cystitis, and vincristine can cause peripheral neuropathy. Radiation therapy produces many adverse effects, such as mucositis, growth retardation, organ dysfunction, and the later development of secondary cancers. Significant therapy-related **late effects** may develop in pediatric cancer patients (Table 154–4).

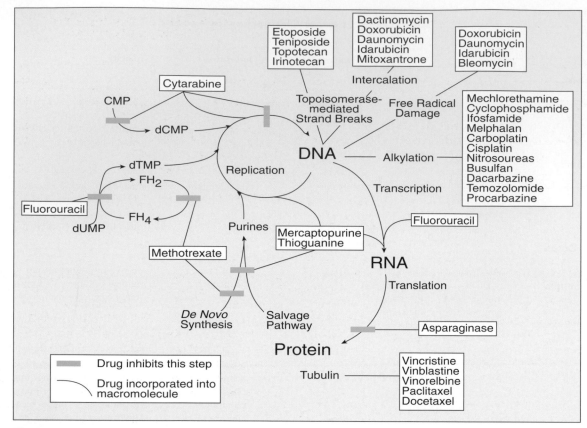

Figure 154–1

Site of action of the commonly used anticancer drugs. CMP, cytidine monophosphate; dCMP, deoxycytidine monophosphate; dTMP, deoxythymidine monophosphate; dUMP, deoxyuridine monophosphate; FH_2, dihydrofolate; FH_4, tetrahydrofolate. (From Balis FM, Holcenberg JS, Blaney SM: General principles of chemotherapy. In Pizzo PA, Poplack DG [eds]: Principles and Practice of Pediatric Oncology, 4th ed. Philadelphia, Lippincott Williams & Wilkins, 2002, p 241.)

TABLE 154–4. Long-Term Sequelae of Cancer Therapy

Problem	Etiology
Infertility	Alkylating agents; radiation
Second cancers	Genetic predisposition; radiation, alkylating agents, VP-16, topoisomerase II inhibitors
Sepsis	Splenectomy
Hepatotoxicity	Methotrexate, 6-mercaptopurine, radiation
Hepatic veno-occlusive disease	High-dose, intensive chemotherapy (busulfan, cyclophosphamide) ± bone marrow transplant
Scoliosis	Radiation
Pulmonary (pneumonia, fibrosis)	Radiation, bleomycin, busulfan
Cardiomyopathy, pericarditis	Adriamycin (doxorubicin), daunomycin, radiation
Leukoencephalopathy	Cranial irradiation ± methotrexate
Cognition/intelligence	Cranial irradiation ± methotrexate
Pituitary dysfunction (isolated growth hormone deficiency, panhypopituitary)	Cranial irradiation
Psychosocial	Stress, anxiety, death of peers; conditioned responses to chemotherapy
Thyroid dysfunction	Radiation
Osteonecrosis	Corticosteroids

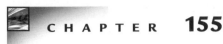

CHAPTER 155

Leukemia

ETIOLOGY

The etiology of childhood leukemia is unknown and is probably multifactorial, with genetics and environmental factors playing important roles. The role of genetics is highlighted by the many recurrent non-random chromosomal translocations in the leukemia cells. A translocation may lead to the formation of a new gene, whose expression may lead to a novel protein with transforming capabilities. In **chronic myelogenous leukemia**, a translocation between chromosome 9 and 22 results in a fusion gene incorporating parts of two genes, *BCR* and *ABL*. The protein formed by this novel gene plays an important role in the development of chronic myelogenous leukemia. Certain constitutional genotypes can predispose a child to the development of acute leukemia. Patients with trisomy 21 (Down syndrome), Fanconi anemia, Bloom syndrome, ataxia-telangiectasia, Wiskott-Aldrich syndrome, and neurofibromatosis type 1 all have an increased risk. Siblings of children with leukemia also are at twofold to fourfold increased risk of developing leukemia, which increases for twin siblings (25% for monozygotic twins). For some patients with leukemia, the unique antigen receptor gene rearrangement or the specific chromosomal translocation characterizing their leukemic clone can be shown in cord blood cells and neonatal blood spots used for screening for metabolic diseases, suggesting a possible in utero etiology. There also have been a few reports of familial leukemia. Environmental factors that may increase the risk of leukemia include ionizing radiation and exposure to certain chemotherapy agents, particularly to topoisomerase II inhibitors.

EPIDEMIOLOGY

Each year, 2500 to 3500 new cases of childhood leukemia occur in the U.S. The disease affects about 40 children per 1 million younger than age 15 years. **Acute lymphoblastic leukemia (ALL)** accounts for approximately 75% of cases. The subtypes of acute myelogenous leukemia (AML) and chronic myelogenous leukemia account for 15% to 20% and less than 5% of cases, respectively. Other chronic leukemias, including juvenile myelomonocytic leukemia, chronic myelomonocytic leukemia, and chronic lymphocytic leukemia, are rare in childhood.

ALL is classified according to cell lineage as either B lineage or T lineage. The incidence of ALL peaks at 2 to 5 years of age and is higher in boys than in girls.

TABLE 155–1. Acute Myelogenous Leukemia Subtypes

Name/Morphology	FAB Classification
Myeloblastic with minimal maturation	M0
Myeloblastic without maturation	M1
Myeloblastic with maturation	M2
Acute promyelocytic leukemia	M3
Acute myelomonocytic leukemia	M4
Acute monocytic leukemia	M5
Acute erythrocytic leukemia	M6
Acute megakaryoblastic leukemia	M7

FAB, French-American-British.

T cell ALL in particular is associated with a male predominance. In the U.S., ALL is more common in white than in African American children.

AML is classified according to the French-American-British system (Table 155–1), which assigns leukemic cells to the myeloid, monocyte, erythroid, or megakaryocytic lineage. The incidence of AML is high in the neonatal period, then declines and stabilizes until adolescence, when there is a slight increase. This increase continues into adulthood, especially beyond 55 years of age. Males and females are equally affected by AML. Hispanic and African American children have slightly higher incidence rates than white children.

CLINICAL MANIFESTATIONS

Signs and symptoms of acute leukemias are related to the infiltration of leukemic cells into normal tissues, resulting in either bone marrow failure (anemia, neutropenia, thrombocytopenia) or specific tissue infiltration (lymph nodes, liver, spleen, brain, bone, skin, gingiva, testes). Common presenting symptoms are fever, pallor, petechiae or ecchymoses, lethargy, malaise, anorexia, and bone or joint pain. **Physical examination** frequently reveals lymphadenopathy and hepatosplenomegaly. Symptomatic CNS involvement is rare at the time of presentation. The testicle is a common extramedullary site for ALL; a painless enlargement of one or both testes may be seen. Patients with T cell ALL are frequently older boys (8 to 10 years) and often have high white blood cell (WBC) counts, anterior mediastinal masses, bulky disease with cervical lymphadenopathy, hepatosplenomegaly, and CNS involvement. In patients with AML, extramedullary soft tissue tumors may be found in various sites. The presence of myeloperoxidase in these tumors may impart a greenish hue; such tumors are known as chloromas.

LABORATORY AND IMAGING STUDIES

The diagnosis of acute leukemia is established by finding immature blast cells on the peripheral blood smear, bone marrow aspirate, or both. With rare exception (a sick patient with hyperleukocytosis and a large anterior mediastinal mass with airway compression), a bone marrow aspirate should be done urgently to confirm the diagnosis. Most patients have abnormal blood counts; anemia and thrombocytopenia are common. The WBC counts may be low, normal, or high; 15% to 20% of patients have WBC count greater than 50,000/mm³. The likely diagnosis of the particular type of leukemia (lymphoid or myeloid) often can be established by evaluating blast morphology on either a peripheral smear or a bone marrow aspirate. To determine definitively the exact diagnosis, the evaluation of cell surface markers (**immunophenotype**) by flow cytometry and cytochemical staining patterns should be evaluated. **Cytogenetic analysis** should be undertaken in all cases of acute leukemia. Certain types of lymphoid and myeloid leukemias have specific chromosomal abnormalities. In ALL, the t(12;21) translocation is most common (approximately 20% of all cases) and is associated with a favorable prognosis. The t(9;22) translocation occurs in less than 5% of cases and is associated with a poor prognosis. The t(4;11) translocation (and other translocations involving the mixed lineage leukemia gene on chromosome 11) often occurs in infants and patients with secondary AML and is associated with a poor prognosis. Fluorescence in situ hybridization or polymerase chain reaction or both are now employed in most cases of leukemia because many chromosomal abnormalities may not be apparent on routine karyotypes. A **lumbar puncture** always should be performed at the time of diagnosis to evaluate the possibility of CNS involvement. A chest x-ray should be obtained in all patients to exclude an anterior mediastinal mass, which is commonly seen in T cell ALL. Electrolytes, calcium, phosphorus, uric acid, and renal and hepatic function should be monitored in all patients.

DIFFERENTIAL DIAGNOSIS

The differential diagnosis of acute leukemia includes nonmalignant and malignant diseases. Infection is probably the most common mimicker of acute leukemia, particularly Epstein-Barr virus infection. Other infectious agents (cytomegalovirus, pertussis, mycobacteria) also can produce signs and symptoms common to leukemia. Noninfectious diagnoses include aplastic anemia, juvenile rheumatoid arthritis, immune thrombocytopenic purpura, and congenital or acquired conditions that lead to neutropenia or anemia. Several malignant diagnoses also can mimic leukemia, including neuroblastoma, rhabdomyosarcoma, and Ewing sarcoma. These all may appear to be small, round, blue cell tumors. Newborns with trisomy 21 (Down syndrome) may have a condition known as **transient myeloproliferative disorder**, which can produce elevated WBC counts with peripheral blasts, anemia, and thrombocytopenia. It usually resolves with supportive care only, but these children have a significantly increased risk (30%) of developing true acute leukemia (ALL or AML) within the next few months and years of life.

Proliferation and accumulation of histiocytes produces the **histiocytoses**, which include Langerhans cell histiocytosis, familial erythrophagocytic lymphohistiocytosis, and infection-associated (Epstein-Barr virus, cytomegalovirus, herpesviruses, malaria, and others) hemophagocytic syndromes. Langerhans cell histiocytosis manifests with varying degrees of bone, skin, lung, liver, and bone marrow (pancytopenia) involvement, whereas familial erythrophagocytic lymphohistiocytosis and infection-associated hemophagocytic syndromes manifest with fever, weight loss, irritability, hepatosplenomegaly, rash, hypertriglyceridemia, cytopenias, and aseptic meningitis. These histiocytic diseases should be included in the differential diagnosis of leukemia.

TREATMENT

Patients with ALL generally receive three- or four-agent **induction chemotherapy** based on their initial risk group assignment. Low-risk and standard-risk patients receive vincristine, prednisone, and asparaginase for 4 weeks; high-risk patients also receive an anthracycline (daunorubicin). During induction, intrathecal instillation of some combination of methotrexate, cytarabine, and hydrocortisone treats existing CNS leukemia or prevents the development of CNS leukemia. After successful remission induction, which is achieved in nearly all patients with ALL, treatment during remission is given as **consolidation chemotherapy** along with **CNS-directed therapy**. Patients with CNS disease detected at diagnosis and T cell ALL receive cranial radiation therapy. High-risk patients in general receive intensive systemic chemotherapy in addition to the CNS-directed therapy during consolidation; this has resulted in significant improvement in overall outcome. Systemic chemotherapy during this phase often includes cyclophosphamide, cytarabine, and 6-mercaptopurine. Most groups treating childhood ALL agree that some form of delayed intensification is needed to optimize outcomes.

After delayed intensification, all patients receive **continuation therapy** for a total length of therapy of 2 to 2.5 years. Continuation therapy generally consists of a monthly dose of vincristine and short courses

(5 to 7 days) of oral steroid therapy, plus daily oral 6-mercaptopurine, and weekly methotrexate (orally or intramuscularly). In most protocols, intrathecal chemotherapy is given approximately every 3 months during continuation therapy.

The **treatment of AML** is quite different from that of ALL because nonmyelosuppressive drugs (vincristine, prednisone, and asparaginase) are not effective. Several cycles of extremely intensive myelosuppressive chemotherapy are necessary to cure childhood AML; there is little evidence that low-dose continuation therapy is helpful in AML (with the possible exception of M3 AML). Induction therapy for AML usually consists of cytarabine, daunomycin, and etoposide (or 6-thioguanine). Induction is most effective for long-term outcome when two courses of drugs are given consecutively (1 to 2 weeks apart) regardless of blood counts, as opposed to waiting for counts to recover after the first course. Because of the poorer outcome when standard chemotherapy is used, most centers recommend that all children with AML who have a matched sibling donor undergo stem cell (bone marrow) transplantation as soon as induction and consolidation therapy is completed. Gemtuzumab ozogamicin, a drug composed of recombinant humanized anti-CD33 antibody and the cytotoxic antibiotic calicheamicin, is being studied as an adjuvant therapy for newly diagnosed childhood AML.

COMPLICATIONS

Major short-term complications associated with the treatment of leukemia result from bone marrow suppression caused by chemotherapy. Patients may have bleeding and significant anemia that necessitates transfusion of platelets or blood. Low neutrophil counts predispose the patient to significant bacterial infection. Cell-mediated immunosuppression increases the risk of *Pneumocystis jiroveci* (*carinii*) pneumonia. Prophylaxis with oral trimethoprim-sulfamethoxazole or aerosolized pentamidine can prevent this complication. Patients who have not previously had varicella or the varicella vaccine are at risk for severe infection. On exposure, a nonimmune patient should receive varicella-zoster immune globulin. Patients with AML have prolonged periods of neutropenia, which increases the risk of bacterial and fungal infections. Prophylaxis with penicillin and fluconazole is frequently instituted. Long-term sequelae of therapy are less common than in previous treatment eras, but are prevalent in long-term survivors treated in the 1980s and earlier. These sequelae include neurocognitive impairment, short stature, obesity, cardiac dysfunction, infertility, second malignant neoplasms, and psychosocial problems (see Table 154–4).

TABLE 155–2. General Prognostic Factors in Acute Lymphoblastic Leukemia

Factor	Favorable (Lower Risk)	Unfavorable (Higher Risk)
Age	1 to <10 yr	<1 yr or ≥10 yr
Initial WBC count	<50,000/mm^3	>50,000/mm^3
CNS disease at diagnosis	Absent	Present
DNA index	>1.16	≤1.16
Cytogenetics	t(12;21)	t(4;11), t(9;22)
Response to therapy	Rapid	Slow

WBC, white blood cell.

PROGNOSIS

Patients with ALL are classified into four prognostic risk groups (low, standard, high, and very high) based on age, initial WBC count, genetic characteristics, and response to induction therapy, although classification systems are complex and evolving (Table 155–2). In general, low-risk patients are patients 1 to 9 years old with an initial WBC count less than 50,000/mm^3 and favorable cytogenetic findings such as t(12;21). High-risk patients are younger than 1 year old or 10 years old or older, have an initial WBC count greater than 50,000/mm^3, have CNS or testicular disease at diagnosis, or have unfavorable cytogenetics such as t(4;11). Very high risk patients have a hypodiploid DNA index, have a t(9;22) translocation, or fail to achieve remission after 4 weeks of therapy. All other patients are considered to have standard-risk ALL. Immunophenotype, minimal residual disease, and early response to therapy are other factors that influence risk stratification. Infants (<1 year old) with ALL generally have a highly undifferentiated immunophenotype, often have a translocation involving the mixed lineage leukemia gene (e.g., t(4;11)), and have a poor prognosis. It was suggested previously that African American, Native American, and Hispanic children have poorer outcomes compared with white and Asian children; these results have not been confirmed in all studies.

The overall **cure rate** for childhood **ALL** with current therapy can be expected to approximate 80%. Relapse of ALL occurs most commonly in the bone marrow, but also may occur in the CNS, testes, or other extramedullary sites. If relapse occurs while the patient is still receiving treatment, the prognosis is worse than if relapse occurs after discontinuation of therapy. Longer first remissions are associated with higher cure rates with salvage therapy compared with shorter first remissions. Stem cell transplant from a matched sibling donor, matched unrelated donor, or cord blood currently is recommended for patients who have a relapse while receiving initial chemotherapy. The current overall **cure rate** for childhood **AML** is approximately 50%. It is higher for patients who receive a matched sibling stem cell transplant in first remission than for patients treated with chemotherapy alone. The prognosis for relapsed AML is poor.

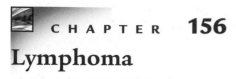

C H A P T E R   156
Lymphoma

ETIOLOGY

Lymphomas, or malignancies of lymphoid tissues, are the third most common malignancy in childhood, behind leukemias and CNS tumors. There are two major types of lymphoma: **Hodgkin disease** and **NHL**. The etiologies of Hodgkin disease and NHL are unknown, but evidence in many cases suggests that Epstein-Barr virus plays a causal role in both conditions.

Almost all cases of NHL in childhood are diffuse and highly malignant and show little differentiation. NHL has three histologic subtypes: small noncleaved cell, lymphoblastic, and large cell. For simplicity, these may be regarded as B cell, T cell, and large cell (which may be of either B cell or T cell origin) (Table 156-1).

Chromosomal translocation may move an oncogene from its normal site to a new, unregulated site, leading to increased expression. In Burkitt lymphoma, a type of NHL, translocation occurs between chromosome 8 (c-*myc* oncogene) and the immunoglobulin gene locus on chromosome 2, 14, or 22, such that the c-*myc* oncogene comes to reside next to an immunoglobulin gene. The c-*myc* gene turns on the immunoglobulin gene, leading to a malignant B cell lymphoma.

EPIDEMIOLOGY

The incidence of Hodgkin disease has a bimodal distribution, with peaks in the adolescent/young adult years and again after age 50; it is rarely seen in children younger than 5. In children, boys are affected more commonly than girls, but in adolescents, the sex ratio is approximately equal. The incidence of NHL increases with age. It is more common in whites than in African Americans and in males than in females. NHL has been described in association with congenital or acquired immunodeficiency states and after organ or stem cell transplantation. Burkitt lymphoma commonly is divided into two forms: a sporadic form commonly seen in North America and an endemic form commonly seen in Africa, which has a strong association with Epstein-Barr virus.

CLINICAL MANIFESTATIONS

Painless, firm lymphadenopathy often confined to one or two lymph node areas, usually the supraclavicular and cervical nodes, is the most common clinical presentation of Hodgkin disease. Mediastinal lymphadenopathy producing cough or shortness of breath is another frequent initial presentation. The presence of one of three **B symptoms** has prognostic value: fever (>38°C for 3 consecutive days), drenching night sweats, and unintentional weight loss of 10% or more within 6 months of diagnosis.

The **sporadic (North American) form** of Burkitt lymphoma more commonly has an abdominal presentation (typically pain), whereas the **endemic (African) form** frequently presents with tumors of the jaw. The anterior mediastinum and cervical nodes are the usual primary sites for T cell lymphomas. These may cause airway or superior vena cava obstruction or pleural effusion or both.

The **diagnosis** of lymphoma is established by results of a tissue biopsy or examination of pleural or peritoneal fluid. Systemic symptoms, such as fever and weight loss, may be present and are particularly prominent in patients with anaplastic large cell lymphoma,

TABLE 156–1.   Subtypes of Non-Hodgkin Lymphoma in Children

Histologic Category	Immunophenotype	Usual Primary Site	Most Common Translocation
Small noncleaved (Burkitt)	Mature B cell (surface immunoglobulin present)	Abdomen (sporadic form); head and neck (endemic form)	t(8;14)(q24;q32) t(2;8)(p11;q24) t(8;22)(q24;q11)
Lymphoblastic	T cell (rarely pre–B cell)	Neck and/or anterior mediastinum	Many
Large cell	T cell, B cell, or indeterminate	Lymph nodes, skin, soft tissue, bone	t(2;5)(p23;q35)

which can be insidious in onset. If the bone marrow contains 25% or greater blasts, the disease is classified as acute leukemia (either B cell ALL or T cell ALL). From prognostic and therapeutic standpoints, this distinction makes little difference because both require aggressive, systemic therapy in addition to CNS-directed therapy.

LABORATORY AND IMAGING STUDIES

Patients suspected to have lymphoma should have a complete blood count, erythrocyte sedimentation rate, and measurement of serum electrolytes, calcium, phosphorus, lactate dehydrogenase, and uric acid. All patients should have a chest x-ray. The diagnosis ultimately requires a pathologic confirmation from tissue or fluid sampling. For staging purposes, a bone marrow aspirate, bone scan, and gallium scan (for Hodgkin disease) also are indicated. The pathologic hallmark of Hodgkin disease is the identification of **Reed-Sternberg cells**. Histopathologic subtypes in childhood Hodgkin disease are similar to those in adults; 10% to 15% have lymphocyte predominant, 50% to 60% have nodular sclerosis, 30% have mixed cellularity, and less than 5% have lymphocyte depletion. All subtypes are responsive to treatment. Staging is according to the Ann Arbor system (Table 156–2). Staging laparotomy, often used in the past, is rarely used in children today because CT scans are helpful in identifying abdominal (nodes, liver, spleen) involvement.

DIFFERENTIAL DIAGNOSIS

The differential diagnosis for lymphomas in children includes leukemia, rhabdomyosarcoma, nasopharyngeal carcinoma, germ cell tumors, and thymomas. Nonmalignant diagnoses include mononucleosis (Epstein-Barr virus infection), branchial cleft and thyroglossal duct cysts, cat-scratch disease, bacterial or viral lymphadenitis, mycobacterial infection, toxoplasmosis, and tinea capitis, all of which can produce significant lymphadenopathy that can mimic lymphoma. Patients with acute abdominal pain from Burkitt lymphoma may be misdiagnosed as having appendicitis.

TREATMENT

The generally accepted treatment for **childhood Hodgkin disease** is a combination of chemotherapy and low-dose, involved-field radiation therapy. Chemotherapy for Hodgkin disease usually consists of some combination of cyclophosphamide, vincristine, procarbazine, doxorubicin, bleomycin, vinblastine, prednisone, and etoposide. In general, four to six courses of combination chemotherapy are given. The successful treatment of selected low-risk patients with

TABLE 156–2. Ann Arbor Staging Classification for Hodgkin Disease*
Stage I
Involvement of a single lymph node region (I), or a single extralymphatic organ or site (I_E)
Stage II
Involvement of ≥2 lymph node regions on the same side of the diaphragm (II), or localized involvement of an extralymphatic organ or site and of ≥1 lymph node regions on the same side of the diaphragm (II_E)
Stage III
Involvement of lymph node regions on both sides of the diaphragm (III), which may be accompanied by localized involvement of an extralymphatic organ or site (III_E), by involvement of the spleen (III_S), or both (III_{SE})
Stage IV
Diffuse or disseminated involvement of ≥1 extralymphatic organs or tissues, with or without associated lymph node enlargement

*Each stage is divided into *A* and *B* categories, in which *A* indicates no systemic symptoms, and *B* indicates the presence of ≥1 of the following: (1) unexplained weight loss >10% of body weight in preceding 6 mo, (2) temperature >38°C for 3 consecutive days, and (3) drenching night sweats.
E, extralymphatic; S, splenic involvement.

chemotherapy alone (without radiation therapy) has been well documented and is being investigated for selected intermediate-risk patients.

Distant, noncontiguous metastases are common in childhood NHL. Systemic chemotherapy is mandatory and should be administered to all children with NHL, even children with clinically localized disease at diagnosis.

T cell lymphoblastic lymphoma and T cell anaplastic large cell lymphoma generally are treated with aggressive multidrug regimens similar to the regimens used in ALL. The main drugs used in the treatment of mature B cell NHL are cyclophosphamide, moderate-dose to high-dose methotrexate, cytarabine, doxorubicin, ifosfamide, and etoposide. Surgery and radiation therapy rarely are used to treat NHL because the disease is rarely localized and is highly sensitive to chemotherapy.

COMPLICATIONS

The short-term complications from the treatment of lymphoma are similar to other pediatric malignancies and commonly include immunosuppression and related sequelae from myelosuppression, nausea, vomiting, and alopecia. **Late adverse effects** include second malignant neoplasms (AML or myelodysplasia, thyroid malignancies, and breast cancer in women), hypothyroidism, impaired soft tissue and bone growth, cardiac dysfunction, and pulmonary fibrosis.

PROGNOSIS

Children and adolescents with **Hodgkin disease** are classified as low, intermediate, or high risk according to stage and nodal bulk. The prognosis is excellent, with an approximately 90% 5-year overall survival, approaching 100% for low-risk patients and 70% to 90% for high-risk patients. For **NHL**, prognosis also is related to stage. The overall 3-year survival rates for B cell, T cell, and large cell NHL are 70% to 90%.

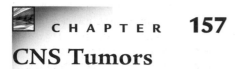

CHAPTER 157

CNS Tumors

ETIOLOGY

Most CNS tumors in children and adolescents are primary tumors (originate in the CNS); in contrast, adults are more likely to have secondary CNS tumors (metastatic from other sites). Childhood brain tumors also differ from tumors in adults in that they are usually low-grade astrocytomas or embryonic neoplasms (medulloblastoma, ependymoma, germ cell tumor), whereas most CNS tumors in adults are high-grade astrocytomas and metastatic carcinomas. CNS tumors also may arise in patients previously treated with radiation therapy. CNS tumors are likely multifactorial in etiology. The classification of CNS tumors is complex and evolving, with the World Health Organization classification the most complete and accurate system (Table 157–1). Children with certain inherited syndromes, including neurofibromatosis (types 1 and 2), Li-Fraumeni syndrome, tuberous sclerosis, Turcot syndrome, and von Hippel–Lindau syndrome, have an increased risk for developing a CNS tumor. Most CNS tumors arise in children with no known underlying disorder or risk factor.

EPIDEMIOLOGY

CNS tumors are the most common solid tumors in children and are second to leukemia in overall incidence. About 1700 new cases occur each year in the

Location	Incidence (%)	5-Year Survival (%)
TABLE 157–1. Location, Incidence, and Prognosis of CNS Tumors in Children		
Infratentorial (Posterior Fossa)	55-60	
Astrocytoma (cerebellum)	20	90
Medulloblastoma	20	50-80
Glioma (brainstem)	15	High grade: 0-5; low grade: 30
Ependymoma	5	50-60
Supratentorial (Cerebral Hemispheres)	40-55	
Astrocytoma	15	50-75
Glioblastoma multiforme	10	0-5
Ependymoma	2.5	50-75
Choroid plexus papilloma	1.5	95
Midline		
Craniopharyngioma	6	70-90
Pineal (germinoma)	1	65-75
Optic nerve glioma	3	90

U.S.; approximately 33 cases per 1 million occur in children younger than age 15 years. The incidence peaks before age 10, then decreases until a second peak after age 70. For medulloblastoma and ependymoma, males are more affected than females; for other tumor types no gender differences exist. In the first 2 to 3 years of life, whites are affected more than nonwhites; otherwise incidence rates are essentially equal for whites and nonwhites.

CLINICAL MANIFESTATIONS

Brain tumors can cause symptoms by impingement on normal tissue, usually cranial nerves, or by an increase in intracranial pressure caused either by obstruction of CSF flow or by a direct mass effect from the tumor. Tumors that obstruct the flow of CSF become symptomatic quickly. Symptoms of **increased intracranial pressure** are lethargy, headache, and vomiting (particularly in the morning on awakening) (see Chapter 184). Irritability, anorexia, poor school performance, and loss of developmental milestones all may be signs of slow-growing CNS tumors. In young children with open cranial sutures, an increase in head circumference may occur. Optic pathway tumors may lead to loss of visual acuity or visual field defects. Inability to abduct the eye as the result of sixth cranial nerve palsy is a common sign of increased intracranial pressure. Cranial nerve deficits other than sixth nerve palsy suggest involvement of the brainstem. Seizures occur in 20% to 50% of patients with supratentorial tumors; focal weakness or sensory changes also may be seen. Pituitary involvement produces neuroendocrine effects (galactorrhea with prolactinoma, excessive growth with growth hormone secretory tumors, precocious puberty). Cerebellar tumors are associated with ataxia and diminished coordination. A history and physical examination are fundamental for evaluation; this should include a careful neurologic assessment, including visual fields and a funduscopic examination (Table 157–2).

LABORATORY AND IMAGING STUDIES

If an intracranial lesion is suspected, **MRI** is the examination of choice, although a CT scan may be more readily obtained, especially in an emergency. Examination of **CSF** by cytocentrifuge histology determines the presence of metastatic disease in primitive neuroectodermal tumors, germ cell tumors, and pineal region tumors. A lumbar puncture should not be performed before a CT scan or MRI has been obtained to evaluate for evidence of increased intracranial pressure. If a tumor is suspected to have metastatic potential (medulloblastoma), MRI of the entire spine should be obtained before surgery to assess for neuraxial dissemination. A postoperative MRI study of the brain (and spine, if not done preoperatively) should be obtained within 24 to 48 hours of surgery to assess the extent of resection. During follow-up, magnetic resonance spectroscopy can help distinguish recurrent tumor from radiation necrosis.

DIFFERENTIAL DIAGNOSIS

In addition to a malignant tumor, the differential diagnosis of a CNS mass lesion should include benign tumor, arteriovenous malformation, aneurysm, brain abscess, cysticercosis, granulomatous disease (tuberculosis, sarcoid), intracranial hemorrhage, pseudotumor cerebri, vasculitis, and rarely metastatic tumor.

TREATMENT

The therapy for children with CNS tumors is individualized and depends on the tumor type, location, size, and associated symptoms. High-dose **dexamethasone** often is administered immediately to reduce tumor-associated edema. Improvements in neurodiagnosis, neurosurgical techniques, chemotherapy regimens, and radiation therapy techniques have improved overall outcome. Surgical objectives are complete excision if possible and maximal debulking if a complete excision is not possible. In children, radiation therapy often is combined with chemotherapy; in young children, radiation therapy often is delayed or avoided altogether if possible. Primitive neuroectodermal tumors (including medulloblastoma) and germ cell tumors are sensitive to chemotherapy; gliomas are less sensitive to chemotherapy. Chemotherapy plays an especially important role, particularly in infants with brain tumors in whom the effects of high-dose CNS radiation may have devastating effects on growth and neurocognitive development.

COMPLICATIONS

Short-term adverse effects of therapy include nausea, vomiting, anorexia, fatigue, immunosuppression, and cushingoid features. Long-term adverse effects include neurocognitive deficits, endocrinologic sequelae, decreased bone growth, ototoxicity, renal insufficiency, cataracts, infertility, and second malignant neoplasms (including myelodysplasia). The neurocognitive deficits can be significant, particularly in infants and young children, and are the primary reason for the continued search for the lowest efficacious radiation therapy dose and the most conformal delivery methods for the radiation therapy boosts. **Cerebellar mutism syndrome** occurs in 25% of patients after resection of a posterior fossa tumor and is characterized by an acute decrease in speech (often mutism), behavioral changes (e.g., irritability or apathy or both), diffuse cerebellar dysfunction, and other neurologic abnormalities. It may begin within hours to days of surgery and is usually self-resolving within weeks to months, although cerebellar ataxia and dysmetria often persist. **Somnolence syndrome**, which is characterized by excessive fatigue and sleepiness, may occur in the months after completion of radiation therapy and is self-limited. **Posterior fossa syndrome** manifests as headache and aseptic meningitis days to weeks after surgery in this area.

PROGNOSIS

The 5-year overall survival rate associated with all childhood CNS tumors (see Table 157–2) is approximately 50% to 60%, resulting in large measure from the high curability of cerebellar astrocytomas and the increasing cure rate for patients with medulloblastoma. Intrinsic brainstem gliomas are nearly universally fatal.

TABLE 157–2. Manifestations and Treatment of Primary CNS Tumors

Tumor and Site	Manifestations	Treatment	Comments
Cerebellar astrocytoma	Onset between 5 and 8 yr of age; ↑ ICP, ataxia, nystagmus, head tilt, intention tremor	Surgical excision plus adjuvant radiotherapy if a solid tumor; corticosteroids to ↓ tumor edema	Symptoms present for 2-7 mo; cystic tumors have favorable outcome
Medulloblastoma Cerebellar vermis and floor of fourth ventricle	Onset between 3 and 5 yr of age; ↑ ICP, obstructive hydrocephalus, ataxia, CSF metastasis, and spinal cord compression	Surgical excision and radiotherapy plus adjuvant chemotherapy,* corticosteroids to ↓ tumor edema	Acute onset of symptoms; tumor is radiosensitive; CSF checked for metastatic cells
Ependymoma Floor of fourth ventricle	↑ ICP, obstructive hydrocephalus; rarely seeds spinal fluid	Surgical excision, radiotherapy, chemotherapy,* corticosteroids to ↓ tumor edema	Onset intermediate between astrocytoma and medulloblastoma
Brainstem glioma	Onset between 5 and 7 yr of age; triad of multiple cranial nerve deficit (VII, IX, X, V, VI), pyramidal tract, and cerebellar signs; skip lesions common; ↑ ICP is late	Excision impossible, radiotherapy is palliative; corticosteroids to ↓ tumor edema; experimental chemotherapy*	Small size but critical location makes this tumor highly lethal
Pinealoma	Paralysis of upward gaze (Parinaud syndrome); lid retraction (Collier sign); hearing loss; precocious puberty; ↑ ICP; may seed spinal fluid	Radiotherapy, chemotherapy; shunting of CSF	Germ cell line; germinoma, dermoid, teratoma, mixed lesions may calcify or secrete HCG or alpha-fetoprotein
Diencephalic glioma Hypothalamus	Onset between 2 and 5 mo of age; alert, euphoric, but emaciated appearance; emesis, optic atrophy, nystagmus	Radiotherapy	Patient may become obese after treatment
Astrocytoma/glioma Cerebral cortex	Onset between 5 and 10 yr of age; personality changes; headache, motor weakness, seizures; ↑ ICP later	Location determines surgical resection or radiotherapy; anticonvulsant and corticosteroids; chemotherapy*	*Differential diagnosis*: Abscess, hydatid or porencephalic cyst; herpes simplex encephalitis, granuloma (TB, *Cryptococcus*); arteriovenous malformation; hematoma; lymphoma
Optic glioma	Onset before 2 yr of age; poor visual acuity, exophthalmos, nystagmus; ↑ ICP; optic atrophy, strabismus	Surgical resection or radiotherapy; chemotherapy*	Neurofibromatosis in 25% of patients
Craniopharyngioma Pituitary fossa	Onset between 7 and 12 yr of age; ↑ ICP, bitemporal hemianopia, sexual and growth retardation; growth hormone and gonadotropic deficiency	Begin cortisol replacement prior to surgery; total excision, adjuvant radiotherapy if extensive	Calcification above sella turcica; diabetes insipidus common postoperatively

*Chemotherapy may delay need for radiotherapy, avoiding treatment-related neurotoxicity.

HCG, human chorionic gonadotropin; ↑ ICP, increased intracranial pressure: headache, vomiting (papilledema, III and VI nerve palsies, wide sutures); TB, tuberculosis.

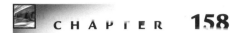

CHAPTER 158

Neuroblastoma

ETIOLOGY

Neuroblastoma is derived from **neural crest cells** that form the adrenal medulla and the sympathetic nervous system. The cause is unknown. Because most cases occur in young children, it is likely that neuroblastoma results from events occurring prenatally and perinatally.

EPIDEMIOLOGY

Neuroblastoma is the most common extracranial solid tumor of childhood and the most common malignancy in infancy. Median age at diagnosis is 20 months. In the U.S., there are approximately 650 new cases of neuroblastoma each year, and the incidence is estimated to be 1 in 7000 live births. The tumor usually occurs sporadically, but in 1% to 2% of cases, there is a positive family history.

CLINICAL MANIFESTATIONS

Neuroblastoma is remarkable for its broad spectrum of clinical prognosis ranging from spontaneous regression to rapid progression and metastasis resulting in death. Children with localized disease are often asymptomatic at diagnosis, whereas children with metastases often appear ill and have systemic complaints, such as fever, weight loss, and pain. The most common presentation is abdominal pain or mass. The mass is often palpated in the flank and is hard, smooth, and nontender. In the abdomen, 45% of tumors arise in the adrenal gland, and 25% arise in the retroperitoneal sympathetic ganglia. Other sites of origin are the paravertebral ganglia of the chest and neck. Paraspinal tumors may invade through the neural foramina and cause spinal cord compression, whereas Horner syndrome sometimes is seen with neck or apical masses. Several **paraneoplastic syndromes**, including secretory diarrhea, profuse sweating, and **opsomyoclonus** ("dancing eyes and dancing feet"), have been associated with neuroblastoma.

Neuroblastoma may metastasize to multiple organs, including the liver, bone, bone marrow, and lymph nodes. If the orbital bones are involved, the patient may present with periorbital ecchymoses. A unique category of neuroblastoma, **stage 4S**, is defined in infants (<1 year old) with a small primary tumor and metastasis limited to skin, liver, or bone marrow. Stage 4S neuroblastoma is associated with a favorable outcome.

LABORATORY AND IMAGING STUDIES

Early studies that may help identify patients with neuroblastoma include complete blood count and plain films. In abdominal neuroblastoma, calcification within the tumor often is observed on plain films of the abdomen. About 90% of neuroblastomas produce **catecholamines (vanillylmandelic acid, homovanillic acid)** that can be detected in increased levels in the urine. Definitive diagnosis of neuroblastoma requires tissue for light microscopic, electron microscopic, or immunohistologic examination. There is an international staging system for neuroblastoma (Table 158–1). Cytogenetic analysis and studies to detect *MYCN* (also known as N-*myc*) amplification provide crucial prognostic information. Diagnostic workup for neuroblastoma involves a CT scan of the chest, abdomen, and pelvis; a bone scan; bilateral bone marrow aspiration and biopsy specimens; and urinary catecholamines. Neuroblastoma cells concentrate metaiodobenzylguanidine (MIBG), a neurotransmitter precursor; MIBG scintigraphy is a sensitive method for detecting metastatic disease.

DIFFERENTIAL DIAGNOSIS

The abdominal presentation of neuroblastoma must be differentiated from Wilms tumor, which also presents as an abdominal flank mass. Ultrasound or CT examination usually is able to differentiate the tumors. Periorbital ecchymoses from orbital metastases sometimes are mistaken for child abuse. Because children with bone marrow involvement may have anemia, thrombocytopenia, or neutropenia, leukemia is often considered in the differential.

TREATMENT

Treatment of neuroblastoma is based on surgical staging and biologic features. Complete surgical excision is the initial treatment of choice for patients with localized neuroblastoma. Children with favorable biology who undergo a gross total resection require no further therapy. In patients with advanced disease, combination chemotherapy usually is given after confirmation of the diagnosis. The most common agents are vincristine, cyclophosphamide, doxorubicin, cisplatin, and etoposide. Delayed resection of the primary tumor is undertaken after numerous courses of chemotherapy. Radiation therapy often is given to the primary tumor bed and areas of metastatic disease. The cure rate for older patients with stage 4 disease had been extremely poor; **high-dose chemotherapy with stem cell rescue** has improved the outcome for some patients. Survival in high-risk patients also has improved with the addition of retinoic acid after maximal reduction of tumor burden with chemotherapy, surgery, and radiation

TABLE 158–1.   International Neuroblastoma Staging System

Stage	Definition	Incidence (%)	Survival at 5 Years[†]
1	Localized tumor with complete gross excision, with or without microscopic residual disease; representative ipsilateral lymph nodes negative for tumor microscopically (nodes attached to and removed with the primary tumor may be positive)	5	≥90%
2A	Localized tumor with incomplete gross excision; representative ipsilateral nonadherent lymph nodes negative for tumor microscopically		
2B	Localized tumor with or without complete gross excision, with ipsilateral nonadherent lymph nodes positive for tumor. Enlarged contralateral lymph nodes must be negative microscopically	10	70%-80%
3	Unresectable unilateral tumor infiltrating across the midline,* with or without regional lymph node involvement; or localized unilateral tumor with contralateral regional lymph node involvement; or midline tumor with bilateral extension by infiltration (resectable) or by lymph node involvement	25	40%-70%
4	Any primary tumor with dissemination to distant lymph nodes; bone, bone marrow, liver, skin, and other organs (except as defined for stage 4S)	60	85%-90% if age at diagnosis is <18 mo 30%-40% if age at diagnosis is >18 mo
4S	Localized primary tumor (as defined for stage 1, 2A, or 2B), with dissemination limited to skin, liver, and bone marrow[‡] (limited to infants <1 yr of age)	5	>80%

*The midline is defined as the vertebral column. Tumors originating on one side and crossing the midline must infiltrate to or beyond the opposite side of the vertebral column.

[†]Survival is influenced by other characteristics such as *MYCN* amplicification. Percentages are approximates.

[‡]Marrow involvement in stage 4S should be minimal (i.e., <10% of total nucleated cells identified as malignant on bone marrow biopsy or on marrow aspirate). More extensive marrow involvement would be considered to be stage 4. The MIBG scan (if performed) should be negative in the marrow.

Modified from Brodeur GM, et al: Revisions of the international criteria for neuroblastoma diagnosis, staging, and response to treatment. J Clin Oncol 11:1466-1477, 1993.

therapy. Retinoic acid induces tumor differentiation in vitro and down-regulates *MYCN* mRNA expression.

COMPLICATIONS

Spinal cord compression from neuroblastoma may cause an irreversible neurologic deficit. Children with opsomyoclonus syndrome may have developmental delay or mental retardation. The aggressive chemotherapy and radiation therapy used to treat high-risk neuroblastoma may result in complications such as ototoxicity, nephrotoxicity, growth problems, and second malignancies.

PROGNOSIS

The age of the patient at presentation of the disease, the stage of the disease, the primary site, the presence or absence of metastasis, cytogenetics, DNA ploidy, amplification of the *MYCN* oncogene (poor prognosis), and histopathology all affect survival. Children with neuroblastoma can be divided into two large groups: children with favorable biology and children with unfavorable biology. Favorable biologic factors are tumor cell differentiation, no amplification of the *MYCN* oncogene, a triploid cytogenetic karyotype, and no loss of genetic material from the short arm of chromosome 1. Patients with favorable biology tend to be younger and often have localized disease. Patients younger than 1 year of age have a better prognosis than older patients, regardless of stage or favorable and unfavorable biologic factors. Older patients with stage 4 disease most commonly have unfavorable biology, and more than 50% relapse as a result of drug-resistant residual disease. Although neuroblastoma represents only 8% of cases of childhood cancer, it is responsible for 15% of cancer deaths in children.

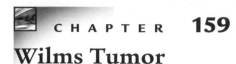

CHAPTER 159

Wilms Tumor

ETIOLOGY

Wilms tumor, also known as nephroblastoma, is thought to arise from primitive, metanephric blastema, the precursor of normal kidney. Although the cause of Wilms tumor is unknown, children with certain congenital anomalies or genetic conditions are at increased risk of developing this cancer.

EPIDEMIOLOGY

Wilms tumor is the most common malignant renal tumor of childhood, with approximately 500 new cases per year in the U.S. The mean age at diagnosis is 3 to 3.5 years of age, and no sex predilection is apparent. A **hereditary** form of Wilms tumor may be associated with bilateral presentation and younger age at onset. Many congenital anomalies are associated with Wilms tumor, including sporadic aniridia, hemihypertrophy, and genitourinary abnormalities (hypospadias, cryptorchidism, horseshoe or fused kidneys, ureteral duplication, and polycystic kidneys). Patients with the **WAGR syndrome** (Wilms tumor, aniridia, genitourinary malformation, and mental retardation) have Wilms tumor as a manifestation of the syndrome itself, resulting from a germline deletion at chromosome 11p. Patients with **Beckwith-Wiedemann syndrome** (hemihypertrophy, omphalocele, macroglossia, Wilms tumor in 3% to 5%) and some other overgrowth syndromes are at increased risk for developing Wilms tumor and should be screened with periodic imaging.

CLINICAL MANIFESTATIONS

Most children with Wilms tumor present with an abdominal mass that is discovered by their parents. Although many children do not have complaints at the time that the mass is first noted, associated symptoms may include abdominal pain, fever, hypertension, and hematuria.

LABORATORY AND IMAGING STUDIES

The first step in diagnosing a potential Wilms tumor is abdominal ultrasound examination, which usually can distinguish an intrarenal mass from a mass in the adrenal gland or other surrounding structures. Evaluation of the inferior vena cava is crucial because tumor may extend from the kidney into the vena cava. Early diagnosis of Wilms tumor may be achieved by ultrasound screening of young children at increased risk for the disease. A complete blood count, urinalysis, liver and renal function studies, and a chest x-ray (to identify pulmonary metastases) should be obtained. In most cases, a CT scan of the chest, abdomen, and pelvis is obtained. The diagnosis is confirmed by histologic examination of the tumor. Although most cases of Wilms tumor are classified as "favorable histology," the presence of anaplasia is predictive of a worse prognosis and is considered "unfavorable." The National Wilms Tumor Study Group has developed a staging system for Wilms tumor (Table 159-1).

DIFFERENTIAL DIAGNOSIS

The differential diagnosis of Wilms tumor includes hydronephrosis and polycystic disease of the kidney; benign renal tumors, such as mesoblastic nephroma and hamartoma; and other malignant tumors, such as renal cell carcinoma, neuroblastoma, lymphoma, and retroperitoneal rhabdomyosarcoma.

TREATMENT

In centers in the U.S., every attempt is made to obtain a complete resection before the initiation of chemotherapy, with or without radiation therapy. In European centers, preoperative chemotherapy is given in an effort to shrink the tumor and make definitive resection easier. In European centers, if a renal tumor has radiographic features of Wilms tumor, no biopsy is performed before initiation of chemotherapy. Patients with no metastases at the time of diagnosis receive vincristine and actinomycin as preoperative therapy; patients with metastases (bone, lung) also receive doxorubicin. The National Wilms Tumor Study Group chemotherapy protocol for Wilms tumor with favorable histology includes vincristine and actinomycin with or without doxorubicin. In patients with stage III or IV disease, the tumor is also treated with radiation therapy. Care must be taken to minimize radiation effects to the liver because radiation hepatotoxicity is potentiated by actinomycin.

Bilateral Wilms tumor is present in about 5% of children on initial presentation, whereas recurrent disease affects the opposite kidney in 4% to 5% of patients. Treatment for each patient with bilateral Wilms tumor should be individualized with a goal of retaining as much functional nephrogenic tissue as possible.

COMPLICATIONS

Patients with bilateral Wilms tumor sometimes are left with inadequate kidney to maintain renal function. Patients who have received irradiation to the abdomen may be short waisted. As women, they may have a small

TABLE 159–1.   National Wilms Tumor Study Group Staging System*

Stage I

The tumor is limited to the kidney and completely excised
The surface of the renal capsule is intact; the tumor is not ruptured before or during removal
No residual tumor is apparent beyond the margins of excision

Stage II

The tumor extends beyond the kidney but is completely excised
Regional extension of the tumor is present (i.e., penetration through the outer surface of the renal capsule into the perirenal soft tissues): vessels outside the kidney substance are infiltrated or contain tumor thrombus; the tumor may have been biopsied or local spillage of tumor confined to the flank has occurred; no residual tumor is apparent at or beyond the margins of excision

Stage III

Residual nonhematogenous tumor confined to the abdomen is present
Any of the following may occur:
  Lymph nodes on biopsy are found to be involved in the hilus, the periaortic chains, or beyond
  Diffuse peritoneal contamination by the tumor has occurred, such as by spillage of tumor beyond the flank before or during surgery, or by tumor growth that has penetrated through the peritoneal surface
  Implants are found on the peritoneal surfaces
  The tumor extends beyond the surgical margins either microscopically or grossly
  The tumor is not completely resectable because of local infiltration into vital structures

Stage IV

Hematogenous metastases; deposits beyond stage III (e.g., lung, liver, bone, and brain)

Stage V

Bilateral renal involvement is seen at diagnosis
An attempt should be made to stage each side according to the above criteria on the basis of extent of disease before biopsy

*The clinical stage is decided by the surgeon in the operating room and is confirmed by the pathologist, who also evaluates the histology. It is done on the basis of gross and microscopic tumor distribution and is the same for tumors with favorable and with unfavorable histologic features. The tumor is characterized, however, by a statement of both criteria (e.g., stage II, favorable histology, or stage II, unfavorable histology).

pelvis and have small infants and an increased requirement for cesarean section. If tumor extends into the renal veins or inferior vena cava, a tumor embolism may cause a life-threatening pulmonary embolism.

PROGNOSIS

The prognosis for patients with Wilms tumor is good. Prognostic factors are tumor stage and tumor histology. Anaplastic variants of Wilms tumor have a significantly poorer outcome than classic Wilms tumor. The 4-year relapse-free survival of patients with tumors of favorable histology is directly related to stage. Cure rates for patients with localized Wilms tumor at diagnosis are greater than 85%, whereas patients with pulmonary metastases have event-free survivals of approximately 70% to 80%.

CHAPTER   160

Sarcomas

ETIOLOGY

Sarcomas are divided into soft tissue sarcomas and bone cancers. Soft tissue sarcomas arise primarily from the connective tissues of the body, such as muscle tissue, fibrous tissue, and adipose tissue. **Rhabdomyosarcoma**, the most common soft tissue sarcoma in children, is derived from mesenchymal cells that are committed to skeletal muscle lineage. Less common nonrhabdomyosarcoma soft tissue sarcomas include fibrosarcoma, synovial sarcoma, and extraosseous **Ewing sarcoma**. The most common malignant bone cancers in children are **osteosarcoma** and Ewing sarcoma. Osteosarcomas derive from primitive bone-forming mesenchymal stem cells, and the Ewing sarcomas are thought to be of neural crest cell origin.

The cause is unknown for most children diagnosed with sarcoma, although a few observations have been made regarding risks. Individuals with **Li-Fraumeni syndrome** (associated with a germline *p53* mutation) and **neurofibromatosis** (associated with *NF1* mutations) are associated with an increased risk of soft tissue sarcomas. There is a 500-fold increased risk for osteosarcoma for individuals with hereditary retinoblastoma. Deletions on the long arm of chromosome 13, which can occur in patients with retinoblastoma, have been found in some patients with osteosarcoma. Li-Fraumeni syndrome and Rothmund-Thomson syndrome are associated with osteosarcoma. Prior treatment for childhood cancer with **radiation therapy** or chemotherapy, specifically alkylating agents, or both increases the risk for osteosarcoma as a second malignancy.

EPIDEMIOLOGY

In the U.S., 850 to 900 children and adolescents younger than 20 years old are diagnosed with soft tissue sarcomas each year, of which approximately 350 are rhabdomyosarcoma. The incidence of rhabdomyosarcoma peaks in children 2 to 6 years old and in adolescents. Two thirds of all cases of rhabdomyosarcoma are diagnosed before 11 years of age. The early peak is associated with tumors in the genitourinary region, head, and neck; the later peak is associated with tumors in the extremities, trunk, and male genitourinary tract. Boys are affected 1.5 times more than girls.

Of the 650 to 700 U.S. children and adolescents younger than 20 years old diagnosed with bone tumors each year, approximately 400 are osteosarcoma and 200 are Ewing sarcoma. Osteosarcoma most commonly affects adolescents, with the peak incidence occurring during the period of maximum growth velocity. The incidence of Ewing sarcoma peaks between ages 10 and 20, but may occur at any age. Ewing sarcoma affects primarily whites; it rarely occurs in African American children or Asian children.

CLINICAL MANIFESTATIONS

The clinical presentation of **rhabdomyosarcoma** varies, depending on the site of origin and subsequent mass effect and presence of metastatic disease. Periorbital swelling, proptosis, and limitation of extraocular motion may be seen with an orbital tumor. Nasal mass, chronic otitis media, ear discharge, dysphagia, neck mass, and cranial nerve involvement may be noted with tumors in other head and neck sites. Urethral or vaginal masses, paratesticular swelling, hematuria, and urinary frequency or retention may be noted with tumors in the genitourinary tract. Trunk or extremity lesions tend to present as rapidly growing masses that may or may not be painful. If there is metastatic disease to bone or bone marrow, limb pain and evidence of marrow failure may be present.

Osteosarcoma often is located at the epiphysis or metaphysis of anatomic sites that are associated with maximum growth velocity (distal femur, proximal tibia, proximal humerus), but any bone may be involved. It presents with pain in a bony site and may be associated with a palpable mass. Because the pain and swelling often are initially thought to be related to trauma, radiographs of the affected region frequently are obtained, which usually reveal a lytic lesion, often associated with calcification in the soft tissue surrounding the lesion. Approximately 75% to 80% of patients with osteosarcoma have apparently localized disease at diagnosis.

Before the availability of chemotherapy, patients with apparently localized osteosarcoma of an extremity were treated with amputation alone. In approximately 80% of these patients, pulmonary metastases developed within 6 months of amputation, indicating that osteosarcoma is characterized by a high incidence of occult micrometastatic disease at diagnosis.

Although **Ewing sarcoma** can occur in almost any bone in the body, the femur and pelvis are the most common sites. In addition to local pain and swelling, clinical manifestations include systemic symptoms, such as fever and weight loss.

LABORATORY AND IMAGING STUDIES

Tissue biopsy is needed for definitive diagnosis of sarcomas. Selection of the biopsy site is important for each patient and has implications for future surgical resection and radiation therapy planning, when indicated. Under the light microscope, rhabdomyosarcoma and Ewing sarcoma appear as **small, round, blue cell tumors**. Osteosarcomas are distinguishable by the presence of **osteoid substance**.

Immunohistochemical staining for muscle-specific proteins, such as actin and myosin, and other muscle-related proteins, such as desmin and vimentin, helps make the diagnosis of rhabdomyosarcoma. Two major histologic variants exist for rhabdomyosarcoma: **embryonal** and **alveolar**. Embryonal histology is most common in younger children with head and neck and genitourinary primary tumors. Alveolar histology occurs in older patients and is seen most commonly in trunk and extremity tumors. Alveolar rhabdomyosarcoma often is characterized by specific translocations: t(2;13) or t(1;13). Metastatic evaluation for patients with rhabdomyosarcoma should include a CT scan of the chest, abdomen, and pelvis; a bone scan; and bone marrow aspiration and biopsy. In patients with a parameningeal primary site (the middle ear, nasopharynx, infratemporal fossa), a lumbar puncture is required.

Definitive diagnosis of osteosarcoma usually is established by carefully placed needle biopsy. The presence of osteoid and immunohistochemical analysis confirms the diagnosis of osteosarcoma. The extent of the primary tumor must be delineated carefully with MRI before starting chemotherapy. Osteosarcoma tends to metastasize to lung (most commonly) and bone; a metastatic evaluation consists of a chest CT scan and a bone scan.

The diagnosis of Ewing sarcoma is established with immunohistochemical analysis and cytogenetic and molecular diagnostic studies of the biopsy material. Ewing sarcoma is characterized by a specific chromosomal translocation, **t(11;22)**, which is seen in 95% of tumors. A variant translocation, t(21;22), is seen in approximately 5% of tumors. MRI of the primary lesion should be performed to delineate extent of the lesion and any associated soft tissue mass. Metastatic evaluation involves a bone scan, chest CT scan, and bone marrow aspiration and biopsy.

DIFFERENTIAL DIAGNOSIS

Patients with Ewing sarcoma often are misdiagnosed as having **osteomyelitis**, whereas children with osteogenic sarcoma often are thought initially to have pain and swelling related to trauma. The differential diagnosis for rhabdomyosarcoma depends on the location of the tumor. Tumors of the trunk and extremities often present as a painless mass and initially may be thought to be benign tumors. Periorbital rhabdomyosarcoma may be misdiagnosed as orbital cellulitis, and other head and neck rhabdomyosarcoma may be confused with chronic infection of ears or sinuses. The differential diagnosis for intra-abdominal rhabdomyosarcoma includes other abdominal malignancies, such as Wilms tumor or neuroblastoma.

TREATMENT

Treatment of rhabdomyosarcoma is based on a staging system that incorporates the primary site and histology. The staging system also involves a local tumor group assessment based on the extent of disease and surgical result. In the intergroup rhabdomyosarcoma studies, the most common chemotherapy agents used are cyclophosphamide, vincristine, and actinomycin. Topotecan and ifosfamide have been studied in the treatment of rhabdomyosarcoma. Radiation is administered to all patients who have residual disease after initial surgery or who have had a biopsy specimen obtained only of the primary tumor.

The treatment of osteosarcoma involves neoadjuvant chemotherapy followed by limb salvage surgery or amputation and further postoperative chemotherapy. Agents effective against osteosarcoma are doxorubicin, high-dose methotrexate, ifosfamide, and platinum drugs (cisplatin, carboplatin).

The treatment for Ewing sarcoma is similar to that for osteosarcoma; preoperative chemotherapy is given, followed by local control measures and further chemotherapy. In contrast to osteosarcoma, Ewing sarcoma is **radiation sensitive**. Chemotherapy includes vincristine, cyclophosphamide, ifosfamide, etoposide, and doxorubicin.

COMPLICATIONS

In addition to the risk of late effects from the chemotherapy, children with sarcomas have potential complications related to local control of the tumor. If the local disease is controlled with surgery, the long-term sequelae may include loss of limb or limitation of function. If local control is accomplished with radiation therapy, the late effects depend on the dose of radiation given, the extent of the site radiated, and the development of the child at the time of radiation therapy. Irradiating tissues interferes with growth and development so that radiation given to a young child can have significant adverse consequences.

PROGNOSIS

For all children with sarcoma, presence or absence of **metastatic disease** at presentation is the most important prognostic factor. The outlook for patients who have distant metastasis from rhabdomyosarcoma, osteosarcoma, or Ewing sarcoma at diagnosis remains quite poor.

Patients with localized rhabdomyosarcomas in favorable sites have an excellent prognosis when treated with surgery followed by vincristine and actinomycin. In patients with osteosarcoma and Ewing sarcoma, another important prognostic factor is the **degree of tumor necrosis** after preoperative chemotherapy. Patients whose tumor specimens show a high degree of necrosis related to the preoperative chemotherapy have an event-free survival rate greater than 80%. Patients who still have large amounts of viable tumor after presurgical chemotherapy have a much worse prognosis. The cure rate for patients with localized osteosarcoma and Ewing sarcoma is approximately 60% to 70%. Patients who have lung metastasis at diagnosis have a cure rate of approximately 30% to 35%. All patients with metastases to other sites have a dismal prognosis.

SUGGESTED READING

Arndt CA, Crist WM: Common musculoskeletal tumors of childhood and adolescence. N Engl J Med 341:342-352, 1999.

Behrman RE, Kliegman RM, Jenson HB (eds): Nelson Textbook of Pediatrics, 17th ed. Philadelphia, WB Saunders, 2004.

Friedman DL, Meadows AT: Late effects of childhood cancer therapy. Pediatr Clin North Am 49:1083-1106, 2002.

Hastings C: The Children's Hospital Oakland Hematology/Oncology Handbook. St Louis, Mosby, 2002.

Lowenberg B, Downing JR, Burnett A: Acute myeloid leukemia. N Engl J Med 341:1051-1062, 1999.

MacDonald TJ, Rood BR, Santi MR, et al: Advances in the diagnosis, molecular genetics, and treatment of pediatric embryonal CNS tumors. Oncologist 8:174-186, 2003.

Nathan DG, Orkin SH, Ginsburg D, Look AT (eds): Nathan and Oski's Hematology of Infancy and Childhood, 6th ed. Philadelphia, WB Saunders, 2003.

Pizzo PA, Poplack DG (eds): Principles and Practice of Pediatric Oncology, 4th ed. Philadelphia, Lippincott Williams & Wilkins, 2002.

Pui CH, Evans WE: Acute lymphoblastic leukemia. N Engl J Med 339:605-615, 1998.

Ries LAG, Eisner MP, Kosary CL, et al (eds): SEER Cancer Statistics Review, 1975-2000. Bethesda, Md, National Cancer Institute. http://seer.cancer.gov/csr/1975_2000.

NEPHROLOGY AND UROLOGY

Karen J. Marcdante

CHAPTER **161**

Assessment

HISTORY

The kidneys maintain body fluid and electrolyte homeostasis and remove metabolic waste products that can be filtered by the glomeruli (see Chapter 32). They have important metabolic (gluconeogenesis) and endocrine functions (vitamin D activation, erythropoietin production). Renal diseases have definable manifestations, but may originate in the kidney or represent a systemic illness (Table 161–1).

A perinatal history is crucial in neonates who present with renal dysfunction. Glomerular filtration begins during the third month of gestation. Fetal urine production contributes to amniotic fluid volume. Renal anomalies are often associated with reduced amniotic fluid volume (oligohydramnios) and rarely with increased amniotic fluid volume (polyhydramnios) (see Chapters 58 and 60).

A history of hypoxia-ischemia increases the risk of compromise from renal vein thrombosis (especially in neonates) or acute tubular necrosis. A detailed family history should be obtained to identify hereditary factors in diseases such as glomerulonephritis, cystic kidney disease, and renal tubular disorders. A history of poor growth may identify children who have underlying renal disease without other overt symptoms.

Fluid balance should be characterized (quantification of intake and output) for evidence of dehydration (see Chapter 33) or renal dysfunction (anuria, oliguria, or polyuria). The presence and quantity of vomiting or diarrhea suggest alterations in fluid status. A history of edema noted on awakening in the morning (as an indicator of protein loss or fluid overload) may be present when edema is not obvious on examination. Questions that delineate the severity of fluid or metabolic imbalance include issues of weight gain (edema) or weight loss (renal insufficiency), respiratory pattern, fatigue or irritability, fever, pallor, and a history of seizures (hypertension, alteration of sodium or calcium levels). The color of the urine may provide clues to underlying glomerular disease, ingestions, or infection.

PHYSICAL EXAMINATION

Many renal diseases are initially asymptomatic and first detected during a routine physical examination. Growth parameters (height and weight) should be measured and plotted. Assessment of hydration status (see Chapter 33) identifies fluid imbalances (dehydration, overhydration). It is important to measure blood pressure because hypertension may be the only sign of underlying renal disease (see Chapter 166). Conversely, orthostatic blood pressure measurements may identify children with intravascular volume depletion. Rashes provide clues to several diseases with renal involvement, including Henoch-Schönlein purpura (purpura) (see Chapter 87), neurofibromatosis (café au lait spots) (see Chapter 186), and systemic lupus erythematosus (malar rash) (see Chapter 90). Preauricular tags and deformities of the external ear sometimes are present in children with congenital renal defects. A careful ophthalmologic examination may detect abnormalities associated with renal disease (keratoconus, aniridia, iridocyclitis, cataracts). A cardiac examination may reveal evidence of volume overload (cardiomegaly), murmurs (cardiac disease, anemia), or a pericardial friction rub (uremia). Rales heard on lung auscultation suggest extravascular fluid from overload or hypoalbuminemia. Palpation and percussion of the abdomen may reveal ascites or masses. Liver enlargement is present in several multisystem diseases (systemic lupus erythematosus, infections, polycystic disease) and in glomerulosclerosis. A distended

TABLE 161–1. Common Manifestations of Renal Disease

	Neonate
Flank mass	Dysplasia, polycystic disease, hydronephrosis, tumor
Hematuria	Asphyxia, malformation, trauma, renal vein thrombosis
Anuria and oliguria	Agenesis, obstruction, asphyxia, vascular thrombosis
	Child and Adolescent
Cola-red colored urine	Hemoglobinuria (hemolysis); myoglobinuria (rhabdomyolysis); pigmenturia (porphyria, urate, beets, drugs); hematuria (glomerulonephritis, Henoch-Schönlein purpura, hypercalciuria)
Gross hematuria	Glomerulonephritis, benign hematuria, trauma, cystitis, tumor, nephrolithiasis
Edema	Nephrotic syndrome, nephritis, acute or chronic renal failure, cardiac or liver disease
Hypertension	Acute glomerulonephritis, acute or chronic renal failure, dysplasia, coarctation of the aorta, renal artery stenosis
Polyuria	Diabetes mellitus, central and nephrogenic diabetes insipidus, hypokalemia, hypercalcemia, psychogenic polydipsia, sickle cell anemia, polyuric renal failure, diuretic abuse
Oliguria	Dehydration, acute tubular necrosis, interstitial nephritis, acute glomerulonephritis, hemolytic uremic syndrome
Urgency	Urinary tract infection, vaginitis, foreign body, hypercalciuria

bladder may be palpated and suggest obstructive causes of renal dysfunction.

RENAL PHYSIOLOGY

Normal renal function depends on intact **glomerular filtration** and **tubular function** (proximal tubule, loop of Henle, and distal tubule). Glomerular filtration and "fine-tuning" of filtrate along the tubules results in **urine formation** (Fig. 161–1). Glomerular filtration results from a net pressure in the glomerulus that favors movement of fluid out of the capillaries. The intraglomerular pressure is regulated by tone of the afferent and efferent arterioles, particularly the latter.

The **proximal tubule** is characterized by isosmotic reabsorption of the glomerular filtrate (see Fig. 161–1). Approximately two thirds of the filtered volume is reabsorbed in the proximal tubule. Solutes, such as glucose and amino acids, are reabsorbed completely. Potassium is reabsorbed nearly completely. Most phosphate is reabsorbed in the proximal tubule. Virtually all of the bicarbonate in the plasma is filtered through the glomerulus; 75% of this is reabsorbed in the proximal tubule. This reabsorption occurs in the presence of a threshold of serum bicarbonate concentration above which the tubule can no longer reabsorb, and bicarbonate is spilled into the urine. When the serum carbon dioxide is less than the threshold, all filtered bicarbonate can be absorbed, and the urine pH is acid. The proximal tubule also secretes compounds, such as organic acids and penicillins.

Further along the tubule, the **loop of Henle** is the site of reabsorption of 25% of sodium chloride that was filtered in the glomerulus (see Fig. 161–1). Active chloride transport is the principal mechanism that "fuels" the countercurrent multiplier and consequently the medullary interstitial hypertonic gradient required for urinary concentration.

The **distal tubule** is composed of the **distal convoluted tubule** and the **collecting ducts**. The distal convoluted tubule is water impermeable and contributes to the dilution of urine by active sodium chloride absorption, driven by a different mechanism than at the loop of Henle. Some of this sodium-potassium exchange (sodium-hydrogen exchange) is regulated by aldosterone. The collecting duct is the primary site of **antidiuretic hormone** activity, which produces a concentrated urine. Active hydrogen ion secretion, which is responsible for the final acidification of the urine, occurs in the collecting duct.

Renal **ammonia** production and intraluminal generation of ammonium (NH_4^+) facilitates hydrogen ion excretion. It is difficult to measure urinary ammonia/ammonium directly, so its presence is inferred by the calculation of the **urinary anion gap**. The principle of electrical neutrality requires equal concentrations of anions and cations. The concentration of chloride, the dominant anion in urine, exceeds the common cations, sodium and potassium. The "gap" largely comprises ammonium. If there is a problem with renal acid excretion or ammonia production, the gap decreases.

There is a developmental aspect to maturation of tubular function, as there is for glomerular function. The maximum **urinary concentrating capacity** in a preterm newborn (approximately 400 mOsm/L) is less than in a full-term newborn (600 to 800 mOsm/L), which is less than in older children and adults (approximately 1200 mOsm/L). Neonates can dilute the urine

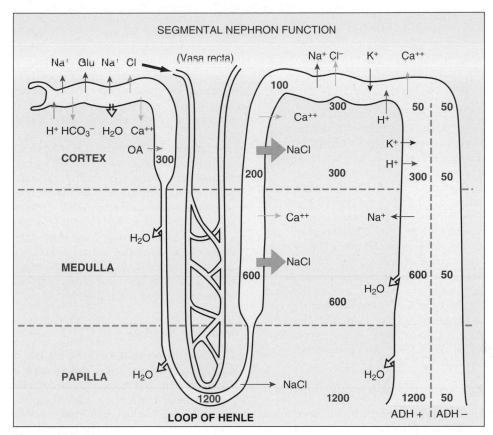

Figure 161–1

Major transport functions of each nephron segment, including representative osmolalities in vasa recta, interstitium, and tubule at different levels within the kidney. ADH, antidiuretic hormone; Glu, glucose; OA, organic acid. (From Andreoli TE, Carpenter CCJ, Plum F, et al [eds]: Cecil Essentials of Medicine. Philadelphia, WB Saunders, 1986.)

to the same degree as adults (75 to 90 mOsm/L), but because the glomerular filtration rate (GFR) is much lower than in adults, the capacity to excrete a water load is quantitatively less. Tubular reabsorption of sodium, potassium, bicarbonate, and phosphate and excretion of hydrogen ions are all reduced in infants relative to adults. Maturation of these functions occurs independently and at different ages, so a neonate rapidly develops the ability to reabsorb sodium, but it takes 2 years for bicarbonate reabsorption to mature.

COMMON MANIFESTATIONS

The wide variety of diseases that affect the kidney can be classified as **primary dysfunction** (diseases originating in the kidney or urinary tract) or **secondary dysfunction** (systemic illnesses that alter renal function) (see Table 161–1). The manifestations of renal disease vary. Primary diseases may present with obvious signs, such as hematuria or edema, or with more subtle signs and symptoms detected on screening examinations (e.g., abdominal or flank mass, hypertension, proteinuria). Fever, irritability, and vomiting may be the presenting symptoms in neonates and infants with **urinary tract infections** (UTIs), whereas frequency and dysuria may be present in older children. Chronic renal disease often is associated with poor growth and feeding difficulties, but may be first detected on screening examinations (hypertension, hematuria). An abnormal urine stream is present in infants with posterior urethral valves and may be present in association with other obstructive lesions.

DIAGNOSTIC TESTS AND IMAGING
Laboratory Studies

The **GFR** is measured most accurately by the infusion of a substance that is freely filtered by the glomerulus but is not metabolized, reabsorbed, or secreted in or by the tubules. The GFR is calculated as follows:

$$GFR = [U]V/[P]$$

where $[U]$ is urine concentration of a substance (mg/dL) used to measure clearance, V is urine flow rate (mL/min), and $[P]$ is serum concentration of the same substance (mg/dL).

By convention, the GFR is corrected to a body surface area of 1.73 m² to allow comparison between people of different sizes. In a full-term newborn, an uncorrected GFR of approximately 4 to 5 mL/min corrects to approximately 40 mL/min/1.73 m². It is easy to compare this value with older children and adults. GFR increases rapidly during the first 2 years of life and achieves adult values (110 to 125 mL/min/1.73 m²) by this age. Subsequently, GFR and body size increase proportionately, and GFR/1.73 m² remains stable.

Creatinine is used to approximate GFR. Plasma creatinine concentration alone is not an adequate measure of renal function because it depends on the size and muscle mass of the child, the state of hydration of the child, and the GFR. To estimate the GFR based on plasma creatinine in a particular child, the correlation between these two values (creatinine and GFR) must be used. The most commonly used formula is:

$$GFR\ (mL/min/1.73\ m^2) = k \times L\ (cm)/P_{Cr}\ (mg/dL)$$

where k is a coefficient derived from the creatinine-length-GFR correlation. The value for k is 0.33 in preterm infants, 0.45 in full-term infants, 0.55 in children and adolescent girls, and 0.7 in adolescent boys. This formula is most useful in infants and children whose body habitus and muscle mass are reasonably normal and whose renal function is relatively stable. **Creatinine clearance** ($[U_{Cr}]V/[P_{Cr}]$) can be used as a rough estimate of glomerular filtration, but often overestimates GFR when renal function is abnormal.

Urinalysis is an easy and useful method of screening for several renal abnormalities. After a visual assessment of the color of the urine, **macroscopic urinalysis** using a urine **dipstick** tests for the presence of protein, blood, and glucose. Protein's ability to bind to the dye used produces a color change. Some low-molecular-weight proteins are unable to bind to the dye, resulting in a false-negative test. Dilute urine also may result in a false-negative result. False-positive tests may occur with extremely alkaline or concentrated urine or if there is a delay in reading the test. Tests for blood are based on the ability of hemoglobin to act as a peroxidase and induce a color change. Dipsticks are exquisitely sensitive to the presence of hemoglobin (or myoglobin) in the urine and yield few, if any, false-negative test results, but many false-positive results. The presence of red blood cells (RBCs) needs to be verified with microscopy for any positive test. Glucosuria is detected using a glucose oxidase-peroxidase reaction.

A **nitrate test** may detect bacteriuria if the bacterium reduces nitrate to nitrite. This reduction requires a relatively long contact time. False-negative results occur with frequent voiding. A low bacterial count may also result in a false-negative test. Gross hematuria or prolonged contact (uncircumcised boys) may result in a false-positive test. The **leukocyte esterase test** detects the presence of white blood cells.

Microscopic urinalysis is used to detect pyuria and verify hematuria (presence of RBCs), casts, and crystals. **Serum creatinine** reflects muscle mass and increases with age. Creatinine is excreted by the kidneys and is often used as a marker of GFR. Creatinine also can be secreted and reabsorbed by renal tubules; this results in a less accurate measure of glomerular filtration, especially in an immature kidney, which shows significant reabsorption of creatinine. **BUN** is also used to estimate renal function, but this test is affected by states of hydration and nutrition.

Imaging Studies

Ultrasound is useful in assessing the urinary tract for anatomic abnormalities. Assessment of kidney presence and size, determination of degree of dilation, and differentiation of cortex and medulla can be accomplished. The bladder also can be visualized. **Pulsed Doppler studies** assess arterial and venous blood flow and can be used to calculate a resistive index within the kidneys.

A **voiding cystourethrogram** (VCUG) involves repeated filling of the bladder to detect vesicoureteral reflux and to evaluate the urethra. An **IV pyelogram** can be used to evaluate kidney structure and function. **CT** and **MRI** have mostly replaced the IV pyelogram.

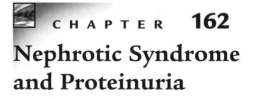

CHAPTER **162**

Nephrotic Syndrome and Proteinuria

ETIOLOGY AND EPIDEMIOLOGY

Proteins and albumin are filtered by the glomerulus. The high concentration of albumin in blood results in albumin appearing in the ultrafiltrate. Most albumin is reabsorbed and catalyzed in the proximal tubule. A small amount of protein is found in the urine of healthy children (<4 mg/m²/hr). **Nephrotic proteinuria** in children is defined as protein greater than 40 mg/m²/hr. Proteinuria between these two levels is abnormal, but not consistent with nephrotic syndrome.

Several mechanisms result in proteinuria. Impaired reabsorption of proteins by the proximal tubule, as seen in **Fanconi syndrome** and drug or heavy metal exposure, may cause significant proteinuria. Factors that increase glomerular permeability also result in proteinuria. These factors include physical damage, abnormal hemodynamics, and hormone-mediated changes.

Nephrotic syndrome is characterized by the presence of heavy **proteinuria** (mainly albuminuria) (>1 g/m^2/24 hr), **hypoproteinemia** (serum albumin <2.5 g/dL), **hypercholesterolemia** (>250 mg/dL), and **edema**. Age, race, and geography affect the incidence of nephrotic syndrome. Certain HLA types (HLA-DR7, HLA-B8, and HLA-B12) are associated with an increased incidence of nephrotic syndrome. The primary disorder is an increase in glomerular permeability to proteins, most likely as a result of the loss of the glomerular basement membrane sialoproteins, which leads to a loss of the normal negative charge. Massive proteinuria results and leads to a decline in serum proteins, especially albumin. Plasma oncotic pressure is diminished, resulting in a shift of fluid from the vascular to the interstitial compartment and a contraction in plasma volume. Renal blood flow and GFR are not usually diminished, and in some instances GFR may be above normal. Edema formation is enhanced by a reduction in effective blood volume and by an increase in tubular sodium chloride reabsorption secondary to activation of the renin-angiotensin-aldosterone system. Most serum lipids (including cholesterol and triglycerides) and levels of lipoprotein are elevated because hypoproteinemia stimulates hepatic lipoprotein synthesis, while lipid metabolism is diminished.

Minimal change nephrotic syndrome (MCNS) is the most common histologic form of nephrotic syndrome, seen in 70% to 80% of cases. Males are affected more frequently than females by a 2:1 ratio. Most children younger than 7 years old with nephrotic syndrome have MCNS. Children 7 to 16 years old with nephrotic syndrome have a 50% chance of having MCNS. A trial of steroid therapy is indicated before biopsy in these older children if the presentation is typical.

The initial presentation of **focal segmental glomerulosclerosis** (FSGS) is usually identical to that of MCNS. FSGS may progress from MCNS or present as a separate entity. A circulating factor that increases glomerular permeability to albumin is found in some patients with FSGS. FSGS accounts for approximately 10% of children with nephrotic syndrome.

Membranous nephropathy is infrequent in childhood. Approximately 1% of children with nephrotic syndrome have this lesion on a kidney biopsy specimen.

It is seen most commonly in adolescents and children with systemic infections, such as hepatitis B, syphilis, malaria, and toxoplasmosis, or receiving drug therapy (gold salts, penicillamine). Hematuria is common.

Congenital nephrotic syndrome is defined as clinical nephrotic syndrome that presents during the first 6 months of life. There are two common types. The Finnish type is an autosomal recessive disorder most common in persons of Scandinavian descent and is due to a mutation in a component protein in the glomerulus filtration slit. The second type is a heterogeneous group of abnormalities including diffuse mesangial sclerosis and conditions associated with drugs or infections. Prenatal diagnosis is suspected if there are elevated levels of maternal alpha-fetoprotein. Secondary forms of nephrotic syndrome may be due to systemic lupus erythematosus and infections (syphilis, hepatitis B).

CLINICAL MANIFESTATIONS

The sudden onset of dependent pitting edema with weight gain or ascites is the most common presentation. Abdominal pain and malaise may be present, especially with significant ascites. Blood pressure is usually normal; circulatory failure rarely develops after a sudden decline in serum albumin levels. Diarrhea (intestinal edema) or respiratory distress (pulmonary edema or pleural effusion) may be present. Typical MCNS is defined as the absence of persistent hematuria, renal insufficiency (elevated BUN and creatinine, oliguria), hypertension, and hypocomplementemia.

DIAGNOSTIC STUDIES

Proteinuria of 1+ or greater on two to three random urine specimens suggests a degree of proteinuria that should be confirmed using a more quantitative method (Table 162–1). The preferred method is a urine protein-to-creatinine ratio on a random sample. The normal ratio generally is less than 0.2 when measured on the first morning specimen.

Most serum lipids (including cholesterol and triglycerides) and levels of lipoprotein are elevated as a result of increased hepatic lipoprotein synthesis and diminished lipid metabolism. In addition to the demonstration of proteinuria, hypercholesterolemia, and hypoalbuminemia, testing may include a serum C3 complement level. A low level of C3 is the most sensitive and specific test that can imply the presence of a lesion other than minimal change disease. If C3 levels are low, a renal biopsy may be indicated before a trial of steroid therapy. Microscopic hematuria may be present (20% of cases), but does not predict response to steroids.

DIFFERENTIAL DIAGNOSIS

Transient proteinuria is seen after vigorous exercise and occasionally in febrile or dehydrated children. The proteinuria usually is mild (protein-to-creatinine ratio <1) and does not indicate renal disease.

Postural (orthostatic) proteinuria is a benign condition defined by normal protein excretion while patients are recumbent, but significant, although moderate, proteinuria when they are upright. "Persistent" proteinuria associated with renal disease has a positional increase during activity, but also is present when recumbent. If proteinuria is persistent, renal disease should be considered.

Glomerular proteinuria is classified by its degree. Intermittent (mild) proteinuria (<0.5 g/m^2/day) is seen in pyelonephritis, renal cystic diseases, obstructive uropathies, and mild glomerulonephritis. Moderate proteinuria (0.5 to 1 g/m^2/day) is seen in acute poststreptococcal glomerulonephritis, mild Henoch-Schönlein nephritis, severe pyelonephritis, chronic glomerulonephritis, and hemolytic uremic syndrome (HUS). Severe proteinuria (>1 g/m^2/day) is characteristically associated with nephrotic syndrome.

TREATMENT

If a child has the typical features of nephrotic syndrome, treatment consists of efforts to reduce edema and therapy with prednisone or equivalent steroids. Because more than 80% of children 1 to 7 years old with typical MCNS respond to corticosteroids, steroid therapy may be undertaken without a renal biopsy. Specific therapy for MCNS is prednisone, 2 mg/kg/day (60 mg/m^2/24 hours) divided into two to four doses per day. Approximately 92% of children who respond to steroids do so within 4 weeks. The optimal duration of steroid therapy for responders is 12 weeks. If a child does not respond to daily prednisone therapy, a renal biopsy is indicated because steroid resistance greatly increases the chance that the underlying pathology is something other than MCNS. Frequent relapses or steroid resistance in MCNS may necessitate immunosuppressive therapy.

No clearly effective therapy for FSGS has been identified yet, although high-dose corticosteroid therapy or immunosuppressive agents or both may produce complete remission in some patients and partial remission in others. More than 80% of patients with FSGS do not respond to corticosteroid therapy.

Aggressive medical therapy of familial congenital nephrotic syndrome, with early nephrectomy, dialysis, and subsequent transplantation, is the only effective approach to this syndrome. Edema due to nephrotic syndrome is treated with restriction of salt intake. Severe edema may require the use of diuretic therapy. Aggressive efforts with diuretics may lead to profound hypovolemia, however. Occasionally, even adding diuretic therapy to salt and water restriction is ineffective in alleviating severe edema. In these situations, cautious parenteral administration of 25% albumin (0.5 g/kg intravenously over 1 to 2 hours) with an IV loop diuretic (furosemide) given during or immediately after albumin usually results in diuresis. The albumin is excreted rapidly, in light of the proteinuria. Effusions may require drainage.

Acute hypertension is treated with β-blockers or calcium channel blockers. Persistent hypertension is often responsive to angiotensin-converting enzyme inhibitors.

COMPLICATIONS

Infection is a major complication in children with the nephrotic syndrome of any type (Table 162–2). **Bacteremia** and **peritonitis** may occur, particularly with *Streptococcus pneumoniae* or *Escherichia coli*. A high index of suspicion and prompt evaluation and antibiotic treatment are indicated in a febrile patient. Side effects of steroids are most common in initial nonresponders and frequently relapsing patients. Hypovolemia may be the result of diarrhea or use of diuretics. The loss of proteins may lead to a hypercoagulable state with a risk of thromboembolism. Warfarin, low-dose aspirin, and dipyridamole all have been used to minimize the risk of clots.

PROGNOSIS

Most children with nephrotic syndrome eventually go into remission. Nearly 80% of children with MCNS experience a relapse of the proteinuria at some point, defined as heavy proteinuria that persists for 3 to 5

TABLE 162–2.	Complications of Nephrotic Syndrome

Spontaneous bacterial peritonitis
Bacteremia
Steroid-related toxicity
Immunosuppression-related toxicity
Acute renal failure
Hypertension
Hypercoagulable state (renal vein thrombosis, pulmonary embolism)

consecutive days. Transient (1 to 2 days) proteinuria may occur with an intercurrent infection in children with MCNS and is not considered a relapse. Steroid therapy usually is rapidly effective for a true relapse. Patients with MCNS who respond to steroid therapy have little risk of chronic renal failure.

Patients with FSGS may be initially responsive to steroids, but become late nonresponders. Many children with FSGS progress to end-stage kidney failure (see Chapter 165). Recurrence of FSGS occurs in 30% of children who undergo renal transplantation.

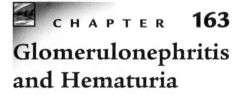

CHAPTER 163

Glomerulonephritis and Hematuria

ETIOLOGY AND EPIDEMIOLOGY

A child with **gross hematuria** requires prompt evaluation. After obtaining a careful history and performing a physical examination, a urinalysis assists with determining the etiology. *Red urine with no blood on a dipstick* implies that the child has ingested foods, medications, or chemicals that led to the color change. In infants, urate crystals, which are orange-red, can be seen on diapers. *Red urine, blood on dipstick, but no blood on microscopy* (when the urine is promptly examined) suggests the presence of free hemoglobin or myoglobin. **Hemoglobinuria** may result from acute intravascular hemolysis, disseminated intravascular coagulation, or any other cause of hemolysis (see Chapter 150). Myoglobin reacts with the "blood-determining" portion of the dipstick and causes a positive result. **Myoglobinuria** results from rhabdomyolysis secondary to crush injury, burns, myositis, or asphyxia (see Chapter 182). *Red urine, blood on dipstick and microscopy, but no RBC casts* suggests urinary tract bleeding from a site beyond the

renal tubules. Examining the morphology of the urinary RBCs is another mechanism for localizing hematuria. Altered RBC morphology is seen in glomerular hematuria (most renal parenchymal disease). The absence of casts or normal RBC morphology does not exclude a glomerular etiology, however. *Red urine, blood on dipstick and microscopy, with RBC casts* suggests one of a variety of glomerular diseases. Glomerular injury may be the result of **immunologic injury** (poststreptococcal acute glomerulonephritis, [PSAGN], **inherited disease** (Alport syndrome), or **vascular injury** (acute tubular or cortical necrosis). Children who have hematuria, with casts and proteinuria less than 1 g/m²/day, are considered to have **nephritis**.

Immune-mediated inflammation is the mechanism for proliferative glomerulonephritis, of which PSAGN is the most common form. PSAGN usually follows a streptococcal pharyngitis or impetigo. An immunologic reaction to the bacteria, mediated by activation of complement, leads to a proliferative glomerulonephritis. Age, gender, socioeconomic status, and genetic predisposition affect the incidence of PSAGN. It occurs most frequently in children 2 to 12 years old. Boys are more frequently affected. Crowded conditions, poor hygiene, malnutrition, and intestinal parasites may result in epidemic outbreaks.

CLINICAL MANIFESTATIONS

PSAGN is associated with hematuria (gross in 65% of cases), edema (75% of cases), and hypertension (50% of cases). Acute renal insufficiency also can occur. Manifestations develop 5 to 21 days (10 days on average) after nephritogenic streptococcal infections (pharyngitis or impetigo). Edema and tea-colored or cola-colored urine are the most common clinical presentations. The GFR is reduced, and distal sodium reabsorption is enhanced, elevating plasma volume and suppressing plasma renin. Renal insufficiency and consequent oliguria and hypertension may lead to complications such as heart failure and encephalopathy. The diagnosis of PSAGN is based on the findings of hematuria with proteinuria, edema, and hypertension.

A **UTI** is the most common identifiable diagnosis made in a child with gross hematuria. Blood without casts is also seen with the hematuria associated with **sickle cell trait** or **disease**, after strenuous **exercise** (in some children), and after renal **trauma**. Coagulopathies can present at times with hematuria. **Hypercalciuria** is an important cause of isolated hematuria in children; 25% to 30% of children with isolated hematuria have elevated urinary calcium excretion. **Urolithiasis** is a cause of painful hematuria. Although believed to be rare in children, urinary tract stones do occur and are often secondary to an identifiable metabolic predisposition or areas of urine stasis or both.

Structural abnormalities of the urinary tract must be considered in patients with gross hematuria. Malignant tumors (Wilms tumor in the kidney, rhabdomyosarcoma in the bladder or prostate) must be considered. Obstruction, cystic disease, and trauma may be accompanied by hematuria.

Microscopic hematuria may be due to well-defined renal parenchymal disorders. **IgA nephropathy** often presents with microscopic hematuria or recurrent gross hematuria shortly after an upper respiratory infection (1 to 2 days). The course of IgA nephropathy is generally benign, but may be associated with recurrent bouts of hematuria after or during respiratory infections. It presents more frequently in boys and in the teens and 20s. Although the prognosis is good in children, progressive renal insufficiency and end-stage renal disease (ESRD) develop in about 25% of adults, particularly patients with proteinuria. No effective therapy has been identified.

Benign familial hematuria is a common, nonprogressive, usually autosomal dominant disorder, often accompanied by thinning of the glomerular basement membrane on electron microscopy. Other family members also have hematuria. **Alport syndrome** initially may cause asymptomatic microscopic hematuria early in life. This genetic disorder has several patterns of inheritance and several mutated genes. It is associated with progressive high-tone bilateral **neurosensory deafness** and progressive renal failure during adolescence and young adulthood, particularly in males. Children with nonfamilial or the non-Alport form of idiopathic familial hematuria have an excellent renal prognosis, but long-term follow-up is required to exclude the progressive forms of familial hematuria.

Rapidly progressive glomerulonephritis (RPGN) is a clinical syndrome of rapidly progressing disease, with a rapid deterioration of kidney function. Signs and symptoms of RPGN include edema, gross hematuria, hypertension, and renal failure. Renal biopsy shows epithelial proliferation typically with **crescent** formation. RPGN is more common in late childhood and adolescence. It may be idiopathic or seen in various conditions, including membranoproliferative glomerulonephritis, PSAGN, IgA nephropathy, antineutrophilic cytoplasmic antibody–induced vasculitis, and Henoch-Schönlein purpura. Therapy depends on the underlying disease and usually involves high-dose corticosteroids. **Acute postinfectious glomerulonephritis** occasionally follows other bacterial and viral infections.

In a child with microscopic hematuria and heavy proteinuria (>40 mg/m²/hr), the proteinuria has reached the level consistent with nephrotic syndrome, and the workup should proceed accordingly (see Chapter 162). Any of the glomerulonephritis conditions described earlier can present with a predominantly nephrotic picture.

LABORATORY AND IMAGING STUDIES

Blood in the urine can present as gross hematuria or microscopic hematuria. Given the sensitivity of a urine dipstick evaluation, a positive result requires microscopic examination. Microscopic hematuria is defined as greater than 3 to 5 RBCs per high-power field in freshly voided and centrifuged urine. The minimal screening evaluation for hematuria is summarized in Table 163–1.

Ultrasound, CT, and rarely IV pyelography of the urinary tract are the most common imaging modalities used in the evaluation of hematuria. Laboratory studies in **PSAGN** reveal hematuria, mild to moderate proteinuria, concentrated urine, and the presence of casts, particularly granular and RBC casts. The BUN and serum creatinine may be transiently elevated as a result of a decreased GFR. Previous streptococcal infection should be documented by the presence of elevated titers of antistreptococcal antibodies in the serum. A reduced serum C3 level shows complement activation, which also is revealed by immunofluorescence on a kidney biopsy specimen (rarely indicated because the clinical picture is often so classic). The C3 returns to normal by 6 to 8 weeks. Hypocomplementemia persisting beyond 8 weeks suggests another condition, most likely mesangiocapillary (also called membranoproliferative) glomerulonephritis. Serum IgG and IgM are usually elevated.

IgA nephropathy is associated with normal complement levels. IgA levels are increased in less than 20% of children with the disease. Urinalysis may reveal micro-

TABLE 163–1. **Basic Workup of a Child with Hematuria**	
History	Present, past, and family
Physical examination	Height, weight, blood pressure, optic fundi, presence or absence of abdominal mass, skin appearance, genitalia, edema, complete physical examination
Laboratory	Urinalysis (including microscopic examination and RBC morphology), urine culture; complete blood count (including platelets); serum electrolytes; creatinine; calcium; streptozyme; serum complement (C3); random urine for total protein, calcium, and creatinine; renal imaging studies

RBC, red blood cell.

scopic hematuria or proteinuria or both. Macroscopic hematuria is seen most often with concurrent infections.

Asymptomatic microscopic hematuria is rarely due to a renal glomerular disorder for which therapies have been identified. Most pediatric nephrologists do not obtain diagnostic kidney biopsy specimens from children with isolated microscopic hematuria.

THERAPY

Specific therapy for PSAGN involves dietary sodium restriction, diuretics, and antihypertensive agents. Proteinuria and edema characteristically decline fairly rapidly (in 5 to 10 days), along with the gross hematuria and renal insufficiency. Microscopic hematuria may persist for months or occasionally years; nonetheless, greater than 95% of children recover completely. Therapy for children with IgA nephropathy is uncertain. Adults have been treated with angiotensin-converting enzyme inhibitors and high-dose IV methylprednisolone; these drugs delay the development of renal failure.

PROGNOSIS AND PREVENTION

PSAGN is a relatively benign disease in children. Complete remission is common, although hypertension and gross hematuria may last for several weeks, and proteinuria may last for several months. Treating the streptococcal infection does not prevent PSAGN. Few children progress to ESRD.

IgA nephropathy results in a variable rate of chronic renal failure. Persistent, heavy proteinuria is a poor prognostic factor in children and adults. Persistent hypertension, reduced GFR at presentation (in adults), and severe glomerular lesions on biopsy specimens also have been associated with poor outcomes. Recurrence of IgA deposits in transplanted kidneys is often observed, but does not alter graft survival significantly. The prognosis for renal recovery in RPGN is uncertain.

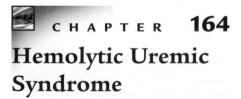

CHAPTER 164
Hemolytic Uremic Syndrome

ETIOLOGY AND EPIDEMIOLOGY

HUS is characterized by a **microangiopathic hemolytic anemia**, **renal cortical injury**, and **thrombocytopenia**. HUS is an important cause of acute renal failure (ARF) in children (see Chapter 165). HUS may be sporadic, epidemic, or endemic. The disease typically occurs in children between the ages of 6 months and 4 years. Verotoxins have been implicated as a major etiology, especially the Shiga-like toxin from *E. coli* O157:H7, which causes the classic prodrome of hemorrhagic enterocolitis. The verotoxin binds to a specific receptor on endothelial cells, producing endothelial swelling. Contamination of meat, fruit, vegetables, and water with verotoxin-producing *E. coli* is responsible for many outbreaks.

HUS presenting without a prodrome of diarrhea may occur at any age and may have a genetic component (often autosomal recessive). Rare familial forms of HUS have been associated with complement factor H, plasminogen-activator inhibitor-1, and other factors involved in the regulation of intravascular clotting and anticoagulation.

CLINICAL MANIFESTATIONS

The classic diarrhea-positive syndrome begins as gastroenteritis, often bloody, followed in 7 to 10 days by weakness, lethargy, irritability, and oliguria or anuria. Physical examination reveals pallor, edema, petechiae, occasionally hepatosplenomegaly, and irritability. The state of hydration varies from normal to dehydration or volume overload. Hypertension may be due to volume overload, or it may be renin mediated. The diagnosis is supported by the presence of microangiopathic hemolytic anemia, thrombocytopenia, and ARF. Seizures may indicate CNS involvement and occur in 20% of cases. Seizures, hemolytic anemia, and thrombocytopenia also suggest a diagnosis of **thrombotic thrombocytopenic purpura**.

LABORATORY STUDIES

Peripheral blood smear reveals schistocytes, helmet and burr cells, and fragmented erythrocytes, all **signs of intravascular hemolysis**. Evidence for disseminated intravascular coagulation is rarely present. The reticulocyte count is elevated, and plasma haptoglobin levels are diminished. Coombs test is negative. Leukocytosis is common. If the child is not anuric, a urinalysis shows microscopic hematuria, proteinuria, and casts. Stool specimens can be cultured, and strains can be serotyped. Diarrhea and excretion of toxin-producing *E. coli* may have ceased by the time the diagnosis of HUS is made.

TREATMENT AND PROGNOSIS

Therapy is supportive with dialysis, control of hypertension, and transfusion of blood products. Antibiotics for the prodromal diarrhea state may result in an increased risk of HUS. Antidiarrheal agents prolong exposure and should be avoided. Most children (approximately 90%) survive the acute phase; more than 50% recover normal renal function. Toxin-induced disease has the best prognosis, whereas familial cases, HUS without diarrhea, and sporadic HUS have poorer outcomes.

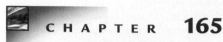

CHAPTER **165**

Acute and Chronic Renal Failure

ACUTE RENAL FAILURE

Etiology and Pathophysiology

ARF is defined as an abrupt and significant decrease in GFR or in tubular function. This is generally associated with a GFR that is reduced sufficiently so that waste products (urea, phosphate) and water cannot be excreted, and body fluid homeostasis is altered. Urine output may be low, normal, or high. Early recognition and management are crucial.

ARF often is subdivided into two forms: **oliguric renal failure** (<1 mL/kg/hr in neonates and infants, <0.5 mL/kg/hr in others) and **nonoliguric renal failure**. Because urine output is maintained in the nonoliguric variant, it can be overlooked easily, but it can be complicated by fluid and electrolyte disturbances, in addition to azotemia. Urinary osmolality is typically similar to serum osmolality in such patients.

The major causes of acute renal insufficiency are listed in Table 165-1. The etiologies are often divided into **prerenal** causes, characterized by renal underperfusion; **intrinsic renal** causes, from vascular, immunologic, ischemic, or toxic injury to the kidney; and **postrenal** causes, which typically relate to urinary tract obstruction. This classification is best applied to the differential diagnosis of oliguric states. If a patient has an acutely elevated serum creatinine and has never had a period of oliguria, the likelihood of a prerenal cause for kidney dysfunction is low. Additionally the categories have few clear boundaries. If a child has renal underperfusion (prerenal) or obstruction (postrenal) for an extended period, there is a high probability of intrinsic renal disease being present.

Acute tubular necrosis is the most common cause of ARF in children and is usually the consequence of renal underperfusion. The hypotensive ischemia (or hypoxia) resulting from poor perfusion is related to early vasoconstriction leading to tubular injury. Toxic injury secondary to drugs, exogenous toxins (ethylene glycol, methanol), or endogenous toxins (myoglobin, hemoglobin) also may result in acute tubular necrosis.

TABLE 165–1. Causes of Acute Renal Failure

Prerenal, Hypovolemic, Hypotension

Dehydration
Septic shock
Heart failure
Hemorrhage
Burns
Peritonitis, ascites, cirrhosis

Postrenal (Obstruction)

Urethral obstruction
  Stricture
  Posterior urethral valves
  Diverticulum
Ureteral obstruction
  Calculi/crystals
  Clot
Ureterocele
Extrinsic tumor compressing bladder outlet
Extrinsic urinary tract tumors
Neurogenic bladder
Tumor lysis syndrome

Intrinsic

Acute tubular necrosis
  Nephrotoxins (drugs)
Acute cortical necrosis
Glomerulonephritis
Interstitial nephritis
Vascular
  Renal vein thrombosis
  Arterial thromboemboli (umbilical artery catheter)
  Disseminated intravascular coagulation
  Immune-mediated (scleroderma)
Pigmenturia
  Hemoglobinuria
  Myoglobinuria

Severe vascular compromise may lead to arterial or venous thrombosis with **acute cortical necrosis**. Acute tubular necrosis is commonly reversible, but acute cortical necrosis represents tissue death; there is usually permanent loss of renal function.

Clinical Manifestations

History, physical examination, and laboratory data are helpful in evaluating a child with ARF (Table 165-2). A precipitating illness associated with vomiting and diarrhea and an inadequate oral intake resulting in hypotension and oliguria are consistent with prerenal causes. Postrenal causes are not associated with hypoperfusion. Urine output can be low, normal, or high. The physical examination may show signs of dehydration (see Chapter 33).

TABLE 165–2.   Laboratory Differential Diagnosis of Renal Insufficiency

	Prerenal		Renal		Postrenal
	Child	Neonate	Child	Neonate	
Urine Na$^+$ (mEq/L)	<20	<20-30	>40	>40	Variable, may be >40
FE$_{Na}$* (%)	<1	<2-5	>2	>2-5	Variable, may be >2
Urine osmolality (mOsm/L)	>500	>300-500	~300	~300	Variable, may be <300
Serum BUN-to-creatinine ratio	>20	≥10	~10	≥10	Variable, may be >20
Urinalysis	Normal		RBCs, WBCs, casts, proteinuria		Variable to normal, possible crystals
Comments	History: diarrhea, vomiting, hemorrhage, diuretics Physical: volume depletion		History: hypotension, anoxia, exposure to nephrotoxins Physical: hypertension, edema		History: poor urine stream and output Physical: flank mass, distended bladder

*FE$_{Na}$, Fractional excretion of sodium (%) = [(urine sodium/plasma sodium) ÷ (urine creatinine/plasma creatinine)] × 100.
RBCs, red blood cells; WBCs, white blood cells.

Flank masses or a distended bladder may be present on examination in obstructive causes; evidence of dehydration is absent. Intrinsic renal failure can be associated with hypertension, cardiac enlargement, or a gallop rhythm, which would suggest volume overload. Urine output characteristically is decreased. Signs of systemic involvement from underlying disease may be noted (systemic lupus erythematosus, Henoch-Schönlein purpura, HUS). Urinalysis usually reveals RBC and granular casts, with mild to moderate proteinuria.

Laboratory Studies and Imaging

To differentiate between prerenal azotemia (where the kidneys are appropriately responding to poor perfusion by maximizing water and salt reabsorption in an effort to increase or maintain vascular volume to enhance perfusion) and intrinsic renal disease with oliguria, the **fractional excretion of sodium** (FE$_{Na}$) was developed. The FE$_{Na}$ is the percent of sodium filtered by the glomeruli that is reabsorbed by the tubules. The FE$_{Na}$ is calculated as follows:

$$[U/P\ Na \div U/P\ creatinine] \times 100$$

where *U* and *P* are the urine and plasma concentrations. Values less than 1% are consistent with prerenal azotemia. Values that exceed 3% are consistent with tubular and intrinsic renal dysfunction. The ratio of serum **BUN** and **creatinine** may also provide some evidence of the type of renal failure.

Urinalysis may identify hematuria, proteinuria, or casts, which direct further studies into the etiology of renal failure. Complement levels and evidence of prior infection also may assist in determining the etiology.

Hyperkalemia can be seen in patients with ARF as a result of increased catabolism and the absence of potassium excretion; it requires immediate attention. **Acidosis** is due to catabolism and the impaired secretion of hydrogen ions. **Hypocalcemia** in ARF is often accompanied by **hyperphosphatemia**.

Ultrasound imaging may reveal increased echogenicity in children with acute tubular necrosis; it may show a loss of corticomedullary differentiation when cortical necrosis is present. Enlarged kidneys are seen when nephritis is the underlying cause of renal failure. Radiologic studies (ultrasound, VCUG, CT, nuclear imaging) are often helpful to determine the cause of obstruction if it is the suspected cause of renal failure.

Renal biopsy, usually performed percutaneously, may be indicated if the presentation is atypical, to assess the severity of systemic disease involvement (systemic lupus erythematosus), guide therapy, or establish a prognosis. Light microscopy should be augmented by special studies (immunofluorescence and electron microscopy).

Treatment

Therapies depend on the cause of acute renal insufficiency, but there are some fundamental steps that apply to all conditions. Determination of fluid balance requires careful assessment of intake and output and should be augmented with measuring weight (at least every 12 hours in severely ill children). Initial fluid and electrolyte therapy is based on providing water to equal insensible losses and water and electrolytes to replace other ongoing losses. If hypovolemia is present, intravascular volume should be expanded by IV administration of physiologic saline (0.9% sodium chloride); 10 mL/kg is usually given intravenously over 30 to 60 minutes. If hypervolemia is present, 2 mg/kg of furosemide, or an equal dose of other loop diuretics, may be attempted. Severe fluid overload in the presence of marked oliguria or anuria is one indication for **dialysis**. Urine output and serum and urine electrolytes levels should be determined frequently during the acute phase.

Foods, fluids, and medications that contain potassium should be restricted until renal function is re-established, the potassium has been brought into the normal range, or dialysis has been initiated. The major risk of hyperkalemia is arrhythmia. An ECG is necessary to identify these rhythm changes (see Chapter 142). Although sodium bicarbonate counteracts acidosis, its administration engenders a risk of fluid overload, hypernatremia, and hypertension.

Treatment of hypocalcemia and hyperphosphatemia primarily involves efforts to lower the serum phosphorus level. Dietary phosphorus restriction and the administration of phosphate binders, calcium acetate, and calcium carbonate are the first therapeutic steps. Symptomatic hypocalcemia can be treated with parenteral calcium, but it must be given cautiously because it may precipitate in the body with circulating phosphorus.

In children with ARF, **dialysis** is indicated to treat three major conditions: (1) hypervolemia unresponsive to fluid restriction or to diuretics, (2) major electrolyte abnormalities unresponsive to medical therapy (hyperkalemia, acidosis) and (3) signs of "uremia." Potential renal replacement therapies in children for ARF include peritoneal dialysis, hemodialysis, and the variations of continuous renal replacement therapy, such as continuous hemofiltration and hemodialysis or continuous venovenous hemodiafiltration. When available, careful monitoring of blood levels of drugs excreted by the kidney and appropriate adjustment of either the total dose or dosage intervals are necessary to prevent complications or further renal injury.

Prognosis

Recovery from an episode of ARF depends on the etiology, the availability of specific treatments for the etiology, and other aspects of the patient's clinical course. Sepsis is a major morbid complication of ARF.

CHRONIC KIDNEY DISEASE
Etiology and Epidemiology

The etiologies of chronic renal disease in childhood relate to the age of the child at the time the kidney disease occurs. Congenital and obstructive abnormalities are the most common causes between birth and 10 years of age. After age 10, acquired diseases, such as FSGS and chronic glomerulonephritis, become more prevalent. The progression to end-stage kidney failure varies. The pubertal growth spurt increases demand on the damaged kidneys, and children often present during late puberty.

Clinical Manifestations

Growth failure in children with chronic renal failure is prominent. The factors associated with growth retardation include undernutrition, osteodystrophy, hormonal abnormalities, medications (steroids), and acidosis. Increased calorie intake leads to a slight increase in growth in some children. Children with chronic renal disease can also have progressive anemia and exhibit severe osteodystrophy. **Renal osteodystrophy** is common in children with chronic renal failure. It is associated with hyperphosphatemia, high serum alkaline phosphatase levels, secondary hyperparathyroidism, and low levels of 1,25-dihydroxyvitamin D. **Anemia** results primarily from a failure of the kidney to produce adequate **erythropoietin** in response to anemia and an impaired response to erythropoietin because of the uremia. Hypertension also may be present.

Treatment

The management of children with chronic renal failure and their complex problems requires a team of pediatric nephrologists, clinical nursing specialists, nutritionists, social workers, psychiatrists, psychologists, child life and occupational therapists, and various other professionals. Children with advanced kidney disease often have **diminished growth** velocity and progressive retardation of bone age before puberty. Undernutrition is a concern, given the poor oral intake common in children with chronic renal disease. With a very low GFR, maintenance dialysis allows protein intake slightly above the recommended daily allowance. Recombinant-produced growth hormone is useful in children with chronic renal failure on or off dialysis. Growth acceleration occurs with pharmacologic doses of human growth hormone. Growth hormone should be used when adequate caloric intake has been established and when treatment of acidosis and osteodystrophy have been undertaken.

In infants, a low-solute formula, used in conjunction with a phosphate binder, may be indicated.

Phosphorus restriction limits dairy and calcium intake; supplemental calcium may be necessary.

When acidosis develops, sodium bicarbonate or sodium citrate is indicated. Unless a child is chronically oliguric, fluid restriction is rarely warranted. Sodium intake depends on the etiology of the renal disease. Many children with congenital renal dysplasias waste sodium in their urine and require supplemental salt. Conversely, children with glomerulonephritis become hypertensive or edematous or both if given excess salt. High-potassium foods should be avoided when renal failure is established.

The initial therapy for **renal osteodystrophy** is to restrict phosphate in the diet. Oral phosphate binders should be initiated. Mildly elevated parathyroid hormone levels are acceptable because tight control of parathyroid hormone has led to a condition known as adynamic bone disease. When the serum phosphorus is under control, therapy with either 1-hydroxylated vitamin D or its analogues is indicated.

Recombinant-produced erythropoietin has resolved much of the anemia formerly seen in chronic renal failure. Erythropoietin rapidly drains adequate iron stores, however, and parenteral iron supplementation is often needed.

The optimal treatment of ESRD is **renal transplantation**. Optimizing medical management of the child and identifying potential live donors should occur before decompensated ESRD forces emergent delivery of renal replacement therapy. Cadaver and living donors have been used extensively for renal transplantation. Live donor transplantation has several advantages and is often the first choice when available. Living donors can be scheduled at the convenience of the donor and the recipient. Additionally, there is slightly improved function in level of GFR and life of the transplanted kidney with live donor kidneys compared with deceased donor kidneys. Children with ESRD should be referred for evaluation to a pediatric renal transplant center.

Maintenance dialysis is effective for a child who is awaiting renal transplantation or in whom renal transplantation is not possible. The development of long-term **peritoneal dialysis** has simplified the delivery of dialysis therapies to even small infants, and it is the most common form of maintenance dialysis prescribed for children by pediatric nephrologists. **Hemodialysis** is used more often for older and larger children, when intravascular access is less of an issue. Infants and children with ESRD have a good prognosis, given the efficacy of dialysis and transplantation.

Prognosis

Kidney transplants have an excellent success rate. More than 93% of transplants of any type (living or deceased donor) are functioning 1 year post-transplant; 50% are still functioning 19 years later. Lifelong immunosuppressive medications are necessary. The major complications of kidney transplant relate to side effects of these medications and include infections and increased risk of malignancy, in particular, a virus-mediated (mostly Epstein-Barr virus) lymphoproliferative disorder that mimics malignant lymphoma. With a high level of suspicion, these conditions usually can be recognized and treated successfully.

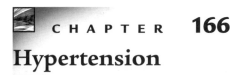

CHAPTER 166

Hypertension

ETIOLOGY

Systolic and diastolic blood pressures normally increase gradually between 1 and 18 years of age. In children, hypertension is a statistical diagnosis, defined as a blood pressure greater than the 95th percentile for age, gender, and height. In adults, hypertension is a risk-defined diagnosis, in which the risk for sequelae of the hypertension increases as blood pressure increases. Hypertension in children is either **primary** ("essential") or most often **secondary**. The secondary causes of hypertension depend on the child's age and other associated features. Hypertension in children may be the result of renal, endocrine, vascular, or neurologic disorders (Table 166–1); drugs or foods (sympathomimetics such as ephedra or pseudoephedrine, or steroids); or skeletal traction. Obese children are more likely to develop essential hypertension than nonobese children.

CLINICAL MANIFESTATIONS

Most children with hypertension have no symptoms; the only way to establish the diagnosis of hypertension is to measure the blood pressure. Blood pressure measurement should be done for all children older than 3 years of age at every medical care encounter. Cuff size selection is crucial in children (see Chapter 139). The history should include a neonatal history (low birth weight or use of umbilical artery catheter); family history of hypertension, stroke, or heart attacks; and dietary history (excessive salt or caffeine, over-the-counter and prescription drugs). Signs and symptoms associated with hypertension are heart failure, stroke, encephalopathy (seizures, headache, coma), polyuria, oliguria, and retinopathy (blurred vision). Additional physical findings include papilledema, abdominal

TABLE 166–1. Causes of Hypertension
Renal Causes
Congenital anomalies
Dysplastic kidney
Polycystic kidney
Obstructive uropathy
Acquired Lesions
Wilms tumor
Glomerulonephritis
Hemolytic uremic syndrome
Reflux nephropathy
Drugs, toxins
Systemic lupus erythematosus
Endocrine Causes
Catecholamine-secreting tumors
Adrenogenital syndrome (11-hydroxylase deficiency)
Cushing syndrome
Hyperaldosteronism
Hyperthyroidism
Diabetic nephropathy
Liddle syndrome (pseudohyperaldosteronism)
Vascular Causes
Coarctation of the aorta
Renal artery embolism
Renal vein thrombosis
Renal artery stenosis
Arteritis (Takayasu, periarteritis nodosa)
Neurologic Causes
Guillain-Barré syndrome
Dysautonomia (Riley-Day syndrome)
Increased intracranial pressure
Quadriplegia
Stress, anxiety
Sympathomimetic drugs
Poliomyelitis
Encephalitis
Neurofibromatosis

LABORATORY STUDIES AND IMAGING

The evaluation of children with hypertension, after several blood pressure measurements have verified its presence, includes (1) assessment for target organ damage (echocardiogram identifies left ventricular hypertrophy), (2) etiologic assessment (urinary catecholamines and metanephrines for a pheochromocytoma, imaging to evaluate for renal artery stenosis), and (3) assessment for the presence of other cardiovascular risk factors, such as hypercholesterolemia. **Renal disease** is the most common cause of hypertension in children; a urinalysis should be performed. A chest radiograph and ECG also should be considered. Initial studies include serum BUN, creatinine, electrolytes, and acid-base balance. A serum uric acid may be elevated in children with essential hypertension. The history, physical examination, mode of presentation, initial laboratory results, and age determine subsequent tests.

TREATMENT

When a diagnosis of hypertension has been established, and it has been determined that there is no curable etiology (e.g., coarctation of the aorta), therapy can be contemplated. For mild hypertension without target organ damage and systemic diseases or other risk factors, therapeutic lifestyle changes (diet, exercise) can be initiated. For moderate to severe hypertension, treatment often begins as the workup is under way. Diuretic therapy may be considered. Calcium channel blockage, angiotensin-converting enzyme inhibitors, β-blockers, or combined α/β-blockers may be used for mild to moderate hypertension. Combined therapy (diuretic and calcium channel blocker or angiotensin-converting enzyme inhibitor) might be appropriate for severe hypertension. Hypertensive emergencies (encephalopathy and acute congestive heart failure) and hypertensive "urgencies" (extreme elevations of blood pressure without neurologic or cardiac symptoms) require prompt hospitalization and usually parenteral antihypertensive treatment with nifedipine, sodium nitroprusside, or labetalol. Renovascular hypertension may be amenable to angioplasty or surgery of the involved blood vessel.

PROGNOSIS

The prognosis depends on the primary disorder. Essential hypertension, when present in adolescents, not associated with morbidity at presentation and untreated, contributes to the cardiovascular, CNS, and renal morbidity associated with hypertension in older patients.

bruits, diminished leg pressure, café au lait spots (neurofibromatosis associated renal artery fibromuscular dysplasia), flank masses (hydronephrosis, neuroblastoma, Wilms tumor), ataxia, opsoclonus (neuroblastoma), tachycardia with flushing and diaphoresis (pheochromocytoma), and truncal obesity, acne, striae, and a buffalo hump (Cushing syndrome). Signs of chronic renal insufficiency also may be present (see Chapter 165).

CHAPTER 167
Vesicoureteral Reflux

ETIOLOGY AND EPIDEMIOLOGY

Vesicoureteral reflux (VUR) is the retrograde flow of urine from the bladder to the ureter or the kidney. It is thought to result from a congenital incompetence of the ureterovesical junction. VUR may be familial; 30% of siblings of a child with reflux also have reflux. VUR may also be secondary to distal bladder obstruction.

Reflux is potentially harmful because of the exposure of the kidney to increased hydrodynamic pressure during voiding. Incomplete emptying of the ureter and bladder predisposes the patient to **UTIs** (see Chapter 114). Without complete emptying of the urinary tract, it is difficult for voiding to prevent bacterial colonization. **Reflux nephropathy** refers to development and progression of gross and histologic renal scarring, particularly if reflux is associated with infection or obstruction (bladder neck obstruction or posterior urethral valves). A single infection may result in renal scarring, although the incidence of scarring is higher in children with recurrent UTIs. Such scarred areas have also been seen in newborns screened because they were siblings of a child with VUR. This finding and genetic studies have suggested that some aspects of reflux nephropathy may also be genetic.

Duplications of the ureters with associated ureteroceles may obstruct the upper collecting system. Often the ureter draining the lower pole of a duplicated renal unit has reflux. The **neurogenic bladder** associated with myelomeningocele is accompanied by reflux in approximately 30% to 50% of affected children. Reflux may also be secondary to increased intravesicular pressure when the bladder outlet is obstructed from inflammation of the bladder (cystitis) or by surgical procedures performed on the bladder.

CLINICAL MANIFESTATIONS

VUR characteristically is discovered during radiologic evaluation after a UTI (see Chapter 114). The younger the patient with a UTI, the more likely reflux is present. No other clinical signs are reliable in differentiating children with UTI with and without reflux. Some patients are noted to have dilated calyces during fetal ultrasonography.

DIAGNOSTIC STUDIES AND IMAGING

A **VCUG** should be performed in all infants and children younger than 8 years old with a documented first UTI, regardless of gender. The VCUG should be

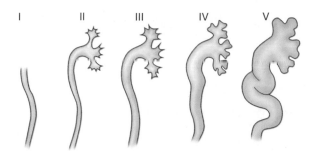

Figure 167–1

International classification of vesicoureteral reflux. Grade I, ureter only. Grade II, ureter, pelvis, and calyces; no dilation, normal calyceal fornices. Grade III, mild to moderate dilation or tortuosity of the ureter and mild to moderate dilation of the renal pelvis; slight or no blunting of the fornices. Grade IV, moderate dilation or tortuosity of the ureter and moderate dilation of the renal pelvis and calyces; complete obliteration of sharp angle of fornices, but maintenance of the papillary impressions in most calyces. Grade V, gross dilation and tortuosity of the ureter; gross dilation of the renal pelvis and calyces. The papillary impressions are no longer visible in most of the calyces. Some authors consider grade IV or V with intrarenal reflux into the collecting ducts a high risk for scarring. (From Duckett JW, Bellinger MF: Cystographic grading of primary reflux as an indicator of treatment. In Johnston JH [ed]: Management of Vesicoureteral Reflux: International Perspectives in Urology, vol 10. Baltimore, Williams & Wilkins, 1984.)

performed after the infection has been treated, but there is no need to wait days or weeks before performing the test. An international grading system has been used to describe reflux (Fig. 167–1). The incidence of renal scarring in patients with low grade VUR is low (15%) and increases with higher grades of reflux (grade IV or V), in which scarring may occur in 65% of the patients. Grade I or II VUR is likely to resolve without surgical intervention, but VUR is less likely to resolve (in fewer than half of the patients) in grade IV or V. **Nuclear renal scanning** best identifies renal scars.

TREATMENT

The presence of VUR is generally an indication for long-term prophylactic antibiotic therapy (trimethoprim-sulfamethoxazole, sulfisoxazole, or nitrofurantoin). **Complications** of reflux nephropathy are hypertension and ESRD. ESRD is predicted by proteinuria (>1 g/day) and is the result of the development of focal and segmental glomerulosclerosis and interstitial scarring. The indications for surgical repair of VUR are controversial and have been made more complex by the development of dextranomer/

hyaluronic acid copolymer, which may allow minimally invasive correction of the reflux.

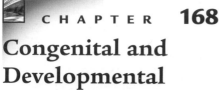

CHAPTER 168
Congenital and Developmental Abnormalities of the Urinary Tract

ETIOLOGY AND EPIDEMIOLOGY

Anomalies of the urinary tract occur in 3% to 4% of infants. **Bilateral renal agenesis**, which occurs in 1 in 4000 births, is the result of failure of development or degeneration of the ureteric bud. Renal agenesis is a component of **Potter syndrome** (flat facies, clubfoot, and pulmonary hypoplasia resulting from oligohydramnios with fetal compression by the uterus). The pulmonary hypoplasia is fatal. **Unilateral renal agenesis** (1:2900 births) is more common in infants of diabetic mothers and in African Americans. It is accompanied by normal or minimally reduced renal function. This condition can also be found with VUR and other anomalies of the genital tract, ear, skeletal system, and cardiovascular system. Unilateral renal agenesis can be a component of the VACTERL (*v*ertebral abnormalities, *a*nal atresia, *c*ardiac abnormalities, *t*racheoesophageal fistula or *e*sophageal atresia, *r*enal agenesis and dysplasia, and *l*imb defects) association, Turner syndrome, and Poland syndrome.

Renal hypoplasia/dysplasia refers to kidneys that are congenitally small or malformed or both, often with increased fibrosis. Over time, affected children progress to chronic renal failure because of the reduced nephron number. The kidneys are often unable to reabsorb sodium and water fully, requiring salt and water supplementation to optimize growth potential.

Multicystic renal dysplasia is a developmental abnormality with abnormal organization and ductal differentiation that affects 1 in 4000 live births. There is no functioning renal tissue in the affected kidney. It is usually unilateral because bilateral disease is lethal. The prenatal and postnatal ultrasound appearance of multicystic renal dysplasia is pathognomonic. There is an association with VUR to the contralateral kidney. Multicystic renal dysplasia often spontaneously involutes over the first few years of life. If the diagnosis, based on imaging, is certain, surgical removal of such a kidney is rarely indicated, unless severe hypertension develops or recurrent UTIs occur.

Polycystic kidney diseases are a group of genetic diseases affecting both kidneys and other tissues. The two major forms are autosomal recessive and autosomal dominant in transmission. Autosomal recessive polycystic kidney disease occurs in 1 in 10,000 to 40,000 children. Autosomal dominant polycystic kidney disease has an incidence of 1 in 1000 births, making it the most common inherited kidney disease. Although there is some overlap clinically, the two conditions differ morphologically. Both may appear in infancy or in older children. The genes responsible for this disorder have been identified. Renal cysts also are observed in other inherited disorders, such as von Hippel–Lindau syndrome and tuberous sclerosis.

Urinary tract obstruction can occur at any anatomic level of the genitourinary system (Table 168–1). Early in gestation, severe obstruction is thought to result in renal dysplasia. Ureteral obstruction later in fetal life or after birth results in dilation of the ureter and collecting system, often with subse-

TABLE 168–1. Site and Etiology of Urinary Tract Obstruction	
Site	**Etiology**
Infundibula/Pelvis	Congenital
	Calculi
	Infection
	Trauma
	Tumor
Ureteropelvic junction	Congenital stenosis*
	Calculi
	Trauma
Ureter	Obstructive megaureter*
	Ectopic ureter
	Ureterocele
	Calculi*
	Retroperitoneal tumor (lymphoma)
	Inflammatory bowel disease
	Retroperitoneal fibrosis
	Chronic granulomatous disease
Bladder	Neurogenic dysfunction*
	Tumor (rhabdomyosarcoma)
	Diverticula
	Ectopic ureter
Urethra	Posterior valves*
	Diverticula
	Strictures
	Atresia
	Ectopic ureter
	Foreign body
	Phimosis*
	Priapism

*Relatively common.

quent renal parenchymal alterations. An obstructed urinary tract is susceptible to infections, which may worsen renal injury further. **Posterior urethral valves** are the most common cause of **bladder outlet obstruction** in males, present in 1 in 50,000 boys. Parents may note a poor urine stream in affected children. These sail-shaped membranes arise from the verumontanum and attach to the urethral wall. The prostatic urethra becomes dilated, VUR may be present, and hypertrophied detrusor muscle develops. Renal dilation varies in severity, and some degree of dysplasia is often present. Severe obstruction may be associated with oligohydramnios, resulting in lethal pulmonary hypoplasia. Rupture of the renal pelvis produces **urinary ascites**, which is the most common cause of ascites in the newborn period.

CLINICAL MANIFESTATIONS

Bilateral renal agenesis results in insufficient lung development, due to oligohydramnios, and characteristic facial features (Potter syndrome). Respiratory distress is severe, and pneumothoraces occur. Unilateral renal agenesis may be asymptomatic because the non-affected kidney undergoes compensatory growth.

Autosomal recessive polycystic kidney disease is characterized by marked enlargement of both kidneys. There are innumerable, relatively small cysts throughout the cortex and medulla, which are dilated collecting ducts. Interstitial fibrosis and tubular atrophy may not be present at birth, but develop with time, frequently progressing to kidney failure. **Hepatic fibrosis** is present and may lead to portal hypertension. Bile duct ectasia and biliary dysgenesis occur. The diagnosis can be made by in utero ultrasound. In some fetuses, massive renal enlargement results in lethal pulmonary hypoplasia. Most affected infants have clinical manifestations such as flank masses, hepatomegaly, pneumothorax, proteinuria, or hematuria.

Autosomal dominant polycystic kidney disease characteristically presents in the 30s or 40s, but can present in infancy or childhood. Infants have a clinical picture similar to that in autosomal recessive polycystic kidney disease, but older children may show a pattern similar to that of adults, with large isolated cysts developing and enlarging. Renal pathology shows glomerular and tubular cysts. Hepatic cysts are often present. Pancreatic, splenic, and ovarian cysts also can be seen. **Cerebral aneurysms** may be present, and the risk of hemorrhage depends on size, blood pressure, and family history of intracranial hemorrhage.

Obstructions may be silent, but usually are discovered during a UTI or with a flank mass (see Chapter 114). In a newborn, abdominal masses, especially in the flank, are most often the result of ureteropelvic junction obstruction. Many obstructive uropathies are detected during fetal ultrasonography (see Chapters 58 and 60).

DIAGNOSTIC IMAGING

Renal ultrasound and **radionuclide renography** (usually with a diuretic administered) are the standard tests for diagnosis of urinary tract obstruction. Renal ultrasound studies facilitate the identification of renal agenesis, renal hypoplasia, and cystic changes in the presence of obstruction, scarring, and dilation. The dilated upper urinary tract may or may not be obstructed. A VCUG is also a part of the evaluation. Many boys with posterior urethral valves are identified by in utero ultrasound. Postnatally the diagnosis and extent of renal damage are established by ultrasonography and VCUG.

TREATMENT

Therapy for polycystic renal disease is limited to conservative measures, renal replacement therapy, and kidney transplantation. Liver transplant is less commonly necessary.

A clearly obstructed ureteropelvic junction necessitates surgery. Ureteral obstruction may also occur at the midureter and the lower ureter in association with a ureterocele or with an ectopic ureteral orifice, which is frequently associated with reflux. Ectopic ureters may drain a single collecting system or may drain the upper portion of a duplicated collecting system. Ectopic ureters are frequently obstructed; when this happens, surgical intervention is required.

Treatment of posterior urethral valves consists of either diversion (usually via vesicostomy) or primary valve ablation, depending on the individual circumstances. Careful follow-up to prevent UTI is essential. Voiding dysfunction and incontinence are common in later childhood.

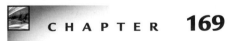

CHAPTER 169
Other Urinary Tract and Genital Disorders

URINARY TRACT STONES
Etiology

Calculi in the urinary tract is called **nephrolithiasis** or **urolithiasis**. Primary bladder stones can be seen in children with recurrent UTIs, children who have undergone bladder surgery (sutures can be a nidus for crystal formation), and children who have had intestinal augmentation to the their bladders. Renal stones in children can result from obstructive anatomic abnormalities, a metabolic predisposition, or both. Most (90%) stones in the urinary tract arise from the kidneys and become symptomatic if they become lodged in the urinary tract (most commonly at the ureteropelvic junction or the ureterovesical junction), causing acute obstruction to the flow of urine. Metabolic causes include hyperoxaluria, uric acid disorders, distal renal tubular acidosis (see Chapter 37), cystinuria (which differs from cystinosis), normocalcemic hypercalciuria, and primary hyperparathyroidism. Each of these conditions has its own specific treatment, and proper diagnosis is crucial. At least 25% of children with an obstructive anatomic abnormality have a coexisting metabolic predisposition.

Clinical Manifestations

The acute obstruction of urine flow is the cause of renal colic, a severe pain that has a classic description in children old enough to describe the symptoms (severe flank pain radiating to the groin). In younger children, the diagnosis can be made only if there is a high index of suspicion. Hematuria may occur, but is not a reliable sign, especially in children younger than 5 years of age. In this age range, nonspecific abdominal pain may be the only clue to the diagnosis.

Laboratory Studies and Imaging

Radiologic imaging of children with abdominal pain often includes ultrasound or CT. Ultrasound may identify stones in the kidney, but can easily miss stones that are more distal. CT can identify stones throughout the urinary tract, but the stones can be obscured by the administration of oral or intravenous contrast material. If there is suspicion of stone disease, the CT scan should be performed before administering any contrast agents. Diagnosis is facilitated when stone material can be obtained and sent for analysis. In the absence of analyzable stone material, urine must be collected and assayed for all the relevant analytes to establish the diagnosis; this usually requires at least one and often two timed urine collections.

Treatment

The acute treatment of urinary calculi consists of hydration and analgesia. The only generic treatment that applies to all metabolic stone conditions (the obstructive abnormalities require repair) is to increase fluid intake markedly. This treatment often requires setting specific goals and measuring 24-hour urine output to see how well the child is complying. An intake that approximates twice the daily "maintenance" requirement is often prescribed. Specific metabolic conditions have their own treatments, some geared at enhancing excretion of soluble metabolic end products and others geared toward decreasing the production of the stone-forming chemical.

Intervention to extract the stone or to break it up with lithotripsy requires consultation with urologists. Surgical repair of the potential obstruction is necessary, but not always sufficient for prevention of recurrent stones.

ANOMALIES OF THE PENIS
Etiology

Hypospadias occurs in approximately 1 in 500 newborn infants. The urethral meatus is located ventrally and proximal to its normal position, an abnormality resulting from a failure of the urethral folds to fuse completely over the urethral groove. The ventral foreskin is also lacking, and the dorsal portion gives the appearance of a hood. Severe hypospadias with undescended testes is a variant of ambiguous genitalia, and the underlying etiologies include congenital adrenal hyperplasia with masculinization of females or an androgen insensitivity syndrome. Other urinary tract anomalies do not occur often in association with hypospadias. Hypospadias may occur alone, but it is usually associated with a **chordee** (a fixed ventral curvature of the penile shaft). Rarely the urethra opens onto the perineum. In this circumstance, the chordee is extreme, and the scrotum is bifid and sometimes extends to the dorsal base of the penis.

In 90% of uncircumcised males, the foreskin becomes retractable by the age of 16 years. Before this age, the prepuce normally may be tight and may not need treatment. After this age, the inability to retract the prepuce is termed **phimosis**. The condition may be congenital or the result of inflammation. **Paraphimosis** occurs when the prepuce has been retracted behind the coronal sulcus and cannot resume its normal position.

Clinical Manifestations and Treatment

The meatal opening in hypospadias may be located anteriorly (on the glans, coronal or distal third of the shaft), on the middle (distal) third of shaft, or posteriorly (near the scrotum). Testes are undescended in 10% of boys with hypospadias. Inguinal hernias are common. Males with hypospadias should not be circumcised, particularly if the meatus is proximal to the glans, because the foreskin may be necessary for later repair. Most pediatric urologists tend to repair hypospadias before the patient is 18 months old.

Phimosis is rarely symptomatic, and parents should be reassured that loosening of the prepuce usually occurs during puberty. Treatment, if needed, is the application of topical steroids. If the narrowing is severe, gentle stretching often results in improvement. Circumcision should be reserved for the most severe cases. **Paraphimosis** results in venous stasis and edema, which leads to severe pain. When paraphimosis is discovered early, reduction of the foreskin may be possible with lubrication. In some cases, circumcision is needed.

DISORDERS AND ABNORMALITIES OF THE SCROTUM AND ITS CONTENTS

Etiology

Undescended testes (cryptorchidism) are found in 0.7% of boys after 1 year of age. It is more common in full-term newborns (3.4%) than in older children. For neonatal cryptorchidism, the percentage increases with shorter gestation (17% in neonates weighing 2000 to 2500 g and 100% in neonates weighing <900 g). Cryptorchidism is bilateral in 30% of reported cases. Spontaneous testicular descent does not occur beyond the age of 1 year, but failure to find one or both testes in the scrotum does not indicate undescended testicles. **Retractile testes**, absent testes, and ectopic testes also may be the cause of cryptorchidism.

Clinical Manifestations

A history of maternal drug use (steroids) and family history are important in the evaluation of a child for cryptorchidism. Whether the testis was ever seen in the scrotum also should be asked. The true undescended testis is found along the normal embryologic path of descent, usually in the presence of a patent processus vaginalis. Unilateral cryptorchidism is twice as common as bilateral cryptorchidism, and the right side is significantly more frequently affected than the left. An undescended testis is often associated with an inguinal hernia; it is also subject to **torsion**. There is a high incidence of infertility in adulthood. When bilateral and untreated, infertility is uniform. There is an increased risk of malignancy in the undescended testis. A malignant tumor in the cryptorchid testis occurs 20% to 44% of the time, usually between the ages of 20 and 30. The greatest risk seems to be in males who are untreated or who underwent surgical correction during or after puberty.

Retractile testes are normal testes that can retract into the inguinal canal from an exaggerated cremasteric reflex. The diagnosis of retractile testes is likely if testes are palpable in the newborn examination but not at a later examination. Frequently the parents describe a retractile testis; they see their son's testes in his scrotum when he is in the bath and see one or both "disappear" when he gets cold.

Complications

Torsion of the testis is an emergency requiring prompt diagnosis and treatment if the affected testis is to be saved. Torsion accounts for approximately 40% of cases of acute scrotal pain and swelling and is the major cause of the acute scrotum in boys younger than 6 years of age. It is thought to arise from abnormal fixation of the testis to the scrotum. On examination, the testicle is swollen and tender, and the cremasteric reflex is absent. The absence of blood flow on nuclear scan or Doppler ultrasound is consistent with torsion.

The differential diagnosis of testicular torsion includes an incarcerated hernia and torsion of the testicular epididymal appendix. Torsion of the appendix testis is associated with point tenderness over the lesion and minimal swelling. In adolescents, the differential diagnosis of testicular torsion also must include **epididymitis**, the most common cause of acute scrotal pain and swelling in older adolescents. Diagnosis is aided by an antecedent history of sexual activity or UTI. Testicular torsion must be considered as the principal diagnosis when severe acute testicular pain is present.

Treatment

The undescended testis is usually histologically normal at birth, but atrophy and poor development are found by the end of the first year of life. Given the high incidence of infertility in adults with unilateral cryptorchidism, the contralateral descended testis also may be abnormal. Surgical correction at an early age results in a greater probability of fertility in adulthood. Administration of human chorionic gonadotropin results in testosterone release from functioning testes and may result in descent of retractile testes.

Orchidopexy usually is undertaken in the second year of life. Most extra-abdominal testes can be brought into the scrotum when the associated hernia is corrected. If the testis is not palpable, ultrasound or MRI may determine its location. The closer the testis is to the internal inguinal ring, the better the chance of successful orchidopexy.

Surgical correction of testicular torsion is called *detorsion and fixation of the testis*. If explored within 6 hours of torsion, the testis survives in 90% of cases. The contralateral testis usually is fixed to the scrotum to prevent its possible future torsion. If torsion of the appendix is found at the time of exploration, removal of the necrotic tissue is indicated.

ACKNOWLEDGEMENT

We gratefully acknowledge the contributions of Dr Bruce Morgenstern, Chief, Division of Nephrology, Phoenix Children's Hospital.

SUGGESTED READING

Avner E, Harmon W, Niaudet P (eds): Pediatric Nephrology, 5th ed. Philadelphia, Lippincott Williams & Wilkins, 2004.

Behrman RE, Kliegman RM, Jenson HB (eds): Nelson Textbook of Pediatrics, 17th ed. Philadelphia, Elsevier, 2003.

Chan JC, Williams DM, Roth KS, et al: Kidney failure in infants and children. Pediatr Rev 23:47-60, 2002.

Diven SC, Travis LB: A practical primary care approach to hematuria in children. Pediatr Nephrol 14:65-72, 2000.

Eddy AA, Symons JM: Nephrotic syndrome in childhood. Lancet 362:629-639, 2003.

Rocchini AP: Pediatric hypertension 2001. Curr Opin Cardiol 17:385-389, 2002.

ENDOCRINOLOGY

Nicholas Jospe

CHAPTER 170

Assessment

The endocrine system regulates vital body functions by means of biochemical messengers (hormones). There are interactions between the endocrine system and the nervous system; hormones can be regulated by nerve cells, and endocrine agents can serve as neural messengers. There is an intimate relationship between the endocrine system and the immune system; autoantibodies may produce an excess or deficiency of a hormone. **Hormones** are defined as circulating messengers, with the location of their action at a distance from the specialized organ (**gland**) of origin of the secretion and production of the hormone. Manifestations of an endocrine disorder may be related to the response of the peripheral tissue to a hormone excess or deficiency. Functioning endocrine tumors produce profound physiologic changes long before the appearance of a tumor mass. Hormone action also may be **paracrine** (acting on adjacent neighboring cells to the cell of origin of the hormone) or **autocrine** (acting on the cell of origin of the hormone itself); agents acting in these ways are called factors rather than hormones (Fig. 170–1). Hormones generally are regulated in a feedback loop so that the production of a hormone is linked to its effect; corticotropin-releasing factor (CRF) from the hypothalamus stimulates adrenocorticotropic hormone (ACTH) in the pituitary gland, which stimulates cortisol in the adrenal gland, which feeds back to suppress CRF and ACTH production so that an equilibrium is reached, and levels of serum cortisol and ACTH remain in the normal range. The set-point of the equilibrium may change with development; in prepuberty, small amounts of sex steroids completely suppress gonadotropin secretion, but during pubertal development, the sensitivity of this feedback loop decreases.

Endocrine disorders generally manifest in one of four ways:

1. By **excess hormone**: In Cushing syndrome, there is an excess of glucocorticoid present; if the excess is secondary to autonomous glucocorticoid secretion by a target organ (cortisol secretion by the adrenal gland), the trophic hormone ACTH is suppressed.
2. By **deficient hormone**: In glucocorticoid deficiency, the level of cortisol is inadequate; if the deficiency is at the target organ (the adrenal gland), the trophic hormone is elevated (ACTH). In type 1 diabetes mellitus (DM1), the insulin secretion is low to absent.
3. By an abnormal **response of end organ** to hormone: In pseudohypoparathyroidism, there is resistance to parathyroid hormone.
4. By **gland enlargement** that may have effects as a result of size rather than function: With a large nonfunction-

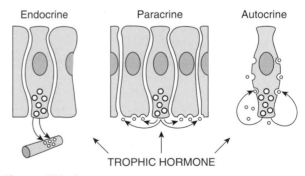

Figure 170–1

Schematic representation of mechanisms of action of hormones and growth factors. Although traditional hormones are formed in endocrine glands and transported to distant sites of action through the bloodstream (endocrine mechanism), peptide growth factors may be produced locally by the target cells themselves (autocrine modality of action) or by neighboring cells (paracrine action). (From Wilson JD, Foster DW [eds]: Williams Textbook of Endocrinology, 8th ed. Philadelphia, WB Saunders, 1992, p 1007.)

ing pituitary adenoma, abnormal visual fields and other neurologic signs and symptoms result even though no hormone is produced by the tumor.

Peptide hormones act through specific cell membrane receptors; when the hormone is attached to the receptor, the complex triggers various second messengers that cause the biologic effects (Fig. 170–2). Peptide hormone receptor number and avidity may be regulated by hormones; continuous, rather than episodic, exposure to gonadotropin-releasing hormone (GnRH) down-regulates GnRH receptor number and receptor activity on pituitary gonadotropes. **Steroid hormones** exert their effects by attachment to intracellular receptors, and the hormone-receptor complex translocates to the nucleus, where it interacts with DNA (hormone response elements upstream to the specific gene), causing appropriate effects (Fig. 170–3).

The interpretation of serum hormone levels must be related to their controlling factors; a given value of parathyroid hormone (PTH) may be normal in a eucalcemic patient, but the same value may be inadequate in a hypocalcemic patient with partial hypoparathyroidism; this same value of PTH may be excessive in a hypercalcemic patient who might have hyperparathyroidism.

HYPOTHALAMIC-PITUITARY AXIS

The **hypothalamus** controls many endocrine systems either directly or through the anterior pituitary gland; higher CNS centers control the hypothalamus. Hypothalamic releasing or inhibiting factors travel down capillaries of the pituitary portal system to control the

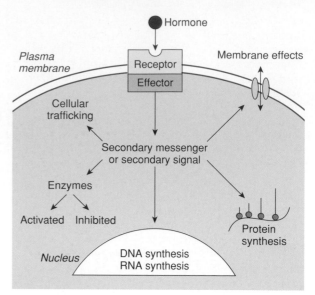

Figure 170–2

A general model for the action of peptide hormones, catecholamines, and other membrane-active hormones. The hormone in the extracellular fluid interacts with the receptor at the cell membrane and activates an associated effector system, which leads to generation of an intracellular signal or second messenger that produces the final effects of the hormone. Abnormalities in the transmembrane domains of the receptors may cause disease (e.g., testotoxicosis). Abnormalities in the secondary messenger region also may cause disease (e.g., McCune-Albright syndrome). (From Wilson JD, Foster DW [eds]: Williams Textbook of Endocrinology, 8th ed. Philadelphia, WB Saunders, 1992, p 92.)

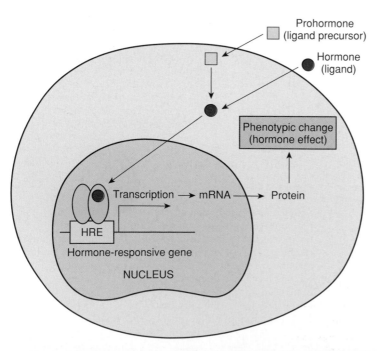

Figure 170–3

The ligand (hormone or prohormone) binds to the nuclear receptor, which binds to the promoter elements in the appropriate gene. Such genes, which are regulated by their ligand, contain specific DNA sequences called hormone response elements (HRE), to which the receptor binds. The nuclear receptor regulates gene transcription. (From Melmed S, Polonsky K, Kronenberg H, Larsen R [eds]: Williams Textbook of Endocrinology, 10th ed. Philadelphia, Elsevier, 2003, p 37.)

anterior pituitary gland, regulating the hormones specific for the factor (Fig. 170–4). The pituitary hormones enter the peripheral circulation and exert their effects on target glands, which produce other hormones that feed back to suppress their controlling hypothalamic and pituitary hormones (insulin-like growth factor-1 [IGF-1], cortisol, sex steroids, and thyroxine [T4] all feed back on the hypothalamic-pituitary system). Prolactin is the only pituitary hormone that is suppressed by a hypothalamic factor, prolactin inhibitory factor (dopamine). Hypothalamic deficiency leads to a decrease in most pituitary hormone secretions, but may lead to an increase in prolactin secretion. The hypothalamus is the location of vasopressin-secreting axons that either terminate in the posterior pituitary gland and exert their effect via vasopressin secretion from this area or terminate in the mediobasal hypothalamus, from which they can exert some effects on water balance, even in the absence of the posterior pituitary gland.

In childhood, **increased pituitary** secretion of various hormones as a result of an adenoma is rare, although cases of pituitary gigantism (growth hormone [GH] excess from a pituitary adenoma) do occur. Destructive lesions of the pituitary gland or hypothalamus are more common in childhood. A **craniopharyngioma**, a tumor of Rathke pouch, may descend into the sella turcica, causing erosion of the bone and destruction of pituitary and hypothalamic tissue. Hypopituitarism is the result of lack of functioning pituitary or hypothalamic cells. Calcification of the tumor on plain radiographic examination of the CNS or on CT scan is common. Acquired hypopituitarism also may result from pituitary infections; from infiltration, such as with Langerhans cell histiocytosis (histiocytosis X), lymphoma, and sarcoidosis; after radiation therapy or trauma to the CNS; and as a consequence of autoimmunity against the pituitary gland.

As a clinical entity, **congenital hypopituitarism** usually is caused by absence of hypothalamic releasing factors rather than anatomic absence of the pituitary gland itself. The pituitary gland does not release its hormones for lack of hypothalamic stimulation, but it can be stimulated by exogenous hypothalamic releasing factors. Exogenous administration is of limited relevance insofar as the end products of the glands themselves are administered in hypopituitarism (thyroid hormone or sex steroids). Congenital defects of pituitary secretion can result from anatomic malformations of the hypothalamus and pituitary hypoplasia or aplasia or from more subtle defects of hormone secretion. Congenital defects associated with hypopituitarism range from **holoprosencephaly** (cyclopia, cebocephaly, orbital hypotelorism), to cleft palate (6% of cases of cleft palate are associated with GH deficiency). **Septo-optic**

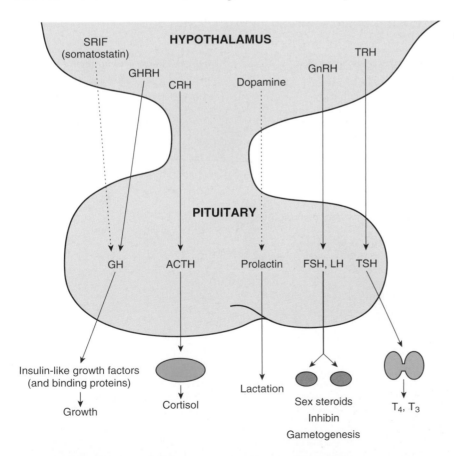

Figure 170–4

Hormonal influences of the hypothalamus and pituitary gland. *Solid line* represents stimulatory influence; *dotted line* represents inhibitory influence. ACTH, adrenocorticotropic hormone; CRH, corticotropin-releasing hormone or CRF; FSH, follicle-stimulating hormone; GH, growth hormone; GHRH, GH–releasing hormone or GRF; GnRH, gonadotropin-releasing hormone or luteinizing hormone releasing factor, LRF or LHRH; LH, luteinizing hormone; SRIF, somatotropin release–inhibiting factor, somatostatin or SS; TRH, thyrotropin-releasing hormone or TRF; TSH, thyroid-stimulating hormone; T3, triiodothyronine; T4, thyroxine.

TABLE 170–1. Diagnostic Evaluation of Hypopituitarism

Manifestation	Cause	Tests*
Growth failure, hypothyroidism, or both	GH deficiency, TRH/TSH deficiency, or both	Provocative GH tests, free T$_4$, bone age, IGF1, IGF BP3
Hypoglycemia	GH deficiency, ACTH insufficiency, or both	Provocative GH tests, test of ACTH secretion, IGF1, IGF BP3
Micropenis, pubertal delay or arrest	Hypogonadotropic hypogonadism or GH deficiency	Sex steroids (E$_2$, testosterone), basal LH and FSH (analyzed by ultrasensitive assays) or after GnRH administration, provocative GH tests, IGF1, IGF BP3
Polyuria, polydipsia	ADH deficiency	Urine analysis (sp. gr.), serum electrolytes, urine and serum osmolality, water deprivation test

*Each patient with hypopituitarism should have CNS MRI as part of evaluation to determine the etiology of the condition.
ADH, antidiuretic hormone; E$_2$, estradiol; FSH, follicle-stimulating hormone; GH, growth hormone; IGF1, insulin-like growth factor; IGF BP3, insulin-like growth factor binding protein 3; LH, luteinizing hormone; sp. gr., specific gravity; T$_4$, thyroxine; TRH, thyrotropin-releasing hormone; TSH, thyroid-stimulating hormone.

dysplasia (optic nerve hypoplasia, absent septum pellucidum, or variations of both, and hypopituitarism) may have significant visual impairment such that pendular nystagmus (to-and-fro nystagmus caused by an inability to focus on a target) results. The MRI findings of congenital hypopituitarism include an ectopic posterior pituitary gland "hot spot" and the appearance of a "pituitary stalk transection" and small pituitary gland.

The assessment of pituitary function may be determined by measuring some of the specific pituitary hormone in the basal state; other assessments require the measurement after stimulation. Indirect assessment of pituitary function can be obtained by measuring serum concentrations of the target gland hormones (Table 170–1). Several tests of pituitary function are listed in Table 170–2.

TABLE 170–2. Anterior Pituitary Hormone Function Testing

Random Hormone Measurements	Provocative Stimulation Test	Target Hormone Measurement
GH (useless as a random determination except in GH resistance or in pituitary gigantism)	Arginine (a weak stimulus) L-Dopa (Useful clinically) Insulin-induced hypoglycemia (a dangerous but accurate test) Clonidine (useful clinically) GRH 12-24-hr integrated GH levels (of questionable utility)	IGF1, IGF BP3 (affected by malnutrition as well as GH deficiency)
ACTH (early AM sample useful only if in high normal range)	Cortisol after insulin-induced hypoglycemia (a dangerous test) 11-Desoxycortisol after metyrapone CRH ACTH stimulation test (may differentiate ACTH deficiency from primary adrenal insufficiency)	AM cortisol 24-hr urinary free cortisol
TSH*	TRH	FT$_4$
LH, FSH*	GnRH (difficult to interpret in prepubertal subjects)	Testosterone Estradiol
Prolactin (elevated in hypothalamic disease and decreased in pituitary disease)	TRH	None

*New supersensitive assays allow determination of abnormally low values found in hypopituitarism.
CRH, corticotropin-releasing hormone; FSH, follicle-stimulating hormone; FT$_4$, free thyroxine; GH, growth hormone; GRH, growth hormone–releasing hormone; IGF1, insulin-like growth factor; IGF BP3, insulin-like growth factor binding protein 3; L-dopa, L-dihydroxyphenylalanine; LH, luteinizing hormone; TRH, thyrotropin-releasing hormone; TSH, thyroid-stimulating hormone.

CHAPTER 171

Diabetes Mellitus

Diabetes mellitus is characterized by hyperglycemia and glycosuria and is an endpoint of a few disease processes (Table 171–1). The most common type occurring in childhood is DM1, which is caused by autoimmune destruction of the insulin-producing beta cells (islets) of the pancreas. Patients with DM1 have permanent insulin deficiency and require insulin. Type 2 diabetes mellitus (DM2) is less common in children and results from insulin resistance and relative insulin deficiency, usually with obesity. In relation to certain ethnic and geographic considerations, however, the incidence of DM2 in the U.S. is increasing. Individuals with DM2 are not dependent on insulin for survival, but they may require insulin to achieve adequate glycemic control. Less common subtypes of DM2 result from genetic defects of the insulin receptor or inherited abnormalities in sensing of ambient glucose concentration by pancreatic beta cells (see Table 171–1).

DEFINITION

A **diagnosis** of diabetes mellitus is made if a fasting serum glucose concentration is greater than 126 mg/dL or a 2-hour postprandial serum glucose concentration is greater than 200 mg/dL on two separate occasions. A patient is considered **glucose intolerant** if fasting serum glucose concentrations are greater than 110 mg/dL but less than 126 mg/dL and if 2 hour postprandial values are greater than 140 mg/dL but less than 200 mg/dL. Sporadic hyperglycemia occurs in children, usually in the setting of an intercurrent illness. When the hyperglycemic episode is clearly related to an illness or other physiologic stress, the probability of incipient diabetes is small (<5%). Sporadic hyperglycemia occurring without a clear precipitating physiologic stress is of more concern because diabetes develops in at least 30%.

INSULIN-DEPENDENT (TYPE 1) DIABETES MELLITUS

Etiology

DM1 results from the autoimmune destruction of the insulin-producing beta cells (islets) of the pancreas. In addition to the presence of diabetes susceptibility genes, an unknown environmental insult presumably occurs to trigger the autoimmune destruction. A variety of cross-sectional, retrospective, and prospective studies have produced conflicting data regarding a host of environmental factors and their etiologic role in DM1. These include cow's milk feeding before age 2 years and viral infectious agents (coxsackie B virus, cytomegalovirus, mumps, and rubella). Potential mechanisms for viral initiation of the autoimmune response include

TABLE 171–1. Classification of Diabetes Mellitus in Children and Adolescents

Type	Comment
Type 1 (Insulin-Dependent)	
Transient neonatal	Presents immediately after birth; lasts 1-3 mo
Permanent neonatal	Other pancreatic defects possible
Classic type 1	Glycosuria, ketonuria, hyperglycemia, islet cell antibody to glutamic acid decarboxylase positive; genetic component
Type 2 (Non–Insulin-Dependent)	
Secondary	Cystic fibrosis, hemochromatosis, drugs (L-asparaginase, tacrolimus)
Adult type (classic)	Associated with obesity, insulin resistance; genetic component
Maturity onset diabetes of youth	Autosomal dominant, onset before 25 years of age; not associated with obesity or autoimmunity; single gene mutations include: hepatocytic nuclear factors 1-β, 1-α, 4-α; glucokinase; insulin promoter factor 1
Mitochondrial diabetes	Associated with deafness and other neurologic defects, maternal transmission—mtDNA point mutations
Other	
Gestational diabetes	Abnormal glucose tolerance only during pergnancy, which reverts to normal post partum; increased risk for later onset of diabetes

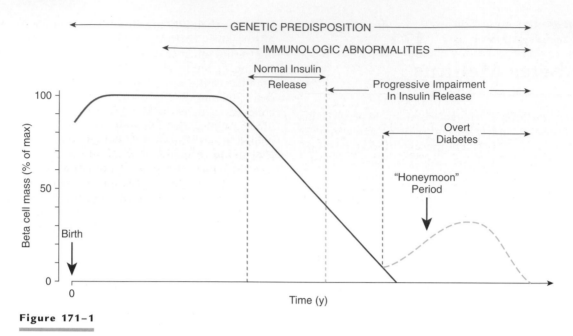

Figure 171–1

Schematic representation of the autoimmune evolution of diabetes in genetically predisposed individuals.

direct beta cell damage through viral infection, antibody cross-reactivity, and polyclonal activation of B lymphocytes. DM1 is thought to be primarily a T cell–mediated disease, however.

Antibodies to islet cell antigens may be seen months to 10 years before the onset of beta cell dysfunction, which most likely indicates an ongoing destructive process (Fig. 171–1). Many different antibodies to beta cell antigens can be detected, including islet cell antibodies, insulin autoantibodies, antibodies to tyrosine phosphatase IA-2, and antibodies to glutamic acid decarboxylase. Studies in family members of patients with DM1 have shown that the risk for diabetes increases with the number of antibodies detected in the serum. In individuals with only one detectable antibody, the risk is only 10% to 15%; in individuals with three or more antibodies, the risk is 55% to 90%. Antibodies to other organs are present and linked to progression to disease; these include antiperoxidase thyroid antibodies leading to **Hashimoto thyroiditis**, tissue transglutaminase antibodies linked with **celiac disease**, and 21-hydroxylase antibodies leading to **Addison disease**. When 80% to 90% of the beta cell mass has been destroyed, the remaining beta cell mass is insufficient to maintain glycemic control, and clinical manifestations of diabetes result (see Fig. 171–1).

Epidemiology

DM1 is the most common pediatric endocrine disorder, affecting approximately 1 in 300 to 500 children younger than 18 years old. The annual incidence in children ranges from a high of 30 in 100,000 among Scandinavian populations to a low of 1 in 100,000 in Japan. In the U.S., the annual incidence is approximately 15 in 100,000. The annual incidence of DM1 is increasing steadily but with significant geographic differences. The prevalence of DM1 in the U.S. is highest in whites and is lower in African Americans and Hispanic Americans.

Genetic determinants play a role in the susceptibility to DM1, although the mode of inheritance is complex and likely multigenic. Siblings or offspring of patients with diabetes have a risk of 3% to 6% for development of diabetes; an identical twin has a 30% to 50% risk. The association of DM1 susceptibility with the HLA region on chromosome 6 is the strongest determinant of susceptibility, accounting for approximately 40% of the familial inheritance of DM1. Specific HLA alleles (HLA DR3 and HLA DR4) have been determined to increase the risk of developing DM1, whereas other specific HLA alleles have been found to exert a protective effect. More than 90% of children with DM1 possess HLA DR3 alleles, HLA DR4 alleles, or both. The insulin gene region VNTR on chromosome 11 also has been linked to DM1 susceptibility; there is some evidence for association of at least 18 other loci with DM1. Genetic factors do not fully account for susceptibility to DM1; environmental factors also play a role.

Clinical Manifestations

When insulin secretory capacity becomes inadequate to support peripheral glucose uptake and to suppress hepatic glucose production, hyperglycemia results. The initial manifestation of insulin deficiency is postprandial hyperglycemia. Fasting hyperglycemia then develops. Ketogenesis is a sign of more complete insulin deficiency. Lack of suppression of gluconeogenesis, glycogenolysis, and fatty acid oxidation contributes to the hyperglycemia and further generation of ketone bodies β-hydroxybutyrate, acetoacetate, and acetone. Protein stores in muscle and fat stores in adipose tissue are metabolized to provide substrates for gluconeogenesis and fatty acid oxidation.

Glycosuria occurs when the serum glucose concentration exceeds the renal threshold for glucose reabsorption (approximately 180 mg/dL). Glycosuria causes an osmotic diuresis (including obligate loss of sodium, potassium, and other electrolytes), leading to dehydration. Polydipsia occurs as the patient attempts to compensate for the excess fluid losses. Weight loss results from the persistent catabolic state and the loss of calories through glycosuria and ketonuria. The classic presentation of DM1 includes polyuria, polydipsia, polyphagia, and weight loss.

Diabetic Ketoacidosis

If the clinical features of DM1 are not detected early, diabetic ketoacidosis (DKA) can occur. DKA also can occur in patients with known diabetes if insulin injections are omitted. DKA also can occur during periods of intercurrent illness when greater insulin requirements go unmet in the presence of elevated concentrations of the counterregulatory hormones glucagon, cortisol, and catecholamines. In the setting of hyperglycemia, DKA can be considered to be present if (1) the arterial pH is less than 7.25, (2) the serum bicarbonate level is less than 15 mEq/L, and (3) ketones are elevated in serum or urine.

Pathophysiology

In the absence of adequate insulin secretion, persistent partial hepatic oxidation of fatty acids to ketone bodies occurs. Two of these three ketone bodies are organic acids, the excess of which results in a metabolic acidosis with an elevated anion gap. Lactic acid also can contribute to the acidosis when severe dehydration results in decreased tissue perfusion. Hyperglycemia causes an osmotic diuresis that is initially compensated for by increased fluid intake. As the hyperglycemia and diuresis worsen, most patients are unable to maintain the large fluid intake, and dehydration occurs. Vomiting as a result of increasing acidosis and increased insensible losses caused by tachypnea worsen the dehydration. Electrolyte abnormalities occur secondary to loss of electrolytes in the urine and transmembrane alterations resulting from acidosis. As hydrogen ions accumulate as a result of ketoacidosis, exchange of hydrogen ions for intracellular potassium occurs. Serum concentrations of potassium increase initially with acidosis, then decrease as serum potassium is cleared by the kidney. Depending on the duration of ketoacidosis, serum potassium concentrations at diagnosis may be increased, normal, or decreased, but intracellular potassium concentrations are depleted. A decreased serum potassium concentration is an ominous sign of total body potassium depletion. Phosphate depletion also can occur as a result of the increased renal phosphate excretion required for elimination of excess hydrogen ions. Sodium depletion also is common in DKA, resulting from renal losses of sodium caused by osmotic diuresis and from gastrointestinal losses from vomiting (Fig. 171–2).

Presentation

Patients with DKA present initially with polyuria, polydipsia, and nausea and vomiting. Abdominal pain occurs frequently and can mimic an acute abdomen. The presence of polyuria, despite a state of clinical dehydration, indicates osmotic diuresis and differentiates patients with DKA from patients with gastroenteritis or other gastrointestinal disorders. Respiratory compensation for acidosis results in tachypnea with deep (**Küssmaul**) respirations. The "fruity" odor of acetone frequently can be detected on the patient's breath. The abdomen may be distended secondary to a paralytic ileus. An altered mental status can occur, ranging from disorientation to coma.

Laboratory studies reveal hyperglycemia, with serum glucose concentrations ranging from 200 mg/dL to greater than 1000 mg/dL. Arterial pH is less than 7.25, and the serum bicarbonate concentration is less than 15 mEq/L. Serum sodium concentrations may be elevated, normal, or low, depending on the balance of sodium and free water losses. The measured serum sodium concentration is artificially depressed, however, because of hyperglycemia (see Chapter 35).

Hyperlipidemia also can contribute to the decrease in measured serum sodium. The level of BUN can be elevated with prerenal azotemia secondary to dehydration. The white blood cell count is usually elevated and can be left-shifted without implying the presence of infection. Fever is unusual, however, and should prompt a search for infectious sources that may have triggered the episode of DKA.

Treatment

Therapy for patients with DKA involves careful replacement of fluid deficits, correction of acidosis and hyperglycemia via insulin administration, correction of electrolyte imbalances, and monitoring for complications of treatment. The optimal approach to management of DKA must strike a balance between adequate

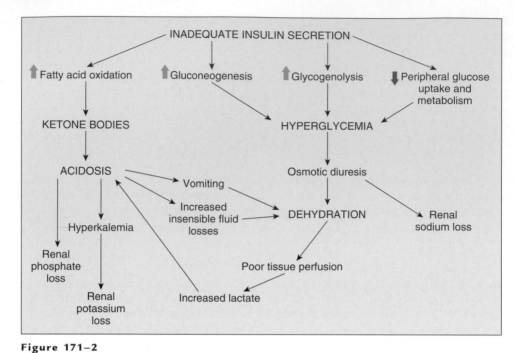

Figure 171–2

Pathophysiology of diabetic ketoacidosis.

correction of fluid losses to avoid complications of severe dehydration and avoidance of rapid shifts in osmolality and fluid balance. The most serious complication of DKA and its treatment is **cerebral edema** and cerebral herniation.

Dehydration. A patient with severe DKA is assumed to be approximately 10% dehydrated. If a recent weight measurement is available, the precise extent of dehydration can be calculated. An initial IV fluid bolus of a glucose-free isotonic solution (normal saline, lactated Ringer's solution) at 10 to 20 mL/kg should be given to restore intravascular volume and renal perfusion. The remaining fluid deficit after the initial bolus should be added to maintenance fluid requirements, and the total should be replaced slowly over 36 to 48 hours. Ongoing losses resulting from osmotic diuresis usually do not need to be replaced, unless urine output is large or signs of poor perfusion are present. Osmotic diuresis is usually minimal when the serum glucose concentration decreases to less than 300 mg/dL. To avoid rapid shifts in serum osmolality, 0.9% sodium chloride can be used as the replacement fluid for the initial 4 to 6 hours, followed by 0.45% sodium chloride.

Hyperglycemia. Fast-acting soluble insulin should be administered as a continuous IV infusion (0.1 U/kg/hr). Serum glucose concentrations should decrease at a rate no faster than 100 mg/dL/hr. When serum glucose concentrations decrease to less than 250 to

300 mg/dL, glucose should be added to the IV fluids. If serum glucose concentrations decrease to less than 200 mg/dL before correction of acidosis, the glucose concentration of the IV fluids should be increased, but the insulin infusion should not be decreased by more than half, and it should never be discontinued.

Acidosis. Insulin therapy lowers glucagon and diminishes its effect on liver, decreases the production of free fatty acids (FFAs) and protein catabolism, and enhances glucose usage in target tissues. These processes correct acidosis. Bicarbonate therapy should be avoided unless severe acidosis (pH <7.0) results in hemodynamic instability, or symptomatic hyperkalemia is present. Potential adverse effects of bicarbonate administration include paradoxical increases in CNS acidosis caused by increased diffusion of carbon dioxide across the blood-brain barrier, potential tissue hypoxia caused by shifts in the oxyhemoglobin dissociation curve, abrupt osmotic changes, and increased risk of development of cerebral edema.

As acidosis is corrected, urine ketone concentrations may appear to rise. β-Hydroxybutyrate, which is not detected in urine ketone assays, is converted with treatment to what the assay most detects, acetoacetate. Urine ketone concentration is not a useful index of the adequacy of therapy.

Electrolyte Imbalances. Regardless of the serum potassium concentration at presentation, total body potassium depletion is likely. Potassium concentrations can decrease rapidly as insulin, and then glucose, therapy improves the acidotic state and potassium is exchanged for intracellular hydrogen ions. When adequate urine output is shown, potassium should be added to the IV fluids. Potassium replacement should be given as 50% potassium chloride and 50% potassium phosphate at a concentration of 20 to 40 mEq/L. This combination provides phosphate for replacement of deficits, but avoids excess phosphate administration, which may precipitate hypocalcemia. If the serum potassium level is greater than 6, potassium should not be added to IV fluids until the potassium level decreases.

Monitoring. A flow sheet should be used to record and monitor fluid balance and laboratory measurements. Initial laboratory measurements should include serum glucose, sodium, potassium, chloride, bicarbonate, BUN, creatinine, calcium, phosphate, and magnesium concentrations; arterial or venous pH; and a urinalysis. Serum glucose measurement should be repeated every hour during therapy, and electrolyte concentrations should be repeated every 2 to 3 hours. Calcium, phosphate, and magnesium concentrations should be measured initially and every 4 to 6 hours during therapy. Neurologic and mental status should be assessed at frequent intervals, and complaints of headache or deterioration of mental status should prompt rapid evaluation for possible **cerebral edema**. Indicative symptoms include a decreased sensorium, sudden severe headache, vomiting, change in vital signs (bradycardia, hypertension, apnea), pupillary changes, ophthalmoplegia, or seizure.

Complications

Clinically apparent **cerebral edema** occurs in 1% to 5% of cases of DKA. Cerebral edema is the most serious complication of DKA, with a mortality rate of 20% to 80%. The pathogenesis of cerebral edema likely involves osmolar shift resulting in fluid accumulation in the intracellular compartment and cell swelling. Subclinical cerebral edema is common in patients with DKA, but the factors that exacerbate this process leading to symptomatic brain swelling and possible cerebral herniation are not clearly defined. Cerebral edema typically occurs 6 to 12 hours after therapy for DKA is begun, often following a period of apparent clinical improvement. Factors that have been found to correlate with increased risk for cerebral edema include higher initial BUN concentration, lower initial PCO_2, failure of the serum sodium concentration to increase as glucose concentration decreases during treatment, and treatment with bicarbonate.

Signs of advanced cerebral edema include obtundation, papilledema, pupillary dilation or inequality, hypertension, bradycardia, and apnea. **Treatment**

involves the rapid use of IV mannitol, endotracheal intubation, and hyperventilation. Other complications of DKA are intracranial thrombosis or infarction, acute tubular necrosis with acute renal failure caused by severe dehydration, pancreatitis, arrhythmias caused by electrolyte abnormalities, pulmonary edema, and bowel ischemia. Peripheral edema occurs commonly 24 to 48 hours after therapy is initiated and may be related to residual elevations in antidiuretic hormone and aldosterone.

Transition to Outpatient Management

When the acidosis has been corrected, and the patient tolerates oral feedings, the IV insulin infusion can be discontinued, and a regimen of SC insulin injections can be initiated. The first SC insulin dose should be given 30 to 45 minutes before discontinuation of the IV insulin infusion. Further adjustment of the insulin dose should be made over the following 2 to 3 days. A patient already diagnosed with DM1 may be restarted on the prior doses if these were adequate. For a patient with new-onset DM1, typical starting doses are approximately 0.7 U/kg/24 hours for prepubertal patients and approximately 1 U/kg/24 hours for adolescents, using a mixed split-dosing regimen including short-acting insulin (regular) or fast-acting insulin (lispro or aspart) in conjunction with long-acting insulin (usually NPH). The dose should be divided into two daily injections, with two thirds of the total daily dose given in the morning, 30 minutes before breakfast if using regular insulin or at breakfast if using lispro or aspart, and one third given in the evening, likewise 30 minutes before dinner if using regular or at dinner if using lispro or aspart (Fig. 171–3). The ratio of insulins in the morning dose should be two-thirds intermediate-acting insulin (NPH or Lente), and one-third short-acting or fast-acting insulin. Regular insulin is used less and less in favor of lispro or aspart insulin. In the evening, one half of the evening insulin dose should be given as intermediate-acting insulin (NPH or Lente), and one half should be given as short-acting or fast-acting insulin.

Another alternative for making the transition to SC insulin is to begin by giving injections of lispro or aspart insulin before each meal and NPH or insulin glargine at bedtime. This regimen can be converted to a twice-daily regimen of NPH and short-acting insulin after the patient is able to tolerate a full diet, and serum glucose concentrations stabilize.

Serum glucose concentrations should be assessed before each meal, at bedtime, and at 2 to 3 AM to provide information for adjustment of the regimen. Patients and their families should begin learning the principles of diabetes care as soon as possible. Demonstration of ability to administer insulin injections and

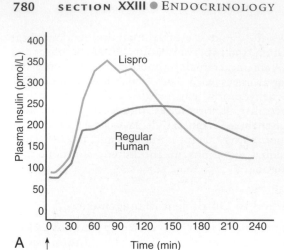

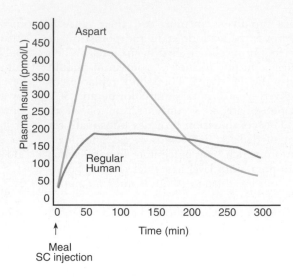

A

Meal
SC injection

Meal
SC injection

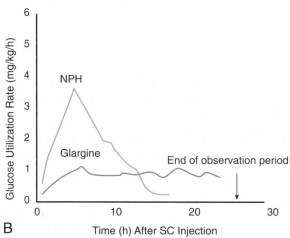

B

Figure 171–3

Representative profiles of insulin effect using combined injection regimens: intermediate-acting insulin (NPH or Lente) and regular (short-acting) insulin. **A,** Short-acting lispro, regular, or aspart insulins. **B,** Long-acting NPH or glargine profiles. (Adapted from Mudaliar SR, Lindberg FA, Joyce M, et al: Insulin aspart [B28 asp-insulin]: A fast-acting analog of human insulin: Absorption kinetics and action profile compared with regular human insulin in healthy nondiabetic subjects. Diabetes Care 22:1501-1506, 1999; and Lepore M, Kurzals R, Pampanelli S, et al: Pharmacokinetics and dynamics of S.C. injection of the long-acting glargine [HOE 901] in T1DM. Diabetes 48[Suppl 1]: A97, 1999.)

test glucose concentrations using a glucometer is necessary before discharge, as is knowledge of hypoglycemia management. Meal planning is crucial to control of glucose in DM1, and nutrition services must be part of the care delivered to the families from the outset.

Honeymoon Period

In patients with new onset of DM1 who do not have DKA, the beta cell mass has not been completely destroyed. The remaining functional beta cells seem to recover with insulin treatment, and they are again able to produce insulin. When this occurs, insulin requirements decrease, and there is a period of stable blood glucose control, often with nearly normal glucose con-

centrations. This phase of the disease, known as the honeymoon period, usually starts in the first weeks of therapy and usually continues for a few months at most, but can last 2 years.

Outpatient Type 1 Diabetes Mellitus Management

Management of DM1 in children requires a comprehensive approach, with attention to medical, nutritional, and psychosocial issues. Therapeutic strategies should be flexible, with the individual needs of each patient and the family taken into account. Optimal care involves a team of diabetes professionals, including a physician, a diabetes nurse educator, a dietitian, and a social worker or psychologist.

Goals

The Diabetes Control and Complications Trial established that intensive insulin therapy, with the goal of maintaining blood glucose concentrations as close to normal as possible, can delay the onset and slow the progression of complications of diabetes (retinopathy, nephropathy, neuropathy). Intensive insulin therapy also resulted in an increase in severe hypoglycemia. One should balance these two features when planning the treatment goals, especially for very young children. The adverse effects of hypoglycemia in young children may be significant because the immature CNS may be more susceptible to glycopenia. Although the risk for diabetic complications increases with duration of diabetes, there is controversy as to whether the rate of increase of risk may be slower in the prepubertal years than in adolescence and adulthood. It is safe to establish goals to achieve tight control of blood glucose concentrations in childhood.

The goals of therapy differ, depending on the age of the patient. For children younger than 5 years old, an appropriate goal is maintenance of blood glucose concentrations between 100 and 200 mg/dL. For school-age children, 80 to 180 mg/dL is a reasonable target range. For adolescents, the goal is 70 to 150 mg/dL. Goals of therapy also should take into account other individual characteristics, such as a past history of severe hypoglycemia and the abilities of the patient and family.

Insulin Regimens

Many types of insulin differ in duration of action and time to peak effect (Table 171–2). These insulins can be used in various combinations, depending on the needs and goals of the individual patient. The most commonly used regimen in school-age children involves two SC injections per day of intermediate-acting insulin (NPH) and short-acting insulin (regular, or lispro or aspart insulin) (see Fig. 171–3). This regimen is preferred because it does not require the patient to give an insulin injection at midday, during school hours. Patients using this regimen must adhere to a meal schedule with consistent breakfast, lunch, and dinner and snacks as needed; this can be difficult to coordinate with variations in daily activities. Other regimens use multiple injections of short-acting insulin given before meals in combination with a long-acting basal insulin (e.g., Ultralente or glargine) or with an intermediate-acting insulin given at bedtime. These regimens provide more flexibility but require the patient to administer many injections per day and are more suitable for adolescents than young children. *Pumps* that provide a continuous SC infusion of short-

TABLE 171–2. Insulin Preparations			
Type of Insulin	**Onset**	**Peak Action**	**Duration**
Very Short-Acting			
Lispro, aspart	10-20 min	30-90 min	3 hr
Short-Acting			
Regular	30 min-1 hr	2-4 hr	6-10 hr
Intermediate-Acting			
NPH	1-4 hr	4-12 hr	16-24 hr
Lente	1-4 hr	4-12 hr	12-24 hr
Long-Acting			
Protamine zinc	4-6 hr	8-20 hr	24-30 hr
Ultralente	4-6 hr	8-20 hr	24-36 hr
Glargine	1-2 hr	No peak	24-30 hr

acting insulin also are available and are being used by children and adolescents who are highly motivated to achieve tight control.

Two insulin analogues are available in which altered amino acid positioning results in rapid absorption. Lispro and aspart insulins are synthetic human insulin analogues in which two amino acid positions are reversed. These alterations in the insulin structure result in faster absorption and onset of action than regular insulin (see Table 171–2). Lispro or aspart insulin can be substituted for regular insulin and may be particularly useful in patients who have problems with postprandial hypoglycemia. Because of the short duration of action, lispro or aspart must be used in combination with an intermediate-acting or long-acting insulin. Glargine is an insulin analogue in which the amino acid glycine is substituted for asparagine in the A-chain of insulin, and two arginine molecules are added to the C-terminus of the B-chain. These alterations result in increased solubility at acidic pH and decreased solubility at physiologic pH. Glargine is injected subcutaneously, precipitates, and is absorbed very slowly. In clinical studies, glargine has been shown to have a duration of greater than 24 hours and to have essentially no peak of activity; it acts as a basal insulin.

Newly diagnosed patients in the honeymoon period may require 0.4 to 0.6 U/kg/24 hours. Prepubertal patients with a duration of diabetes longer than 1 to 2 years typically require 0.5 to 1 U/kg/24 hours. During middle adolescence, when elevated GH concentrations produce relative insulin resistance, insulin requirements increase by 40% to 50%, and doses of 1 to 2 U/kg/24 hours are typical.

Nutrition

Balancing the daily meal plan with the dosages of insulin is crucial for maintaining serum glucose concentrations within the target range and avoiding hypoglycemia or hyperglycemia. The content and schedule of meals varies according to the type of insulin regimen used; it is recommended that carbohydrates contribute 50% to 65% of the total calories; protein, 12% to 20%; and fat, less than 30%. Saturated fat should contribute less than 10% of the total caloric intake, and cholesterol intake should be less than 300 mg/24 hours. High fiber content is recommended.

Children using a combination of intermediate-acting and short-acting insulins given twice a day need to maintain a relatively consistent meal schedule so that peaks of carbohydrate absorption correspond with peaks in insulin action. A typical meal schedule for a patient using this type of regimen involves three meals and three snacks daily. The total carbohydrate content of the meals and snacks should be kept constant. Patients using multiple injection regimens or the insulin pump can maintain a more flexible meal schedule with regard to the timing of meals and the carbohydrate content. These patients give an injection of insulin before each meal, with the total dose calculated according to the carbohydrate content of the meal. Further adjustments in the dose can be made based on the measured serum glucose concentration and plans for exercise during the day.

Blood Glucose Testing

Blood glucose should be routinely monitored (with rapid, portable glucose meters) before each meal and at bedtime. Hypoglycemia during the night or excessive variability in the morning glucose concentrations should prompt additional testing at 2 or 3 AM to ensure that there is no hypoglycemia leading to the Somogyi effect or rebound hyperglycemia at the morning (before breakfast) sample. During periods of intercurrent illness or when blood glucose concentrations are greater than 300 mg/dL, urine ketones also should be tested.

Long-Term Glycemic Control

Measurements of glycohemoglobin or hemoglobin A_{1c} reflect the average blood glucose concentration over the preceding 3 months and provide a means for assessing long-term glycemic control. Glycohemoglobin should be measured four times a year, and the results should be used for counseling of patients. Table 171–3

TABLE 171–3. Biochemical Indices of Glycemic Control		
Poor Control	**Average Control**	**Intensive Control**
HgbA$_{1c}$ >10% Average blood glucose >240 mg/dL	HgbA$_{1c}$ >8-10% Average blood glucose 180-240 mg/dL	HgbA$_{1c}$ 6-8% Average blood glucose 120-180 mg/dL

HgbA$_{1c}$, Hemoglobin A$_{1c}$.

summarizes the correlation between hemoglobin A_{1c} or glycohemoglobin and daily blood glucose measurements. Measurements of glycohemoglobin or hemoglobin A_{1c} are inaccurate in patients with hemoglobinopathies. Glycosylated albumin or fructosamine can be used in these cases.

Complications

Patients with DM1 of greater than 3 to 5 years' duration should receive an annual ophthalmologic examination for retinopathy. Urine should be collected annually for assessment of microalbuminuria; if present, microalbuminuria suggests early renal dysfunction and indicates a high risk of progression to nephropathy. *Treatment* with angiotensin-converting enzyme inhibitors may halt the progression of microalbuminuria. In children with DM1, annual cholesterol measurements and periodic assessment of blood pressure are recommended. Early detection of hypertension and hypercholesterolemia with appropriate intervention can help to limit future risk of coronary disease.

Other Disorders

Chronic lymphocytic thyroiditis is particularly common and can result in hypothyroidism. Because symptoms can be subtle, thyroid function tests should be performed annually. Other disorders that occur with increased frequency in children with DM1 include celiac disease, IgA deficiency, Addison disease, and peptic ulcer disease.

Special Problems

Hypoglycemia

Iatrogenic hypoglycemia occurs commonly in patients with DM1. Patients in adequate or better control of DM1 using conventional insulin therapy have an average of one episode per week of mild symptomatic hypoglycemia, and patients on intensive regimens have an average of two episodes per week. Severe episodes of hypoglycemia, resulting in seizures or coma or requiring assistance from another person, occur in 10% to 25% of these patients per year.

Hypoglycemia in patients with DM1 results from a relative excess of insulin in relation to the serum glucose concentration. This excess can be caused by alterations in the dose, timing, or absorption of insulin; alterations of carbohydrate intake; or changes in insulin sensitivity resulting from exercise. Defective counterregulatory responses also contribute to hypoglycemia. Abnormal glucagon responses to falling serum glucose concentrations develop within the first few years of the disease, and abnormalities in epinephrine release occur after a longer duration.

Lack of awareness of hypoglycemia occurs in approximately 25% of patients with diabetes. Recent episodes of hypoglycemia may play a role in the pathophysiology of hypoglycemia unawareness; after an episode of hypoglycemia, autonomic responses to subsequent episodes are reduced. A return of symptoms of hypoglycemia can be exhibited in these patients after 2 to 3 weeks of strict avoidance of hypoglycemic episodes.

Symptoms of hypoglycemia include symptoms resulting from neuroglycopenia (headache, visual changes, confusion, irritability, or seizures) and symptoms resulting from the catecholamine response (tremors, tachycardia, diaphoresis, or anxiety) (see Chapter 172). Mild episodes can be treated with administration of rapidly absorbed oral glucose (glucose gel or tablets, fruit juices, and nondiet or non–artificially sweetened sodas). More severe episodes that result in seizures or loss of consciousness at home should be treated with glucagon injections. IV glucose should be given in hospital settings.

Early Morning Hyperglycemia

A variety of situations can lead to early morning hyperglycemia. The most frequent assumption is that the evening dose of intermediate-acting insulin is inadequate, but this is not always the case. Hypoglycemia that occurs during the night can result in increased secretion of counterregulatory hormones and rebound hyperglycemia, a situation known as the **Somogyi phenomenon**. Patients experiencing nighttime hypoglycemia also may experience headache on awakening, diaphoresis, and nightmares.

In some children, the evening intermediate-acting insulin is given early, and the dose wanes by the early morning, resulting in an increase in glucose concentrations. Increased secretion of GH during the early morning hours also can contribute to morning hyperglycemia, particularly during middle adolescence. This situation is known as the **dawn phenomenon**. Testing of blood glucose concentrations at 2 or 3 AM can

distinguish between these possibilities. Depending on the results, the evening intermediate-acting insulin dose may need to be changed or given at bedtime.

Prognosis

Long-term complications of DM1 include retinopathy, nephropathy, neuropathy, and macrovascular disease. Evidence of organ damage caused by hyperglycemia is rare in patients with duration of diabetes of less than 5 to 10 years, and clinically apparent disease rarely occurs before 10 to 15 years' duration. The eventual morbidity and mortality attributable to these disorders are substantial. Some degree of diabetic retinopathy eventually occurs in nearly 100% of patients with DM1 and is the cause of approximately 5000 new cases of blindness in the U.S. yearly. Nephropathy eventually occurs in 30% to 40% and accounts for approximately 30% of all new adult cases of end-stage renal disease. Neuropathy occurs in 30% to 40% of postpubertal patients with DM1 and leads to sensory, motor, or autonomic deficits. Macrovascular disease results in an increased risk of myocardial infarction and stroke among individuals with diabetes.

Intensive control of diabetes, employing frequent blood glucose testing and multiple daily injections of insulin or an insulin pump, can reduce substantially the development or progression of diabetic complications. Intensive management resulted in a 76% reduction of risk for retinopathy, a 39% reduction in microalbuminuria, and a 60% reduction in clinical neuropathy. For pubertal and adult patients, these benefits of intensive therapy likely outweigh the increase in risk for hypoglycemia. For younger patients, in whom the risks for hypoglycemia are greater, and the benefits of tight glucose control may be lower, a less intensive regimen may be appropriate.

NON–INSULIN-DEPENDENT (TYPE 2) DIABETES MELLITUS

Pathophysiology

DM2 can occur as the result of various pathophysiologic processes; however, the most common form results from peripheral insulin resistance with failure of the pancreas to maintain compensatory hyperinsulinemia (see Table 171-1). The precise defects underlying the insulin-resistant state and the eventual pancreatic beta cell failure are complex and poorly understood. Other subtypes of DM2 also can occur in children. **Maturity-onset diabetes of youth (MODY)** comprises a group of dominantly inherited forms of relatively mild diabetes. Insulin resistance does not occur in these patients; instead the primary abnormality is an insufficient insulin secretory response to glycemic stimulation. DM2 in childhood also can result from rare inherited defects in **mitochondrial genes**. Other rare subtypes of DM2 are syndromes of severe insulin resistance caused by mutations in the insulin receptor gene and diabetes resulting from the secretion of abnormal forms of insulin.

Epidemiology

DM2 was thought to be uncommon in childhood; the prevalence of this disorder in children is increasing in parallel with the increased prevalence of childhood obesity. The prevalence is highest in children of ethnic groups with a high prevalence of DM2 in adults, including Native Americans, Hispanic Americans, and African Americans. Obesity, the metabolic syndrome, and a family history of DM2 are risk factors.

Clinical Manifestations and Differential Diagnosis

As with DM1, a **diagnosis** of diabetes mellitus can be made if a fasting serum glucose concentration is greater than 126 mg/dL or a 2-hour postprandial serum glucose concentration is greater than 200 mg/dL on two separate occasions. A patient is considered **glucose intolerant** if fasting serum glucose concentrations are greater than 110 mg/dL but less than 126 mg/dL and if 2-hour postprandial values are greater than 140 mg/dL but less than 200 mg/dL. The diagnosis of DM2 may be suspected on the basis of polyuria and polydipsia and in a background of the metabolic syndrome. Differentiating DM2 from DM1 in children sometimes can be challenging. The possibility of DM2 should be considered in patients who are obese, have a strong family history of DM2, have other characteristics of the metabolic syndrome and acanthosis nigricans on physical examination, or have absence of antibodies to beta cell antigens at the time of diagnosis of diabetes. **Acanthosis nigricans** is a dermatologic manifestation of hyperinsulinism that presents as hyperkeratotic pigmentation in the nape of the neck and in flexural areas. Although ketoacidosis occurs far more commonly in DM1, it also can occur in patients with DM2 under conditions of physiologic stress and cannot be used as an absolute differentiating factor. The diagnosis of DM2 can be confirmed by evaluation of insulin or C-peptide responses to stimulation with oral carbohydrate.

Therapy

DM2 is the result of a combination of insulin resistance and insulin hyposecretion. Asymptomatic patients with mildly elevated glucose values (slightly >126 mg/dL for fasting or slightly >200 mg/dL for random glucose) may be managed initially with lifestyle modifications, including nutrition therapy (dietary adjustments) and increased exercise. Exercise has been shown to decrease insulin resistance. In most children with new-onset uncomplicated DM2, oral hypoglycemic agents are usually the first line of therapy. These medications include insulin secretagogues and insulin sensitizers. The most common treatment is either metformin or one of the thiazolidinediones. A rare side effect of metformin is lactic acidosis, which occurs mainly in patients with compromised renal function. The most common side effect is gastrointestinal upset. If ketonuria or ketoacidosis occurs, insulin treatment is necessary at first, but may be switched within weeks to oral medications. Insulin can be used in children with DM2, but may lead to continued weight gain. Oral drugs may be used as combinations.

Because DM2 may have a long preclinical course, early diagnosis is possible, including prevention in subjects at risk who have the **metabolic syndrome**. Data are emerging indicating that treatment with insulin sensitizers may delay or prevent development of the full-blown disease. As in adults, significant lifestyle modifications, such as improved eating habits and increased exercise, have a role in preventing or decreasing the morbidity of DM2.

CHAPTER 172
Hypoglycemia

Hypoglycemia in infancy and childhood can result from a large variety of hormonal and metabolic defects (Table 172-1). Hypoglycemia occurs most frequently in the early neonatal period, often as a result of inadequate energy stores to meet the disproportionately large metabolic needs of premature or small for gestational age newborns. Hypoglycemia in the first few days of life in an otherwise normal newborn is less frequent and warrants concern (see Chapter 6). After the initial 2 to 3 days of life, hypoglycemia is far less common and is more frequently the result of endocrine or metabolic disorders.

DEFINITION

Serum glucose concentrations less than 45 mg/dL are considered to be abnormal and necessitate treatment. Serum glucose concentrations less than 55 mg/dL occasionally can occur in normal individuals, especially with prolonged fasting, but should be considered suspect, particularly if there are concurrent symptoms of hypoglycemia (Table 172-2). The **diagnosis** of

TABLE 172–1. Classification of Hypoglycemia in Infants and Children

Abnormalities in the Hormonal Signal Indicating Hypoglycemia

Counterregulatory Hormone Deficiency

Panhypopituitarism
Isolated growth hormone deficiency
ACTH deficiency
Addison disease
Glucagon deficiency
Epinephrine deficiency

Hyperinsulinism

Infant of a diabetic mother
Infant with erythroblastosis fetalis
Persistent hyperinsulinemic hypoglycemias of infancy
Beta cell adenoma (insulinoma)
Beckwith-Wiedemann syndrome
Anti-insulin receptor antibodies

Inadequate Substrate

Prematurity/small for gestational age infant
Ketotic hypoglycemia
Maple syrup urine disease

Disorders of Metabolic Response Pathways

Glycogenolysis

Glucose-6-phosphatase deficiency
Amylo-1,6-glucosidase deficiency
Liver phosphorylase deficiency
Glycogen synthase deficiency

Gluconeogenesis

Fructose-1,6-diphosphatase deficiency
Pyruvate carboxylase deficiency
Phosphenolpyruvate carboxykinase deficiency

Fatty Acid Oxidation

Long, medium, or short chain fatty acid acyl-CoA dehydrogenase deficiency
Carnitine deficiency (primary or secondary)
Carnitine palmitoyltransferase deficiency

Other

Enzymatic defects
  Galactosemia
  Hereditary fructose intolerance
  Propionicacidemia
  Methylmalonic acidemia
  Tyrosinosis
  Glutaric aciduria
Global hepatic dysfunction
Reye syndrome
Hepatitis
Heart failure
Sepsis, shock
Carcinoma/sarcoma (IGF-2 secretion)
Malnutrition-starvation
Hyperviscosity syndrome

Drugs/Intoxications

Oral hypoglycemic agents
Insulin
Alcohol
Salicylates
Propranolol
Valproic acid
Pentamidine
Ackee fruit (unripe)
Quinine
Trimethoprim-sulfamethoxazole (with renal failure)

IGF, insulin-like growth factor.

hypoglycemia should be made on the basis of a low serum glucose concentration, symptoms compatible with hypoglycemia, and resolution of the symptoms after administration of glucose.

Clinical Manifestations

The symptoms and signs of hypoglycemia result from direct depression of the CNS owing to lack of energy substrate and the counterregulatory response to low glucose via catecholamine secretion (see Table 172–2). The manifestations in infants differ compared with the manifestations in older children. Symptoms and signs of hypoglycemia in infants are relatively nonspecific and include jitteriness, feeding difficulties, pallor, hypotonia, hypothermia, episodes of apnea and bradycardia, depressed levels of consciousness, and seizures. In older children, symptoms and signs include confusion, irritability, headaches, visual changes, tremors, pallor, sweating, tachycardia, weakness, seizures, and coma.

Failure to recognize and treat severe prolonged hypoglycemia can result in serious long-term morbidity, including mental retardation and nonhypoglycemic seizures. Younger infants and patients with more severe or prolonged hypoglycemia are at greatest risk for adverse outcomes.

Pathophysiology

Normal regulation of serum glucose concentrations requires appropriate interaction of numerous hormonal signals and metabolic pathways. An overview of

TABLE 172–2.   Symptoms and Signs of Hypoglycemia

Features Associated with Epinephrine Release*	Features Associated with Cerebral Glycopenia
Perspiration	Headache
Palpitation (tachycardia)	Mental confusion
Pallor	Somnolence
Paresthesia	Dysarthria
Trembling	Personality changes
Anxiety	Inability to concentrate
Weakness	Staring
Nausea	Hunger
Vomiting	Convulsions
	Ataxia
	Coma
	Diplopia
	Stroke

*These features may be blunted if the patient is receiving β-blocking agents.

these pathways is presented in Figure 172–1. The components required for glycemic regulation include hormonal signals, energy stores, and metabolic pathways.

HORMONAL SIGNAL

In a normal individual, a decrease in serum glucose concentrations leads to suppression of insulin secretion and increased secretion of the counterregulatory hormones (GH, cortisol, glucagon, and epinephrine). This hormonal signal promotes the release of amino acids (particularly alanine) from muscle to fuel gluconeogenesis and the release of triglyceride from adipose tissue stores to provide FFAs for hepatic ketogenesis. FFAs and ketones serve as alternate fuels. This hormonal signal also stimulates the breakdown of hepatic glycogen and promotes gluconeogenesis. Failure of any of the components of this hormonal signal can lead to hypoglycemia.

Hyperinsulinemia

Failure of suppression of insulin secretion in response to low serum glucose concentrations can occur in infants, but is uncommon beyond the neonatal period. In neonates, this situation arises most frequently in infants of diabetic mothers who have been exposed to high concentrations of maternally derived glucose in utero, resulting in fetal islet cell hyperplasia. The hyperinsulinemic state is transient, usually lasting hours to days.

Hyperinsulinism that persists beyond a few days of age can result from a condition previously referred to as nesidioblastosis, but more appropriately called **persistent hyperinsulinemic hypoglycemia of the newborn**. In these infants, hyperplasia of the pancreatic islet cells develops in the absence of excess stimulation by maternal diabetes. Some patients with persistent hyperinsulinemic hypoglycemia of the newborn have genetic abnormalities of the sulfonylurea receptor or other genetic defects that alter the function of the ATP-sensitive potassium channel that regulates insulin secretion. Hyperinsulinism also can

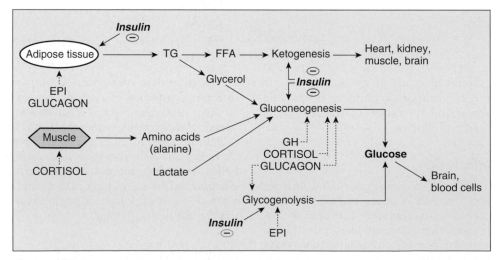

Figure 172–1

Regulation of serum glucose. ⊖ represents inhibitions. EPI, epinephrine; FFA, free fatty acid; GH, growth hormone; TG, triglyceride.

occur in **Beckwith-Wiedemann syndrome**, a condition characterized by neonatal somatic gigantism: macrosomia, macroglossia, omphalocele, visceromegaly, and earlobe creases.

Regardless of the cause, neonates with hyperinsulinism are characteristically large for gestational age (see Chapter 60). Hypoglycemia is severe and frequently occurs within 1 to 3 hours of a feeding. Glucose requirements are increased, often two to three times the normal basal glucose requirement of 4 to 8 mg/kg/min. The *diagnosis* of hyperinsulinism is confirmed by the detection of serum insulin concentrations greater than 5 µU/mL during an episode of hypoglycemia. The absence of serum and urine ketones at the time of hypoglycemia is an important diagnostic feature, distinguishing hyperinsulinism from defects in counterregulatory hormone secretion.

Treatment initially involves the infusion of IV glucose at high rates and of diazoxide to suppress insulin secretion. If this therapy is unsuccessful, long-acting somatostatin analogues can be tried. Often, medical therapy for persistent hyperinsulinemic hypoglycemia of the newborn is unsuccessful, and subtotal (90%) pancreatectomy is required to prevent long-term neurologic sequelae of hypoglycemia.

In children, hyperinsulinemia is rare and usually results from an **islet cell adenoma**. Children with this condition characteristically have a voracious appetite, obesity, and accelerated linear growth. As in infants, *diagnosis* requires demonstration of insulin concentrations greater than 5 µU/mL during an episode of hypoglycemia. CT or MRI of the pancreas should be attempted, but visualization of an adenoma is usually difficult. Surgical removal of the adenoma is curative.

Factitious Hyperinsulinemia

In rare cases, insulin or a hypoglycemic medication is administered by a parent or caregiver to a child as a form of child abuse, which is a condition referred to as **Munchausen syndrome by proxy**. This *diagnosis* should be suspected if extremely high insulin concentrations are detected (>100 µU/mL). C-peptide concentrations are low or undetectable, which confirms that the insulin is from an exogenous source.

Defects in Counterregulatory Hormones

Abnormalities in the secretion of counterregulatory hormones that produce hypoglycemia usually involve GH, cortisol, or both. Deficiencies in glucagon and epinephrine secretion are rare. GH and cortisol deficiency occur as a result of hypopituitarism. Hypopituitarism results from congenital hypoplasia or aplasia of the pituitary or more commonly from deficiency of hypothalamic releasing factors (see Chapter 173). Clues to

this diagnosis in infants include the presence of hypoglycemia in association with midline facial or neurologic defects (e.g., cleft lip and palate or absence of the corpus callosum), pendular nystagmus (indicating visual impairment from possible abnormalities in the development of the optic nerves, which can occur in septo-optic dysplasia), and the presence of microphallus and cryptorchidism in boys (indicating abnormalities in gonadotropin secretion). Jaundice and hepatomegaly also can occur, simulating neonatal hepatitis. Despite the presence of GH deficiency, these infants are usually of normal size at birth. Older children with hypopituitarism usually have short stature and a subnormal growth velocity.

Deficient cortisol secretion also can occur in primary adrenal insufficiency resulting from a variety of causes. In infants, primary adrenal insufficiency often results from congenital adrenal hyperplasia (CAH), most frequently as a result of 21-hydroxylase deficiency (see Chapter 177). In older children, primary adrenal insufficiency is seen most frequently in **Addison disease**, but it also can occur in adrenoleukodystrophy and other disorders (see Chapter 178). Addison disease should be suspected if there is hyperpigmentation of the skin, a history of salt cravings, hyponatremia, and hyperkalemia.

Confirmation of GH or cortisol deficiency as the cause of hypoglycemia requires the detection of low serum GH and cortisol concentrations during an episode of hypoglycemia or after other stimulatory testing. In contrast to hyperinsulinism, serum and urine ketones are positive at the time of hypoglycemia, and FFAs are elevated. Treatment involves supplementation of the deficient hormones in physiologic doses.

ENERGY STORES

Sufficient energy stores in the form of glycogen, adipose tissue, and muscle are necessary to respond appropriately to hypoglycemia. Deficiencies in these stores are a common cause of hypoglycemia in neonates who are small for gestational age or premature (see Chapter 60). Beyond the early neonatal period, energy stores are usually sufficient to meet the metabolic requirements except in malnourished children. Release of substrate from energy stores is thought to be abnormal in one common form of childhood hypoglycemia, ketotic hypoglycemia.

Ketotic Hypoglycemia

Ketotic hypoglycemia is usually seen in children between 18 months and 5 years of age. It is the most common cause of new-onset hypoglycemia in children older than 2 years of age. Patients have symptoms of hypoglycemia after a period of prolonged fasting, often in the setting of an intercurrent illness with decreased feeding. Children with this disorder are often thin and small and may have a history of being small for gestational age. Defective mobilization of alanine from muscle to fuel gluconeogenesis is thought to be the cause, although the condition may derive mostly from being a small child and having lower fuel reserves. Because there are no specific diagnostic tests for this disorder, ketotic hypoglycemia is a *diagnosis of exclusion*.

Treatment involves avoidance of fasting and frequent feedings of a high-protein, high-carbohydrate diet. Patients may require hospitalization for IV glucose infusion if they cannot maintain adequate oral intake during a period of illness. The disorder usually resolves spontaneously by 7 to 8 years of age.

METABOLIC RESPONSE PATHWAYS

Maintenance of normal serum glucose concentrations in the fasting state requires glucose production via glycogenolysis and gluconeogenesis and the production of alternative energy sources (FFAs and ketones) via lipolysis and fatty acid oxidation.

Glycogenolysis

Glycogen storage diseases occur in a variety of subtypes that differ in severity (see Chapter 52). Among the subtypes that result in hypoglycemia, the most severe form is glucose-6-phosphatase deficiency. This subtype is characterized by severe hypoglycemia, massive hepatomegaly, growth retardation, and lactic acidosis. In contrast, deficiencies in the glycogen phosphorylase enzymes may cause isolated hepatomegaly with or without hypoglycemia.

The *diagnosis* of glycogen storage disease is suggested by a finding of hepatomegaly without splenomegaly. Ketosis occurs with hypoglycemic episodes. Confirmation of the diagnosis requires specific biochemical studies of leukocytes or liver biopsy specimens. *Treatment* involves frequent high-carbohydrate feedings during the day and continuous feedings at night via nasogastric tube. Feedings of uncooked cornstarch during bedtime are sufficient to maintain serum glucose concentrations in some patients.

Gluconeogenesis

Defects in gluconeogenesis are uncommon and include fructose-1,6-diphosphatase deficiency and phosphoenolpyruvate carboxykinase deficiency. Affected patients exhibit fasting hypoglycemia, hepatomegaly caused by fatty infiltration, lactic acidosis, and hyperuricemia. Ketosis occurs, and FFA and alanine concentrations are high. *Treatment* involves frequent high-carbohydrate, low-protein feedings (see Chapter 52).

Fatty Acid Oxidation

Fatty acid oxidation disorders of ketogenesis include the fatty acid acyl-coenzyme A (CoA) dehydrogenase deficiencies; long chain, medium chain, and short chain acyl-CoA dehydrogenase deficiencies; and hereditary carnitine deficiency (see Chapter 55). Of these disorders, medium chain acyl-CoA dehydrogenase deficiency is the most common; it occurs in 1 in 9000 to 15,000 live births. Patients often are well in infancy and have the first episode of hypoglycemia at 2 years of age or older. Episodes of hypoglycemia usually occur with prolonged fasting or during episodes of intercurrent illness.

Mild hepatomegaly may be present along with mild hyperammonemia, hyperuricemia, and mild elevations in hepatic transaminases. Ketone concentrations are low or undetected. The *diagnosis* is confirmed by the finding of elevated concentrations of dicarboxylic acids in the urine. *Treatment* involves avoidance of fasting.

Other Metabolic Disorders

Many metabolic disorders can lead to hypoglycemia, including galactosemia, hereditary fructose intolerance, and disorders of organic acid metabolism (see Table 172–1). Hypoglycemia in these disorders is usually a reflection of global hepatic dysfunction secondary to the buildup of hepatotoxic intermediates. Many of these disorders present with low concentrations of ketone bodies because ketogenesis also is affected. The finding of non–glucose-reducing substances in the urine suggests a diagnosis of galactosemia or hereditary fructose intolerance. Occurrence of symptoms after ingestion of fructose or sucrose **suggests hereditary fructose intolerance**. *Treatment* requires dietary restriction of the specific offending substances.

MEDICATIONS AND INTOXICATION

Hypoglycemia can occur as an adverse effect of numerous medications, including insulin, oral hypoglycemic agents, and propranolol, and as a result of salicylate intoxication. Valproate toxicity can cause a disorder similar to that seen in the fatty acid oxidation defects. Ethanol ingestion also can cause hypoglycemia, especially in younger children, because the metabolism of ethanol results in the depletion of cofactors necessary for gluconeogenesis.

REACTIVE HYPOGLYCEMIA

The term *reactive hypoglycemia* has been used to describe hypoglycemia occurring 2 to 3 hours after a meal. This condition can occur in patients who have the *dumping syndrome* as a consequence of gastric surgery. Rapid gastric emptying results in a rapid increase of serum glucose and excess stimulation of insulin secretion.

Rarely, transient reactive hypoglycemia can occur in patients who later have DM1. Delayed insulin secretion in response to elevations in serum glucose concentrations is thought to be responsible for this phenomenon.

Diagnosis

Because the list of causes of hypoglycemia is long and complex, establishing the *etiology* in a particular patient can be difficult. Frequently, it is difficult to make an accurate diagnosis until one can obtain a *critical sample* of blood and urine at the time of the hypoglycemic episode. In a child with unexplained hypoglycemia, a serum sample should be obtained before treatment for the measurement of glucose and insulin, GH, cortisol, FFAs, and β-hydroxybutyrate. Measurement of serum lactate levels also should be considered. A urine specimen should be obtained for measuring ketones and reducing substances. Hypoglycemia without ketonuria suggests hyperinsulinism or a defect in fatty acid oxidation. The results of this initial testing can establish whether endocrine causes are responsible and, if not, provide initial information regarding which types of metabolic disorders are most likely. Whenever possible, additional samples of blood and urine should be frozen for further analysis if necessary.

Emergency Management

Acute care of a patient with hypoglycemia consists of rapid administration of IV glucose (2 mL/kg of 10% dextrose in water). After the initial bolus of glucose, an infusion of IV glucose should be established to provide approximately 1.5 times the normal hepatic glucose production rate (8 to 12 mg/kg/min in infants, 6 to 8 mg/kg/min in children). Higher infusion rates may be needed for hyperinsulinemic states. This infusion allows for suppression of the catabolic state and prevents further decompensation in patients with certain metabolic disorders. If adrenal insufficiency is suspected, stress doses of glucocorticoids should be administered.

CHAPTER 173
Short Stature

GROWTH

Normal growth is the final common pathway of many factors, including endocrine, environmental, nutritional, and genetic influences (see Chapter 5). Maintenance of a normal linear growth pattern is good evidence of overall health and can be considered a "bioassay" for the well-being of the whole child. The effects of certain hormones on growth and ultimate height are listed in Table 173-1. Just as various factors influence stature, stature itself influences psychological, social, and potentially economic well-being. Parental concern about the psychosocial consequences of abnormal stature is a common factor that causes a family to seek medical attention. There is an increased bias toward "heightism," particularly among males, and the physician must be sensitized to the overall context of a particular youngster's attention to stature.

Growth Hormone Physiology

GH secretion is stimulated by hypothalamic GH-releasing factor (GRF) and inhibited by GH release inhibitory factor (somatostatin, SRIF), which interact with their individual receptors on the somatotrope in a noncompetitive manner. GH circulates with a GH-binding protein (GHBP) that is the proteolytic product of the extracellular domain of the membrane-bound GH receptor; GHBP abundance reflects the abundance of GH receptors. GH secretion causes production and secretion of IGF-1 and IGF-2 in many tissues of the body, including the liver. IGF-1 is most closely associated with postnatal growth, and serum concentrations of IGF-1 follow serum concentration of GH. IGF-1 production also is decreased in states of malnutrition in which, paradoxically, GH secretion is increased; in malnutrition, the abundance of GH receptors decreases and unlinks the relationship between increasing GH and increasing IGF-1 production. In obesity, the opposite happens, and GH secretion decreases to low levels, but IGF-1 concentrations remain normal. GH also stimulates the production of six different IGF binding proteins in the liver, kidney, and other tissues. Some IGF binding proteins are inhibitory, and some increase IGF activity. There are at least four proteins with lesser affinity for IGF-1, called *IGFBP-related proteins*. IGF BP3 is measurable in clinical assays and is itself GH dependent, but less influenced by nutrition and age than is IGF-1; measuring IGF-1 and IGF BP3 is useful in evaluating GH adequacy.

IGF-1 acts primarily as a paracrine and autocrine agent, so the IGF-1 measured in the peripheral circulation is far removed from the site of action and is an imperfect reflection of IGF-1 physiology. IGF-1 resembles insulin in structure, and the IGF-1 receptor resembles the insulin receptor, so cross-reaction of one agent, if present in excess, can cause physiologic effects usually attributed to the other agent. This has been referred to as specificity spillover. When IGF-1 attaches to its membrane-bound receptor, second messengers are stimulated to change the physiology of the cell and produce growth effects.

TABLE 173–1.   Hormonal Effects on Growth

Hormone	Bone Age	Growth Rate	Adult Height*
Androgen excess	Advanced	Increased	Diminished
Androgen deficiency	Normal or delayed	Normal or decreased	Increased slightly or normal
Thyroxine excess	Advanced	Increased	Normal or diminished
Thyroxine deficiency	Retarded	Decreased	Diminished
Growth hormone excess	Normal or advanced	Increased	Excessive
Growth hormone deficiency	Retarded	Decreased	Diminished
Cortisol excess	Retarded	Decreased	Diminished
Cortisol deficiency	Normal	Normal	Normal

*Effect in most patients with treatment.
Adapted from Underwood LE, Van Wyk JJ: Normal and aberrant growth. In Wilson JD, Foster DW (eds): Textbook of Endocrinology, 8th ed. Philadelphia, WB Saunders; 1992.

MEASUREMENT OF GROWTH

Accurate measurements of height, or length, and weight should be plotted on the Centers for Disease Control and Prevention growth charts for the timely diagnosis of growth disorders (see Chapter 5; the charts can be downloaded at http://www.cdc.gov/growthcharts/). The correct measurement of an infant's length requires one adult to hold the infant's head still and another adult to extend the feet with the soles perpendicular to the lower legs. A caliper-like device such as an infantometer is used, or the movable plates on an infant scale are slid until one rests at the top of the infant's head and the other at the bottom of the infant's feet perpendicular to a ruler so that the exact distance between the two plates can be determined. It is never accurate to measure an infant lying on a sheet of paper on the examining table by making a mark at the moving head and another at the moving feet and determining the distance between the two. If this technique is used, a true disorder of growth may be missed, or a disorder of growth may be suspected in a normal child.

After 2 years of age, the height of a child should be measured in the standing position. A decrease of roughly 1.25 cm in height measurement may occur when the child is measured in the standing position rather than in the lying position; many children who appear to be "not growing" are referred to a subspecialist, when all that has changed is the position of the child at the time of measurement. Children measured in the standing position should be barefoot against a hard surface, where they can place the back with legs straight, bare feet together, and all aspects of the body pressed as far back as possible against the upright surface. A Harpenden stadiometer or equivalent device is optimal for the measurement of stature, but the flexible bars that extend upward on some health scales are unreliable and may be misleading.

Measurement Marfan or **arm span** is essential when the diagnosis of Marfan or Klinefelter syndrome, short-limbed dwarfism, or other dysmorphic conditions is considered. Arm span is measured as the distance between the tips of the fingers when the patient holds both arms outstretched horizontally while standing against a solid surface. The **upper-to-lower segment ratio** is the result of the ratio of the upper segment (determined by subtraction of the measurement from the symphysis pubis to the floor [known as the lower segment] from the total height) to the lower segment. This ratio changes with age. A normal term infant has an upper-to-lower ratio of 1.7:1, a 1-year-old has a ratio of 1.4:1, and a 10-year-old has a ratio of 1:1. Conditions of hypogonadism, not commonly discerned or suspected until after the normal age for onset of puberty, lead to greatly decreased upper-to-lower ratio in an adult, whereas long-lasting and untreated hypothyroidism leads to a high upper-to-lower ratio in the child.

ENDOCRINE FACTORS AFFECTING GROWTH

GH, or somatotropin, is a 191-amino acid protein secreted by the pituitary gland under the control of GRF and SRIF (see Fig. 170–4). GH secretion is enhanced by α-adrenergic stimulation, hypoglycemia, starvation, exercise, early stages of sleep, and stress. GH secretion is inhibited by β-adrenergic stimulation, hyperglycemia, and GH treatment itself. GH has direct effects (e.g., diabetogenic activity) and indirect effects (many aspects of growth) mediated by the IGFs. Serum concentrations of GH are low throughout the day except for occasional peaks within the 24-hour period, most often in the middle of the night or early morning. The ascertainment of GH deficiency on the basis of a single determination of a random GH concentration is impossible. Adequacy of GH secretion may be determined by a stimulation test to measure peak GH secretion (see Table 170–2). A normal response is a vigorous secretory peak after stimulation, whereas the lack of such a peak is consistent with GH deficiency. However, there is a high false-positive rate (on any day, about 10% or more of normal children may not reach the normal GH peak after even two stimulatory tests and would be labeled inappropriately as GH deficient). Indirect measurements of GH secretion, such as serum concentrations of IGF1 and IGFBP3, are replacing GH stimulatory tests.

Most of the effects of GH on stature are the result of GH-stimulated production of IGFs. Serum IGF-1 values are related to GH secretion, rising in GH excess and decreasing in GH deficiency. Because malnutrition, such as protein calorie malnutrition or anorexia nervosa, decreases IGF-1 levels even though it increases GH secretion, IGF-1 is not an infallible reflection of GH secretion. IGF-2 levels decrease in GH deficiency but do not rise above normal values in GH excess. IGF-2 seems to have a prominent role in fetal growth.

The factors responsible for postnatal growth are not the same as the factors that mediate fetal growth. **Thyroid hormone** is essential for normal postnatal growth, although a thyroid hormone–deficient fetus achieves a normal birth length; similarly, a GH-deficient fetus has a normal birth length, although in IGF-1 deficiency resulting from GH resistance (**Laron dwarfism**), fetuses are shorter than controls. Adequate thyroid hormone is necessary to allow the secretion of GH. Hypothyroid patients may appear falsely to be GH deficient; with thyroid hormone repletion, GH secretion normalizes. Gonadal steroids are important in the pubertal growth spurt. The effects of other hormones on growth are noted in Table 173–1.

ABNORMALITIES OF GROWTH
Short Stature of Nonendocrine Causes

Short stature is defined as subnormal height relative to other children of the same sex and age, taking family heights into consideration. The Centers for Disease Control and Prevention growth charts use the 3rd percentile of the growth curve as the demarcation of the lower limit, but pathologic short stature is usually 3.5 SDs below the mean, which is far below the 3rd percentile; growth charts that show curves down to these low limits are rare. **Growth failure** denotes a slow growth rate regardless of stature. Ultimately a slow growth rate leads to short stature, but a disease process is detected sooner if the decreased growth rate is noted before the stature becomes short. Height velocity may be plotted on special charts. Plotted on a growth chart, growth failure appears as a curve that crosses

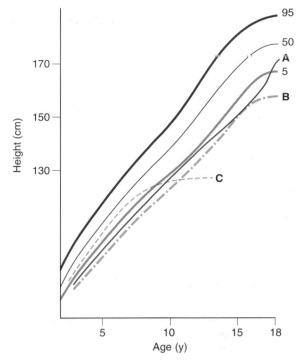

Figure 173–1

Patterns of linear growth. Normal growth percentiles (5th, 50th, and 95th) are shown along with typical growth curves for **A**, constitutional delay of growth and adolescence (short stature with normal growth rate for bone age, delayed pubertal growth spurt, and eventual achievement of normal adult stature); **B**, familial short stature (short stature in childhood and as an adult); and **C**, acquired pathologic growth failure (e.g., acquired untreated primary hypothyroidism). (See Chapter 5.)

percentiles and is associated with a height velocity below the 5th percentile of height velocity for age (Fig. 173-1). A corrected mid-parental, or genetic target, height helps determine if the child is growing well for the family; it is calculated by finding the average height of the parents and adding 6.5 cm (2.5 inches) for a male patient or subtracting 6.5 cm from a female patient to correct for the average difference between adult height of men and women in the U.S. of 13 cm (5 inches). To determine a range of normal height for the family under consideration, the corrected mid-parental height is bracketed by 2 SDs, which for the U.S. is approximately 10 cm (4 inches). The range limited by 10 cm (4 inches) above and 10 cm (4 inches) below the corrected mid-parental height represents a range of expected adult height for the child, or the target height. The presence of a height 3.5 SDs below the mean, a height velocity below the 5th percentile for age, or a height below the target height corrected for mid-parental height requires a diagnostic evaluation.

Nutrition is the most important factor affecting growth on a worldwide basis (see Chapter 28). Failure to thrive may develop in the infant as a result of **maternal deprivation** (nutritional deficiency or aberrant psychosocial interaction) or as a result of organic illness (anorexia, nutrient losses through a form of malabsorption, or hypermetabolism caused by hyperthyroidism) (see Chapter 21). Psychological difficulties also can affect growth, as in **psychosocial** or **deprivation dwarfism**, in which the child develops functional temporary GH deficiency and poor growth as a result of psychological abuse; when placed in a different, healthier psychosocial environment, GH physiology normalizes, and growth occurs.

The common condition known as **constitutional delay in growth or puberty or both** is a variation of normal growth, caused by a delayed tempo, or cadence, of physiologic development and not a disease (Table 173-2; see also Fig. 173-1). Usually a family member had delayed growth or puberty (a mother who had late onset of puberty or menarche or a father who started to shave late or grew in stature into his 20s), but achieved a near-normal final height. The bone age is delayed more than 2 SDs from normal, but the growth rate remains mostly within the lower limits of normal. Constitutional delay usually leads to a delay in secondary sexual development. Genetic or familial short stature (Table 173-3) refers to the stature of a child of short parents, who is expected to reach a lower than average height and yet normal for these parents. If the parents were malnourished as children, grew up in a zone of war, or suffered famine, the heights of the parents are less predictive. The combination of constitutional growth delay and genetic short stature leads to more obvious short stature and brings the child to medical attention earlier and more frequently than a child who simply has one of the conditions. Although there are differences in height associated with ethnic differences, the most significant difference in stature between ethnic groups is the result of nutrition. Growth curves exist for Asian children.

Phenotypic features suggesting an underlying chromosomal disorder can occur in a host of syndromes, and these can be suspected by attending to arm spans and upper-to-lower segment ratios. Recognizable physical syndromes of short stature often combine obesity and decreased height, whereas otherwise normal obese children are usually taller than average and have advanced skeletal development and physical maturation (see Table 173-2). The **Prader-Willi syndrome** includes fetal and infantile hypotonia, small hands and feet (acromicria), postnatal acquired obesity with an insatiable appetite, developmental delay, hypogonadism, almond-shaped eyes, and abnormalities of the SNRP portion of the 15th chromosome at 15q11-q13. Most cases have deletion of the paternal sequence, but about 20% to 25% have uniparental disomy, in which both chromosomes 15 derive from the mother; if both chromosomes 15 come from the father, Angelman syndrome develops. **Laurence-Moon-Bardet-Biedl syndrome** is characterized by retinitis pigmentosa, hypogonadism, and developmental delay with autosomal dominant inheritance pattern. Laurence-Moon syndrome is associated with spastic paraplegia, however, and Bardet-Biedl syndrome is associated with obesity and polydactyly. **Pseudohypoparathyroidism** leads to short stature and developmental delay with short fourth and fifth digits (Albright hereditary osteodystrophy phenotype), with resistance to PTH and resultant hypocalcemia and elevated levels of serum phosphorus.

SHORT STATURE CAUSED BY GROWTH HORMONE DEFICIENCY

Etiology and Epidemiology

Classic congenital or **idiopathic GH deficiency** occurs in about 1 in 4000 to 10,000 children. Idiopathic GH deficiency is a hypothalamic disease of inadequate GRF; the pituitary gland can manufacture GH, but does not secrete it for lack of trophic stimulation. Less often, GH deficiency is caused by anatomic defects of the pituitary gland; in genetic forms, any number of gene defects can occur. Hereditary forms of GH deficiency have been described that affect pituitary differentiation, that result in heterogeneous defects of the gene for GH or of the GRF receptor or of the GH receptor. *Classic GH deficiency* is the term that refers to very reduced to absent secretion of GH; numerous short children may have intermediate forms of decreased GH secretion (partial GH deficiency or neurosecretory disorder). Acquired GH deficiency causing late-onset growth failure suggests the possibility of a **tumor** of the hypothalamus or pituitary (Table 173-4).

Clinical Manifestations

Infants with congenital GH deficiency achieve a normal or near-normal birth length and weight at term, but the growth rate slows after birth, most noticeably after age 2 to 3 years, as these children become progressively shorter for age. They also tend to have an elevated weight-to-height ratio and appear chubby and short. Careful measurements in the first year of life may suggest the diagnosis, but most patients elude diagnosis until several years of age because of inaccurate height measurements and lack of suspicion. A patient with classic GH deficiency has the appearance of a cherub (a chubby, immature appearance), with a high-pitched voice resulting from an immature larynx. Unless severe hypoglycemia occurred or dysraphism

TABLE 173–2. Causes of Short Stature

Variations of Normal	Syndromes of Short Stature
Constitutional (delayed bone age) Genetic (short familial heights)	Turner syndrome (syndrome of gonadal dysgenesis) Noonan syndrome (pseudo–Turner syndrome) Autosomal trisomy 13, 18, 21 Prader-Willi syndrome
Endocrine Disorders	Laurence-Moon-Bardet-Biedl syndrome Autosomal abnormalities Dysmorphic syndromes (e.g., Russell-Silver, Cornelia

GH deficiency
Congenital
  Isolated GH deficiency
  With other pituitary hormone deficiencies
  With midline defects
  Pituitary agenesis
  With gene deficiency
	de Lange)
	Pseudohypoparathyroidism
	
	Chronic Disease

Acquired
  Hypothalamic/pituitary tumors
  Histiocytosis X (Langerhans cell histiocytosis)
  CNS infections and granulomas
  Head trauma (birth and later)
  Hypothalamic/pituitary radiation
  CNS vascular accidents
  Hydrocephalus
  Autoimmune
  Psychosocial dwarfism (functional GH deficiency)
  Amphetamine treatment for hyperactivity*
	Cardiac disorders
	  Left-to-right shunt
	  Congestive heart failure
	Pulmonary disorders
	  Cystic fibrosis
	  Asthma
	Gastrointestinal disorders
	  Malabsorption (e.g., celiac disease)
	  Disorders of swallowing
	  Inflammatory bowel disease
	Hepatic disorders

Laron dwarfism (increased GH and decreased IGF1)
Pygmies (normal GH and IGF2 but decreased IGF1)
Hypothyroidism
Glucocorticoid excess
  Endogenous
  Exogenous
Diabetes mellitus under poor control
Diabetes insipidus (untreated)
Hypophosphatemic vitamin D–resistant rickets
Virilizing congenital adrenal hyperplasia (tall child,
  short adult)
P-450$_{c21}$, P-450$_{c11}$ deficiencies
	Hematologic disorders
	  Sickle cell anemia
	  Thalassemia
	Renal disorders
	  Renal tubular acidosis
	  Chronic uremia
	Immunologic disorders
	  Connective tissue disease
	  Juvenile rheumatoid arthritis
	  Chronic infection
	  AIDS
	Hereditary fructose intolerance

Skeletal Dysplasias	**Malnutrition**
Osteogenesis imperfecta Osteochondroplasias	Kwashiorkor, marasmus Iron deficiency Zinc deficiency
Lysosomal Storage Diseases	Anorexia caused by chemotherapy for neoplasms
Mucopolysaccharidoses Mucolipidoses	

IGF, insulin-like growth factor.
*Only if caloric intake severely diminished.
Modified from Styne DM: Growth disorder. In Fitzgerald PA (ed): Handbook of Clinical Endocrinology. Norwalk, Conn, Appleton & Lange, 1986.

(midline defects) of the head includes a CNS defect that affects mentation, the patient has normal intellectual growth and age-appropriate speech. Male neonates with isolated GH deficiency with or without gonadotropin deficiency may have a microphallus (a stretched penile length of <2 cm [normal is 3 to 5 cm])

and fasting hypoglycemia. Patients who lack ACTH in addition to GH may have more profound hypoglycemia because cortisol is another hormone that stimulates gluconeogenesis.

GH resistance or GH insensitivity is caused by abnormal number or function of GH receptors or a

TABLE 173–3. Differential Diagnosis and Therapy of Short Stature

	Hypopituitarism GH Deficiency (Possibly with GnRH, CRH, or TRH Deficiency)	Constitutional Delay	Familial Short Stature	Deprivational Dwarfism	Turner Syndrome	Hypothyroidism	Chronic Disease
Family history positive	Rare	Frequent	Always	No	No	Variable	Variable
Gender	Both	Males more than females	Both	Both	Female	Both	Both
Facies	Immature or with midline defect (e.g., cleft palate or optic hypoplasias)	Immature	Normal	Normal	Turner facies or normal	Coarse (cretin if congenital)	Normal
Sexual development	Delayed	Delayed	Normal	May be delayed	Female prepubertal	Usually delayed, may be precocious if hypothyroidism is severe	Delayed
Bone age	Delayed	Delayed	Normal	Usually delayed; growth arrest lines present	Delayed	Delayed	Delayed
Dentition	Delayed	Normal; delay usual	Normal	Variable	Normal	Delayed	Normal or delayed
Hypoglycemia	Variable	No	No	No	No	No	No
Karyotype	Normal	Normal	Normal	Normal	45,X or partial deletion of X chromosome or mosaic	Normal	Normal
Free T$_4$	Low (if TRH-deficient) or normal	Normal	Normal	Normal or low	Normal: hypothyroidism may be acquired	Low	Normal
Stimulated GH	Low	Normal for bone age	Normal	Possibly low, or high if malnourished	Usually normal	Low	Usually normal
Insulin-like growth factor I	Low	Normal or low for chronologic age	Normal	Low	Normal	Low	Low or normal (depending on nutritional status)
Therapy	Replace deficiencies	Reassurance; sex steroids to initiate secondary sexual development in selected patients	None	Change or improve environment	Sex hormone replacement, GH; oxandrolone may be useful	T$_4$	Treat malnutrition, organ failure (e.g., dialysis, transplant, cardiotonic drugs, insulin)

ACTH, adrenocorticotropic hormone; CRH, corticotropin-releasing hormone; GH, growth hormone; GnRH, gonadotropin-releasing hormone; T$_4$, thyroxine; TRH, thyrotropin-releasing hormone.

TABLE 173–4. Growth Failure: Screening Tests

Test	Rationale
CBC	*Anemia:* nutritional, chronic disease, malignancy *Leukocytosis:* inflammation, infection *Leukopenia:* bone marrow failure syndromes *Thrombocytopenia:* malignancy, infection
ESR, CRP	Inflammation of infection, inflammatory diseases, malignancy
Metabolic panel (electrolytes, liver enzymes, BUN)	Signs of acute or chronic hepatic, renal, adrenal dysfunction; hydration and acid-base status
Carotene, folate, and prothrombin time; celiac antibody panel	Assess malabsorption; detect celiac disease
Urinalysis with pH	Signs of renal dysfunction, hydration, water and salt homeostasis; renal tubular acidosis
Karyotype	Determines Turner (XO) or other syndromes
Cranial imaging (MRI)	Assesses hypothalamic-pituitary tumors (craniopharyngioma, glioma, germinoma) or congenital midline defects
Bone age	Compare with height age, and evaluate height potential
IGF1, IGF BP3	Reflects growth hormone status or nutrition
Free thyroxine	Detects panhypopituitarism or isolated hypothyroidism
Prolactin	Elevated in hypothalamic dysfunction or destruction, suppressed in pituitary disease

CBC, complete blood count; CRP, C-reactive protein; ESR, erythrocyte sedimentation rate; IGF BP3, insulin-like growth factor binding protein 3.

postreceptor defect. Patients with the autosomal recessive **Laron syndrome**, with mutations of the GH receptor, have a prominent forehead, blue sclerae, delayed dentition and bone maturation, and low blood glucose. They have elevated serum GH concentrations, although serum IGF-1 and IGF BP3 concentrations are low. The characteristic decrease in the number of GH receptors is reflected in the decreased serum concentration of GH-binding protein. The patients do not respond to the administration of GH with an increase in growth or an increase in serum concentrations of IGF-1 or IGF BP3. Subjects with Laron syndrome have been treated experimentally with recombinant human IGF-1 with variable degrees of success. Malnutrition or severe liver disease may cause acquired GH resistance because serum GH is elevated, and IGF-1 is decreased.

Diagnosis

If family or other medical history does not provide a likely diagnosis, screening tests should include a metabolic panel to evaluate kidney and liver function, a complete blood count to rule out anemia, and a celiac panel with antibodies to tissue transglutaminase to rule out celiac disease and carotene and folate levels to reflect nutrition and rule out malabsorption. A urinalysis aids in evaluation of renal function, and urinary pH and serum bicarbonate can be obtained to ascertain whether renal tubular acidosis is present. In a girl without another explanation for short stature, a karyotype may be obtained to rule out **Turner syndrome**.

After chronic disease or familial short stature is ruled out, and routine laboratory testing is completed and normal (see Table 173–4), two GH stimulatory tests are commonly performed (see Table 170–2). GH testing should be offered to a patient who is short (<5th percentile and usually >3.5 SDs below the mean), who is growing poorly (<5th percentile growth rate for age), or whose height projection, based on current height and skeletal maturation as assessed by bone age, is below the target height when corrected for family height.

Classic GH-deficient patients do not show an increase in serum GH levels after stimulation by various secretagogues. Some patients release GH in response to secretagogue testing, but cannot release GH spontaneously during the day or night. Measuring serum IGF-1 and IGF BP3 is helpful but not consistently helpful in establishing a diagnosis of GH deficiency and the basis for growth-promoting therapy. Tests for GH deficiency are insensitive, in that these do not consistently allow segregation of GH-sufficient from GH-deficient. In equivocal cases, an operational definition of GH deficiency might be that patients who require GH grow significantly faster when administered a normal dose of GH than before treatment.

Treatment

GH deficiency is treated with biosynthetic recombinant DNA–derived GH; preparations differ as to form (powder that needs diluent versus premixed preparation), injection device (syringes, pen devices, needleless device), and frequency of administration (daily, six times per week, or every 2 to 4 weeks using a depot form of GH). Dosage also is titrated to the growth rate. Treatment with GH carries the risk of an increased incidence of slipped capital femoral epiphysis, especially in rapidly growing adolescents, and pseudotumor cerebri.

Human cadaver–derived pituitary GH is no longer used because of the risk of contamination with the neurodegenerative infectious Jakob-Creutzfeldt agent or prions.

Administration of GH to patients with normal GH responsiveness to secretagogues is controversial, but as noted earlier, diagnostic tests are imperfect; if the patient is growing extremely slowly without alternative explanation, GH therapy is sometimes used. GH is effective in increasing the growth rate and final height in Turner syndrome and in chronic renal failure; GH also is used for treatment of short stature and muscle weakness of Prader-Willi syndrome. Other indications include children born small for gestational age who have not exhibited catch-up growth by 2 years of age and the long-term treatment of idiopathic short stature with height 2.25 SDs or less below the mean. This condition also is called non–GH-deficient short stature.

Psychological support of children with severe short stature is important because they may become the object of ridicule by classmates. Although there is controversy, marital status, satisfaction with life, and vocational achievement may be decreased in children of short stature who are not given supportive measures.

CHAPTER 174
Disorders of Puberty

The staging of pubertal changes and the sequence of events are discussed in Chapter 67 (see also Chapter 68). The onset of puberty is marked by pubarche and gonadarche. **Pubarche** results from adrenal maturation or adrenarche, which is the appearance of pubic hair. Other features are oiliness of hair and skin, acne, axillary hair, and body odor. Adrenarche does not include breast development in females or testicular enlargement in males. **Gonadarche** is characterized by increasing secretion of gonadal sex steroids as a result of the maturation of the hypothalamic-pituitary-gonadal axis. These sex steroids differ by gender, consisting of testosterone from the testes and estradiol and progesterone from the ovaries. In males, physical signs are pubic hair, axillary hair, facial hair, increased muscularity, deeper voice, increased penile size, and increased testicular volume. In females, the physical signs are breast development, development of the female body habitus, increased size of the uterus, and menarche with regular menstrual cycles. The third component is the growth spurt of puberty.

Hypothalamic GnRH, produced by cells in the arcuate nucleus, is secreted from the median eminence of the hypothalamus into the pituitary portal system and reaches the membrane receptors on the pituitary gonadotropes to cause the production and release of luteinizing hormone (LH) and follicle-stimulating hormone (FSH) into the circulation. In females, FSH stimulates the ovarian production of estrogen and later in puberty causes the formation and support of corpus luteum. In males, LH stimulates the production of testosterone from the Leydig cells; later in puberty, FSH stimulates the development and support of the seminiferous tubules. The gonads also produce the protein inhibin. Both sex steroids and inhibin suppress the secretion of gonadotropins. The interplay of the products of the gonads and GnRH modulates the serum concentrations of gonadotropins. GnRH is released in episodic pulses that vary during development and during the menstrual period. These pulses ensure that gonadotropins are released in a pulsatile manner. With the onset of puberty, the amplitude of the pulses of gonadotropins increases, first at night and then throughout the day. Sex steroids are secreted in response, first during the night and then throughout the day. This endocrine change of puberty may be shown by obtaining frequent blood samples or by the administration of exogenous GnRH. The hypothalamic-pituitary-gonadal axis is active in the fetus and newborn, but is suppressed in the childhood years until activity increases again at the onset of puberty.

Adrenarche occurs several years earlier than gonadarche and is heralded by increasing circulating dehydroepiandrosterone (DHEA) or androstenedione. Serum DHEA increases years before the appearance of its effects, such as the development of pubic or axillary hair.

DELAYED PUBERTY

Puberty is delayed when there is no sign of pubertal development by age 13 years in girls and 14 years in boys living in the U.S. (Tables 174–1 and 174–2).

Constitutional Delay in Growth and Adolescence

Patients with short stature secondary to constitutional delay exhibit a significantly delayed bone age (2 SDs below the mean, which is equal to a 1.5- to 2-year delay as a teenager). The height of the patient should remain close to the genetic potential, based on the parental heights, when reinterpreted for that bone age (see Table 174–2 and Chapter 173). The bone age should be consistent with the somatic maturity of the patient. Usually, height gain is below, although fairly parallel to, the normal percentiles on the growth curve. The prepubertal nadir, or deceleration before their pubertal growth spurt, is prolonged or protracted. These patients have delayed onset of pubertal development.

TABLE 174–1. Classification of Delayed Puberty and Sexual Infantilism

Constitutional delay in growth and puberty
Hypogonadotropic hypogonadism
  CNS disorders
    Tumors (craniopharyngioma, germinoma, glioma, prolactinoma)
    Congenital malformations
    Radiation therapy
    Other causes
  Isolated gonadotropin deficiency
    Kallmann syndrome (anosmia-hyposmia)
    Other disorders
  Idiopathic and genetic forms of multiple pituitary hormone deficiencies
  Miscellaneous disorders
    Prader-Willi syndrome
    Laurence-Moon-Bardet-Biedl syndrome
    Functional gonadotropin deficiency
      Chronic systemic disease and malnutrition
      Hypothyroidism
      Cushing disease
      Diabetes mellitus
      Hyperprolactinemia
      Anorexia nervosa
      Psychogenic amenorrhea
      Impaired puberty and delayed menarche in female athletes and ballet dancers (exercise amenorrhea)
Hypergonadotropic hypogonadism
  Klinefelter syndrome (syndrome of seminiferous tubular dysgenesis) and its variants
  Other forms of primary testicular failure
  Anorchia and cryptorchidism
  Syndrome of gonadal dysgenesis and its variants (Turner syndrome)
  Other forms of primary ovarian failure
  XX and XY gonadal dysgenesis
    Familial and sporadic XX gonadal dysgenesis and its variants
    Familial and sporadic XY gonadal dysgenesis and its variants
  Pseudo-Turner syndrome
  Galactosemia

Modified from Grumbach MM, Styne DM: Puberty. In Wilson JD, Foster DW (eds): Williams Textbook of Endocrinology, 9th ed. Philadelphia, WB Saunders, 1998.

A family history of delayed puberty in a parent or sibling is reassuring. Spontaneous puberty usually begins in these patients by the time the bone age reaches 12 years in boys and 11 years in girls. Other causes of delayed puberty must be eliminated before a diagnosis of constitutional delay in puberty is made. In boys and girls with constitutional delay, observation and reassurance are appropriate. Spontaneous progression into puberty occurs when the bone age reaches 12 to 13 years, and an adult height normal for the genetic potential is attained. In some cases, boys may be treated with low-dose testosterone for a few months if the bone age is at least 12 years. Treatment is not required for longer than 4 to 8 months because endogenous hormone production usually ensues. No similar form of therapy for constitutional delay is available for girls. Young women with delayed puberty may need to be evaluated for primary amenorrhea (absent puberty), as outlined subsequently.

Hypogonadotropic Hypogonadism

As a cause of delayed or absent puberty, hypogonadotropic hypogonadism is particularly challenging, and it may be difficult to distinguish from constitutional delay (see Tables 174–1 and 174–2). Hypogonadotropic hypogonadism is a condition that precludes spontaneous entry into gonadarche; adrenarche usually occurs to some degree. Throughout childhood and in early puberty, patients with hypogonadotropic hypogonadism have normal proportions and growth. When these patients reach adulthood, eunuchoid proportions may ensue because their long bones grow for longer than normal, producing an upper-to-lower ratio below the lower limit of normal of 0.9 and an arm span greater than their height. If a patient has concurrent GH deficiency, however, stature is exceptionally short, and the condition may have been diagnosed in infancy with a microphallus.

Isolated Gonadotropin Deficiency

Disorders that can cause hypogonadism include congenital hypopituitarism, tumors, infiltrative disease (hemochromatosis), and many syndromes, including Lawrence-Moon-Bardet-Biedl, Prader-Willi, and Kallmann syndromes. If there is an inability to release gonadotropins, but no other pituitary abnormality, the patient has isolated gonadotropin deficiency (almost universally a result of absent GnRH). Patients grow normally until the time of the pubertal growth spurt, when they fail to experience the accelerated growth characteristic of the normal growth spurt.

Kallmann syndrome combines isolated gonadotropin deficiency with disorders of olfaction. There is genetic heterogeneity; some patients have a decreased sense of smell, others have abnormal reproduction, and some have both. This disorder is caused by mutations in the KAL gene at Xp 22.3 (X chromosome). The mutation causes the GnRH neurons to remain ineffectually located in the primitive nasal area, rather than migrating to the correct location at the medial basal hypothalamus as occurs normally. Olfactory bulbs and olfactory sulci are often absent on MRI. Other symptoms include disorders of the hand, with one hand

TABLE 174–2.   Differential Diagnostic Features of Delayed Puberty and Sexual Infantilism

	Stature	Plasma Gonadotropins	GnRH Test: LH Response	Plasma Gonadal Steroids	Plasma DHEAS	Karyotype	Olfaction
Constitutional delay in growth and adolescence	Short for chronologic age, usually appropriate for bone age	Prepubertal, later pubertal	Prepubertal, later pubertal	Prepubertal, later normal	Low for chronologic age, appropriate for bone age	Normal	Normal
Hypogonadotropic hypogonadism							
Isolated gonadotropin deficiency	Normal, absent pubertal growth spurt	Low	Prepubertal or no response	Low	Appropriate for chronologic age	Normal	Normal
Kallmann syndrome	Normal, absent pubertal growth spurt	Low	Prepubertal or no response	Low	Appropriate for chronologic age	Normal	Anosmia or hyposmia
Idiopathic multiple pituitary hormone deficiencies	Short stature and poor growth since early childhood	Low	Prepubertal or no response	Low	Usually low	Normal	Normal
Hypothalamopituitary tumors	Decrease in growth velocity of late onset	Low	Prepubertal or no response	Low	Normal or low for chronologic age	Normal	Normal
Primary gonadal failure							
Syndrome of gonadal dysgenesis and variants	Short stature since early childhood	High	Hyperresponse for age	Low	Normal for chronologic age	XO or variant	Normal
Klinefelter syndrome and variants	Normal to tall	High	Hyperresponse at puberty	Low or normal	Normal for chronologic age	XXY or variant	Normal
Familial XX or XY gonadal dysgenesis	Normal	High	Hyperresponse for age	Low	Normal for chronologic age	XX or XY	Normal

DHEAS, dehydroepiandrosterone sulfate; GnRH, gonadotropin-releasing hormone; LH, luteinizing hormone.
From Grumbach MM, Styne DM: Puberty. In Wilson JD, Foster DW (eds): Williams Textbook of Endocrinology, 9th ed. Philadelphia, WB Saunders, 1997.

copying the movements of the other hand and short-ened fourth metacarpal bone, and an absent kidney.

Abnormalities of the Central Nervous System

CNS tumors, including pituitary adenoma, germinoma, glioma, prolactinoma, or craniopharyngioma, are important causes of gonadotropin deficiency. Craniopharyngiomas have a peak incidence in the teenage years and may cause any type of anterior or posterior hormone deficiency. Craniopharyngiomas usually calcify, erode the sella turcica when they expand, and may impinge on the optic chiasm, leading to bitemporal hemianopsia and optic atrophy. Germinomas are noncalcifying hypothalamic or pineal tumors that frequently produce human chorionic gonadotropin (HCG), which may cause sexual precocity in boys who are of a prepubertal age (HCG cross-reacts with the LH receptor because of the similarity of structure between LH and HCG). Other tumors that may affect pubertal development include astrocytomas and gliomas.

Idiopathic Hypopituitarism

Congenital absence of various combinations of pituitary hormones may produce idiopathic hypopituitarism. Although this disorder may occur in family constellations, after X-linked or autosomal recessive patterns, sporadic types of congenital idiopathic hypopituitarism are more common. Congenital hypopituitarism may manifest in a male with GH deficiency, with associated gonadotropin deficiency with a microphallus, or with hypoglycemia with seizures, especially if ACTH and GH deficiency occurs as well.

Syndromes of Hypogonadotropic Hypogonadism

Weight loss resulting from voluntary dieting, malnutrition, or chronic disease leads to decreased gonadotropin function when weight decreases to less than 80% of ideal weight. **Anorexia nervosa** is characterized by striking weight loss and psychiatric disorders (see Chapter 70). Primary or secondary amenorrhea frequently is found in affected girls, and pubertal development is absent or minimal, depending on the level of weight loss and the age of onset. Regaining weight to the ideal level may not immediately reverse the condition. Increased physical activity, even without weight loss, can lead to decreased menstrual frequency and gonadotropin deficiency in **athletic amenorrhea**; when physical activity is interrupted, menstrual function may return. Chronic or systemic illness can lead to pubertal delay or to amenorrhea from hypothalamic dysfunction. Examples include cystic fibrosis, diabetes mellitus, inflammatory bowel disease, and hematologic disease. **Hypothyroidism** inhibits the onset of puberty and delays menstrual periods. Conversely, severe primary hypothyroidism may lead to precocious puberty.

Hypergonadotropic Hypogonadism

Hypergonadotropic hypogonadism is characterized by elevated gonadotropin and low sex steroid levels resulting from primary gonadal failure. This is a permanent condition almost always diagnosed at the time of lack of entry into gonadarche and one that would not have been suspected throughout childhood. Gonadotropins do not increase to greater than normal until around the normal time of puberty.

Ovarian Failure

Turner syndrome or the syndrome of gonadal dysgenesis is a common cause of ovarian failure and short stature. The karyotype is classically 45,XO, but other abnormalities of the X chromosome or mosaicism are possible. The incidence of Turner syndrome is 1 in 2000 to 5000 births. The features of a girl with Turner syndrome need not be evident on physical examination or by history, and the diagnosis must be considered in any girl who is short without a contributory history. Patients with other types of gonadal dysgenesis and galactosemia and patients treated with radiation therapy or chemotherapy for malignancy may have ovarian failure (see Table 174–2).

Testicular Failure

Klinefelter syndrome (seminiferous tubular dysgenesis) is the most common cause of testicular failure. The karyotype is 47,XXY, but variants with more X chromosomes are possible. The incidence is approximately 1 in 500 to 1000 in males. Testosterone levels may be close to normal, at least until mid-puberty, because Leydig cell function may be spared; however, seminiferous tubular function characteristically is lost, causing infertility. The common observation is that LH levels may be normal to elevated, whereas FSH levels are usually more unequivocally elevated. The age of onset of puberty is usually normal, but secondary sexual changes may not progress because of inadequate Leydig cell function.

Primary Amenorrhea

When it is determined that no secondary sexual development is present after the upper age limits of normal pubertal development, serum gonadotropin levels should be obtained to determine whether the patient has a hypogonadotropic or hypergonadotropic hypogonadism (see Table 174–2). Based only on gonadotropin measurements, the differentiation between constitutional delay in growth and hypogonadotropic hypogonadism is difficult because the gonadotropins levels are low in both conditions. Sometimes observation for months or years is necessary before the diagnosis is confirmed.

Differential Diagnosis. Lack of menstruation in the presence of normal pubertal development might be the result of physiologic variation, in which 5 years might pass before regular menstrual periods are established. The entities leading to **hypogonadism** include congenital hypopituitarism; tumors such as a pituitary adenoma, germinoma, glioma, prolactinoma, and craniopharyngioma; infiltrative disease; and Laurence-Moon-Biedl, Prader-Willi, and Kallmann syndromes. In females, stress, competitive athletics, or inadequate nutrition from chronic or systemic illness or from an eating disorder can lead to extreme pubertal delay, or amenorrhea on the basis of hypothalamic dysfunction. Hypogonadotropic hypogonadism manifesting as primary amenorrhea may be difficult to distinguish from constitutional delay. When primary amenorrhea occurs, an anatomic defect may be responsible; the Mayer-Rokitansky-Kuster-Hauser syndrome of congenital absence of the uterus occurs in 1 in 4000 to 5000 female births. Anatomic obstruction by imperforate hymen or vaginal septum also presents with normal secondary sexual development without menstruation. The complete syndrome of **androgen insensitivity** includes normal feminization, absence of pubic or axillary hair, and primary amenorrhea. In this syndrome, all müllerian structures, including ovaries, uterus, fallopian tubes, and upper third of the vagina, are lacking; the karyotype is 46,XY, and subjects have intra-abdominal testes. Undiagnosed Turner syndrome is another relatively common cause of amenorrhea, resulting from abnormal ovarian function. Secondary sexual development also is absent or minimal.

Treatment

If a permanent condition is apparent, replacement with sex steroids is indicated. Females are given low-dose ethinyl estradiol (5 to 10 µg) or conjugated estrogens in low daily doses until breakthrough bleeding occurs, at which time cycling is started with a dose on the first 25 days of the month; on days 20 to 25 of the month, a progestational agent, such as medroxyprogesterone acetate (5 mg), is added to mimic the normal increases in gonadal hormones and to induce a normal menstrual period. In males, testosterone enanthate or cypionate (50 mg monthly with a progressive increase to 100 to 200 mg) is given intramuscularly once every 4 weeks. Transdermal administration also is possible. Oral agents are not used for fear of hepatotoxicity. This starting regimen is appropriate for patients with either hypogonadotropic or hypergonadotropic hypo-

gonadism, and doses are increased gradually to adult levels. Patients with apparent constitutional delay in puberty who have by definition passed the upper limits of normal onset of puberty may be given a 3-month course of low-dose, sex-appropriate gonadal steroids and be observed to see if spontaneous puberty occurs. This course of therapy might be repeated once more without undue advancement of bone age. All patients with any form of delayed puberty are at risk for decreased bone density; adequate calcium intake is essential. Patients with hypogonadotropic hypogonadism may be able to achieve fertility by the administration of gonadotropin therapy or pulsatile hypothalamic-releasing hormone therapy administered by a programmable pump on an appropriate schedule. Subjects with hypergonadotropic hypogonadism, whether Turner syndrome or Klinefelter syndrome, have by definition a primary gonadal problem and are unlikely to achieve spontaneous fertility.

In subjects with Turner syndrome, the goals of therapy include promoting growth with exogenous human GH supplementation and induction of the secondary sexual characteristics and of menses with low-dose cyclic estrogen replacement therapy, with progestagen added at the end of each cycle. Patients with Turner syndrome have had successful pregnancies after in vitro fertilization with a donor ovum and endocrine support.

SEXUAL PRECOCITY

Classification

Sexual precocity (precocious puberty) is classically defined as secondary sexual development occurring before the age of 9 years in boys or 8 years in girls (Tables 174–3 and 174–4). The lower limit of normal puberty may be 7 years in white girls and 6 years in African American girls. At present, the mean age at which girls exhibit Tanner II breast development (thelarche) is approximately 10 years for white girls and 9 years for African American girls (normal range 8 to 13 years). The mean age at which girls exhibit Tanner II pubic hair development is 9 years for white girls and 10.5 years for African American girls. Menarche usually occurs at 12.2 and 12.9 years (range 10 to 15 years). The normal developmental sequence is **thelarche** followed closely by **pubarche** and finally **menarche** 2 to 3 years later. In boys, the first normal event is enlargement of testes followed by appearance of pubic hair (long diameter of the testis >2.5 cm, volume >4 mL).

The first distinction regarding puberty is that of central versus peripheral. The condition is **central precocious puberty** if it emanates from premature activation of the hypothalamic-pituitary-gonadal axis (GnRH-dependent); it is **peripheral** when the

TABLE 174–3.   **Classification of Sexual Precocity**

True precocious puberty or complete isosexual precocity
  Idiopathic true precocious puberty
  CNS tumors
   Hamartomas (ectopic GnRH pulse generator)
   Other tumors
  Other CNS disorders
  True precocious puberty after late treatment of
   congenital virilizing adrenal hyperplasia
**Incomplete isosexual precocity (GnRH-independent
  sexual precocity)**
  Males
   Chorionic gonadotropin-secreting tumors (HCG-
    dependent sexual precocity)
   CNS tumors (e.g., germinoma, chorioepithelioma,
    and teratoma)
   Tumors in locations outside the CNS (hepatoblastoma)
   LH-secreting pituitary adenoma
   Increased androgen secretion by adrenal or testis
    Congenital adrenal hyperplasia (21-OH deficiency,
     11-OH deficiency)
    Virilizing adrenal neoplasm
    Leydig cell adenoma
    Familial testotoxicosis (familial premature
     gonadotropin-independent Leydig cell and germ
     cell maturation)
  Females
   Estrogen-secreting ovarian or adrenal neoplasms
   Ovarian cysts
  Males and females
   McCune-Albright syndrome
   Primary hypothyroidism
   Peutz-Jeghers syndrome
  Iatrogenic sexual precocity
Variations of pubertal development
  Premature thelarche
  Premature menarche
  Premature adrenarche
  Adolescent gynecomastia
Contrasexual precocity
  Feminization in males
   Adrenal neoplasm
   Increased extraglandular conversion of circulating
    steroids to estrogen
  Virilization in females
   Congenital adrenal hyperplasia
   P-450$_{C21}$ deficiency
   P-450$_{C11}$ deficiency
   3β-ol deficiency
  Virilizing adrenal neoplasms
  Virilizing ovarian neoplasms (e.g., arrhenoblastomas)

From Grumbach MM, Styne DM: Puberty. In Wilson JD, Foster DW
(eds): Williams Textbook of Endocrinology, 9th ed. Philadelphia, WB
Saunders, 1998.
GnRH, gonadotropin-releasing hormone; HCG, human chorionic
gonadotropin; LH, luteinizing hormone.

hypothalamic-pituitary-gonadal axis is not involved in the process (GnRH-independent). The second distinction is that of **isosexual** versus **heterosexual** (or contrasexual) puberty. Isosexual precocity is virilization in a boy and feminization in a girl, whereas heterosexual precocity is virilization in a girl and feminization in a boy. A boy may have incomplete isosexual precocious puberty as a result of autonomous production of testosterone or other androgens from the testes or adrenal glands or as a result of a tumor that produces HCG, stimulating the testes. A girl might have isosexual precocious puberty as a result of autonomous production of estrogens from the ovaries or heterosexual puberty from androgens from the adrenal glands. These terms are confusing, and it is adequate to use the terms *feminization in boys* or *masculinization in girls* to designate heterosexual puberty.

Central Precocious Puberty (Constitutional or Familial Precocious Puberty)

In **central precocious puberty**, every endocrine and physical aspect of pubertal development is normal but too early; this includes tall stature, advanced bone age, increased sex steroid and increased pulsatile gonadotropin secretion, and increased response of LH to GnRH. Individuals who begin puberty only a few months early may have **constitutional** or **familial precocious puberty**, in which members of some families enter puberty before the lower age limits of normal. Individuals who enter puberty much earlier have other forms of central precocious puberty. The clinical course of central precocious puberty may wax and wane. If no cause can be determined, the diagnosis is idiopathic precocious puberty; this condition occurs much more often in girls than in boys. Obese girls have earlier menarche than normal weight girls, and the current epidemic of overweight and obesity in developed countries is contributing to a shift to earlier entry into puberty. Boys with precocious puberty have a higher incidence of CNS disorders, such as tumors and hamartomas, precipitating the precocious puberty. Affected boys always must be investigated for the possibility of harboring a tumor. Almost any condition that affects the CNS, including hydrocephalus, meningitis, encephalitis, suprasellar cysts, head trauma, and irradiation, can precipitate central precocious puberty. Children with epilepsy and mental retardation also have an increased prevalence of precocious puberty.

A CNS tumor or disease must be considered in all children with precocious puberty before the condition is diagnosed as idiopathic. **Hamartomas** of the tuber cinereum have a characteristic appearance on CT or MRI; biopsy is rarely required. The mass of GnRH neurons may act as an unrestrained ectopic

TABLE 174–4.   Differential Diagnosis of Sexual Precocity

	Serum Gonadotropin Concentration*	LH Response to GnRH	Serum Sex Steroid Concentrations	Gonadal Size	Miscellaneous
True precocious puberty	Pubertal values	Pubertal	Pubertal values of testosterone or estradiol	Normal pubertal testicular enlargement or ovarian and uterine enlargement (by sonography)	MRI scan of brain to rule out CNS tumor or other abnormality; bone scan for McCune-Albright syndrome
Incomplete sexual precocity (pituitary gonadotropin–independent)					
Males					
Chorionic gonadotropin–secreting tumor in males	High HCG (low LH)	Prepubertal (suppressed)	Pubertal values of testosterone	Slight to moderate uniform enlargement of testes	Hepatomegaly suggests hepatoblastoma; MRI scan of brain if chorionic gonadotropin–secreting CNS tumor suspected
Leydig cell tumor in males	Suppressed	Suppressed	Very high testosterone	Irregular asymmetric enlargement of testes	
Familial testotoxicosis	Suppressed	Suppressed	Pubertal values of testosterone	Testes symmetric and >2.5 cm but smaller than expected for pubertal development; spermatogenesis may occur	Familial; probably sex-limited, autosomal dominant trait
Premature adrenarche	Prepubertal	Prepubertal	Prepubertal testosterone; DHEAS values appropriate for pubic hair stage 2	Testes prepubertal	Onset usually after 6 yr of age; more frequent in brain-injured children
Females					
Granulosa cell tumor (follicular cysts may present similarly)	Suppressed	Suppressed	Very high estradiol	Ovarian enlargement on physical examination, MRI, CT, or sonography	Tumor often palpable on abdominal examination
Follicular cyst	Suppressed	Suppressed	Prepubertal to very high estradiol values	Ovarian enlargement on physical examination, MRI, CT, or sonography	Single or repetitive episodes; exclude McCune-Albright syndrome (e.g., perform skeletal survey and inspect skin)
Feminizing adrenal tumor	Suppressed	Suppressed	High estradiol and DHEAS values	Ovaries prepubertal	Unilateral adrenal mass
Premature thelarche	Prepubertal	Prepubertal	Prepubertal or early pubertal estradiol	Ovaries prepubertal	Onset usually before 3 yr of age
Premature adrenarche	Prepubertal	Prepubertal	Prepubertal estradiol; DHEAS values appropriate for pubic hair stage 2	Ovaries prepubertal	Onset usually after 6 yr of age; more frequent in brain-injured children

*In supersensitive assays.

DHEAS, dehydroepiandrosterone sulfate; GnRH, gonadotropin-releasing factor; HCG, human chorionic gonadotropin; LH, luteinizing hormone.
Modified from Grumbach MM, Styne DM: Puberty. In Wilson JD, Foster DW (eds): Williams Textbook of Endocrinology, 9th ed. Philadelphia, WB Saunders, 1997.

hypothalamus that secretes GnRH and causes precocious puberty. These hamartomas are not true neoplasms because they do not grow; however, they may require neurosurgical attention, such as ventriculoperitoneal shunting, if they lead to increased intracranial pressure. The resulting precocious puberty is responsive to medical therapy with GnRH agonists, and surgery is rarely indicated.

Other masses that cause precocious puberty are not benign. **Optic** or **hypothalamic gliomas** (with or without neurofibromatosis), astrocytomas, and ependymomas may cause precocious puberty by disrupting the negative restraint of the areas of the CNS that normally inhibit pubertal development throughout childhood. These tumors may require radiotherapy, which contributes to a significant risk for hypopituitarism. Growth is greater than that found in agematched controls, but less than in GH-replete patients with precocious puberty. The GH deficiency is not as obvious as in GH-deficient patients without precocious puberty. With GnRH treatment, the precocious puberty is controlled, and the growth rate decreases to that of a GH-deficient child. GH is additional therapy.

Gonadotropin-Releasing Hormone–Independent Precocious Puberty

The most common cause of GnRH-independent precocious puberty, **McCune-Albright syndrome**, more frequent in girls than boys, includes precocious gonadarche, a bone disorder with polyostotic fibrous dysplasia, and a skin disorder consisting of hyperpigmented cutaneous macules (café au lait spots). The precocious gonadarche results from ovarian hyperfunction and sometimes cyst formation, leading to episodic estrogen secretion. This disorder results from a somatic mutation in the G protein intracellular signaling system (specifically $G_{s\alpha}$, which leads to unregulated constitutive activation of adenylate cyclase); several endocrine organs may autonomously hyperfunction despite the absence of their stimulating trophic hormones. There also may be hyperthyroidism, hyperadrenalism, or acromegaly. **Adrenal carcinomas** usually secrete adrenal androgens, such as DHEA; **adrenal adenomas** may virilize a child as a result of the production of androgen or may feminize a child as a result of the production of estrogen.

Boys may have precocious gonadarche on the basis of a rare entity called **familial GnRH-independent sexual precocity with premature Leydig cell maturation**, which is a condition with germ cell maturation caused by an X-limited dominant defect producing constitutive activation of the LH receptor, which leads to continuous production and secretion of testosterone without requiring the presence of LH or HCG. Outside of the pituitary, gonadotropins can originate from a tumor. HCG-secreting tumors stimulate LH receptors and increase testosterone secretion. These tumors may be found in various places, including the pineal gland (dysgerminomas, which are radiosensitive) or the liver (hepatoblastoma, which may lead to death in just a few months after diagnosis).

Ovarian cysts may occur once or may be recurrent. High serum estrogen values may mimic ovarian tumors. CAH is a cause of virilization in girls and is discussed in the following sections.

Evaluation of Sexual Precocity

The first step in evaluating sexual precocity is to determine by physical examination which characteristic of normal puberty is apparent (see Chapter 67) and whether only estrogen effects or only androgen effects or both are present (see Table 174–4). In girls, androgen effect manifests as adult odor, pubic and axillary hair, and facial skin oiliness and acne, whereas estrogen effect manifests as breast development, uterine increase, and eventually menarche. In boys, androgen effect manifests as adult odor, pubic and axillary hair, and facial skin oiliness and acne; it is also important to note whether the testes are enlarged more than 2.5 cm in length, which implies gonadarche. If the testes are not enlarged, but virilization is progressing, the source of the androgens may be the adrenal glands or exogenous sources. If the testes are slightly enlarged but not consistent with the stage of pubertal development, ectopic production of HCG or familial Leydig and germ cell maturation may be the cause. Most of the enlargement of testes during puberty is the result of seminiferous tubule maturation. If only Leydig cells are enlarged as in these conditions, the testes make considerable testosterone, but show only minimal enlargement.

Laboratory examinations include determination of sex steroid (testosterone, estradiol, or DHEA) and baseline gonadotropin concentrations. The inherent nature of gonadotropin secretion is characterized by low secretory rates throughout childhood and pulsatile secretion in adolescents and adults. If baseline gonadotropin values are elevated into the normal pubertal range, central precocious puberty is likely. If baseline gonadotropins are low, however, no immediate conclusion may be drawn as to GnRH-dependent versus GnRH-independent precocious puberty. This distinction often requires assessment of gonadotropin responsiveness to GnRH stimulation. A prepubertal GnRH response is FSH predominant, whereas a pubertal response is more LH predominant. Thyroid hormone determination also is useful because severe primary hypothyroidism can cause incomplete precocious puberty. If there is a suggestion of a CNS anomaly or a tumor (CNS, hepatic, adrenal, ovarian, or testicular), CT or MRI of the appropriate location is indicated. The diagnosis of central precocious puberty mandates that MRI of the CNS be performed.

Treatment

Long-acting, superactive analogues of GnRH are the treatment of choice for central precocious puberty because they suppress gonadotropin secretion by down-regulating GnRH receptors in the pituitary gonadotropes (Table 174–5). After a brief (2 to 3 days) increase in gonadotropin secretion and, rarely, some withdrawal bleeding in girls, values decrease, and the pubertal process reverts to the prepubertal state. The early sexual development and increased height of a patient with precocious puberty mandate psychological support or even counseling for children and families. Boys with GnRH-independent premature Leydig cell and germ cell maturation do not respond to GnRH analogues, but require treatment with an inhibitor of testosterone synthesis (e.g., ketoconazole), an anti-androgen (e.g., spironolactone), or an aromatase inhibitor (e.g., testolactone). Patients with precocious puberty from a hormone-secreting tumor require surgical removal, if possible. The precocious puberty of the McCune-Albright syndrome is GnRH independent and unresponsive to therapy with GnRH analogue. Therapy is provided with testolactone and antiandrogens or antiestrogen, such as tamoxifen. After successful therapy for the latter conditions, central precocious puberty may develop secondarily; GnRH agonist administration is effective therapy.

VARIATIONS IN PUBERTAL DEVELOPMENT

Isolated Premature Thelarche (Premature Breast Development)

Benign **premature thelarche** is the isolated appearance of unilateral or bilateral breast tissue in girls, usually at ages 6 months to 3 years. There are no other signs of puberty and no evidence of excessive estrogen effect (vaginal bleeding, thickening of the vaginal secretions, increased height velocity, or bone age acceleration). Ingestion or dermal application of estrogen-containing compounds must be excluded. Laboratory investigations are not usually necessary, but a pelvic ultrasound study rarely may be indicated to exclude ovarian pathology. Girls with this condition should be re-evaluated at intervals of 6 to 12 months to ensure that apparent premature thelarche is not the beginning of progression into precocious puberty. The prognosis is excellent; if no progression occurs, no treatment other than reassurance is necessary. There is no indication for a breast biopsy in a patient with established premature thelarche.

Gynecomastia

In males, breast tissue is termed *gynecomastia,* and it may occur to some degree in 45% to 75% of normal pubertal boys (see Chapter 67). Androgens normally are converted to estrogen by aromatization; in early puberty, only modest amounts of androgens are

---

TABLE 174–5. Pharmacologic Therapy of Sexual Precocity

Disorder	Treatment	Action and Rationale
GnRH-dependent true or central precocious puberty	GnRH agonists	Desensitization of gonadotropes; blocks action of endogenous GnRH
GnRH-independent incomplete sexual precocity		
Girls		
Autonomous ovarian cysts	Medroxyprogesterone acetate	Inhibition of ovarian steroidogenesis; regression of cyst (inhibition of FSH release)
McCune-Albright syndrome	Medroxyprogesterone acetate*	Inhibition of ovarian steroidogenesis; regression of cyst (inhibition of FSH release)
	Testolactone* or fadrozole	Inhibition of P-450 aromatase; blocks estrogen synthesis
Boys		
Familial testotoxicosis	Ketoconazole*	Inhibition of P-450$_{c17}$ (mainly 17,20-lyase activity)
	Spironolactone* or flutamide *and* testolactone or fadrozole	Antiandrogen Inhibition of aromatase; blocks estrogen synthesis
	Medroxyprogesterone acetate*	Inhibition of testicular steroidogenesis

*If true precocious puberty develops, a GnRH agonist can be added.
FSH, follicle-stimulating hormone; GnRH, gonadotropin-releasing hormone.
Modified from Grumbach MM, Kaplan SL: Recent advances in the diagnosis and management of sexual precocity. Acta Paediatr Jpn 30(Suppl):155, 1988.

produced, and the estrogen effect can overwhelm the androgen effects at this stage. Later in pubertal development, the androgen production is so great that there is little effect from the estrogen produced by aromatization. Gynecomastia also can suggest the possibility of Klinefelter syndrome as puberty progresses. Prepubertal gynecomastia suggests an unusual source of estrogen either from exogenous sources (oral or dermal estrogen administration is possible from contamination of food or ointments) or from endogenous sources (from abnormal function of adrenal gland or ovary or from increased peripheral aromatization).

Isolated Premature Adrenarche (Pubarche)

The isolated appearance of pubic hair before age 6 to 7 years in girls or before age 9 years in boys is termed **premature pubarche**, usually results from adrenarche, and is relatively common. If the pubic hair is associated with any other feature of virilization (clitoral or penile enlargement or advanced bone age) or other signs (acne, rapid growth, or voice change), a detailed investigation for a pathologic cause of virilization is indicated to rule out a life-threatening cause, such as an adrenocortical carcinoma. Measurements of serum testosterone, 17-hydroxyprogesterone (17-OHP), and DHEA in basal and ACTH-stimulated states are indicated in heavily virilized patients to investigate the possibility of **CAH**. Ultrasound studies may reveal a hyperplastic adrenal gland or a virilizing adrenal or ovarian tumor. Most patients with isolated pubic hair do not have these abnormal signs of progressive virilization and simply have premature adrenarche (*pubarche*) resulting from premature activation of DHEA secretion from the adrenal gland. The skeletal maturation as assessed by bone age may be slightly advanced, and the height slightly may be increased, but testosterone concentrations are normal. DHEA levels usually are high for prepuberty, but are consistent with Tanner (sexuality maturity rating) stages II and III.

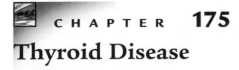

CHAPTER 175
Thyroid Disease

THYROID PHYSIOLOGY AND DEVELOPMENT

Thyrotropin-releasing hormone (TRH), a tripeptide synthesized in the hypothalamus, stimulates the release of pituitary thyroid-stimulating hormone (TSH). Pituitary TSH is a glycoprotein that stimulates the synthesis and release of thyroid hormones by the thyroid gland. Plasma concentrations of TSH above the normal range indicate primary hypothyroidism, and concentrations below the normal range most often indicate the presence of hyperthyroidism, although other possibilities include hypothalamic or pituitary deficiency or suppression of TSH secretion. Thyroid function develops in three stages:

1. Embryogenesis begins on the floor of the primitive oral cavity, and the gland descends to its definitive position in the anterior lower neck by the end of the first trimester. Thyroid glands that do not reach the normal location are ectopic but may retain function; however, the glands most often become insufficient by early to mid childhood to support full thyroid secretion (a lingual or sublingual site or even tissue found in a thyroglossal duct cyst may be the only functioning thyroid gland).
2. The hypothalamic-pituitary-thyroid axis becomes functional in the second trimester.
3. Peripheral metabolism of thyroid hormones matures in the third trimester.

T_4, triiodothyronine (T_3), and TSH do not cross the placenta in significant amounts, so concentrations in fetal serum reflect primarily fetal secretion and metabolism. Antithyroid antibodies, thyroid-stimulating immunoglobulins (TSIs), iodides (including radioactive iodides), and medications given to mothers to treat hyperthyroidism (e.g., propylthiouracil and methimazole) do cross the placenta, however, and affect fetal thyroid function. An infant born prematurely or with intrauterine growth retardation may have an interruption of the normal maturational process and appear to have hypothyroidism by standard tests. It is controversial as to whether treatment is indicated in such situations.

The thyroid gland (1) concentrates iodine and (2) attaches it (organifies it) to tyrosine molecules to produce either monoiodotyrosine or diiodotyrosine, with subsequent (3) coupling of two tyrosines, T_4 or T_3. The major fraction of circulating **T_3 (approximately two thirds) is derived from peripheral deiodination of T_4** to T_3, but some is produced by the thyroid gland itself. In Graves disease, a larger fraction originates in the thyroid gland. The conversion of T_4 to T_3 requires the removal of one iodine from the outer ring of tyrosine; removing an iodine from the inner ring results in reverse T_3, which has little biologic effect. Preferential conversion of T_4 to reverse T_3 rather than T_3 occurs in utero and in all forms of severe illness, including respiratory distress syndrome, fevers, anorexia, cachexia, and starvation. Conversion from T_4 to T_3 increases immediately after birth and throughout life. T_4 and T_3 are noncovalently bound to a specific serum carrier protein, **T_4-binding globulin**, and, to a lesser extent, albumin. Only small (<0.02%) fractions of T_4 and T_3 are not bound; free T_4 (as it is converted to free T_3) and free T_3 are biologically active. Free T_3 exerts metabolic effects and negative feedback on TSH release (Fig. 175–1).

Serum TSH increases just after birth, but soon reaches lower values considered normal for later life. T_4 secretion increases after birth, partially as a result of the peak in TSH and partially because of maturation of thyroid metabolism. Serum thyroid hormone concentrations decrease, but only slowly reach values routinely found in adults. It is important to refer to age-adjusted normative data to interpret thyroid function tests properly, whether relative to making diagnoses of hyperthyroidism or hypothyroidism or when adjusting therapy. Free T_4 is the test of choice because it eliminates the effects of variation in protein binding, which can be substantial.

Table 175–1 summarizes laboratory test results in various types of thyroid abnormalities. Although a thyroid scan rarely is indicated in the evaluation of pediatric thyroid disease, the presence of thyroid agenesis or of ectopic thyroid tissue and the diagnoses of hyperfunctioning "hot" nodules or of nonfunctioning "cold" nodules may be detected by this test. A thyroid scan performed with the short-lived isotope radioactive iodine (^{123}I) indicates the size, shape, and location of the thyroid gland and iodine concentrating ability. A solitary nodule is a source of concern for the possibility of cancer, especially if it is solid and nonfunctional. Ultrasound may determine whether it is cystic or solid. If the nodule is solid, a ^{123}I scan indicates its functional status. Excisional biopsies usually are performed on

solitary nodules. Scans are rarely indicated in the diagnosis of Hashimoto thyroiditis or thyrotoxicosis.

THYROID DISORDERS

Hypothyroidism

Hypothyroidism is diagnosed by a decreased serum free T_4. Hypothyroidism might be the result of disease of the thyroid gland (primary hypothyroidism) or of abnormalities of the pituitary gland (secondary) or the result of abnormality of the hypothalamus (tertiary). Hypothyroidism is congenital or acquired and may be associated with a goiter (Table 175–2).

Congenital Hypothyroidism

Congenital hypothyroidism occurs in approximately 1 in 4000 live births and usually is caused by dysgenesis: disorders of embryogenesis (agenesis, aplasia, ectopia). Thyroid tissue usually is not palpable in these sporadic nongoitrous conditions. Dyshormonogenesis, disorders of intrathyroid metabolism or goitrous congenital hypothyroidism, occurs in about 1 in 30,000 live births. The goiter reflects an inborn error of metabolism in the pathway of iodide incorporation or thyroid hormone biosynthesis or reflects the transplacental passage of antithyroid drugs given to the mother. The free T_4 concentration is low, and the TSH level is elevated, proving primary hypothyroidism. Routine neonatal screening programs to measure cord blood or heel-stick TSH values occur in every state in the U.S. An immediate confirmatory serum sample should be obtained from any infant having a positive result on a **screening test** (low T_4 and high TSH confirms the finding).

Isolated secondary or tertiary hypothyroidism is rare, occurring in 1 in 100,000 live births; the free T_4 is normal to low. When tertiary or secondary hypothyroidism is detected, assessment of other pituitary hormones and investigation of pituitary-hypothalamic anatomy via MRI are indicated. Although not a hypothyroid condition, **congenital T_4-binding globulin deficiency** occurs in about 1 in 10,000 live births and is associated with a low serum total T_4 concentration, a normal TSH and serum free T_4, and a euthyroid status. This entity does not require treatment with thyroid hormone because it is merely a binding protein abnormality and is commonly X-linked dominant.

Clinical manifestations of congenital hypothyroidism in the immediate newborn period usually are subtle, but become more evident weeks or months after birth. By then, however, it is late to ensure that already there is not a detriment to the infant's cognitive development. Newborn screening is crucial to make an early diagnosis and initiate thyroid replacement therapy by

---

TABLE 175–1. Laboratory Test Results in Various Types of Thyroid Function Abnormalities in Children*

	Serum Total T_4	Free T_4	Serum TSH	Serum TBG
Primary hypothyroidism	↓	↓	↑	N
Hypothalamic (TRH) tertiary hypothyroidism	↓	↓	↓	N
Pituitary (TSH) secondary hypothyroidism	↓	↓	↓	N
TBG deficiency	↓	N	N	↓
TBG excess	↑	N	N	↑

*TSH may be slightly elevated.

N, normal; ↓, decreased; ↑, increased; T_3, triiodothyronine; T_4, thyroxine; TBG, thyroid-binding globulin; TRH, thyrotropin-releasing hormone; TSH, thyroid-stimulating hormone.

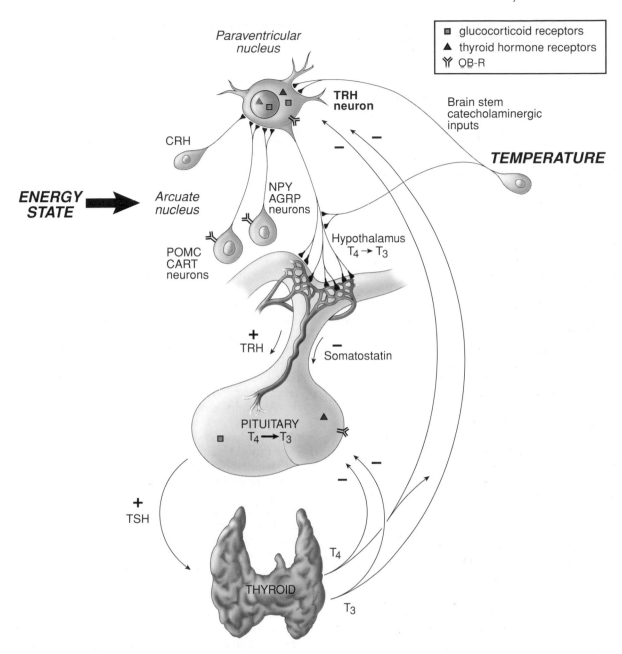

Figure 175–1

Interrelationships of the hypothalamic-pituitary-thyroid axis. Thyroid-stimulating hormone (TSH) from the pituitary gland stimulates the secretion of thyroxine (T_4) and triiodothyronine (T_3) from the thyroid gland. These act at the pituitary gland level to control secretion of TSH by a negative feedback mechanism. In addition, T_4 is metabolized to the potent T_3 within the pituitary gland by a monoiodinase. Secretion of TSH is stimulated by thyrotropin-releasing hormone (TRH) from the hypothalamus and inhibited by somatostatin. Thyroid hormone acts at the hypothalamus to stimulate secretion of somatostatin (somatostatin acts as a negative signal to the pituitary secretion of TSH). CRH, corticotropin-releasing hormone; OB-R, leptin receptor. (From Melmed S, Polonsky K, Kronenberg H, Larsen R [eds]: Williams Textbook of Endocrinology, 10th ed. Philadelphia, Elsevier, 2003, p 101.)

TABLE 175–2.   Causes of Hypothyroidism in Infancy and Childhood

Age	Manifestation	Cause
Newborn	No goiter	Thyroid gland dysgenesis or ectopic location Exposure to iodides TSH deficiency TRH deficiency
	Goiter	Inborn defect in hormone synthesis* or effect Maternal goitrogen ingestion, including propylthiouracil, methimazole, iodides Severe iodide deficiency (endemic)
Child	No goiter	Thyroid gland dysgenesis Cystinosis Hypothalamic-pituitary insufficiency Surgical after thyrotoxicosis or other thyroid surgery
	Goiter	Hashimoto thyroiditis: chronic lymphocytic thyroiditis Inborn defect in hormone synthesis or effect Goitrogenic drugs Infiltrative (sarcoid, lymphoma)

*Impaired iodide transport, defective thyroglobulin iodination, defective iodotyrosine dehalogenase, defective thyroglobulin, or its coupling to iodotyrosines.
TRH, thyrotropin-releasing hormone; TSH, thyroid-stimulating hormone.

younger than 1 month of age and in the absence of definitive signs. Findings at various stages after birth include gestation greater than 42 weeks, birth weight greater than 4 kg, hypothermia, acrocyanosis, respiratory distress, large posterior fontanel, abdominal distention, lethargy and poor feeding, jaundice more than 3 days after birth, edema, umbilical hernia, mottled skin, constipation, large tongue, dry skin, and hoarse cry. Thyroid hormones are crucial for maturation and differentiation of tissues such as bone (the bone age is often delayed at birth because of intrauterine hypothyroidism) and brain (most thyroid-dependent brain maturation occurs 2 to 3 years after birth) (Table 175–3).

When **treatment** is initiated within 1 month or less after birth, the prognosis for normal intellectual development is excellent; screening programs usually offer therapy within 1 to 2 weeks of birth. If therapy is instituted after 6 months, when the signs of severe hypothyroidism are present, the likelihood of normal intellectual function is markedly decreased. Growth improves after thyroid replacement even in late diagnosed cases. The dose of T_4 changes with age; 10 to 15 μg/kg of T_4 is used for a newborn, but about 3 μg/kg is used later in childhood. In neonatal hypothyroidism, the goal is to bring the serum free T_4 rapidly into the upper half of the range of normal. Suppression of TSH is not seen in all cases and is not necessary in all cases because such suppression may lead to excessive doses of T_4.

Acquired Hypothyroidism

The **etiology** of acquired hypothyroidism is presented in Table 175–2, and the **clinical manifestations** are summarized in Table 175–3. The signs and symptoms may be subtle, and hypothyroidism should be suspected in any child who has a decline in growth velocity, especially if not associated with weight loss. The most common cause of acquired hypothyroidism in older children in the U.S. is lymphocytic autoimmune thyroiditis (**Hashimoto thyroiditis**). In many areas of the world, iodine deficiency is the etiology of endemic goiter (**endemic cretinism**). The failure of the thyroid gland may be heralded by an increase of TSH before T_4 levels decrease. In contrast to untreated congenital hypothyroidism, acquired hypothyroidism is not a cause of permanent developmental delay.

Hashimoto Thyroiditis

Also known as autoimmune or *lymphocytic thyroiditis,* Hashimoto thyroiditis is a common cause of goiter and acquired thyroid disease in older children and adolescents. A family history of thyroid disease is present in 25% to 35% of patients, suggesting a genetic predisposition. The *etiology* is an autoimmune process targeted against the thyroid gland with lymphocytic infiltration and lymphoid follicle and germinal center formation preceding fibrosis and atrophy.

Clinical manifestations include a firm, nontender euthyroid, hypothyroid, or, rarely, hyperthyroid (hashitoxicosis) diffuse goiter with a pebble-like feeling; an insidious onset after 6 years of age (the incidence peaks in adolescence, with a female predominance); and sometimes a pea-sized Delphian lymph node above the thyroid isthmus. Associated autoimmune diseases include DM1, adrenal insufficiency

TABLE 175–3. Symptoms and Signs of Hypothyroidism

Ectodermal	Poor growth
	Dull facies: thick lips, large tongue, depressed nasal bridge, periorbital edema
	Dry scaly skin
	Sparse brittle hair
	Diminished sweating
	Carotenemia
	Vitiligo
Circulatory	Sinus bradycardia/heart block
	Cold extremities
	Cold intolerance
	Pallor
	ECG changes: low-voltage QRS complex
Neuromuscular	Muscle weakness
	Hypotonia: constipation, potbelly
	Umbilical hernia
	Myxedema coma (carbon dioxide narcosis, hypothermia)
	Pseudohypertrophy of muscles
	Myalgia
	Physical and mental lethargy
	Developmental delay
	Delayed relaxation of reflexes
	Paresthesias (nerve entrapment: carpal tunnel syndrome)
	Cerebellar ataxia
Skeletal	Delayed bone age
	Epiphyseal dysgenesis, increased upper-to-lower segment ratio
Metabolic	Myxedema
	Serous effusions (pleural, pericardial, ascites)
	Hoarse voice (cry)
	Weight gain
	Menstrual irregularity
	Arthralgia
	Elevated CPK
	Macrocytosis (anemia)
	Hypercholesterolemia
	Hyperprolactinemia
	Precocious puberty in severe cases

CPK, creatine phosphokinase.

(Schmidt syndrome), and hypoparathyroidism. Autoimmune polyglandular syndrome type I consists of hypoparathyroidism, Addison disease, mucocutaneous candidiasis, and often hypothyroidism. Autoimmune polyglandular syndrome type II consists of Addison disease, DM1, and frequently autoimmune hypothyroidism. Trisomy 21 and Turner syndrome predispose to the development of autoimmune thyroiditis.

The **diagnosis** may be confirmed by serum antithyroid peroxidase (previously antimicrosomal) and antithyroglobulin antibodies. Neither biopsy nor thyroid scan is indicated in Hashimoto thyroiditis, although the thyroid scan and uptake may differentiate hashitoxicosis from Graves disease.

Treatment with thyroid hormone sufficient to suppress TSH to a normal level is indicated for hypothyroidism in Hashimoto thyroiditis. Patients without manifestation of hypothyroidism require periodic thyroid function testing (serum TSH and free T_4) every 6 to 12 months to detect the later development of hypothyroidism. Goiter with a normal TSH usually is not an indication for treatment.

Hyperthyroidism

Graves Disease

Most children with hyperthyroidism have Graves disease, the autonomous functioning of the thyroid caused by autoantibodies stimulating the thyroid gland (TSIs). The resulting excessive synthesis, release, and peripheral metabolism of thyroid hormones produce the clinical features. Hashimoto thyroiditis and thyrotoxicosis are on a continuum of autoimmune diseases; there is overlap in their immunologic findings. Antimicrosomal and antithyroglobulin antibodies may be present in thyrotoxicosis, although the values are usually lower than in Hashimoto thyroiditis. Exceptionally high titers of antibodies may indicate that the patient has the thyrotoxic phase of Hashimoto thyroiditis (hashitoxicosis caused by the release of preformed thyroid hormone), with the subsequent development of permanent hypothyroidism. In Graves disease, serum T_4 or T_3 or both levels are elevated, whereas TSH is suppressed. Rare causes of hyperthyroidism include McCune-Albright syndrome, thyroid neoplasm, TSH hypersecretion, subacute thyroiditis, and iodine or thyroid hormone ingestion.

Clinical Manifestations. Graves disease presents as hyperthyroidism (Table 175–4). In children, Graves disease is about five times more common in girls than in boys, with a peak incidence in adolescence. Personality changes, mood instability, and poor school performance are common presenting problems. The tremor, anxiety, inability to concentrate, and weight loss may be insidious and confused with a psychological disorder until thyroid function tests reveal the elevated serum free T_4 level. Serum T_4 may be near-normal, whereas serum T_3 is selectively elevated (T_3 toxicosis, a rare entity). A firm, homogeneous goiter is usually present. Many patients complain of neck fullness and, in older subjects, a change in the size of their shirt collars. Thyroid gland enlargement is best visualized with the neck only slightly extended and with the

TABLE 175–4.   Clinical Manifestations of Hyperthyroidism

Increased catecholamine effects	Nervousness
	Palpitations
	Tachycardia
	Atrial arrhythmias
	Systolic hypertension
	Tremor
	Brisk reflexes
Hypermetabolism	Increased sweating
	Shiny, smooth skin
	Heat intolerance
	Fatigue
	Weight loss—increased appetite
	Increased bowel movement (hyperdefecation)
	Hyperkinesis
Myopathy	Weakness
	Periodic paralysis
	Cardiac failure—dyspnea
Miscellaneous	Proptosis, stare, exophthalmos, lid lag, ophthalmopathy
	Hair loss
	Inability to concentrate
	Personality change (emotional lability)
	Goiter
	Thyroid bruit
	Onycholysis
	Painful gland*
	Acute thyroid storm (hyperpyrexia, tachycardia, coma, high-output heart failure, shock)

*Unusual except in subacute thyroiditis with hyperthyroid phase.

examiner lateral to the patient; palpation of the thyroid gland is best performed with the examiner's hands around the neck from the back. The patient swallows so that the examiner can feel the size, consistency, nodularity, and motion of the gland. The examiner should watch the patient swallow to note any discernible enlargement or asymmetry or both of the thyroid lobes. The thickness is estimated, and the dimensions of each lobe are measured vertically and laterally. Auscultation may reveal a bruit over the gland, which needs to be differentiated from a carotid bruit.

Treatment. Three treatment choices are available: pharmacologic, surgical, and radioactive iodine.

Drugs. Medical therapy to block thyroid hormone synthesis consists of propylthiouracil (5 to 7 mg/kg/24 hours orally in divided doses every 8 hours) or methimazole (0.5 to 0.7 mg/kg/24 hours orally in divided doses every 8 to 12 hours). Both medications are equally effective; methimazole may be easier to manage and titrate. Propranolol is started if symptoms are severe (2 to 3 mg/kg/24 hours orally) to control cardiac manifestations and is tapered as the propylthiouracil or methimazole takes effect. Propylthiouracil usually is continued for 1 to 2 years because the remission rate is approximately 25% per year. In patients complying with the treatment regimen, the 2-year course of treatment can be repeated. Propylthiouracil should suppress thyroid function to normal, without the need to add thyroid hormone replacement to normalize serum free T_4. Complications of propylthiouracil are lupus-like syndrome, rash, granulocytopenia, and jaundice. The granulocytopenia is an idiosyncratic complication of rapid onset, which is observed only in the early months after institution of antithyroid medication and which must be attended to promptly by obtaining a complete blood count. If a suppressed white blood cell count is observed, antithyroid therapy must be discontinued; this is potentially lethal (more rarely, thrombocytopenia or aplastic anemia) and is a rare complication that affects 3 in 10,000 users a year and is extremely unlikely later on during the course of therapy. After resolution, the other of the two antithyroid medications can be started because there is usually less than a 50% chance of a similar reaction from the other medication. These side effects are sometimes severe and usually reversible after discontinuation of antithyroid therapy; failure to monitor and then discontinue propylthiouracil when complications arise may be fatal. Iodine administration may suppress thyroid function, but it becomes ineffective in a few weeks. It is sometimes used as a preparation for surgery but never for long-term therapy.

Surgery. Surgical treatment consists of partial or complete thyroidectomy. Risks associated with thyroidectomy include the use of anesthesia and the possibility that the thyroid removal will be excessive, causing hypothyroidism, or that it will be inadequate, resulting in persistent hyperthyroidism. In addition, keloid formation, recurrent laryngeal nerve palsy, and hypoparathyroidism (transient postoperative or permanent) may occur. Thyroid storm caused by the release of large amounts of preformed hormone is a serious but rare complication. Even with optimal immediate postoperative results, patients may become hypothyroid within 10 years.

Radioiodine. Radioiodine (^{131}I) is slower in exerting therapeutic effects, may require repeated dosing, and is likely to cause permanent hypothyroidism. Ultimately, hypothyroidism is the desired outcome because it is easier and safer to treat than continued hyperthyroidism. Although studies reveal no long-term consequences, concern remains about possible sequelae in children. This method of treatment is entering the mainstream for adolescents and adults. Radioiodine given to a pregnant teenager renders the fetus hypothyroid and is contraindicated.

Thyroid Storm

Thyroid storm (see Table 175–4) is a rare medical emergency consisting of tachycardia and hyperthermia. *Treatment* includes reducing the hyperthermia with a cooling blanket and administering propranolol to control the tachycardia, hypertension, and autonomic hyperfunction symptoms. Iodine may be given to block thyroid hormone release. Cortisol may be indicated for relative adrenal insufficiency, and therapy for heart failure includes diuretics and digoxin.

Congenital Hyperthyroidism

This disorder results from transplacental passage of maternal TSIs. The *clinical* manifestations in the neonate may be masked for several days until the short-lived effects of transplacental maternal antithyroid medication wear off (assuming the mother was receiving such medication), at which time the effects of TSIs are observed. Irritability, tachycardia (often with signs of cardiac failure simulating "cardiomyopathy"), polycythemia, craniosynostosis, bone age advancement, poor feeding and, later, failure to thrive are the clinical hallmarks. This condition may be anticipated if the mother is known to be thyrotoxic in pregnancy so that timely therapy can be offered. If the mother was cured of hyperthyroidism before pregnancy by surgery or radioiodine treatment, which limits or curtails T$_4$ production but not the underlying immune disturbance producing TSIs, the infant still may be affected.

Treatment for a severely affected neonate includes oral propranolol, 2 to 3 mg/kg/24 hours in divided doses, and propylthiouracil, approximately 5 mg/kg/24 hours orally in three divided doses. Because the half-life of the immunoglobulin is several weeks, spontaneous resolution of neonatal thyrotoxicosis resulting from transplacental passage of TSIs usually occurs by 2 to 3 months of age. Observation without treatment is indicated in patients who are minimally affected.

TUMORS OF THE THYROID

Carcinoma of the thyroid is rare in children, but papillary and follicular carcinomas represent 90% of children's thyroid cancers. A history of therapeutic head or neck irradiation or radiation exposure from nuclear accidents predisposes a child to thyroid cancer. Carcinoma usually presents as a firm to hard, painless, nonfunctional solitary nodule and may spread to adjacent lymph nodes. Rapid growth, hoarseness (recurrent laryngeal nerve involvement), and lung metastasis may

be present. If the nodule is solid on ultrasound, is "cold" on radioiodine scanning, and feels hard, the likelihood of a carcinoma is high. Excisional biopsy usually is performed, but fine needle aspiration biopsy also may be diagnostic.

Treatment includes total thyroidectomy, selective regional node dissection, and radioablation with ^{131}I for residual or recurrent disease. The **prognosis** is usually good if the disease is diagnosed early.

Medullary carcinoma of the thyroid may be asymptomatic except for a mass. *Diagnosis* is based on the presence of elevated calcitonin levels, either in the basal state or after pentagastrin stimulation, and histology. This tumor most often occurs with multiple endocrine neoplasia 2a or 2b, pheochromocytoma, or alone, possibly in a familial pattern. The presence of mutations of the *RET* proto-oncogene is predictive of the development of medullary carcinoma of the thyroid in some families. Screening the other members of the family is indicated after a proband is recognized, and prophylactic thyroidectomy is indicated for the family members with the same allele.

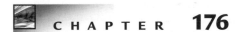

CHAPTER 176

Disorders of Parathyroid Bone and Mineral Endocrinology

PARATHYROID HORMONE AND VITAMIN D

Calcium and phosphate are regulated mainly by diet and three hormones: PTH, vitamin D, and calcitonin. PTH is secreted in response to a decrease in serum ionized calcium level. PTH attaches to its membrane receptor, then acts via adenylate cyclase to mobilize calcium from bone into the serum and to enhance fractional reabsorption of calcium by the kidney while inducing phosphate excretion, all of which increase the serum calcium concentration and decrease serum phosphate. Lack of PTH effect is heralded by low serum calcium in the presence of elevated phosphate for age. PTH stimulates vitamin D secretion by increasing renal 1α-hydroxylase activity and acts indirectly to elevate serum calcium concentration by stimulating the production of 1,25-dihydroxyvitamin D from 25-hydroxyvitamin D. Calcitonin increases the deposition of calcium into bone; in normal states, the effect is subtle, but calcitonin may be used to suppress extremely elevated serum calcium values.

1,25-Dihydroxyvitamin D enhances calcium absorption from the gastrointestinal tract, resulting in increased serum calcium levels and increased bone mineralization. Vitamin D, derived from exposure of the skin to UV rays (usually via the sun) or from oral ingestion, must be modified sequentially first to 25-hydroxyvitamin D in the liver and then 1α-hydroxylated to the metabolically active form (1,25-dihydroxyvitamin D) in the kidney. The serum concentration of 25-hydroxyvitamin D is a better reflection of vitamin D sufficiency than the measurement of 1,25-hydroxyvitamin D. See Chapter 31 for additional information.

HYPOCALCEMIA

The **clinical manifestations** of hypocalcemia (ionized calcium <4.5 mg/dL; total calcium <8.5 mg/dL if serum protein is normal) result from increased neuromuscular irritability and include muscle cramps, carpopedal spasm (tetany), weakness, paresthesia, laryngospasm, or seizure-like activity (patient is often awake and aware during these episodes, in contrast to many episodes of epilepsy). Latent tetany can be detected by the *Chvostek sign* (facial spasms are produced by lightly tapping over the facial nerve just in front of the ear) or by the *Trousseau sign* (carpal spasms are exhibited when arterial blood flow to the hand is occluded for 3 to 5 minutes with a blood pressure cuff inflated to 15 mm Hg above systolic blood pressure). Total serum calcium concentration is usually measured, although a determination of serum ionized calcium (approximately half the total calcium in normal circumstances), the biologically active form, is preferable. Albumin is the major reservoir of protein-bound calcium. Disorders that alter plasma pH or serum albumin concentration must be considered when circulating calcium concentrations are being evaluated. The fraction of ionized calcium is inversely related to plasma pH; **alkalosis** can precipitate hypocalcemia by lowering ionized calcium without changing total serum calcium. Alkalosis may result from hyperpnea caused by anxiety or from hyperventilation related to physical exertion. Hypoproteinemia may lead to a false suggestion of hypocalcemia because the serum total calcium level is low even though the ionized Ca^{2+} remains normal. It is best to measure serum ionized calcium if hypocalcemia or hypercalcemia is suspected.

Primary hypoparathyroidism causes hypocalcemia, but does not cause rickets. The etiology of primary hypoparathyroidism includes the following:

1. Congenital malformation (DiGeorge syndrome) resulting from developmental abnormalities of the third and fourth branchial arches, leading to hypoparathyroidism and mandibular hypoplasia; hypertelorism; short philtrum; low-set and mal-

formed ears; and malformations of the heart and great vessels, such as ventricular and atrial septal defects, right aortic arch, interrupted aortic arch, and truncus arteriosus (see Chapters 143 and 144)
2. Surgical procedures, such as thyroidectomy or parathyroidectomy, in which parathyroid tissue is removed either deliberately or as a complication of surgery for another goal
3. Autoimmunity, which may destroy the parathyroid gland

Pseudohypoparathyroidism may occur in one of three forms, all with hypocalcemia and hyperphosphatemia, as follows:

1. *Type Ia*—an abnormality of the $G_{s\alpha}$ protein linking the PTH receptor to adenylate cyclase; biologically active PTH is secreted in great quantities, but exerts no effect because there is no way for PTH to stimulate its receptor
2. *Type Ib*—normal $G_{s\alpha}$ with other abnormalities in the production of adenylate cyclase
3. *Type II*—normal production of adenylate cyclase, but a distal defect eliminates the effects of PTH

Pseudohypoparathyroidism is an autosomal dominant condition that may present at birth or later. Other *clinical manifestations* of pseudohypoparathyroidism associated with **Albright hereditary osteodystrophy** include short stature, stocky body habitus, round facies, short fourth and fifth metacarpals, calcification of the basal ganglia, subcutaneous calcification, and often developmental delay. Albright hereditary osteodystrophy may be inherited separately from pseudohypoparathyroidism so that a patient may have a normal appearance with hypocalcemia or may have the Albright hereditary osteodystrophy phenotype with normal serum calcium, phosphate, PTH, and response to PTH (pseudopseudohypoparathyroidism).

During the first 3 days after birth, serum calcium concentrations normally decline in response to withdrawal of the maternal calcium supply via the placenta. Sluggish PTH response in a neonate may result in a transient hypocalcemia. Hypocalcemia caused by attenuated PTH release is found in infants of mothers with hyperparathyroidism and hypercalcemia; the latter suppresses fetal PTH release, causing **transient hypoparathyroidism** in the neonatal period.

Normal serum magnesium concentrations also are required for normal parathyroid gland function and action. **Hypomagnesemia** may cause a secondary hypoparathyroidism, which responds poorly to therapies other than magnesium replacement.

Neonatal tetany resulting from excessive phosphate consumption classically occurs in a 1-week-old to 1-month-old infant who is fed cow's milk. The resultant hyperphosphatemia drives down the serum calcium level, causing symptomatic hypocalcemia. Cow's milk contains more calcium than human milk, but also has more phosphorus. Excessive phosphate retention, as occurs in patients with renal failure, also produces hypocalcemia.

The **etiology of hypocalcemia** usually can be discerned by combining features of the clinical presentation with determinations of serum ionized calcium, phosphate, alkaline phosphatase, PTH (preferably at a time when the calcium is low), magnesium, and albumin. X-rays of the long bones and hands and knees are important if the problem occurs after the neonatal period. If the PTH concentration is not elevated appropriately relevant to a low serum calcium, hypoparathyroidism (transient, primary, or caused by hypomagnesemia) is present. Vitamin D stores can be estimated by measuring serum 25-hydroxyvitamin D and renal function assessed by a serum creatinine measurement or determination of creatinine clearance (Table 176-1).

Treatment of severe tetany or seizures resulting from hypocalcemia consists of IV calcium gluconate (1 to 2 mL/kg of 10% solution) given slowly over 10 minutes, while cardiac status is monitored by ECG for bradycardia, which can be fatal. Long-term treatment of hypoparathyroidism involves administering vitamin D, preferably in the form of 1,25-dihydroxyvitamin D, and calcium. Therapy is adjusted to keep the serum calcium in the lower half of the normal range to avoid episodes of hypercalcemia that might produce nephrocalcinosis, which can be monitored by renal ultrasound, and pancreatitis.

RICKETS

Rickets is defined as decreased or defective bone mineralization in growing children; **osteomalacia** is the same condition in adults. The proportion of osteoid (the organic portion of the bone) is excessive. As a result, the bone becomes soft, and the metaphyses of the long bones widen. Poor linear growth, bowing of the legs on weight bearing (often painful), thickening at the wrists and knees, and prominence of the costochondral junctions (rachitic rosary) of the rib cage occur. At this stage, the x-ray findings are diagnostic.

In **nutritional vitamin D deficiency**, calcium is not absorbed adequately from the intestine (see Chapter 31). Poor vitamin D intake (food fads or poor maternal diet affecting breast milk vitamin D) or avoidance of sunlight in infants exclusively breastfed may contribute to the development of rickets. Vitamin D–deficiency rickets occurs predominantly in African American or Asian infants who are breastfed and have inadequate exposure to sun because of illness or parental choice. Fat malabsorption resulting from hepatobiliary disease (biliary atresia, neonatal hepatitis) or other causes also may produce vitamin D deficiency because vitamin D is a fat-soluble vitamin. Defects in vitamin D metabolism by the kidney (renal failure, autosomal recessive deficiency of 1α-hydroxylation, **vitamin D–dependent rickets**) or liver (defect in 25-hydroxylation) also can cause rickets. Very low birth weight infants have an increased incidence of rickets of prematurity.

In **familial hypophosphatemic rickets**, the major defect in mineral metabolism is failure of the kidney to reabsorb filtered phosphate adequately so that serum phosphate decreases, and urinary phosphate is high. The *diagnosis* of this X-linked disease usually is made within the first few years of life. Disease typically is more severe in males.

The **etiology** of rickets usually can be determined by assessment of the mineral and vitamin D (25-hydroxyvitamin D <8 ng/mL suggests nutritional vitamin D deficiency) status as outlined for the different disorders (see Table 176-1). Further testing of mineral balance or measurement of other vitamin D metabolites may be required in more difficult cases.

Several chemical forms of vitamin D can be used for **treatment** of the different rachitic conditions, but their potencies vary widely, and required dosages depend on the condition being treated (see

TABLE 176-1.   Important Physiologic Changes in Bone and Mineral Diseases

Condition	Calcium	Phosphate	Parathyroid Hormone	25(OH)D
Primary hypoparathyroidism	↓	↑	↓	Nl
Pseudohypoparathyroidism	↓	↑	↑	Nl
Vitamin D deficiency	Nl(↓)	↓	↑	↓
Familial hypophosphatemic rickets	Nl	↓	Nl (sl↑)	Nl
Hyperparathyroidism	↑	↓	↑	Nl
Immobilization	↑	↑	↓	Nl

Nl, normal; sl, slight; ↑, high; ↓, low; 25(OH)D, 25-hydroxyvitamin D.

Chapter 31). Rickets usually is treated with 1,25-hydroxyvitamin D and supplemental calcium. In hypophosphatemic rickets, phosphate supplementation (not calcium) must accompany vitamin D therapy, which is given to suppress secondary hyperparathyroidism. Adequate therapy restores normal skeletal growth and produces resolution of the radiographic signs of rickets. Nutritional rickets is treated with vitamin D in one large dose or multiple smaller replacement doses. Surgery may be required to straighten legs in untreated patients with long-standing disease.

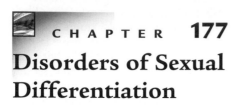

CHAPTER 177
Disorders of Sexual Differentiation

NORMAL SEXUAL DEVELOPMENT

Gender is determined by a combination of karyotype (genotypic or chromosomal sex), which usually determines the morphology of internal organs and gonads (gonadal sex); the appearance of the external genitalia and the form of secondary sex characteristics (phenotypic sex); the self-perception of the individual (gender identity); and the perception of the individual by others (gender role). In most children, these features blend and conform, but in some patients, one or more features may not follow this sequence, leading to an intersex condition (see Chapter 23).

Ambiguous genitalia in a newborn must be attended to with as little delay as possible and with informed sensitivity to the psychosocial context as required. To offset the risk of lifelong pattern of gender uncertainty in the patient and confusion in the parents, the healthcare providers must help families come to an appropriate closure and gender choice. Complicating matters, the laboratory evaluations required might take days or weeks to complete, delaying a sex assignment and naming of the infant, such that choice often precedes diagnosis.

Diagnosis and treatment of disorders of sex differentiation are best understood in terms of the embryology and hormonal control of normal sex differentiation. The internal and external genitalia are formed between 9 and 13 weeks of gestation. Regardless of karyotype, a fetal gonad is bipotential and has the capacity to support development of a normal male or female phenotype. A female phenotype develops unless specific "male" influences alter development. The male or female phenotype develops internally from bipotential gonads and ducts and externally from

bipotential anlage (Fig. 177–1). In the presence of a gene called *SRY* for sex-determining region on the Y gene on the Y chromosome, the primitive fetal gonad differentiates into a testis (Fig. 177–2). The testis secretes testosterone, which has direct effects (stimulation of development of the wolffian ducts), but also is locally converted to dihydrotestosterone (DHT) by the 5α-reductase enzyme for other effects. DHT causes enlargement, rugation, and fusion of the labioscrotal folds into a scrotum; fusion of the ventral surface of the penis to enclose a penile urethra; and enlargement of the phallus with ultimate development of male external genitalia. Testicular production and secretion of müllerian-inhibitory substance cause the regression and disappearance of the müllerian ducts and their derivatives, such as the fallopian tubes and uterus. In the presence of testosterone, the wolffian ducts develop into the vas deferens, seminiferous tubules, and prostate.

In the absence of *SRY,* an ovary spontaneously develops from the bipotential, primitive gonad. In the absence of fetal testicular secretion of müllerian-inhibitory substance, a normal uterus, fallopian tubes, and posterior third of the vagina develop out of the müllerian ducts, and the wolffian ducts degenerate. In the total absence of androgens, the external genitalia appear female.

A child with ambiguous genitalia may have a male karyotype or a female karyotype. In the female pseudohermaphrodite, the genotype is 46,XX, and the gonads are ovaries, but the external genitalia are virilized. In the male pseudohermaphrodite, the genotype is 46,XY, and the external genitalia are undervirilized. Reasons can include abnormal development of the testes; defects of sex steroid biosynthesis, including testosterone or DHT; or androgen receptor defects. On physical examination, it is essential to note where the urethral opening lies and whether there is fusion of the posterior portion of the labioscrotal folds. Endogenous excessive production of androgen (as in CAH) in a female fetus between 9 and 13 weeks of gestation leads to ambiguous genitalia. If the vaginal opening is normal, and there is no fusion, but the clitoris is enlarged without ventral fusion of the ventral urethra, the patient had later exposure to androgens. A patient with a fully formed scrotum, even if small, and a normally formed but small penis, termed a *microphallus,* must have had normal exposure to and action of androgen during 9 to 13 weeks of gestation.

ABNORMAL SEXUAL DEVELOPMENT
Virilization of the 46,XX Female (Female Pseudohermaphroditism)

Masculinization of the external genitalia of genotypic females (except for isolated enlargement of the clitoris,

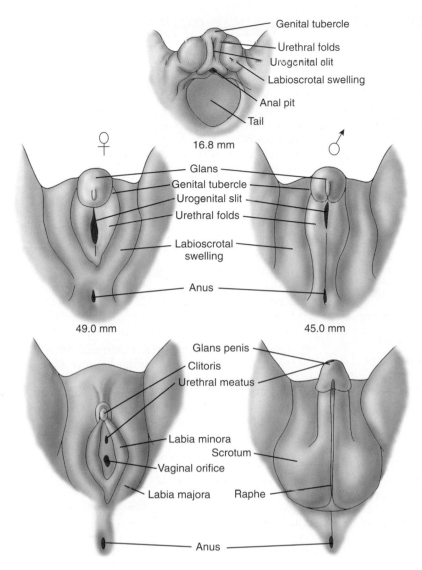

Genital tubercle
Urethral folds
Urogenital slit
Labioscrotal swelling
Anal pit
Tail

16.8 mm

♀

Glans
Genital tubercle
Urogenital slit
Urethral folds
Labioscrotal
swelling
Anus

♂

49.0 mm

45.0 mm

Glans penis
Clitoris
Urethral meatus

Labia minora
Scrotum
Vaginal orifice
Labia majora
Raphe

Anus

Figure 177-1

Differentiation of male and female external genitalia as proceeding from a common embryonic anlage. Testosterone acts at 9 to 13 weeks of gestation to virilize the bipotential anlage. In the absence of testosterone action, the female phenotype develops. (From Grumbach MM, Conte FA: Disorders of sexual differentiation. In Wilson JD, Foster DW [eds]: Textbook of Endocrinology, 8th ed. Philadelphia, WB Saunders, 1990, p 873. Adapted from Spaulding MH: Contrib Embryol Instit 13:69-88, 1921.)

which can occur from later androgen exposure) is always caused by the presence of excessive androgens during the critical period of development (8 to 13 weeks of gestation) (Table 177-1). The magnitude of the changes reflects the quantity and duration of exposure to androgens. The degree of virilization can range from mild clitoral enlargement to the appearance of a "male" phallus with a penile urethra and fused scrotum with raphe. Congenital virilizing adrenal hyperplasia is the most common cause of ambiguous genitalia; it is most commonly the result of an adrenal enzyme deficiency that impairs aldosterone and cortisol synthesis, but does not affect androgen production. The impaired cortisol secretion leads to ACTH hypersecretion, which stimulates hyperplasia of the adrenal

cortex and excessive adrenal production of androgens (see Chapter 178).

Inadequate Masculinization of the 46,XY Male (Male Pseudohermaphroditism)

Underdevelopment of the male external genitalia occurs because of a relative deficiency of testosterone production or action (Table 177-2). The penis is small, with various degrees of hypospadias (penile or perineal) and associated chordee or ventral binding of the phallus; unilateral, but more often bilateral, cryptorchidism may be present. The testes should be sought carefully in the inguinal canal or labioscrotal folds by palpation or ultrasound. Rarely a palpable

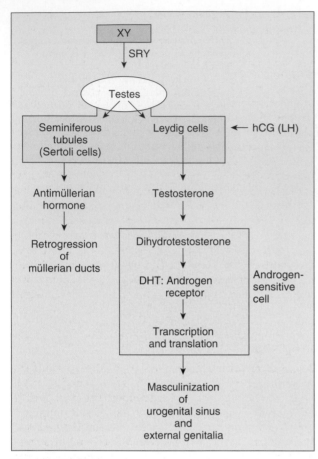

Figure 177–2

A diagrammatic scheme of male sex determination and differentiation. DHT, dihydrotestosterone; *SRY,* the gene for the testis-determining factor. *SRY* is the master gene controlling male sex differentiation, but there are many other genes and their products that control male and female sexual differentiation. (From Wilson JD, Foster DW [eds]: Williams Textbook of Endocrinology, 8th ed. Philadelphia, WB Saunders, 1992, p 918.)

gonad in the inguinal canal or labioscrotal fold represents a herniated ovary, or an ovotestis in a hermaphrodite. The latter patients have ovarian and testicular tissue and usually an XX genotype and ambiguous external genitalia. Production of testosterone by a gonad implies that testicular tissue is present and that at least some cells carry the *SRY* gene.

Testosterone production can be reduced by specific deficiencies of the enzymes needed for androgen biosynthesis or by dysplasia of the gonads. In the latter, if müllerian-inhibiting substance production also is reduced, a rudimentary uterus and fallopian tubes are present. Enzyme defects in testosterone biosynthesis, which also block cortisol production, produce adrenal

TABLE 177–1. Causes of Virilization in the Female

Condition	Additional Features
P-450$_{c21}$ deficiency	Salt loss in some
3β-Hydroxysteroid dehydrogenase deficiency	Salt loss
P-450$_{C11}$ deficiency	Salt retention/hypertension
Androgenic drug exposure (e.g., progestins)	Exposure between 9th and 12th wk gestation
Mixed gonadal dysgenesis or mosaic Turner syndrome	Karyotype = 46,XY/45,X
True hermaphrodite	Testicular and ovarian tissue present
Maternal virilizing adrenal or ovarian tumor	Rare, positive history

hyperplasia. Hypopituitarism with LH deficiency does not result in ambiguous genitalia because placental HCG in the fetal circulation stimulates fetal gonadal testosterone synthesis during the critical 9 to 13 weeks of gestation to allow development of a normal male

TABLE 177–2. Causes of Inadequate Masculinization in the Male

Condition	Additional Features
P-450$_{scc}$ (STAR) deficiency	Salt loss
3β-Hydroxysteroid dehydrogenase deficiency	Salt loss
P-450$_{c17}$ deficiency	Salt retention/hypokalemia/ hypertension
Isolated P-450$_{c17}$ deficiency with 17,20-desmolase deficiency	Adrenal function normal
17β-Hydroxysteroid oxidoreductase deficiency	Adrenal function normal
Dysgenetic testes	Possible abnormal karyotype
Leydig cell hypoplasia	Rare
Complete androgen insensitivity or testicular feminization	Female external genitalia, absence of müllerian structures
Partial androgen insensitivity	As above with ambiguous external genitalia
5α-Reductase deficiency	Autosomal recessive, virilization at puberty

phallus. Later in gestation, fetal LH is needed to stimulate the testes to produce adequate androgen to enlarge the fetal penis. Congenital gonadotropin deficiency may produce a normally formed but small penis (microphallus without hypospadias); this condition is often combined with deficiencies of GH and ACTH in neonatal hypopituitarism, causing neonatal hypoglycemia. Microphallus caused by this etiology responds to testosterone treatment, resulting in an enlargement of the penis.

The complete form of **androgen resistance** or **androgen insensitivity syndrome** is the most dramatic example of resistance to hormone action by defects in the androgen receptor. Affected patients have a **46,XY** karyotype, normally formed testes (usually located in the inguinal canal or labia majora), and feminine-appearing external genitalia with a short vagina and no internal müllerian structures. At the time of puberty, testosterone concentrations increase to or above the normal male range. Because a portion of the testosterone is normally converted to estradiol in peripheral tissues, and the estrogen cannot be opposed by the androgen, breast development ensues at the normal age of puberty without growth of pubic, facial, or axillary hair or the occurrence of menstruation. Gender identity and gender role are unequivocally **female**.

5α-Reductase deficiency presents at birth with predominantly female phenotype or with ambiguous genitalia, including perineoscrotal hypospadias. The defect is in 5α reduction of testosterone to its metabolite DHT. At puberty, spontaneous secondary male sexual development occurs, and the individual, raised as a girl until this age, in most cases converts to a male gender identity and male gender role. The interpretation of this change is controversial, but is said by some to indicate that gender role, classically thought to be set by 2 to 4 years of age, can change much later in life. Others state that the child is recognized at birth as being different than a normal female and propose that the change in gender is culturally acceptable.

APPROACH TO THE INFANT WITH GENITAL AMBIGUITY

The major goal is a rapid identification of any life-threatening disorders (salt loss and shock caused by the salt-losing form of CAH). The decision of sex assignment is crucial, but is rendered more complex by the realization that prenatal androgen exposure (in an individual without complete androgen resistance) causes a tendency toward a male gender identity and male gender role. Although the classic approach to sex assignment has been based on the feasibility of genital reconstruction and potential fertility rather than on karyotype or gonadal histology, the effects of prenatal androgen must be considered. It may be inappropriate to raise a female infant who is severely virilized from virilizing CAH as a male; in most reported cases, sex assignment and adult gender role remain female. If surgically corrected as a female, she will likely retain fertility because the internal organs are female. A 46,XY male with ambiguous genitalia and an extremely small phallus that does not increase in size with androgen therapy (partial androgen resistance) traditionally has been raised as a female because surgical construction of a fully functional phallus is difficult. Some of these patients frequently revert spontaneously, however, to a male gender identity. Present management of ambiguous genitalia involves extensive open discussion with parents involving the biology of the infant and the likely prognosis. Treatment should be individualized and managed by a team including an experienced pediatric endocrinologist, a urologist or gynecologist, and the family physician or pediatrician of the affected infant.

Diagnosis

The first step toward diagnosis is to determine if the disorder represents virilization of a genetic female (androgen excess) or underdevelopment of a genetic male (androgen deficiency) (see Fig. 177–2). Inguinal gonads that are evident on palpation usually are testes and indicate that incomplete development of a male phenotype has occurred; this pattern is not consistent, and ovaries and ovotestes may feel similar. Similarly, absence of female internal genitalia (detected by ultrasound) implies that müllerian-inhibiting substance was present and secreted by fetal testes. Karyotype determination is only one of many factors in deciding the sexual identity for purposes of rearing; the *SRY* gene may be found on chromosomes other than the Y chromosome, and conversely a Y chromosome may lack an *SRY* gene (it may have been translocated to an X chromosome, leading to the development of a 46,XX male).

Statistically, most virilized females have CAH, and 90% of these females have 21-hydroxylase deficiency. The diagnosis is established by measuring the plasma concentration of 17-OHP (see Chapter 178), which typically is hundreds of times above the normal range. Other enzymatic defects also may be diagnosed by quantifying the circulating levels of the steroid precursor proximal to the defective enzyme block.

Establishing an accurate diagnosis is more difficult in underdeveloped males. When certain types of adrenal hyperplasia coexist with defects in androgen production of the testes, excessive ACTH secretion elevates levels of specific adrenal steroid precursors substantially, allowing diagnosis. If the defect is restricted to testosterone biosynthesis, the measurement of testosterone and its precursors in the basal state and after stimulation by HCG may be required. Patients with normal levels of testosterone either have persistent androgen resistance (they lack a response to exogenous testosterone) or have had an interruption of normal morphogenesis of the genitalia. Abnormalities of the sex chromosomes may be associated with dysgenetic gonads, which may be associated with persistence of müllerian structures.

Treatment

Treatment consists of replacing deficient hormones (cortisol in adrenal hyperplasia or testosterone to increase phallic size and facilitate puberty in a child with androgen biosynthetic defects who will be raised as male), surgical restoration to make the individual look more appropriate for the sex of rearing, and psychological support of the whole family. Gonads and internal organs discordant for the sex of rearing are removed. Dysgenetic gonads with Y-genetic material always should be removed because **gonadoblastomas** or **dysgerminomas** subsequently may develop in the organ. Reconstructive surgery usually has been started by 2 years of age so that genital structure reflects sex of rearing. This recommendation for reconstructive surgery is controversial; some advocate that surgery not be performed in infancy or early childhood so that the child or young adolescent can be involved in the decision. A decision for sex of rearing is recommended from birth, however, and the knowledge that the intersexed person may change gender later on is shared with parents from the outset.

CHAPTER 178
Adrenal Gland Dysfunction

The adrenal gland consists of an outer cortex, responsible for the synthesis of steroids, and an inner medulla derived from neuroectodermal tissue, which synthesizes catecholamines. The *adrenal cortex* consists of three zones: an outer glomerulosa whose end product is the mineralocorticoid aldosterone, which regulates sodium and potassium balance; a middle zone, the fasciculata, whose end product is cortisol; and an inner reticularis, which synthesizes sex steroids. The general scheme of these synthetic steps is shown in Figure 178–1.

Hypothalamic corticotropin-releasing hormone (CRH) stimulates the release of pituitary ACTH, derived by selective processing from pro-opiomelanocortin. ACTH governs the synthesis and release of cortisol and adrenal androgens. Primary adrenal insufficiency or cortisol deficiency from any defect in the adrenal gland results in an oversecretion of ACTH; cortisol deficiency also may occur from ACTH (secondary) or CRH (tertiary) deficiency, causing low serum ACTH concentrations and low cortisol. Endogenous (or exogenous) glucocorticoids feed back to inhibit ACTH and CRH secretion. The renin-angiotensin system and potassium regulate aldosterone secretion; ACTH has little effect on aldosterone production except in excess, when it may increase aldosterone secretion.

Steroids that circulate in the free form (not bound to cortisol-binding protein [transcortin]) may cross the placenta from mother to fetus, but ACTH does not. The placenta plays an important role in steroid biosynthesis in utero, acting as a metabolic mediator between mother and child. Because the fetal CRH-ACTH-adrenal axis is operational in utero, deficiencies in cortisol synthesis lead to excessive ACTH secretion. If a virilizing adrenal enzyme defect is present, such as 21-hydroxylase deficiency, the fetal adrenal gland secretes androgens, virilizing the fetus.

The normal variation of serum cortisol and ACTH levels leads to values that are high early in the morning and lower at night. This normal diurnal variation may not be established until the child is 1 to 4 years old.

ADRENAL INSUFFICIENCY

The **clinical manifestations** of inadequate adrenal function result from the inadequate secretion or action of glucocorticoids, mineralocorticoids, or both (Table 178–1). In addition, in the case of enzyme defects that affect the gonad and the adrenal gland, overproduction or underproduction of potent androgens can occur, depending on the site of enzyme blockade (see Fig. 178–1). Progressive prenatal virilization of the external genitalia may occur in females; incomplete virilization may occur in males. Ambiguity of the external genitalia is a common manifestation of disordered fetal adrenal enzyme function. Precise *diagnosis* is essential for the prescription of appropriate therapy, long-term outlook, and genetic counseling. Table 178–2 presents a diagnostic classification of adrenal insufficiency in infancy and childhood. In patients with enzyme ·defects, an elevation in the precursor steroid is present proximal to the enzyme block, a deficiency of steroids is present subsequent to the block, and an excess of precursor is metabolized through remaining normal alternate enzyme pathways. Enzyme kinetics may be exploited in the diagnosis and treatment of CAH.

The dominant clinical features of adrenal insufficiency in infancy are related to mineralocorticoid

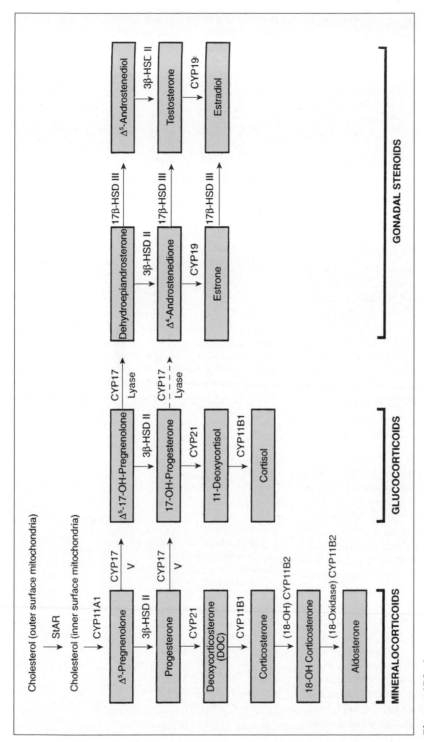

Figure 178–1

Diagram of the steroid biosynthetic pathways and the biosynthetic defects that result in congenital hyperplasia. The defect in patients with lipoid adrenal hyperplasia is not (except for one reported case) in the CYP11A1 (cholesterol side-chain cleavage) enzyme, but in StAR, the steroidogenic acute regulatory protein. This protein is involved in the transport of cholesterol from the outer mitochondrial membrane to the inner membrane, where the CYP11A1 enzyme is located. CYP11B1 (11β-hydroxylase) catalyzes 11β-hydroxylation of deoxocorticosterone and 11β-deoxycortisol primarily. CYP17 (17α-hydroxylase/17,20-lyase) catalyzes 17α-hydroxylation and splitting of the 17,20 bond, but for the latter it has preferential Δ⁵-17,20-lyase activity (see text). CYP19 (aromatase) catalyzes the conversion of corticosterone to aldoste-one. 3β-HSD I and 3β-HSD II, 3β-hydroxysteroid dehydrogenase/Δ⁴,⁵-isomerase types I and II; CYP21 (P450₂₁), 21-hydroxylase; 17β-HSD 3, 17β-hydroxysteroid dehydrogenase type 3. In the human, deletion of a homozygous null mutation of CYP11A (P450ₛcc) is probably lethal in utero, but a heterogeneous mutation caused congenital lipoid adrenal hyperplasia. (From Melmed S, Polonsky K, Kronenberg H, Larsen R [eds]: Williams Textbook of Endocrinology, 10th ed. Philadelphia, Elsevier, 2003, p 917.)

TABLE 178–1. Clinical Manifestations of Adrenal Insufficiency

Cortisol deficiency
  Hypoglycemia
  Inability to withstand stress
  Vasomotor collapse
  Hyperpigmentation (in primary adrenal insufficiency
    with excess of adrenocorticotropic hormone)
  Apneic spells
  Muscle weakness, fatigue
Aldosterone deficiency
  Hyponatremia
  Hyperkalemia
  Vomiting
  Urinary sodium wasting
  Salt craving
  Acidosis
  Failure to thrive
  Volume depletion
  Hypotension
  Dehydration
  Shock
  Diarrhea
  Muscle weakness
Androgen excess or deficiency (caused by adrenal
    enzyme defect)
  Ambiguous genitalia in certain conditions

alkalosis is present. This distinction may be lifesaving in preventing unnecessary investigations or inappropriate therapy.

Not all forms of adrenal hyperplasia present at birth; the spectrum of disorder ranges from severe, or

TABLE 178–2. Causes of Adrenal Insufficiency in Infancy and Childhood

Congenital adrenal hypoplasia
  Secondary to ACTH deficiency
  Autosomal recessive
  X-linked
Adrenal hemorrhage, necrosis, thrombosis
Congenital adrenal hyperplasia
  STAR deficiency
  3β-Hydroxysteroid dehydrogenase deficiency
  P-450$_{c21}$ (21-hydroxylase) deficiency
  P-450$_{c11}$ (11β-hydroxylase) deficiency
  P-450$_{c17}$ (17-hydroxylase) deficiency
Isolated deficiency of aldosterone synthesis
  P-450$_{c11}$ (18-hydroxylase) deficiency
  P-450$_{c11}$ (18-hydroxysteroid dehydrogenase) deficiency
Pseudohypoaldosteronism—end-organ unresponsiveness
    to aldosterone
Congenital adrenal unresponsiveness to ACTH
Addison disease
  Autoimmune adrenal insufficiency*
  Infections of the adrenal gland
    Tuberculosis
    Histoplasmosis
    Meningococcosis
  Infiltration of the adrenal gland
    Sarcoidosis
    Hemochromatosis
    Amyloidosis
    Metastatic cancer, lymphoma
  Adrenoleukodystrophy
Secondary—pituitary-hypothalamic
  Craniopharyngioma
  Histiocytosis
  Empty sella syndrome
  Pituitary irradiation
  Sarcoidosis
  Hypothalamic lesions
  Postpartum pituitary necrosis
  Head trauma
Drugs (suppress adrenal steroidogenesis)
  Acute withdrawal of steroid therapy given for
    >7-10 days
  Metyrapone
  Ketoconazole

*Isolated or as part of polyglandular syndrome type I (adrenal, hypoparathyroidism, mucocutaneous candidiasis) or type II (adrenal, thyroid, insulin-dependent diabetes).
ACTH, adrenocorticotropic hormone.

deficiency; these develop only if there is impairment of mineralocorticoid secretion or action. Serum electrolyte measurement reveals hyponatremia and hyperkalemia usually developing by 5 to 7 days after birth but not usually immediately after birth. Vomiting, dehydration, and acidosis soon follow, as do shock and death, if the affected subject remains undiagnosed and untreated. In females, the ambiguity of the external genitalia, resulting from excessive androgen secretion, implies that mineralocorticoid deficiency must be ruled out, as occurs in the setting of salt-losing CAH, although not in simple virilizing CAH. Clinically, these forms cannot be distinguished such that all presentations of ambiguous genitalia should involve evaluation for mineralocorticoid deficiency. In males, the most common form of CAH, 21-hydroxylase deficiency, does not cause abnormal genitalia such that there is no obvious physical clue to the potential for salt loss. There may be hyperpigmentation of the scrotal skin, but this is a subtle sign likely to have been overlooked. In all infants, the diagnosis of adrenal insufficiency may be overlooked or confused with pyloric stenosis. In pyloric stenosis, in contrast to salt-losing CAH, vomiting hydrochloric acid in stomach contents results in hypochloremia, serum potassium is normal or low, and

classic, to mild, or late-onset, or nonclassic. Milder forms may manifest in childhood, adolescence, or even young adulthood, not as glucocorticoid or mineralo-corticoid deficiencies, but as androgen excess. In patients with congenital adrenal hypoplasia or adrenal hemorrhage, the secretion of all adrenal steroids is low. In contrast, CAH leads to a diagnostic steroid pattern in blood and urine (see Fig. 178-1). Deficiency of 21-hydroxylase is the most common form (95%) and serves as a paradigm for these disorders.

21-HYDROXYLASE DEFICIENCY

The incidence of classic 21-hydroxylase deficiency is about 1 in 12,000 among various white populations. A higher incidence occurs in Yupik Eskimos, Yugosla-vians, and Ashkenazi Jews. Nonclassic CAH may occur with an incidence of 1 in 50 in certain populations. The gene for 21-hydroxylase lies on the short arm of chro-mosome 6; if there is an affected proband, the genotype may be determined, permitting prenatal diagnosis in a subsequent pregnancy.

Deficient 21-hydroxylase activity (P-450$_{c21}$ defi-ciency) impairs the conversion of 17-OHP to 11-deoxycortisol and, in the salt-losing form, of proges-terone to deoxycorticosterone, a mineralocorticoid proximal in the pathway to the production of aldos-terone. The decreased production of cortisol causes hypersecretion of ACTH, which stimulates the synthe-sis of steroids immediately proximal to the block and causes shunting of precursors to the androgen pathway, leading to the overproduction of androgens. The primary clinical manifestation is the virilization of the external genitalia of the affected female fetus, in whom the development of the uterus, ovaries, and fallopian tubes remains unaffected by the androgens. The degree of virilization varies, ranging from mild clitoromegaly to complete fusion of labioscrotal folds, with severe clitoromegaly simulating a phallus (see Chapter 177). A male infant with this defect appears normal at birth, although penile enlargement may be apparent thereafter. The deficiency in aldosterone, found in about 75% of patients, causes salt wasting with shock and dehydration until the diagnosis is established and appropriate treatment is given.

Inadequately treated, 21-hydroxylase activity defi-ciency (assuming salt loss does not lead to serious complications) exhibits postnatal virilization, causing excessive height gain and skeletal advance, early appearance of pubic hair, and progressive penile or cli-toral enlargement. Although there is excessive linear growth initially, progressive advancement in the bone age is accompanied by early epiphyseal fusion, ulti-mately yielding jeopardy of adult height potential. Late-onset CAH is noted years after birth, and affected subjects have milder manifestations without ambigu-ous genitalia, but they do have acne, hirsutism, and, in girls, irregular menstrual cycles or amenorrhea. Late-onset CAH in girls may be confused with ovarian hyperandrogenism polycystic ovarian disease.

Biochemical diagnostic studies show elevated levels of serum 17-OHP, the substrate for the defective 21-hydroxylase enzyme activity. In newborns with CAH, the values are elevated a hundredfold to a thou-sandfold, but in late-onset CAH, an ACTH stimulation test is necessary to show an abnormally high response of 17-OHP. Serum cortisol and aldosterone levels (in salt losers) are low, whereas the testosterone level is elevated because it is derived from 17-OHP.

The goals of treatment are to achieve normal linear growth and bone age advancement. Long-term therapy consists of providing glucocorticoids at a dose of approximately 13 to 18 mg/m^2/24 hours in three divided doses of oral hydrocortisone or its equivalent. Mineralocorticoid therapy for salt losers consists of fludrocortisone (Florinef) at a dose of 0.1 to 0.2 mg/24 hours often with sodium chloride supplementation in infancy and early childhood. Surgical correction of ambiguous external genitalia begins by 1 to 2 years of life to permit normal development of gender identity. The adequacy of glucocorticoid replacement therapy often is monitored by determining serum concentra-tions of adrenal precursors, including androstene-dione and 17-OHP for 21-hydroxylase deficiency. In addition, the assessment of linear growth and skele-tal age, by bone age determination, is required as a reflection of appropriate therapy. To avoid adrenal insufficiency, threefold higher doses of glucocorti-coids are given during stressful states, such as febrile illnesses and surgery, and SC glucocorticoid (Solu-Cortef) is used in severe emergencies. Mineralocorti-coid therapy is monitored with serum sodium and potassium and plasma renin activity levels. Prenatal treatment with dexamethasone to suppress fetal ACTH-induced androgen production can reduce or eliminate the ambiguity of the external genitalia in affected female fetuses, if begun at approximately 7 weeks of gestation.

OTHER ENZYME DEFECTS

Other enzyme defects are rare in contrast to 21-hydroxylase deficiency. In 11-hydroxylase deficiency, the next most common cause of CAH, virilization occurs with salt retention and hypokalemia, as a result of the buildup of deoxycorticosterone (see Fig. 178-1), which is a potent mineralocorticoid. Hypertension develops as a result of excessive mineralocorticoid pro-duction. Table 178-3 summarizes the clinical and bio-chemical features of adrenal insufficiency in infancy.

TABLE 178–3. Clinical and Biochemical Features in Newborn Adrenal Insufficiency

		Ambiguous Genitalia		Serum					Urine		
	Electrolyte Disturbance*	Virilized Female	Undervirilized Male	Cortisol	11-Deoxycortisol	17-OHP	DHEA	Aldosterone	17-OHCS	17-KS	Pregnanetriol
Hypoplasia	Severe	No	No	D	D	D	D	D	D	D	D
Hemorrhage	Moderate to severe	No	No	D	D	D	D	D	D	D	D
STAR deficiency	Severe	No	Yes	D	D	D	D	D	D	D	D
3β-HSD	Severe	Yes	Yes	D	D	D	I	D	D	I	D
P-450$_{21}$ deficiency	Absent to severe	Yes	No	D	D	I	I	D	D	I	I
Aldosterone synthesis block	Severe	No	No	Nl	Nl	Nl	Nl	D	Nl	Nl	Nl
Pseudohypoaldosteronism	Severe	No	No	Nl	Nl	Nl	Nl	I	Nl	Nl	Nl
P-450$_{11}$ deficiency	None	Yes	No	D	I	Nl or I	Nl	D	I	I	Nl–sl I
P-450$_{17}$ deficiency	†	No	Yes	D	Nl–D	D	D	Nl–D	D	D	D
Unresponsiveness to ACTH	†	No	No	D	Nl–D	Nl–D	Nl–D	Nl–D	D	D	Nl–D

*Usually manifested after 5 days of age.
†High normal Na$^+$ and low normal to low K$^+$.
ACTH, adrenocorticotropic hormone; D, decrease; HSD, hydroxysteroid dehydrogenase; I, increase; Nl, normal; 17-KS, 17-ketosteroid; 17-OHCS, 17-hydroxycorticosteroid.

ADDISON DISEASE

Addison disease is a rare acquired disorder of childhood, usually associated with autoimmune destruction of the adrenal cortex. It is a form of primary adrenal insufficiency, and there is absence of glucocorticoid and mineralocorticoid.

Clinical manifestations are hyperpigmentation, salt craving, postural hypotension, fasting hypoglycemia, and episodes of shock during severe illness. Baseline and ACTH-stimulated cortisol values are subnormal, confirming the diagnosis; hyponatremia, hyperkalemia, and elevated plasma renin activity indicate mineralocorticoid deficiency. Addison disease may occur within the context of autoimmune polyglandular syndrome type I, consisting as well of hypoparathyroidism, mucocutaneous candidiasis, and often hypothyroidism. Associated autoimmune disorders include oophoritis, pernicious anemia and malabsorption, chronic hepatitis, vitiligo, and alopecia (see Table 178-2).

Replacement **treatment** with 13 to 18 mg/m^2/24 hours of hydrocortisone is indicated, with supplementation during stress at three times the normal maintenance dosage or the use of subcutaneous glucocorticoid (see earlier for CAH). The dose is titrated to allow a normal growth rate. Mineralocorticoid replacement with fludrocortisone is monitored by plasma renin activity and serum sodium and potassium determinations.

CUSHING SYNDROME

Classic **clinical manifestations** of Cushing syndrome in children include progressive central or generalized obesity, marked failure of longitudinal growth, hirsutism, weakness, a nuchal fat pad (buffalo hump), acne, striae, hypertension, and often hyperpigmentation when ACTH is elevated. The most frequent etiology is exogenous glucocorticoid administration in the context of numerous conditions requiring administration of long-term pharmacologic doses of glucocorticoids. Endogenous causes include adrenal adenoma, carcinoma, nodular adrenal hyperplasia, an ACTH-secreting pituitary microadenoma resulting in bilateral adrenal hyperplasia (Cushing disease), or an extremely rare ACTH-secreting tumor. The high-dose dexamethasone suppression test (20 μg/kg orally every 6 hours for 48 hours) suppresses glucocorticoid secretion in Cushing disease, but not in autonomous adrenal production of cortisol or in an ectopic ACTH-secreting tumor. Parenteral glucocorticoid therapy is necessary during and immediately after surgical treatment to avoid acute adrenal insufficiency.

Spontaneous Cushing syndrome is rare in childhood. Iatrogenic Cushing syndrome is far more common, produces similar clinical manifestations, and may be induced by the use of potent glucocorticoids for chronic inflammatory, neoplastic, and collagen vascular disorders and for suppression of the immune response. Depending on the potency of glucocorticoid used and its duration of use, adrenal gland size and secretory ability and pituitary ACTH production and secretion are suppressed. Recovery of pituitary ACTH secretion precedes that of adrenal gland function. Glucocorticoids should be withdrawn gradually over many weeks rather than cut abruptly when phasing out long-term treatment. Specifically, a taper is accomplished safely by bringing the patient's dose, when clinically safe, down to approximately 25 mg/m^2/24 hours in three divided doses of oral hydrocortisone, then progressively to zero over 6 to 8 weeks. During this tapering process, any emergency requires glucocorticoid therapy at triple the physiologic dose. After the taper, the ability of the adrenal gland to respond to ACTH with a doubling of plasma cortisol to levels of at least 15 to 20 μg/dL indicates recovery of pituitary-adrenal function; this test is rarely required.

Treatment of Cushing syndrome is directed to the etiology. Treatment may include excision of autonomous adrenal, pituitary, or ectopic ACTH-secreting tumors. Rarely, adrenalectomy or adrenal ablative agents (mitotane) are needed to control the symptoms.

SUGGESTED READING

Allen DB, Fost N: hGH for short stature: Ethical issues raised by expanded access. J Pediatr 144:648-652, 2004.

Arlt W, Allolio B: Adrenal insufficiency. Lancet 361:1881-1892, 2003.

Behrman RE, Kliegman RM, Jenson HB (eds): Nelson Textbook of Pediatrics, 17th ed. Philadelphia, WB Saunders, 2003.

Cooper DS: Combined T$_4$ and T$_3$ therapy—back to the drawing board. JAMA 290:3002-3004, 2003.

Cooper DS: Hyperthyroidism. Lancet 362:459-468, 2003.

Cutler GB Jr: Treatment of hypopituitary children. J Pediatr 144:415-416, 2004.

Devendra D, Liu E, Eisenbarth GS: Type 1 diabetes: Recent developments. BMJ 328:750-754, 2004.

Dunger DB, Sperling MA, Acerini CL, et al: European Society for Paediatric Endocrinology/Lawson Wilkins Pediatric Endocrine Society consensus statement on diabetic ketoacidosis in children and adolescents. Pediatrics 113:e133-e140, 2004.

Eisenbarth GS, Gottlieb PA: Autoimmune polyendocrine syndromes. N Engl J Med 350:2068-2079, 2004.

Elder J: Ambiguous genitalia. In Kliegman RM, Greenbaum LA, Lye PS (eds): Practical Strategies in Pediatric Diagnosis and Therapy. Philadelphia, WB Saunders, 2004, pp 517-532.

Frader J, Alderson P, Asch A, et al: Health care professionals and intersex conditions. Arch Pediatr Adoles Med 158:426-429, 2004.

Gahagan S, Silverstein J: Prevention and treatment of type 2 diabetes mellitus in children with special emphasis on American Indian and Alaskan Native children. Pediatrics 112:e328-e347, 2003.

Hoppu S, Ronkainen MS, Kimpimaki T, et al: Insulin autoantibody isotypes during the prediabetic process in young children with increased genetic risk of type 1 diabetes. Pediatr Res 55:236-242, 2004.

MacLaughlin DT, Donahoe PK: Sex determination and differentiation. N Engl J Med 350:367-378, 2004.

Ogilvy-Stuart AL: Neonatal thyroid disorders. Arch Dis Child Fetal Neonatal Educ 87:F165-F171, 2002.

Rangecroft L: Surgical management of ambiguous genitalia. Arch Dis Child 88:799-801, 2003.

Roberts CGP, Landenson PW: Hypothyroidism. Lancet 363:793-802, 2004.

Speiser PW, White PC: Congenital adrenal hyperplasia. N Engl J Med 349:776-788, 2003.

Stanhope R: Gonadotrophin-dependent precocious puberty and occult intracranial tumors: Which girls should have neuroimaging? J Pediatr 143:426-427, 2003.

CHAPTER **179**

Assessment

The process and interpretation of the neurologic examination vary with age. The examination of a newborn is unique with transient and primitive reflex patterns. The examination of an adolescent is similar to that of an adult.

HISTORY

Gathering neurologic history follows the traditional steps of medical history taking with two additions: the **pace** of the process and the **localization** of problem within the neuraxis. The pace or evolution of symptoms provides clues to the nature of the disease process. Symptom evolution is defined as **progressive**, **static**, **intermittent**, or **salutatory**. Progressive symptoms may evolve suddenly or hyperacutely (seizures or stroke), acutely over minutes or hours (extradural hemorrhage), subacutely over days or weeks (brain tumor), or symptoms may follow an indolent, chronic course (hereditary neuropathies). Static neurologic abnormalities are observed in the first few months of life and do not change in character over time (cerebral palsy). They are often caused by congenital abnormalities of brain or brain injury sustained during the prenatal or neonatal period. Intermittent, recurrent, or brief symptoms suggest epileptic or migraine syndromes. Salutatory disorders, characterized by periods of symptoms followed by partial recovery, are seen with demyelinating and vascular diseases.

PHYSICAL EXAMINATION

Because the brain and skin have the same embryonic origin from the ectoderm, abnormalities of hair, skin, teeth, and nails are frequent accompaniments of congenital brain disorders (neurocutaneous disorders).

Café au lait macules are flat, light brown areas of skin greater than 0.5 cm in size. **Adenoma sebaceum**, fibrovascular lesions that look like acne on the nose and malar face regions, is commonly seen in older children and adults with tuberous sclerosis.

The **head circumference** is measured in its largest occipitofrontal circumference and plotted against appropriate standard growth curves (see Chapter 5). **Microcephaly** is an occipitofrontal circumference 2 SDs below the mean. **Microcephaly** is an occipitofrontal circumference 2 SDs above the mean. Measurements plotted over time may show an accelerating pattern (hydrocephalus) or a decelerating pattern, indicating brain injury or degenerative neurologic disorder. The anterior fontanel is slightly depressed and pulsatile when a calm infant is placed in the sitting position. A tense or bulging fontanel may indicate increased intracranial pressure (ICP) but also may be seen in a crying infant or an infant with fever. Premature closure of one or more of the sutures (**craniosynostosis**) results in an unusual shape of the head. Abnormal shape, location, and condition of the face, eyes, nares, or ears are found in many genetic syndromes.

A careful **ocular examination** is an essential component of a complete neurologic assessment and should include a search for epicanthal folds, coloboma, conjunctival telangiectasias, or cataracts. A direct ophthalmoscopic examination helps assess the status of the optic discs and macula. A complete examination of the retina requires dilating the pupil and using an indirect ophthalmoscope.

Examination of the hands and feet reveals the presence of abnormal creases, polydactyly, or syndactyly (see Chapters 50 and 199). The neck and spine should be examined for midline defects that may be obvious (spina bifida with myelomeningocele) or subtle (cutaneous dimples, sinus tracts, tufts of hair, or subcutaneous lipomas). Kyphosis and scoliosis may result from abnormalities of the CNS or peripheral nervous system (see Chapter 202).

NEUROLOGIC EXAMINATION OF A NEONATE

The neurologic examination of a neonate is used to assess the function of the basal ganglia, brainstem, and more caudal structures. The results of the examination should be used cautiously in predicting developmental outcome.

Reflexes

Numerous **primitive reflexes**, present at birth, assess the functional integrity of the brainstem and basal ganglia (Table 179–1). They are symmetric and disappear at 4 to 6 months of age, indicating the normal maturation of descending inhibitory cerebral influences (Moro reflex). The **grasp** and **rooting** reflexes are inhibited by maturation of frontal lobe structures and may reappear later in life with frontal lobe lesions. The **Landau** and **parachute** reflexes become apparent after the newborn period, indicating proper maturation of appropriate brain structures. Asymmetry or persistence of the primitive reflexes may indicate focal brain or peripheral nerve lesions.

Posture

Posture is the position that an infant naturally assumes when placed supine. An infant at 28 weeks of gestation shows an extended posture. By 32 weeks, there is a slight trend toward increase in tone of the lower extremities with more lower extremity flexion. At 34 weeks, the lower extremities are flexed, and the upper extremities are extended. At term, the infant flexes lower and upper extremities. **Recoil** is defined as a liveliness with which an arm or leg springs back to its original position after passive stretching and release. Recoil is essentially absent in a small premature infant but is brisk at term.

Movement and Tone

Spontaneous movements of a small premature infant are slow and writhing. Spontaneous movements of a

TABLE 179–1. CNS Reflexes of Infancy

Reflex	Description	Age of Appearance	Age of Disappearance	Origin in CNS
Moro	Sudden head extension causes extension followed by flexion of the arms and legs	Birth	4-6 mo	Brainstem vestibular nuclei
Grasp	Placing a finger in palm results in flexing of the infant's fingers, accompanied by flexion at elbow and shoulder	Birth	4-6 mo	Brainstem vestibular nuclei
Rooting	Tactile stimulus about the mouth results in the infant's mouth pursuing the stimulus	Birth	4-6 mo	Brainstem trigeminal system
Trunk incurvation	Stroking the skin along the edge of the vertebrae produces curvature of the spine with the apex opposite to the direction of the stroke	Birth	4-6 mo	Spinal cord
Placing	Infant places foot on examining surface when dorsum of foot is brought into contact with the edge of the surface	Birth	4-6 mo	Cerebral cortex
Crossed extension	One leg held firmly in extension and the dorsum and sole of the foot stimulated results in a sequence of flexion, extension, and adduction, followed by toe fanning of the opposite leg	Birth	4-6 mo	Spinal cord
Tonic neck	With the infant supine, turning of the head results in ipsilateral extension of the arm and leg in a "fencing" posture	Birth	4-6 mo	Brainstem vestibular nuclei
Parachute	With the infant sitting, tilting to either side results in extension of the ipsilateral arm in a protective fashion	6-8 mo	Never	Brainstem vestibular nuclei
Landau	With the infant held about the waist and suspended, extension of the neck produces extension of the arms and legs	6-8 mo	15 mo-2 yr	Brainstem

term infant are more rapid. The popliteal angle, heel-to-ear maneuver, scarf maneuver, and head control are used in assessing muscle tone and estimating gestational age (see Chapter 58).

NEUROLOGIC EXAMINATION OF A CHILD

The purpose of the neurologic examination is to "localize" or identify the region within the neuraxis from which the symptoms are arising. The **mental status examination** assesses various zones of the cerebral cortex. The **cranial nerve examination** evaluates the integrity of the brainstem. The **motor examination** evaluates upper and lower motor neuron function. The **sensory examination** assesses the peripheral sensory receptors and their central reflections. The **deep tendon reflexes** assess the upper and lower motor connections. The **gait** assessment puts the motor system into a dynamic state for better functional assessment.

Mental Status Evaluation

Alertness is assessed in infants by observing spontaneous activities, feeding behavior, and visual ability to fix and follow the movement of objects. Response to tactile, visual, and auditory stimuli is noted. In circumstances of altered consciousness, the response to painful stimuli is noted. Toddlers are expected to play at a level appropriate for their age. Older children can be tested for orientation to time, place, person, and purpose.

The best way to assess intellectual abilities is through language skills. **Language function** is receptive (understanding speech or gesture) and expressive (speech and the use of gestures). Abnormalities of language resulting from disorders of the cerebral hemispheres are referred to as **dysphasia** or **aphasias**. Anterior, expressive, or *Broca aphasia* is characterized by sparse, nonfluent language. Posterior, receptive, or *Wernicke aphasia* is characterized by an inability to understand language. Speech is fluent but nonsensical. Global aphasia refers to impaired expressive and receptive language.

Many simple bedside measures exist to evaluate age-appropriate language and social skills (see Chapter 7). In addition to expressive and receptive language function, older children can be tested for reading, writing, numerical skills, fund of knowledge, abstract reasoning, judgment, humor, and memory.

CRANIAL NERVE EVALUATION

The evaluation of cranial nerve function depends on the stage of brain maturation and the ability to cooperate.

Cranial Nerve I

The sense of smell can be assessed in verbal, cooperative children 2 to 3 years old. Aromatic substances, such as perfumes and vanilla, should be used, not volatile substances (e.g., ammonia), which irritate the nasal mucosa and do not test smell.

Cranial Nerve II

Full-term newborns in the quiet awake state follow a human face, a light in a dark room, or a large, optico-kinetic strip. Visual acuity has been estimated to be 20/200 in newborns and 20/20 in infants 6 months old. Standard visual charts that display pictures instead of letters assess visual acuity in toddlers. Peripheral vision is tested by surreptitiously bringing objects into the visual field from behind. A reduced pupillary reaction to light suggests lesions of the anterior visual pathways, including the retina, optic nerves, chiasm, and tract. Unilateral optic nerve lesions are identified by the "swinging flashlight test." Both pupils constrict when a light is shone in the normal eye. When the light is swung over to the abnormal eye, both pupils dilate inappropriately; this is called an afferent pupillary defect or **Marcus Gunn pupil**. Lesions of the posterior visual pathway, including the lateral geniculate, optic radiations, and occipital cortex, have normal pupillary light reactions, but are expressed by loss of visual fields.

Cranial Nerves III, IV, and VI

Extraocular movements are assessed by observation of spontaneous, pursuit, and saccadic eye movements. Pursuit movements are slow and occur when the eyes are tracking an object. Saccadic movements are quick, conjugate eye movements and occur when the eyes move from fixation on one object to fixation on a different object. Pursuit and saccadic eye movements are controlled by different CNS mechanisms. Rotating the head or spinning the infant can help assessment of oculocephalic vestibular reflexes (**doll's head maneuver**). The oculocephalic reflex is said to be uninhibited when turning of the head in one direction elicits an immediate movement of the eyes in the opposite direction. This response is normal in a newborn. An uninhibited response in a child indicates that the cortex is not functioning properly to inhibit the brainstem. Multiple, random saccadic eye movements as the head is turned are normal. The oculocephalic response is said to be incomplete when the eyes do not move fully and conjugately in response to head turning. An incomplete response indicates dysfunction of the brainstem.

Cranial nerve III (oculomotor nerve) innervates the pupil; levator palpebrae superioris; medial, superior, and inferior recti; and inferior oblique muscles. Cranial nerve IV (trochlear nerve) innervates the superior oblique muscle. Cranial nerve VI (abducens nerve) innervates the lateral rectus muscle. Abnormalities of these cranial nerves that control eye movement may cause diplopia. Because cranial nerve VI has a long intracranial route within the subarachnoid space, failure of abduction of one or both eyes is a frequent but nonspecific sign of increased ICP.

The pupillary light reaction is present by 30 weeks of gestation. Lesions of the third cranial nerve produce a dilated, mydriatic pupil. Lesions of the facial sympathetic fibers produce a constricted, meiotic pupil. Third nerve lesions may be associated with incomplete eye movements. Interruption of the sympathetic innervation of the pupil and lid may produce **Horner syndrome** with meiosis, ptosis, and unilateral facial anhidrosis. Anticholinergic and sympathomimetic drugs dilate the pupil, and cholinergic, narcotic, and sedative drugs constrict the pupil.

Cranial Nerve V

The muscles of mastication can be observed as an infant sucks and swallows. The masseter muscles may be palpated directly. In later childhood, as cooperation improves, pterygoid function may be assessed by voluntary jaw deviation. The left pterygoid muscle moves the jaw to the right. The **corneal reflex** can be tested (cranial nerves V and VII) at any age. Facial sensation of light touch and pain can be determined with cotton gauze and pinprick.

Cranial Nerve VII

The facial muscles are assessed by observing the face at rest, with crying, and with blinking. At older, cooperative ages, children can be asked to smile, blow out their cheeks, blink forcibly, and furrow their foreheads. Weakness of all muscles of the face, including the forehead, eye, and mouth, indicates a lesion of the facial nerve. If the facial weakness affects only the lower face and mouth, sparing the forehead and eye closure, an ipsilateral lesion of upper motor neuron in the brain (tumor, stroke, abscess) must be considered because the upper third of the face receives bilateral cortical innervation.

Cranial Nerve VIII

Lesions of cranial nerve VIII cause deafness, tinnitus, and vertigo. Alert neonates blink in response to a bell. Four-month-old infants turn their head and eyes to localize a sound stimulus. Hearing can be tested in a verbal child by whispering a word in one ear while covering or masking the opposite ear. Tuning fork testing at 512 Hz can distinguish conductive and sensorineural losses. In **Rinne testing**, a tuning fork is placed alternately with the tines next to the pinna and with the stem on the mastoid process. Air conduction should sound louder and last longer than bone conduction. If bone conduction produces a better quality sound than air conduction, middle ear disease is likely. In **Weber testing**, the stem of the tuning fork is placed on the middle of the forehead. The sound should be equal in the two ears. If the sound is heard better in one ear, the problem is either a sensorineural loss in the opposite ear or a conductive loss in that ear. A conductive loss produces less air masking and an apparent improved bone conduction in the involved ear.

Lesions of the vestibular component of cranial nerve VIII produce symptoms of vertigo, nausea, vomiting, diaphoresis, and nystagmus. Nystagmus is an involuntary beating eye movement with a rapid phase in one direction and a slow phase in the opposite direction. By convention, the direction of the nystagmus is defined by the fast phase and may be horizontal, vertical, or rotatory.

Cranial Nerves IX and X

The gag reflex is brisk at all ages except in a very immature neonate. An absent gag reflex suggests a lower motor neuron lesion of the brainstem, cranial nerves IX or X, neuromuscular junction, or pharyngeal muscles. Uvula deviation toward one side suggests palsy of cranial nerves IX or X on the opposite side. Weak, breathy, or nasal speech; weak sucking; drooling and inability to handle secretions; and gagging and nasal regurgitation of food are additional symptoms of cranial nerve X dysfunction.

Cranial Nerve XI

Observing the infant's posture and spontaneous activity assesses the functions of the trapezius and sternocleidomastoid muscles. Head tilt and drooping of the shoulder suggest lesions involving cranial nerve XI. In later childhood, strength in these muscles can be tested directly and individually.

Cranial Nerve XII

Atrophy and fasciculation of the tongue, usually indicating a lesion of the anterior horn cells (e.g., spinal muscular atrophy [SMA]), can be observed at any age and are assessed most reliably when the infant is asleep. By 1 year of age, having the child follow a lollipop with the tongue can assess specific tongue movements. The tongue deviates toward the weak side in unilateral lesions.

MOTOR EXAMINATION

Power

Power in infants is assessed by observation of sponta-neous movements and movements against gravity. Arm and leg movements should be symmetric, seen best when the infant is held supine with one hand sup-porting the buttocks and one supporting the shoul-ders. The limbs should be lifted easily off the bed. Power is graded on a 5-point scale with 5 being normal; 4, weak but able to provide resistance; 3, able to move against gravity but not against resistance; 2, unable to move against gravity; 1, minimal movement; and 0, complete paralysis.

Strength in toddlers is assessed by functional abili-ties. The child should be able to reach high above his or her head, wheelbarrow walk, run, hop, easily go up and down stairs, and arise from the ground. Subtle asymmetry can be detected when the child extends his or her arms out in front with the palms upward and eyes closed. The hand on the weaker side cups and begins to pronate slowly, called a **pronator drift**. Cooperative children can undergo individual muscle strength testing. Lower motor neuron disease is detected by weakness, whereas upper motor neuron disease appears as stiffness. When the corticospinal pathway is interrupted, the affected limb still can move, but movements are coarse, slow, and stiff. Extrapyramidal motor pathway lesions may produce similar symptoms or may produce movement disor-ders, such as tremor, chorea, or athetosis. **Muscle fas-ciculations** indicate denervation from disease of the anterior horn cell or peripheral nerve.

Tone

Tone represents the dynamic resistance of muscles to movement across a joint (stretch) or to gravity. In infants, two types of tone are assessed: active (stretch) and passive (gravity). Passive tone is the resistance to stretch felt as the limb is flexed and extended. Lower motor lesions produce decreased passive tone. Chronic upper motor lesions produce increased passive tone. Active tone is the posture that an infant adopts when he or she is placed in a particular position. When the hands are grasped, and the infant is pulled from supine to sitting, the infant's arms should pull on the exam-iner's fingers, and the head should not lag behind the shoulders. When the child is held upright with the examiner's hands in the infant's axillae, the infant's shoulders should exert downward force on the exam-iner's hands. The infant's legs should be extended and pushing down on the examining table. When the child is held carefully above the table in prone or supine sus-pension, the child should have no difficulty raising the limbs and head above the plane of the body. In upper

motor lesions, the infant exhibits abnormal postures, such as standing on tiptoes instead of flatfooted and hands constantly fisted with the thumb within the fist. An older child with pyramidal disease has increased resistance to passive movement that is velocity depend-ent, suddenly giving way at a critical point (**clasped knife response or spasticity**). In extrapyramidal disease, an increase in resistance is present throughout passive movement of a joint (**cogwheel rigidity**).

Bulk

Muscle bulk represents the volume of muscle tissue. Observation, palpation, and comparison with con-tralateral extremities are necessary to assess muscle bulk. In many lower motor neuron conditions (neu-ropathies or SMA), muscle bulk is diminished or atrophic. Excessive muscle bulk is seen in myotonia congenita (baby Hercules) and Duchenne muscular dystrophy, in which muscle tissue is replaced with exu-berant fibrosis ("pseudohypertrophy").

Coordination

Lack of coordination of movement is termed **ataxia**. The cerebellum and its associated pathways modulate volitional movement. If either the afferent (joint posi-tion senses) or efferent cerebellar connections (cere-bellum through thalamus to cerebral cortex) are disturbed, the patient has ataxia. Truncal ataxia reflects disturbances of the midline cerebellar vermis (medul-loblastoma, acute postinfectious cerebellar ataxia, or ethanol intoxication). Appendicular ataxia reflects disturbances of the ipsilateral cerebellar hemisphere (cystic cerebellar astrocytoma). Observation and func-tional analysis help assess coordination in infants and toddlers. Watching the child sit or walk assesses truncal stability. Exchanging toys or objects with the child permits assessment of intention tremor and dys-metria, signs of cerebellar dysfunction. Cooperative children can do repetitive finger or foot tapping to test rapid alternating movements. Cerebellar and corti-cospinal tract dysfunction produce slow, rapidly alter-nating movements. The finger or foot tapping test alone cannot distinguish between the two.

Gait

Watching an infant creep, crawl, or cruise or a child walk or crawl may be the best global assessment for how the motor and coordination systems are func-tioning (see Chapter 196). Subtle deficits in power, tone, or balance may be seen, and subtle asymmetries may be observed. The toddler gait is normally wide-based and unsteady. The base narrows with age. By 6 years old, a child is able to tandem walk and walk high on the toes and heels. Cerebellar dysfunction results in a broad-based, unsteady gait accompanied by difficulty in executing turns. Corticospinal tract dysfunction produces a stiff, scissoring gait and toe walking. Arm swing is decreased, and the arm is flexed across the body. Extrapyramidal dysfunction produces a slow, shuffling gait with dystonic postures. There also may be choreoathetotic movements. Lower motor neuron disease results in either a waddling gait (if the proximal muscles are weak) or a steppage gait (if the distal muscles are weak). Analysis of gait, similar to analysis of speech, is frequently extremely difficult because these are complex patterns with inputs from every part of the nervous system.

Reflexes

Deep tendon reflexes at the triceps, biceps, brachioradialis, knee, and ankle are elicited by sudden tendon stretch and can be obtained at any age. These reflexes are decreased in lower motor neuron disease and increased with the development of clonus in chronic upper motor neuron disease. The **Babinski response** or extensor plantar reflex with an upward movement of the great toe and flaring of the toes on noxious stimulation of the side of the foot is a sign of corticospinal tract dysfunction. This reflex is unreliable in the neonates except when asymmetric because the "normal" response at this age varies. The plantar response is consistently flexor (toes down) after 18 months of age.

SENSORY EXAMINATION

The sensory examination of newborns and infants is limited to observing the response to light touch or gentle sterile pinprick. Stimulation of the limb should produce a facial grimace. A spinal reflex alone may produce withdrawal movement of the limb. In a cooperative child, the senses of pain, touch, temperature, vibration, and joint position can be tested individually. The cortical areas of sensation must be intact to identify by touch an object placed in the hand (**stereognosis**), a number written in the hand (**graphesthesia**) or to distinguish between two sharp objects applied simultaneously and closely on the skin (**two-point discrimination**).

SPECIAL DIAGNOSTIC PROCEDURES

Cerebrospinal Fluid Analysis

Analysis of CSF is essential when CNS infection is suspected and provides important clues to various other diagnoses (Table 179–2). Differentiating a hemorrhagic CSF caused by a traumatic lumbar puncture

TABLE 179–2.   Analysis of Cerebrospinal Fluid

Normal Cerebrospinal Fluid	Newborn	>1 Month Old
Cell count	10-25/mm^3	5/mm^3
Protein	<65-150 mg/dL	<40 mg/dL
Glucose	>2/3 blood glucose or >40 mg/dL	>2/3 blood glucose or >60 mg/dL

Increased Polymorphonuclear and Decreased Cerebrospinal Fluid Glucose

Bacterial infection
Partially treated bacterial meningitis
Brain or parameningeal abscess
Parasitic infection
Leak of dermoid contents

Increased Lymphocytes and Decreased Cerebrospinal Fluid Glucose

Mycobacterial infection (tuberculosis)
Fungal infection
Carcinomatous meningitis
Sarcoidosis

Increased Lymphocytes and Normal Cerebrospinal Fluid Glucose

Viral meningitis
Postinfectious disease (ADEM)
Vasculitis

Increased Cerebrospinal Fluid Protein

Infection
Venous thrombosis
Hypertension
Spinal block (Froin syndrome)
Guillain-Barré syndrome
Meningeal carcinomatosis

Mild Cerebrospinal Fluid Pleocytosis

Tumor
Infarction
Multiple sclerosis
Subacute bacterial endocarditis

Bloody Cerebrospinal Fluid

Subarachnoid hemorrhage
Subdural hemorrhage
Intraparenchymal hemorrhage
Hemorrhagic meningoencephalitis (group B streptococcus, HSV)
Trauma
Vascular malformation
Coagulopathy

ADEM, acute disseminated encephalomyelitis; HSV, herpes simplex virus.

(LP) from a true subarachnoid hemorrhage may be difficult. In most cases of traumatic LP, the person performing the LP has a sense of whether the tap was traumatic, and the fluid clears significantly over time. Caution must be exercised before performing an LP to limit risk of cerebral herniation when there is clinical evidence of increased ICP (papilledema, depression of consciousness, or focal neurologic deficits). A CT scan should be performed before the LP if increased ICP is suspected. If increased ICP is present, it must be treated before an LP is performed.

Electroencephalography

The electroencephalogram (EEG) records electrical activity generated by the cerebral cortex. EEG rhythms mature throughout childhood. There are three key features present: background, symmetry, and presence or absence of epileptiform patterns. The EEG background of a premature infant is discontinuous and accompanied by a predominance of slower frequencies (2 to 4 Hz) until 36 weeks of gestation, when the waking portion of the record is continuous. Sleep remains characterized by a discontinuous pattern (trace alternans). In later childhood, the occipital background of the EEG is characterized by 8- to 12-Hz activity (alpha frequency), whereas faster rhythms (13 to 30 Hz) (beta) are seen anteriorly. There should be general symmetry between the backgrounds of the two hemispheres without a localized area of higher amplitude or slower frequencies (focal slowing). Fixed slow wave foci (1 to 3 Hz) delta rhythms suggest an underlying structural abnormality (brain tumor, abscess, or stroke). Bilateral disturbances of brain activity (increased ICP or metabolic encephalopathy) must be suspected when there is diffuse slow wave activity (delta frequency). Spikes, polyspikes, and spike-and-wave abnormalities, either in a localized region (focal) or distributed bihemispherically (generalized), indicate an underlying seizure tendency.

Evoked Responses

Evoked responses are computer-analyzed CNS responses to afferent stimuli. The stimulus (a click for auditory testing, a flash or pattern stimulus for visual testing, and a vibratory stimulus for somatosensory testing) is applied, and the CNS response is monitored over the scalp. Repetitive stimuli are computer averaged, and a response pattern is obtained. Abnormalities of the components of the response pattern can be localized to specific areas of the CNS. Somatosensory responses are of value in assessing peripheral nerve, spinal cord, and cerebral hemispheric function. Visual and auditory responses are valuable in assessing hearing, central auditory function, and abnormalities of visual acuity and the visual pathways. Auditory evoked responses, also known as brainstem-evoked responses, assess auditory pathways at the level of the brainstem. Evoked responses are of particular value in small infants and patients with altered consciousness.

Electromyography and Nerve Conduction Studies

Electromyography (EMG) and nerve conduction velocities (NCV) assess abnormalities of the neuromuscular apparatus, including anterior horn cells, peripheral nerves, neuromuscular junctions, and muscles. Normal muscle is electrically silent at rest. Spontaneous discharge of motor fibers (**fibrillations**) or groups of muscle fibers (**fasciculation**) indicates denervation, revealing dysfunction of anterior horn cells or peripheral nerves. Abnormal muscle responses to repetitive nerve stimulation are seen with diseases of the neuromuscular junction, such as myasthenia gravis and botulism. The amplitude and duration of the muscle compound action potential are decreased in primary diseases of muscle. NCV assess the transmission along peripheral nerves. NCV are slowed in demyelinating neuropathies (Guillain-Barré syndrome). The amplitude of the signal is diminished in axonal neuropathies.

Neuroimaging

Imaging the brain and spinal cord is accomplished predominantly using CT and MRI. Ultrasonography is a noninvasive bedside procedure that can visualize the brain and ventricles of infants and young children with open fontanels; ultrasonography also may visualize the spinal cord in infants.

CHAPTER 180
Headache and Migraine

ETIOLOGY AND EPIDEMIOLOGY

Headache is a common symptom in children and adolescents. Most headaches are related to intercurrent viral illnesses and fever. Headache can be the first symptom of serious conditions, however, such as meningitis or brain tumors, so a systematic approach is necessary.

Migraine and **tension-type headache** are the most common causes of acute recurrent headaches in children and adults (Table 180-1). The pathogenesis of migraine is incompletely understood, but there is a

TABLE 180–1. Primary Headaches in Children and Adolescents: Migraine and Tension-Type

Migraine	Tension-Type
≥5 attacks	≥10 attacks
1- to 72-hr duration	30-min to 7-day duration
Pounding quality	Pressing/tightening quality (nonpulsing)
Moderate to severe intensity	Mild to moderate intensity
Photophobia or phonophobia or both	Absence of photophobia or phonophobia
Unilateral or bifrontal	Bilateral location
Nausea/vomiting	Absence of nausea/vomiting
Aura (flashes of light, wavy or zigzag lines, enlarging scotoma surrounded by luminous changes)	
Aggravated by activity	Not aggravated by usual activities
Family history of migraine	

that flicker in one or both visual fields. Migraine auras may also consist of brief episodes of unilateral or perioral numbness, unilateral weakness, or even vertigo. Sometimes patients with migraine have episodes of neurologic deficits that persist for hours, then resolve completely. These episodes are called **complicated migraine** and typically consist of hemiparesis, monocular blindness, ophthalmoplegia, or confusion. These unusual forms of migraine require diagnostic investigations including neuroimaging, EEG, and appropriate metabolic studies.

Tension-type headaches in children are generally milder and less disruptive to the patient's lifestyle. The pain is more global and squeezing in character, but can last for many hours or days. These headaches can be acute and related to environmental stresses or can be chronic and a symptom of underlying psychiatric illness, such as anxiety neurosis, hysterical neurosis, or depression. Tension headaches have a different clinical profile than that of migraine (see Table 180–1).

"migraine generator" within the brainstem, which produces paroxysmal hyperexcitability along the sensory pathways of cranial nerve V, followed by release of a cascade of inflammatory mediators to the pial and dural vasculature. These inflammatory peptides produce a phase of vasoconstriction. Simultaneously, there is a spreading wave of neuronal depolarization that produces transient disturbances of cerebral function, the most common of which is the visual aura, but other somatosensory symptoms and signs also may occur.

CLINICAL MANIFESTATIONS

The temporal pattern of the headache must be clarified. Each pattern (acute, acute recurrent, chronic progressive, and chronic nonprogressive) has its own differential diagnosis (Table 180–2).

Migraine frequently begins in childhood. Infants and toddlers who are unable to verbalize the source of their discomfort may exhibit spells of irritability, sleepiness, pallor, and vomiting. Young children with migraine frequently lack many of the typical features. Periodic headaches in children accompanied by nausea or vomiting and relieved by rest are likely to be migraine. Migraine headaches in children are stereotyped attacks of frontal, bitemporal, or unilateral intense pounding or throbbing pain lasting 1 to 48 hours. Nausea, vomiting, pallor, photophobia, phonophobia, and an intense desire to seek a quiet dark room for rest accompany the pain. A characteristic but inconsistent symptom of childhood migraine is the visual aura that immediately precedes the headache and persists for 15 to 30 minutes. The visual aura consists of spots, flashes, or lines of light

TABLE 180–2. Four Temporal Patterns of Childhood Headache

Acute

Single episode of head pain without prior history. In adults, the "first and worst" headache raises concerns for aneurysmal subarachnoid hemorrhage, but in children, this pattern is commonly due to *febrile illness* related to upper respiratory tract infection

Acute Recurrent

Pattern of attacks of head pain separated by symptom-free intervals. Primary headache syndromes, such as *migraine or tension-type* headache, usually cause this pattern. Infrequently recurrent headaches are attributed to epileptic syndromes (e.g., benign occipital epilepsy), substance abuse, or recurrent trauma

Chronic Progressive

Most *ominous* of the temporal patterns, implies a gradually increasing frequency and severity of headache. The pathologic correlate is *increasing intracranial pressure*. Causes of this pattern include pseudotumor cerebri, brain tumor, hydrocephalus, chronic meningitis, brain abscess, and subdural collections

Chronic Nonprogressive or Chronic Daily

Pattern of frequent or constant headache. CDH generally is defined as ≥4 mo history of ≥15 headaches/month with headaches lasting ≥4 hr. Affected patients have normal neurologic examinations; usually interwoven psychological factors and great anxiety about underlying organic causes

DIAGNOSTIC STUDIES

If the general physical or neurologic examinations reveal any abnormalities, cranial CT or MRI should be considered. Localized disturbances of function, alteration of consciousness, or chronic progressive patterns warrant imaging. Conversely a normal neurologic examination in a child with recurrent headache is reassuring, and CT or MRI is not likely necessary. Sometimes the neurologic examination yields equivocal findings, or the history is so compelling for serious intracranial pathology that CT or MRI is required, despite a normal examination. Worrisome headaches are headaches that are most severe on awakening, awaken the patient in the middle of the night, are severely exacerbated by coughing or bending, are acute without a previous history of headache, are present daily and getting progressively more severe in a crescendo pattern, or are accompanied by vomiting with or without nausea. Physical signs of increased ICP necessitate immediate therapy and imaging.

TREATMENT

The treatment of migraine requires an individually tailored regimen to reflect the frequency, severity, and disability produced by the headache. Many families visit a physician only for reassurance that there is no serious underlying disease and thereafter are content to treat the headache symptomatically. Intermittent or "symptomatic" analgesics are the mainstay for treatment of infrequent, intense episodes of migraine. Symptomatic therapy requires early administration of the analgesic, rest, and sleep in a quiet dark room. Administration of oral medication often is limited because of nausea and vomiting. The "triptan" agents, available in injectable, nasal spray, oral disintegrating, and tablet form, are serotonin receptor agonists that may alleviate migraine symptoms within 15 to 20 minutes.

Many children experience such severe or frequent attacks to justify the daily use of preventive agents. Daily prophylactic medications not may only reduce attack frequency and severity, but may also enhance the effectiveness of symptomatic medications taken during attacks to reduce their intensity and duration (Table 180–3). Prophylactic medications are used when headaches occur frequently and interfere with activities of daily living. Before initiating daily medications, lifestyle modifications must be put into place to regulate sleep, establish routines including exercise, and identify any precipitating or aggravating influences, eliminating as many as possible (e.g., caffeine, stress, missed meals). Other treatment options include psychological support or counseling, stress management, and biofeedback. In addition to mild analgesics, treatment options for tension headaches include psycho-

TABLE 180–3.   Treatment of Pediatric and Adolescent Migraine

Biobehavioral

Regular sleep schedules
Regular dietary schedule (avoid missing meals)
Eliminate precipitating factors
Reassurance
Biofeedback
Psychotherapy

Acute Therapy

Analgesics
Acetaminophen
Nonsteroidal anti-inflammatory drugs
  Ibuprofen
  Naproxen

5-Hydroxytryptamine Agonists
  Sumatriptan
  Zolmitriptan
  Rizatriptan
  Almotriptan
  Frovatriptan
  Eletriptan

Antiemetics
Metoclopramide
Promethazine

Prophylactic Agents

Tricyclic antidepressant (amitriptyline)
Cyproheptadine
Anticonvulsants (topiramate, valproic acid, gabapentin)
β-Adrenergic blocker (propranolol)
Calcium channel blocker (verapamil)
Serotonin reuptake inhibitor (fluoxetine)

logical support or counseling, biofeedback, antidepressants, and psychiatric intervention.

CHAPTER 181

Seizures (Paroxysmal Disorders)

Paroxysmal disorders of the nervous system result in sudden, reversible changes in mental status or somatosensory function that tend to be stereotyped and repetitive in nature. They have a variable duration from seconds to minutes (rarely hours), end abruptly, and are followed by a gradual return to baseline. There

TABLE 181–1.   Paroxysmal Disorders of Childhood

Seizure disorders
Migraine and variants
    Paroxysmal torticollis
    Paroxysmal vertigo (benign)
Syncope and vasovagal events
    Breath-holding spells
Transient ischemic attack
Metabolic disorders
    Hypoglycemia
Sleep disorders
    Narcolepsy, cataplexy
    Night terrors
Paroxysmal dystonia or choreoathetosis
Shudder attacks
Pseudoseizures

TABLE 181–2.   Causes of Seizures

Perinatal Conditions

Cerebral malformation
Intrauterine infection
Hypoxic-ischemic*
Trauma
Hemorrhage*

Infections

Encephalitis*
Meningitis*
Brain abscess

Metabolic Conditions

Hypoglycemia*
Hypocalcemia
Hypomagnesemia
Hyponatremia
Hypernatremia
Storage diseases
Reye syndrome
Degenerative disorders
Porphyria
Pyridoxine dependency and deficiency

Poisoning

Lead
Cocaine
Drug toxicity (see Chapter 45)
Drug withdrawal

Neurocutaneous Syndromes

Tuberous sclerosis
Neurofibromatosis
Sturge-Weber syndrome
Klippel-Trenaunay-Weber syndrome
Linear sebaceous nevus
Incontinentia pigmenti

Systemic Disorders

Vasculitis (CNS or systemic)
SLE
Hypertensive encephalopathy
Renal failure
Hepatic encephalopathy

Other

Trauma*
Tumor
Febrile*
Idiopathic*
Familial

*Common.
SLE, systemic lupus erythematosus.

may be a warning before (aura) or a state of altered awareness afterward (postictal state). The **differential diagnosis** of transient paroxysmal disorders in childhood includes seizures, migraine, transient ischemic attack, syncope, vertigo, hypoglycemia, breath-holding spells, tics, and conversion reactions (Table 181–1). A thorough medical history extracted from the patient and primary witnesses is the most reliable tool for establishing the exact diagnosis.

The **EEG** is the most useful neurodiagnostic test in distinguishing seizure from nonepileptic paroxysmal disorders. The EEG must be interpreted in the context of the clinical history because many normal children have epileptiform EEG patterns. Children with seizures may have normal EEGs between attacks. When the diagnosis is still unclear, more sophisticated EEGs with prolonged simultaneous video and EEG monitoring of the patient to capture a spell may be necessary to make a definitive diagnosis.

ETIOLOGY AND EPIDEMIOLOGY

Seizures represent the abnormal and excessive discharging of the neural-glial network. A diverse group of disturbances of cerebral function or homeostasis can lead to seizures (Table 181–2). **Epilepsy** is defined as recurrent, unprovoked seizures. Epileptic seizures are generally separated on the basis of the mechanism of the electrical phenomena into seizures that arise from one region of the cortex (focal, partial, or localization related) and seizures that arise from both hemispheres simultaneously (generalized). The epileptic syndromes represent clinical entities wherein the clinical event, EEG pattern, natural history, and prognosis are consistent and uniform. The clinical seizure

TABLE 181–3. Classification of Seizures and Epileptic Syndromes

Partial Seizures

Simple partial (consciousness not impaired)
  Motor signs
  Special sensory (visual, auditory, olfactory, gustatory, vertiginous, or somatosensory)
  Autonomic
Complex partial (consciousness impaired)
  Psychic (déjà vu, fear, and others)
  Impaired consciousness at onset
  Development of impaired consciousness
Secondarily generalized seizures
  "Jacksonian" seizures

Generalized Seizures

Absence
  Typical
  Atypical
Tonic
Clonic
Tonic-clonic
Minor motor
  Atonic
  Myoclonic

Epileptic Syndromes

Benign focal epilepsy (benign rolandic epilepsy, benign centrotemporal epilepsy)
Juvenile myoclonic epilepsy
Infantile spasms (West syndrome)
Lennox-Gastaut syndrome
Acquired epileptic aphasia (Landau-Kleffner syndrome)
Benign neonatal convulsions

---

classification describes individual events, whereas epileptic syndromes consider age of onset, etiology (often genetic), and association of seizure types (Table 181–3).

Partial seizures constitute 40% to 60% of the classifiable epilepsies of childhood. Focal brain lesions (tumors, infarct, dysgenesis) may cause partial epilepsies, but most partial seizures in children are due to genetic influences (rolandic seizures).

Tonic, clonic, and biphasic tonic-clonic seizures are common during childhood. Although it is often difficult to distinguish primary generalized tonic and clonic seizures from secondarily generalized partial seizures on purely clinical grounds, this distinction is important. Most children with exclusively primary generalized tonic-clonic seizures have genetic epilepsy, whereas partial seizures frequently may be associated with focal brain lesions. The presence of an aura indicates a focal origin of the attack. Young children often are unaware of an aura or focal onset of their seizure, and caregivers frequently witness only the generalized aspects of the event.

Approximately 6% to 20% of epileptic children have typical generalized absence seizures (petit mal epilepsy). There is a 75% concordance rate in monozygotic twins, which suggests a genetic etiology. Approximately 40% to 50% of children with absence seizures have associated generalized seizures; 60% occur before and 40% occur after the onset of absence seizures.

Myoclonic, tonic, atonic, and atypical absence seizures compose 10% to 15% of childhood epilepsies. These seizures frequently are associated with underlying structural brain disease and are difficult to treat and classify. They often occur in combination with each other and with generalized tonic-clonic seizures. The peak age of occurrence of myoclonic absence seizures is within the first year (37%), and status epilepticus is the first ictal manifestation in 77% of patients.

CLINICAL MANIFESTATIONS

Partial Seizures

Simple partial seizures arise from a specific anatomic focus. Clinical symptoms include motor, sensory, psychic, or autonomic abnormalities, but consciousness is preserved. Location and direction of spread of the seizure focus determine the clinical symptoms. Complex partial seizures are similar, but in addition, consciousness is impaired. When partial seizures spread to involve the whole brain and produce a generalized tonic-clonic seizure, they show secondary generalization ("jacksonian" seizures). Partial seizures that manifest only with psychic or autonomic symptoms can be difficult to recognize. Uncinate seizures arising from the medial temporal lobe manifest with an olfactory hallucination of an extremely unpleasant odor (burning rubber). Gelastic seizures originating from hypothalamic tumors are spells of uncontrolled laughter. Lip-smacking seizures arise from the anterior temporal lobe and episodes of macropsia, micropsia, altered depth perception, and vertigo from the posterior temporal lobe. Limbic temporal lobe discharges result in dreamlike states (déjà vu and bizarre psychic abnormalities). Episodic autonomic phenomena, such as fever, tachycardia, shivering, and increased gastrointestinal motility, may rarely be seizures of temporal lobe origin.

Generalized Seizures

Generalized Tonic, Clonic, and Tonic-Clonic Seizures (Generalized Major Motor Seizures)

Tonic, clonic, and biphasic tonic-clonic seizures are common during childhood. They may occur alone or be associated with other seizure types. Typically the attack begins abruptly, but occasionally is preceded by a series of myoclonic jerks. During a tonic-clonic seizure, consciousness and control of posture are lost, followed by tonic stiffening and upward deviation of the eyes. Pooling of secretions, pupillary dilation, diaphoresis, hypertension, and piloerection are common. Clonic jerks follow the tonic phase, then the child is briefly tonic again. Thereafter, the child remains flaccid and urinary incontinence may occur. As the child awakens, irritability and headache are common. During an attack, the EEG shows repetitive synchronous bursts of spike activity followed by periodic paroxysmal discharges. Brief seizures of any type are not believed to produce brain damage directly. Generalized tonic-clonic activity lasting longer than 20 minutes is defined as **status epilepticus** and may lead to irreversible brain injury.

Absence Seizures

The clinical hallmark of absence seizures is a brief loss of environmental awareness accompanied by eye fluttering or simple automatisms, such as head bobbing and lip smacking. Seizures usually begin between 4 and 6 years of age. Neurologic examination and brain imaging are normal. The characteristic EEG patterns consist of synchronous **3-Hz spike-and-wave activity** with frontal accentuation. The clinical seizure invariably is accompanied by the electrical discharge, and both are provoked by hyperventilation or strobe light stimulation. Staring spells can be either primary generalized absence (petit mal) or complex partial seizures (temporal lobe epilepsy). Differentiating absence epilepsy from partial complex staring seizures can be difficult. Both seizure types are characterized by stoppage of activity, staring, and alteration of consciousness and may include automatisms. The automatisms of partial complex seizures are usually more complicated and may involve repetitive swallowing, picking of the hands, or walking in nonpurposeful circles. Partial complex seizures are often followed by postictal confusion. Absence seizures are not. Absence seizures are provoked by hyperventilation and usually last a few seconds. Partial complex seizures occur spontaneously and usually last several minutes. Children may have dozens of absence seizures per day. They rarely have more than one or two partial complex seizures in a day.

Myoclonic, Tonic, Atonic, and Atypical Absence Seizures

Atypical absence seizures manifest as episodes of impaired consciousness with automatisms, autonomic phenomena, and motor manifestations, such as eye opening, eye deviation, and body stiffening. The EEG shows slow spike-and-wave activity at 2 to 3 Hz. Myoclonus is a lightning-like jerk of part of the body. The phenomenon is epileptic if the EEG shows epileptiform discharges during the jerk and nonepileptic if it does not. Nonepileptic myoclonus may originate in the basal ganglia, brainstem, or spinal cord. It may be benign, as in sleep myoclonus, or indicate serious pathology. Myoclonic epilepsy usually is associated with multiple seizure types. The underlying illness producing myoclonic epilepsy may be developmental and static or progressive and associated with neurologic deterioration (neuronal ceroid lipofuscinosis, Lafora body, and Univerricht-Lundborg disease). Myoclonic absence refers to the body jerks that commonly accompany absence seizures and atypical absence seizures. Bilateral massive epileptic myoclonus is symmetric and varies in intensity.

Epileptic Syndromes

Benign focal epilepsy, also known as **rolandic epilepsy**, usually begins between ages 5 and 10 years. The incidence may be 21 per 100,000, comprising 16% of all afebrile seizures in children younger than age 15 years. They are usually focal motor seizures involving the face and arm and tend to occur only during sleep or on awakening in more than half of patients. Symptoms commonly include abnormal movement or sensation around the face and mouth with drooling and a rhythmic guttural sound. Speech and swallowing are impaired. A family history of similar seizures is found in 13% of patients. The disorder is called benign because seizures usually respond promptly to anticonvulsant therapy; intellectual outcome and brain imaging are normal, and epilepsy resolves after puberty. Continued treatment is not needed.

Benign neonatal convulsions are an autosomal dominant genetic disorder localized to chromosome 20. Generalized clonic seizures occur toward the end of the first week of life ("3-day fits" or familial 5th day fits). Response to treatment varies, but the outlook generally is favorable.

Juvenile myoclonic epilepsy ("of Janz") occurs in adolescence and is an autosomal dominant disorder localized on chromosome 6 with variable penetrance. The patient may have absence, generalized tonic or clonic, and myoclonic seizures. The hallmark is morning myoclonus occurring predominantly within 90 minutes of awakening. Seizures usually resolve promptly with therapy with valproic acid, but therapy must be maintained for life.

Infantile spasms (West syndrome) are brief contractions of the neck, trunk, and arm muscles, followed by a phase of sustained muscle contraction lasting 2 to 10 seconds. The initial phase consists of flexion and extension in various combinations such that the head may be thrown either backward or forward. The arms and legs may be either flexed or extended. Spasms occur most frequently when the child is awakening from or going to sleep. Each jerk is followed by a brief period of relaxation, then repeated multiple times in clusters of unpredictable and variable duration. Many clusters occur each day. The EEG during the waking state, **hypsarrhythmia**, is dramatically abnormal, consisting of high-voltage slow waves, spikes, and polyspikes accompanied by background disorganization. Burst suppression patterns are seen during sleep. The peak age of onset is 3 to 8 months, and 86% of infants experience the onset of seizures before age 1 year. In circumstances in which flexion of the thighs and crying are prominent, the syndrome often is mistaken for colic. Infantile spasms have a poor prognosis. The etiology is not determined in 40% of children. This idiopathic or "cryptogenic" group (normal development before seizures; no etiology) has a better response to therapy than the group with a clear etiology, and 40% have a good intellectual outcome. Etiology is determined in 60% (Table 181–4). This symptomatic group

responds poorly to anticonvulsant therapy and has a poor intellectual prognosis. **Tuberous sclerosis** is the most common recognized cause. Treatment of infantile spasms includes adrenocorticotropic hormone, oral corticosteroids, benzodiazepines, and valproic acid. Irritability, swelling, hypertension, glycosuria, and severe infections are complications to be anticipated with steroid therapy. The Food and Drug Administration has not yet approved vigabatrin, a promising drug available in Europe and Canada, because it can cause visual field deficits.

Lennox-Gastaut syndrome is an epileptic syndrome with variable age of onset. Most children present before age 5 years. Multiple seizure types—including atonic-astatic, partial, atypical absence, and generalized tonic, clonic, or tonic-clonic varieties—characterize the disorder. Many children have underlying brain injury or malformations. These seizures usually respond poorly to treatment, but some patients have a good response to valproic acid.

Astatic-akinetic or **atonic seizures** have their onset between 1 and 3 years of age. The seizures last 1 to 4 seconds and are characterized by a loss of body tone, with falling to the ground, dropping of the head, or pitching forward or backward. A tonic component usually is associated. The seizures frequently result in repetitive head injury if the child is not protected with a hockey or football helmet. They are most frequent on awakening and on falling asleep; 50 or more daily seizures are usual. Children with astatic-akinetic seizures usually have mental retardation and underlying brain abnormalities. **Tuberous sclerosis** is a frequent cause.

Acquired epileptic aphasia (Landau-Kleffner syndrome) is characterized by the abrupt loss of previously acquired language in young children. The language disability is an acquired cortical auditory deficit (auditory agnosia). Some patients develop partial and generalized epilepsy. The EEG is highly epileptiform in sleep, the peak area of abnormality often being in the dominant perisylvian region (language areas). It is unclear whether frequent temporal lobe seizures cause the language disability or whether unknown, perhaps inflammatory temporal lobe pathology is responsible for the seizures and language loss.

Rasmussen encephalitis is a chronic, progressive focal inflammation of the brain of unknown origin. An autoimmune origin and focal viral encephalitis have been postulated. The usual age of onset is 6 to 10 years. The disease begins with focal, persistent motor seizure activity, including epilepsia partialis continua. Over months, the child develops hemiplegia and cognitive deterioration. EEG shows focal spikes and slow wave activity. Brain imaging studies are initially normal, then show atrophy in the involved area. Hemispherectomy has been the only successful therapy as measured

TABLE 181–4. Etiologies of Infantile Spasms (West Syndrome)

Metabolic
  Phenylketonuria
  Biotinidase deficiency
  Maple syrup urine disease
  Isovalericacidemia
  Ornithine accumulation
  Nonketotic hyperglycinemia
  Pyridoxine dependency
  Hypoglycemia
  Lipidosis
Developmental malformations
  Polymicrogyria
  Lissencephaly
  Schizencephaly
  Down syndrome and other chromosomal disorders
Aicardi syndrome
Organoid nevus syndrome
Neurocutaneous syndromes
  Tuberous sclerosis
  Sturge-Weber syndrome
Congenital infections
  Toxoplasmosis
  Cytomegalovirus
  Syphilis
Encephalopathies
  Post-asphyxia
  Post-traumatic
  Posthemorrhagic
  Postinfectious

by seizure eradication and prevention of cognitive deterioration, but permanent hemiparesis is an inevitable consequence.

Special Conditions

Febrile seizures may be caused by infection of the nervous system (meningitis, encephalitis, or brain abscess), unrecognized epilepsy triggered by fever, or **simple febrile convulsions**. The last-mentioned represent a common genetic predisposition to seizures in infancy that is precipitated by a rapid increase in body temperature. They occur in 2% to 4% of children between ages 6 months and 6 years. More than half occur between ages 1 and 2 years (mean age 22 months). Uncomplicated or benign febrile seizures are generalized major motor convulsions lasting less than 15 minutes that occur only once in a 24-hour period in a neurologically and developmentally normal child. If there are focal features, the seizures last longer than 15 minutes, the child has preexisting neurologic challenges, or the seizures occur multiple times within one febrile event, the seizure is referred to as a **complex** or **atypical febrile seizure**.

The prognosis of children with simple febrile seizures is excellent. Intellectual achievements are normal. Many children have further febrile seizures, but the development of epilepsy (afebrile seizures) is rare. Febrile seizures recur in 50% of children who have their first febrile seizure at younger than 1 year of age and in 28% of children who have their first seizure at older than 1 year of age. About 10% of children with febrile seizures have three or more recurrences. The risk of multiple recurrences is greater in infants with onset in the first year. Children with complex febrile seizures have only a 7% risk of having further complicated febrile seizures. The risk of epilepsy in most children with febrile seizures is no greater than the general population (approximately 1%). Factors that increase the risk for the development of epilepsy include abnormal neurologic examination or development, family history of epilepsy, and complex febrile seizures. The probability of developing epilepsy is 2% if one risk factor is present and 10% if two or three risk factors are present.

Because febrile seizures are brief, and the outcome is benign, most children require no treatment. Rectal diazepam can be administered during a seizure to abort a prolonged event. Daily administration of phenobarbital or valproic acid prevents febrile seizures, but the potential for serious side effects limits the use of these agents. Phenobarbital is ineffective when given at the onset of a febrile illness because a therapeutic level cannot be achieved rapidly enough. Intermittent treatment with oral diazepam three to four times per day during a febrile illness has shown variable effectiveness.

Status epilepticus is defined as ongoing seizure activity for greater than 20 minutes or repetitive seizures without return of consciousness for greater than 30 minutes. The Epilepsy Foundation of America defines status epilepticus as two or more sequential seizures without full recovery of consciousness between seizures or more than 30 minutes of continuous seizure activity. Functionally, any convulsive seizure associated with reductions in oxygen saturations and cortical perfusion produces a risk for irreversible brain injury and may be managed as status epilepticus. About 25% of children presenting with status epilepticus have an acute brain injury, such as purulent or aseptic meningitis, encephalitis, electrolyte disorder, or acute anoxia. Twenty percent have a history of brain injury or congenital malformation. In 50%, there is no definable etiology, but in 50% of this group, status is associated with fever. Sudden cessation of anticonvulsant medication is another frequent cause. Overall the mortality rate of status epilepticus is less than 10% and related to the etiology of the seizure pattern.

IMMEDIATE TREATMENT

The first priority of treatment is to ensure an adequate airway and to assess the cardiovascular status (see Chapter 38). The child's oropharynx should be cleared and suctioned, and the airway should be secured. Oxygen is administered. If there is any doubt concerning the adequacy of the airway, the child should be intubated. If violent muscle activity impairs ventilation, muscle paralysis and sedation should be instituted. An IV infusion should be started, and laboratory evaluation should be undertaken. Hypoglycemia and electrolyte abnormalities must be addressed. Several pharmacologic options exist for management of status epilepticus (Fig. 181–1). Initial management is usually with a benzodiazepine. Lorazepam (0.05 to 0.1 mg/kg), diazepam (0.1 to 0.3 mg/kg), and midazolam (0.2 mg/kg) all are effective agents. Diazepam distributes rapidly to the brain, but has a short duration of action. Alternatively, or even simultaneously, administration of either phenytoin (10 to 15 mg/kg) or fosphenytoin (10 to 20 mg/kg) at a rate of 1 mg/kg/min is effective. Phenytoin and fosphenytoin distribute more slowly but have a much longer duration of action. If the seizures do not stop with these measures, a continuous IV infusion of diazepam, loading dose of 10 to 20 mg/kg of phenobarbital, or IV valproic acid at a dose of 20 mg/kg is appropriate (Table 181–5). If this approach is ineffective, preparations for general anesthesia are undertaken. While awaiting anesthesia, continuously infused diazepam or pentobarbital is recommended. When status epilepticus stops, maintenance therapy is initiated with the appropriate anticonvulsant.

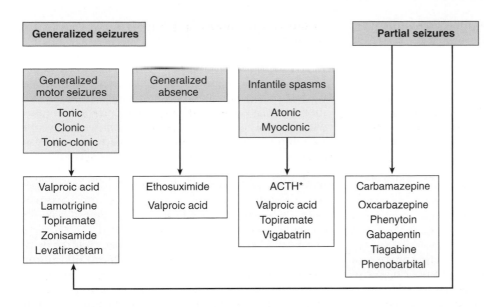

Figure 181–1

Treatment for epilepsy. ACTH, adrenocorticotropic hormone. *, for infantile spasms.

TABLE 181–5.	**Management of Status Epilepticus**

Stabilization

ABCs (airway, breathing, circulation)
ECG monitoring
Oxygen and pulse oximetry
IV access
Immediate laboratory tests
 Glucose
 Basic metabolic panel (sodium, calcium, magnesium)
 Antiepileptic drug levels
 Toxicologies

Pharmacologic Management

Benzodiazepine
 Lorazepam 0.05-0.2 mg/kg
 Diazepam 0.2-0.5 mg/kg
 Midazolam 0.2 mg/kg
Fosphenytoin 10-20 mg/kg (phenytoin equivalents)
Phenobarbital 10-20 mg/kg
Valproic acid 20 mg/kg
General anesthesia

Pseudoseizures may occur in children with hysteria or malingering. Children with genuine seizure disorders consciously or subconsciously may exhibit activity that simulates their own seizures. Although the clinical differentiation can be difficult, pseudoseizures differ from epileptic seizures in that movement is tremulousness or thrashing rather than true tonic-clonic activity. Verbalization and pelvic thrusting are seen more commonly in pseudoseizures; urinary and fecal continence is preserved, and injury does not occur. Pseudoseizures are more likely to be initiated or terminated by suggestion. An EEG performed during pseudoseizure activity does not show typical epileptiform patterns.

LABORATORY AND DIAGNOSTIC EVALUATION OF SEIZURES

A complete laboratory evaluation of a child with the new onset of seizures includes a complete blood count; measurement of blood chemistries, including glucose, calcium, sodium, potassium, chloride, bicarbonate, urea nitrogen, creatinine, magnesium, and phosphorus; blood or urine toxicology screening; analysis of CSF; and EEG and brain imaging (MRI). Neonates also may require testing of blood ammonia and for inborn errors of metabolism, CSF glycine, lactate and herpes simplex polymerase chain reaction, urine and stool culture of viruses (especially cytomegalovirus and enterovirus), and a clinical trial of pyridoxine. Analysis of CSF is not necessary if the patient is afebrile and has no other neurologic signs or if the history does not suggest a meningeal infection or subarachnoid hemorrhage. Children with **simple febrile seizures** who have recovered completely may require little or no laboratory evaluation other than studies necessary to evaluate the source of the fever.

MRI is superior to CT in showing brain pathology, but in the emergency department setting, CT may be desirable because it can be performed rapidly and shows acute intracranial hemorrhage more clearly than MRI. MRI is likely to be normal in patients with the primary generalized epilepsies, such as typical absence and myoclonic epilepsy of Janz. Lesions (tumors, arteriovenous malformations, cysts, strokes, gliosis, or focal atrophy) in 25% of other patients may be identified even when the clinical examination and EEG do not suggest focal features. Identification of some static lesions, such as cortical dysplasia, hamartoma, and mesial temporal sclerosis, may allow consideration of surgical correction of medically refractory epilepsy.

LONG-TERM THERAPY

The decision to institute daily seizure medications for a first unprovoked seizure must be based on the likelihood of recurrence balanced with the risk of long-term drug therapy. Determination of the recurrence risk is based on the clinical history and results of neurodiagnostic testing. Absence seizures, infantile spasms, atypical absence seizures, and astatic-akinetic seizures are universally recurrent at the time of diagnosis, indicating the need for therapy. The overall risk of recurrence for children whose first seizure is generalized tonic-clonic is approximately 50%. It seems reasonable to wait for recurrence before therapy is instituted. An otherwise healthy child with a single unprovoked partial seizure with a normal neurodiagnostic evaluation, including a normal EEG, may have a recurrence risk of 25%. In such a case, it is reasonable to educate family members regarding first aid techniques for seizures and to withhold daily antiepileptic agents. Conversely a child with preexisting neurologic abnormality and an abnormal EEG may have a recurrence risk of 75%, in which case institution of a daily antiepileptic agent may be justified after the first seizure.

When treatment is initiated, the goal is to maintain an optimal functional state. Medication toxicity should be weighed against the risk of seizure itself. Initial drug selection is based on the mechanism of the seizure (see Fig. 181-1). A single agent should be chosen to limit toxicity, contain cost, and improve compliance. Approximately 50% of children obtain satisfactory seizure control with the initial drug. If seizure control is not achieved with confirmed therapeutic anticonvulsant levels, addition of a second drug must be considered. When available, measuring anticonvulsant blood levels is helpful in adjusting medication and monitoring compliance, but the levels should be interpreted in light of the patient's clinical state. Antiepileptic drug levels should be drawn at trough, usually early in the morning before the morning doses. When hepatic or renal disease is present, drug binding is likely to be altered. In this instance, free and bound anticonvulsant levels can be

helpful. Treatment is not necessary for benign febrile seizures.

The duration of anticonvulsant treatment varies with seizure type. Children with generalized tonic, clonic, and tonic-clonic seizures; absence seizures; and certain partial seizures may not require therapy for more than 2 to 4 years. The risk of recurrence is higher with partial onset seizures. Children with juvenile myoclonic epilepsy, progressive myoclonic epilepsy, atypical absence seizures, and Lennox-Gastaut syndrome usually require treatment for life. As a rule, children who are neurologically abnormal, have seizures that were initially difficult to control, and have persistently epileptiform EEGs are at highest risk for recurrence when therapy is discontinued.

General guidance for families with children with epilepsy is to be careful with heights, head injury, and swimming. Children with epilepsy have a greater risk of submersion accidents. This risk can be minimized by maintaining therapeutic anticonvulsant drug levels and by appropriate adult supervision.

CHAPTER **182**

Weakness and Hypotonia

ETIOLOGY AND EPIDEMIOLOGY

The corticospinal tract and its neurons from the cerebral cortex through the spinal cord that subserve voluntary motor activity are known as the **upper motor neuron**. The anterior horn cells, their motor roots, peripheral motor nerves, neuromuscular junctions, and muscles represent the **lower motor neuron**. Maintenance of normal tone and coordination of agonist, antagonist, synergistic, and fixating muscle groups involve an integrated communication between the motor nuclei of the cerebral cortex, spinal cord, cerebellum, brainstem, thalamus, basal ganglia, and motor cortex of the cerebrum. The cerebellum and basal ganglia facilitate volitional movement. The cerebellum provides dynamic feedback regarding joint position, and the basal ganglia modulate agonists and antagonistic muscle groups.

Destruction of the upper motor neuron causes loss of voluntary control, but not total loss of movement. Motor nuclei of the basal ganglia, thalamus, and brainstem have their own tracts that innervate anterior horn cells and produce simple or complex stereotyped patterns of movement. Destruction of the spinal cord leaves simple, stereotyped reflex movements coordinated by local spinal reflexes below the level of the lesion intact. Destruction of the lower motor neuron

TABLE 182–1. Clinical Distinction between Upper Motor Neuron versus Lower Motor Neuron Lesions

Clinical Sign	Upper Motor Neuron (Corticospinal tract)	Lower Motor Neuron (Neuromuscular)
Tone	Increased (spastic)	Decreased
Reflexes	Increased	Decreased
Babinski reflex	Present	Absent
Atrophy	Absent	Possible
Fasciculations	Absent	Possible

leads to total absence of movement because it is the final common pathway producing muscle activity.

CLINICAL MANIFESTATIONS

Weakness caused by upper motor neuron disease or corticospinal tract lesions is different in quality from weakness produced by the lower motor unit (Table 182–1). The former results in a loss of dexterous movements. The corticospinal tract permits fine motor activity and is best tested by asking the patient to perform rapid alternating movements of the distal extremities. Mild dysfunction produces slowed, stiff motions. More severe dysfunction produces stiff, abnormal postures (spasticity) that do not respond to voluntary command. The posture in corticospinal tract disease consists of the forearm being flexed at the elbow and wrist and adducted close to the chest, with the leg extended and adducted. Disease of the lower motor unit produces progressive loss of strength with hypotonia and no abnormality of posture. Function is best tested by measuring the strength of individual muscle groups or, in a young child, by observing the ability to perform tasks requiring particular muscle groups (walk up or down stairs, arise from the ground, walk on toes or heels, raise the hands above the head, and squeeze a ball).

DISEASE OF THE UPPER MOTOR NEURON
Etiology and Epidemiology

Tumors, trauma, infections, demyelinating syndromes, infarction, metabolic diseases, and degenerative diseases may injure the corticospinal tract, producing an upper motor neuron pattern of weakness coupled with increased deep tendon reflexes, spasticity, and extensor plantar responses (Babinski sign).

Clinical Manifestations

The distribution of weakness depends on the location of the lesion. A tumor in the left parietal region may produce a right hemiparesis. A brainstem glioma may produce a slowly progressive quadriparesis. Compression of the spinal cord in the thoracic region from a tumor, such as neuroblastoma or lymphoma, would produce a spastic paraparesis, affecting only the legs. A disorder of myelin synthesis, such as a leukodystrophy, would produce a progressive symmetric quadriparesis.

DISEASES OF THE SPINAL CORD

Acute spinal cord lesions, such as infarction or compression, may produce a **flaccid, areflexic paralysis** that mimics lower motor neuron disease. A child who exhibits an acute or subacute flaccid paraparesis is most likely to have either an acute cord syndrome or Guillain-Barré syndrome. The acute cord syndrome may be the result of transverse myelitis, a cord tumor, infarction, demyelination, or trauma. The hallmarks of spinal cord disease are a sensory level, a motor level, disturbance of bowel and bladder function, and local spinal pain or tenderness. **Transverse myelitis**, an acute postinfectious demyelinating disorder of the spinal cord, is treated with high-dose steroids. Trauma and tumors necessitate immediate neurosurgical management to preserve vital function.

DISEASES OF THE LOWER MOTOR NEURON

Each anterior horn cell in the spinal cord and brainstem gives rise to a single myelinated axon that extends to muscle. After numerous branchings, each axon twig terminates in a synapse with a single muscle fiber. The presynaptic axon terminal releases acetylcholine, which traverses the synaptic cleft, binds to receptors on the muscle membrane, initiates muscle contraction, and is inactivated by acetylcholinesterase. The lower motor unit consists of all of these components. Neuromuscular disease affects any component of the lower motor neuron unit. The distribution of muscle weakness can point toward specific diseases (Table 182–2). Diseases may affect each component of the motor unit (Table 182–3).

DISEASES OF THE ANTERIOR HORN CELL
Spinal Muscular Atrophy
Etiology

Progressive degeneration of anterior horn cells is the key manifestation of SMA, a genetic illness that may

TABLE 182–2. Topography of Neuromuscular Diseases

Proximal Muscle Weakness

Muscular dystrophy
  Duchenne
  Limb-girdle
Dermatomyositis; polymyositis
Kugelberg-Welander disease (late-onset spinal muscular
  atrophy)

Distal Limb Weakness

Polyneuropathy (Guillain-Barré syndrome)
Hereditary motor sensory neuropathy I
Hereditary motor sensory neuropathy II
Myotonic dystrophy
Distal myopathy

Ophthalmoplegia and Limb Weakness

Myasthenia gravis
Botulism
Myotonic dystrophy
Congenital structural myopathy
Miller Fisher variant of Guillain-Barré syndrome

Facial and Bulbar Weakness

Myasthenia gravis
Botulism
Polio
Miller Fisher variant of Guillain-Barré syndrome
Myotonic dystrophy
Congenital structural myopathy
Facioscapulohumeral dystrophy

TABLE 182–3. Neuromuscular Disorders in Children and Adolescents

Anterior Horn Cell

Spinal muscular atrophy*
Poliomyelitis (natural or vaccine)
Enteroviruses

Peripheral Nerve

Guillain-Barré syndrome
Tick paralysis
Hereditary*
Vitamin E, B_{12}, and B_1 deficiencies
Toxins
  Lead, thallium, arsenic, mercury
  Hexane
  Acrylamide
  Organophosphates
Diphtheria
Collagen vascular disease
Porphyria
Paraneoplastic
Drugs
  Amitriptyline
  Dapsone
  Hydralazine
  Isoniazid
  Nitrofurantoin
  Vincristine

Neuromuscular Junction

Myasthenia gravis
  Acquired
  Neonatal transitory*
  Neuromuscular junction
  Congenital*
Botulism*
Aminoglycosides

Muscle

Dystrophy
  Duchenne
  Becker
  Limb-girdle
  Facioscapulohumeral
  Myotonic*
  Congenital*
Myositis (viral, polymyositis)
Congenital structural myopathy (see Table 182–4)

Metabolic, Endocrine, and Mineral

Glycogen storage disease II (Pompe disease)
Carnitine metabolism abnormalities
Mitochondrial abnormalities
Thyroid excess or deficiency
Cortisol excess or deficiency
Hyperparathyroidism; calcium excess
Potassium excess or deficiency (periodic paralysis)

*Infants.

begin in intrauterine life or anytime thereafter and may progress at a rapid or slow pace. The earlier in life the process starts, the more rapid the progression. Infants who are affected at birth or who become weak within the first several months of life usually progress to flaccid quadriplegia with bulbar palsy, respiratory failure, and death within the first year of life. This early fulminant form of the illness is called **Werdnig-Hoffmann disease**. A mild form of the illness, **Kugelberg-Welander syndrome**, begins in late childhood or adolescence with proximal weakness of the legs and progresses slowly over decades. Variants of SMA between these age extremes occur with unpredictable courses.

SMA is one of the most frequent autosomal recessive diseases, with a carrier frequency of 1 in 50. All types of SMA are caused by mutations in the survival motor neuron gene (*SMN1*). There are two almost identical copies, *SMN1* and *SMN2,* present on chromosome

5q13. Only homozygous absence of *SMN1* is responsible for SMA, whereas homozygous absence of *SMN2*, found in about 5% of controls, has no clinical phenotype. The number of *SMN2* copies modulates the SMA phenotype.

Clinical Manifestations

SMA may begin between 6 months and 6 years of age and may progress rapidly or slowly or may progress rapidly initially, then seemingly plateau. The clinical manifestations include progressive proximal weakness, decreased spontaneous movement, and floppiness. Atrophy may be marked. Head control is lost. With time, the legs stop moving altogether, and the children play only with toys placed in their hands. The range of facial expression diminishes, and drooling and gurgling increase. The eyes remain bright, open, mobile, and engaging. Weakness is flaccid, with early loss of reflexes. **Fasciculations** sometimes can be seen in the tongue and are best identified when the child is asleep. Infants have normal mental, social, and language skills and sensation. Breathing becomes rapid, shallow, and predominantly abdominal. In an extremely weak child, respiratory infections lead to atelectasis, pulmonary infection, and death.

Laboratory and Diagnostic Studies

The level of creatine phosphokinase may be mildly elevated. The EMG shows fasciculations, fibrillations, positive sharp waves, and high-amplitude, long-duration motor units. Muscle biopsy specimens show grouped atrophy. The diagnosis is established by DNA probe for SMA.

Treatment

No treatment for SMA exists. Symptomatic therapy is directed toward minimizing contractures, preventing scoliosis, aiding oxygenation, preventing aspiration, and maximizing social, language, and intellectual skills. Respiratory infections are managed early and aggressively with pulmonary toilet, chest physical therapy, oxygen, and antibiotics. The use or nonuse of artificial ventilation must be individualized for each patient in each stage of the illness.

Poliomyelitis

Poliomyelitis is an acute enteroviral illness with prodromal vomiting and diarrhea associated with an aseptic meningitis picture during which the patient experiences the evolution of an **asymmetric flaccid weakness** as groups of anterior horn cells become infected (see Chapter 101).

PERIPHERAL NEUROPATHY

The principal peripheral nerve diseases in childhood are (1) Guillain-Barré syndrome, (2) hereditary motor sensory neuropathy (HMSN) (Charcot-Marie-Tooth disease), and (3) tick paralysis. Peripheral neuropathy produced by diabetes mellitus, alcoholism, chronic renal failure, amyloid, exposure to industrial or metal toxins, vasculitis (often as **mononeuritis multiplex**), or the remote effects of neoplasm is a common cause of weakness and sensory loss in adults but is rare in children.

Guillain-Barré Syndrome

Etiology

Guillain-Barré syndrome is a postinfectious autoimmune peripheral neuropathy that often occurs after a respiratory or gastrointestinal infection. Infection with *Campylobacter jejuni* is associated with a severe form of the illness.

Clinical Manifestations

The characteristic symptoms are areflexia, flaccidity, and relatively symmetric weakness beginning in the legs and ascending to involve the arms, trunk, throat, and face. Progression can occur rapidly, in hours or days, or more indolently, over weeks. Typically the child complains of numbness or paresthesia in the hands and feet, then experiences a "heavy," weak feeling in the legs, followed by inability to climb stairs or walk. Deep tendon reflexes are absent even when strength is relatively preserved. Objective signs of sensory loss are usually minor compared with the dramatic weakness. Progression to bulbar and respiratory insufficiency may occur rapidly. Close monitoring of respiratory function is essential. **Dysfunction of autonomic** nerves can lead to hypertension, hypotension, orthostatic hypotension, tachycardia, and other arrhythmias; urinary retention or incontinence; stool retention; or episodes of abnormal sweating, flushing, or peripheral vasoconstriction. This polyneuropathy can be difficult to distinguish from an acute spinal cord syndrome. Preservation of bowel and bladder function, loss of arm reflexes, absence of a sensory level, and lack of spinal tenderness would point more toward Guillain-Barré syndrome. A cranial nerve variant of Guillain-Barré syndrome called the **Miller Fisher variant** manifests with ataxia, partial ophthalmoplegia, and areflexia.

Porphyria and tick paralysis may simulate Guillain-Barré syndrome. Other causes of peripheral neuropathy include vasculitis, heredity, nutritional deficiency (vitamins B_1, B_{12}, and E), endocrine disorders, infections (diphtheria, Lyme disease), and toxins (organophosphate, lead).

The illness may resolve spontaneously, and 75% of patients recover normal function within 1 to 12 months. Twenty percent of patients are left with mild to moderate residual weakness in the feet and lower legs. The mortality rate is 5%, and death is caused by autonomic dysfunction (hypertension-hypotension, tachycardia-bradycardia, and sudden death), respiratory failure, complications of mechanical ventilation, cardiovascular collapse, or pulmonary embolism.

Laboratory and Diagnostic Studies

The CSF in Guillain-Barré syndrome is often normal in the first days of the illness, then shows elevated protein levels without significant pleocytosis. NCV and EMG also may be normal early in the disease, but then show delay in motor NCV and decreased amplitude and temporal dispersion of the evoked compound motor action potential.

Treatment

Children with moderate or severe weakness or rapidly progressive weakness should be cared for in a pediatric ICU. Endotracheal intubation should be performed electively in patients who exhibit early signs of hypoventilation, accumulation of bronchial secretions, or obtunded pharyngeal or laryngeal reflexes. Before mechanical ventilation, respiratory sufficiency is monitored by frequent spirometric studies, including vital capacity and maximum inspiratory force. Therapy is symptomatic and rehabilitative and directed at hypertension, hypotension, and cardiac arrhythmia; pulmonary embolism; nutrition, fluids, and electrolytes; pain; skin, cornea, and joints; bowel and bladder; infection; psychological support; and communication. Plasma exchange and IV immunoglobulin are beneficial in rapidly progressive disease. Most patients are treated initially with IV immunoglobulin (total dose 1 to 2 g/kg/day given for 4 to 5 days).

Hereditary Motor Sensory Neuropathy (Charcot-Marie-Tooth Disease)

Etiology

HMSN, commonly called Charcot-Marie-Tooth disease, is a chronic, genetic polyneuropathy characterized by weakness and wasting of distal limb muscles. The most common form (Charcot-Marie-Tooth type 1A) is due to a duplication of DNA at 17p11.2-12, a region containing the peripheral myelin protein (*PMP 22*) gene. A deletion in this region gives rise to a much milder condition, known as hereditary neuropathy with liability to pressure palsies. An X-linked form of HMSN is caused by mutations of the gap junction protein, connexin 32. HMSN type II is a neuronal form with normal or mildly decreased NCV and no hyper-

trophic changes. Type I HMSN and type II HMSN are inherited as autosomal dominant traits with variable expressivity.

Clinical Manifestations

Most often, complaints begin in the preschool years with **pes cavus deformity of feet** and weakness of the ankles with frequent tripping (see Chapter 201). Examination shows high-arched feet, bilateral weakness of foot dorsiflexors, and normal sensation despite occasional complaints of paresthesia. Progression of HMSN is slow, extending over years and decades. Eventually, patients develop weakness and atrophy of the entire lower legs and hands and mild to moderate sensory loss in the hands and feet. Some patients never have more than a mild deformity of the feet, loss of ankle reflexes, and electrophysiologic abnormalities. Others in the same family may be confined to a wheelchair and have difficulties performing everyday tasks with their hands.

Laboratory and Diagnostic Studies

HMSN type I is a demyelinating illness with severely decreased NCV and hypertrophic changes on nerve biopsy.

Treatment

Specific treatment for HMSN is not available, but braces that maintain the feet in dorsiflexion can improve function measurably. Early surgery is contraindicated because progression of the disease destabilizes even a good repair.

Tick Paralysis

Tick paralysis produces an acute lower motor neuron pattern of weakness clinically similar to Guillain-Barré syndrome. An attached female tick releases a toxin, similar to botulism, that blocks neuromuscular transmission. Affected patients present with a severe generalized flaccid weakness, including ocular, papillary, and bulbar paralysis. A methodical search, particularly in hairy areas, for an affixed tick must be made in any child with acute weakness. Removal of the tick results in a prompt return of motor function.

NEUROMUSCULAR JUNCTION

Myasthenia Gravis

Etiology and Epidemiology

Myasthenia gravis is an autoimmune condition in which antibodies to the acetylcholine receptors at the neuromuscular junction block and, through complement-mediated pathways, damage the neuromuscular junction.

Clinical Manifestations

Classic myasthenia gravis may begin in the teenage years with the onset of ptosis, diplopia, ophthalmoplegia, and weakness of extremities, neck, face, and jaw. Fluctuating and generally minimal symptoms are present on awakening in the morning and gradually worsen as the day progresses or with exercise. In some children, the disease never advances beyond ophthalmoplegia and ptosis (ocular myasthenia). Others have a progressive and potentially life-threatening illness that involves all musculature, including that of respiration and swallowing (systemic myasthenia).

Diagnostic Studies

The diagnosis is confirmed with IV edrophonium chloride (Tensilon), which transiently improves strength and decreases fatigability. Antiacetylcholine receptor antibodies often can be detected in the serum. Repetitive nerve stimulation shows a decremental response at 1 to 3 Hz.

Treatment

Treatment includes acetylcholine esterase inhibitors (pyridostigmine [Mestinon]), thymectomy, prednisone, plasmapheresis, and immunosuppressive agents. When respiration is compromised, immediate intubation and admission to an ICU are indicated.

Neonatal Transitory Myasthenia Gravis

A transitory myasthenic syndrome develops in 10% to 20% of neonates born to mothers with myasthenia gravis. Symptoms persist for 1 to 10 weeks (mean 3 weeks). Almost all infants born to mothers with myasthenia have antiacetylcholine receptor antibody, but neither antibody titer nor extent of disease in the mother predicts which neonates have clinical disease. Symptoms and signs include ptosis, ophthalmoplegia, weak facial movements, poor sucking and feeding, hypotonia, and variable extremity weakness. The diagnosis is made by showing clinical improvement lasting approximately 45 minutes after IM administration of neostigmine methylsulfate, 0.04 mg/kg. Treatment with oral pyridostigmine or neostigmine 30 minutes before feeding is continued until spontaneous resolution occurs.

Congenital Myasthenic Syndrome

A variety of rare disorders of the neuromuscular junction have been reported that are not autoimmune mediated. The conditions manifest as hypotonic infants with feeding disorders and variable degrees of weakness. Some of the identified variants include abnormalities of the presynaptic region (familial infantile myasthenia), synaptic defects (congenital end plate acetylcholinesterase deficiency), or postsynaptic disorders (slow channel myasthenic syndrome).

MUSCLE DISEASE
Duchenne Dystrophy
Etiology

Muscular dystrophy is a common sex-linked recessive trait appearing in 20 to 30 per 100,000 boys. The disease results from absence of a large protein called **dystrophin** that is associated with the muscle fiber plasma membrane. **Becker muscular dystrophy** arises from an abnormality in the same gene locus that results in the presence of dystrophin that is abnormal in either amount or molecular structure. It has the same clinical symptoms as Duchenne dystrophy, but onset is later, and progression is slower.

Clinical Manifestations

At about 2 to 3 years of age, boys develop an awkward gait and an inability to run properly. Some have an antecedent history of mild slowness in attaining motor milestones, such as walking and climbing stairs. Examination shows firm calf hypertrophy and mild to moderate proximal leg weakness exhibited by a hyperlordotic, waddling gait and inability to arise from the ground easily. The child typically arises from a lying position on the floor by using his arms to "climb up" his legs and body (**Gower sign**). Arm weakness is evident by 6 years of age, and most boys are confined to a wheelchair by 12 years of age. By age 16, little mobility of arms remains, and respiratory difficulties increase. Death is caused by pneumonia or congestive heart failure resulting from myocardial involvement.

Laboratory and Diagnostic Studies

Serum creatine phosphokinase levels are always markedly elevated. Muscle biopsy specimen shows muscle fiber degeneration and regeneration accompanied by increased intrafascicular connective tissue. Diagnosis is established by DNA probe for Duchenne muscular dystrophy. Prenatal diagnosis of both diseases is possible by genetic testing. Approximately one third of cases represent new mutations.

Treatment

Supportive care includes physical therapy, bracing, proper wheelchairs, and prevention of scoliosis. A multidisciplinary approach is recommended.

Limb-girdle dystrophy is usually an autosomal recessive disease presenting with proximal leg and arm weakness. The genetic defect lies within one of the many muscle proteins that compose the muscle fiber plasma membrane cytoskeleton complex. The clinical manifestations are similar to the manifestations of Duchenne dystrophy, but are seen in an older child or teenager and progress slowly over years. By midadulthood, most patients are wheelchair bound.

Facioscapulohumeral dystrophy is usually an autosomal dominant disease presenting in teenagers with facial and proximal arm weakness. Genetic diagnosis is possible by finding a characteristic 4q35 deletion. The child has mild ptosis, a decrease in facial expression, inability to pucker the lips or whistle, neck weakness, difficulty in fully elevating the arms, scapular winging, and thinness of upper arm musculature. Progression is slow, and most patients retain excellent functional capabilities for decades.

Myotonic Dystrophy

Etiology and Epidemiology

Myotonic dystrophy is an autosomal dominant genetic disease caused by progressive expansion of a triplet repeat, GCT, on chromosome 19q13.2-13.3 in a gene designated myotonin protein kinase (*MP-PK*).

Clinical Manifestations

Myotonia is a disorder of muscle relaxation. Patients grasp onto an object and have difficulty releasing their grasp, "peeling" their fingers away slowly. Myotonic dystrophy presents either at birth, with severe generalized hypotonia and weakness, or in adolescence, with slowly progressive facial and distal extremity weakness and myotonia. The adolescent type is the classic illness and is associated with cardiac arrhythmias, cataracts, male pattern baldness, and infertility in males (hypogonadism). The facial appearance is characteristic, with hollowing of muscles around temples, jaw, and neck; ptosis; facial weakness; and drooping of the lower lip. The voice is nasal and mildly dysarthric.

Some mothers with myotonic dystrophy give birth to infants with the disease who are immobile and hypotonic, with expressionless faces, tented upper lips, ptosis, absence of sucking and Moro reflexes, and poor swallowing and respiration. Often, weakness and atony of uterine smooth muscle during labor lead to associated hypoxic-ischemic encephalopathy and its sequelae. The presence of congenital contractures, clubfoot, or a history of poor fetal movements indicates intrauterine neuromuscular disease.

TABLE 182–4.   Congenital Myopathies
Congenital structural myopathy
Central core
Nemaline rod
Centronuclear
Congenital fiber type of disproportion
Congenital muscular dystrophy
Miscellaneous types
Metabolic, endocrine, and mineral
Glycogen storage disease II (Pompe disease)
Carnitine metabolism abnormalities
Mitochondrial abnormalities

Congenital Myopathies

Etiology

Congenital myopathies are a group of congenital, often genetic, nonprogressive or slowly progressive myopathies characterized by abnormal appearance of the muscle biopsy specimen (Table 182–4).

Clinical Manifestations

A child with a congenital myopathy is profoundly hypotonic with moderately diffuse weakness involving limbs and face. Associated conditions include congenitally dislocated hips, a high-arched palate, clubfoot, and contractures at hips, knees, ankles, or elbows secondary to intrauterine weakness. The attainment of motor milestones is moderately to severely delayed. The clinical course is either static or slowly progressive. Progressive kyphoscoliosis represents a significant problem in some children. Reflexes are diminished.

Laboratory and Diagnostic Studies

Creatine phosphokinase levels may be mildly elevated. EMG may show a nonspecific "myopathic" pattern or may be normal. The definitive diagnosis is made by muscle biopsy; the characteristic features include nemaline rods, fiber-type disproportion, and central core changes.

Dermatomyositis

Etiology and Epidemiology

The etiology and epidemiology of dermatomyositis are discussed in Chapter 91.

Clinical Manifestations

The clinical features include progressive proximal muscle weakness coupled with dermatologic features, including erythematous rash around the eyes (**heliotrope**) and plaques on the knuckles (**Gottron rash**) and on the extensor surfaces of the knees, elbows, and toes. Subcutaneous calcinosis is a late finding (see Chapter 91).

Diagnostic Studies and Therapy

Myositis-specific autoantibodies may be identified in the serum. Diagnostic testing includes measurement of serum creatine phosphokinase levels, EMG, MRI of muscle, and muscle biopsy. See Chapter 91 for therapy.

Metabolic Myopathies

Glycogen storage disease type II (Pompe disease) and muscle carnitine deficiency are discussed in Chapter 52. **Mitochondrial myopathies** are characterized by muscle biopsy specimens that display ragged red fibers, representing collections of abnormal mitochondria (see Chapter 57). Typical symptoms include hypotonia, ophthalmoplegia, and progressive weakness, but the phenotype of these disorders is broad. **Endocrine myopathies**, including hyperthyroidism, hypothyroidism, hyperparathyroidism, and Cushing syndrome, are associated with proximal muscle weakness. Hypokalemia and hyperkalemia produce fluctuating weakness (periodic paralysis) and loss of tendon jerks.

Treatment of Neuromuscular Diseases

The major complications of neuromuscular disorders are the development of joint contractures, scoliosis, and pneumonia. Prevention and treatment of contractures with active range of motion exercises and bracing are important because contractures can be painful or inhibit function even when strength is adequate. Surgery to release contractures or to realign tendons is most helpful in nonprogressive or in very slowly progressive conditions. Kyphoscoliosis produces loss of function, disfigurement and, when severe, life-threatening decrease of ventilatory reserve. Prevention or delay in the development of these complications can be achieved by maintaining ambulation for as long as possible, ensuring a properly fitted wheelchair, bracing, and surgery. Pneumonia may be associated with thick secretions that are difficult to clear, progressive atelectasis, and respiratory failure. Anticipatory treatment with antibiotics, hospitalization, chest physical therapy, oxygen, and ventilatory support helps in most cases.

Laboratory and Diagnostic Studies

See Table 182–5 and text for individual disorders.

TABLE 182–5. Evaluation of Neuromuscular Disease

Complete medical history
Complete family history
Complete neurologic examination
Complete blood count, differential, ESR
Electrolytes, BUN, creatinine, glucose, calcium, phosphate, alkaline phosphatase, magnesium
Muscle chemistries: CPK, aldolase
Metabolic studies: lactate, pyruvate
Chest x-ray
ECG
Stool: botulism culture and toxin, *Campylobacter* culture
CSF (protein, cells)
Tensilon test, neostigmine test, acetylcholine receptor antibodies
EMG-NCV
Muscle biopsy
MRI of spinal cord

CPK, creatine phosphokinase; EMG, electromyogram; ESR, erythrocyte sedimentation rate; NCV, nerve conduction velocity.

Malignant Hyperthermia

Patients with Duchenne muscular dystrophy, central core myopathy, and other myopathies are susceptible to the life-threatening syndrome of **malignant hyperthermia**. Malignant hyperthermia is manifested as a rapid increase of body temperature and PCO_2, muscle rigidity, cyanosis, hypotension, arrhythmias, and convulsions. This syndrome may occur during administration of anesthesia consisting of succinylcholine or inhalation agents such as halothane. Malignant hyperpyrexia can also occur in children without muscle disease as an autosomal dominant genetic disorder. A family history of unexplained death during operations is often noted. Diagnosis of idiopathic malignant hyperthermia is possible with genetic testing or the in vitro muscle contraction test. Excessive tonic contracture on exposure to halothane and caffeine in vitro indicates susceptibility. Treatment with IV dantrolene, sodium bicarbonate, and cooling is helpful.

Neonatal and Infantile Hypotonia

The clinical distinction between upper and lower motor neuron disorders in infants is blurred because incomplete myelinization of the developing nervous system limits expression of many of the cardinal signs, such as spasticity. Neuromuscular and cerebral disorders may produce hypotonia in a young child or infant. The two critical clinical points are whether the child is weak and presence or absence of the deep tendon reflexes. Hypotonia and weakness coupled with depressed or absent reflexes suggest a neuromuscular disorder. A stronger child with brisk reflexes suggests an upper motor neuron source for the hypotonia.

Hypotonia without Significant Weakness (Central Hypotonia)

Some infants who appear to move well when supine in their cribs are "floppy" when handled or moved. When placed on their backs, these infants are bright-eyed, have expressive faces, and can lift their arms and legs without apparent difficulty. When lifted, their heads flop, they "slip through" at the shoulders, do not stand upright on their legs, and form an "inverted U" in prone suspension (**Landau posture**). When placed prone as neonates, they may lie flat instead of having their arms and legs tucked underneath them. Passive tone is decreased, but reflexes are normal. This clinical picture may be associated with significant cerebral disease or may be a benign phenomenon that is outgrown.

Prader-Willi syndrome presents with severe neonatal hypotonia; severe feeding problems leading to failure to thrive; small hands and feet; and, in boys, small penis, small testicles, and cryptorchidism. Severe hyperphagia and obesity develop in early childhood. Approximately 60% to 70% of affected individuals have an interstitial deletion of paternal chromosome 15q11q13. Many other syndromes also present with severe neonatal floppiness and mental dullness (Table 182-6).

Infants who have a connective tissue disorder, such as **Ehlers-Danlos syndrome**, **Marfan syndrome**, or familial laxity of the ligaments, may exhibit marked passive hypotonia, "double jointedness," and increased skin elasticity. They have normal strength and cognition and achieve motor and mental milestones normally. They have peculiar postures of their feet or an unusual gait.

Infants with **benign congenital hypotonia** typically exhibit the condition at 6 to 12 months old, with delayed gross motor skills. They are unable to sit, creep, or crawl, but have good verbal, social, and manipulative skills and an intelligent appearance. Strength appears normal, and the infants can kick arms and legs briskly and bring their toes to their mouths. The children display head lag, slip-through in ventral suspension, and floppiness of passive tone. Parents may remember that the infant has seemed floppy from birth. The differential diagnosis includes upper and motor neuron disorders and connective tissue diseases. Extensive laboratory investigation is often unrevealing and of questionable value. A complete physical examination, complete blood count, electrolytes, bicarbonate, BUN, creatinine, calcium, creatine phosphokinase,

---

TABLE 182–6.   Approach to Differential Diagnosis of the Floppy Infant

Hypotonia with Weakness

Awareness Intact

Neuromuscular disease
  Spinal muscular atrophy*
  Myasthenic syndromes
  Congenital neuropathy or myopathy
Spinal cord disease (cervical cord trauma or compression)
  Tumor
  Spinal cord infarct
  Malformation
  Spina bifida
  Syringomyelia

Consciousness Depressed

Severe brain illness*
Structural (hydrocephalus)
Infectious
Metabolic (e.g., anoxia or hypoglycemia)
Intoxication through mother
  Magnesium sulfate
  Barbiturates
  Narcotics
  Benzodiazepines
  General anesthesia
Metabolic abnormality
  Hypoglycemia
  Kernicterus

Hypotonia without Weakness

Acute systemic illness*
Mental retardation
Specific syndromes
  Down syndrome*
  Cerebrohepatorenal (Zellweger peroxisomal disorder)
  Oculocerebrorenal (Lowe syndrome)
  Kinky hair disease (Menkes syndrome—copper metabolism disorder)
  Neonatal adrenal leukodystrophy
  Prader-Willi syndrome
Connective tissue disorder
  Ehlers-Danlos syndrome
  Marfan syndrome
  Congenital laxity of ligaments
Nutritional-metabolic disease
  Rickets
  Renal tubular acidosis
  Celiac disease
  Biliary atresia
Congenital heart disease
Benign congenital hypotonia

*Common.

bilirubin, alanine aminotransferase, aspartate amino-transferase, thyroid function studies, and urinalysis are generally necessary and sufficient. Most of these children "catch up" to their peers and appear normal by 3 years of age. Often, other family members have exhibited a similar developmental pattern.

STROKE IN CHILDHOOD
Etiology

Cerebrovascular infarction or hemorrhage is uncommon in children. The incidence is 2.5 to 10 per 100,000 children and is higher in neonates. A wide spectrum of conditions can produce stroke in childhood (Table 182–7). The most common causes are congenital heart disease (cyanotic), sickle cell anemia (SS), meningitis, and hypercoagulable states.

Heart disease and its complications (endocarditis) may give rise to thromboses in cerebral arteries or veins or to emboli in cerebral arteries. Cerebral venous and arterial thromboses occur in 1% to 2% of infants with unrepaired cyanotic congenital heart disease and probably are related to local congestion of blood flow, failure of passage of blood through the lungs (right-to-left cardiac shunting), and polycythemia. Predisposing factors include acute episodes of severe cyanosis, febrile illnesses, dehydration, hyperventilation, and iron deficiency anemia. Sources of emboli include mural thrombi from dilated, poorly contracting cardiac chambers, bacterial endocarditis, nonbacterial endocarditis, valvular disease, atrial myxoma, cardiac catheterization, and cardiac surgery. Septic emboli producing cerebral infarcts occur in 10% to 20% of patients who develop bacterial endocarditis.

Clinical Manifestations

Cerebral embolization characteristically occurs without warning, produces its full deficit within seconds (hyperacute), and may be associated with focal deficits, focal seizures, sudden headache, and hemorrhagic infarction. The most common sources of cerebral emboli are the heart and the carotid artery. Cerebral thrombosis may be preceded by transient ischemic attacks that resolve completely. The deficits themselves evolve over hours in a stepwise or stuttering progression. The sudden emergence of neurologic deficits implies cerebrovascular disease, and the site of occlusion is suggested by the neurologic deficits.

Occasionally a thorough evaluation of a child with a stroke fails to reveal the etiology. Angiography or magnetic resonance angiography may disclose the site of vascular occlusion, but the pathogenetic mechanism remains unknown. This condition is termed **acute hemiplegia of childhood**.

TABLE 182–7. Causes of Stroke in Childhood
Cardiac or other embolic source
Endocarditis
Cyanotic congenital heart disease
Valvular disease
Patent foramen ovale
Infectious
Bacterial meningitis
Encephalitis
Chickenpox
Vasculitis or vasculopathy
Arterial dissection
Traumatic
Spontaneous
Moyamoya disease
Sickle cell anemia
Neurofibromatosis
Vasculitis
Coagulopathies
Hypocoagulation (hemophilia, von Willebrand, thrombocytopenia)
Hypercoagulation
Factor V Leiden deficiency
Protein C deficiency
Protein S deficiency
Antiphospholipid antibodies
Antithrombin III deficiency
Sickle cell disease
Disseminated intravascular pathology
Head or neck trauma
Carotid or vertebral dissections
Atlantoaxial dislocation
Fibromuscular dysplasia
Atherosclerosis
Drugs or toxins
Amphetamine-cocaine abuse
Pregnancy/oral contraceptive pills
Hypertension
Hemolytic-uremic syndrome
Nephrotic syndrome
Malignancy
Carcinomatous meningitis
Leukemic meningitis
Chemotherapy (asparaginase)
Liver disease
Inborn error of metabolism
Homocystinuria
Neonatal
Emboli from dead twin
Emboli from involuting umbilical vessels
Polycythemia

Congenital hemiplegia becomes apparent in infants 4 to 6 months old with decreased use of one side of the body, early "handedness," or ignoring one side. CT reveals an area of encephalomalacia in the contralateral cerebral hemisphere. The details of the child's intrauterine, labor, delivery, and postnatal history often are unremarkable. Some neonates present with focal seizures. The timing of the injury is unknown, but the injury may represent an embolus from the fetal-placental unit.

Diagnostic Tests and Imaging

If clinical assessment does not reveal the cause of the stroke, a complete laboratory investigation should be undertaken promptly based on suspected etiologies (see Table 182–7). An evolving stroke is distinguished from an attack of migraine by abnormal findings on diffusion-weighted MRI.

Treatment

There is no treatment to repair the neurologic injury after the stroke, so prevention of future stroke must be the focus in children if the etiology can be identified. One therapeutic dilemma involves strokes that present "in evolution," recurrent transient ischemic attacks, or ongoing cerebral embolization. The role of anticoagulants (IV heparin, subcutaneous low-molecular-weight heparin, and oral warfarin), platelet antiaggregants (aspirin and dipyridamole), thrombolysis via arterial or venous catheters, or surgery to enlarge stenosed channels, excise sources of emboli, or provide alternative sources of intracerebral blood flow is controversial.

CHAPTER 183

Ataxia and Movement Disorders

ETIOLOGY

Ataxia is an impairment of coordination or balance of voluntary movement. With few exceptions, this condition represents a disturbance of cerebellar pathways, including the cerebellar peduncles within the brainstem, spinocerebellar tract in the spinal cord, thalamic nuclei, and cortical reflections. The most common causes of acute ataxia in childhood are postinfectious acute cerebellar ataxia and drug intoxications. The **differential diagnosis** includes other disorders within the posterior fossa, such as tumors (medulloblastoma, ependymoma, cerebellar astrocytoma), multiple sclerosis, strokes, and hemorrhages. Other causes of recurrent or progressive ataxia, such as the paraneoplastic opsoclonus-myoclonus syndrome associated with neuroblastoma, inborn errors of metabolism, labyrinthine dysfunction, head trauma, epilepsy, postictal state, and

migraine, can be difficult to diagnose and require special diagnostic testing for their identification. Congenital disorders also may produce chronic, nonprogressive ataxia (Table 183–1).

CLINICAL MANIFESTATIONS

The usual symptoms are a broad-based, unsteady gait (truncal ataxia) and intention tremor or dysmetria. An intention tremor worsens as the arm approaches the target. Overshooting or undershooting of the target is termed **dysmetria** (abnormality of distance). Classically, these symptoms stem from disorders of the cerebellar pathways, but peripheral nerve lesions causing loss of proprioceptive inputs to the cerebellum (Miller Fisher variant of Guillain-Barré syndrome) may present with similar symptoms.

Postinfectious acute cerebellar ataxia may follow chickenpox, infectious mononucleosis, or a mild respiratory or gastrointestinal viral illness by about 1 week. The pathogenesis of the syndrome is uncertain and may represent either a direct viral infection of the cerebellum or an autoimmune response directed to the cerebellar white matter and precipitated by the preceding viral infection. Symptoms begin abruptly, causing staggering and frequent falling. Symptoms can progress to difficulty with standing and sitting. Truncal ataxia may be the only symptom or dysmetria of the arms, dysarthria, nystagmus, vomiting, irritability, and lethargy may be present. Symptoms usually peak within 2 days, then stabilize and resolve over 1 to 2 weeks. CSF examination sometimes shows a mild lymphocytic pleocytosis or mild elevation of protein content. Brain imaging is usually normal. No specific therapy is available except to prevent injury during the ataxic phase. Recovery is usually complete.

DRUG INTOXICATION

Overdosage with any sedative-hypnotic agent can produce acute ataxia and lethargy, but ataxia without lethargy usually results from intoxication with alcohol, phenytoin, or carbamazepine. It is important to ask whether anyone in the household or a house that the child visits (grandparent, sitter) is taking anticonvulsant or antipsychotic medications. Treatment is supportive, and the toxic agent is removed.

POSTERIOR FOSSA TUMORS

Brain tumors are the second most common neoplasm in children. About 50% arise from within the posterior fossa. Tumors that arise in this area of the cerebellum or the brainstem produce progressive ataxia with headache that may be acute or gradual in onset. When these symptoms begin, there is a progressive worsening

TABLE 183–1. Causes of Ataxia

Neoplasm	**Demyelinative**
Medulloblastoma*	Multiple sclerosis
Ependymoma	Acute disseminated encephalomyelitis
Cystic cerebellar astrocytoma*	**Structural or Congenital**
Brainstem glioma	Cerebellar hypoplasia
Paraneoplastic	Vermal aplasia
Neuroblastoma (opsoclonus-myoclonus-ataxia)	Dandy-Walker malformation
Infectious	Joubert syndrome
Encephalitis	Arnold-Chiari malformation
Brainstem encephalitis	Hydrocephalus
Meningitis	**Hereditary**
Postinfectious	Episodic ataxia (acetazolamide responsive)
Acute cerebellar ataxia*	Friedreich ataxia
Guillain-Barré syndrome (Miller Fisher variant)	Machado-Joseph disease
Migrainous	Ramsay Hunt syndrome
Basilar migraine*	Spinocerebellar ataxia 1
Trauma	Spinocerebellar ataxia 2
Cerebellar hemorrhage	Ataxia-telangiectasia
Cerebellar contusion	Marinesco-Sjögren syndrome
Concussion	**Metabolic**
Postconcussive syndrome*	Metachromatic leukodystrophy
Toxic Ingestion*	Adrenoleukodystrophy
Antihistamines	Maple syrup urine disease
Ethanol	Hartnup disease
Anticonvulsants	GM_2 gangliosidosis (juvenile)
Vascular	Refsum disease
Cerebellar hemorrhage or infarction	Vitamin E deficiency
Vertebral artery dissection	Leigh disease
	Wilson disease
	Abetalipoproteinemia
	Sea-blue histiocytosis

*Common.

over days, weeks, or months. The ataxia and dysmetria may result from primary cerebellar invasion or from obstruction of the CSF pathways (aqueduct of Sylvius or fourth ventricle) with resultant hydrocephalus. The most common tumors in this region include medulloblastoma, ependymoma, cerebellar astrocytoma, and brainstem glioma.

PARANEOPLASTIC OPSOCLONUS-MYOCLONUS SYNDROME

Rarely a neuroblastoma located in the adrenal medulla or anywhere along the paraspinal sympathetic chain in the thorax or abdomen is associated with degeneration of Purkinje cells and the development of severe ataxia,

dysmetria, irritability, **myoclonus**, and **opsoclonus**. An immunologic reaction directed toward the tumor may be misdirected to attack also Purkinje cells and other neuronal elements. The myoclonic movements are irregular, lightning-like movements of a limb or the head. Opsoclonus is a rapid, multidirectional, conjugate movement of the eyes, which suddenly dart in random directions. The presence of this sign in infants and toddlers should prompt a vigorous search for an occult neuroblastoma, including urine testing of the adrenergic metabolites (vanillylmandelic acid and homovanillic acid), chest x-ray, abdominal ultrasound, and MRI with contrast enhancement of the entire sympathetic chain. These tumors tend to be localized and curable by surgical resection. Treatment with corticosteroids often relieves the acute neurologic symptoms, but 64% of children are left with persistent cerebellar deficits, and 36% have intellectual deficits.

INBORN ERRORS OF METABOLISM

Several rare inborn errors of metabolism can present with intermittent episodes of ataxia and somnolence. These include Hartnup disorder, branched chain ketoaciduria (maple syrup urine disease), multiple carboxylase deficiency (biotinidase deficiency), disorders of the urea cycle, and abnormalities of pyruvate metabolism.

LABYRINTHINE DYSFUNCTION

Difficulty walking with a severe staggering gait is one manifestation of labyrinthine dysfunction, but the diagnosis usually is clarified by the associated symptoms of a severe sense of spinning dizziness (vertigo), nausea and vomiting, and associated signs of pallor, sweating, and nystagmus.

MOVEMENT DISORDERS

Movement disorders or **dyskinesias** are a diverse group of clinical entities associated with abnormal excessive, exaggerated, chaotic, or explosive movements of voluntary muscles. They are generally the result of abnormalities of the extrapyramidal system or the basal ganglia and its connections. Symptoms may be one of two types. **Bradykinesia** and **hypokinesia** describe the slow gait, halting speech patterns, apparent inactivity, and paucity of facial expression seen in adults with Parkinson disease and in some children with extrapyramidal disorders. Movement disorders that are excessive or **hyperkinetic** patterns are activated by stress and fatigue and often disappear in sleep. The abnormal movements are typically diffuse and migratory, but may be isolated to specific muscle groups (segmental myoclonus, palatal myoclonus) and may not disappear in sleep.

Chorea is a hyperkinetic, rapid, unsustained, irregular, purposeless, nonpatterned movement. Muscle tone is decreased. Choreiform movement abnormalities may be congenital, familial, metabolic, vascular, toxic, infectious, or neoplastic in origin. The movements may occur alone or as part of a more extensive neurologic disorder (Sydenham chorea, Huntington chorea, cerebral palsy, Wilson disease, or reactions to toxins and drugs). Fidgety behavior, inability to sit still, clumsiness, dysarthria, and an awkward gait may occur. The exact mechanism of dysfunction within the extrapyramidal system is unknown.

Athetosis is a hyperkinetic, slow, coarse, writhing movement that is more pronounced in distal muscles. Muscle tone may be increased. Athetosis is seen fre-

quently in combination with chorea (choreoathetosis) and usually is present in conjunction with other neurologic signs. It may be seen in virtually all the disorders mentioned for chorea, but the most prominent cause is encephalopathy. Athetosis is a prominent feature of Hallervorden-Spatz disease, Wilson disease, and Pelizaeus-Merzbacher dystrophy. Many children with mixed forms of cerebral palsy have spasticity and choreoathetosis.

Dystonia is a hyperkinetic, sustained, slow, twisting motion (torsion spasm) that may progress to a fixed posture and can be activated by repetitive movement (action dystonia). It has many causes and associated neurologic signs. Dystonia usually begins in the legs when appendicular muscles are involved and in the neck or trunk when axial muscles are involved. Tardive dyskinesia usually is associated with antipsychotic drug use. Darting tongue movements, incessant flexion and extension of the distal muscles, standing and marching in place, and a perception of restlessness are common.

Tremor is a hyperkinetic, rhythmic, oscillatory movement caused by simultaneous contractions of antagonistic muscles. The amplitude and frequency are regular. In children, tremor is usually due to physiologic, familial, or cerebellar origin, but it may be seen in association with other disease processes (thyrotoxicosis, hypoglycemia, or Wilson disease) or drugs (e.g., bronchodilators, amphetamines, or tricyclic antidepressants).

Myoclonus is a hyperkinetic, brief flexion contraction of a muscle group, resulting in a sudden jerk. Myoclonus may be epileptic or nonepileptic. Nonepileptic myoclonus is distinguished from tremor in that it is a simple contraction of an agonist muscle, whereas tremor is a simultaneous contraction of agonist and antagonist muscles. Myoclonus is seen as a manifestation of various epilepsies and of infectious, toxic, and metabolic encephalopathies.

Tics are rapid, purposeless, involuntary, stereotyped movements and typically involve the face, eyes, shoulder, and arm. Most tic disorders in children are transient and not intrusive into the child's life, but they often are a source of great parental anxiety. Occasionally, tics are "unmasked" by stimulant agents. Persistent motor tics (>12 months) in association with vocal tics are characteristic of **Tourette syndrome**, a chronic tic disorder that usually begins before age 7 years. The prevalence is at least 5 in 10,000, with a male-to-female ratio of 4:1. The pathophysiology underlying the tics is unknown, but a family history of tics is elicited in more than 50% of cases. The severity and pattern of the tics vary over months and years. Vocal tics begin later in the clinical course. The motor tics vary from muscle twitches (simple motor tic) and grunts (simple vocal tic) to complex stereotyped movement patterns (e.g., orchestrated movements). Comorbid features, such as obsessive-compulsive disorder and attention-deficit/hyperactivity syndrome, may be present in half of children with Tourette disorder (see Chapters 13 and 19). Tic disorders are clinical diagnoses, and neurodiagnostic studies have limited value. Many children with tic disorders or Tourette syndrome are unperturbed by their tics and require no therapy. Others are quite disabled and may benefit from psychological support and pharmacologic therapy with α-adrenergic receptor agonists (clonidine) or neuroleptics (pimozide, haloperidol, risperidone). The natural history of Tourette disorder is favorable with about two thirds of children experiencing a significant reduction of tics or complete remission.

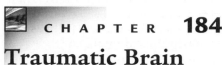

CHAPTER 184

Traumatic Brain Injury and Coma

Children with head trauma may have depression of consciousness and neurologic deficits or may be completely alert without any immediate signs of neurologic injury. The former necessitates immediate management, and the latter necessitates vigilant observation. Most serious trauma results from motor vehicle crashes, sports, recreation-related injuries, and violence.

PATIENTS WITH NEUROLOGIC DEFICITS

Victims of head trauma with neurologic deficits may have awakened after the injury (lucid interval) and then undergone a depression of mental status or may have remained unconscious from the moment of injury. Some progressively deteriorate and require immediate neurosurgical care. See Chapter 41 for the management of head trauma. Skull and cervical spine radiographs and cranial CT are obtained as soon as possible. Syndromes of post-traumatic hemorrhage are summarized in Table 184–1.

Children with cerebral contusion who survive the acute cerebral swelling may improve rapidly or slowly or remain vegetative. Children who show daily improvement starting within days of the injury often recover completely. Maximal recovery may take weeks, months, or even a year. Caution must be used in providing families with a prognosis. Coma lasting for weeks after head trauma still is compatible with an ultimately good outcome, although the risk of late sequelae is increased. Patients who remain in a vegetative state for months after head injury are unlikely to improve.

TABLE 184–1. Syndromes of Post-traumatic Intracranial Hemorrhage

Syndrome	Clinical and Radiologic Characteristics	Treatment
Epidural	Onset over minutes to hours Uncal herniation with third nerve palsy and contralateral hemiparesis Lens-shaped extracerebral hemorrhage compressing brain	Surgical evacuation or observation Prognosis good
Acute subdural	Onset over hours Uncal herniation Focal neurologic deficits Crescentic extracranial hemorrhage compressing brain	Surgical evacuation Prognosis guarded
Chronic subdural	Onset over weeks to months Anemia, macrocephaly Seizures, vomiting Crescentic, low-density mass on CT	Subdural taps or subdural shunt as necessary Prognosis good
Intraparenchymal	Depressed consciousness Focal neurologic deficits Additional multiple contusions	Supportive care Prognosis guarded
Subarachnoid	Stiff neck Late hydrocephalus	Supportive care Prognosis variable
Contusion	Focal neurologic deficits Brain swelling with transtentorial herniation CT: multifocal low-density areas with punctate hemorrhages	Medical treatment of elevated intracranial pressure* Prognosis guarded

*Mannitol, elevate head of bed, diuresis, hyperventilation, steroids.

CONCUSSION

Concussion is a brief period of altered consciousness, lasting seconds to minutes, that occurs immediately after head trauma. Amnesia often follows concussion. **Retrograde amnesia** is the inability to remember events immediately before the trauma and may extend backward in time for minutes, hours, days, or weeks. Usually, retrograde memory is regained gradually, and permanent amnesia lasts only for the few minutes immediately before the injury. **Antegrade amnesia** is the inability to form new memories and becomes manifested by the patient incessantly repeating the same questions shortly after they have been answered ("Where am I?" "Why am I here?"). This state often persists for hours. The period of retrograde and antegrade amnesia usually correlates with the severity of the trauma.

The pathophysiology of concussion is thought to be a shearing phenomenon of white matter tracts as the brain undergoes torsional changes within the cranium, resulting in a temporary failure of axon conduction. If loss of consciousness is maintained for longer than 1 hour or if recovery of consciousness is slow and accompanied by focal neurologic deficits, the pathophysiology is likely to include contusion and laceration, which may lead to focal or generalized **cerebral edema**.

Repeated concussions, especially within a short time frame, such as days or weeks, carry a significant risk of permanent brain injury. A commonly used guideline is that children who sustain a sports-related concussion can resume participation 4 weeks after the injury if they have been asymptomatic at rest and with exertion for 2 weeks.

Malignant Post-traumatic Cerebral Swelling

Occasionally, epidural, subdural, or intracranial hemorrhage or a rapid, life-threatening increase in ICP develops unexpectedly in children after head trauma, who had appeared stable initially. The **Glasgow Coma Scale** is a valuable tool for monitoring the course of patients after trauma for signs of deterioration (see Chapter 42). Management includes ensuring an appropriate airway, breathing, and circulation. Emergent surgical intervention for decompression and drainage of the blood collection may be needed. Increased ICP may require monitoring, placement of a ventricular drain, and aggressive medical management, including intubation and ventilation, osmotic therapy, and sedation.

Transient neurologic disturbances sometimes develop a few minutes after minor or severe head trauma and last for minutes to hours before clearing. The most common symptoms are cortical blindness and a confusional state, but hemiparesis, ataxia, or any other neurologic deficit may appear. These symptoms may represent a trauma-triggered migraine precipitated in susceptible children, but care must be exercised to exclude intracranial pathology.

Post-traumatic seizures are divided into one of three patterns: impact seizures, early post-traumatic seizures, and late post-traumatic seizures. Impact seizures occur within seconds of the injury and are presumed to reflect a direct mechanical stimulation to the cortex. The prognosis is excellent, and likelihood of later epilepsy is negligible. Occasionally, pallid breath-holding spells can occur after head injury, mimicking impact seizures. Early post-traumatic seizures occurring within the first week of the head injury are likely the result of a localized area of cerebral contusion or edema. The long-term prognosis for these is quite favorable. Late post-traumatic seizures arise more than a week after the trauma (≤2 years) and most likely indicate an area of cortical gliosis or scarring that will be a source for long-term epilepsy. These patients often require long-term antiepileptic drug therapy.

Drowsiness, **headache**, and **vomiting** are common after head trauma. They are not by themselves of concern if consciousness is preserved, the clinical trend is one of improvement, and results of the neurologic examination are normal. Children are especially susceptible to somnolence after head trauma but should be easily arousable. If these symptoms worsen or persist for more than 1 to 2 days, neuroimaging may be indicated to look for subdural hematoma or cerebral edema.

Skull fractures may be linear, diastatic (spreading the suture), depressed (an edge displaced inferiorly), or compound (bone fragments breaking the skin surface). Linear and diastatic fractures necessitate no treatment, but indicate severe trauma capable of producing an underlying hematoma. Small, depressed fractures have the same significance as linear fractures, but if the depression is more than 0.5 to 1 cm, surgical elevation of bone fragments and repair of associated dural tears are generally recommended. Compound fractures or penetrating injuries necessitate emergent surgical débridement but not prophylactic antibiotic therapy. Tetanus prophylaxis must be ensured. The risk of local brain contusion and early seizures is high.

Skull fractures may present with localized bogginess and pain, subcutaneous bleeding over the mastoid process (**Battle sign**) or around the orbit (**raccoon eyes**), blood behind the tympanic membrane (**hemotympanum**), or CSF leak from the nose (rhinorrhea) or ear (**otorrhea**). Rarely, after linear skull fractures, a soft, pulsatile scalp mass is palpable within a few weeks to months. Radiographically the fracture edges are separated by a soft tissue mass that consists of fibrotic tissue and accumulated brain and meningeal tissue and perhaps a **leptomeningeal cyst**. The recommended treatment involves surgical excision of abnormal tissue and dural repair.

CSF leak occurs when a skull fracture tears adjacent dura, creating communications between the subarachnoid space and the nose, paranasal sinuses, mastoid air cells, or middle or external ear. Clear fluid that leaks from the nose or ear after head trauma is presumed to be CSF until proved otherwise. The presence of air within the subdural, subarachnoid, or ventricular space also indicates a dural tear and open communication between the nose or paranasal sinuses and brain. In most cases, the dura heals spontaneously when the patient's head is kept elevated. Patients with CSF leaks are at risk for the development of meningitis (pneumococcal) or extradural abscesses. If the leak persists or recurs or if meningitis supervenes, the fracture site is identified, and the dura is surgically repaired.

Cranial nerve palsies, after head injury secondary to a laceration or contusion to one of the cranial nerves, may result from a skull fracture and may be transitory or permanent. Longitudinal fracture of the petrous bone produces a conductive hearing loss and facial palsy, which begin hours after the injury and usually resolve spontaneously. Transverse petrous fractures produce sensorineural hearing loss and immediate facial palsy with a poor prognosis for spontaneous recovery. Disruption of the ossicular chain can cause hearing loss and may necessitate surgery. Vestibular disturbances, producing prolonged post-traumatic vertigo, are extremely common. Permanent loss of olfaction after a head injury is the result of a vibrational rupture of the thin olfactory nerves within the cribriform plate. Disruption of cranial nerves III, IV, or VI produces ophthalmoplegia, diplopia, and head tilt. Even seemingly minor head injuries can produce sixth nerve palsy with medial deviation of one eye.

Cervical spine injuries must be suspected in any unconscious child, especially if bruises are present on the head, neck, or back. In conscious children, findings of neck or back pain, burning or stabbing pains radiating to the arms, paraplegia, quadriplegia, or asymmetric motor or sensory responses of arms or legs indicate spinal cord injury. Cervical spine injury (displaced or fractured vertebra) may result in complete transection of the cord with spinal shock, loss of sensation, and flaccid paralysis. A contused cord (without vertebral abnormality) may be exhibited in a similar manner. Any patient with a clinical or radiologic abnormality of the spine requires immediate spine and cardiopulmonary stabilization and neurosurgical consultation. High-dose (30 mg/kg bolus, then 5.4 mg/kg/hr for 23 hours) IV methylprednisolone is indicated in cases of spinal cord trauma and improves the ultimate degree of recovery of function.

Postconcussive Syndrome

Many children complain of headache, dizziness, forgetfulness, inability to concentrate, slowing of response time, mood swings, irritability, and other subtle aberrations of cerebral function for days or weeks after an uncomplicated concussion. These deficits resolve spontaneously, but may require weeks or months for full recovery. Children may require brief periods of special schooling, home tutoring, and reassurance.

Evaluation and Treatment

Children who have been unconscious from a head injury or who have amnesia after a blow to the head should be evaluated in an emergency department. High-risk patients include those with persistent depressed level of consciousness, focal neurologic signs, decreasing level of consciousness, penetrating skull injury, or depressed skull fractures. These patients warrant care in a skilled trauma center and CT or MRI examination.

The observation period should increase with the severity of the injury. There should be no hesitation to admit children without neurologic deficits who have sustained a concussion to the hospital for observation. If the child appears well after several hours and is discharged home, parents should be instructed to call their physician for any change in alertness, orientation, or neurologic functioning. An increase in somnolence, headache, or vomiting is cause for concern and neuroimaging.

Prognosis

Children with concussion without subsequent neurologic deficits have a favorable long-term prognosis, and late sequelae are rare. Children with moderate contusions usually make good recoveries even when neurologic signs persist for weeks. Long-term sequelae may include poor memory and slowing of motor skills or a generalized decrease in cognitive skills, behavioral alterations, and attention deficits. Language function, especially in a young child, frequently makes a good recovery. Rehabilitation programs with physical therapy, behavioral management, and appropriate education may be necessary. Poor prognostic signs include a Glasgow Coma Scale score of less than 4 on admission without improvement in 24 hours, absent pupillary light reflexes, and persistent extensor plantar reflexes. Extracranial trauma also contributes to the morbidity of these patients (aspiration pneumonia, acute respiratory distress syndrome, sepsis, and emboli).

DISORDERS OF CONSCIOUSNESS

Consciousness represents awareness of self and environment (place and time). **Arousal** represents the system that initiates consciousness. Consciousness is mediated by the cerebral cortex, and arousal is mediated by the reticular activating system (RAS) within the brainstem. The RAS is a network of neurons located in the core of the brainstem extending from the mid pons through the midbrain and hypothalamus to the thalamus. The RAS projects widely to the cerebral cortex serving a general arousal function ("switch").

Coma is defined as a state of unresponsive unconsciousness. Coma is caused by dysfunction of the cerebral hemispheres (bilaterally), the brainstem (herniation syndromes), or both simultaneously. Depression of consciousness may be acute, chronic, transitory, or recurring.

Acute Disorders of Consciousness

Acute changes in consciousness vary in degree from mild lethargy and confusion to deep coma. In childhood, the most common causes of coma are infections, hypoxia-ischemia (cardiac arrest, near-drowning), intoxication, head trauma, and an "ictal" (subclinical status epilepticus) or postictal state (Table 184–2).

TABLE 184–2. Causes of Coma and Diagnostic Approach

Causes

Metabolic derangements
  Hypoglycemia
  Hyponatremia or its correction
  Hypernatremia or its correction
  Hyperosmolarity or its correction
  Hypercapnia
  Uremia
  Hyperammonemia
  Hepatic failure
  Reye syndrome
  Urea cycle enzyme deficiency
  Fatty acid/acyl-coenzyme A dehydrogenase deficiency
  Methylmalonicaciduria
  Propionicaciduria
  Idiopathic hyperammonemia of prematurity
  Mitochondrial diseases
  Diabetes mellitus–ketoacidosis or hypoglycemia
  Lead intoxication
Hypertensive encephalopathy
Infection (see Table 179–2)
  Meningitis
  Encephalitis
  Brain abscess
  Toxic shock syndrome
  Cat-scratch disease
  Postinfectious (acute disseminated encephalomyelitis)
  Postimmunization syndrome (hypotonic-
    hyporesponsive spells)
Stroke
  Infarction
  Hemorrhage
  Subarachnoid hemorrhage
Trauma
  Shaken baby syndrome
  Epidural hemorrhage
  Subdural hemorrhage
  Subarachnoid hemorrhage

Concussion
Hypoxia-ischemia
  Postdrowning
  Post–cardiopulmonary arrest
  Carbon monoxide intoxication
Neoplasm
  Brain tumor
Structural
  Hydrocephalus
Toxins
  Ethanol
  Narcotics
  Antihistamines
  Iron
  Acetaminophen
  Aspirin
  "Recreational" drugs
  Lead poisoning
  Drug intoxication or withdrawal
  Cerebral edema
Epilepsy
  Subclinical status epilepticus
  Postictal states
Migraine
Miscellaneous
  Gastrointestinal (intussusception)
  HUS-TTP
  Vasculitis (systemic lupus erythematosus)

Diagnostic Approach

Glucose, Na$^+$, K$^+$, Cl$^-$, CO$_2$, BUN, creatinine, AST, ALT,
  PT, PTT, blood gas, ammonia, lead level, pyruvate,
  lactate, urinalysis, and urine amino and organic acids
CT, MRI, MRA, MRV, angiogram
CSF analysis
EEG
Blood and urine analyses for toxic substances

ALT, alanine aminotransferase; AST, aspartate aminotransferase; EEG, electroencephalogram; HUS, hemolytic uremic syndrome; PT, prothrombin time; PTT, partial thromboplastin time; TTP, thrombotic thrombocytopenic purpura.

Assessment

Airway, breathing, and circulation are addressed first. Vital signs, including pulse oximetry, must be assessed. The most common cause of long-term morbidity in a patient with depressed consciousness is hypoxia. General physical examination searches for clues as to the cause of depressed consciousness, such as dehydration, unusual odors, needle tracts, trauma, or signs of organ system failure. Breathing patterns may provide important clues to the depth, localization, and etiology of the depressed consciousness. Some patterns of respiration have specific anatomic correlates. **Cheyne-Stokes respiration** is a central neurogenic hyperventilation and gasping respiration. In Cheyne-Stokes respiration, a period of hyperventilation with a crescendo-decrescendo pattern alternates with a shorter period of apnea. Cerebral, thalamic, or hypothalamic modulation of respiration has been lost, but brainstem control is intact. This pattern also can be seen in patients with metabolic disorders, heart failure, or primary respiratory disease. A midbrain lesion yields **central neurogenic hyperventilation**, which consists of sustained rapid deep breathing. **Gasping** respirations are irregularly irregular and indicate dysfunction of the low brainstem-medulla. This pattern of respiration is ominous and usually is followed by terminal apnea.

The neurologic examination begins with a formal assessment of the degree of consciousness. One system for following the level of consciousness is the **Glasgow Coma Scale** (Table 184–3). Unresponsive patients are assessed regarding their best verbal responses, best motor response, and eye opening to stimulation with a score of 3 to 15 points. Depression of consciousness also can be documented (Table 184–4).

The detailed neurologic examination of a comatose patient focuses on the integrity of the brainstem because the RAS lies within the brainstem. Pupillary responses assess the midbrain function (Table 184–5). Eye movements are observed or elicited with the **doll's head maneuver** (oculocephalic response) or cold caloric stimulation (**oculovestibular response**) (Fig. 184–1). The doll's head maneuver should not be performed until it is clear that there is no cervical spine injury. An awake patient can move the eyes voluntarily by either saccadic (quick) or pursuit (slow) eye movements. In a comatose patient, the oculocephalic response to head turning elicits uninhibited eye movements if the brainstem is intact. With uninhibited eye movements, the eyes move opposite to the direction of head movement at exactly the same pace, as if they were freely floating "ball bearings" within the orbits. If the brainstem has been injured, this maneuver reveals incomplete or absent eye movements. If the oculocephalic responses are not elicited or unclear, cold water is flushed into the external ear canal. In a conscious person, this maneuver elicits nystagmus to the opposite side and extreme vertigo with vomiting. Cold water placed in the ear of a comatose patient elicits tonic eye deviation toward the ear irrigated. With complete loss of oculomotor function, the eyes remain in the center of the orbit, as if they are "painted on," regardless of any stimulation.

Body posture at rest and after noxious stimulation can indicate the anatomic level responsible for the alteration of consciousness. Mild depression may be manifested by a comfortable "sleeping" posture, with

TABLE 184–3.   Glasgow Coma Scale

Response	Score
Best Motor Response	
Nil (flaccid)	1
Extensor response	2
Abnormal flexion	3
Withdrawal	4
Localization of pain	5
Obeys commands	6
Best Verbal Response	
Nil	1
Incomprehensible sounds	2
Inappropriate words	3
Confused conversation	4
Oriented, fluent speech	5
Best Eye Opening Response	
Nil	1
To pain	2
To speech	3
Spontaneous	4

TABLE 184–4.   Stages of Depressed Consciousness

Stage	Manifestations
Lethargy	Sleepy, poor attention, fully arousable
Confusion	Poor orientation
Delirium	Agitated confusion, hallucinations, autonomic abnormalities (e.g., excess sweating, tachycardia, hypertension)
Obtundation	Arousable to noxious stimulation
Stupor	Arousable momentarily with noxious stimulation, localizes pain
Coma	Unarousable, does not localize pain

TABLE 184–5.　Effect of Coma-Producing Toxins on Pupillary Size

Pupils Small

Narcotics (except meperidine)
Sedatives
Barbiturates
Alcohol
Major tranquilizers
Phenothiazines
Cholinergic agonists
Organophosphate insecticides
Nicotine
Certain plants and mushrooms

Pupils Large

Anticholinergics
Antihistamines
Tricyclic antidepressants
Phenothiazines
Glutethimide

Pupils Normal

Salicylates
Acetaminophen

limbs slightly flexed, body tilted to one side, and eyes fully closed. Frequent spontaneous readjustments of position, yawns, and sighs are observed. Patients who lie in a flat, extended, unvarying position with eyes half-open exhibit a deeper coma. An asymmetric posture suggests motor dysfunction of one side. Posture changes with noxious stimulation may indicate more serious neurologic conditions. **Decorticate posturing** consists of rigid extension of the legs and feet, flexion and supination of the arms, and fisting of the hands. It occurs when the midbrain and red nucleus control body posture without inhibition by diencephalon, basal ganglia, and cortical structures. **Decerebrate posturing** consists of rigid extension of legs, arms, trunk, and head with hyperpronation of lower arms. It indicates pontine and vestibular nucleus control of posture without inhibition from more rostral structures. These postures may be exhibited unilaterally or bilaterally, indicating equal or unequal dysfunction of the two sides of the brain.

Etiology

Recognition of the pace or evolution of the change in consciousness is an important clue to the etiology. A detailed history and physical examination usually provide sufficient clues to differentiate among the three major diagnostic categories producing coma: **metabolic** or **toxic**, **infectious**, and **structural**. In most clinical situations, the cause of the coma is readily identified.

Metabolic derangements are common causes of disorders of consciousness. Disturbances of blood chemistries (glucose, sodium, calcium, bicarbonate, BUN, and ammonia) may produce depressed mental status. Metabolic causes of acute coma are suggested by spontaneous fluctuations in the level of consciousness, tremors, myoclonus, asterixis, visual and tactile hallucinations, and deep coma with preservation of pupillary light reflexes. Acute metabolic or toxic disorders usually produce a hypotonic, limp state, but hypertonia, rigidity, and decorticate and decerebrate posturing are observed sometimes in coma caused by hypoglycemia, hepatic encephalopathy, and short-acting barbiturates. A subacute course of somnolence progressing to deep, unarousable "sleep" (stupor) over hours suggests drug intoxication or organ system failure, such as renal or hepatic failure, producing a metabolic encephalopathy. Care must be taken to investigate background chronic medical conditions or their treatment (diabetes mellitus, insulin administration, and leukemia) that may produce a decline in consciousness. Intoxication and ingestion are common causes of acute alteration of consciousness, and a thorough history must be taken to search for the offending agent (see Chapter 45).

CNS infection, such as meningitis or encephalitis, causes abrupt alteration of mental status. The presence of fever, petechiae, chills, and sweats suggests infection. Prodromal photophobia and pain on movement of the head or eyes are symptoms of meningeal irritation, but meningeal signs may be absent in a child with depressed mental status. Premonitory symptoms, such as abdominal pain, diarrhea, sore throat, conjunctivitis, cough, or rash, point toward viral encephalitis or a postinfectious syndrome as the cause of the altered consciousness.

Structural processes, such as hemorrhage, stroke, or acute hydrocephalus, are infrequent, sudden causes of depressed consciousness in children. If trauma or immersion injuries are suspected, neck manipulation should be avoided until the cervical spine films exclude vertebral fracture or subluxation. An evolution of headache and morning vomiting suggests increased ICP. A gradual fading of alertness or declining school performance over preceding weeks suggests an expanding intracranial mass, subdural effusion or hematoma, or chronic infection (tuberculous meningitis, HIV). A history of social and emotional difficulties, drug abuse, or depression raises concern for self-inflicted injury or toxic ingestion.

Clinical Manifestations

Papilledema or paralysis of cranial nerves III or VI in a patient with depressed consciousness is strong

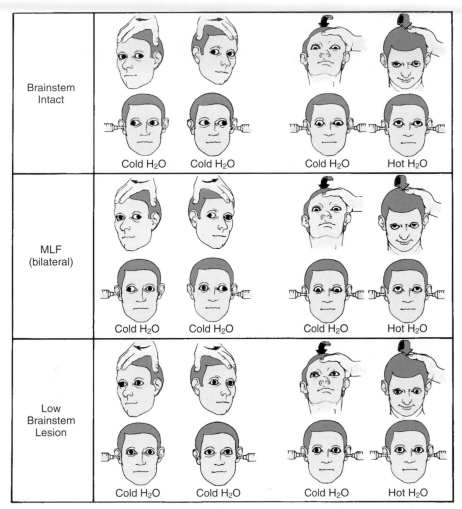

Figure 184–1

Ocular reflexes in unconscious patients. *Top,* Oculocephalic *(above)* and oculovestibular *(below)* reflexes in an unconscious patient whose brainstem ocular pathways are intact. Horizontal eye movements are illustrated on the left, and vertical eye movements are illustrated on the right. Lateral conjugate eye movements *(upper left)* to head turning are full and opposite in direction to the movement of the face. A stronger stimulus to lateral deviation is achieved by irrigating cold water against the tympanic membrane. There is tonic conjugate deviation of both eyes toward the stimulus; the eyes usually remain tonically deviated for 1 minute or more before slowly returning to the midline. Because the patient is unconscious, there is no nystagmus. Extension of the neck in a patient with an intact brainstem produces conjugate deviation of the eyes in the downward direction, and flexion of the neck produces deviation of the eyes upward. Bilateral cold water against the tympanic membrane likewise produces conjugate downward deviation of the eyes, whereas hot water ($\leq$44°C [$\leq$111.2°F]) causes conjugate upward deviation of the eyes. *Middle,* Effects of bilateral medial longitudinal fasciculus (MLF) lesions on oculocephalic and oculovestibular reflexes. The left portion illustrates that oculocephalic and oculovestibular stimulation deviates the appropriate eye laterally and brings the eye that normally would deviate medially only to the midline because the MLF, with its connections between the abducens and oculomotor nuclei, is interrupted. Vertical eye movements often remain intact. *Bottom,* Effects of a low brainstem lesion. On the left, neither oculovestibular nor oculocephalic movements cause lateral deviation of the eyes because the pathways are interrupted between the vestibular nucleus and the abducens area. Likewise, on the right, neither oculovestibular nor oculocephalic stimulation causes vertical deviation of the eyes. Rarely, particularly with low lateral brainstem lesions, oculocephalic responses may be intact even when oculovestibular reflexes are abolished. (From Plum F, Prosner J: The Diagnosis of Stupor and Coma, 3rd ed. Philadelphia, FA Davis, 1980, p 54.)

TABLE 184–6. Progression of Stages and Anatomic Levels of Transtentorial Central Herniation

Signs	Thalamus	Midbrain	Medulla*
Consciousness	Confusion; stupor	Coma	Coma
Respirations	Sighs; Cheyne-Stokes type	Central neurogenic hyperventilation	Gasping; absent
Pupils	Small, reactive	3-5 mm, fixed	Unreactive
Extraocular movements	Roving; uninhibited	Incomplete, dysconjugate	Absent
Motor response	Spastic; decorticate	Decerebrate	Flaccid

*Uncal herniation with unilateral oculomotor nerve palsy or hemiplegia is another sign of severe increased intracranial pressure.

evidence of elevated ICP, a medical and neurosurgical emergency. A progressive loss of consciousness accompanied by a characteristic progression of motor, oculomotor, pupillary, and respiratory signs (Table 184-6) indicates incipient transtentorial herniation. "Uncal herniation" implies the mesial temporal lobe is shifting across the tentorial edge, producing a unilateral third nerve palsy and contralateral hemiparesis. Medical therapy (hyperventilation, osmotic agents, steroids) must be instituted, emergency cranial CT performed, and urgent neurosurgical consultation obtained.

To cause a depression of consciousness, unilateral cerebral lesions must directly compress and distort the diencephalon and brainstem, increase ICP by their bulk and associated edema, or block CSF pathways producing hydrocephalus. Focal midbrain and diencephalic lesions that impair the RAS also can depress consciousness. Space-occupying lesions include tumors, abscesses, hemorrhages, cysts, and inflammatory masses.

Deprivation of oxygen to the brain, caused by either deficient oxygen in the blood (hypoxemia) or deficient delivery of blood to the brain (ischemia), impairs consciousness (Table 184-7). Severe ischemia produces loss of consciousness within seconds and permanent brain damage within a few minutes. Deterioration in functioning may occur for several hours after a severe hypoxic-ischemic insult. The development of circulatory failure from anoxic cardiac injury, disseminated intravascular coagulation, or cerebral edema may compound the initial injury.

Rarely, patients experience delayed **postanoxic encephalopathy**. An initial hypoxic-ischemic event causes stupor or coma. The patients awaken in 24 to 48 hours, but several days to weeks later they become irritable, apathetic, and confused. A spastic quadriplegia accompanied by pseudobulbar palsy then develops. Pathologic and radiologic studies reveal severe bilateral leukoencephalopathy. The pathogenesis is unknown. Patients may die, recover completely, or remain in a vegetative state. The prognosis of cerebral hypoxic-ischemic injury is extremely variable in children. Short duration of coma (hours to 1 to 2 days) and presence of intact brainstem function on admission to the hospital indicate a good prognosis. The most common permanent neurologic sequelae are spasticity, ataxia, choreoathetosis, parkinsonian syndrome, intention or action myoclonus, memory loss, visual agnosia, and impairments of learning and attention. Improvement can occur for several months to 1 year after the insult. Treatment involves physical therapy, occupational therapy, rehabilitative services, and education.

Primary subarachnoid hemorrhage usually is caused by rupture of a saccular **berry aneurysm** of one of the major cerebral arteries in the circle of Willis.

TABLE 184–7. Causes of Hypoxia and Ischemia

Hypoxia (Decreased Oxygen Levels)

PO_2 Decreased

Pulmonary disease
Cardiac disease; right-to-left shunt
Hypoventilation
Exogenous (e.g., drowning, choking, suffocation)
Neuromuscular disease
Central respiratory drive decreased

PO_2 Normal; Decreased Oxygen Content

Severe anemia
Carbon monoxide poisoning
Methemoglobinemia

Ischemia (Decreased Perfusion)

Cardiac disease (decreased cardiac output)
Myocardial infarction
Arrhythmia
Valvular disease
Pericarditis
Pulmonary embolism
Hypotension, shock
Hanging, strangulation
Extensive cerebrovascular disease

These aneurysms are presumed to result from localized developmental defects in the arterial walls and are associated with cystic kidney disease and coarctation of the aorta. Aneurysmal hemorrhage is uncommon in childhood. The usual clinical manifestations are the sudden onset of intense headache followed by collapse and loss of consciousness. Focal neurologic deficits vary, but nuchal rigidity almost invariably is present. Retinal or subhyaloid hemorrhages are common. Treatment should take place in an ICU and consists of bed rest, sedation, and therapy to eliminate vascular spasm until surgical or endovascular elimination of the aneurysm is feasible.

Postinfectious syndromes (**acute disseminated encephalomyelitis**) closely resemble episodes of viral meningoencephalitis, but are the consequence of acute multifocal, immunologically mediated demyelination rather than of direct viral invasion of the brain. Fever, stiff neck, depression of consciousness, and focal neurologic deficits occur a few days after a benign systemic viral syndrome. The course is variable, but most children recover without sequelae within a few days to weeks. Systemic viral infection seems to trigger the syndrome by an unknown mechanism. These syndromes were first described after measles, mumps, rubella, and chickenpox and after vaccination against smallpox and rabies.

Laboratory and Diagnostic Imaging

Head CT remains the preferred imaging technique in emergency situations because it can be performed rapidly and accurately identifies acute hemorrhages, large space-occupying lesions, edema, and shifts of the midline. The initial head CT scan is done without contrast material to identify blood and calcifications. Contrast material can be administered to identify inflammatory and neoplastic lesions. Several metabolic derangements give rise to severe elevations of ICP without producing recognizable CT abnormalities. These derangements include hepatic encephalopathy, Reye syndrome, hyponatremia, lead encephalopathy, trauma, treatment of diabetic ketoacidosis, and global or multifocal hypoxic-ischemic injury. LP in a patient with impending transtentorial herniation should be avoided.

Examination of the CSF may be needed to establish the cause of the alteration of consciousness. Care must be exercised, and appropriate neuroimaging should be performed to ensure that no added injury is inflicted with LP. The presence of red blood cells in the CSF suggests primary subarachnoid hemorrhage, parenchymal hemorrhage, or hemorrhagic infection (herpes simplex virus, group B streptococcus, *Neisseria meningitidis*). White blood cells in the CSF usually denote infectious meningitis or meningoencephalitis,

but may also be associated with subacute bacterial endocarditis, vasculitis, carcinomatous meningitis, or a parainfectious syndrome.

Treatment

The etiology of coma determines the treatment. Ingestions may necessitate gastric lavage, charcoal administration, forced diuresis, dialysis, or specific antidotes (see Chapter 45). Infections are treated with appropriate antibiotics or antiviral agents (see Chapter 95). Structural brain lesions may necessitate surgical excision or medical treatment of increased ICP.

Prognosis

The outcome of coma relates to many variables, including the etiology. Intoxication carries a good prognosis, whereas hypoxia carries a bad prognosis. Other prognostic factors include the duration of coma and the age of the patient (children have a better outcome than adults). The Glasgow Coma Scale on admission also projects outcome. Complete recovery from traumatic coma of several days' duration is possible in children. Some survivors of severe coma are left in a persistent vegetative state, however, or with severe neuropsychiatric disability.

Brain Death

Brain death means irreversible cessation of all cortical and brainstem functions. Guidelines that are generally accepted as death for children and adolescents exclude neonates (Table 184–8). In certain clinical situations, demonstration of a total absence of cerebral blood flow on four-vessel intracranial angiography or nuclide brain scanning may be required as definitive confirmation of brain death. Application of the criteria of brain death is particularly problematic in premature and newborn infants.

Transient, Recurrent Depression of Consciousness

Episodic alteration or depression of consciousness with full recovery is usually due to seizure, migraine, syncope (e.g., cardiac arrhythmia), or metabolic abnormality (hypoglycemia). Consciousness can be impaired during **seizures** or in the postictal state. Nonconvulsive status epilepticus that is either generalized or partial complex can directly impair consciousness for extended periods. Some patients may have a prolonged postictal state after an unrecognized seizure.

Basilar artery or **confusional migraine** attacks can last hours and be accompanied by agitation, ataxia, cortical blindness, vertigo, or cranial nerve palsies.

TABLE 184–8. Guidelines for Determination of Brain Death*

Two physicians must be present
  The treating physician
  A board-eligible or board-certified neurologist, neurosurgeon, internist, pediatrician, surgeon, or anesthesiologist
Body temperature ≥33°C
No confounding drug intoxication (e.g., barbiturates with levels > therapeutic)
No spontaneous movements, communication, or interaction with the environment
No supraspinal response to externally applied stimuli (pain, touch, light, sound)
Absence of brainstem reflexes including
  Pupillary light
  Oculocephalic
  Oculovestibular
  Corneal
  Oropharyngeal—gag
  Tracheal—cough
Apnea test (includes at least a 10-minute preoxygenation with 100% oxygen) allowing the PaCO$_2$ to increase to >60 mm Hg, with no spontaneous breaths
Electrocerebral silence on electroencephalogram
Absent cerebral perfusion (e.g., nuclear perfusion scan)

*All of the criteria listed should be present on multiple examinations at least 6 to 24 hours after the onset of coma and apnea. There must be documented absence of drug intoxication (including sedatives and neuromuscular blocking agents), hypothermia, and cardiovascular shock. A cause of coma sufficient to account for the loss of brain function should be established.

Headache may precede or follow the neurologic signs.

Syncope is one of the most common causes of abrupt, episodic loss of consciousness. Neurocardiogenic syncope, cardiac arrhythmia, or an obstructive cardiomyopathy (septal hypertrophy, left atrial myxoma, or critical aortic stenosis) can cause recurrent episodes of loss of consciousness. Two thirds of children with syncope have irregular, myoclonic movements as they lose consciousness (anoxic seizures). Children with unexplained syncope require a complete cardiac examination (see Chapter 140).

Metabolic derangements, particularly **hypoglycemia**, give rise to recurrent episodes of lethargy, confusion, seizures, or coma. Autonomic symptoms, such as anxiety, excess sweating, tremulousness, and hunger, often herald attacks. A typical spell usually can be aborted by feeding the child orange juice or other sugar-containing solutions. Several other metabolic disorders cause recurrent bouts of **hyperammonemia** (see Chapter 53). Symptoms include nausea, vomiting, lethargy, confusion, ataxia, hyperventilation, and coma.

INCREASED INTRACRANIAL PRESSURE

Etiology

When the cranial sutures are fused, the skull becomes a rigid container enclosing a fixed volume, including the brain (80% to 85%), CSF (10% to 15%), and blood (5% to 10%). There is an exponential relationship between the volume within a closed container and pressure so that as intracranial volume increases, there is a massive increase in ICP. The brain can accommodate increased ICP initially by expelling CSF and blood from the intracranial compartment into the spinal subarachnoid space. When the limits of this accommodation are reached, the brain itself begins to shift in response to the continuing elevation of ICP. There are compartments bounded by dural extensions (falx cerebri and tentorium cerebelli) within the skull. Brain shifts across these dural or skull barriers are called **herniations** and may occur under the falx, through the tentorial notch, or into the foramen magnum. Supratentorial masses produce a downward transtentorial herniation. Infratentorial masses produce foramen magnum herniation. Unilateral frontal masses produce transfalcial herniation. Transtentorial herniation is more likely to occur with a unilateral hemispheric lesion than with diffuse supratentorial brain swelling. Transtentorial and foramen magnum herniations are immediately life-threatening and indicate critically increased ICP (Table 184–9). Herniation sequences also compress vascular supply, leading to infarction of vital thalamic and brainstem structures. Extreme caution should be exercised before attempting LP in the presence of increased ICP because withdrawal of CSF in the thecal sac can change pressures between the intracranial compartments promoting brainstem shifts and herniations. The causes of increased ICP can be categorized broadly as follows: mass lesion, hydrocephalus, and brain swelling (Table 184–10).

Clinical Manifestations

The symptoms and signs of increased ICP include headache, vomiting, lethargy, irritability, sixth nerve palsy, strabismus, diplopia, and papilledema. Infants who have an open fontanel usually do not develop papilledema or abducens palsy. Specific signs of increased ICP in infants consist of a bulging fontanel, suture diastasis, distended scalp veins, a persistent downward deviation of the eyes ("sunsetting"), and rapid growth of head circumference. Specific signs of increased ICP in the infratentorial compartment (posterior fossa) include stiff neck and head tilt.

Focal neurologic deficits reflect the site of the lesion that is producing the increased ICP and may include hemiparesis from supratentorial lesions and ataxia

TABLE 184–9.   Herniation Syndromes

Location	Etiology	Description	Clinical Findings
Transtentorial			
Unilateral (uncal)	Tumor	Temporal lobe structures shift below tentorium compressing midbrain, cranial nerve III, and PCA	Hemiparesis
	Stroke		Enlarged pupil
	Hemorrhage		Coma
	Abscess		
	Unilateral edema		
Bilateral (central)	Cytotoxic edema	Downward displacement of both temporal lobes compressing the diencephalons and midbrain	Posture—decorticate, decerebrate
	Anoxia		Pupils—small, reactive
	Trauma		Respirations—Cheyne-Stokes
Cerebellar	Diffuse mass lesions	*Upward* movement, midbrain compression	Pupils dilated
	Cerebellar mass lesions	*Downward* movement, medulla through foramen	Respiration irregular
	Diffuse CNS edema		
			Coma
			Cranial nerve palsies
			Apnea
			Bradycardia
			Death

PCA, posterior cerebral artery.

from infratentorial lesions. The major specific sign of critically increased ICP is dilation and poor reactivity of one or both pupils. The **Cushing triad** of elevated blood pressure, decreased pulse, and irregular respirations is a late sign of critically elevated ICP.

Laboratory and Diagnostic Studies

The cause of increased ICP is determined by brain imaging with either CT or MRI. CT usually is preferred because it is rapid, readily available, and provides clear visualization of an acute hemorrhage. Mass lesions, hydrocephalus, and trauma are easily recognized. Diffuse brain swelling produced by hypoxic-ischemic injury, meningitis, encephalitis, metabolic abnormalities, or toxins may be more difficult to recognize. The best evidence of severely increased ICP on CT scan consists of effacement of the dorsal perimesencephalic cisterns.

Treatment

The treatment of increased ICP includes rigorous support of the vital signs and the following specific interventions. Immediate endotracheal intubation and hyperventilation produces the most rapid reduction in ICP by cerebral vasoconstriction, leading to decreased cerebral blood volume. Mannitol (0.25 to 1 g/kg) is used acutely to produce an osmotic shift of fluid from the brain to the plasma. A ventricular catheter is used to remove CSF and to monitor the ICP continuously. Pentobarbital-induced coma reduces pressure by severely suppressing cerebral metabolism and cerebral blood flow. Acetazolamide and furosemide may transiently decrease CSF production.

All treatments for increased ICP are temporary measures intended to prevent critical herniations until the underlying disease process either is treated or resolves spontaneously. Timely intervention can reverse the vicious cycle of cerebral herniation. A complete neurologic recovery is possible even after clear signs of transtentorial or foramen magnum herniation have begun. When these signs are completed, however, with bilaterally dilated, unreactive pupils, absent eye movements, and flaccid quadriplegia, recovery is no longer possible.

Increased Intracranial Pressure *with* Focal Lesions on Computed Tomography

Brain abscess or any mass lesion may produce increased ICP not only by virtue of large size, but also by blockage of CSF pathways, blockage of venous

TABLE 184–10.   Causes of Increased Intracranial Pressure

Abnormal CT or MRI

Mass Effect
Hydrocephalus
Infarction with edema
Hemorrhage
Tumor
Abscess
Cyst
Inflammatory mass

Diffuse Edema
Hypoxic-ischemic injury
Trauma
Infection
Meningitis
Encephalitis
Hypertension
Metabolic derangement or toxin
Hyponatremia
Diabetic ketoacidosis
Dialysis dysequilibrium syndrome
Reye syndrome
Fulminant hepatic encephalopathy
Pulmonary insufficiency with hypercarbia
Lead intoxication

No Definable Imaging Abnormality

Idiopathic intracranial hypertension (pseudotumor
  cerebri)
 Intracranial venous sinus thrombosis
 Drugs
 Vitamin A, retinoic acid
 Tetracycline, nalidixic acid
Endocrinologic disturbance
 Withdrawal of long-term steroid administration
 Addison disease
 Hypoparathyroidism
Obesity in women with menstrual irregularities
Iron deficiency anemia
Catch-up growth in infants with malnutrition (e.g.,
  cystic fibrosis)
High-altitude brain edema

outflow, or production of cerebral edema. This vasogenic edema is produced by leakage of plasma proteins and fluid through a damaged blood-brain barrier at the level of the endothelial cell. Brain abscesses usually present as mass lesions, producing focal neurologic signs and increased ICP. Symptoms of infection, including fever, malaise, anorexia, and stiff neck, may be subtle or absent. Brain edema around an abscess is usually severe and extends into the surrounding white matter. The diagnosis of brain abscess is suspected in children with chronic cardiac or pulmonary disease that may embolize infected material to their brains. Caution must be exercised before LP in a patient with a brain abscess because the risks of transtentorial herniation are high as a result of the extensive unilateral white matter edema.

Hydrocephalus usually produces a slowly evolving syndrome of increased ICP extending over weeks or months. Enlarging ventricles and interstitial edema in the periventricular white matter exert pressure. The edema is created by transudation of CSF through the ependymal barrier. CSF is an ultrafiltrate of plasma continuously produced by the choroid plexus within the lateral, third, and fourth ventricles. The normal volume of CSF is approximately 50 mL in neonates and 150 mL in adults. CSF normally flows from the lateral ventricles through the intraventricular foramen of Monro to the third ventricle. From the third ventricle, it passes through the cerebral aqueduct to the fourth ventricle. CSF exits the fourth ventricle from the single midline foramen of Magendie and the two lateral foramina of Luschka. Subarachnoid flow occurs superiorly to the cisterns of the brain and inferiorly to the spinal subarachnoid space. Absorption of CSF is accomplished predominantly by the arachnoid villi, which are microtubular invaginations into the large dural sinuses and are most concentrated along the superior sagittal sinus.

Hydrocephalus is due to the obstruction of CSF flow anywhere along its course (Table 184–11). **Obstructive hydrocephalus** is caused by a block before the CSF flows to the subarachnoid space, usually within the fourth ventricle or at the level of the aqueduct. Impairment of CSF flow within the subarachnoid space or impairment of absorption is known by the misnomer **"communicating" hydrocephalus**, where there is actually extraventricular obstruction of CSF flow (external hydrocephalus). Hydrocephalus caused by overproduction of CSF without true obstruction is seen in choroid plexus papillomas, which account for 2% to 4% of childhood intracranial tumors and manifest in early infancy.

Ventricular distention and increased ICP cause the clinical manifestations of hydrocephalus. Dilation of the lateral ventricles results in stretching of the corticopontocerebellar and corticospinal pathways, which sweep around the lateral margins of these ventricles to reach the cerebral peduncles. This stretching results in ataxia and spasticity that initially are most marked in the lower extremities because the leg fibers are closest to the ventricles. Distention of the third ventricle may compress the hypothalamic regions and result in endocrine dysfunction. The optic nerves, chiasm, and tracts also are in proximity to the anterior third ventricle, and visual dysfunction results when these structures are compressed. Dilation of the cerebral aqueduct

TABLE 184–11. Causes of Hydrocephalus
Obstruction of CSF pathways
Intraventricular foramina (Monro)
Parasellar mass (e.g., craniopharyngioma, germinoma
or pituitary tumor)
Intraventricular tumor (e.g., ependymoma)
Tuberous sclerosis
Aqueduct of Sylvius (cerebral aqueduct)
Aqueductal stenosis
Midbrain or pineal region tumor
Postinfectious or postinflammatory
Posthemorrhagic
Impaired flow from the fourth ventricle foramina of
Luschka and Magendie
Basilar impression
Platybasia
Dandy-Walker malformation
Arnold-Chiari malformation
Congenital bone lesions of the cranial base
Achondroplasia, rickets
Overproduction of CSF
Choroid plexus papilloma
Defective reabsorption of CSF (e.g., extraventricular
obstruction or communicating hydrocephalus)
Hypoplasia of the arachnoid villi
Postinfectious or posthemorrhagic (destruction of
arachnoid villi or subarachnoid fibrosis)
Superior sagittal sinus occlusion (preventing
absorption of CSF)

compresses the surrounding periaqueductal vertical gaze center, causing paresis of upward gaze (sunsetting eyes or Parinaud syndrome). Manifestations of increased ICP may evolve slowly when obstruction to CSF flow is not complete, and there is time for transependymal absorption of CSF into the veins of the white matter, or rapidly when obstruction is abrupt and complete (as in subarachnoid hemorrhage), and compensation cannot occur.

The **treatment** of hydrocephalus may be either medical or surgical, depending on the etiology. After subarachnoid hemorrhage or meningitis, the flow or absorption of CSF may be transiently impaired. In this circumstance, the use of agents, such as acetazolamide, which transiently decreases CSF production, may be beneficial. Surgical management consists of removing the obstructive lesion (tumor, cyst, or arteriovenous malformation) or placing a shunt or both. A shunt consists of polyethylene tubing extending usually from a lateral ventricle to the peritoneal cavity (**ventriculoperitoneal shunt**). Shunts carry the hazards of infection (*Staphylococcus epidermidis* or *Corynebacterium*) or sudden occlusion with signs and symptoms of acute hydrocephalus.

Increased Intracranial Pressure *without* Focal Lesion on Computed Tomography

Altered Mental Status

Diffuse brain swelling in an acutely ill child usually results from hypoxic-ischemic injury, trauma, infection, metabolic derangement, or toxic ingestion. Hypoxic-ischemic injury produces cytotoxic edema, which consists of swelling of neurons, glia, and endothelial cells because of damage to the cellular metabolic machinery.

Bacterial meningitis may produce increased ICP by blockage of CSF pathways, toxic cerebral edema, increase in cerebral blood flow, or multifocal cerebral infarctions (see Chapter 100). Most children with bacterial meningitis can undergo LP safely because the brain swelling is diffuse and distributed evenly throughout the brain and spinal CSF compartments. A few patients with meningitis show transtentorial herniation, however, within a few hours of LP. Focal neurologic signs, poorly reactive pupils, and a tense fontanel are contraindications to LP in an infant or child with suspected bacterial meningitis. Children with bacterial meningitis and depression of consciousness should be examined frequently within the first 12 hours after LP. If the pupils dilate, or other evidence of increased ICP becomes evident, immediate treatment must be undertaken and may be lifesaving.

Increased Intracranial Pressure with Normal Mental Status

Idiopathic intracranial hypertension (pseudotumor cerebri) is a common "benign" cause of increased ICP, but herniation does not occur. Patients do not appear critically ill. They exhibit a daily debilitating headache associated with diplopia, abducens palsy, and papilledema. Brain imaging studies are usually normal. This syndrome has been associated with the ingestion of certain drugs (tetracycline, vitamin A, oral contraceptive agents), endocrine disturbances (thyroid disease, Addison disease), chronic sinopulmonary diseases, and intracranial venous sinus thrombosis. Most commonly, this condition is idiopathic and affects children who are otherwise perfectly well except for being overweight. When the diagnosis is established after appropriate neuroimaging and documentation of an elevated opening pressure with LP, idiopathic intracranial hypertension gradually resolves over several weeks or months. **Treatment** with acetazolamide, several LPs, or a short course of corticosteroids is generally sufficient. Rarely, chronic papilledema from persistent pseudotumor cerebri produces visual impairment, and more aggressive management is required (optic nerve fenestration).

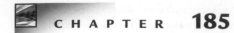

CHAPTER 185

Neurodegenerative Disorders (Childhood Dementia)

Children typically acquire developmental milestones in a variable but predictable sequence (see Chapter 7). Rarely, children present with stagnation of development or frank loss of previously acquired skills. These entities are referred to as neurodegenerative disorders. A variety of medical or surgical disorders can have deleterious effects on normal development. It is essential that a thorough investigation be undertaken to exclude these conditions because some are readily reversible.

Primary degenerative diseases of the nervous system are usually hereditary or metabolic processes. Their onset is often insidious with gradual progression over weeks, months, or years. Typically, they are symmetric in their manifestations. Symptoms may target either gray matter structures or white matter tracts.

ACQUIRED ILLNESSES MIMICKING DEGENERATIVE DISEASES

Children with poorly controlled epilepsy may be continuously in either an ictal or a postictal state. They may appear stuporous. The antiepileptic regimen may be contributing to the lack or loss of developmental abilities. Antiepileptic drugs that are sedating or affect mood, memory, motivation, or attention may contribute to school failure. Use of high doses or use of multiple anticonvulsants may compound this problem. In this situation, readjustment of medications or achievement of better control returns the child to his or her previous level of functioning.

Other chronic drug use or overuse (sedatives, tranquilizers, anticholinergics, anticonvulsants) can bring about progressive mental confusion, lethargy, and ataxia (see Chapter 45). Intoxications with metals, such as lead, may cause chronic learning difficulties or may present acutely with irritability, listlessness, anorexia, and pallor, progressing to fulminant encephalopathy. Vitamin deficiency of thiamine, niacin, vitamin B_{12}, and vitamin E can produce encephalopathy, peripheral neuropathy, and ataxia. Congenital and acquired hypothyroidism impairs intelligence and retards developmental progress. Unrecognized congenital hypothyroidism produces irreversible damage if it is not treated immediately after birth (see Chapter 175).

Structural brain diseases, such as hydrocephalus and slowly growing tumors, may mimic dementia. Certain indolent brain infections, such as rubeola (measles causing subacute sclerosing panencephalitis), rubella (German measles), syphilis, prion disease, and some fungi, cause mental and neurologic deterioration over months and years. Congenital HIV infection causes failure of normal development and regression of acquired skills and may be the leading identifiable cause of developmental regression in the U.S.

Emotional disorders, such as severe psychosocial deprivation in infancy, can give rise to apathy and failure to attain developmental milestones (see Chapter 21). Children with pervasive developmental disorder (autistic spectrum) typically go through a phase of developmental stagnation or disintegration at about 12 to 18 months of age after a period of early normal milestones. Depression in older children can lead to blunting of affect, social withdrawal, and poor school performance, which raise the question of encephalopathy and dementia.

HEREDITARY AND METABOLIC DEGENERATIVE DISEASES

Degenerative diseases may affect gray matter (**neuronal degenerative disorders**), white matter (**leukodystrophies**), or specific, focal regions of the brain. Many white and gray matter degenerative illnesses result from enzymatic disorders within subcellular organelles, including lysosomes, mitochondria, and peroxisomes. Disorders of lysosomal enzymes typically impair metabolism of brain sphingolipids and gangliosides. These enzyme deficiencies have classic patterns of expression with specific names, such as Niemann-Pick disease, Gaucher disease, and Tay-Sachs disease. The same apparent deficiencies can produce unusual clinical syndromes that differ greatly from the classic patterns. The age of onset, rate of progression, and neurologic signs may be entirely different. For this reason, any patient with a degenerative neurologic condition of unknown cause should have leukocytes or skin fibroblasts harvested for measurement of a standard battery of lysosomal, peroxisomal, and mitochondrial enzymes (see Chapters 56 and 57).

Gray matter degeneration (neuronal degeneration) is characterized early by **dementia** and **seizures**. This group of gray matter disorders, which cause slowly progressive loss of neuronal function, is separated into disorders with and disorders without accompanying visceromegaly (hepatosplenomegaly). Most are autosomal recessive traits except for Hunter syndrome (sex-linked recessive), Rett syndrome (sex-linked dominant), and the mitochondrial encephalopathies (nuclear or mitochondrial DNA defects).

Gray Matter Degenerative Diseases with Visceromegaly

Mucopolysaccharidoses are caused by defective lysosomal hydrolases. Mucopolysaccharides are important matrix constituents of connective tissue, skin cartilage, bone, and cornea. In these diseases, they accumulate within lysosomes. Abnormally large amounts are excreted in the urine. The clinical manifestations include dwarfism, kyphoscoliosis, coarse facies, hepatosplenomegaly, cardiovascular abnormalities, and corneal clouding. Neurologic involvement is seen in mucopolysaccharidosis types I H (**Hurler syndrome**), II (**Hunter syndrome**), III (**Sanfilippo syndrome**), and VII. Children with Hurler syndrome, the most severe of these illnesses, appear normal during the first 6 months of life, then develop the characteristic skeletal and neurologic features. Mental deficiency, spasticity, deafness, and optic atrophy are progressive. Hydrocephalus frequently occurs because of obstruction to CSF flow by thickened leptomeninges.

Mucolipidosis II (I-cell disease), **mucolipidosis III, GM$_1$ gangliosidosis, fucosidosis**, and **mannosidosis** resemble Hurler syndrome clinically but do not exhibit excess excretion of mucopolysaccharides and involve different disorders in lysosomal hydrolases. The diagnosis is confirmed by analysis of enzymes in white blood cells, serum, and skin fibroblasts.

Classic **Niemann-Pick disease** is caused by a deficiency of the enzyme sphingomyelinase. Sphingomyelin accumulates in foam cells of the reticuloendothelial system of the liver, spleen, lungs, and bone marrow. It also distends neurons of the brain. Intellectual retardation and regression, myoclonic seizures, hypotonia, hepatosplenomegaly, jaundice, and sometimes retinal cherry-red spots are noted within the first year of life. The diagnosis is confirmed by finding foam cells in the bone marrow and sphingomyelinase deficiency in leukocytes and skin fibroblasts.

Although the most common form of **Gaucher disease** is an indolent illness of adults, there is a rapidly fatal infantile form featuring severe neurologic involvement caused by deficiency of the enzyme glucocerebrosidase. Glucoceramide accumulates in the liver, spleen, and bone marrow. The characteristic neurologic signs are neck retraction, extraocular movement palsies, trismus, difficulty swallowing, apathy, and spasticity. Gaucher cells are found in bone marrow, and the level of serum acid phosphatase is increased.

Gray Matter Degenerative Disease without Visceromegaly

Tay-Sachs disease (GM$_2$ gangliosidosis) occurs commonly in Jewish children of eastern European background. It is caused by deficiency of hexosaminidase A and results in the accumulation of GM$_2$ ganglioside in cerebral gray matter and cerebellum. Infants are normal until 6 months of age, when they develop listlessness, irritability, hyperacusis, intellectual retardation, and a retinal cherry-red spot. The ganglion cells of the retina and macula are distended with ganglioside and appear as a large area of white surrounding a small red fovea that is not covered by ganglion cells. Within months, blindness, convulsions, spasticity, and opisthotonos develop.

Rett syndrome is a common neurodegenerative disorder affecting only females with onset at about 1 year of age. It is characterized by the loss of purposeful hand movements and communication skills; social withdrawal; gait apraxia; stereotypic repetitive hand movements that resemble washing, wringing, or clapping of the hands; and acquired microcephaly. The illness plateaus for many years before seizures, spasticity, and kyphoscoliosis develop. The etiology is a mutation on an X chromosome gene coding for a transcription factor called *methyl-CpG-binding protein 2*. The exact phenotype is influenced by whether the mutation is missense or truncating and on the pattern of X chromosome inactivation in the individual patient.

Neuronal ceroid lipofuscinosis is a family of genetic diseases characterized histologically by the accumulation of autofluorescent hydrophobic material, consisting of hydrophobic proteins and esterified dolichol lipopigments in lysosomes. Pathogenesis at the molecular level is now being elucidated. The original infantile form of neuronal ceroid lipofuscinosis (NCL1) is palmitoyl protein thioesterase deficiency (gene at the 1p32 locus), the late infantile form (NCL2) is pepstatin-resistant proteinase deficiency (gene at the 11p15.5 locus), and the original juvenile form (NCL3) is a defect in a gene (locus 16p11.2-12.3) whose product, the NCL3 protein, still lacks functional characterization. The clinical features are dementia, retinal degeneration, and severe myoclonic epilepsy. Visceral symptoms, despite the presence of the storage process, are absent. The disease may present at any age.

Mitochondrial diseases represent a clinically heterogeneous group of disorders that fundamentally share a disturbance in oxidative phosphorylation (ATP synthesis) (see Chapter 57). Specific genetic diagnoses are often difficult to identify because clinical features are pleotropic within individual defects and overlap between different defects and because analysis of mitochondrial protein function is technically demanding. Specific syndromes include **MELAS** (*m*itochondrial myopathy, *e*ncephalopathy, *l*actic *a*cidosis, and *s*troke-like episodes); **MERRF** (*m*yoclonus, *e*pilepsy, and *r*agged *r*ed *f*ibers), which includes dementia, hearing loss, optic nerve atrophy, ataxia, and loss of deep sensation; and **NARP** (*n*europathy, *a*taxia, and *r*etinitis *p*igmentosa).

Degenerative Diseases of the White Matter (Leukodystrophies)

The prominent signs of diseases affecting primarily white matter are spasticity, ataxia, optic atrophy, and peripheral neuropathy. Seizures and dementia are late manifestations. Life expectancy ranges from months to a few years.

Metachromatic leukodystrophy is an autosomal recessive lipidosis caused by deficiency of the enzyme arylsulfatase. Demyelination of the CNS and peripheral nervous system occurs. Children present between 1 and 2 years of age with stiffening and ataxia of gait, spasticity, optic atrophy, intellectual deterioration, absent reflexes, upgoing toes, increased CSF protein, and slowing of motor NCV.

Krabbe disease (globoid cell leukodystrophy) is an autosomal recessive lipidosis and is caused by a deficiency of the enzyme galactocerebrosidase. It presents a similar clinical picture that begins at 6 months of age and includes extreme irritability, macrocephaly, hyperacusis, and seizures. Demyelination of the CNS and peripheral nervous system results in upper and lower motor neuron signs.

Adrenoleukodystrophy is a sex-linked, recessively inherited disorder associated with progressive central demyelination and adrenal cortical insufficiency (see Chapter 178). It is caused by an impaired capacity of a subcellular organelle, the peroxisome, to degrade saturated unbranched very long chain fatty acids, particularly hexacosanoate (C26:0). The most common presentation is in boys in early school years who develop subtle behavioral changes and intellectual deterioration, followed by cortical visual and auditory deficits and a stiff gait. Later, spastic quadriparesis, coma, and seizures supervene. Symptomatic adrenocortical insufficiency with fatigue, vomiting, and hypotension develops in 20% to 40% of patients, usually at the same time as the neurologic illness. The disease also can present with slowly progressive paraplegia in young men, which is called adrenomyeloleukodystrophy. The diagnosis is established by finding an elevated hexacosanoate level in plasma lipids and typical abnormalities of neuroimaging.

Degenerative Diseases with Focal Manifestations

Some neurodegenerative disorders have predilections to target specific regions or systems within the neuraxis, producing symptoms referable to the affected region. Ataxia indicates disease of the cerebellum or spinocerebellar pathways. Abnormalities of extraocular movement or respiration indicate disease of the brainstem. Choreoathetosis or dystonia indicates disease of the motor basal ganglia. Paraplegia indicates disease of the spinal cord. Hereditary degenerative diseases can cause ataxia (see Table 183–1).

Cerebellar Pathways

Friedreich ataxia is a relentlessly progressive, autosomal recessive disorder that becomes manifested in the early teenage years with ataxia, dysmetria, dysarthria, pes cavus, hammer toes, diminished proprioception and vibration, diminished or absent reflexes, upgoing toes, kyphoscoliosis, nystagmus, and a hypertrophic cardiomyopathy. It is caused by a homozygous GAA expansion of 120 to 1700 trinucleotide repeats of the first intron of the frataxin gene on chromosome 9. The GAA repeats are unstable on transmission. The size of the GAA expansion determines the frequency of cardiomyopathy and loss of reflexes in the upper limbs.

Ataxia-telangiectasia is an autosomal recessive genetic disorder of DNA repair that produces a neurologic disorder, immunologic deficiency, lymphoid malignancy, and gonadal dysgenesis (see Chapter 73). The basic pathologic defect is an inability to respond properly to homologous double-stranded DNA breaks by either DNA repair or induction of apoptosis. The disorder is caused by a lack of the ATM protein, a DNA-binding protein kinase related to kinases involved in cell cycle progression and response to DNA damage. The ATM gene is a large gene on 11q22-23. Most mutations of the gene are unique and nonsense. Most patients are compound heterozygotes. In 80% of cases, a genetic diagnosis can be made by failure to detect the ATM protein on Western blot.

The neurologic symptoms manifest between 1 and 2 years of age with progressive ataxia, dystonia, chorea, swallowing difficulty, poor facial movements, and severe abnormalities of saccadic and pursuit eye movements. Most characteristically, patients develop oculomotor apraxia, a disorder in which the child visually tracks by making head movements to compensate for the inability to generate saccadic eye movements. Intellect is preserved. Patients are wheelchair bound in childhood. The external hallmark of the disease, **conjunctival telangiectasia**, does not manifest until about 5 years of age. Telangiectases also develop on the ear, malar face, neck, elbow, knee, hands, and feet. In addition, prematurely gray hair and atrophic skin develop in patients. Recurrent sinopulmonary infections are a problem in some patients from infancy. Thirty percent of patients die of lymphoreticular cancers. Laboratory clues to the diagnosis include elevation of blood alpha-fetoprotein levels and depression of blood IgA and circulating T cell levels. Patients with IgA deficiency are at risk of anaphylaxis after blood transfusion that includes IgA. There is presently no therapy for the disease or the neurologic symptoms.

Lesch-Nyhan syndrome is a sex-linked recessive disorder caused by deficiency of hypoxanthine-guanine phosphoribosyltransferase, leading to the formation of excess uric acid. Infants appear normal until late in the first year of life, when they exhibit psychomotor retardation, choreoathetosis, spasticity, and severe self-mutilation. These patients never achieve ambulation. Gouty arthritis and renal calculi with renal failure also occur. The hyperuricemia and renal complications are treated with allopurinol, a xanthine oxidase inhibitor, but no effective treatment for the neurologic disease is available.

Wilson disease is a treatable, degenerative condition that exhibits signs of cerebellar and basal ganglia dysfunction. It is an autosomal recessive inborn error of copper metabolism. Serum ceruloplasmin levels are low. Abnormal copper deposition is found in the liver, producing cirrhosis; in the peripheral cornea, producing a characteristic green-brown (Kayser-Fleischer) ring; and in the CNS, producing neuronal degeneration and protoplasmic astrocytosis. Neurologic symptoms characteristically begin in the early teenage years with dysarthria, dysphasia, drooling, fixed smile, tremor, dystonia, and emotional lability. MRI shows abnormalities of the basal ganglia. Treatment is with a copper-chelating agent, such as oral penicillamine.

Brainstem

Subacute necrotizing encephalomyelopathy, or Leigh disease, is a neuropathologically defined, degenerative inherited CNS disease primarily involving the periaqueductal region of the brainstem, caudate, and putamen. Symptoms usually begin before 2 years of age and consist of hypotonia, feeding difficulties, respiratory irregularity, weakness of extraocular movements, and ataxia. Blood and CSF lactate and pyruvate levels are elevated. Different disorders of mitochondrial function can produce this clinical syndrome. Decreased pyruvate carboxylase or pyruvate dehydrogenase activity, biotinidase deficiency, and cytochrome *c* oxidase deficiency have been identified as causative in some cases. Vitamin therapies have been attempted but with little success except in children with biotinidase deficiency.

Many degenerative encephalopathies defy diagnosis despite extensive laboratory analysis. The diagnosis of leukodystrophy usually can be made confidently on the basis of extensive cerebral white matter changes on CT or MRI. The diagnosis of hereditary or metabolic gray matter encephalopathy when histologic and biochemical studies are normal is much less secure. Acquired lesions (infectious, inflammatory, vascular, or toxic) are difficult to exclude completely. Brain biopsy is not likely to be helpful, unless specific lesions are shown on neuroimaging.

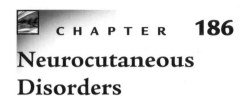

CHAPTER 186

Neurocutaneous Disorders

The skin, teeth, hair, nails, and brain are derived embryologically from ectoderm. Abnormalities of these surface structures may indicate abnormal brain development. The term **phakomatosis** means "mother spots" or "birthmarks" and refers to tuberous sclerosis and neurofibromatosis. Not all of the so-called neurocutaneous disorders have characteristic cutaneous lesions, however, and not all are of ectodermal origin. von Hippel–Lindau disease does not have characteristic cutaneous lesions. von Hippel–Lindau disease and Sturge-Weber disease are of mesenchymal rather than ectodermal origin. Neurofibromatosis, tuberous sclerosis, Sturge-Weber disease, von Hippel–Lindau disease, and ataxia-telangiectasia are the most common of the more than 40 neurocutaneous disorders.

NEUROFIBROMATOSIS
Etiology

There are two distinct genetic types of neurofibromatosis. **Neurofibromatosis type 1 (NF1)**, also known as von Recklinghausen disease, is an autosomal-dominant disorder with an incidence of approximately 1 in 3000. It is caused by mutations of the *NF1* gene, located at chromosome 17q11.2 and coding for a tumor suppressor gene, neurofibromin. Spontaneous new mutations occur in 30% to 50% of cases. Neurofibromin is a major negative regulator of a key signal transduction pathway in cells, the Ras pathway, which transmits mitogenic signals to the nucleus. Loss of neurofibromin leads to increased levels of activated Ras (bound to GTP) and increased downstream mitogenic signaling. Somatic mosaicism, in which an abnormality in one copy of the *NF1* gene is present in some cells but not others, indicates a postzygotic mutation, and is called **segmental neurofibromatosis**. NF2 is an autosomal-dominant disorder with an incidence of 1 in 33,000. Half the cases have no family history. The *NF2* gene is a tumor suppressor gene on chromosome 22 that codes for a protein called *merlin*. Merlin is similar to a family of proteins that serve as linkers between integral membrane proteins and the cytoskeleton and are involved in Rho-mediated signal transduction.

Clinical Manifestations

The cardinal features of neurofibromatosis are café au lait spots, axillary freckling, cutaneous neurofibromas, and iris hamartomas (Lisch nodules). **Café au lait spots** are present in more than 90% of patients who have NF1. They typically appear in the first few years of life and increase in number and size over time. The presence of six or more spots larger than 5 mm suggests the diagnosis. **Lisch nodules** also increase in frequency with age and are present in more than 90% of adults who have NF1. Approximately 25% of children exhibit these iris nodules.

Neurofibromas are composed of various combinations of Schwann cells, fibroblasts, mast cells, and vascular elements. Dermal neurofibromas are nearly universal and consist of discrete, small, soft lesions that lie within the dermis and epidermis and move passively with the skin. They rarely cause any symptoms. Plexiform neurofibromas are large, occasionally nodular, subcutaneous lesions that lie along the major peripheral nerve trunks. They often cause symptoms including pain, weakness, and invasion of adjacent viscera or spinal cord. Sarcomatous degeneration may occur. Surgical treatment is attempted, but results are often unsatisfactory. Other tumors that occur in NF1 are optic nerve gliomas, astrocytomas of brain and spinal cord, and malignant peripheral nerve tumors.

NF2 predisposes patients to multiple intracranial and spinal tumors, including bilateral vestibular schwannomas, schwannomas of other cranial and spinal nerves, meningiomas, and gliomas. Peripheral nerve tumors, including schwannomas and neurofibromas, are uncommon. The average life span is less than 40 years. Posterior capsular or cortical cataracts are common, but Lisch nodules, café au lait spots, and axillary freckling are not features of the disease.

Common complications are learning disability, scoliosis, macrocephaly, headache, and optic gliomas. Other skeletal complications include sphenoid wing dysplasia and cortical thinning of the long bones with pseudarthrosis. Systemic complications, including peripheral nerve malignancy, pheochromocytoma, renovascular hypertension, and epilepsy, are individually rare. Hyperintense lesions on T2-weighted MRI (hamartomas) in the basal ganglia, internal capsule, thalamus, cerebellum, and brainstem are common and distinctive for the disease. They are benign and disappear in adulthood. The average life expectancy of patients with NF1 may be reduced by 10 to 15 years, and malignancy is the most common cause of death. Genetic and psychological counseling are important components of care for this chronic disorder.

TUBEROUS SCLEROSIS
Etiology

Tuberous sclerosis, an autosomal dominant disorder, is characterized by hamartomas in many organs, especially the brain, eye, skin, kidneys, and heart. The incidence is 1 in 10,000 births. Two thirds of cases are sporadic and thought to represent new mutations. Germline mosaicism is uncommon, but explains how parents who apparently do not have the disease can have multiple children with tuberous sclerosis. Mutations affecting either of the presumed tumor suppressor genes *TSC1* (chromosome 9) or *TSC2* (chromosome 16) cause tuberous sclerosis. The *TSC1* and *TSC2* genes encode distinct proteins, hamartin and tuberin, which are widely expressed in the brain. These proteins may interact as part of a cascade pathway that modulates cellular differentiation, tumor suppression, and intracellular signaling. Tuberin has a GTPase-activating, protein-related domain that may contribute to a role in cell cycle passage and intracellular vesicular trafficking. Somatic loss or intragenic mutation of the corresponding wild-type allele is seen in the associated hamartomas. Among sporadic tuberous sclerosis cases, mutations in *TSC2* are more frequent and often accompanied by more severe neurologic deficits.

Clinical Manifestations

The classic clinical features are facial angiofibromas (formerly referred to as **adenoma sebaceum**), mental retardation, and severe epilepsy. Less than 50% of patients with tuberous sclerosis exhibit all three features. Other major signs are ungual fibromas, retinal hamartomas, hypopigmented macules, shagreen patches, renal angiomyolipoma, cardiac rhabdomyoma, brain tubers, and brain subependymal nodules and astrocytomas. Facial angiofibromas do not develop until 2 to 5 years of age, but hypomelanotic macules, called **ash-leaf spots**, are present in infancy and best detected with a Wood lamp under UV light. **Shagreen patches** are elevated, rough plaques of skin with a predilection for the lumbar and gluteal regions that develop in late childhood or early adolescence. Cardiac rhabdomyomas are largest during prenatal life and infancy and are rarely symptomatic. Occasionally, they may cause arrhythmias or cardiac outflow obstruction. Renal angiomyolipomas may undergo malignant transformation and are the most common cause of death in adults with tuberous sclerosis. Tubers in the cerebral cortex are areas of cerebral dysplasia that, in combination with other microscopic areas of abnormal development, are responsible for the symptoms of mental retardation and epilepsy. Subependymal nodules are hamartomas that may mutate into a growth phase and become subependymal giant cell astrocytomas causing obstruction of CSF outflow and hydrocephalus. These brain lesions can be detected directly by MRI and indirectly by CT, which shows periventricular calcifications within the nodule, especially around the foramen of Monro.

Tuberous sclerosis is one of the most common causes of infantile spasms. These children often develop intractable epilepsy, with myoclonic, atonic, partial, and grand mal seizures; mental retardation; autism; and hyperactivity.

STURGE-WEBER SYNDROME

The Sturge-Weber syndrome is characterized by angiomas of the leptomeninges overlying the cerebral cortex in association with an ipsilateral facial port-wine nevus that, at the least, covers part of the forehead and upper eyelid. The nevus may have a much more extensive and even bilateral distribution. This nevus flammeus is an ectasia of superficial venules, not a hemangioma, because it has no endothelial proliferation. Ocular defects of Sturge-Weber syndrome include glaucoma and hemangiomas of the choroid, conjunctiva, and episclera. Glaucoma is present in 30% to 50% of patients and may be progressive. Sturge-Weber syndrome is sporadic and not genetic.

The most common associated neurologic abnormality is seizures. Seizures develop because of ischemic injury to the brain underlying the meningeal angiomas. Angiomas, most commonly located in the posterior parietal, posterior temporal, and anterior occipital lobes, consist of thin-walled veins within the pia mater. They produce venous engorgement and presumably stasis within the involved areas. Positron emission tomography has shown hypoperfusion and hypometabolism in these areas. In some children with Sturge-Weber syndrome, progressive ischemia of the underlying brain develops, resulting in hemiparesis, hemianopia, intractable focal seizures, and dementia. Calcium is detectable in the gyri of the brain underlying the angioma, and, as the intervening sulci are spared, the radiologic picture of "tram track" or "railroad track" calcifications is seen in about 60% of cases. Many children with Sturge-Weber syndrome are intellectually normal, and seizures are well controlled with standard anticonvulsants. Hemispherectomy has been proposed for infants whose seizures begin early in life and are difficult to control. Intellectual and motor outcome seems improved, but the surgical risks of the procedure are considerable. Laser surgery is the most promising therapeutic option for cosmetic management of the facial nevus flammeus. Expert ophthalmologic management of glaucoma and choroidal hemangiomas is required.

CHAPTER 187

Congenital Malformations of the Central Nervous System

The precursor of the nervous system is the neural plate of the embryonic ectoderm, which develops at 18 days of gestation. The neural plate gives rise to the neural tube, which forms the brain and spinal cord, and the neural crest cells, which form the peripheral nervous system, meninges, melanocytes, and adrenal medulla. The neural tube begins to form on day 22 of gestation. The rostral end forms the brain, and the caudal region forms the spinal cord. The lumen of the neural tube forms the ventricles of the brain and the central canal of the spinal cord. Most brain malformations can be produced by a variety of injuries occurring during a vulnerable period of gestation. Precipitating factors include chromosomal, genetic, and metabolic abnormalities; infections (toxoplasmosis, rubella, cytomegalovirus, herpes); and exposure to irradiation, certain drugs, and maternal illness during pregnancy.

CONGENITAL ANOMALIES OF THE SPINAL CORD
Etiology and Clinical Manifestations

Defective closure of the caudal neural tube at the end of week 4 of gestation results in anomalies of the lumbar and sacral vertebrae or spinal cord called **spina bifida**. These anomalies range in severity from clinically insignificant defects of the L5 or S1 vertebral arches to major malformations of the spinal cord that lies uncovered by skin or bone on the infant's back. The latter severe defect, called a **meningomyelocele**, results in total paralysis and loss of sensation in the legs and incontinence of bowel and bladder. In addition, affected children usually have an associated anomaly of the brainstem, an **Arnold-Chiari malformation** that may result in hydrocephalus and weakness of face and swallowing. In a **meningocele**, the spinal canal and cystic meninges are exposed on the back but the underlying spinal cord is anatomically and functionally intact. In **spina bifida occulta**, the skin of the back is apparently intact, but defects of the underlying bone or spinal canal are present. These defects include tethering of the cord to a thick filum terminale, a lipoma or dermoid cyst, or a tiny epithelial tract extending from the skin surface to the meninges. A small dimple or tuft of hair may be present over the affected vertebra.

Patients with spina bifida occulta may have difficulties controlling bowel or bladder, weakness and numbness in the feet, and recurrent ulcerations in the areas of numbness. Bladder dysfunction may result in repeated episodes of urinary tract infections, reflux nephropathy, and renal insufficiency. An epithelial tract may predispose to recurrent episodes of meningitis.

Diagnostic Studies

Meningomyelocele in the fetus is suggested by an elevated **alpha-fetoprotein** in the mother's blood and confirmed by ultrasound examination and high concentrations of alpha-fetoprotein and acetylcholinesterase in the amniotic fluid.

Treatment and Prevention

Neonates with meningomyelocele must undergo operative closure of the open spinal defects and treatment of hydrocephalus by placement of a ventriculoperitoneal shunt. Toddlers and children with lower spinal cord dysfunction require physical therapy and bracing of the lower extremities and intermittent bladder catheterization. Children with meningomyelocele who do not have associated brain anomalies are likely to have normal intelligence.

The spina bifida malformation can be prevented in many cases by **folate** administration to the pregnant mother. Because the defect occurs so early in gestation, all women of childbearing age are advised to take 0.4 mg of oral folate every day.

Diastematomyelia

In diastematomyelia, a bone spicule or fibrous band divides the spinal cord into two longitudinal sections. An associated lipoma that infiltrates the cord and tethers it to the vertebrae may be present. Symptoms include weakness and numbness of the feet and urinary incontinence. Reflexes in the feet are diminished or absent. Surgical treatment to free the cord prevents further neurologic deterioration and may improve preexisting symptoms.

CRANIAL DEFECTS

Defective closure of the rostral neural tube produces anencephaly or encephalocele. Neonates with anencephaly have a rudimentary brainstem or midbrain, but no cortex or cranium. This is a rapidly fatal condition. Patients with encephalocele usually have a skull defect and exposure of meninges alone or meninges and brain. Occasionally the defect can produce protrusion of frontal lobe into the nose without a noticeable skull or skin defect. The recurrence risk in subsequent

pregnancies for either cranial or spinal neural tube defects is 10%. Within a family, an anencephalic birth may be followed by the birth of a second child affected with a lumbosacral meningomyelocele. The inheritance of neural tube defects is polygenic.

CONGENITAL MALFORMATIONS OF THE BRAIN

Macrocephaly and Microcephaly

Macrocephaly represents a head circumference above the 97th percentile and may be the result of **macrocrania** (increased skull thickness), **hydrocephalus** (enlargement of the ventricles), or **megalencephaly** (enlargement of the brain). Diseases of bone metabolism or hypertrophy of the bone marrow resulting from hemolytic anemia cause macrocrania. Megalencephaly may be the result of an embryologic disorder causing abnormal proliferation of brain tissue (neurofibromatosis, tuberous sclerosis, Sotos syndrome, Riley-Smith syndrome, and hemimegalencephaly) or accumulation of abnormal metabolic substances (e.g., Alexander disease, Canavan disease, Tay-Sachs disease, and mucopolysaccharidoses).

Microcephaly represents a head circumference below the 3rd percentile. Myriad syndromes and metabolic disorders are associated with microcephaly, some of which are hereditary (Table 187–1). In most instances, a small head circumference is a reflection of a small brain. Brain growth is rapid during the perinatal period, and any insult (e.g., infectious, metabolic, toxic, or vascular disorder) sustained during this period or early infancy is likely to impair brain growth and result in microcephaly. Rarely a small head is the result of premature closure of one or more skull sutures called **craniosynostosis**. This diagnosis is readily made by the abnormal shape of the skull. **Microcephaly vera** is an autosomal recessive disorder that produces severe hypoplasia of the frontal regions of the brain and skull. These children are severely mentally retarded. As a rule, macrocephaly and microcephaly raise a concern about cognitive ability, but head circumference alone should never be used to establish a prognosis for intellectual development.

Holoprosencephaly represents varying degrees of failure of the primary cerebral vesicle to divide and expand laterally and often is associated with midline facial defects (hypotelorism, cleft lip, and cleft palate). This anomaly may occur in an isolated fashion or be associated with a chromosomal or genetic disorder. The prognosis for infants with severe holoprosencephaly is uniformly poor.

Hydrocephalus represents enlargement of the ventricular system. In all types of congenital hydrocephalus, the degree of ventricular enlargement corre-

TABLE 187–1. Causes of Microcephaly

Primary Microcephaly

Microcephaly vera
Chromosomal disorders
  Trisomy 21
  Trisomy 13
  Trisomy 18
  $5P^-$
  Angelman syndrome
  Prader-Willi syndrome
CNS malformation
  Holoprosencephaly
  Encephalocele
  Hydranencephaly
CNS migrational disorder
  Lissencephaly
  Schizencephaly
  Pachygyria
  Micropolygyria
  Agenesis of the corpus callosum
Sex-linked microcephaly
Syndromes
  Smith-Lemli-Opitz syndrome
  Cornelia de Lange syndrome
  Seckel dwarfism syndrome
  Cockayne syndrome
  Rubinstein-Taybi syndrome
  Hallermann-Streiff syndrome

Secondary (Acquired) Microcephaly

Infections (congenital)
  Rubella
  Cytomegalovirus
  Toxoplasmosis
  Syphilis
  HIV
Infections (noncongenital)
  Meningitis
  Encephalitis
Stroke
Toxic
  Radiation of the fetus
  Fetal alcohol syndrome
  Maternal phenylketonuria
Hypoxic-ischemic or other severe brain injury
  Periventricular leukomalacia
Systemic disease
  Chronic cardiac or pulmonary disease
  Chronic renal disease
  Malnutrition
Craniosynostosis totalis

lates roughly with outcome, but examples of neonates with severe hydrocephalus who receive ventriculoperitoneal shunts and then have normal development are well known. Children with congenital hydrocephalus often have associated defects in the closure of the neural tube.

Hydranencephaly is a condition in which the brain presumably develops normally, but then is destroyed by an intrauterine, probably vascular, insult. The result is a virtual absence of the cerebrum with an intact skull. The thalamus, brainstem, and some occipital cortex are present. The child may have a normal outward appearance but does not achieve developmental milestones.

Many malformations result from the failure of normal migration of neurons from the germinal matrix zone around the ventricle to the cortical surface at 1 to 5 months of gestation. Often, multiple malformations exist in the same patient. Neurologic development with all of these anomalies, described subsequently, varies and depends on the type and extent of the malformations.

Schizencephaly is characterized by symmetric bilateral clefts within the cerebral hemispheres that extend from the cortical surface to the ventricular cavity. Clinical manifestations include severe mental and motor retardation. Some children have unilateral schizencephaly manifested by hemiparesis and mild mental impairment.

Lissencephaly indicates smooth brain with absence of sulcation. The normal six-layered cortex does not develop. Affected children have seizures and profound developmental retardation. This anomaly most commonly is part of a genetic or chromosomal disorder.

In **macrogyria**, the gyri are few in number and too broad. In **polymicrogyria**, the gyri are too many and too small. Sometimes macrogyria and polymicrogyria affect an entire hemisphere, producing enlargement of that hemisphere and a clinical syndrome of severe, medically intractable seizures that begin in early infancy. Hemispherectomy is required to stop the seizures. Gray matter heterotopias are abnormal islands within the central white matter of neurons that have never completed the migratory process.

Agenesis of the corpus callosum may be partial or complete and may occur in an isolated fashion or in association with other anomalies of cellular migration. **Dandy-Walker malformation** is diagnosed on the basis of the classic triad: complete or partial agenesis of the vermis, cystic dilation of the fourth ventricle, and enlarged posterior fossa. There may be associated hydrocephalus, absence of the corpus callosum, and neuronal migration abnormalities. Intelligence may be normal or impaired, depending on the degree of associated cerebral neuronal defects.

Megalencephaly, or large brain, is diagnosed by finding a large head with radiographically normal-appearing intracranial contents. Most often this is a familial trait of no clinical significance. Sometimes it is associated with disorders of neuronal migration and a clinical syndrome of developmental retardation. Neurofibromatosis and Sotos syndrome (cerebral gigantism) are two genetic syndromes associated with megalencephaly and sometimes with mental retardation. Megalencephaly is also a feature of numerous metabolic diseases that produce a progressive, degenerative encephalopathy.

PSYCHOMOTOR RETARDATION

Mental Retardation

Clinical Manifestations

Mental retardation is a global cognitive deficiency with accompanying disturbances in language, behavior, and socialization. Generally, individuals with mental retardation (IQ <70) score 2 SDs below the mean on standard psychometric testing. Associated with subaverage mental abilities, affected patients exhibit limitations of adaptive behavior, including language, social or interpersonal skills, self-help skills, and academic skills. The history and general physical examination in most children with mental retardation are unremarkable. The usual presenting feature is lack of language development. No focal neurologic deficits are present, and laboratory evaluation is unrevealing. Most children with idiopathic mental retardation probably have microscopic aberrations of CNS development (microdysgenesis) involving the structure of neurons or neuronal organelles, aggregation of neurons, myelinization of white matter, synapse formation, or interneuronal connections.

Evaluation of a child with mental retardation includes a thorough history of prenatal, perinatal, and postnatal health. Specific questioning about maternal health and habits, including alcohol and drug use, must be explored. History of infections during the pregnancy must be addressed. Even a seemingly innocuous upper respiratory infection syndrome in the midtrimester may suggest cytomegalovirus infection. Perinatal history must be reviewed. Although families often attribute their child's developmental disability to forceps trauma or an umbilical cord problem, these are rare causes of later developmental disturbances. A perinatal insult sufficient to produce long-term neurologic injury typically is associated with a neurologic syndrome including depressed consciousness, seizures and abnormal tone, systemic acidosis, and multisystem dysfunction (e.g., cardiovascular and renal). Physical examination should include occipitofrontal circumference, thorough search for neurocutaneous markers, and a complete neurologic examination.

Laboratory and Diagnostic Studies

Laboratory investigation may include chromosomal analysis, molecular fragile X testing, fluorescence in situ hybridization probes, and metabolic studies (glucose, uric acid, ammonia, lactate, and cholesterol). Thyroid function studies and lead levels are often included as part of the initial investigation. If there is suggestion of loss or stagnation of skills, more comprehensive investigations may be considered. Neuroimaging is warranted in the presence of microcephaly or macrocephaly, neurocutaneous markers, asymmetry on examination, or dysmorphic features.

Treatment

Early infant stimulation and educational programs and management of comorbid behavioral disturbances should be provided, but no specific treatment program can increase inherent learning capacity.

Chromosomal Disorders

Many chromosomal abnormalities, such as **trisomy 21**, are associated with mental retardation (see Chapter 49). The most common form of familial mental retardation, affecting 1 in 1250 males, is the **fragile X syndrome**. The syndrome is caused by expansion of a trinucleotide repeat, CGG, and abnormal methylation of a CpG island of the *FMR-1* gene at chromosome position Xq27.3. The features are varying degrees of mental retardation, autistic behavior, large ears, macroorchidism, and an elongated, narrow face. Females may be affected, but usually not as severely as males.

Two other syndromes associated with mental retardation are caused by deletions of the same region of the long arm of chromosome 15. **Angelman syndrome** is caused by the loss of the maternal allele and is manifested by severe mental retardation, intractable seizures, tremulousness, a characteristic facies, and a happy external demeanor. **Prader-Willi syndrome** is caused by the loss of the paternal allele and is manifested by severe hypotonia and feeding difficulties in the neonatal period, cryptorchidism, small hands and feet, mild mental retardation, and almond-shaped eyes. The difference in phenotype, depending on loss of the maternal or paternal allele, supports the genetic phenomenon of **imprinting**.

SUGGESTED READING

Behrman RM, Kliegman RE, Jenson HB (eds): Nelson Textbook of Pediatrics, 17th ed. Philadelphia, WB Saunders, 2003.

Booth CM, Boone RH, Tomlinson G, et al: Is this patient dead, vegetative, or severely neurologically impaired? Assessing outcome for comatose survivors of cardiac arrest. JAMA 291:870-879, 2004.

Campbell C, Sherlock R, Jacob P, et al: Congenital mytonic dystrophy: Assisted ventilation duration and outcome. Pediatrics 113:811-816, 2004.

Chang BS, Lowenstein DH: Epilepsy. N Engl J Med 349:1257-1266, 2003.

Digre KB: Not so benign intracranial hypertension. BMJ 326:613-614, 2003.

Emery AE: The muscular dystrophies. Lancet 359:687-696, 2002.

Greenbaum LA: Delirium and coma. In Kliegman RM, Greenbaum LA, Lye PS (eds): Practical Strategies in Pediatric Diagnosis and Therapy, 2nd ed. Philadelphia, WB Saunders, 2004, pp 705-726.

Gupta A, Cohen BH: Headaches in childhood. In Kliegman RM, Greenbaum LA, Lye PS (eds): Practical Strategies in Pediatric Diagnosis and Therapy, 2nd ed. Philadelphia, WB Saunders, 2004, pp 633-649.

Hardart MKM, Truog RD: Spinal muscular atrophy—type 1. Arch Dis Child 88:848-850, 2003.

Hirtz D, Berg A, Bettis D, et al: Practice parameter: Treatment of the child with a first unprovoked seizure. Neurology 60:166-175, 2003.

Hughes RAC: Treatment of Guillain-Barré syndrome with corticosteroids: Lack of benefit? Lancet 363:181-182, 2004.

Hughes RAC: Peripheral neuropathy. BMJ 324:466-469, 2002.

Kaye EM: Update on genetic disorders affecting white matter. Pediatr Neurol 24:11-24, 2001.

LaRoche SM, Helmers SL: The new antiepileptic drugs. JAMA 291:615-620, 2004.

Lewis D, Ashwal S, Hershey A, et al: Practice parameter: Pharmacological treatment of migraine headache in children and adolescents: Report of the American Academy of Neurology Quality Standards Subcommittee and the Practice Committee of the Child Neurology Society. Neurology 63:2215-2224, 2004.

Lewis D, Ashwal S, Dahl G, et al: Practice parameter: Evaluation of children and adolescents with recurrent headaches: Report of the Quality Standards Subcommittee of the American Academy of Neurology and the Practice Committee of the Child Neurology Society. Neurology 59:490-498, 2002.

McDonald JW, Sadowsky C: Spinal-cord injury. Lancet 359:417-424, 2002.

Malik SL, Painter MJ: Hypotonia and weakness. In Kliegman RM, Greenbaum LA, Lye PS (eds): Practical Strategies in Pediatric Diagnosis and Therapy, 2nd ed. Philadelphia, WB Saunders, 2004, pp 651-673.

Rivkin M: Stroke in childhood. In Kliegman RM, Greenbaum LA, Lye PS (eds): Practical Strategies in Pediatric Diagnosis and Therapy, 2nd ed. Philadelphia, WB Saunders, 2004, pp 727-742.

Schoenen J, Sandor PS: Headache with focal neurological signs or symptoms: A complicated differential diagnosis. Lancet 3:237-245, 2004.

Shevell M, Ashwal S, Donley D, et al: Practice parameter: Evaluation of the child with global developmental delay: Report of the Quality Standards Subcommittee of the American Academy of Neurology and The Practice Committee of the Child Neurology Society. Neurology 60:367-380, 2003.

Silberstein SD: Migraine. Lancet 363:381-391, 2004.

Zafeiriou DI, Pitt M, de Sousa C: Clinical and neurophysiological characteristics of congenital myasthenic syndromes presenting in early infancy. Brain Dev 26:47-52, 2004.

CHAPTER **188**

Assessment

Approximately one of three Americans of any age has at least one recognizable skin disorder at any time. The most common cutaneous diseases encountered in community settings, in relative order of frequency, are dermatophytosis, acne, seborrheic dermatitis, atopic dermatitis (eczema), verrucae (warts), tumors, psoriasis, vitiligo, and infections such as herpes simplex and impetigo. In children attending pediatric dermatology clinics, atopic dermatitis, impetigo, tinea capitis, acne vulgaris, verrucae vulgaris, and seborrheic dermatitis account for most diagnoses. More African American children are diagnosed with atopic dermatitis or tinea capitis, whereas more white children are diagnosed with acne vulgaris or verrucae vulgaris, perhaps reflecting inherent racial differences in the incidence or distribution of, or susceptibility to, these diseases.

HISTORY

The history is an essential component in the evaluation of a skin lesion (Table 188–1). The age of the patient, onset, duration, progression, associated cutaneous symptoms (pain, pruritus), and associated systemic signs or symptoms (fever, malaise, weight loss) are important clues. The skin is readily available for self-diagnosis and self-treatment; patients and parents frequently institute presumptive therapy before seeking medical opinion. Over-the-counter remedies may alter the appearance of a rash dramatically. Obtaining an accurate description of the **original lesion** improves diagnostic accuracy. Patients often do not consider a topical antibiotic or anti-itch medication as "treatment"; a severe contact dermatitis to neomycin may be missed if the patient does not admit to applying a topical antibiotic. Other important historical information includes a history of allergies, environmental exposure, travel history, previous treatment, and family history.

PHYSICAL EXAMINATION

A careful examination of the skin requires a visual and a tactile assessment. Examination of the skin over the entire body must be performed systematically. The body parts must be separated into segments, with careful attention to each segment. Mucous membranes, hair, nails, and teeth, all of ectodermal origin, also may be involved in cutaneous disorders and should be assessed.

COMMON MANIFESTATIONS

A descriptive nomenclature of skin lesions helps not only with generating a differential diagnosis, but also with communication between healthcare providers. Determination of the primary or secondary nature of the lesion is the cornerstone of dermatologic diagnosis. A **primary lesion** is defined as the basic lesion that arises de novo and is most characteristic of the disease process (Table 188–2 and Fig. 188–1). A primary lesion is not the first lesion the patient notices; two different types of primary lesions may be present. In most cases, **secondary lesions** are the residue, or result, of the effects of the primary lesion, which may be created by scratching or infection and rarely may be seen in the absence of a primary lesion (Table 188–3).

The color, texture, configuration, location, and distribution of the lesion should be recorded. Detailed evaluation of color is important because even subtle variation may imply different diagnoses. Evaluation of lesion color must take into consideration the

TABLE 188–1. Evaluation of Patient with a Skin Lesion

Demographic Data

What are the age, gender, and race of the patient?

Morphology (Primary and Secondary Lesion)

What did the lesion or rash look like when it was first noted?
How has it changed?
Is the appearance of the lesion today typical (e.g., a good day or bad day)?
Has the lesion blistered, bled, or drained?

Chronologic Course of Eruption or Lesion

When was the lesion or eruption first noticed?
How long does an individual lesion last?
Do the lesions or eruptions appear in crops?
If transient, is the eruption seasonal?
Is the eruption worse at one particular time of the day?

Distribution

Where did the eruption begin?
How did it spread?
Is there a pattern to the spreading?
Does it occur on the face?
Does it occur on the palms or soles?
Any changes in hair, nails, or teeth?

Symptoms

Does the lesion or eruption itch?
Is the lesion or eruption painful?
Have there been any associated fevers?
Are there any symptoms of temperature instability?
What seems to trigger the lesion or eruption?
What seems to help alleviate symptoms?
Are there are other symptoms (review of related systems)?

Treatment and Skin Care

Have any prescription creams, ointments, or gels been applied?
Have any prescription or over-the-counter medications been given orally (e.g., prednisone, antibiotics, antihistamines, or antifungals)?
What over-the-counter creams, ointments, gels, lotions, or powders have been applied (e.g., topical antibiotics, steroids, antifungals, or emollients)?

Medical History

Has the patient had any prior skin disorders?
Does the patient have a history of chronic or recurrent infections (cutaneous, otitis media, sinusitis, pneumonia)?
Does the patient have a history of atopy (e.g., asthma, environmental, food, or seasonal allergies)?
Does the patient have a history of drug allergies?

Family History

Does the family have a history of skin disease?
Does the family have a history of skin cancer?
Does the family have a history of atopy (asthma, seasonal allergies, drug allergies, or atopic dermatitis)?

Social History

Who lives with the patient?
Who are the caregivers?
Does the patient attend daycare?
Has the patient had any contacts with similar eruptions or lesions?

Sexual Activity

Is the patient sexually active?
Is there any disease or similar symptoms in sexual partners?

---

background pigmentation of the patient. In deeply pigmented patients, redness is masked, and subsequent assessment of the severity of the eruption may be greatly diminished. A detailed observation of configuration (Table 188–4) and distribution is important. A localized or grouped eruption may suggest a cutaneous infection, whereas widespread, symmetric involvement of extensor surfaces may suggest a primary skin disorder, such as psoriasis. More than one type of lesion may be present at one time and may reflect the evolution of the disease. Lesions on mucous membranes are usually short-lived, and lesions in thick-skinned areas, such as the palms and soles, may be particularly difficult to characterize.

The configuration of skin lesions and pattern of distribution are often characteristic. Herpesvirus lesions are usually grouped lesions. Linear lesions suggest trauma or excoriation. Annular lesions may suggest Lyme disease, syphilis, and fungal infections.

Skin lesions may appear different on diverse skin colors. Erythema is often subtle on darkly pigmented skin and may be missed. Hyperpigmentation is a common response to inflammation and often appears red on lightly pigmented skin, but may appear dark brown or have a bluish or violet color on dark skin. Residual hyperpigmentation or hypopigmentation may persist in dark skin after inflammation has resolved.

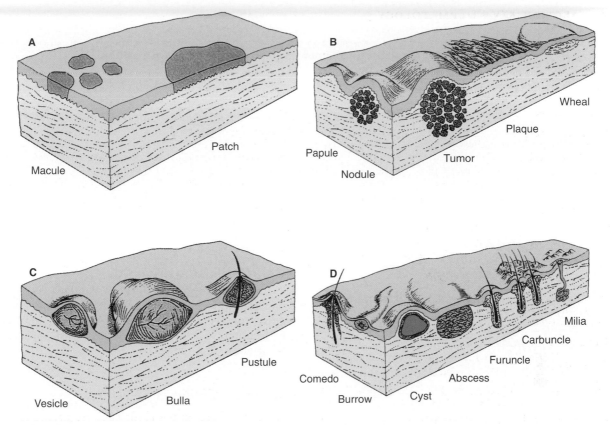

Figure 188–1

Morphology of primary skin lesions. A, Macules are flat and nonpalpable. **B,** Papules are palpable, elevated, and solid. **C,** Vesicles are palpable, elevated, and fluid-filled. **D,** Special primary lesions. (From Swartz MH: Textbook of Physical Diagnosis: History and Examination. Philadelphia, WB Saunders, 1989.)

TABLE 188–2. Descriptive Terminology of Primary Skin Lesions

Macule	Flat, well-circumscribed lesion <1 cm in diameter distinguished from surrounding skin by color only, with variable size and shape, which may be erythematous, pigmented, or purpuric
Patch	Similar to macule, but >1 cm in diameter
Papule	Elevated, circumscribed solid lesion <1 cm in diameter, which may be scaly or ulcerated or may become pustular
Plaque	Similar to papule, but >1 cm in diameter
Nodule	Large, palpable papule that extends 2 cm deep into the dermis or subcutaneous tissue
Tumor	Similar to nodule, but extends >2 cm into the dermis or subcutaneous tissue
Vesicle	Small fluid-filled (usually clear or straw-colored) epidermal lesion <1 cm in diameter
Bulla	Similar to vesicle, but >1 cm in diameter, which may be flaccid or tense, reflecting depth within the skin
Purpura	Macule resulting from extravasated blood into the skin; does not blanch with pressure
Petechia	Small, red-to-purple circumscribed macule resulting from extravasated blood measuring a few millimeters in diameter
Ecchymosis	Larger, hemorrhagic patches or plaques resulting from extravasated blood
Palpable purpura	Papule resulting from extravasated blood; characteristic of leukocytoclastic vasculitis, which may occur in various conditions, including infection, collagen vascular disorders, serum sickness, and drug eruptions
Pustule	Papule that contains purulent exudate (pus), which may have an initial papular phase and often is surrounded by erythema
Wheal (hive)	Transient, rounded or flat-topped edematous plaque; varies greatly in size and may have an annular or gyrate configuration
Telangiectasia	Dilated superficial blood vessels
Milia	Superficial, white, small epidermal keratin cyst
Comedo	Plug of keratin and sebum within the orifice of a hair follicle, which can be open (whitehead) or closed (blackhead) and is the characteristic lesion of acne vulgaris
Cyst	Papule or nodule with an epidermal lining composed of fluid or solid material

TABLE 188–3. Descriptive Terminology of Secondary Skin Lesions	
Scale	Results from abnormal keratinization; may be fine or sheetlike
Crust	Dried collection of serum and cellular debris
Erosion	Moist, shallow epidermal depression with loss of the superficial epidermis
Ulcer	Circumscribed, depressed, focal loss of entire epidermis into dermis; heals with scarring
Atrophy	Shallow depression that results from thinning of epidermis or dermis
Scar	Thickened, firm, and discolored collection of connective tissue that results from dermal damage; initially pink, but lightens with time
Sclerosis	Circumscribed or diffuse hardening of skin; usually forms in a plaque
Lichenification	Accentuated skin lines/markings that result from thickening of the epidermis
Excoriation	Superficial linear erosion that is caused by scratching
Fissure	Linear break within the skin surface that is usually painful

DIFFERENTIAL DIAGNOSIS

Although the skin is readily available for examination, the description of hundreds of distinct cutaneous lesions and the dynamic evolution of lesions often complicates diagnosis. Cutaneous bacterial, fungal, and viral infections (see Chapter 98); atopic dermatitis (see Chapter 80); allergic reactions to foods (see Chapter 84) and drugs (see Chapter 85); and rheumatic diseases are commonly included in the differential diagnosis of primary skin disorders.

Numerous systemic diseases have cutaneous manifestations (Table 188–5). Many diseases are characterized by exanthems consisting primarily of macular erythema, including scarlet fever; staphylococcal scalded skin syndrome, and toxic shock syndrome. An erythematous, maculopapular exanthem is the rash most commonly associated with rheumatic diseases, allergic drug reactions (see Chapter 85), Kawasaki disease, graft-versus-host disease, and many infections, especially viral. Target lesions are the hallmark of erythema multiforme (EM), Stevens-Johnson syndrome (SJS), and toxic epidermal necrolysis (TEN). Petechiae or purpura may be the manifestation of disseminated intravascular coagulopathy or other bleeding diatheses (see Chapter 151). Wheals (hives) suggest an allergic etiology (see Chapter 81).

DISTINGUISHING FEATURES

Erythema nodosum presents as symmetric, tender, red, 1- to 5-cm discrete nodules and plaques over the shins and occasionally with lesions on the thighs, ankles, knees, arms, face, and neck. It is a cell-mediated hypersensitivity reaction associated with a wide range of systemic diseases, including tuberculosis, group A streptococcus, inflammatory bowel disease, invasive fungal infections, and certain drugs (oral contraceptives), although in many cases no etiology is identified. Erythema nodosum can occur at any age, but the highest incidence is between the ages of 20 and 30.

TABLE 188–4. Descriptive Terminology of Configuration of Skin Lesions	
Linear	Lesions arranged in straight lines, which may imply external insult or developmental anomaly occurring along embryonic lines (lines of Blaschko)
Nummular	Round, coin-sized, and coin-shaped
Annular	Circular or ringlike with central clearing; there are polycyclic/serpiginous variations and confluence of individual annular lesions
Target lesion (iris or targetoid)	Erythematous papule or plaque with a characteristic configuration of a red-to-violaceous dusky center surrounded by a raised, edematous, pale ring and a red periphery, creating a target-like impression
Grouped	Clustered
Reticular	Lacy or netlike
Maculopapular	Generalized eruption of small papules mixed with erythematous macules, which is characteristic of the rash of measles (morbilliform)
Dermatomal	Following dermatomal distribution
Zosteriform	Grouped vesicles in a dermatomal distribution, which is characteristic of the rash of zoster
Erythema nodosum	Symmetric, tender, red, 1- to 5-cm discrete nodules and plaques characteristically over the shins

TABLE 188–5. Characteristics of Cutaneous Signs of Systemic Diseases

Disease	Age of Onset	Skin Lesions	Distribution
Systemic lupus erythematosus	Any	Erythematous patches; palpable purpura; livedo reticularis; Raynaud phenomenon; thrombocytopenic and nonthrombocytopenic purpura	Photodistribution; malar
Discoid lupus	Adolescents	Annular, scaly plaques; atrophy; dyspigmentation	Photodistribution
Neonatal lupus erythematosus	Newborn to 6 mo	Annular, erythematous, scaly plaques	Photodistribution; head/neck
Juvenile dermatomyositis	Any	Erythematous-to-violaceous, scaly macules; discrete papules overlying knuckles	Periocular, face; shoulder girdle; extensor extremities; knuckles; palms
Henoch-Schönlein purpura	Children and adolescents	Purpuric papules and plaques	Buttocks; lower extremities
Kawasaki disease	Infants, children	Erythematous, maculopapular-to-urticarial plaques; acral and groin erythema, edema, and desquamation	Diffuse
Inflammatory bowel disease	Children and adolescents	Aphthae; erythema nodosum; pyoderma gangrenosum; thrombophlebitis	Oral ulcers; perianal fissures
Sweet syndrome	Any	Infiltrated erythematous, edematous plaques	Diffuse
Graft-versus-host disease	Any	Acute: erythema; papules; vesicles; bullae	Head and neck; palms/soles; diffuse
Hypersensitivity reaction	Any	Erythema; urticarial macules and plaques	Diffuse
Serum sickness–like reaction	Any	Edematous, purpuric plaques	Acral; diffuse

Women are affected three times more often than men; in children, girls are only slightly more affected than boys. The erythema usually evolves into a brownish red or bluish bruiselike color 1 to 2 weeks after initial onset; the lesions usually resolve in 3 to 6 weeks without scarring. The diagnosis is based on the characteristic physical findings. Definitive diagnosis requires a deep skin biopsy that includes the subcutaneous fat. Chest radiograph, complete blood count, purified protein derivative, antistreptolysin O titer, throat culture, and possibly fungal antigen skin tests should be performed. Treatment is based on the identification and management of the underlying disorder.

Alopecia, or hair loss (Table 188–6), may be patchy (**alopecia areata**), diffuse over the scalp (**alopecia totalis**), or diffuse over the scalp and entire body (**alopecia universalis**). Alopecia may be categorized for diagnostic purposes into scarring and nonscarring disorders; the latter are rare in children, but are associated most commonly with prolonged tinea capitis and kerion (see Chapter 98). Alopecia also may result from seborrheic dermatitis, malnutrition and nutritional deficiencies (iron, zinc), genetic inheritance, autoimmune disorders (lupus erythematosus, Hashimoto thyroiditis, Addison disease), and illness within the preceding 3 months. Physical examination includes evaluation of the scalp for scaling, erythema, or scarring, which suggests hair loss from a primary skin disease of the scalp, and of the hair shafts for broken, frayed tips (**"black dots"**), which suggests traumatic breakage from tight braids (**traction alopecia**) or compulsive pulling and breaking of hair (**trichotillomania**). Examination of the nails is helpful because most disease processes affect the hair and the nails.

Vesiculobullous lesions may be congenital, hereditary, or acquired. These lesions may be classified by the cleavage plane on skin biopsy specimen (Fig. 188–2). Common disorders are secondary to toxins, infections, or hypersensitivity reactions (Table 188–7).

INITIAL DIAGNOSTIC EVALUATION AND SCREENING TESTS

The initial diagnostic evaluation is a thorough history and physical examination, which is usually sufficient for diagnosis because of the visibility of the skin. Screening tests may be indicated based on the history and physical examination findings. It is usually unnecessary to perform laboratory or imaging studies. Initial tests that may be indicated include potassium hydroxide examination for fungi and dermatophytes, skin scrapings for scabies, Gram stain for bacterial

TABLE 188-6.   Differential Diagnosis of Hair Loss

Disease	Age of Onset	Clinical Features	Associated Findings	Prognosis
Alopecia areata	Variable	Discrete 2- to 5-cm round, coin-shaped patches of hair loss; may progress to total alopecia	May see loss of eyebrows, eyelashes; nail pits	Variable
Monilethrix	Infancy	Dull, dry brittle hair that breaks easily	Follicular keratosis	May improve slightly with age
Tinea capitis	2-7 yr	Ill-defined, round patches of hair loss with scaling and crusting of the scalp	May have tinea infection of face or neck; posterior cervical lymphadenopathy	Complete recovery after antifungal treatment
Telogen	Variable, more prominent in toddlers	Diffuse thinning of hair, without discrete patches of alopecia; scalp is normal	Follows severe illness or high fever by 3-6 mo	Resolves spontaneously over several months
Loose anagen syndrome	6 mo-6 yr	Seen in fair, blond children; presenting complaint is that the hair is easily and painlessly pulled from the scalp in clumps; scalp is normal	None	Improves with age
Trichotillomania	10-16 yr	Circumscribed, irregular areas of hair loss with broken or frayed hair shafts; excoriations in scalp	Obsessive-compulsive disorder in older children	Improves with behavioral modification
Traction alopecia	2-8 yr	Patchy, thinning of hair with broken hair shafts; scalp is normal	Trauma (e.g., tight braiding of the hair)	Improves slightly with age

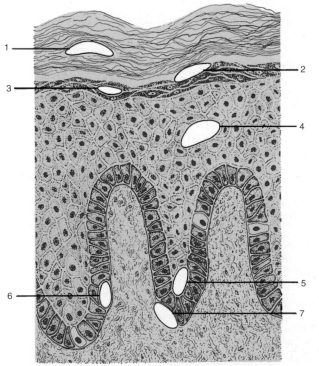

Figure 188-2

Blister cleavage sites in the skin. *1,* Intracorneal; *2,* subcorneal; *3,* granular layer; *4,* intraepidermal; *5,* suprabasal; *6,* junctional (between the basal cell membrane and basement membrane); *7,* subepidermal. (From Nopper AJ, Rabinowotz RG: Rashes and skin lesions. In Kliegman RM [ed]: Practical Strategies in Pediatric Diagnosis and Therapy. Philadelphia, WB Saunders, 1996.)

TABLE 188–7.   Vesiculobullous Eruptions

Entity	Clinical Clues
Hereditary	
Epidermolysis bullosa (AR, AD)	Bullae at birth in more severe forms Localized or widespread Dystrophic nails in some forms Bullae induced by trauma, friction; may occur spontaneously Mucosal involvement in severe forms
Incontinentia pigmenti (X-linked recessive)	Crops of blisters at birth or early infancy Often linear May have coexistent streaky hyperpigmentation Eosinophilia Associated CNS, dental, ocular, cardiac, skeletal abnormalities Females affected; males may have Klinefelter syndrome
Porphyria cutanea tarda (AD or acquired)	On dorsal hands, other sun-exposed skin Heal with milia formation Increased fragility of skin Hypertrichosis
Epidermolytic hyperkeratosis (bullous congenital ichthyosiform erythroderma) (AR)	Verruciform scales in flexural surfaces Bullae within first week of life Hyperkeratosis after third month Collodion membrane at birth in some cases
Autoimmune	
Linear IgA disease (chronic bullous disease of childhood)	Onset usually before 6 yr of age Sites of predilection: perioral, periocular, lower abdomen, buttocks, anogenital region Annular or rosette configuration of tense blisters—"cluster of jewels" Mucous membranes commonly involved Spontaneous remission DIF shows linear deposits of IgA at DEJ
Bullous pemphigoid	Large, tense subepidermal bullae Lower abdomen, thighs, face, flexural areas Oral lesions common DIF shows linear deposits of C3 and IgG at DEJ
Pemphigus vulgaris	Flaccid bullae, persistent erosions Seborrheic distribution Mucosal involvement common, usually the initial manifestation Positive Nikolsky sign DIF with intercellular (desmosomal) deposits of IgG, C3
Pemphigus foliaceus	Small flaccid bullae or shallow erosions with scaling, crusting Back, scalp, face, upper chest, abdomen Oral lesions uncommon May resemble a generalized exfoliative dermatitis DIF shows intercellular deposition of IgG, C3 in superficial epidermis
Dermatitis herpetiformis	Intensely pruritic Associated with gluten-sensitive enteropathy Extensor surfaces: elbows, knees, buttocks, shoulders, neck Hemorrhagic lesions on palms and soles DIF shows granular deposition of IgA in dermal papillae
Infectious	
Bacterial	
Staphylococcal scalded skin syndrome	Generalized, tender erythema Positive Nikolsky sign Occasionally associated with underlying infection such as osteomyelitis, septic arthritis, pneumonia Desquamation, moist erosions observed More common in children younger than 5 years of age
Bullous impetigo	Localized benign staphylococcal scalded skin syndrome

Continued

TABLE 188–7.   Vesiculobullous Eruptions—cont'd

Entity	Clinical Clues
Viral	
Herpes simplex virus	Grouped vesicles on erythematous base
	May be recurrent in same site—lips, eyes, cheeks, hands
	Reactivated by fever, sunlight, trauma, stress
	Positive Tzanck smear, herpes culture
Varicella	Crops of vesicles on erythematous base—"dewdrops on rose petal"
	Highly contagious
	May see multiple stages of lesions simultaneously
	Associated with fever
	Positive Tzanck smear, varicella-zoster culture
Herpes zoster	Grouped vesicles on erythematous base limited to one or several adjacent dermatomes
	Usually unilateral
	Burning, pruritus
	Positive Tzanck smear, varicella-zoster culture
	Thoracic dermatomes most commonly involved in children
Hand-foot-mouth syndrome (coxsackievirus)	Prodrome of fever, anorexia, sore throat
	Oval blisters in acral distribution, usually few in number
	Shallow oval oral lesions on erythematous base
	Highly infectious
	Peak incidence in late summer and in fall
Hypersensitivity	
Erythema multiforme major (Stevens-Johnson syndrome)	Prodrome of fever, headache, malaise, sore throat, cough, vomitting, dirarrhea
	Involvement of 2 mucosal surfaces, usually see hemorrhagic crusts on lips
	Target lesions progress from central vesiculation to extensive epidermal necrosis; may have sheets of denuded skin
	Associated with infections and drugs
Toxic epidermal necrolysis	Possible extension of erythema multiforme major involving >30% of body surface
	Severe exfoliative dermatitis
	Older children and adults
	Frequently related to drugs (e.g., sulfonamides, anticonvulsants)
	Positive Nikolsky sign
Extrinsic	
Contact dermatitis	Irritant or allergic
	Distribution dependent on the irritant or allergen
	Distribution helpful in establishing diagnosis
Insect bites	Occur occasionally following flea or mosquito bites
	May be hemorrhagic bullae
	Often in linear or irregular clusters
	Very pruritic
Burns	Irregular shapes and configurations
	May be suggestive of abuse
	Vary from first to third degree, bullae with second and third degree
Friction	Usually on acral surfaces
	May be related to footwear
	Often activity related
Miscellaneous	
Urticaria pigmentosa	Positive Darier sign
	Coexistent pigmented lesions
	Usually presents during infancy
	Dermatographism commonly seen
Miliaria crystallina	Clean, 1- to 2-mm superficial vesicles occurring in crops, rupture spontaneously
	Intertriginous areas, especially neck and axillae

AD, autosomal dominant; AR, autosomal recessive; DEJ, dermoepidermal junction; DIF, direct immunofluorescence.
From Nopper AJ, Rabinowotz RG: Rashes and skin lesions. In Kliegman RM (ed): Practical Strategies in Pediatric Diagnosis and Therapy. Philadelphia, WB Saunders, 1996.

infections, cytology (Tzanck test) for herpesvirus and varicella-zoster virus infection, and Wood light examination for the yellowish gold fluorescence of tinea versicolor. The most definitive dermatologic test is the skin biopsy, which is required only occasionally. The biopsy specimen can be accomplished by punch biopsy, a simple, relatively painless procedure. Other definitive tests useful to diagnose underlying diseases with cutaneous manifestations include patch testing of suspected allergens, dark-field examination for syphilis, and blood tests.

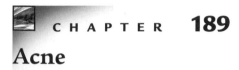

CHAPTER 189
Acne

ETIOLOGY

Acne vulgaris is a chronic inflammatory disorder of pilosebaceous units that affects areas with the greatest concentration of sebaceous glands, such as the face, chest, and back. The pathogenesis of acne is multifactorial with gender, age, genetic factors, and environment all major contributing factors. The **primary event** is the obstruction of the sebaceous follicle with lamellated keratin from abnormal keratinization, increased sebum production from sebaceous glands, and overgrowth of normal skin flora. Androgens are a potent stimulus of the sebaceous gland. The subsequent inflammatory component and pustule formation results from proliferation of *Propionibacterium acnes,* coagulase-negative staphylococci, and the yeast *Malassezia furfur.* Each of these organisms possesses lipolytic enzymes, although *P. acnes* is primarily responsible for formation of free fatty acids. Chemotactic factors released by bacteria attract neutrophils that ingest the bacteria and release hydrolytic enzymes, which contributes to further inflammation and the development of pustules and nodulocystic lesions, eventually leading to scarring.

EPIDEMIOLOGY

Acne is the most common skin disorder in adolescents, occurring in 85% of teenagers. The incidence is similar in both sexes, although boys often are more severely affected. Acne may begin at 8 years of age and even earlier in patients treated with systemic corticosteroids.

CLINICAL MANIFESTATIONS

Superficial plugging of the pilosebaceous unit with keratinous material, lipid, and bacteria results in non-inflammatory small (2 to 3 mm) **open (blackhead)** and **closed (whitehead) comedones**. Comedones are the earliest lesion of acne and typically are found over the nose, chin, and central forehead. An open comedo is less likely to become inflammatory than a closed comedo. Rupture of a comedo into adjacent dermis induces a neutrophilic inflammatory response and development of inflammatory **papules** and **pustules** in the same distribution. Larger (1 to 3 cm), skin-colored or red cysts and nodules represent deeper plugging and usually are found over the cheeks, around the nose, and on the back. Increased and persistent inflammation, especially with **cystic acne** and rupture of a deep cyst, increases the risk of scarring.

Pomade acne results from use of oily hair products and is characterized by lesions, predominantly closed comedones, on the forehead. **Steroid-induced acne** may occur after a few weeks of therapy. The lesions tend to be monomorphic and clustered on the trunk, shoulders, and upper arms. Prolonged use of topical corticosteroids can cause a similar eruption.

Neonatal acne occurs in about 20% of normal newborns at 2 to 4 weeks of age and is thought to be a response to maternal androgens. The primary lesions are pinpoint, red, inflammatory closed comedones found on the lateral cheeks and forehead and occasionally on the chest or back. These lesions usually resolve spontaneously over months. Neonatal acne must be differentiated from more common and benign cutaneous disorders presenting in newborns, such as milia or **miliaria rubra (prickly heat)**.

Infantile acne occurs in infants 3 to 16 months old and may persist for months, but usually resolves by 3 years of age. Boys are more commonly affected. These children have typical lesions of acne, including comedones, papules, and cysts. Cyst formation may be dramatic, with severe facial pitted scarring occurring in 10% to 15%. The lesions of infantile acne must be differentiated from adenoma sebaceum, the lesions associated with tuberous sclerosis. Topical treatment with benzoyl peroxide gel and tretinoin is usually effective within a few weeks; oral erythromycin also may be necessary.

LABORATORY AND IMAGING STUDIES

Laboratory studies, such as bacterial and fungal cultures, and imaging studies are not necessary to diagnose acne.

DIFFERENTIAL DIAGNOSIS

The diagnosis of acne is usually not difficult because of the characteristic and chronic lesions. Acne must be differentiated from rosacea and folliculitis. **Rosacea** is a cutaneous vascular disorder of adults, usually involving the cheeks and nose, which produces erythema, telangiectasias, and rhinophyma. **Folliculitis** is caused by superficial infection with *Escherichia coli* and *Pseudomonas* and follows exposure, such as in a contaminated hot tub. Severe or refractory acne in young children may be a sign of congenital adrenal hyperplasia or a virilizing tumor.

TREATMENT

The mainstay of treatment of acne is topical keratolytic agents and topical antibiotics. The vehicle for medication delivery is important to consider in prescribing these agents. Creams are appropriate for patients with sensitive or dry skin. Patients with oily skin may benefit from gels, which have a drying effect. Gels may cause irritation and local erythema. Lotions can be used with any skin type and have the advantage of spreading well over hair-bearing skin. The propylene glycol in lotions may induce a burning sensation or a drying effect. Topical antibiotics are delivered as solutions, usually in alcohol; solutions work best in patients with oily skin.

The keratolytic agents (2.5% to 10% benzoyl peroxide, 2% salicylic acid, 20% azelaic acid, 0.025% to 0.1% tretinoin, 0.1% adapalene, 0.05% to 0.1% tazarotene) produce superficial desquamation and subsequently relieve the follicular obstruction. Keratolytic agents are available in several different formulations that have varying degrees of efficacy. There is a direct relationship between the potency of the keratolytic cream or gel and the degree of associated irritation. Several topical antibiotics (2% erythromycin, 1% clindamycin, 2.2% tetracycline) are available. Oral antibiotics (tetracycline, erythromycin) should be administered for deeper cystic lesions. Tetracyclines are the most effective antibiotics because they also have significant anti-inflammatory activity. They also cause photosensitivity, however, and sunscreen should be prescribed along with tetracyclines to minimize this adverse effect.

For recalcitrant or severe nodulocystic acne, oral isotretinoin (1 mg/kg/day for a 20-week period) may be instituted. Isotretinoin, an oral analogue of vitamin A, normalizes follicular keratinization, reduces sebum production, and decreases 5α-dihydrotestosterone formation and androgen receptor–binding capacity. Isotretinoin has an approximately 80% response rate, but has a high incidence of adverse effects and should be used only by physicians familiar with all the potential adverse effects. Isotretinoin therapy requires careful patient selection, pretreatment counseling, and monthly laboratory monitoring. Isotretinoin is **teratogenic** and must not be used immediately before and during pregnancy.

COMPLICATIONS

Although not associated with a high degree of clinical morbidity, acne has significant and frequently devastating effects on an adolescent's body image and self-esteem. There may be little correlation between severity and psychosocial impact. Even mild cases of acne require thorough assessment and continued monitoring.

PROGNOSIS

Classically, acne lasts 3 to 5 years; some individuals may have disease for 15 to 20 years. Only early treatment with isotretinoin has been shown to alter the natural course of acne. Acne lesions often heal with temporary postinflammatory erythema and hyperpigmentation. Depending on the severity, chronicity, and depth of involvement, pitted, atrophic, or hypertrophic scars may develop. **Cystic acne** has the highest incidence of scarring because rupture of a deep cyst induces the greatest inflammation of the dermis and subcutaneous tissues. In susceptible individuals, scarring may follow pustular or even comedonal acne. Certain areas, such as the glabellar region of the forehead and the lateral areas of the cheeks, appear to scar more frequently.

PREVENTION

Greasy hair and cosmetic preparations should be avoided because they exacerbate preexisting acne. There are no effective means for preventing acne. There is little evidence that diet is associated with acne. Improvement often is noted during summer months, which may be related to climate or to reduced stress from school. Repetitive cleansing with soap and water or use of astringents or abrasives removes only surface lipids. Their use makes the skin appear less oily, but does not prevent formation of microcomedones; their use may be damaging because of the irritation and dryness they cause.

CHAPTER 190
Contact Dermatitis

ETIOLOGY

Inflammation in the top layers of the skin caused by direct contact with a substance is divided into two subtypes: contact irritant dermatitis and contact allergic dermatitis. **Contact irritant dermatitis** is common and observed after the skin surface is exposed to an irritating chemical or undergoes repeated exposure to a substance that dries the skin. **Allergic contact dermatitis** is a cell-mediated immune reaction that can be divided into two phases, the **sensitization phase** and the **elicitation phase** (see Chapter 77). The antigens involved in allergic contact dermatitis, haptens, readily penetrate the epidermis and are bound by Langerhans cells, the antigen-presenting cells of the epidermis. The hapten is presented to T lymphocytes, and an immune cascade follows.

EPIDEMIOLOGY

Contact diaper dermatitis is a common problem that affects approximately 10% of infants between birth and 2 years of age.

CLINICAL MANIFESTATIONS

Contact irritant dermatitis is characterized by ill-defined red patches and plaques with secondary scales. The eruption is localized to skin surfaces that are exposed to the irritant. Irritant diaper dermatitis is distributed in the perianal region and on the buttocks, areas that are exposed repeatedly to urine and feces. Contact irritant dermatitis is observed frequently on the dorsal surface of the hands in patients who repeatedly wash their hands with an irritating soap.

Contact allergic dermatitis is usually an acute and severe reaction limited to exposed sites. The initial lesions are bright red, pruritic patches, often in linear or sharply marginated, bizarre configurations. Within the patches are clear vesicles and bullae with sero-sanguineous drainage. Signs and symptoms of the disease may be delayed for 7 to 14 days after exposure if the patient has not been sensitized previously. On re-exposure, symptoms begin within hours and are usually more severe. The eruption may persist for weeks.

LABORATORY AND IMAGING STUDIES

The diagnosis is established by clinical presentation and history of exposure to a recognized irritant or allergen. *Candida* dermatitis, if suspected, can be confirmed by a potassium hydroxide preparation of skin scrapings to identify the presence of budding yeast.

DIFFERENTIAL DIAGNOSIS

Distribution of the dermatitis and a detailed exposure history are the most useful diagnostic tools. Involvement of the lower legs and distal arms suggests exposure to plants of the *Rhus* species (poison ivy or poison oak). Dermatitis of the ears (earrings), wrist (bracelet or watch), or periumbilical region (buckle of jeans or pants) suggests a metal allergy to nickel. Distribution on the dorsal surface of the feet indicates a shoe allergy, usually to dyes, rubber, or leather. Topical antibiotics (neomycin) and fragrances (soap, perfumes, cosmetics) are frequent causes of allergic contact dermatitis.

Diaper rashes caused by *Candida* are quite common. *Candida* is environmentally ubiquitous and thrives in warm, moist conditions. Infections usually begin as an intensely erythematous, nontender macule with irregular but distinct borders, differentiating it from cellulitis. Subsequently, **satellite lesions**, which are smaller red discrete papules that are adjacent to but separate from the primary lesion, develop and spread. The eruption may spread to include the entire perineum, including the scrotum and penis in boys and the labia and vagina in girls. Oral candidiasis (**thrush**) is often present. Contact irritant dermatitis primarily affects the prominent, exposed surfaces, whereas *Candida* primarily affects intertriginous areas. **Treatment** consists of topical nystatin cream or ointment, clotrimazole 1% cream, or miconazole 2% ointment. Systemic antifungal agents are unnecessary for immunocompetent patients. Concurrent oral thrush should be treated with nystatin suspension or topically applied gentian violet. Lesions associated with significant inflammation can be treated adjunctively with a short course (1 to 2 days) of topical 1% hydrocortisone. More potent topical steroids are contraindicated to avoid atrophic skin changes.

Psoriasis, **seborrheic dermatitis**, and **Langerhans cell histiocytosis** can present with an erythematous rash in the diaper area. Referral to a dermatologist should be considered for any child with diaper rash that does not respond to conventional therapy or with severe rash.

TREATMENT

Topical steroids are effective in treatment of allergic and irritant contact dermatitis. High potency steroids may be necessary for severe reactions of allergic contact dermatitis. Oral antihistamines or oral steroids may be required to control itching.

COMPLICATIONS

Inflamed skin, especially macerated skin from urine and feces irritation, is prone to injury from friction and to bacterial or candidal superinfection. *Candida albicans* is present in 70% of cases of diaper dermatitis.

PREVENTION

It is controversial whether diaper rash is more frequent with use of absorbent disposable diapers or with cloth diapers. Occlusion, such as with plastic pants, should be avoided because it predisposes the skin to maceration. Every effort should be made to identify the trigger of contact dermatitis because re-exposure often leads to increasingly severe reactions.

CHAPTER 191
Seborrheic Dermatitis

ETIOLOGY

Seborrheic dermatitis is a chronic inflammatory disease that has different clinical presentations at different ages. Areas prone to seborrheic dermatitis include the scalp and scalp margins, eyebrows, base of eyelashes, nasolabial folds, external ear canals, and posterior auricular folds. Seborrheic dermatitis classically presents in infants as **cradle cap** and in adolescents as **dandruff**. Genetic and environmental factors influence the onset and clinical course, which parallels the distribution, size, and activity of sebaceous glands, although their role is uncertain. *M. furfur* seems to play a causative agent role.

EPIDEMIOLOGY

Seborrheic dermatitis is common in children, especially in infants as cradle cap and in adolescents as dandruff, paralleling the activity of the sebaceous glands.

CLINICAL MANIFESTATIONS

Seborrheic dermatitis in infants presents as **cradle cap**, which may begin during the first month and persist during the first year of life. It is usually asymptomatic other than the appearance. Cradle cap describes the thick, waxy, yellow-white scaling and crusting of the scalp with greasy adherent scale. It is usually prominent on the vertex of the skull, but it may be diffuse. A greasy, scaly, erythematous, nonpruritic papular dermatitis may extend to the face, posterior auricular folds, and diaper area and may involve the entire body. Diaper and intertriginous areas can have sharply demarcated erythematous patches with yellowish, greasy, or waxy-appearing scale. Significant erythema may be present, particularly if the eruption spreads onto the face and torso. Postinflammatory hypopigmentation may persist after the inflammation has faded. The eruption is usually asymptomatic, which helps to differentiate it from infantile atopic dermatitis, which is pruritic.

Classic seborrheic dermatitis during adolescence usually is localized to the scalp and intertriginous areas and may include blepharitis and involvement of the external auditory canal. **Dandruff** is a fine, white, dry scaling of the scalp with minor itching. Scalp changes vary from diffuse, brawny scaling to focal areas of thick, oily, yellow crusts with underlying erythema. Pruritus may be minimal or severe. Seborrheic plaques on the extremities appear similar to eczema and less erythematous and less well demarcated.

LABORATORY AND IMAGING STUDIES

Laboratory studies and imaging studies are not necessary to diagnose cradle cap or dandruff. Atypical or resistant cases should have fungal cultures and potassium hydroxide studies for *Trichophyton tonsurans* (see Chapter 98).

DIFFERENTIAL DIAGNOSIS

The differential diagnosis includes secondary syphilis, drug eruptions, atopic dermatitis (see Chapter 80), and cutaneous fungal infections (see Chapter 98). Seborrheic dermatitis with pronounced scaling may resemble psoriasis. Intractable, severe generalized seborrheic dermatitis suggests histiocytosis, and intractable seborrheic dermatitis accompanied by chronic diarrhea and failure to thrive suggests Leiner disease or AIDS (see Chapter 105).

Pityriasis rosea must be considered in the differential diagnosis and is a benign, self-limited eruption that may occur at any age, with peak incidence during adolescence. A solitary 2- to 5-cm, pink, round patch that often has a hint of central clearing, the so-called **herald patch**, is the first manifestation of the eruption. The herald patch typically is found on the breast, lower torso, or proximal thigh and is often misdiagnosed as fungal or eczematous in origin. One to 2 weeks later, multiple 0.5- to 2-cm, oval to oblong, red or tan ("fawn"-colored) macules with a fine, branlike scale erupt on the torso and proximal extremities in a characteristic arrangement parallel to skin tension lines (**"Christmas tree" pattern**). Papular and papulovesicular variants may be seen in infants and young children. Rarely the eruption may have an inverse distribution involving the axillae and groin. Usually the condition is asymptomatic, but mild prodromal symptoms may be present with the appearance of the herald patch; pruritus is present in 25% of cases. The eruption lasts 4 to 14 weeks, with gradual resolution. Residual hyperpigmentation or hypopigmentation can take additional months to clear. The etiology is unknown. Treatment is unnecessary. Pruritus can be managed with oral antihistamines, phototherapy, and low potency topical corticosteroids.

Psoriasis is a common papulosquamous condition characterized by well-demarcated, erythematous, scaling papules and plaques. Psoriasis occurs at all ages, including infancy, with onset of 30% of cases during childhood. The disease is characterized by a chronic and relapsing course, although spontaneous remissions can occur. Infections, stress, trauma, and medications may cause disease exacerbations. The disease also tends to worsen during the fall and winter, probably secondary to decreased humidity within the environment. Various subtypes of psoriasis exist. The most common variety is **plaque-type psoriasis (psoriasis vulgaris)**, which can be localized or generalized. The lesions consist of round, well-demarcated, red plaques measuring 1 to 7 cm with **micaceous scale**, which is distinctive in its thick, silvery appearance with pinpoint bleeding points revealed on removal of the scales (**Auspitz sign**). The lesions of psoriasis have a distinctive distribution involving the extensor aspect of the elbows and knees, posterior occipital scalp, periumbilical region, lumbosacral region, and intergluteal cleft. Children often have facial lesions involving the upper inner aspect of the eyelids. Nail plate involvement is common and includes pitting, onycholysis, subungual hyperkeratosis, and "oil staining" (reddish brown subungual macular discoloration).

Guttate (droplike) psoriasis occurs exclusively in children and young adults. Numerous 0.5- to 2-cm, oval or lancet-shaped, scaling, red papules and small plaques distributed over the upper torso and proximal extremities typify this form of psoriasis. Guttate psoriasis may be related to streptococcal infections, and the possibility of concurrent streptococcal infections (including streptococcal perianal dermatitis) should be investigated in cases of new onset and flares of guttate psoriasis.

Inverse psoriasis describes the presence of marginated, bright red, macerated, scaling patches and plaques in the axillary and inguinal regions. This condition can be differentiated from seborrheic dermatitis, candidiasis, and noninfectious intertrigo by the well-delineated nature of the patches and plaques. The typical psoriatic scale is not seen in this variant.

Erythrodermic and pustular forms of psoriasis are severe and potentially fatal, generalized forms of psoriasis that are uncommon in children. These forms may be associated with fever, leukocytosis, temperature instability, electrolyte and fluid abnormalities, and rarely high-output cardiac failure. Erythrodermic psoriasis is characterized by acute onset of generalized erythema with subsequent exfoliative scaling. Pustular psoriasis is characterized by spreading, bright red plaques with the sudden onset of fine, 2- to 3-mm sterile pustules at the periphery of the lesions.

The cornerstone of therapy is topical corticosteroids. Treatment of psoriasis with oral systemic corticosteroids can induce pustular psoriasis and should be avoided. Because of the risk of atrophy, striae, and telangiectases, especially when potent fluorinated corticosteroid preparations are administered long-term, the goal is to use the least potent corticosteroid. Topical calcipotriene, a vitamin D analogue, is a useful adjuvant to topical corticosteroids. Guttate psoriasis is generally quite difficult to treat with topical agents, and phototherapy usually is instituted in affected patients. Generalized erythrodermic psoriasis and pustular psoriasis may necessitate systemic treatments or Goeckerman therapy involving UVB irradiation and tar.

Lichen planus is an uncommon dermatosis in childhood. The primary lesion is a pruritic, flat-topped, polygonal, and violaceous papule that most often arises on the flexor wrists, knees, feet, anterior shins, and shaft of the penis. Close inspection of the surface of the papule reveals a fine, whitish reticulation or streaking (**Wickham striae**). Mucous membranes are involved in 50% of cases with lacy, white plaques on the buccal mucosa and infrequently on the palate, lips, and tongue. The oral and genital lesions may become erosive and extremely painful. Characteristic nail findings include plate ridging, dystrophy, subungual hyperkeratosis, and pterygia. Variants of lichen planus are bullous, annular, linear, and hypertrophic lichen planus. Typically, lichen planus is a chronic disorder lasting an average of about 12 to 15 months; it may be cyclic, recurring 7 to 8 years later. Chronic cases can persist for years, with episodes of remissions and exacerbations. The underlying etiology of lichen planus is unknown; rarely, systemic medications have been associated with lichen planus–like eruptions. Treatment includes the use of systemic antihistamines (hydroxyzine, diphenhydramine) for pruritus and the use of corticosteroids (topical, intralesional, systemic).

TREATMENT

Minor amounts of scale of seborrheic dermatitis can be removed easily by frequent shampooing. For all ages, daily shampooing with zinc pyrithione (Head & Shoulders, DHS Zinc), selenium sulfide 1% to 2.5%, or salicylic acid (T-Sal) can treat scalp scale. Seborrheic dermatitis with inflamed lesions responds rapidly to treatment with low potency steroids two to four times daily for 3 to 5 days. Wet compresses should be applied to the moist or fissured plaques before application of the corticosteroid ointment.

COMPLICATIONS

The response to treatment is usually rapid. Secondary bacterial infection can occur, but is uncommon. Intractable disease and other complications warrant further evaluation for other etiologies.

PROGNOSIS

Cradle cap is self-limited and resolves during the first year of life. Postinflammatory hypopigmentation may persist after the inflammation has faded. Seborrheic dermatitis does not cause permanent hair loss. Continued use of an antiseborrheic shampoo is often required for control of dandruff.

PREVENTION

Frequent shampooing, especially with early signs of seborrheic dermatitis, may help prevent progression.

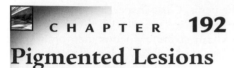

CHAPTER 192
Pigmented Lesions

DERMAL MELANOSIS (MONGOLIAN SPOT)

The most frequently encountered pigmented lesion is dermal melanosis (mongolian spot), which occurs in 70% to 96% of African American, Asian, and Native American infants and in approximately 5% of white infants. This is a heritable, developmental lesion caused by entrapment of melanocytes in the dermis during their migration from the neural crest into the epidermis. The dendritic melanocytes contain melanosomes expressing variable amounts of pigment and are located in the reticular dermis. Although most of these lesions are found in the lumbosacral area, they also occur at other sites, such as the buttocks, flank, extremities, or, rarely, the face. The lesion is macular and gray-blue, lacks a sharp border, and may cover an area of 10 cm or larger in length. Most lesions gradually disappear during the first few years of life; aberrant lesions in unusual sites are more likely to persist. Dermal melanosis has been associated with cleft lip, spinal meningeal tumor, and melanoma, but is usually a benign finding without associated morbidity.

CAFÉ AU LAIT MACULES

Café au lait spots are pigmented macules with smooth borders, resembling the "coast of California," which may be present in a newborn but tend to develop during childhood. They range in color from very light brown to a chocolate brown. Five café au lait macules are found in 1.8% of newborns and 25% to 40% of normal children and have no significance. Children with six or more café au lait macules (>0.5 cm in length), especially when accompanied by "freckling" in the flexural creases, should be evaluated carefully for additional stigmata of neurofibromatosis type 1 (see Chapter 186). The axillary and inguinal freckles represent tiny café au lait macules. Café au lait spots are usually the first cutaneous lesions to appear in a

TABLE 192–1.   NIH Consensus Criteria for Neurofibromatosis Type 1*
≥6 café au lait macules >0.5 cm (children) or >1.5 cm (adults)
≥2 neurofibromas or 1 plexiform neurofibroma
Axillary or inguinal freckling
Optic glioma
≥2 Lisch nodules of the iris
Distinctive bone changes
First-degree relative with neurofibromatosis type 1
*Definitive diagnosis requires at least two criteria.

patient with neurofibromatosis, but additional genetic and clinical investigations may be needed to establish a diagnosis (Table 192–1). The pigmented patches of **McCune-Albright syndrome** (polyostotic bone dysplasia, café au lait spots, and multiple endocrine disorders) also are referred to as café au lait macules; however, they are usually unilateral, elongated, and large (>10 cm) and often have a ragged, irregular border, resembling the "coast of Maine." Other important conditions associated with café au lait spots as a minor feature include **Fanconi anemia** (mental retardation, aplastic anemia, orthopedic abnormalities, and risk for subsequent development of malignancy) and **tuberous sclerosis**, a neurocutaneous syndrome manifesting developmental delay or cognitive impairment, hypopigmented macules (**ash-leaf spots**), facial angiofibromas, and **shagreen patches** (skin-colored or yellowish plaque resembling shark or pig skin, usually located on the back and especially in the lumbosacral region).

CONGENITAL MELANOCYTIC NEVI

Approximately 1% to 2% of newborns have melanocytic nevi. Small lesions (as opposed to giant pigmented nevi) are flat or slightly elevated plaques, often with an oval or lancet configuration. Most lesions are dark brown; scalp lesions may be red-brown at birth. The pigmentation within an individual lesion is often variegated or speckled with an accentuated epidermal surface ridge pattern. Textural changes, deeper pigmentation, and elevation help to differentiate these lesions from café au lait macules. Thick, dark, coarse hair frequently is associated with congenital melanocytic nevi. These lesions vary in site, size, and number, but are most often solitary. Histologically, they are characterized by the presence of nevus cells in the dermis; most have nevus cells extending into the deeper dermis. These lesions pose a slightly increased risk for the development of malignant melanoma, mostly developing during adulthood. For

TABLE 192–2.   Common Birthmarks

Color/Lesion	Birthmark	Location	Other Features
Brown/macule or patch	Café au lait macule	Variable, trunk	Associated with neurofibromatosis
Brown (<20 cm)/plaque (see text)	Congenital melanocytic nevus	Scalp, trunk	Possible increased risk of melanoma
Brown (>20 cm)/plaque (see text)	Giant melanocytic nevus	Trunk most common	3%-7% risk of melanoma, neurocutaneous melanosis
Brown–flesh-colored/ plaque	Epidermal nevus	Variable, trunk and neck	
Red/patch	Port-wine stain (nevus flammeus)	Variable, face most common	Associated with Sturge-Weber syndrome
Red/papule or plaque	Hemangioma	Variable, head and neck most common	Facial lesions (beard distribution) associated with airway lesions
Red-purple/plaque	Lymphatic malformation	Variable, trunk, proximal leg	Often have a vesicular appearance
Gray-blue/patch	Dermal melanosis (mongolian spot), nevus of Ito	Buttocks, lower trunk	Usually resolve spontaneously
Gray-blue/patch	Nevus of Ota	Forehead and eyelids	Ocular pigmentation
Gray-blue/patch	Nevus of Ito	Posterior shoulder	
Blue/nodule	Dermoid cyst	Scalp, face, neck	May connect to CNS if midline
Blue-purple/nodule	Cephalohematoma	Scalp	
Blue-purple/plaque	Venous malformation	Variable	Enlarge slowly over time
Yellow-orange/plaque	Nevus sebaceus	Scalp, face, neck	Basal cell carcinoma may arise within lesion
Yellow-orange/nodule	Congenital juvenile xanthogranuloma	Trunk	
Yellow-brown/papule or nodule	Mastocytoma	Variable	May become urticarial or blister
Hypertrichosis/plaque	Congenital melanocytic nevus	Scalp, trunk	
Hypertrichosis/tumor	Plexiform neurofibroma	Trunk most common	Associated with neurofibromatosis
Hypertrichosis/plaque	Smooth muscle hamartoma	Trunk	
White/patch	Nevus anemicus	Variable	
White/patch	Nevus depigmentosus	Variable	

this reason, many dermatologists advise removal of these lesions before or near the time of puberty. Should the family elect to observe rather than excise the nevus, periodic evaluation of the lesion for surface changes and associated symptoms should be performed. Excisional biopsy is indicated in instances in which malignant change is suspected. The differential diagnosis is listed in Table 192–2.

CONGENITAL GIANT MELANOCYTIC NEVI

Giant congenital nevi are defined as nevi that would be approximately 20 cm in length in adulthood (but smaller in a newborn, approximately 5 to 12 cm in length). These nevi may occupy 15% to 35% of the body surface, most commonly involving the trunk or head and neck region. The pigmentation often is variegated from light brown to black. The affected skin may be smooth, nodular, or leathery. Prominent, dark hypertrichosis is often present. Numerous smaller (1 to 5 cm) light brown patches (**satellite nevi**) are diffusely distributed. **Malignant melanoma** develops in the nevus in approximately 2% to 10% of affected patients over a lifetime.

Neurocutaneous melanosis is rarely associated with giant congenital melanocytic nevi in an axial distribution; affected patients have hydrocephalus and seizures, and death results from an intracranial melanoma in early childhood. Because of the significant incidence of malignant degeneration, the extensive deformity, and the intense pruritus that may accompany these lesions, staged surgical excision usually is attempted. The use of tissue expansion techniques has greatly improved the capability for surgical removal of large lesions.

PEUTZ-JEGHERS SYNDROME

The cutaneous lesions of the Peutz-Jeghers syndrome consist of brown to blue-black macules (darker than freckles) that develop around the nose and mouth. These may be present at birth or develop soon thereafter. The lips and oral mucosa are often involved, as are the hands, fingertips, and toes. Macular hyperpigmentation is the only visible sign of this autosomal dominant disorder until adolescence. In adolescence, intussusception, bleeding, and subsequent anemia develop; this is evidence of coexisting small bowel polyposis.

POSTINFLAMMATORY HYPERPIGMENTATION

Hyperpigmentation may be secondary to any inflammatory process in the skin and has many causes, including primary irritant dermatitis, infections, panniculitis, and hereditary diseases such as epidermolysis bullosa. The hyperpigmentation may result from enhanced melanosome production, larger melanin deposits in basal cells, greater numbers of keratinocytes, an increase in the thickness of the stratum corneum, or deposits of melanin in dermal melanophages.

ACQUIRED NEVI

Acquired melanocytic nevi or **moles** are common skin lesions. Melanocytic nevi may occur at any age; however, the lesions seem to develop most rapidly in prepubertal children and teenagers. Melanocytic nevi are well-delineated, round-to-oval, brown papules. Lesions are most common on the face, chest, and upper torso. Family history, skin type, and sun exposure are considered major risk factors. Irregular pigmentation, rapid growth, bleeding, and a change in configuration or borders suggest signs of malignant degeneration. Surgical excision and histologic examination are indicated in moles that have such features or are changing.

Malignant melanoma is rare in childhood; however, there is an alarming increase in incidence in adolescence. Education of parents and children regarding the risks of sun exposure, appropriate sun protection, and observation of changes in moles that are suggestive of malignancy is important.

Blue nevi are rare, oval, dome-shaped, blue or deep black papules or tumors 1 to 3 cm in size found on the upper half of the body. They grow slowly and have little tendency to become malignant, but may be difficult to differentiate clinically from vascular tumors or atypical melanocytic nevi. If the diagnosis is in question, excisional biopsy is diagnostic and curative.

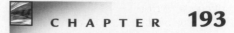

CHAPTER **193**

Hemangiomas and Vascular Malformations

Birthmark is a term that describes congenital anomalies of the skin. It should not be used as a definitive diagnosis because congenital skin lesions vary greatly in their appearance and prognosis (see Table 192–2).

Vascular lesions can be divided into two major categories: hemangiomas and vascular malformations. **Hemangiomas** are benign tumors resulting from proliferation of cells of the vascular endothelium and are characterized by a growth phase, marked by endothelial proliferation and hypercellularity, and by an involutional phase. Malformations are developmental defects derived from the capillary, venous, arterial, or lymphatic vessels. These lesions remain relatively static; growth is commensurate with growth of the child. Differentiating between these two entities is important because they have different prognoses and clinical implications. **Vascular malformations** are congenital abnormalities that are composed of anomalous capillaries, veins, lymphatics, or any combination of the three.

HEMANGIOMAS

Hemangiomas are the most common soft tissue tumors of infancy, occurring in approximately 5% to 10% of 1-year-old infants. True hemangiomas are characterized by a growth phase, marked by endothelial proliferation and hypercellularity, and by an involutional phase. Hemangiomas are heterogeneous; their appearance is dictated by the depth and location in the skin and by the stage of evolution. In newborns, hemangiomas may originate as a pale white macule with threadlike telangiectasia. When the tumor proliferates, it assumes its most recognizable form, a bright red, slightly elevated, noncompressible plaque. Hemangiomas that lie deeper in the skin are soft, warm masses with a slightly bluish discoloration. Frequently, hemangiomas have a superficial and a deep component. They range from a few millimeters to several centimeters in diameter and are usually solitary; 20% involve multiple lesions. Hemangiomas occur predominantly in females (3:1) and have an increased incidence in premature infants. Approximately 55% are present at birth; the rest develop in the first weeks of life. Superficial hemangiomas reach their maximal size by 6 to 8 months, but deep hemangiomas may grow for 12 to 14 months. They then undergo slow, spontaneous resolution, which takes 3 to 10 years.

Despite the benign nature of most cutaneous hemangiomas, there may be the risk of functional compromise or permanent disfigurement depending on the location and extent. Ulceration, the most frequent complication, can be painful and increases the risk of infection, hemorrhage, and scarring.

The **Kasabach-Merritt** phenomenon, a complication of a rapidly enlarging vascular lesion, is characterized by hemolytic anemia, thrombocytopenia, and coagulopathy. These massive tumors are usually a deep red-blue color, are firm, grow rapidly, have no sex predilection, and tend to proliferate for a longer period (2 to 5 years). Most patients with Kasabach-Merritt phenomenon do not have typical hemangiomas, but have other proliferative vascular tumors, usually kaposiform hemangioendotheliomas or tufted angiomas. The Kasabach-Merritt phenomenon necessitates aggressive (often multimodality) treatment and carries a significant mortality rate.

Periorbital hemangiomas pose considerable risk to vision (amblyopia) and should be monitored carefully. Hemangiomas involving the ear may decrease auditory conduction, which ultimately may cause speech delay. Multiple cutaneous (diffuse hemangiomatosis) and large facial hemangiomas may be associated with visceral hemangiomas. **Subglottic hemangiomas** are manifested as hoarseness and stridor; progression to respiratory failure may be rapid. Approximately 50% of affected infants have associated cutaneous hemangiomas; "noisy breathing" in an infant with a cutaneous hemangioma involving the chin, lips, mandibular region, and neck warrants direct visualization of the airway. Symptomatic airway hemangiomas develop in greater than 50% of infants with extensive facial hemangiomas in the "beard" distribution.

Extensive cervicofacial hemangiomas may be associated with multiple anomalies, including *p*osterior fossa malformations, *h*emangiomas, *a*rterial anomalies, *c*oarctation of aorta and cardiac defects, and *e*ye abnormalities (**PHACE syndrome**). This syndrome has marked female predominance (9:1) and is thought to represent a developmental field defect that occurs during weeks 8 to 10 of gestation. Strokes are common. **Lumbosacral hemangiomas** suggest an occult spinal dysraphism with or without anorectal and urogenital anomalies. Imaging of the spine is indicated in all patients with midline cutaneous hemangiomas in the lumbosacral area. Most hemangiomas do not necessitate medical intervention and involute spontaneously; however, if complications arise, and treatment is warranted, oral systemic corticosteroids are the mainstay of therapy.

Pyogenic Granuloma

A pyogenic granuloma is an acquired, benign vascular tumor seen in toddlers and young children. They occur on the face in the periocular region and on the oral mucosa, hands, fingers, proximal upper extremity, and shoulders. Initially the lesions appear to be inconsequential, pink-red papules that often appear after minor trauma. The lesions grow slowly over a period of months to produce a bright red, vascular, often pedunculated papule measuring 2 to 10 mm. The lesions often have the appearance of granulation tissue and are very friable. When traumatized, these lesions may bleed profusely, often requiring emergent medical attention. Pulsed dye laser therapy or surgical excision is the most definitive treatment option.

VASCULAR MALFORMATIONS

As already stated, vascular malformations are congenital abnormalities that are composed of anomalous capillaries, veins, lymphatics, or any combination of the three.

Port-Wine Stain (Nevus Flammeus)

Port-wine stains (nevus flammeus) are malformations of the superficial capillaries of the skin. These lesions are present at birth and should be considered permanent developmental defects. Port-wine stain lesions may be only a few millimeters in diameter or may cover extensive areas, occasionally involving half the body surface. They do not proliferate after birth; any apparent increase in size is caused by growth of the child. A port-wine stain may be localized to any body surface, but facial lesions are the most common. Port-wine stains are pink-red, sharply demarcated macules and patches in infancy. With time, they darken to a purple or "port-wine" color and may develop a pebbly or slightly thickened surface. The most successful treatment modality in use is the pulsed dye laser, which is usually effective in fading these lesions. Treatment is more effective if undertaken in infancy.

Most port-wine stains occur as isolated defects and do not indicate systemic malformations. Rarely, they may suggest ocular defects or specific neurocutaneous syndromes. Children with facial port-wine stains involving skin innervated by the V1 branch of the trigeminal nerve are at risk for **Sturge-Weber syndrome** and should have a thorough ophthalmologic and neuroimaging evaluation in infancy (see Chapter 186). Sturge-Weber syndrome (encephalotrigeminal angiomatosis) consists of a facial port-wine stain, usually in the cutaneous distribution of the first branch of the trigeminal nerve; a leptomeningeal angiomatosis; mental retardation; seizures; hemiparesis contralateral to the facial lesions; and ipsilateral intracortical calcification. Ocular manifestations are frequent and include buphthalmos, glaucoma, angioma of the choroid, hemianoptic defects, and optic atrophy.

Radiographs of the skull of an older child show pathognomonic "tram-line," double-contoured calcifications in the cerebral cortex on the same side as the port-wine stain. MRI or CT may identify the calcifications in a younger child before they are apparent on radiographs. The prognosis depends on the extent of cerebral involvement, rapidity of progression, and response to treatment. Anticonvulsant therapy and neurosurgical procedures have been of value in some patients.

Klippel-Trénaunay-Weber syndrome is characterized by the triad of cutaneous capillary and venous malformations (usually a port-wine stain), venous varicosities, and hyperplasia of the soft tissues—and often bone—of the involved area. The lower limb is most commonly affected. Complications include severe edema, phlebitis, thrombosis, ulceration of the affected area, and vascular malformations involving the viscera. Port-wine stains also occur with moderate frequency in **Beckwith-Wiedemann syndrome** with macroglossia, omphalocele, macrosomia, hyperinsulinemic hypoglycemia, and cytomegaly of the fetal adrenal gland; in **Cobb syndrome** (cutaneomeningospinal angiomatosis), with arteriovenous or venous angioma of the spinal cord; and occasionally in **von Hippel–Lindau disease**, with cerebellar hemangioblastoma.

Transient Macular Stains (Salmon Patches)

Transient macular stains (salmon patches, stork bite, angel's kiss) are variants of nevus flammeus that are present in 70% of normal newborns. They are red, irregular, macular patches resulting from dilation of dermal capillaries and usually are found on the nape of the neck, the eyelids, and the glabella. Most of the facial lesions fade by 1 year of age, but lesions on the neck may persist for life. Surveys of adult populations confirm the persistence of the nuchal lesions in approximately 25% of the population.

Venous and Lymphatic Malformations

Venous malformations present as soft, blue, compressible plaques and nodules that may occur on any skin surface. They appear at birth and enlarge slowly with time secondary to engorgement of the anomalous vessels. Venous malformations may be quite small and of minimal concern or extremely large lesions that can be severely disfiguring and may be complicated by thrombosis, infection, and edema of surrounding tissue. **Lymphatic malformations (lymphangiomas)** are composed of dilated lymph channels that are lined by normal lymphatic endothelium. They may be superficial or deep and often are associated with anomalies of the regional lymphatic vessels.

The term **lymphangioma circumscriptum** is used to describe the most common type of lymphatic malformation, which may be present at birth or appear in early childhood. Areas of predilection are the oral mucosa, the proximal limbs, and the joint flexures. These lesions consist of clustered red-to-purple, gelatinous papules measuring 2 to 5 mm in size.

Cystic hygroma is a benign, congenital, multilocular mass of anomalous cystic lymph vessels. It usually is found in the neck region. Surgical excision or sclerotherapy is the available treatment option for venous and lymphatic malformations. The tumors tend to increase in size and should be treated by surgical excision.

Epidermal Nevi

Epidermal nevi are a group of lesions that are found in the neonatal period. Most consist of an overgrowth of keratinocytes that often have an identifiable differentiation toward one of the cutaneous appendages. They vary considerably in size, clinical appearance, histologic characteristics, and evolution, depending on topographic location. Lesions occurring in sites normally rich in sebaceous glands (the scalp) may look like sebaceous nevi, whereas others that are found in areas where the epidermis is thick (the elbow) look primarily warty in nature.

The most common type of epidermal nevus in a newborn is the nevus sebaceus, a hairless, papillomatous, yellow or pink, slightly elevated plaque on the scalp, forehead, or face. These lesions have a characteristic shape, often being oval or lancet shaped. Because a significant incidence of basal cell epitheliomas occurs in these lesions after puberty, they should be removed surgically.

CHAPTER **194**

Erythema Multiforme, Stevens-Johnson Syndrome, and Toxic Epidermal Necrolysis

EM minor, SJS (or EM major), and TEN are acute hypersensitivity reactions characterized by cutaneous and mucosal necrosis. These disorders may represent a continuum of a clinical spectrum ranging from the well-localized lesions of EM to the serious and life-threatening extensive desquamation of TEN. These syndromes represent a T cell–mediated hypersensitivity reaction to a precipitating cause, usually infectious organisms or drugs. Infectious agents are associated more closely with eruptions of EM minor and SJS, whereas drugs are implicated with the more severe reactions of TEN.

Other common vesiculobullous diseases include varicella and herpes simplex (see Chapter 98) and rarely epidermolysis bullosa and pemphigus (see Table 188–7). **Epidermolysis bullosa** is a group of rare, hereditary, blistering disorders characterized by blister formation caused by minor trauma. There are three major forms based on the level of skin separation, the pattern of inheritance, and the development of scarring. **Epidermolysis bullosa simplex** is a nonscarring, autosomal dominant disorder caused by defective keratin elements. **Junctional epidermolysis bullosa** is an autosomal recessive mechanobullous disorder with subepidermal blistering occurring within the dermal-epidermal junction. **Dystrophic epidermolysis bullosa** has autosomal dominant and recessive patterns with blister formation below the dermal-epidermal junction in the superficial papillary dermis. Systemic involvement may be severe, with gastrointestinal complications being the most common. The management of all forms of epidermolysis bullosa is symptomatic and palliative, consisting of good wound care, prevention of trauma, and treatment of secondary infection. Intact bullae should be drained because this increases comfort and prevents extension of the blister when it is compressed.

Pemphigus is a rare autoimmune disease caused by circulating autoantibodies to desmoglein 1 and 3, desmosomal proteins involved in the intercellular adhesion of epithelial cells, resulting in intraepidermal separation and blister formation. The disease is serious, but the prognosis in children is relatively good with appropriate treatment, usually long-term corticosteroids.

ERYTHEMA MULTIFORME MINOR

EM minor is a common, self-limiting, acute hypersensitivity syndrome characterized by the abrupt onset of 1- to 3-cm, oval or round, deep red, well-demarcated, flat macules with a dusky gray or bullous center. Some of the lesions have a wheal-like appearance; in contrast to urticaria, these are fixed and represent epidermal cell necrosis rather than the transient tissue edema of urticaria. The classic **target lesion** consists of three concentric rings; the outermost is red, the intermediate is white, and the center is a dusky red or blue. If blistering occurs, it is mild and involves less than 10% of the body surface area. Mucous membrane involvement tends to be minimal and affects no more than one mucosal surface. Cutaneous lesions are symmetric and involve the upper extremities, with the dorsal hands, palms, and extensor surfaces most commonly involved.

EM minor is less severe than SJS and accounts for nearly 80% of EM cases. Most EM cases in children are precipitated by herpes simplex virus infection and may recur with each episode of inapparent herpes infection. A positive clinical history of herpes labialis is obtained in 50% of cases. Herpes simplex virus DNA is detected in 80% of children with EM, suggesting that it is the primary cause of EM minor in children. Symptomatic treatment is usually sufficient. Oral antihistamines help suppress the pruritus, stinging, and burning. The use of systemic steroids is controversial and usually not indicated. Children with recurrent lesions associated with documented herpes simplex virus infections may be candidates for prophylactic oral acyclovir. The prognosis is excellent, with most lesions lasting no more than 2 weeks. Healing occurs without scarring.

STEVENS-JOHNSON SYNDROME (ERYTHEMA MULTIFORME MAJOR)

Stevens-Johnson syndrome is a severe, life-threatening, blistering hypersensitivity reaction. It is usually preceded by a febrile respiratory illness 1 to 14 days before the onset of cutaneous lesions. Involvement of at least two mucous membrane surfaces is required for diagnosis and is a distinguishing characteristic from EM minor. Children have extreme irritability, anorexia, and fever. The upper and lower lips are swollen and bright red with erosions and hemorrhagic crusts. Erosions of the tongue, buccal mucosa, and gingival margin may be seen. The eyelids are usually swollen. Early in the disease process, there is bilateral conjunctival injection; however, this usually progresses to conjunctival erosions. There may be erosions of the vaginal or perianal mucosa. Urogenital, esophageal, and tracheal surfaces may be involved in the most severe cases. The extent of skin involvement varies. There may be mucosal lesions only or a combination of mucosal and skin lesions. Red macules and target-like lesions appear suddenly and tend to coalesce into large patches, with a predominant distribution over the face and trunk. Skin lesions evolve rapidly into frank bullae and areas of necrosis. The extent of epidermal detachment is 10% to 20% of the body surface area.

Drugs and *Mycoplasma pneumoniae* infections are the most common causes of SJS in children. Herpes simplex virus seems to have no role in the pathogenesis of SJS. Other precipitating factors are other viral infections, bacteria, syphilis, and deep fungal infections. The most common drugs implicated are nonsteroidal anti-inflammatory drugs (NSAIDs), followed by sulfonamides, anticonvulsants, penicillins, and tetracycline derivatives.

SJS occurs in children 2 to 18 years old and seems to be more common in younger patients than EM. The diagnosis of SJS is clinical; there are no diagnostic tests. Confusion with potentially toxin-mediated diseases (Kawasaki disease, scarlet fever, toxic shock syndrome, and staphylococcal scalded skin syndrome) and rheumatologic disorders (Behçet disease) may occur. Patients with Kawasaki disease have conjunctival injection and hyperemia of the mucous membranes (see Chapter 88). Necrosis of the mucosal surfaces does not occur; blistering, erosions, and severe crusting are not observed. The mucosal changes of staphylococcal scalded skin syndrome are minor, and frank erosions are not present. The blistering of the skin is superficial and involves larger areas of the face and intertriginous regions. Rheumatologic disorders usually can be excluded by their chronic, less abrupt course.

SJS is a serious illness with a 5% to 15% mortality rate. Discontinuation of the offending agent, pain management, and supportive care are the mainstays of therapy. Children often require prolonged hospitalization. They have severe intraoral pain, resulting in poor oral intake. Parenteral or nasogastric feeding should be instituted early because this may accelerate the healing process. Careful fluid management and monitoring of electrolytes are essential. Skin cultures for potential infections should be performed, and appropriate parenteral antibiotics should be given if warranted. Systemic steroids have not been shown to be beneficial; they may increase morbidity and mortality.

The most common serious long-term sequelae of SJS involve ocular complications. Keratitis, corneal ulcerations, uveitis, severe conjunctivitis, and panophthalmitis may occur, leading to partial or complete blindness. An ophthalmology consultation with close follow-up is essential.

TOXIC EPIDERMAL NECROLYSIS

TEN is a severe, life-threatening condition characterized by extensive skin necrosis equivalent to a second-degree burn. It is distinguished from EM minor and SJS by larger body surface area involvement (>30%) and massive, sheetlike denudation of skin. Typically, greater than 50% body surface area is affected. Individual lesions overlap with lesions of EM, but are more abrupt in occurrence and evolution. An upper respiratory prodrome may have been present 1 to 3 days before skin manifestations. Patients with TEN present with high fever, severe irritability, and abrupt onset of diffuse, deep red or dusky discoloration of the skin. Intraepidermal blistering is suggested by the **Nikolsky sign**, which is elicited when there is an absence of cohesion between the keratinocytes of the superficial epidermis so that the separated layers easily slip laterally with minimal pressure. The children have exquisite pain of their skin and seem to have a toxic condition. The dusky redness rapidly progresses into sheetlike peeling of the entire epidermis, leaving deep erosions. Mucous membrane involvement is usually less than that of SJS; significant overlap can occur.

Drugs (nonsteroidal anti-inflammatory drugs, particularly ibuprofen and naproxen) are the most common precipitating factors. Sulfonamides, anticonvulsants, penicillins, and tetracyclines also have been reported to cause TEN. Infectious organisms are not associated with the development of TEN. TEN is a severe disease with a mortality of 30% to 50%. Supportive care with aggressive fluid and electrolyte management, wound care, and pain control results in decreased morbidity and mortality. Superinfection and respiratory failure are the major causes of death. Severely affected children may benefit from the wound care expertise of a burn unit. The use of systemic corticosteroids is controversial and is thought to increase the risk of infection and decrease wound healing. IV immunoglobulin and cyclosporine have been used with some encouraging results; controlled studies have not been performed.

CHAPTER 195
Cutaneous Infestations

Arthropods are common in the environment. Although many can bite or sting humans, only a few infest humans. Arachnids (mites) are the most common, parasitizing humans and animals by burrowing into the skin and depositing eggs within the skin.

SCABIES
Etiology

Scabies is caused by the mite *Sarcoptes scabiei*. The female mite burrows into the epidermis and deposits her eggs, which mature in 10 to 14 days. The disease is highly contagious because infested humans do not manifest the typical signs or symptoms for 3 to 4 weeks, facilitating transmission. An immunocompetent person with scabies typically harbors 10 to 20 mites.

Epidemiology

Scabies is the most common human infestation and is estimated to affect at least 300 million persons worldwide.

Clinical Manifestations

The clinical presentation varies depending on the age of the patient, the duration of infestation, and the immune status of the patient. Severe and paroxysmal itching is the hallmark, with complaints of itching that is frequently worse than the eruption would suggest. Most children exhibit an eczematous eruption composed of red, excoriated papules and nodules. The classic linear papule or burrow is often difficult to find. Distribution is the most diagnostic finding; the papules are found in the axillae, umbilicus, groin, penis, instep of the foot, and web spaces of the fingers and toes. Infants infested with scabies have diffuse erythema, scaling, and pinpoint papules. Pustules and vesicles are much more common in infants and are found in the axillae and groin and on the palms and soles. The face and scalp usually are spared in adults and older children, but these areas are usually involved in infants. Chronic lesions may develop a malodorous, scaly crust. Immunocompromised or neurologically impaired persons may develop a severe form of the disease known as **Norwegian** or **crusted scabies**, with infestation of 2 million live mites at one time.

Laboratory and Imaging Studies

The diagnosis of scabies can be confirmed by microscopic visualization of the mite, eggs, larvae, or feces in scrapings of papules or burrows examined under oil immersion. Skin biopsy is rarely necessary but may be useful if lesions have become nodular.

Differential Diagnosis

The diagnosis of scabies should be considered in any child with severe itching, and a thorough search for an infested contact should be undertaken.

Treatment

Curative treatment is achieved by a 12-hour (overnight) application of permethrin 5% cream applied to the entire body. Gamma benzene hexachloride should be avoided in young children because of a small risk of CNS toxicity. Parents and all caregivers should be treated simultaneously. Itching persists for 7 to 14 days after the mites have been killed. Bed linens, towels, pajamas, and clothes worn for the previous 2 days before treatment should be machine-washed in hot water and machine-dried using high heat. Heat is the most effective scabicide. Items that are not washable may be dry-cleaned or placed in a sealed plastic bag for 24 hours.

Complications

Secondary bacterial infection may occur, but is uncommon. Scabies can be much more severe among immunocompromised persons. In contrast to the pediculoses, scabies is not a vector for infections.

Prognosis

Pruritus may persist for 7 to 14 days after successful therapy because of a prolonged hypersensitivity reaction, which does not indicate treatment failure. Inadequate treatment or reinfestation should be suspected if new lesions develop after treatment.

Prevention

The family should be educated about the mode of scabies transmission. Mites live only a short time off the body, and extensive fumigation is not necessary.

PEDICULOSES

Etiology

Three species of lice infest humans: *Pediculus humanus capitis,* the **head louse**; *Pthirus pubis,* the **pubic louse** or **crab louse**; and *Pediculus humanus humanus,* (also known as *Pediculus humanus corporis*), the **body louse**. Lice are wingless insects 2 to 4 mm in length that cannot fly or jump. Transmission usually occurs by direct contact with the head of another infested individual. Indirect spread through contact with fomites or personal belongings of an infested individual, such as hairbrushes, combs, or caps, is much less frequent.

Pediculosis differs from scabies infestation in that the louse resides on the hair or clothing and intermittently feeds on the host by piercing the skin. The "bite" causes small urticarial papules and itching. Head lice live close to the skin and may live for 30 days, depositing 100 to 400 eggs as **nits** on hair shafts, usually within 6 mm of the scalp.

Epidemiology

Head lice infestations are unrelated to hygiene. Head lice are seen most frequently in early school-age children but are not more common among children with long hair or with dirty hair. It is estimated that 6 to 12 million persons in the U.S. and 1% to 3% of persons in developed countries are infested with head lice each year. In the U.S., head lice infestation is rare among African Americans and may be more common in girls, which is attributed to their tendency to play more closely with one another than boys do.

Pubic lice are transmitted by sexual contact. Their presence in children may be a sign of child abuse. Body lice are firm evidence of poor hygiene, such as infrequent washing and clothing changes.

Clinical Manifestations

Itching, if present, is the primary symptom. Pediculosis capitis usually causes pruritus behind the ears or on the nape of the neck or a crawling sensation in the scalp. Pediculosis pubis usually causes mild to severe pruritus in the groin. Eyelash involvement in children may cause crusting and blepharitis. Pediculosis corporis causes pruritus that, because of repeated scratching, may result in lichenification or secondary bacterial infection. Excoriations and crusting, with or without associated regional lymphadenopathy, may be present.

Laboratory and Imaging Studies

No laboratory or imaging studies are necessary.

Differential Diagnosis

Infestation with the head louse may be asymptomatic and has little morbidity. The diagnosis can be confirmed by visualizing a live louse. A fine-toothed comb to trap lice is more effective than simply looking at the hair. Wet combing is more time-consuming, but dry combing produces static that may propel the lice away from the comb.

Nits represent the outer casing of the louse ova. **Brown nits** located on the proximal hair shaft suggest active infestation. **White nits** located on the hair shaft 4 cm or further from the scalp indicate previous infestation. Because nits remain stuck in the hair for weeks to months after an infestation has resolved, many children with nits do not have active lice infestation.

Treatment

The treatment of head lice is controversial because resistance to many established options has been shown. Over-the-counter permethrin (1%) and pyrethrin-based products (0.17% to 0.33%) are the first choices of therapy. Because 20% to 30% of eggs may survive one treatment, a second treatment should be applied in 7 to 10 days. The prevalence of drug resistance has not been determined. Malathion (0.5%) lotion may be used as an alternative for resistant cases, but most treatment failures are likely due to misdiagnosis or misapplication of the medications.

Everyone in the family should be checked for head lice and treated if live lice are found, to reduce the risk of reinfestation. Bed linens, towels, pajamas, and clothes worn for the previous 2 days before treatment should be machine-washed in hot water and machine-dried using high heat. Items that are not washable may be dry-cleaned or placed in a sealed plastic bag for 24 hours. Brushes and combs should be soaked in dish detergent or rubbing alcohol for 1 hour. Rugs, furniture, mattresses, and car seats should be vacuumed thoroughly.

The finding of active lice infestation indicates their presence for 1 month or more. Manual removal of nits after treatment is not necessary to prevent spread.

Children treated for head lice should return to school immediately after completion of the first effective treatment or first wet combing, regardless of the presence of remaining nits. There is no evidence that "no nit" or "nit-free" policies reduce transmission of head lice. If required for return to school, nit removal is best achieved by wetting the hair and combing with a fine-toothed metal comb.

Complications

Excoriations can become secondarily infected with skin bacteria, usually *Staphylococcus* and *Streptococcus*. The body louse functions as a vector for potentially serious infectious diseases, including **epidemic typhus**, caused by *Rickettsia prowazekii*; **louse-borne relapsing fever**, caused by *Borrelia recurrentis*; and **trench fever**, caused by *Bartonella quintana*. These louse-borne infections are rare in the U.S. In contrast to body lice, head lice and pubic lice are not associated with transmission of other infections.

Prognosis

Pediculicide treatment along with appropriate disinfestation measures of fomites is highly effective. Reinfestation from untreated contacts or fomites, especially for pediculosis corporis, is more likely than primary treatment failure.

Prevention

Families, school nurses, and other healthcare professionals need to be educated about the mode of transmission and precise diagnosis before treatment of contacts is instituted. There is no evidence that group screening is effective.

SUGGESTED READING

Barbagallo JS, Kolodzieh MS, Silverberg NB, Weinberg JM: Neurocutaneous disorders. Dermatol Clin 20:547-560, 2002.

Behrman RE, Kliegman RM, Jenson HB (eds): Nelson Textbook of Pediatrics, 17th ed. Philadelphia, WB Saunders, 2003.

Bhumbra NA, McCullough SG: Skin and subcutaneous infections. Prim Care 30:1-24, 2003.

Bruckner AL, Frieden IJ: Hemangiomas in infancy. J Am Acad Dermatol 48:477-493, 2003.

James WD: Clinical practice: Acne. N Engl J Med 352:1463-1472, 2005.

Nopper AJ, George ME: Rashes and skin lesions. In Kliegman RM, Greenbaum LA, Lye PS (eds): Practical Strategies in Pediatric Diagnosis and Therapy, 2nd ed. Philadelphia, WB Saunders, 2004, pp 1017-1058.

Spergel JM, Paller AS: Atopic dermatitis and the atopic march. J Allergy Clin Immunol 112(6 Suppl):S118-S127, 2003.

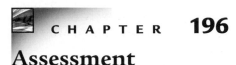

CHAPTER **196**

Assessment

Multiple congenital and acquired mechanisms may produce orthopedic problems specific to childhood; other pathologic mechanisms are common to all age groups (Table 196–1).

IN UTERO POSITIONING

The in utero position produces joint and muscle contractures and affects torsional and angular alignment of long bones, especially of the lower extremities (Fig. 196–1). All normal full-term newborns have 20- to 30-degree hip and knee flexion contractures. These contractures decrease to neutral by 4 to 6 months of age. The newborn hip externally rotates in extension 80 to 90 degrees and has limited internal rotation of 0 to 10 degrees. The normal newborn foot also may reflect the in utero position. Most commonly, in utero the feet are in the tucked-under position, which can be observed after birth. On inspection, the forefoot appears adducted or deviated inwardly with respect to the hindfoot, the heel may be inverted, and the foot tends to be in equinus or pointed down at the ankle. If the foot can be positioned so that the lateral border is straight, the heel slightly everted, and the foot dorsiflexed to above a right angle, the clinical diagnosis of normal in utero positioning is validated.

The face may be distorted by in utero positioning, whereas the spine and upper extremities are less affected. The effects of normal in utero position are physiologic in origin but produce parental concern. The child may be 3 to 4 years old before the intrauterine effects completely resolve.

DEVELOPMENTAL MILESTONES AND NEUROLOGIC MATURATION

Neurologic maturation, marked by the achievement of motor milestones at the regular intervals, is important for normal musculoskeletal development (see Section II). A trophic relationship exists between skeletal form and gross motor development. Normal neurologic development must be included in the definition of a normal musculoskeletal system. Any process that produces a neurologic abnormality secondarily may cause an aberration of musculoskeletal growth. Any disorder that primarily affects skeletal muscle may produce abnormalities of skeletal growth and development.

GAIT

Disturbances of gait, including **limp**, are common manifestations of pediatric orthopedic disorders (Tables 196–2 and 196–3). Understanding the normal developmental aspects of gait is helpful in distinguishing maturational from pathologic processes. Normal gait (walking on level ground) is composed of a stance phase and a swing phase. The gait cycle is the interval between stance phases on the same limb. The stance phase (60% of gait) is performed when the foot, which bears weight, contacts the ground; it begins with the heel-strike and ends with the toe-off. In the swing phase (40%), the foot is off the ground. A toddler's (12 to 18 months old) gait is quite hesitant and inconsistent. The gait is broad based and characterized by rapid cadence, short steps, flatfoot initial ground contact, and nonaccompaniment by the reciprocal arm swing. A 2-year-old has increased velocity and step length and a diminished cadence. Normal adult gait is achieved by 3 to 7 years old.

Limping is either painless or painful (see Table 196–2). A painful limp is characterized by acute onset

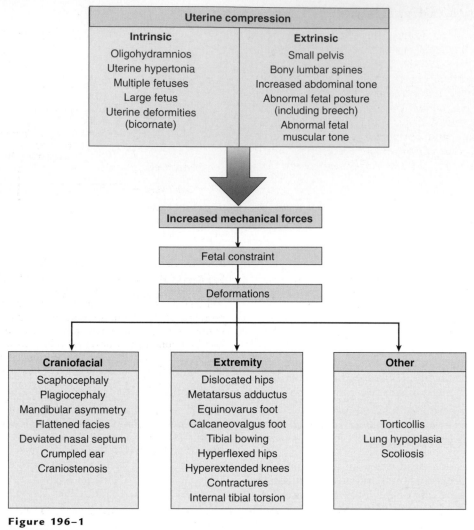

Figure 196–1

Deformation abnormalities resulting from uterine compression.

and usually is caused by trauma, infection (septic arthritis and osteomyelitis), or acquired disorders (see Table 196–3). Stance phase and stride length are shortened in an attempt to decrease standing on the involved limb. Trunk shift to the opposite side also decreases stress and maintains balance; this is referred to as an **antalgic gait**. A painless limp is characterized by normal stance phase, but a persistent trunk sway. This type of gait is called a **Trendelenburg gait**.

Painless limping may be associated with neuromuscular disorders producing muscle weakness about the hip, especially in the gluteus medius muscle, the major hip abductor. This muscle stabilizes the pelvis during stance phase and prevents a pelvic drop to the opposite side. Trauma or weakness of this muscle and inflammatory hip disorders are the most common causes of limping. Disorders that have bilateral involvement produce a **waddling gait**.

Knee pathology, usually from trauma, can produce a limp by limiting knee flexion and causing the child to circumduct the leg and elevate the pelvis during swing phase. It also produces a shortened stance phase. Poor dorsiflexion of the foot resulting from weakness (peroneal nerve injury or peripheral neuropathy) or trauma causes increased knee flexion for toe clearance during the swing phase, resulting in a **drop-foot gait**. **Toe-walking**, which is common in early walkers, may be the result of habit, leg length discrepancy, underlying neuromuscular disorder (cerebral palsy), or a congenital contracture of the gastrocnemius and soleus muscles (Achilles tendon or heel cord).

GROWTH AND DEVELOPMENT

During the growing years, the ends of long bone contain a much greater proportion of cartilage than after maturity (Fig. 196–2). The high cartilage content (articular and physeal) leads to a unique vulnerability from trauma and metaphyseal infections. The infections may involve the metaphysis, joint space, or both.

Special anatomic features within the child's skeletal system stimulate and support the various kinds of skeletal growth that continuously occur in the immature skeleton (Fig. 196–3). The epiphyseal growth plate,

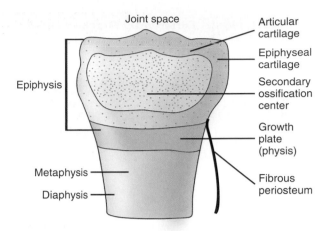

Figure 196–3

Schematic of long bone structure. The shaft, or diaphysis, is adjacent to the metaphysis, which is the closest extension of endochondral bone. The epiphyseal growth plate (physis) is the avascular cartilage between the articular surface and the metaphyseal bone. The growth plate is the region of longitudinal bone growth. The contribution to eventual bone length varies: 80% for proximal humerus, 20% for the distal ulna, 70% for the distal femur, 57% for the proximal tibia, and 60% for the proximal fibula. When growth is complete, the epiphyseal growth plate is ossified or closed. The cartilaginous epiphyseal plate is supported by internal interdigitation with the metaphyseal bone and externally by the insertion of the fibrous periosteum. (Modified from Shapiro F: Epiphyseal Disorders. N Engl J Med 317:1702, 1987.)

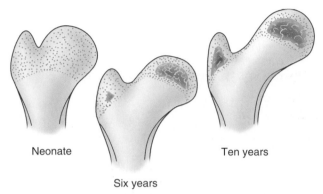

Figure 196–2

Lightly stippled areas represent cartilage composition, whereas heavily darkened areas are zones of ossification. (From Tachjidan MO: Congenital Dislocation of the Hip. New York, Churchill Livingtone, 1982, p 105.)

Category	Mechanism	Example
TABLE 196–1. Mechanisms of Common Pediatric Orthopedic Problems		
Congenital		
Malformation	Teratogenesis before 12 wk gestation	Spina bifida
Disruption	Amniotic band constriction	Extremity amputation
	Fetal varicella infection	Limb scar/atrophy
Deformation	Leg compression	Developmental dysplasia of the hip (DDH)
	Neck compression	Torticollis
Dysplasia	Abnormal cell growth or metabolism	Osteogenesis imperfecta
		Skeletal dysplasias
Acquired		
Infection	Pyogenic-hematogenous spread	Septic arthritis, osteomyelitis
Inflammation	Antigen-antibody reaction	Systemic lupus erythematosus
	Immune mediated	Juvenile rheumatoid arthritis
Trauma	Mechanical forces, overuse	Child abuse, sports injuries, unintentional injury, fractures, dislocations, tendinitis
Tumor	Primary bone tumor	Osteosarcoma
	Metastasis to bone from other site	Neuroblastoma
	Bone marrow tumor	Leukemia, lymphoma

TABLE 196–2. Differential Diagnosis of Gait Disturbances (Limping)

Early Walker (1-3 Years Old)

Painful Limp

Septic arthritis and osteomyelitis
Transient monarticular synovitis
Occult trauma ("toddler's fracture")
Intervertebral discitis

Painless Limp

Developmental dysplasia of the hip
Neuromuscular disorder
Cerebral palsy
Lower extremity length inequality

Child (3-10 Years Old)

Painful Limp

Septic arthritis and osteomyelitis
Transient monarticular synovitis
Trauma
Rheumatologic disorders
  Juvenile rheumatoid arthritis
Intervertebral discitis

Painless Limp

Developmental dysplasia of the hip
Legg-Calvé-Perthes disease
Lower extremity length inequality
Neuromuscular disorder
  Cerebral palsy
  Muscular dystrophy (Duchenne)

Adolescent (11 Years Old to Maturity)

Painful Limp

Septic arthritis and osteomyelitis
Trauma
Rheumatologic disorder
Slipped capital femoral epiphysis: acute; unstable

Painless Limp

Slipped capital femoral epiphysis: chronic; stable
Developmental dysplasia of the hip: acetabular
  dysplasia
Lower extremity length inequality
Neuromuscular disorder

(rickets), regional soft tissue processes, inborn errors of metabolism (mucopolysaccharidosis, mucolipidosis, Gaucher disease, and disorders of collagen or cartilage synthesis), and other metabolic processes (oxalosis, renal tubular acidosis, uremia, and endocrine excess or deficiencies) may affect each of these processes,

TABLE 196–3. Mechanisms of Gait Disturbances with or without Pain

Mechanical

Trauma, fracture, sprain
Sports injury; overuse injury
Child abuse
Developmental dysplasia of the hip

Osseous

Legg-Calvé-Perthes disease
Slipped capital femoral epiphysis
Osteomyelitis
Discitis
Osteoid osteoma

Articular

Septic arthritis
Toxic synovitis
Rheumatic disease (JRA, SLE)
Hemophilia

Neurologic

Guillain-Barré syndrome (other peripheral neuropathies)
Intoxication
Cerebellar ataxia
Brain tumor
Lesion occupying spinal cord space
Myopathy
Hemiplegia
Sympathetic reflex dystrophy

Hematologic

Sickle cell pain crisis
Leukemia
Metastatic tumor
Bone tumor
Langerhans cell histiocytosis

Other

Kawasaki disease
Conversion reaction
Gaucher disease
Scurvy
Rickets
Psoas abscess

JRA, juvenile rheumatoid arthritis; SLE, systemic lupus erythematosus.

---

also called the **physis**, provides for longitudinal growth of the bones. Articular cartilage provides for enlargement of the bone ends and for growth of some of the small bones largely covered by articular cartilage, such as the carpals and tarsals. The perichondrium and the periosteum provide appositional growth or circumferential growth of the cartilage and skeletal structures. Trauma, infection, nutritional deficiency

TABLE 196–4. Glossary of Orthopedic Terminology

Abduction	Movement away from the midline
Adduction	Movement toward and possibly across the midline
Anteversion	Increased angulation of the femoral head and neck with respect to the knee in the frontal plane
Apophysis	Bone growth center that is not a growth plate and that has a strong muscle insertion (e.g., greater trochanter of femur)
Arthroplasty	Surgical reconstruction of a joint
Arthrotomy	Surgical incision into a joint
Calcaneus	Dorsiflexion of hindfoot
Cavovarus	High longitudinal or medial arch of foot with plantar-flexed supinated forefoot and hindfoot varus
Cavus	High longitudinal arch of the foot (usually plantar-flexed forefoot)
Dislocation	Complete loss of contact between 2 joint surfaces
Equinus	Plantar flexion of the forefoot, hindfoot, or entire foot
Extension	Means to straighten, and is the reverse of flexion
External rotation	External rotation, away from the midline
Flexion	Means to bend
Internal rotation	Inward rotation, toward the midline
Osteotomy	Surgical division of a bone
Subluxation	Incomplete loss of contact between 2 joint surfaces
Valgum	Angulation of a bone or joint in which the apex is toward the midline; genu valgum or knock-knee
Varum	Angulation of a bone or joint away from the midline; genu varum or bowleg

producing a distinct aberration in the particular growth function.

The terminology used in orthopedics to describe position, motion, and function can be confusing. Some common orthopedic terms are presented in Table 196–4.

CHAPTER 197
Musculoskeletal Trauma

Fractures in children account for 10% to 15% of all childhood injuries. Children's skeletal systems have anatomic, biomechanical, and physiologic differences from those of adults. These differences result in different fracture patterns, including epiphyseal injuries, problems of diagnosis, and variation in management techniques.

The anatomic differences in the pediatric skeleton include the presence of preosseous cartilage, physes, and thicker, stronger periosteum that produces callus more rapidly and in greater amounts. Biomechanically, the pediatric skeletal system can absorb more energy before deformation and fracture than adult bone can. This increased absorbency has been attributed to lower ash content and greater porosity of young bone. As maturation occurs, the porosity decreases, and the cortical bone becomes thicker and stronger. The thick periosteum of a child's bone is a major determinant in

whether a fracture becomes displaced. The thick periosteum also can act as an impediment to closed reduction because of the hinging phenomenon. Conversely, it can help stabilize a fracture after reduction.

UNUSUAL FEATURES
Fracture Remodeling

Remodeling occurs by a combination of periosteal resorption and new bone formation. Anatomic alignment in certain pediatric fractures is not always necessary. The major factors affecting fracture remodeling are the child's age, the proximity of the fracture to a joint, and the relationship of the fracture to the plane of joint motion. The amount of remaining musculoskeletal growth provides the basis for remodeling; the younger the child, the greater the remodeling potential. Certain physes also have a relatively greater growth potential than others. Fractures adjacent to a physis undergo the greatest amount of remodeling, provided that the residual deformity is in the plane of motion of that joint. Fracture remodeling is not effective in displaced intra-articular fractures, diaphyseal fractures, malrotation, and fracture displacement or deformity not in the plane of joint motion. The amount of remodeling is significantly diminished as a child approaches skeletal maturity.

Overgrowth

Overgrowth, especially in long bones such as the femur, is the result of the increased blood flow associated with fracture healing. Femoral fractures in children younger than 10 years old frequently overgrow 1 to 3 cm. This accounts for the concept of *bayonet apposition* to compensate for the overgrowth that may occur over the next 1 to 2 years. After 10 years of age, overgrowth is less of a problem, and end-on alignment is recommended.

Progressive Deformity

Injuries to a physis can result in complete or partial closure. As a consequence, angular deformity, shortening, or both can occur. The magnitude depends on the bone involved and the amount of remaining growth. Growth arrest most commonly occurs in the distal femur, distal tibia, and proximal tibia.

Healing Rate

Fractures heal more quickly in children than in adults. This effect is due to their growth potential and thicker, more metabolically active periosteum. As older children and adolescents mature, the rate of healing slows and approaches that of adults.

PEDIATRIC FRACTURE PATTERNS
Nonepiphyseal Fractures
Complete

Complete fractures occur when both sides of the bone are fractured. This is the most common fracture type. These fractures may be classified as spiral, transverse, oblique, or comminuted, depending on the direction of the fracture line.

Buckle or Torus Fracture

Compression of bone produces a buckle or torus fracture. These fractures typically occur in the metaphyseal areas in young children, especially the distal radius. They are inherently stable and usually heal in 2 to 3 weeks with simple immobilization.

Greenstick

When a bone is angulated beyond the limits of plastic deformation, a greenstick fracture may occur. This type of fracture represents bone failure on the tension side and compression or bend deformity on the opposite side. The energy has been insufficient to result in a complete fracture.

Bowing or Bend Fractures

Traumatic bowing or bend deformities are due to plastic deformation of bone. The bone was angulated beyond its limit of plastic deformation, but did not fracture. No fracture line is visible radiographically.

Epiphyseal Fractures

Fractures involving the physes are common, constituting 15% to 20% of all children's fractures. There is a male-to-female ratio of 2:1, and the upper extremity is involved twice as frequently as the lower. The peak incidence in boys is 13 to 14 years and in girls is 11 to 12 years. The distal radius is the most common site, followed by the distal tibia.

Ligaments frequently insert into epiphyses. As a consequence, traumatic forces supplied to an extremity may be transmitted to the physis. The strength of the physes is enhanced by their shape and by the perichondrial ring. The physis still is not as strong biomechanically, however, as the metaphyseal or diaphyseal bone. The physis is most resistant to traction and least resistant to torsional or angular forces.

Classification

Salter and Harris classified epiphyseal injuries into five groups (Fig. 197–1):

- *Type I*—epiphyseal separation through the physis
- *Type II*—fracture through a portion of the physis, but exiting across the metaphysis
- *Type III*—fracture through the physis, but exiting across the epiphysis into the joint
- *Type IV*—a fracture line extending across the metaphysis, physis, and epiphysis
- *Type V*—a crush injury to the physis

This classification allows generalized prognostic information regarding the risk for premature physeal closure and the indications for treatment. A *type VI* injury (injury to the perichondral ring that often results in a peripheral bony bridge and rapid angular deformities) also has been suggested.

Treatment

Types I and II fractures usually can be managed by closed reduction techniques and do not require perfect alignment. A major exception is type II fractures of the distal femur. Fractures in this location have a poor prognosis, unless almost anatomic alignment is obtained by either closed or open methods. Types III and IV epiphyseal fractures require anatomic alignment because of displacement of the physis and the articular surfaces. Type V fractures usually are recognized in retrospect and invariably result in premature growth plate closure.

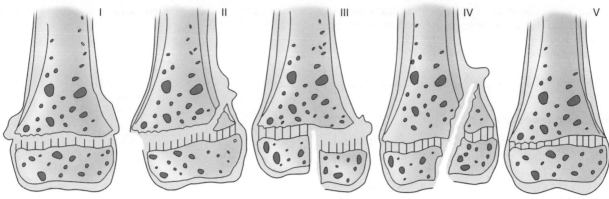

Figure 197–1

The types of growth plate injury as classified by Salter and Harris. (From Salter RB, Harris WR: Injuries involving the epiphyseal plate. J Bone Joint Surg Am 45:587, 1963.)

MANAGEMENT OF PEDIATRIC FRACTURES

Most pediatric fractures can be managed by closed methods. Some fractures have a better prognosis if the fractures are reduced, by either open or closed techniques, and then internally fixed. Approximately 3% to 4% of pediatric fractures require internal fixation. Common indications for internal fixation in children and adolescents with open physes include the following:

- Displaced epiphyseal fractures
- Displaced intra-articular fractures
- Unstable fractures
- Fractures in the multiply injured child
- Open fractures

In children, the goals of surgery and type of internal fixation device used are different. The goals of surgery are not rigid internal fixation, but rather attainment and maintenance of anatomic alignment. Simple fixation with the use of Steinmann pins, Kirschner wires, and small cortical screws is indicated. Fractures subsequently are protected with external immobilization, usually a plaster cast, until satisfactory healing has occurred. All internal fixation devices are removed after fracture healing to prevent incorporation into the callus formation and bone and to prevent physeal damage if a physis has been transgressed by a smooth wire or pin.

External fixation also has been successful for certain pediatric fractures. The major indications are pelvic and open extremity fractures, especially fractures with extensive soft tissue loss, burns, or vascular and nerve repairs.

SPECIAL PROBLEMS

Neurovascular Injuries

The most common sites of neural or vascular injuries are the distal humerus, in which supracondylar fractures occur, and the knee, in which dislocations and physeal fractures or dislocations occur. Careful neurovascular examination is necessary for all fractures and should be documented in the patient's medical record.

Compartment Syndromes

Hemorrhage and soft tissue swelling within tight fascial compartments may result in muscle ischemia and neurovascular compromise unless decompressed surgically. This condition is called **compartment syndrome**. The forearm and lower leg are the major sites, and these syndromes tend to occur after supracondylar fractures at the distal humerus and tibial shaft fractures. Common findings are tense compartments, severe pain, decreased sensation in the nerves that transverse the involved compartment, and pain with passive stretch (fingers or toes) of involved muscles. In addition, when an injured extremity is placed in a cast, it is possible that a cast-induced compartment syndrome may develop. It is the responsibility of the treating physician to ensure that parents understand the signs of ischemia and appreciate that it is an emergency. The parents must contact the physician or return to the hospital immediately.

Toddler's Fracture

An oblique fracture of the distal one third of the tibia without a fibula fracture can occur with minimal trauma in children 1 to 3 years old and occasionally up to 6 years old. Limping or inability to bear weight is a common complaint. These fractures may not be visible radiographically, but occasionally oblique radiographs may be helpful. A physical examination may show minimal soft tissue swelling, pain, and slight warmth.

Child Abuse

Fractures attributable to child abuse constitute a special issue that constantly must be considered in trauma assessment of infants and young children, especially children 3 years old or younger (see Chapter 22). Multiple fractures that are visible radiographically at different stages of healing are a classic sign. If a child has been shaken, frequently areas adjacent to the epiphysis on the metaphyseal side fracture, producing the appearance of metaphyseal "corner" fractures. Long bone fractures, especially spiral fractures of the humeral, tibial, or femoral shaft, suggest that someone has forcefully twisted the extremity. When there is any suspicion of abuse, the child should be admitted to the hospital for full assessment. Radiographs of a specific area are appropriate, but a bone scan may be more helpful in identifying other, old and new fractures. A thorough physical examination focusing on soft tissues, the skeletal system, and the cranium, along with a careful examination of the retina for hemorrhage or detachment, is important.

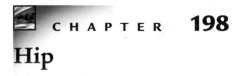

CHAPTER 198

Hip

The hip is a ball (femoral head) and socket (acetabulum) joint that provides the skeleton with structural balance and stability. The femoral head and acetabulum have a trophic relationship and are interdependent for normal growth and development (Fig. 198–1). When this trophic relationship is interrupted, abnormal hip development follows. Muscle balance and activity related to appropriate gross motor development are essential to normal development of the hip. The blood supply to the capital femoral epiphysis (CFE) or femoral head is unique because the CFE and femoral neck lie intracapsularly, but the blood supply from the retinacular vessels is extraosseous, lying on the surface of the femoral neck and entering the epiphysis peripherally. The blood supply to the femoral head is vulnerable to damage from septic arthritis, trauma, and other vascular insults. **Avascular necrosis** or **osteonecrosis**, either as an idiopathic process or secondary to other disorders, is common in children.

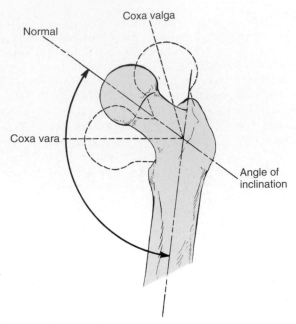

Figure 198–1

Coxa vara and coxa valga. The neck-shaft angle is measured on an anteroposterior radiograph. This angle is formed by a line drawn through the femoral shaft center and one bisecting the head and neck. Normally the value of this angle decreases with age. A reasonably accurate neck-shaft angle measurement may be made on an anteroposterior pelvic radiograph by placing the patient's hips in maximal internal rotation. Otherwise, because of the illusion caused by anteversion or external rotation on a one-plane radiograph, the measured neck-shaft angle value may be considerably larger than the true value. Internal femur rotation has a negligible effect on the neck-shaft angle. (From Chung SMK: Hip Disorders in Infants and Children. Philadelphia, Lea & Febiger, 1981, p 85.)

DEVELOPMENTAL DYSPLASIA OF THE HIP

Developmental dysplasia of the hip (DDH) represents abnormal development or dislocation of the hip; at birth, the hips usually are not dislocated, but rather "dislocatable." Dislocations tend to occur after delivery. Because dislocations are not truly congenital in origin, the term DDH is more appropriate than congenital dysplasia or dislocation of the hip. DDH is classified into two major groups: **typical**, in a neurologically normal infant, and **teratologic**, when an underlying neuromuscular disorder (myelodysplasia or arthrogryposis multiplex congenita) or syndrome complex is present. The teratologic type of dislocation occurs in utero. Typical DDH is the most common form.

Etiology

The causes of DDH are multifactorial. *Physiologic* factors are a positive family history (in 20% of cases), generalized ligamentous laxity, maternal estrogen and other hormones associated with pelvic ligament relaxation, and female predominance (9:1). *Mechanical* factors are primigravida, breech presentation, oligohydramnios, and postnatal positioning. The positive family history and the generalized ligamentous laxity are related factors. Maternal estrogens and other hormones associated with pelvic relaxation also result in further, although temporary, relaxation of the newborn hip joint.

Approximately 60% of children with typical DDH are firstborn, and 30% to 50% are in a breech position. In this presentation, the fetal pelvis is positioned in the maternal pelvis, which results in extreme hip flexion and limitation of hip motion. Increased hip flexion results in stretching of the already lax capsule and ligamentum teres. It also produces posterior uncoverage of the femoral head. This position and decreased hip motion alter the normal trophic relationship of the hip, resulting in abnormal development of the cartilaginous acetabulum.

The sex ratio of infants with DDH who are breech is 2:1 female to male. The gender change substantiates the importance of the mechanical factors of the breech position in the development of DDH. Congenital muscular torticollis (14% to 20% of cases) and metatarsus adductus (1% to 10%) also are associated with DDH. The presence of either of these two conditions necessitates a careful examination of the hips.

Postnatal factors also are important. Maintaining the hips in the position of adduction and extension is a major factor leading to dislocation. Placing the extremities in this position puts the unstable hip under pressure as a result of the normally present hip flexion and abduction contractures. As a consequence, the femoral head can be displaced from the acetabulum over several days, weeks, or perhaps months.

Clinical Manifestations

Particular test results and other physical findings are common in infants with DDH. The **Barlow test** is the most important maneuver in examination of the newborn hip. This is a provocative test that attempts to dislocate an unstable hip. The examiner stabilizes the infant's pelvis with one hand, then flexes and adducts the opposite hip and applies a posterior force (Fig. 198-2). If the hip is dislocatable, this is usually readily felt. After release of the posterior pressure, the hip usually relocates spontaneously. It has been estimated that 1 in 100 newborns has clinically unstable

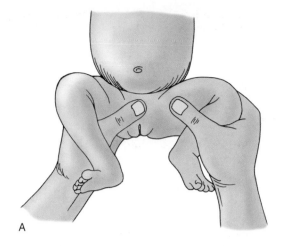

A

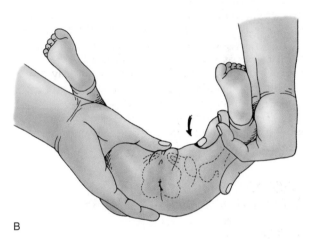

B

Figure 198-2

Barlow (dislocation) test. Reverse of Ortolani test. If the femoral head is in the acetabulum at the time of examination, the Barlow test is performed to discover any hip instability. **A,** The infant's thigh is grasped as shown and adducted with gentle downward pressure. **B,** Dislocation is palpable as the femoral head slips out of the acetabulum. Diagnosis is confirmed with the Ortolani test.

hips (subluxation or dislocation), but only 1 in 800 to 1000 infants develops a persistent dislocation.

The **Ortolani test** is a maneuver to reduce a recently dislocated hip. The result is most likely to be positive in infants 1 to 2 months old because adequate time must pass for the true dislocation to have occurred. In this test, the infant's thigh is flexed and abducted, and the femoral head is lifted anteriorly toward the acetabulum (Fig. 198-3). If reduction is possible, the relocation is felt as a "clunk," not as a "click." After 2 months

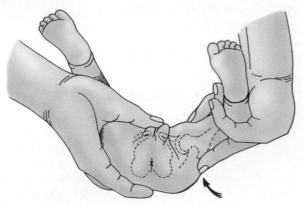

Figure 198-3

Ortolani (reduction) test. With the infant relaxed and content on a firm surface, the hips and knees are flexed to 90 degrees. The hips are examined one at a time. The examiner grasps the infant's thigh with the middle finger over the greater trochanter and lifts the thigh to bring the femoral head from its dislocated posterior position to opposite the acetabulum. Simultaneously the thigh is gently abducted, reducing the femoral head in the acetabulum. In a positive finding, the examiner senses reduction by a palpable, nearly audible "clunk."

of age, manual reduction of a dislocated hip is not usually possible because of the development of soft tissue contractures.

Limitation of hip abduction indicates soft tissue contractures and may indicate DDH (Fig. 198-4). Conversely, hip abduction contractures may indicate dysplasia of the contralateral hip.

An **asymmetric number of thigh skin folds** and apparent shortening of an extremity (uneven knee levels) when the supine infant's feet are placed together on the examining table with the hips and knees flexed (**positive Galeazzi sign**) suggest DDH because these findings indicate proximal displacement of the femoral head. In older or walking children, complaints of limping, waddling (bilateral DDH), increased lumbar lordosis (swayback), toe-walking, and in-toeing may be associated with an unrecognized DDH.

A common concern regarding an unstable hip is the presence of a hip "click." This click is usually not pathologic and is secondary to breaking the surface tension across the hip joint, snapping of gluteal tendons, patellofemoral motion, or femorotibial (knee) rotation.

Radiographic Evaluation

Ultrasonography is used for initial evaluation and to follow the results of conservative treatment in newborns and infants (<3 months old) with DDH. Hip stability and acetabular development usually can be assessed accurately. Ultrasonography is expensive and requires considerable experience to perform accurately.

Radiographic evaluation is useful in older infants (>3 months old) and includes anteroposterior and Lauenstein (frog-leg) position lateral radiographs of the pelvis. The ossific nucleus does not appear until 4 to 6 months of age and may be delayed further in infants with DDH. Line measurements usually are made to determine the relationship of the femoral head to the acetabulum. Arthrography, CT, and MRI may be beneficial in select or difficult cases.

Figure 198-4

Hip abduction test. Place the infant supine, flex the hips 90 degrees, and fully abduct. Although the normal abduction range is broad, hip disease should be suspected in any patient who lacks more than 30 to 45 degrees of abduction. (From Chung SMK: Hip Disorders in Infants and Children. Philadelphia, Lea & Febiger, 1981, p 69.)

ABDUCTION TEST

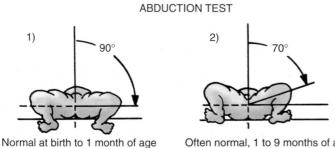

1) 90°
Normal at birth to 1 month of age

2) 70°
Often normal, 1 to 9 months of age

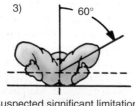

3) 60°
Suspected significant limitation

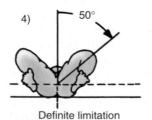

4) 50°
Definite limitation

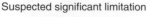

Treatment

The treatment of DDH is individualized and depends on the child's age at diagnosis. The goal is a concentric and stable reduction that results in normal growth and development of the hip. When an unstable hip is recognized at birth, maintenance of the hip in the position of flexion and abduction ("human" position) for 1 to 2 months usually is sufficient. This position maintains reduction of the femoral head and allows for tightening of the ligamentous structures and for stimulation of normal growth and development of the acetabulum. Usually, double or triple diapers are sufficient in neonates. Treatment usually is continued until clinical stability of the hip is seen and the radiographic or ultrasound measurements are within normal limits. Between 1 and 6 months of age, the Pavlik harness is indicated. This device places the hips in the human position by flexing the hips more than 90 degrees (preferably 100 to 110 degrees) and providing gentle abduction. This positioning redirects the femoral head toward the acetabulum. Usually, spontaneous relocation of the femoral head occurs within 3 to 4 weeks. The Pavlik harness is approximately 95% successful in dysplastic or subluxated hips and 80% successful in true dislocations.

If a reduction does not occur, a surgical closed reduction is attempted. This reduction consists of preliminary skin traction for 1 to 3 weeks to stretch the soft tissue contractures, percutaneous adductor tenotomy, closed reduction, and application of a hip spica cast in the "human" position. In an older infant (6 to 18 months old), surgical closed reduction is the major method of treatment. If the hip shows significant residual instability at the time of closed reduction, an open reduction may be indicated. Beyond 18 months of age, the dysplastic changes are so advanced that open reduction followed by pelvic or femoral osteotomy, or both, is usually necessary.

Complications

The most important and severe complication of DDH is iatrogenic avascular necrosis (osteonecrosis) of the CFE. Reduction of the femoral head under pressure produces cartilaginous compression, which can lead to occlusion of the intra-articular, extra-osseous epiphyseal vessels and produce partial or total CFE infarction. Revascularization follows, but abnormal growth and development may occur, especially if the physis is severely damaged. The hip is most vulnerable to this complication before the development of the ossific nucleus (4 to 6 months). Redislocation and subluxation of the femoral head and residual acetabular dysplasia are other common complications.

SEPTIC ARTHRITIS AND OSTEOMYELITIS

▶ SEE CHAPTERS 117 AND 118.

TRANSIENT MONARTICULAR SYNOVITIS

Transient synovitis of the hip is a common cause of limping in young children and is characterized by acute onset of pain, limp, and mild restriction of hip motion, especially abduction and internal rotation. This is a diagnosis of exclusion because septic arthritis or osteomyelitis of the hip must be excluded.

Etiology

The etiology of transient synovitis is uncertain. Possible causes have included active or recent viral infection and hypersensitivity. Approximately 70% of involved children have a nonspecific viral upper respiratory infection 7 to 14 days before the onset of hip symptoms.

Diagnosis

Biopsy specimens from the hip joints of patients with transient synovitis are unnecessary but have shown synovial hypertrophy secondary to nonspecific inflammatory reaction. Hip joint aspirations, if necessary, are negative, although a small effusion is common. The differential diagnosis includes septic arthritis, juvenile rheumatoid arthritis, fractures, psoas abscess, leukemia and other malignancies, osteonecrosis, and other disorders that are listed in Tables 196–2 and 196–3.

Clinical Manifestations

The mean age of onset is 6 years; most patients are 3 to 8 years old. The male-to-female ratio is 2:1. The acute onset of pain is felt in the groin, anterior thigh, or knee. Any child with nontraumatic anterior thigh or knee pain must be evaluated carefully for hip pathology because this is the site of referred pain. Patients usually are ambulatory, and the hip is not usually held in the flexed, abducted, and externally rotated position typical of bacterial infection unless a significant effusion is present. Children are usually afebrile, and the white blood cell count and erythrocyte sedimentation rate (ESR) are normal or slightly elevated. Patients at high risk for septic arthritis usually have temperature greater than 38.5°C, an ESR greater than 20 mm/hr, leukocytosis, severe pain, tenderness to palpation, spasm, and refusal to walk.

Radiographic Evaluation

Anteroposterior and frog-leg lateral radiographs of the pelvis are usually normal. Ultrasound examination of the hip may be useful in showing the hip joint effusion. Aspiration of fluid may improve symptoms and improve local blood flow. Bone scans may help differentiate a septic process.

Treatment

The treatment of choice includes bed rest and non-weight bearing until the pain resolves, followed by limited activities (for 1 to 2 weeks). This regimen sometimes is difficult because children want to return to normal activities when their symptoms resolve. If the child returns to normal activities too early, exacerbation of symptoms can occur. Nonsteroidal anti-inflammatory drugs are helpful. Lack of improvement necessitates further evaluation for more serious disorders.

LEGG-CALVÉ-PERTHES DISEASE

Legg-Calvé-Perthes disease (LCPD) is idiopathic avascular necrosis (osteonecrosis) of the CFE and the associated complications in a growing child. This disorder is caused by an interruption of the CFE blood supply. It is more common in boys (4-5:1) and is bilateral in approximately 20% of patients. Children with LCPD have delayed bone ages, disproportionate growth, and mild short stature. Some patients have a hypercoagulable state (factor V Leiden), hyperviscosity, synovitis, or venous congestion.

Clinical Manifestations

The clinical onset occurs between ages 2 and 12 years (mean age 7 years). Mild or intermittent pain in the anterior thigh and a limp may be present. The classic presentation is a "painless" limp. The pertinent early physical findings include antalgic gait; muscle spasm and mild restriction of motion, especially abduction and internal rotation; proximal thigh atrophy; and mild shortness of stature.

Radiographic Evaluation

Radiographic assessment is necessary to determine the extent of CFE involvement, follow disease progression, and assess sphericity of the femoral head, the possibility of CFE collapse and extrusion, and the response to treatment. Anteroposterior and frog-leg lateral pelvic radiographs usually are adequate, but occasionally additional procedures, such as arthrography, bone scans, and MRI, may be useful. Bone scans and MRI are helpful in recognizing early LCPD, but are of limited value in assessing the extent of CFE involvement or following the disease progression.

Prognosis

The short-term prognosis concerns femoral head deformity at the completion of the healing stage. The long-term prognosis involves the potential for osteoarthritis of the hip in adulthood. The prognostic factors for the development of late degenerative arthritis include femoral head deformity and age at clinical onset. Older children with significant residual femoral head deformity are at risk for development of degenerative arthritis. The incidence is essentially 100% in children who are 10 years old or older at onset. This rate is in contrast to a negligible risk in children 5 years old or younger and a 38% risk when onset occurs between 6 and 9 years old. Additional prognostic features are femoral head containment, hip range of motion, and premature CFE closure.

Treatment

LCPD is a local, self-healing disorder. Prevention of femoral head deformity and secondary osteoarthritis is the only justification for treatment. There are four basic treatment goals:

- Elimination of hip irritability
- Restoration and maintenance of a good range of hip motion
- Prevention of CFE collapse, extrusion, or subluxation
- Attainment of a spherical femoral head at healing

Treatment uses the concept of **containment**; the femoral head is contained within the acetabulum so that the latter acts as a mold for the reossifying CFE. Containment is indicated for children 6 years old (perhaps 5 years old in girls) or older in whom more than one half of the CFE is involved. Nonsurgical containment uses abduction casts and orthoses, or surgical containment is accomplished with proximal femoral varus osteotomy, with or without derotation, and pelvic osteotomies to redirect the acetabulum and contain the femoral head in the position of weight bearing. The long-term results of surgical containment treatment are 85% to 90% satisfactory (round or oval femoral head).

SLIPPED CAPITAL FEMORAL EPIPHYSIS

Etiology

Slippage of the CFE (SCFE) is the most common adolescent hip disorder. The etiology is unknown. An endocrine basis has been suggested because SCFE frequently occurs in adolescents who either are obese and have delayed skeletal maturation or are tall and thin and following a recent growth spurt. In obese children, a low level of sex hormones has been postulated; in tall, thin children, an overabundance of growth hormone is implicated. Sex hormones and growth hormones alter the rate of proliferation of the cartilage cells in the physis and the rate of skeletal growth. SCFE also can occur as a complication of an underlying endocrine disorder, such as hypothyroidism, pituitary disorders, pseudohypoparathyroidism, and treatment with recombinant growth hormone. When a SCFE occurs before puberty, a hormonal abnormality or systemic disorder should be suspected. Nonetheless, the histopathology of SCFE indicates mechanical factors as the ultimate cause of slippage. Obesity produces high shear forces across the weakened and obliquely oriented growth plate.

Radiographic Evaluation

Anteroposterior and frog-leg lateral radiographs of the pelvis are used to assess the hips. The earliest sign of SCFE is widening of the physis without slippage. This is considered a preslip condition. As slippage occurs, the CFE stays in the acetabulum, and the femoral neck rotates anteriorly and occasionally superiorly, resulting in a varus, retroverted femoral head and neck (Fig. 198–5). The degree of slippage between the CFE and the femoral neck can be classified as mild (0 to 33%), moderate (34% to 50%), and severe (>50%) by radiographic measurements. Slippage resulting in a valgus deformity is rare except in metabolic disorders, such as renal osteodystrophy and Marfan syndrome, and as a sequela to radiation therapy.

Classification

SCFE is classified as stable or unstable depending on the continuity between the CFE and femoral neck.

Stable Slipped Capital Femoral Epiphysis

Continuity and stability are seen between the CFE and femoral neck. The deformity occurs as a slow slippage through the physis. Initially the physis is wide; this is a preslip condition. The patient may have mild discomfort, but the physical findings are usually normal. Preslips frequently are seen in the opposite hip of an adolescent with a previous SCFE. As slippage occurs, symptoms increase; this now represents a chronic SCFE, the most common type. The patient usually has a history of symptoms lasting several months. Because of continuity between the femoral neck and CFE, however, the symptoms are not severe, and the child is

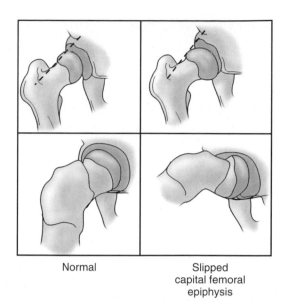

Normal   Slipped capital femoral epiphysis

Figure 198–5

Klein's line and slipped capital femoral epiphysis (SCFE). Klein's line extends along the lateral femur neck and normally passes through a small part of the lateral femoral head. In SCFE, the line does not pass through the head or may just touch its lateral margin. A frog-leg lateral, rather than an anteroposterior, projection gives the clearest view of SCFE. (From Chung SMK: Hip Disorders in Infants and Children. Philadelphia, Lea & Febiger, 1981, p 85.)

able to walk, albeit with a mildly antalgic, externally rotated gait.

Unstable Slipped Capital Femoral Epiphysis

In unstable SCFE, the continuity between the CFE and femoral neck is disrupted, producing instability and acute symptoms. Usually, antecedent symptoms are absent or mild, such as pain and limp for less than 3 weeks. Slippage occurs suddenly, with or without significant trauma; the pain is so severe that the child usually is unable to stand or bear weight.

An unstable SCFE also can occur on an existing chronic or stable SCFE. Affected adolescents have had previous symptoms (pain, limp, out-toed gait) for several months. Trauma, usually mild, is a potential underlying factor that results in the sudden slippage.

Clinical Manifestations

The physical findings in SCFE depend on the degree of slippage and stability of the CFE. In an unstable SCFE, the physical examination is limited by pain with any attempted hip motion. In stable, chronic SCFE, the patient has an antalgic gait, and the affected extremity is externally rotated. Hip range of motion shows a lack of internal rotation and increased external rotation. As the hip is flexed, it becomes progressively externally rotated. Limitation of flexion and abduction also may be present as a result of a varus deformity of the proximal femur. Adolescents, especially obese adolescents, with nontraumatic knee pain (referred pain) should be evaluated carefully for SCFE.

Treatment

The goals of treatment for SCFE are prevention of further slippage and minimization of complications. These are accomplished by epiphysiodesis of the CFE. The technique selected depends on CFE stability and the severity of the slippage. Current methods include in situ internal fixation with pins or screws (single or multiple), open bone graft epiphysiodesis, closed bone graft epiphysiodesis, osteotomies of the femoral neck or subtrochanteric regions to realign the proximal femur, and hip spica cast immobilization.

Complications

The two serious complications in SCFE are avascular necrosis and chondrolysis. Avascular necrosis occurs as a result of injury to the retinacular vessels. This injury can be caused by forced manipulation of an unstable slip, compression from intracapsular hematoma, or direct injury during surgery. Partial forms of avascular necrosis also may occur after internal fixation as a result of disruption of the intraepiphyseal blood vessels. Chondrolysis occurs when there is destruction of the articular cartilage of the hip joint. The etiologic mechanism of this complication is unclear, but has been shown to be associated with more severe slips, black race, pins or screws protruding out of the femoral head, and female gender.

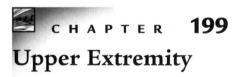

CHAPTER 199
Upper Extremity

SHOULDER

The shoulder joint has minimal geometric stability because of the relatively small glenoid fossa that articulates with a proportionately large hemispheric humeral head. A large range of motion is gained at the expense of intrinsic stability; consequently the musculature about the shoulder, particularly the muscles of the rotator cuff, must function with normal gleno-

humeral contact. Scapulothoracic movement greatly expands the range of motion possible at the shoulder area; the scapula, just as is the case with the glenohumeral joint, requires strong coordinated musculature to function with stability.

Sprengel Deformity

Failure of the scapula to descend to its normal location is **Sprengel deformity**, which occurs with varying degrees of severity. The scapula is located abnormally high with respect to the child's neck and thorax. Webbing of the neck or skin of the neck and a low posterior hairline may be associated findings. In the severe form, a bone (omovertebral) may connect the scapula with the lower cervical spine, and virtually no scapulothoracic movement may be possible; often, associated muscle anomalies are present that further limit strength and stability of the shoulder girdle. In the mild form, the scapula is slightly high riding, with less than normal motion. Association with congenital cervical vertebral anomalies, particularly the **Klippel-Feil anomaly**, occurs and suggests the possibility of significant problems in other organ systems. The best outcome in severe Sprengel deformities is achieved in early childhood by surgically repositioning and occasionally partially resecting the scapula. This procedure improves cosmesis and motion, especially shoulder abduction.

Brachial Plexus (Obstetric) Palsy

▶ SEE CHAPTER 60.

Dislocation of the Shoulder

Dislocation of the shoulder is uncommon in childhood but becomes more frequent in adolescence. The younger the individual at the time of the initial dislocation, the more likely that recurrent dislocation will develop. The chances of redislocation are so high that many orthopedic surgeons now favor early reconstruction rather than instituting conservative treatment and awaiting further dislocations.

Epiphysiolysis of the Proximal Humeral Epiphysis

A child who engages regularly in a throwing sport is at risk for traumatic epiphysiolysis of the proximal humeral physis. This disorder is a fatigue separation through the physis; it heals with rest and avoidance of repetitive throwing. Pain about the shoulder is the usual presenting complaint.

Overuse Syndromes

Overuse syndromes, inflammatory responses in tendons and bursae subjected to repetitive mild trauma, are uncommon in childhood but may be seen in adolescents. Subacromial **bursitis** occurs in tennis players and swimmers. Bicipital **tendinitis** is uncommon in children, but may produce a sensation of something snapping in the shoulder or shoulder pain when the bicipital groove is shallow, and the tendon can subluxate from it. In these types of inflammatory responses, direct tenderness over the involved anatomic structure is diagnostic.

ELBOW

The elbow joint consists of three articulations: the ulna and the humerus, the radius and the humerus, and the proximal radius and ulna. Collectively, these articulations provide for a hinge-type joint that allows for a palm-up (supination) and a palm-down (pronation) positioning of the wrist and hand. The elbow has great geometric stability, and the musculature moving the joint provides primarily flexion and extension at the elbow joint, but there are smaller muscles that primarily serve to rotate the radius about its long axis.

Nursemaid's Elbow

The radial head is not as bulbous in infants as in older children. During infancy, the annular ligament that passes around its base can partially slip off the head with traction across the elbow. When the ligament slips, the entity is known as nursemaid's elbow, or subluxation of the annular ligament (Fig. 199–1). The sub-

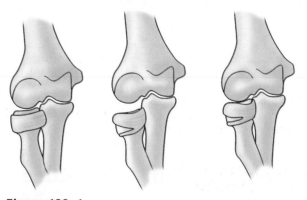

Figure 199–1

The pathology of pulled elbow. The annular ligament is torn when the arm is pulled. The radial head moves distally, and when traction is discontinued, the ligament is carried into the joint. (From Rang M: Children's Fractures. Philadelphia, JB Lippincott, 1974, p 121.)

luxation is initiated by a jerk on the extended elbow when a child falls with the hand being held or when a child is forcefully lifted by the hand. When the subluxation occurs, the hand typically is held in a palm-down position, and the child may refuse to use the hand or may cry when the elbow is moved. Moving the hand to a palm-up position with pressure over the radial head usually reduces the ligament subluxation and restores full normal use of the extremity. The parents should be educated about the mechanism of injury and should be encouraged to avoid picking the child up by holding the hand or forearm. When subluxation has occurred, there is a propensity for subsequent episodes. The problem generally resolves with maturation.

Panner Disease

Panner disease is an osteochondrosis that involves the ossific nucleus of the capitellum, the lateral portion of the distal humeral epiphysis. It is most common in adolescents, especially adolescents involved in throwing activities. They complain of pain and may have crepitation and loss of motion. Anteroposterior, lateral, and oblique radiographs; CT; or MRI may be helpful. In the absence of a loose osteocartilaginous body, **treatment** is conservative; if such a body is present, surgery is indicated.

Throwing Injuries

The elbow is especially vulnerable to throwing injuries in a skeletally immature child. The most common pathology results from abnormal compressive forces acting across the radial side of the joint. In addition to Panner disease, the radial head may become asymmetric compared with the opposite side or may be fragmented. Some irregularity in shape of the cartilaginous radial head is present. Additionally, there may be irregularity of the capitellum. Rarely, small pieces of bone and cartilage (loose bodies) from the capitellum or radial head become entrapped in the joint. Before the problem becomes established or severe, the child complains of an aching pain about the elbow, which generally is worse after throwing than during the time spent at the throwing activity. On physical examination, an early loss of supination (the palm-up position of the hand) can be detected. Children in whom these lesions develop generally have a high emotional investment in their particular sport, most commonly baseball, and nonparticipation is a difficult option for them to accept. Avoidance of pitching until the elbow is normal on physical examination with follow-up radiograph is the best solution. Often, switching the baseball player to another position allows the child to avoid pitching. Behind such highly motivated youngsters is usually an overzealous parent or coach in need of appropriate counseling.

WRIST AND HAND

Multiple small joints, a delicately balanced intrinsic muscle system, a powerful extrinsic muscle system, dense sensory innervation, and specialized skin combine to make the hand a highly mobile, sensitive, and delicate yet powerful anatomic part. The extrinsic muscles, whose muscle origin is in the forearm and that motor the hand via tendons that pass to it, provide great power, whereas the intrinsic muscles, which are located in the hand itself, modulate the effects of the powerful extrinsic musculature and provide for delicate coordinated movement. Asking the patient to open the hand, extend and spread the fingers and thumb, and clench the hand to a fist yields much insight because these maneuvers require coordinated function of the intrinsic and extrinsic musculature and full range of motion in the small joints of the hand. After this maneuver, having the individual squeeze the examiner's fingers gives further information about the strength of the hand.

Finger Abnormalities

Extra digits (**polydactyly**) occur as simple and complex varieties (Table 199-1). Skin tags and digit remnants typically seen near the metacarpophalangeal joint of the small finger or of the thumb that do not have palpable bone in their base or possess voluntary movement may be excised while the child is still in the nursery. Varieties of polydactyly more complex than this should be referred for amputation.

Syndactyly also occurs in simple and complex patterns (Table 199-2). There always is concern about the sharing of common important structures between the digits and about the tethering effect of the syndactyly on the growth of the affected digits. Referral for delineation of the specific pathology and development of a treatment strategy are indicated when the condition is recognized.

Isolated thickening in the flexor pollicis longus tendon may produce a **trigger thumb**. As the nodule enlarges, it may snap or trigger as it passes through the first pulley that prevents bow stringing of the tendon.

TABLE 199–1. Syndromes Associated with Polydactyly

Ellis–van Creveld syndrome
Rubinstein-Taybi syndrome
Carpenter syndrome
Meckel-Gruber syndrome
Polysyndactyly
Trisomy 13
Orofaciodigital syndrome

TABLE 199–2. Syndromes Associated with Syndactyly

Apert syndrome
Carpenter syndrome
de Lange syndrome
Holt-Oram syndrome
Orofaciodigital syndrome
Polysyndactyly
Fetal hydantoin syndrome
Laurence-Moon-Biedl syndrome
Fanconi pancytopenia
Trisomy 21
Trisomy 13
Trisomy 18

Ultimately, it may not pass through at all, producing a flexion deformity at the interphalangeal joint. The nodule is usually palpable at the level of the metacarpophalangeal joint on the volar surface. These children should be referred because many need surgery, release of the first pulley, to correct the triggering or the contracture.

Ganglion

Ganglion, which is a synovial fluid–filled cyst about the wrist, is common in childhood. The usual site is the dorsum of the wrist near the radiocarpal joint, and a secondary site is over the volar radial aspect of the wrist. The essential pathology is a defect in one of the joint capsules; with wrist use, synovial fluid is pumped into the soft tissue, where it becomes walled off by reactive fibrous tissue. Often, in a skeletally immature child, the process is benign and tends to disappear with the passage of time. In the event that a ganglion is sufficiently large to cause pain or interfere with normal tendon function, aspiration and injection of the cyst are sometimes helpful. In refractory cases, surgical excision of the cyst accompanied by removal of the tract that extends into the joint is curative.

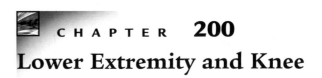

CHAPTER **200**

Lower Extremity and Knee

Torsional (in-toeing and out-toeing) and angular (physiologic bowlegs and knock-knees) variations of the lower extremities are common reasons parents seek medical attention for a child. Most of these complaints do not necessitate active treatment because they are physiologic and resolve with normal growth. It is important to understand the natural history to reassure a concerned family.

ANGULAR VARIATIONS

Reasons for angular deformities can be either physiologic (**variations**) or pathologic (**deformities**). Physiologic torsional and angular variations are the most common. These occur predominantly in the tibia. The femur is less commonly involved.

Physiologic Bowlegs (Genu Varum)

The lower extremities of newborns and infants (<1 year old) commonly have mild to moderate bowing and internal rotation (Fig. 200–1). This condition is caused by in utero positioning, in which the hips are flexed, abducted, and externally rotated; the knees are flexed and lower legs are internally rotated; and the feet are in slight equinus, supination, and contact with the posterolateral aspect of the opposite thigh. This position produces hip flexion, abduction, and external rotation contractures; knee flexion contractures and internal tibial torsion; and mild supination of the feet. The bowed appearance is actually a torsional combination from the external rotation of the hip (tight posterior

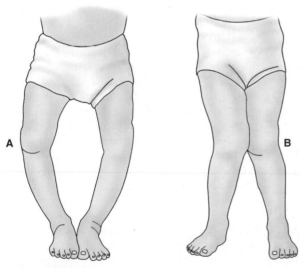

Figure 200–1

Bowleg and knock-knee deformities. A, Bowleg deformity. Bowlegs are referred to as varus angulation (genu varum) because the knees are tilted away from the midline of the body. **B,** Knock-knee or valgus deformity of the knees. The knee is tilted toward the midline. (From Scoles P: Pediatric Orthopedics in Clinical Practice. Chicago, Year Book Medical Publishers, 1982, p 84.)

capsule) and the internal tibial torsion. With the onset of standing and independent walking, the bowing spontaneously corrects over 6 to 12 months. Significant improvement does not occur during the first year of life. The typical infant has 15 degrees of genu varum or bowleg configuration. This decreases to approximately 10 degrees by 1 year of age. By 2 years of age, most children have straight or neutrally aligned lower extremities. **Treatment** may be indicated for children 2 to 3 years old or older in whom there has been no documented improvement with growth, but this is rarely necessary.

Physiologic Knock-Knees (Genu Valgum)

As the spontaneous correction of physiologic bowlegs continues, there is typically an overcorrection, of variable degree, into mild genu valgum or knock-knee (see Fig. 200–1). This physiologic angular variation commonly is seen between 3 and 4 years of age, but resolves spontaneously between 5 and 8 years. As with physiologic bowlegs, **treatment** rarely is indicated.

TORSIONAL VARIATIONS

In-Toeing

Internal Femoral Torsion or Anteversion

Internal femoral torsion or anteversion is the most common cause of in-toeing in children 2 years of age or older (Table 200–1). It occurs more commonly in girls than boys (2:1). Most children with this condition have generalized ligamentous laxity. The **etiology** of femoral torsion is controversial; it may be congenital (persistent infantile femoral anteversion) or acquired secondary to abnormal sitting habits.

Clinical Manifestations. The primary clinical feature of internal femoral torsion is an in-toed gait.

TABLE 200–1. Common Causes of In-Toeing and Out-Toeing
In-Toeing
Internal femoral torsion or anteversion Internal tibial torsion Metatarsus adductus Talipes equinovarus (clubfoot)
Out-Toeing
External femoral torsion External tibial torsion Calcaneovalgus feet Hypermobile pes planus (flatfoot)

While watching the undressed child walk, the examiner notes the entire lower leg to be internally rotated. The hip has 80 to 90 degrees of internal rotation in the extended position; as a result, external rotation is limited to 0 to 10 degrees. Generalized ligamentous laxity, resulting in elbow and finger hyperextension, knee recurvatum, and hypermobile flatfeet (pes planus), is present. These children sit almost exclusively in the "television" or "W" position. This position may allow the lower leg to act as a lever, producing the torsional change in the "biologically plastic" femur. Although this condition is also called **femoral anteversion**, which implies an abnormality of the proximal femur, it is actually a torsional abnormality throughout the femoral shaft that results in a change in the normal alignment between the hip and knee.

Radiographic Evaluation. Radiographic evaluation for internal femoral torsion is not routinely necessary. Clinical measurements usually are accurate. CT of the hip and knee can be used to measure precisely the degree of torsion radiographically, but is usually not necessary.

Treatment. Management consists primarily of observation. It was incorrectly believed that internal femoral torsion was associated with bunions, back pain, degenerative osteoarthritis of the hip and knee, and difficulty with athletic ability. Correction of abnormal sitting habits usually allows this torsional variation to resolve with normal growth and development. It can take 1 to 3 years for complete correction to occur, however. Children older than 10 years of age and young adolescents may not have enough remaining musculoskeletal growth for spontaneous correction to occur. After these children have been followed for 1 to 2 years without improvement, and if there is significant cosmetic or functional disability, surgical correction may be beneficial.

Internal Tibial Torsion

Internal or medial tibial torsion is the most common cause of in-toeing in children younger than 2 years old and is the result of normal in utero positioning. This condition may be associated with metatarsus adductus. It also is the major component of physiologic bowlegs.

Clinical Manifestations. The degree of tibial torsion can be measured by the supine or prone thigh-foot angle. In both tests, the child's knee is flexed to 90 degrees to neutralize the normal tibiofemoral rotation, and the foot is placed in a neutral or simulated weight-bearing position. The long axis of the foot is compared with the long axis of the thigh (prone test) or tibia (supine test). An inwardly rotated foot is assigned a negative value and represents internal tibial torsion. The measurements must be recorded on each visit to document improvement. Radiographic measurements usually are of no value in assessment of internal tibial torsion.

Treatment. Internal tibial torsion is a physiologic condition, and spontaneous resolution with normal growth and development can be anticipated. If there has been no documented improvement by 2 years of age, a nighttime orthosis, such as a Denis Browne splint, may be considered. There are no prospective studies documenting the efficacy of an orthosis. Rarely, persistent internal tibial torsion in an older child or adolescent may necessitate surgical derotation.

Out-Toeing

External tibial torsion is common and usually associated with a calcaneovalgus foot (see Chapter 201; Table 200–1). Both are the result of a variation in normal in utero position. When these two conditions are combined with the normally externally rotated hip (tight posterior hip capsule), a very externally rotated or out-toed appearance is the result. External tibial torsion is physiologic and undergoes spontaneous resolution with normal growth similar to internal tibial torsion.

PATHOLOGIC GENU VARUM

Tibia Vara (Blount Disease)

Idiopathic tibia vara, or Blount disease, is the most common pathologic disorder producing a progressive genu varum deformity. It is characterized by abnormal growth of the medial aspect of the proximal tibial epiphysis, resulting in a progressive varus angulation below the knee. Tibia vara can occur at any age in a growing child. It is classified according to the age at clinical onset, as follows: infantile (1 to 3 years), juvenile (4 to 10 years), and adolescent (≥11 years). The infantile group is the most common; the juvenile and adolescent forms typically are combined as late-onset tibia vara, which occurs much less frequently.

Etiology

Although the exact cause of tibia vara is unknown, it seems to be secondary to growth suppression from increased compressive forces across the medial aspect of the knee.

Clinical Manifestations

The characteristics of infantile tibia vara include predominance of black race, female gender, marked obesity, approximately 80% bilateral involvement, a prominent medial metaphyseal beak, internal tibial torsion, and lower extremity length inequality. Characteristics of the juvenile and adolescent (late-onset) form are black race, predominance of males, marked obesity, approximately 50% bilateral involvement, slow progressive genu varum deformity, pain rather than deformity as the primary initial complaint, no palpable proximal medial metaphyseal beak, minimal internal tibial torsion, mild medial collateral ligament laxity, and mild lower extremity length inequality.

The differences between the three tibia vara groups seem to be related primarily to the age at clinical onset, the amount of remaining growth, and the magnitude of the medial compression forces on the involved side. The infantile-onset group has the potential for the greatest deformity, and the adolescent-onset group has the least.

Radiographic Evaluation

Standing anteroposterior and lateral radiographs of the lower extremities are necessary to assess pathologic genu varum deformities. Radiographically, fragmentation with a protuberant step deformity and beaking of the proximal medial tibial metaphysis are considered the major features of infantile tibia vara. The changes of the proximal medial tibia are less conspicuous in the late-onset forms and are characterized by wedging of the medial portion of the epiphysis, a mild posteromedial articular depression, a serpiginous cephalad curved physis of variable width, and mild or no fragmentation or beaking of the proximal medial metaphysis.

The major deformity that must be differentiated from infantile tibia vara is the physiologic genu varum deformity. It is difficult to differentiate radiographically between these two disorders in children younger than 2 years old.

Treatment

When the radiographic findings confirm the diagnosis, treatment should begin immediately. Orthotic management may be considered for children 3 years or younger with a mild deformity. Approximately 50% of children with this criterion may achieve adequate correction using orthoses. Conservative management in the late-onset forms of tibia vara is contraindicated. The children are too large, compliance is poor, and the remaining growth is too small to allow for adequate correction.

The indications for surgical treatment in infantile tibia vara include 4 years of age or older, failure of orthotic management, and moderate to severe deformity. Proximal tibial valgus osteotomy with associated fibular diaphyseal osteotomy is the procedure of choice.

LOWER EXTREMITY LENGTH DISCREPANCIES

Length discrepancies in the femur, tibia, or both are common problems. The *differential diagnosis is extensive;* some common causes are listed in Table 200–2.

Normal Growth and Development

Approximately 65% of the growth of the entire lower extremity comes from the distal femoral (38%) and proximal tibial (27%) physeal plates. Growth disturbances about the knee can have the most adverse effect on lower extremity length, depending on the amount of remaining growth.

Methods of Limb Length Measurement

Clinical Measurements

Clinical measurements are less accurate than radiographic techniques. A common clinical measurement is from the anterior superior iliac spine to the medial malleolus. This minimizes measurement error secondary to pelvic obliquity. The most accurate clinical

TABLE 200–2. Common Causes of Lower Extremity Length Inequality
Congenital
Proximal femoral focal deficiency
Coxa vara
Hemiatrophy and hemihypertrophy (anisomelia)
Developmental
Developmental dislocation of the hip (DDH)
Legg-Calvé-Perthes disease (LCPD)
Neuromuscular
Polio
Cerebral palsy (hemiplegia)
Infectious
Pyogenic osteomyelitis with physeal damage
Trauma
Physeal injury with premature closure
Overgrowth
Malunion (shortening)
Tumor
Physeal destruction
Radiation-induced physeal injury
Overgrowth

method for measuring limb length involves leveling the pelvis. Blocks of various thicknesses may be placed beneath the foot on the involved side until the iliac crests are level. The height of the blocks indicates the amount of discrepancy.

Radiographic Measurements

Radiographic evaluations are the most accurate method of assessment of leg length. The *teleoradiograph* is a single exposure of both lower extremities. The primary indication is for young children (usually <5 years old). A small amount of magnification error is present, but this type of measurement has the advantage of showing angular deformities.

The *orthoradiograph* consists of three separate, slightly overlapping exposures of the hips, knees, and ankles on a long cassette. Bone length is measured directly on the radiograph. Less magnification is present, and angular deformities are shown. It has the disadvantage of being bulky and difficult to handle.

The *scanogram* is the most accurate method and consists of three narrow exposures of the hips, knees, and ankles on a standard cassette with a radiographic ruler next to the extremity. Minimal magnification is present, and accurate measurements can be made. Angular deformities cannot be visualized fully, however, which may lead to errors in interpretation. Currently, *CT scanogram* techniques are being used with the best accuracy.

The measured discrepancy is followed with the Moseley and Green-Anderson graphs. An anteroposterior radiograph of the left hand and wrist for bone age determination is necessary to assess maturation.

Treatment

Issues in management include etiology of the discrepancy, skeletal age, ultimate discrepancy, anticipated adult height, neuromuscular status of the extremities, joint involvement, and psychological aspects of the child and parents. Discrepancies of greater than 2 cm at maturity usually necessitate treatment. Equalization can be achieved by nonsurgical and surgical methods. Nonsurgical methods include orthotic and prosthetic devices; surgical methods include shortening of the longer extremity, lengthening of the shorter extremity, or a combination of both. Discrepancies of 2 to 5 cm are treated by epiphysiodesis (surgical physeal closure) of the affected side, and discrepancies greater than 5 cm are treated by lengthening.

KNEE

The knee joint is unique because the movement of the tibiofemoral articulation is constrained only by soft tissues rather than by the usual geometric fit between the

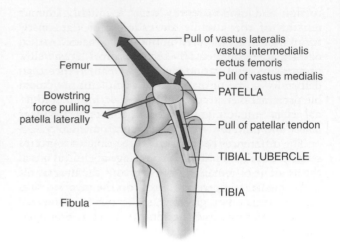

Figure 200–2

Diagram of the knee extensor mechanism. The major force exerted by the quadriceps muscle tends to pull the patella laterally out of the intercondylar sulcus. The vastus medialis muscle pulls medially to keep the patella centralized. (From Smith JB: Knee problems in children. Pediatr Clin North Am 33:1439, 1986.)

ends of articulating bone (Fig. 200–2). Paramount among these constraints are the medial and lateral collateral ligaments, the anterior and posterior cruciate ligaments, and the medial and lateral menisci. Weight is transmitted by load path that includes the points of articular cartilage and the menisci. A second clinically important area, the patellofemoral joint, is part of the knee and a common site of problems, especially in adolescents.

Accumulation of fluid (**effusion**) in the knee is common during childhood and adolescence. When fluid accumulates rapidly after an injury, blood is usually in the joint (**hemarthrosis**); this may indicate an occult fracture or an injury to one of the ligaments or menisci. If there has been repeated trauma, an accumulation of synovial fluid may indicate a chronic internal derangement, usually a tear of a meniscus. Unexplained accumulation of fluid may occur with **arthritis** (septic, viral, postinfectious, Lyme, juvenile rheumatoid arthritis, or systemic lupus erythematosus), with ligamentous laxity (hypermobile joint syndrome), and with overactivity. In addition to the evaluation of other systemic manifestations and the clinical history (fever, hemophilia, rash, or trauma), analysis of an aspiration of fluid from the joint generally is indicated and expedites precise diagnosis.

Discoid Lateral Meniscus

Each meniscus is semilunar in shape, but occasionally the lateral meniscus persists as a solid disc, an entity referred to as *discoid lateral meniscus.* A normal meniscus is attached about its periphery and glides anteriorly and posteriorly with knee motion, but a discoid meniscus is less mobile and may become torn. Occasionally, there is no peripheral attachment about its posterolateral aspect. During knee flexion, the entire discoid meniscus suddenly may displace anteriorly to produce a loud audible "click" or "clunk." Most commonly, the patient comes to clinical attention during late childhood and early adolescence (11 to 15 years old). Anteroposterior radiographs may show widening of the lateral aspect of the knee joint. Arthroscopy, arthrography, and MRI are diagnostic. **Treatment** in most cases involves excision of tears and reshaping of the meniscus arthroscopically. Peripheral reattachment is performed when possible.

Popliteal Cyst

A popliteal cyst (**Baker cyst**) commonly is seen during the middle childhood years (Fig. 200–3). The cause is distention of the gastrocnemius and semimembranosus bursa along the posteromedial aspect of the knee by synovial fluid from the tendon sheaths. In childhood, the cysts usually are benign and resolve with time, although several years may be required. Knee

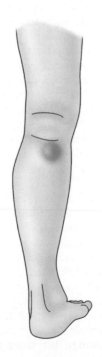

Figure 200–3

Diagram of popliteal cyst location shows posterior and medial aspect of knee, usually inferior to knee crease. (From Ferguson A: Orthopedic Surgery in Infancy and Childhood, 5th ed. Baltimore, Williams & Wilkins, 1981.)

radiographs are normal; the **diagnosis** is confirmed by ultrasound or aspiration. **Treatment** should be directed at reassurance because surgery is rarely indicated.

Osteochondritis Dissecans

Osteochondritis dissecans commonly involves the knee and occurs when an area of bone adjacent to the articular cartilage becomes avascular and separates from the underlying bone. In an older child or young adolescent, this condition usually affects the lateral portion of the medial femoral condyle. Anteroposterior, lateral, and "tunnel" radiographs of the knee are diagnostic and are used to follow the course of the disease. In the young patient, the overlying articular cartilage usually remains intact, and the area of avascular necrosis revascularizes and heals spontaneously. With increasing age, the risk increases for fracture of the articular cartilage and separation of the bony fragment. MRI is helpful in determining the integrity of the articular cartilage. In a young adolescent, the physician must decide whether to follow the lesion expectantly or to attempt to stimulate healing surgically. When cartilage fracture takes place, surgical treatment is necessary; this may consist of arthroscopic excision, drilling of the lesion to promote revascularization and healing, and possible internal fixation.

Osgood-Schlatter Disease

The portion of the patellar ligament inserted into the tibial tubercle, an extension of the proximal tibial epiphysis, is vulnerable to microfracture during late childhood and early adolescence. This condition, Osgood-Schlatter disease, is more common in boys. The natural history is usually benign, with activity-related pain persisting for 12 to 24 months. Physical examination shows swelling and prominence of the tibial tubercle and exquisite local tenderness. Radiographs are necessary to rule out other lesions. Frequently, bony enlargement of the tibial tubercle is a consequence of the healing response. Rest, restriction of activities, and occasionally a knee immobilizer may be necessary, combined with an isometric exercise program. Anti-inflammatory medications also may be beneficial.

Patellofemoral Disorders

The patellofemoral joint depends on a subtle balance among restraining ligaments, muscle forces, alignment, and articular anatomy for normal function (see Fig. 200–2). On its deep surface, the patella has a V-bottom shape; it moves through a matching groove in the distal femur called the *trochlea.* The force of the muscle pulling through the quadriceps tendon and the patellar ligament does not act in a straight line because the patellar ligament inclines in a slightly lateral direction with respect to the line of the quadriceps tendon. This lateral movement, coupled with the movement of the restraining ligaments, tends to move the patella in a lateral direction. The vastus medialis muscle functions to counteract the laterally acting forces. An abnormality of any one or a group of these factors makes the patellofemoral joint function abnormally; the usual clinical manifestation is knee pain.

Idiopathic anterior knee pain is common in adolescents. This condition previously was called **chondromalacia patellae**, but this term is incorrect because the joint surfaces of the patella are normal. Abnormal mechanics and variables associated with puberty are possible etiologic factors. The condition is assessed easily by directly palpating the extended knee and by compressing the patellofemoral joint. To perform the maneuver, the physician merely exerts manual pressure over the patella with the knee extended. Crepitus may be elicited. Radiographs are rarely helpful. Running and climbing stairs elicit pain when the knee is flexed. The pain usually is perceived maximally as the knee comes to within 15 to 20 degrees of full extension. It is reasonable to treat recent or mild cases empirically with anti-inflammatory medication and an exercise program aimed at developing strength and bulk in the vastus medialis muscle; persistent or refractory cases should be referred to an orthopedist. Patellofemoral pain is particularly prevalent among young athletes (participating in running, basketball, and soccer) and in adolescent girls.

Recurrent **patellar subluxation** and **dislocation** resulting from similar muscle imbalance also can occur in late childhood and early adolescence. Several other predisposing factors are known, including generalized ligamentous laxity, internal femoral torsion, genu valgum, and lateral femoral condyle hypoplasia. Acute traumatic dislocations can occur in a normal knee. Initial **treatment** is nonoperative, with a vigorous physical therapy program to strengthen predominantly the quadriceps muscles. If this fails, surgical correction is necessary.

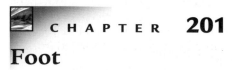

CHAPTER 201
Foot

In newborns and nonambulatory infants, the difference between posturing and deformity must be remembered. *Posturing* is the habitual position in which the infant holds the foot; passive range of motion is normal. *Deformity* produces an appearance similar to posturing, but the motion is restricted. Most pediatric foot disorders are painless. Foot pain does occur, however, especially in older children. The **differential diagnosis** of foot pain in children is presented in Table 201–1.

METATARSUS ADDUCTUS

Congenital metatarsus adductus is a common problem of infants and young children. It also is called *metatarsus varus* if the forefoot is supinated and adducted. The condition occurs equally in boys and girls and is bilateral in 50% of patients. Metatarsus adductus has hereditary tendencies and is more common in firstborn than in later children because of the molding effect from the smaller primigravida uterus and abdominal wall. Approximately 10% of children with metatarsus adductus have DDH; careful examination of the hips is necessary.

Clinical Manifestations

The forefoot is adducted and occasionally supinated. The hindfoot and the midfoot are normal. The lateral border of the foot is convex, and the base of the fifth metatarsal appears prominent. The medial border of the foot is concave. The interval between the first and second toes is usually increased, with the great toe being held in a greater varus position. Ankle dorsiflexion and plantar flexion are normal. Forefoot flexibility varies from flexible to rigid. To perform an assessment, the examiner stabilizes the hindfoot and midfoot in a neutral position and applies pressure over the first metatarsal head. In a walking child with an uncorrected metatarsus adductus deformity, an in-toed gait is noted. Abnormal shoe wear also commonly is seen.

Radiographic Evaluation

Routine radiographs of the foot usually are not necessary for metatarsus adductus because they do not show mobility. Anteroposterior weight-bearing radiographs show adduction of the metatarsals at the tarsometatarsal articulation and an increased intermetatarsal angle between the first and second metatarsals.

Treatment

The feet may be classified into three groups, depending on forefoot flexibility, as follows:

- *Type I* deformities concern flexible feet that can achieve the overcorrected (abducted) position actively and passively. Voluntary correction can be

TABLE 201–1. Differential Diagnosis of Foot Pain by Age

0-6 Years Old	6-12 Years Old	12-20 Years Old
Poor-fitting shoes	Poor-fitting shoes	Poor-fitting shoes
Foreign body	Sever disease	Stress fracture
Fracture	Juvenile rheumatoid arthritis	Foreign body
Osteomyelitis	Foreign body	Ingrown toenail
Juvenile rheumatoid arthritis	Accessory tarsal navicular	Metatarsalgia
Leukemia	Tarsal coalition	Plantar fasciitis
Puncture wound	Ewing sarcoma	Osteochondritis dissecans
Dactylitis	Hypermobile flatfoot	Avascular necrosis of metatarsal (Freiberg infarction) or navicular bone (Köhler disease)
	Trauma (fractures; sprains)	Sever disease
	Puncture wound	Achilles tendinitis
		Trauma (fractures; sprains)
		Plantar warts
		Tarsal coalition
		Accessory ossicles (navicular, os trigonum)

elicited by stroking the lateral border of the foot to stimulate the peroneal musculature. Usually, no treatment is needed.

- *Type II* deformities concern feet that can be corrected to the neutral position passively and actively. These feet may benefit from a trial of corrective shoes, such as straight-last or reversed-last shoes. These shoes are worn full-time (22 hr/day), and the child is re-evaluated in 4 to 6 weeks. If the condition has improved, treatment can be continued. If no improvement occurs, serial plaster casts are necessary.
- *Type III* deformities are rigid and cannot be corrected. These feet are treated with serial casts that are changed at intervals of 1 to 2 weeks. Usually, complete correction can be obtained in 4 to 6 weeks, depending on the child's age and the severity of deformity. The best results are obtained when casting is initiated before the child is 8 months old.

For metatarsus adductus deformities persisting or presenting after 4 years of age, surgical intervention is usually required. Children 4 to 6 years old with a fixed deformity usually are considered for soft tissue release. Older children usually do not benefit from the soft tissue release and require metatarsal osteotomies.

CALCANEOVALGUS FEET

The calcaneovalgus foot is a relatively common finding in newborns and seems to be secondary to in utero positioning. This condition is manifested by a hyperdorsiflexed foot with forefoot abduction and heel valgus and usually is associated with external tibial torsion. These variations usually are unilateral, but may be bilateral. In utero, the plantar surface of the foot was against the wall of the uterus, forcing it into a hyperdorsiflexed, abducted, and externally rotated position. When calcaneovalgus feet and external tibial torsion are combined with the normal newborn external rotation of the hip (tight posterior capsule), an excessively externally rotated lower extremity is the result.

Clinical Manifestations

The infant typically has an externally rotated extremity. The dorsum of the foot can be brought into contact with the anterior aspect of the tibia, and the forefoot has an abducted appearance. The most common condition that must be distinguished from the calcaneovalgus foot is a congenital vertical talus. The differentiation usually can be made clinically because a vertical talus is a rigid deformity.

Radiographic Evaluation

Simulated weight-bearing anteroposterior and lateral radiographs of the feet may be necessary to differentiate between the calcaneovalgus foot and a congenital vertical talus. In a calcaneovalgus foot, the radiographs either are normal or show a slight increase in hindfoot valgus. In congenital vertical talus, the hindfoot is in equinus, and the midfoot is dorsally displaced (rocker-bottom deformity).

Treatment

The typical calcaneovalgus foot requires no treatment. The hyperdorsiflexion of the foot resolves during the first 3 to 6 months of life. The external tibial torsion persists, however, and follows the same natural history as internal tibial torsion. Spontaneous improvement does not occur until the child begins to pull to stand and walk independently. Most affected infants have normally aligned feet and lower extremities by 2 years of age.

TALIPES EQUINOVARUS (CLUBFOOT)

A clubfoot is a deformity of not only the foot, but also the entire lower leg. Clubfoot can be congenital, teratologic, or positional. Congenital clubfoot is usually an isolated abnormality, whereas the teratologic form is associated with a neuromuscular disorder, such as spina bifida, arthrogryposis multiplex congenita, or a syndrome complex. Positional clubfoot is a normal foot that has been held in a deformed position in utero.

Etiology

The cause of congenital clubfoot is unknown. Inheritance may be multifactorial, with a major influence possibly from a single autosomal dominant gene. Biopsy studies of the extrinsic muscles of the calf have suggested a nonprogressive neuromuscular etiology.

Clinical Manifestations

Congenital clubfoot, which constitutes 75% of cases, is characterized by the absence of other congenital abnormalities, variable rigidity of the foot, mild calf atrophy, and mild hypoplasia of the tibia, fibula, and bones of the foot. It occurs more commonly in boys (2 : 1) and is bilateral in 50% of cases. The probability of random occurrence is approximately 0.1%, but within involved families, the probability is approximately 3% for subsequent siblings and 20% to 30% for offspring of involved parents.

Examination of the infant clubfoot shows hindfoot equinus, hindfoot varus, forefoot adduction, and variable rigidity. All are secondary to the medial dislocation of the talonavicular joint. In an older child, the calf and foot atrophy is more obvious than in the infant, regardless of how well corrected or functional the foot. These findings are the result of the neuromuscular etiology of clubfoot.

Radiographic Evaluation

Anteroposterior and lateral standing or simulated weight bearing and maximal dorsiflexion lateral radiographs are used to assess clubfoot (Fig. 201-1). Useful measurements in assessing clubfoot are the anteroposterior talocalcaneal angle, the lateral talocalcaneal angle, and the talocalcaneal overlap. The navicular, which is the primary site of deformity, does not ossify until 3 years of age in girls and 4 years of age in boys.

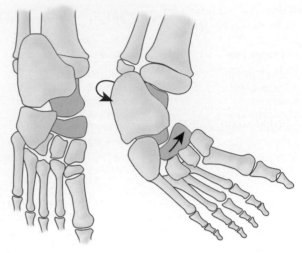

Figure 201-1

Diagram of anteroposterior radiograph of a normal foot and talipes equinovarus. (From Tachdjian MO: Pediatric Orthopedics. Philadelphia, WB Saunders, 1972.)

Line measurements are necessary to determine the position of the unossified navicular.

Treatment

Conservative Management

Conservative methods of treatment are taping and use of malleable splints and serial plaster casts. Taping and malleable splints are particularly useful in premature infants until they attain an appropriate size for casting. Serial plaster casts are the major method of treatment. The technique described by Ponseti is highly effective in providing long-term satisfactory results. The use of this technique is one of the most important recent changes in pediatric orthopedics.

Surgical Management

Most infants treated by the Ponseti technique require a percutaneous tendo Achilles lengthening to correct the equinus component of the deformity. Approximately 20% later require transfer of the tibialis anterior tendon to correct dynamic supination. The need for comprehensive complete soft tissue releases is now less common.

HYPERMOBILE PES PLANUS (FLEXIBLE FLATFEET)

Hypermobile or pronated feet are common sources of parental concern. The affected child is usually asymptomatic and has no limitations of activities. Flexible flatfeet are common in neonates and toddlers as a result of associated ligamentous laxity and fat in the area of the medial longitudinal arch; significant improvement is noted by 6 years of age. In older children, flexible flatfeet usually are secondary to generalized ligamentous laxity.

Clinical Manifestations

In the non–weight-bearing position in an older child with a flexible flatfoot, the normal medial longitudinal arch is present; in the weight-bearing position, the foot becomes pronated, with varying degrees of pes planus and heel valgus. Subtalar motion is normal or slightly increased. Loss of subtalar motion may indicate a rigid flatfoot. Common causes of **rigid flatfeet** include a tight Achilles tendon (heel cord), tarsal coalitions, and neuromuscular abnormalities (with cerebral palsy). Rigid flatfeet also may be a familial trait.

Radiographic Evaluation

Radiographs of asymptomatic flexible flatfeet usually are not indicated.

Treatment

The treatment of flexible flatfeet is conservative; the diagnosis is not possible until after 6 years of age. Treatment is indicated only for persistent symptoms not attributable to other causes or abnormal shoe wear. Feet that are symptomatic with vigorous physical activities usually respond readily to the use of a commercially available medial longitudinal arch support.

PERONEAL SPASTIC FLATFOOT (TARSAL COALITION)

Peroneal spastic flatfoot is a common disorder. It is characterized by a painful, rigid valgus deformity of the midfoot and hindfoot (flatfoot) and peroneal (lateral calf) muscle spasm, without true spasticity. Peroneal spastic flatfoot usually is synonymous with tarsal coalition, a congenital fusion or (more likely) failure of segmentation between two or more tarsal bones. Any condition that alters the normal gliding and rotary motion of the subtalar joint may produce the appearance of a peroneal spastic flatfoot, however. Congenital malformations, arthritis or inflammatory disorders, infection, neoplasms, and trauma are potential, although uncommon, causes.

The most common tarsal coalitions occur at the middle talocalcaneal (subtalar) facet and between the calcaneus and navicular bones (calcaneonavicular coalition). Coalitions can be fibrous, cartilaginous, or osseous. Tarsal coalitions are bilateral in approximately 50% of affected children.

Clinical Manifestations

The onset of symptoms usually occurs during the second decade of life. Although mild limitation of subtalar motion and a valgus deformity are present beginning in early childhood, the onset of symptoms varies with the age at which the fibrous or cartilaginous bar begins to ossify and further decrease motion. The talonavicular coalitions ossify between 3 and 5 years; the calcaneonavicular coalitions, between 8 and 12 years; and the medial facet talocalcaneal coalitions, between 12 and 16 years. The pain typically is felt laterally in the hindfoot and radiates proximally along the lateral malleolus and distal fibula (peroneal muscle spasm). Symptoms frequently are aggravated by sports or by walking on uneven ground. The foot is pronated in the weight-bearing and the non–weight-bearing positions. Subtalar or midtarsal joint motion is diminished or absent, and attempts at motion produce pain. Frequent ankle "sprains" may occur.

Radiographic Evaluation

The diagnosis of tarsal coalition is confirmed radiographically by anteroposterior, lateral weight-bearing, and oblique radiographs of the foot. Beaking of the anterior aspect of the talus on the lateral view suggests a tarsal coalition. Axial views through the posterior and middle talocalcaneal joints can be useful in the diagnosis of the middle facet talocalcaneal coalition. CT is the procedure of choice in the evaluation of tarsal coalitions, especially coalitions involving the middle facet.

Treatment

The treatment of symptomatic tarsal coalition varies according to the type of coalition, the age of the patient, the extent of the coalition, the presence or absence of degenerative osteoarthritis, and the degree of disability. Nonoperative treatment consists of cast immobilization, shoe inserts, or orthotics. When these approaches fail, excision of the coalition and soft tissue interposition to prevent hematoma formation and reossification of the coalition are effective in relieving pain, improving subtalar motion, and allowing resumption of normal activities.

CAVUS FEET

Cavovarus foot, an exaggerated medial longitudinal arch associated with a varus alignment of the hindfoot, often appears during the middle childhood years

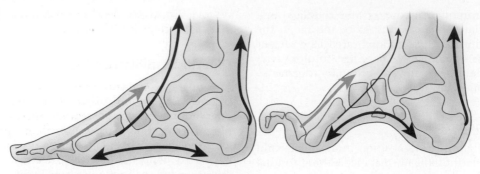

Figure 201–2

Normal muscular balance of the foot and weakness. *Left,* The normal muscular balance of the foot is shown. A right triangle of muscle forces is generated by the gastrocnemius-soleus muscle group posteriorly, the plantar muscles inferiorly, and the tibialis anterior muscle. *Right,* Weakness causes imbalance in the foot with resultant pes cavus. (Redrawn from Chuinard E, Baskin M: Claw-foot deformity. Treatment by transfer of the long extensors into the metatarsals and fusion of the interphalangeal joints. J Bone Joint Surg Am 55:351, 1973.)

(Fig. 201–2). Idiopathic and neuromuscular types may be seen; in either instance, cavovarus is usually a progressive deformity leading to considerable compromise of foot function. In hypermobile pes planus, the foot rotates externally; in high arch or cavovarus posture, however, the foot rotates internally. The cavovarus foot also tends to be rigid. Aggressive treatment is warranted and usually involves reconstructive surgery. Special shoes and shoe modifications are not helpful, but sometimes may be warranted for symptomatic treatment. Because a neuromuscular etiologic mechanism is possible whenever such a deformity of the foot exists, careful assessment of the patient's neurologic function is mandatory. Spinal cord pathology, poliomyelitis, and peripheral neuropathy (**Charcot-Marie-Tooth disease**) always must be considered.

CONGENITAL VERTICAL TALUS

Congenital vertical talus is an uncommon foot deformity producing a rigid, rocker-bottom shape to the foot. The talus is vertically oriented, with dorsal displacement of the navicular. Hindfoot equinovalgus, a convex plantar surface, midfoot and forefoot dorsiflexion and abduction, and rigidity are present. Most affected children have an underlying syndrome, such as spina bifida, arthrogryposis multiplex, or a congenital or chromosomal abnormality (trisomy 18). The diagnosis is confirmed radiographically with anteroposterior and lateral weight bearing or simulated weight-bearing views. A maximal plantar flexion lateral radiograph shows the inability to align the forefoot and midfoot with the hindfoot.

Treatment is similar to that for a congenital clubfoot. Serial manipulations and casts are attempted in infancy, but are only occasionally successful. Most children need surgical intervention with an extensive soft tissue release. The navicular must be reduced onto the head of the talus. Occasionally, transfer of the tibialis anterior tendon to the neck of the talus is necessary to support the talus and prevent recurrence.

OSTEOCHONDROSES

The tarsal navicular (**Köhler disease**) and the head of the second metatarsal (**Frieberg disease**) may undergo idiopathic avascular necrosis. These conditions are relatively uncommon, and both produce pain in the affected site on activity or weight bearing. The pathologic process involves infarction and subsequent revascularization, resorption, and reformation of the affected bone. Symptomatic treatment based on the severity of the child's complaints is appropriate.

As the child enters the adolescent growth spurt, the insertion of major muscle groups to bone is vulnerable to microfracture through the fibrocartilage, resulting in inflammatory and healing responses. The usual site of microfracture in the foot is at the attachment of the triceps surae to the os calcis, producing **Sever disease**. Symptoms wax and wane, depending on the level of activity, until skeletal maturity is achieved. The usual residual manifestation, if any, is some bony enlargement at the tendon insertion site when the cartilage, which proliferated as part of the healing response, undergoes its normal maturation to become bone. **Treatment** is symptomatic and includes the use of anti-inflammatory agents, rest, icing, and elevation.

The major cause of adolescent heel pain is a tight Achilles tendon (heel cord) caused by rapid growth. A stretching exercise program is usually effective in relieving symptoms. **Enthesitis** secondary to juvenile rheumatoid arthritis also must be considered.

ADOLESCENT BUNIONS

Bunions, or hallux valgus deformities, are common in adolescents. Typically the family has a positive history of the condition. The deformity is usually bilateral and occurs predominantly in girls. Most commonly, a congenital malalignment of the first metatarsal (metatarsus primus varus) is present. The hallux valgus deformity, enlargement of the medial aspect of the first metatarsal head, and symptoms usually begin in early adolescence. *Radiographs* of the feet are necessary to assess the deformity; the anteroposterior and lateral weight-bearing views are selected.

Treatment is directed toward relief of symptoms. Initially this consists of appropriately fitting shoes with a wide toe-box and occasionally orthotics if there is associated pes planus. If this measure fails, surgical realignment is necessary. Surgery is effective in relieving symptoms, although it usually does not restore the appearance of the foot to normal.

TOE DEFORMITIES

The most common lesser toe deformity of childhood is **curly toes**. Flexion is present at the proximal interphalangeal joint with lateral rotation. The fourth and fifth toes are most commonly involved. The deformity is caused by tightness of the flexor digitorum longus and brevis tendons. Observation is recommended for infants and young children because 25% to 50% of cases resolve spontaneously. Deformities persisting after 3 to 4 years of age are treated by open tenotomies of the flexor tendons.

Extra toes (**polydactyly**) usually are recognized at birth, and it is appropriate to decide on a management strategy at that time. When the extra toe is attached to the foot by only a tag of skin and soft tissue, as commonly occurs adjacent to the fifth toe, simple amputation or ligation through the stalk is effective. When the abnormality involves the great toe or the middle toes or when there is some rudiment of cartilage or bone connecting it with the foot proper, delayed surgical treatment targeted at the specific abnormality is indicated. Malformation syndromes may be associated with polydactyly (see Table 199–1). Fusing of the toes (**syndactyly**) is more common than polydactyly and is usually a benign cosmetic problem that does not

warrant treatment. Syndromes also may be associated with syndactyly (see Table 199–2).

PUNCTURE WOUNDS

Puncture wounds of the foot are common and generally trivial. For most injuries, cleaning the wound, ensuring prophylaxis for tetanus infection, and administering broad-spectrum oral antibiotic prophylaxis are all that is needed. When infection occurs despite these measures, *Pseudomonas aeruginosa* and *Staphylococcus aureus* are the offending organisms in most cases of osteomyelitis or osteochondritis, supposedly because these organisms normally colonize the skin surface of the foot as a result of the moist environment in an athletic shoe.

Treatment of these infections involves débriding the wound to remove necrotic tissue, which invariably is present, and administering parenteral antibiotics, initially with methicillin and gentamicin. Subsequent antibiotic treatment should be based on culture and sensitivity studies. After surgery, parenteral antimicrobial therapy is required for 10 to 14 days.

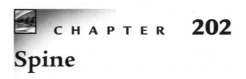

CHAPTER 202

Spine

CLINICAL EXAMINATION

A simplified classification of the common spinal abnormalities is presented in Table 202–1. A complete physical examination is necessary for any child or adolescent with a spinal deformity because the deformity may indicate an underlying disease. The back is examined with the patient in the standing position and viewed from behind (Fig. 202–1). The levelness of the pelvis is assessed first. Lower extremity length inequality results in pelvic obliquity and can produce the appearance of *scoliosis,* termed *compensatory scoliosis.* When the pelvis is level or has been leveled with wood blocks placed under the foot, the spine is examined for symmetry. The back is observed for areas of deformity, spinal curvature, cutaneous lesions (hemangioma or hair tuft), and areas of tenderness.

After the spine is examined for levelness, the patient is asked to bend forward with the hands directed between the feet (**Adams forward bend test**). A tangential view of the spine while standing behind (thoracic area) and in front (lumbar area) allows the observer to determine the symmetry of the back. The

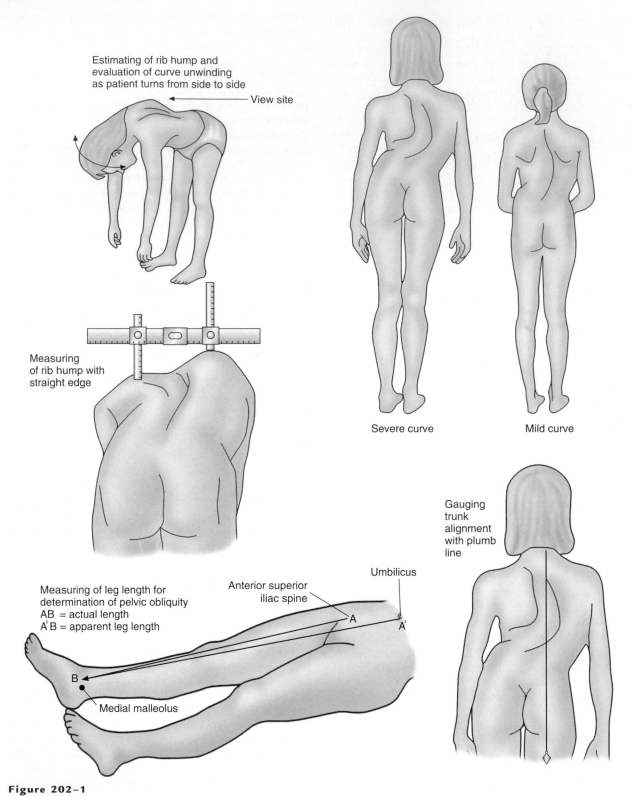

Estimating of rib hump and
evaluation of curve unwinding
as patient turns from side to side

View site

Measuring
of rib hump with
straight edge

Severe curve

Mild curve

Gauging
trunk
alignment
with plumb
line

Measuring of leg length for
determination of pelvic obliquity
AB = actual length
A'B = apparent leg length

Anterior superior
iliac spine

Umbilicus

A

A'

B

Medial malleolus

Figure 202–1

Clinical evaluation of a patient with scoliosis.

TABLE 202–1.   Classification of Spinal Deformities
Scoliosis
Idiopathic
Infantile
Juvenile
Adolescent
Congenital
Failure of formation
Wedge vertabrae
Hemivertebrae
Failure of segmentation
Unilateral bar
Bilateral bar
Mixed
Neuromuscular
Neuropathic diseases
Upper motor neuron
Cerebral palsy
Spinocerebellar degeneration
Friedreich ataxia
Charcot-Marie-Tooth disease
Syringomyelia
Spinal cord tumor
Spinal cord trauma
Lower motor neuron
Myelodysplasia
Poliomyelitis
Spinal muscular atrophy
Myopathic diseases
Duchenne muscular dystrophy
Arthrogryposis
Other muscular dystrophies
Syndromes
Neurofibromatosis
Marfan syndrome
Compensatory
Leg length inequality
Kyphosis
Postural roundback
Scheuermann disease
Congenital kyphosis

Adapted from the Terminology Committee of the Scoliosis Research Society, 1975.

presence of a hump is the hallmark of a scoliotic deformity. The corresponding area opposite the hump typically is depressed. The reason for these "humps and valleys" is *spinal rotation*. Scoliosis represents a rotational malalignment of one vertebra on another; this results in rib elevation when the curve is in the thoracic area and paravertebral muscle elevation when the curve is in the lumbar region. When the trunk is viewed from the side with the patient still in the forward flexed position, the degree of roundback can be ascertained. A sharp, abrupt forward angulation in the midline thoracic or thoracolumbar region indicates a **kyphotic deformity**. In a patient with scoliosis, other areas of the body also must be examined, including the skin (hairy patches, nevi, and lipomas suggest **spinal dysraphism**, and café au lait spots suggest neurofibromatosis), the extremities (skeletal dysplasia), the heart (murmurs indicate Marfan syndrome), and the neurologic system, to determine whether the scoliosis is truly idiopathic or possibly secondary to an underlying neuromuscular disorder or producing neurologic complications.

Radiographic Evaluation

Initial radiographs of the spine include a posteroanterior and lateral standing radiograph of the entire spine to assess for scoliosis, kyphosis, lordosis, congenital malformations, and, if the iliac crests are visible, the skeletal maturity of the patient. The degree of curvature is measured from the most tilted or end vertebra of the curve superiorly and inferiorly using the *Cobb method* (Fig. 202–2).

SCOLIOSIS

Alterations in normal spinal alignment that occur in the anteroposterior or frontal plane are termed *scoliosis*. Most scoliotic deformities are idiopathic (of unknown causation). Others can be congenital, secondary to an underlying neuromuscular disorder, or compensatory from a lower extremity length inequality.

Idiopathic Scoliosis

Idiopathic scoliosis is the most common form of scoliosis. It occurs in healthy, neurologically normal children, and its etiology is unknown. The incidence is only slightly higher in girls, but the condition is more likely to progress and necessitate treatment in girls. Hereditary tendencies are associated with the condition; approximately 20% of patients have other family members with the same condition.

Idiopathic scoliosis is classified into three age groups: infantile (birth to 3 years), juvenile (4 to 10 years), and adolescent (≥11 years). *Idiopathic* adolescent scoliosis (found in 80% of cases) is the most common cause of spinal deformity. The right thoracic curve is the most common pattern. *Infantile* scoliosis is rare in the U.S. but is common in England. *Juvenile* scoliosis is not common, but many children with the diagnosis of

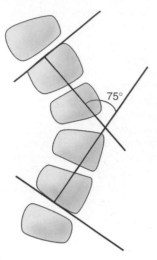

Figure 202–2

Cobb method of scoliotic curve measurement. Determine which are the end vertebrae of the curve: They are at the upper and lower limits of the curve and tilt most severely toward the concavity of the curve. Draw two perpendicular lines, one from the bottom of the lower body and one from the top of the upper body. Measure the angle formed. This is the accepted method of curve measurement according to the Scoliosis Research Society. Curves of 0 to 20 degrees are mild; 20 to 40 degrees, moderate; and greater than 40 degrees, severe.

adolescent scoliosis actually had the juvenile-onset type, but the diagnosis was not made until later.

Clinical Manifestations

Idiopathic scoliosis is usually a painless disorder. Any child with scoliosis and back pain requires a careful neurologic examination. Left thoracic curves and back pain are associated with an increased incidence of intraspinal pathology, such as a syrinx or tumor. These children should be evaluated by MRI of the spine.

Treatment

Treatment of idiopathic scoliosis is based on the maturation of the patient and whether the curve is progressive or nonprogressive. No treatment is necessary for nonprogressive deformities. The possibility for progression varies based on several factors, including sex, age, curve location, and curve magnitude. The risk for progression is much higher for girls (5 : 1). The younger the child, the higher the risk for progression. Treatment of progressive idiopathic adolescent scoliosis involves observation, an orthosis, or surgery; exercises alone are ineffective. Typically, curves less than 25 degrees are observed. Progressive curves between 25 and 45 degrees in a skeletally immature patient are managed by an orthosis. Curves greater than 45 degrees generally necessitate surgery.

Congenital Scoliosis

Abnormalities of vertebral formation during the first trimester may lead to structural deformities of the spine that are evident at birth or in early childhood. Congenital scoliosis can be classified as (1) partial or complete failure of vertebral formation (wedge vertebrae or hemivertebrae), (2) partial or complete failure of segmentation (unsegmented bars), or (3) mixed (Fig. 202–3). The condition may occur as a single anomaly or in combination with other bone, neural, or soft tissue abnormalities of the axial or appendicular skeleton. Congenital genitourinary malformations occur in 20% of children with congenital scoliosis. Unilateral renal agenesis is the most common abnormality, but 6% of affected children may have a silent, obstructive uropathy. Overall, 30% to 34% have extravertebral anomalies or syndromes, such as VATER syndrome (*v*ertebral defects, imperforate *a*nus, *t*racheoesophageal fistula, and *r*adial and *r*enal dysplasia) or Klippel-Feil syndrome.

Renal ultrasound is performed in all patients to assess for possible genitourinary problems. Congenital heart disease may be found in 10% to 15% of patients. Spinal dysraphism occurs in approximately 20% of patients with congenital scoliosis. This includes tethered spinal cord, intradural lipomas, syringomyelia, diplomyelia, and diastematomyelia. These abnormalities frequently are associated with cutaneous lesions of the back (e.g., hairy patches, skin dimples, and hemangiomas) and abnormalities of the feet and lower extremities (e.g., cavus feet, calf atrophy, asymmetric foot size, and neurologic changes). MRI of the spine is the procedure of choice for evaluation of possible spinal dysraphism.

The risk of progression of spinal deformity in a child with congenital scoliosis varies, depending on the growth potential of the malformed vertebra. Defects such as a block vertebra have little growth potential, whereas unilateral unsegmented bars typically produce progressive deformities. Seventy-five percent of involved patients show some progression that continues until skeletal growth stops; approximately 50% require treatment. Rapid progression can be expected during periods of rapid growth, before 2 years and after 10 years of age. Thoracolumbar curves and multiple hemivertebrae are associated with rapid progression, whereas nonsegmented hemivertebra is the least likely to progress.

Early **diagnosis** and prompt **treatment** of progressive curves are essential elements in the care of congenital spinal deformity. Orthotic treatment is of

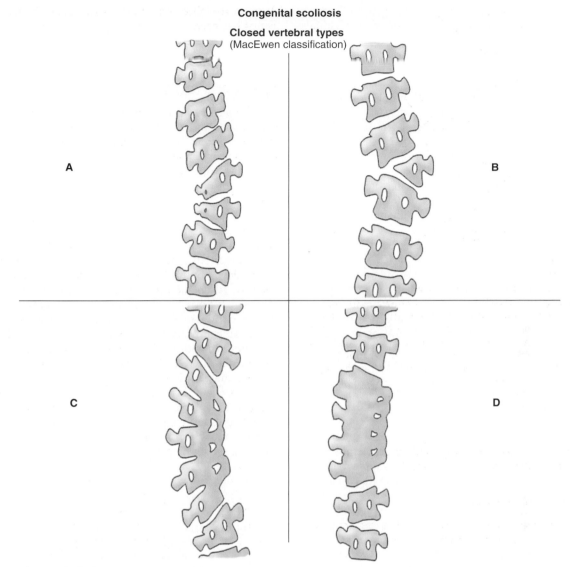

Congenital scoliosis

Closed vertebral types
(MacEwen classification)

A

B

C

D

Figure 202–3

Types of closed vertebral and extravertebral spinal anomalies that result in congenital scoliosis. A, Partial unilateral failure of formation (wedge vertebra). **B,** Complete unilateral failure of formation (hemivertebra). **C,** Unilateral failure of segmentation (congenital bar). **D,** Bilateral failure of segmentation (block vertebra).

limited value because these curves tend to be rigid. A spinal fusion without instrumentation is the most common procedure. If severe, the scoliosis may produce deformity, pulmonary restriction (cor pulmonale), and neurologic compression.

Neuromuscular Scoliosis

Progressive spinal deformity is a common and potentially serious abnormality associated with many neuro-muscular disorders, such as cerebral palsy, Duchenne muscular dystrophy, spinal muscular atrophy, and spina bifida. Progression is usually continuous when scoliosis begins. The magnitude of the deformity depends on the severity and pattern of weakness, whether the disease process is progressive, and the amount of remaining musculoskeletal growth. In non-ambulatory patients, the curves tend to be long and sweeping, produce pelvic obliquity, involve the cervical spine, and alter pulmonary function, producing restrictive lung disease. As these curves progress, sitting balance can be lost, and the affected individuals must use their arms to support an upright position. Spinal alignment must be part of the routine examination of a child with a neuromuscular disorder. Ambulatory patients have a much lower incidence of spinal deformity than nonambulatory or more severely involved patients. The standing or sitting forward bending test can be used to assess the symmetry of spinal alignment.

Any asymmetry is an indication for **radiographic evaluation**, which should include a posteroanterior and lateral standing or anteroposterior and lateral sitting view of the entire spine. If the child or adolescent cannot sit unsupported, a supine anteroposterior radiograph may be necessary.

The goal of **treatment** is to prevent progression and loss of function. Nonambulatory patients usually are more comfortable, are more independent, and have better respiratory function when they are able to sit erect without external support. Orthotic management or bracing is not usually effective; surgery is necessary in most cases. The current instrumentation systems are sufficiently strong and distribute the corrective forces such that postoperative immobilization is usually not necessary.

Compensatory Scoliosis

Adolescents with lower extremity length inequality may have a positive screening examination for scoliosis. With a pelvic obliquity, the patient's spine curves in the same direction as the obliquity. The magnitude of the lower extremity length discrepancy can be measured radiographically by a scanogram of the lower extremities. Distinguishing between a structural and a compensatory spinal deformity is important.

KYPHOSIS

The term *kyphosis* refers to a roundback deformity or to an increased angulation in the thoracic or thoracolumbar spine in the sagittal plane. Roundback deformities can be postural, structural (**Scheuermann kyphosis**), or congenital in origin.

Postural Roundback

Postural kyphosis is secondary to bad posture and is a common concern of parents. Postural kyphosis is voluntarily corrected in the standing and prone positions. Radiographically, no vertebral abnormalities are present. There may be some increase in the normal kyphosis of the thoracic region, but a supine hyperextension film shows complete correction. The child

is responsible for correcting posture. Active **treatment** is not indicated.

Scheuermann Disease

Scheuermann disease is common and second only to idiopathic scoliosis as a cause of pediatric spinal deformity. It occurs equally among male and female adolescents. Its *etiology* is unknown; hereditary factors are present, but with no definite pattern of inheritance. The differentiation between postural kyphosis and Scheuermann disease is determined by clinical and radiographic evaluation.

Clinical Manifestations

A patient with Scheuermann disease cannot correct the kyphosis in either the standing or the prone, hyperextended position. When viewed from the side in the forward flexed position, patients with Scheuermann disease usually show an abrupt angulation in the mid to lower thoracic region (Fig. 202–4). A patient with a postural roundback shows a smooth, symmetric contour. In both conditions, the normal lumbar lordosis is increased when the patient stands erect. Approximately 50% of patients with Scheuermann disease have apical back pain, especially with thoracolumbar kyphosis. The classic **radiographic findings** of Scheuermann kyphosis include narrowing of disc space; loss of the normal anterior height of the involved vertebra, producing wedging of 5 degrees or more in

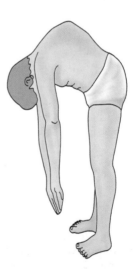

Figure 202–4

Note the sharp break in the contour of a child with kyphosis. (From Behrman RE [ed]: Nelson Textbook of Pediatrics, 14th ed. Philadelphia, WB Saunders, 1992.)

three or more vertebrae; irregularities of the end plates; and Schmorl nodes.

Treatment

Treatment of Scheuermann kyphosis is similar to that for scoliosis and depends on the maturation age of the patient, the degree of deformity, and the presence or absence of pain in the apical region. Nonoperative treatment consists of a corrective plaster cast followed by an orthosis. Permanent correction of the kyphotic deformity can be achieved with nonoperative management. Surgical treatment in Scheuermann disease rarely is necessary and is indicated for patients who have completed growth, who have a severe deformity, or who have chronic, intractable pain.

Congenital Kyphosis

Congenital kyphosis includes congenital failure of the formation of all or part of the vertebral body (but with preservation of the posterior elements) or failure of anterior segmentation of the spine (anterior unsegmented bar), or both. More severe deformities usually are recognized at birth and rapidly progress thereafter. Less obvious deformities may not appear until years later. When the progression begins, it does not cease until the end of growth. The most important factor regarding congenital kyphosis is that a progressive deformity in the thoracic spine can result in *paraplegia*. This usually is associated with the failure of vertebral body formation. **Treatment**, when necessary, is operative. Orthotic management is ineffective.

SPONDYLOLYSIS AND SPONDYLOLISTHESIS

Spondylolysis is a defect in the pars interarticularis without forward slippage of the involved vertebra onto the one below. *Spondylolisthesis* refers to the forward slippage or displacement of the involved vertebra. The lesions are not present at birth, but occur in 5% of children by 6 years of age. Children involved in certain sports, such as gymnastics, have an even higher incidence of spondylolysis. This increased incidence has been attributed to repetitive hyperextension stresses resulting in a fatigue fracture of the pars interarticularis.

Spondylolisthesis is classified according to the degree of slippage of one vertebra on the other: grade 1, less than 25%; grade 2, 25% to 50%; grade 3, 50% to 75%; grade 4, 75% to 100%; and grade 5, complete displacement. The most common location of spondylolisthesis is the fifth lumbar vertebra on the sacrum (first sacral vertebra).

Clinical Manifestations

Physical examination for spondylolysis or spondylolisthesis is similar to that for any disorder of the spine. A palpable "step-off" at the lumbosacral area and a vertically oriented sacrum indicate severe spondylolisthesis. A neurologic examination must be performed because nerve root involvement can occur, especially with severe displacement.

Radiographic Evaluation

Radiographic evaluation should include standing posteroanterior and lateral views of the entire spine, with an oblique radiograph of the lumbar spine. MRI may be required in patients with neurologic findings.

Treatment

Children and adolescents with asymptomatic spondylolysis require periodic evaluation during growth to assess for possible slippage; treatment rarely is required. Painful spondylolysis may benefit from orthotic management. If this does not relieve pain, surgical intervention with an in situ posterior spinal fusion may be required.

Adolescents with spondylolisthesis may require treatment, which depends on age, type of defect, degree of the slippage, and associated malalignment in the involved area:

- *Grade 1*—Usually no treatment is required unless there is chronic pain. Conservative management may be tried initially; if this fails, surgical intervention may be necessary.
- *Grade 2*—Usually a spinal fusion is required because of the high risk for further progression.
- *Grades 3 and 4*—Usually fusion is required to prevent further deformity.

DISC SPACE INFECTION (DISCITIS)

A disc space infection may be regarded as an infection of the disc without producing an acute osteomyelitis of the vertebral body. The most common organism is *S. aureus*. The infection can occur at any age. The disc space at times may be sterile. Children may have back pain, but they also may have abdominal or pelvic pain, irritability, and refusal to walk.

Clinical Manifestations

The child typically maintains the spine in a straight, stiff, or splinted position and refuses to flex the lumbar spine. The normal lumbar lordosis is reversed, and there may be paravertebral muscle spasms. Compared with other conditions (osteomyelitis), however, there are inconsistent systemic symptoms, such as fever and an elevated white blood cell count. The ESR typically is elevated.

Radiographic Evaluation

The radiographic features vary according to the interval between the onset of symptoms and delay in diagnosis. Anteroposterior, lateral, and oblique radiographs of the lumbar spine or thoracic spine, depending on the location of symptoms, usually are necessary to make the diagnosis. Typically the disc space is narrowed, with irregularity of the adjacent vertebral body end plates. In early cases, bone scan or, more often, MRI studies may be helpful because they may be positive before routine radiographic changes are present; MRI can be used to differentiate discitis from the distinct, more serious condition of vertebral osteomyelitis.

Treatment

The treatment of disc space infection usually is antibiotic therapy. Blood cultures occasionally may be helpful in establishing a precise organism. Aspiration needle biopsy of the disc space is reserved for children who do not respond to initial treatment with antistaphylococcal antibiotics. Immobilization of the spine may be used on a symptomatic basis. In most children, however, symptoms resolve rapidly with IV antibiotics. IV antibiotics are continued for 1 to 2 weeks and followed by oral antibiotics for an additional 4 weeks.

TORTICOLLIS

The literal definition of torticollis is twisted neck, but the traditional definition is shortening of one sternocleidomastoid muscle. Shortening and secondary contractures can be a primary abnormality of the sternocleidomastoid muscle (muscular torticollis) or secondary to CNS or upper cervical spine abnormalities.

Infants and young children with muscular torticollis have the ear pulled down toward the clavicle on the ipsilateral side. The face looks upward toward the contralateral side. Early in infancy, a "tumor" or thickening is palpated in the lower to mid portion of the sternocleidomastoid muscle. This thickening represents swelling or fibrosis of the central portion of the muscle and often is a precursor of the subsequent contracture. Skull and facial asymmetry or plagiocephaly may be present in congenital cases.

Etiology

In infants, in utero malposition, birth trauma, sternocleidomastoid muscle compartment syndrome, and heredity have been implicated as etiologic factors. In acquired torticollis in children, CNS mass lesions, abnormalities of the cervical spine, and local head and neck infections are more likely. Psychiatric causes may occur during adolescence.

Diagnosis

A thorough neurologic examination should be performed, and anteroposterior and lateral radiographs of the cervical spine should be obtained. A CT scan or MRI of the head and neck is necessary for any patient with persistent neck pain or with neurologic signs and symptoms.

Treatment

Treatment goals include ruling out an underlying disorder, increasing range of motion of the neck, and correcting the cosmetic deformity. Some infants with muscular torticollis may respond to nonoperative measures, which include range of motion exercises of the head and neck and stretching of the restrictive muscles several times daily. General indications for nonoperative management include age younger than 1 year, positive response to stretching exercise over several weeks, and no underlying cervical spine abnormalities or CNS findings.

Principles of surgical management of patients with muscular torticollis include identifying and releasing all restricting bands involving the sternocleidomastoid muscle and other neck structures, moving the head through a full range of motion before completion of the surgery, and resuming physical therapy within 2 weeks of operation to prevent recurrent contracture.

BACK PAIN IN CHILDREN

Back pain in children is unusual and should be viewed with concern. In contrast to adults, in whom back pain frequently is mechanical or psychological in origin, back pain in children is usually the result of organic causes, especially in preadolescents. Back pain lasting more than a few days requires careful investigation. Approximately 85% of children with back pain of more than 2 months have a specific lesion: 33% post-traumatic (occult fracture, spondylolysis), 33% developmental (kyphosis, scoliosis), and 18% infection or tumor. In the remaining 15%, the diagnosis remains undetermined.

Clinical Manifestations

The history should include the onset and duration of symptoms; antecedent factors; general health; family history; location, character, and radiation of pain; and

TABLE 202–2. Differential Diagnosis of Back Pain

Inflammatory Diseases

Discitis (common before 6 years old)
Vertebral osteomyelitis (pyogenic or tuberculous)
Spinal epidural abscess
Pyelonephritis
Pancreatitis

Rheumatologic Diseases

Pauciarticular juvenile rheumatoid arthritis
Reiter syndrome
Juvenile ankylosing spondylitis
Psoriatic arthritis
Inflammatory bowel disease

Developmental Diseases

Spondylolysis
Spondylolisthesis
Scheuermann syndrome
Scoliosis (especially left thoracic)

Mechanical Trauma and Abnormalities

Hip and pelvic anomalies
Herniated disc
Overuse syndromes (common with athletic training and
  in gymnasts and dancers)
Vertebral stress fractures
Compression fracture (steroids, sickle cell anemia)
Upper cervical spine instability

Neoplastic Diseases

Primary vertebral bone tumors (osteogenic sarcoma)
Metastatic tumor (neuroblastoma)
Primary spinal tumor (neuroblastoma, astrocytoma)
Malignancy of bone marrow (ALL, lymphoma)
Benign tumors (eosinophilic granuloma, osteoid
  osteoma)

Other

After lumbar puncture
Conversion reaction
Juvenile osteoporosis

ALL, acute lymphocytic leukemia.

neurologic symptoms, such as muscle weakness, sensory changes, and bowel or bladder dysfunction. Physical examination should include a complete musculoskeletal and neurologic evaluation. Spinal alignment, mobility, muscle spasm, and areas of tenderness should be evaluated and recorded. Muscle strength, sensory assessment (e.g., pain and light touch), deep tendon reflexes, and pathologic reflexes (e.g., Babinski sign) are tested. The danger signs in childhood back

pain are persistent or increasing pain; systemic symptoms, such as fever, malaise, or weight loss; neurologic findings; bowel or bladder dysfunction; young age, especially younger than 4 years (suspect tumor); and painful left thoracic spinal curvatures.

Radiographic Evaluation

The first diagnostic procedure is posteroanterior and lateral standing films of the entire spine with right and left oblique views of the involved area. Other radiographs may be necessary, depending on the location of the pain and the differential diagnoses. These include bone scans, CT scan, and MRI. MRI is especially useful when intraspinal pathology is suspected.

Laboratory Evaluation

Laboratory studies, such as complete blood count, ESR, and tests for the juvenile forms of arthritis (juvenile rheumatoid arthritis and ankylosing spondylitis), may be necessary.

Differential Diagnosis

The differential diagnosis in pediatric back pain is extensive (Table 202–2).

Treatment

The treatment of back pain is based on the specific diagnosis. If no definite diagnosis is established, an initial trial of physical therapy is recommended.

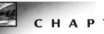

CHAPTER 203

Bone Tumors and Cystic Lesions

Benign bone tumors and cystic lesions are common in childhood. Some represent fibrous dysplasia, and others are benign tumors, whereas subacute osteomyelitis (**Brodie abscess**) and eosinophilic granuloma represent lesions unrelated to abnormal osseous or cartilage growth (Table 203–1). Many of these lesions produce pain, pathologic fractures, or limp; others may be incidental findings on radiographic examination. The **prognosis** usually is excellent. **Treatment** is summarized in Table 203–1. Malignant bone tumors are discussed in Chapter 160.

TABLE 203–1. Benign Bone Tumors and Cysts

Disease	Characteristics	Radiography	Treatment	Prognosis
Osteochondroma (osteocartilaginous exostosis)	Common; distal metaphysis of femur, proximal humerus, proximal tibia; painless, hard, nontender mass	Bony outgrowth, sessile or pedunculated	Excision, if symptomatic	Excellent; malignant transformation rare
Multiple hereditary exostoses	Osteochondroma of long bones; bone growth disturbances	As above	As above	Recurrences
Osteoid osteoma	Pain relieved by aspirin; femur and tibia; predominantly found in boys	Dense sclerosis surrounds small radiolucent nidus, <1 cm	As above	Excellent
Osteoblastoma (giant osteoid osteoma)	As above, but more destructive	Osteolytic component; size >1 cm	As above	Excellent
Enchondroma	Tubular bones of hands and feet; pathologic fractures, swollen bone; Ollier disease if multiple lesions are present	Radiolucent diaphyseal or metaphyseal lesion; may calcify	Excision or curettage	Excellent; malignant transformation rare
Nonossifying fibroma	Silent; rare pathologic fracture; late childhood, adolescence	Incidental radiographic finding; thin sclerotic border, radiolucent lesion	None or curettage with fractures	Excellent; heals spontaneously
Eosinophilic granuloma	Age 5-10 yr; skull, jaw, long bones; pathologic fracture; pain	Small, radiolucent without reactive bone; punched out lytic lesion	Biopsy, excision rare; irradiation	Excellent; may heal spontaneously
Brodie abscess	Insidious local pain; limp; suspected as malignancy	Circumscribed metaphyseal osteomyelitis; lytic lesions with sclerotic rim	Biopsy; antibiotics	Excellent
Unicameral bone cyst (simple bone cyst)	Metaphysis of long bone (femur, humerus); pain, pathologic fracture	Cyst in medullary canal, expands cortex; fluid-filled unilocular or multilocular cavity	Curettage; steroid injection into lesion	Excellent; some heal spontaneously
Aneurysmal bone cyst	As above; contains blood, fibrous tissue	Expands beyond metaphyseal cartilage	Curettage, bone graft	Excellent

SUGGESTED READING

Behrman RE, Kliegman RM, Jenson HB (eds): Nelson Textbook of Pediatrics, 17th ed. Philadelphia, WB Saunders, 2003.

Biermann JS: Common benign lesions of bone in children and adolescents. J Pediatr Orthop 22:268-273, 2002.

Brown R, Hussain M, McHugh K, et al: Discitis in young children. J Bone Joint Surg Br 83:106-111, 2001.

Committee on Quality Improvement, Subcommittee on Developmental Dysplasia of the Hip: Clinical practice guidelines: Early detection of developmental dysplasia of the hip. American Academy of Pediatrics. Pediatrics 105(4 Pt 1):896-905, 2000.

Cummings RJ, Davidson RS, Armstrong PF, Lehman WB: Congenital clubfoot. Instr Course Lect 51:385-400, 2002.

Do TT: Transient synovitis as a cause of painful limps in children. Curr Opin Pediatr 12:48-51, 2000.

Gerbino PG: Elbow disorders in throwing athletes. Orthop Clin North Am 34:417-426, 2003.

Gomez JE: Upper extremity injuries in youth sports. Pediatr Clin North Am 49:593-626, 2002.

Herman MJ, Pizzutillo PD, Cavalier R: Spondylolysis and spondylolisthesis in the child and adolescent athlete. Orthop Clin North Am 34:461-467, 2003.

Leet AI, Skaggs DL: Evaluation of the acutely limping child. Am Fam Physician 61:1011-1018, 2000.

Lincoln TL, Suen PW: Common rotational variations in children. J Am Acad Orthop Surg 11:312-320, 2003.

Loder RT, Aronsson DD, Dobbs MB, Weinstein SL: Slipped capital femoral epiphysis. Instr Course Lect 50:555-570, 2001.

Mankin HJ, Mankin CJ: Metabolic bone disease: An update. Instr Course Lect 52:769-784, 2003.

Masso PD, Meeropol E, Lennon E: Juvenile-onset scoliosis followed up to adulthood: Orthopaedic and functional outcomes. J Pediatr Orthop 22:279-284, 2002.

Prahinski JR, Polly DW, McHale KA, et al: Occult intraspinal anomalies in congenital scoliosis. J Pediatr Orthop 20:59-63, 2000.

Roach JW: Adolescent idiopathic scoliosis. Orthop Clin North Am 30:353-365, 1999.

Scherl SA: Common lower extremity problems in children. Pediatr Rev 25:52-62, 2004.

Schwend RM, Drennan JC: Cavus foot deformity in children. J Am Acad Orthop Surg 11:201-211, 2003.

Thompson GH: Gait disturbances. In Kliegman RM (ed): Practical Strategies in Pediatric Diagnosis and Therapy, 2nd ed. Philadelphia, WB Saunders, 2004.

Thompson GH: Angular deformities of the lower extremities in children. In Chapman MN (ed): Operative Orthopaedics, 3rd ed. Philadelphia, JB Lippincott, 2004.

Thompson GH, Price CT, Roy D, et al: Legg-Calve-Perthes disease: Current concepts. Instr Course Lect 51:367-384, 2002.

Tortolani PJ, McCarthy EF, Sponseller PD: Bone mineral density deficiency in children. J Am Acad Orthop Surg 10:57-66, 2002.

GLOSSARY OF ABBREVIATIONS

AAP American Academy of Pediatrics

ABG arterial blood gas

ACD anticonvulsant drug

ACE angiotensin-converting enzyme

ACIP Advisory Committee on Immunization Practices

ACTH adrenocorticotropic hormone

ADEM acute demyelinating encephalomyelopathy

ADHD attention-deficit/hyperactivity disorder

AFP alpha-fetoprotein

AFSF anterior fontanel soft and flat

AIDS acquired immunodeficiency syndrome

ALC absolute lymphocyte count

ALL acute lymphoblastic leukemia

ANA antinuclear antibody

ANC absolute neutrophil count

ANCA antineutrophil cytoplasmic antibody

AOM acute otitis media

APACHE II Acute Physiology and Chronic Health Evaluation II

aPTT activated partial thromboplastin time

ARDS acute respiratory distress syndrome; adult respiratory distress syndrome

ARF acute renal failure

ASD atrial septal defect

BAL bronchoalveolar lavage

BCG bacille Calmette-Guérin

BMT bone marrow transplant

BOM bilateral otitis media

BP blood pressure

BPD bronchopulmonary dysplasia

BSA bovine serum albumin

BUN blood urea nitrogen

CAH congenital adrenal hyperplasia

CBC complete blood count

CBG capillary blood gas

CC chief complaint

CCAM congenital cystic adenomatoid malformation

CDC Centers for Disease Control and Prevention

CF cystic fibrosis

CGD chronic granulomatous disease

CH50 total hemolytic complement

CHF congestive heart failure

CMV cytomegalovirus

CMV-IG cytomegalovirus immunoglobulin

CNS central nervous system

CP cerebral palsy

CPP cerebral perfusion pressure

CPR cardiopulmonary resuscitation

CPS child protective services

CRP C-reactive protein

CRT capillary refill time

CSD cat-scratch disease

CSF cerebrospinal fluid

CSF colony-stimulating factor

CT computed tomography

CTA clear to auscultation

CVA cerebrovascular accident

CVL central venous line

CVP central venous pressure

CXR chest x-ray

DDH developmental dysplasia of hip

DDX differential diagnosis

DI diabetes insipidus

DIC disseminated intravascular coagulopathy

DKA diabetic ketoacidosis

DM diabetes mellitus

DNA deoxyribonucleic aid

DNR do not resuscitate order

EBV Epstein-Barr virus

ECG electrocardiogram

EEG electroencephalogram

EIA enzyme immunoassay

EITB enzyme-linked immuno-transfer blot or Western blot

ELISA enzyme-linked immunosorbent assay (see EIA)

EM erythema multiforme

EMG electromyography

EOMI extraocular muscles intact

EPO erythropoietin

ERCP endoscopic retrograde cholangiopancreatography

ESR erythrocyte sedimentation rate

ESRD end-stage renal disease

ETT endotracheal tube

FDA United States Food and Drug Administration

FEL familial erythrophagocytic lymphohistiocytosis

FENa fractional excretion of sodium

FEV$_1$ forced expiratory volume in 1 second

FHR fetal heart rate

FISH fluorescent in situ hybridization

FSH follicle-stimulating hormone

FTT failure to thrive

FUO fever of unknown origin

GABHS group A beta-hemolytic streptococcus

GCS Glasgow Coma Scale

G-CSF granulocyte colony-stimulating factor

GERD gastroesophageal reflux disease

GFR glomerular filtration rate

GH growth hormone

GI gastrointestinal

GM-CSF granulocyte-macrophage colony-stimulating factor

GNRH gonadotropin-releasing hormone

GVHD graft-versus-host disease

HAART highly active antiretroviral therapy (a combination HIV treatment regimen usually comprising two nucleoside reverse transcriptase inhibitors and a protease inhibitor)

HAV hepatitis A virus

HbA hemoglobin (adult)

HB$_e$Ag hepatitis B e antigen

HbF hemoglobin (fetal)

HBIG hepatitis B immunoglobulin

HbS hemoglobin (sickle cell)

HB$_s$Ag hepatitis B surface antigen

HBV hepatitis B virus

HCG human chorionic gonadotropin

HCT hematocrit

HCV hepatitis C virus

HDV hepatitis D virus

HEENT head, eyes, ears, nose, throat

HEV hepatitis E virus

HGV hepatitis G virus

HHV6 human herpesvirus 6

HHV7 human herpesvirus 7

HHV8 human herpesvirus 8

HIE hypoxic-ischemic encephalopathy

HIV human immunodeficiency virus

HLA human histocompatibility leukocyte antigen

HLH hemophagocytic lymphohistiocytosis

HMD hyaline membrane disease

hpf high power field

HPI history of present illness

HPV human papillomavirus

HR heart rate

HSM hepatosplenomegaly

HSP Henoch-Schönlein purpura

HSV herpes simplex virus

HUS hemolytic uremic syndrome

IBD inflammatory bowel disease

ICP intracranial pressure

IDM infant of diabetic mother

IFA immunofluorescence assay

IFN interferon (e.g., IFN-α, IFN-β, IFN-γ)

Ig immunoglobulin

IgA immunoglobulin A

IgD immunoglobulin D

IgE immunoglobulin E

IgG immunoglobulin G

IgM immunoglobulin M

IHA indirect hemagglutination assay

IL interleukin (e.g., IL-1, IL-2)

IPV inactivated poliovirus vaccine

IQ intelligence quotient

ITP idiopathic (immune) thrombocytopenic purpura

IUGR intrauterine growth retardation

IV intravenous

IVF intravenous fluids

IVH intraventricular hemorrhage

IVIG intravenous immunoglobulin

JRA juvenile rheumatoid arthritis

KOH potassium hydroxide

KS Kawasaki syndrome

LA latex agglutination

LAD leukocyte adhesion deficiency

LBW low birth weight

LCPD Legg-Calvé-Perthes disease

LES lower esophageal sphincter

LGV lymphogranuloma venereum

LH luteinizing hormone

LP lumbar puncture

LPS lipopolysaccharide

MAC *Mycobacterium avium* complex

MBC minimum bactericidal concentration

MCV mean cell volume

MDI metered-dose inhaler

MELAS mitochondrial encephalomyopathy lactic acidosis and strokelike episodes

MEN multiple endocrine neoplasia

MHC major histocompatibility complex

MIC minimum inhibitory concentration

MMR measles-mumps-rubella

MMM moist mucous membranes

MPV mean platelet volume

MRI magnetic resonance imaging

mRNA messenger RNA

MRSA methicillin-resistant *Staphylococcus aureus*

MSUD maple syrup urine disease

MU million units

NAD no acute distress

NCAT normocephalic atraumatic

NDNT nondistended nontender

NEC necrotizing enterocolitis

NICU neonatal intensive care unit

NIF negative inspiratory force

NK cells natural killer cells

NKDA no known drug allergies

NSAID nonsteroidal anti-inflammatory drug

OFC occipital frontal circumference

OI osteogenesis imperfecta

OME otitis media with effusion

OPV oral poliovirus vaccine

ORS oral rehydration solution

PCOS polycystic ovarian syndrome

PCP *Pneumocystis carinii* pneumonia

PCR polymerase chain reaction

PDA patent ductus arteriosus

PE physical examination

PE pulmonary embolism

PEF peak expiratory flow

PEM protein energy malnutrition

PERRLA pupils equal, round, reactive to light and accommodation

PET positron emission tomography

PFO patent foramen ovale

pfu plaque-forming units

PGE prostaglandin E

PICU pediatric intensive care unit

PID pelvic inflammatory disease

PKU phenylketonuria

PML progressive multifocal leukoencephalopathy

PPD purified protein derivative (for tuberculin skin test)

PPHN primary pulmonary hypertension of the newborn

PT prothrombin time

PTH parathyroid hormone

PTSD post-traumatic stress disorder

PUD peptic ulcer disease

PVC premature ventricular contraction

RAST radioallergosorbent test

RBC red blood cell

RDA recommended daily allowance

RDS respiratory distress syndrome

RIA radioimmunoassay

RID radioimmunodiffusion

RIG rabies immunoglobulin

RMSF Rocky Mountain spotted fever

RNA ribonucleic acid

ROP retinopathy of prematurity

RPR rapid plasma reagin (a nontreponemal serologic test for syphillis)

RR respiratory rate

RRR regular rate and rhythm

RSD reflex sympathetic dystrophy

RSV respiratory syncytial virus

RSV-IG respiratory syncytial virus immunoglobulin

RTA renal tubular acidosis

RT-PCR reverse transcriptase polymerase chain reaction

SBE subacute bacterial endocarditis

SCFE slipped capital femoral epiphysis

SCID severe combined immunodeficiency disease

SD standard deviation

SGA small for gestational age

SIADH syndrome of inappropriate secretion of antidiuretic hormone

SIDS sudden infant death syndrome

SLE systemic lupus erythematosus

STD sexually transmitted disease

SVT supraventricular tachycardia

TBI total body irradiation

TEF tracheoesophageal fistula

TEN toxic epidermal necrolysis

TGV transposition of great vessels

TIG tetanus immunoglobulin

TMP-SMZ trimethoprim-sulfamethoxazole

TNF tumor necrosis factor

TOA tubo-ovarian abscess

TPN total parenteral nutrition

TSH thyroid-stimulating hormone

TSST-1 toxic shock syndrome toxin-1

TTN transient tachycardia of the newborn

TTP thrombotic thrombocytopenic purpura

TU tuberculin unit

UA urinalysis

UC ulcerative colitis

URI upper respiratory tract infection

UTI urinary tract infection

VAHS virus-associated hemophagocytic syndrome

VCA viral capsid antigen

VCUG voiding cystourethrography

VDRL Venereal Disease Research Laboratory (nontreponemal serologic test for syphilis)

VIG vaccinia immunoglobulin

VLBW very low birth weight

VMA vanillylmandelic acid

VS vital signs

VSD ventricular septal defect

VT ventricular tachycardia

vWD von Willebrand disease

VZIG varicella-zoster immunoglobulin

VZV varicella-zoster virus

WBC white blood cell

WHO World Health Organization

XLP X-linked lymphoproliferative syndrome

Note: Page numbers followed by *t* and *f* represent tables and figures, respectively.

O